# Textbook of
# Critical Care Nursing

# Textbook of
# Critical Care Nursing

**Sasmita Das** PhD
Associate Dean
SUM Nursing College
Siksha 'O' Anusandhan (SOA) (Deemed University)
Bhubaneswar, Odisha, India

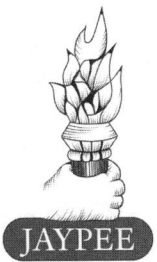

## JAYPEE BROTHERS MEDICAL PUBLISHERS
*The Health Sciences Publisher*
New Delhi | London

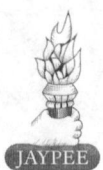
**Jaypee Brothers Medical Publishers (P) Ltd**

**Headquarters**
Jaypee Brothers Medical Publishers (P) Ltd
EMCA House, 23/23-B
Ansari Road, Daryaganj
New Delhi 110 002, India
Landline: +91-11-23272143, +91-11-23272703
+91-11-23282021, +91-11-23245672
Email: jaypee@jaypeebrothers.com

**Corporate Office**
Jaypee Brothers Medical Publishers (P) Ltd
4838/24, Ansari Road, Daryaganj
New Delhi 110 002, India
Phone: +91-11-43574357
Fax: +91-11-43574314
Email: jaypee@jaypeebrothers.com

**Overseas Office**
J.P. Medical Ltd
83 Victoria Street, London
SW1H 0HW (UK)
Phone: +44 20 3170 8910
Fax: +44 (0)20 3008 6180
Email: info@jpmedpub.com

Website: www.jaypeebrothers.com
Website: www.jaypeedigital.com

© 2024, Jaypee Brothers Medical Publishers

The views and opinions expressed in this book are solely those of the original contributor(s)/author(s) and do not necessarily represent those of editor(s) and publisher of the book.

All rights reserved. No part of this publication may be reproduced, stored or transmitted in any form or by any means, electronic, mechanical, photocopying, recording or otherwise, without the prior permission in writing of the publishers.

All brand names and product names used in this book are trade names, service marks, trademarks or registered trademarks of their respective owners. The publisher is not associated with any product or vendor mentioned in this book.

Medical knowledge and practice change constantly. This book is designed to provide accurate, authoritative information about the subject matter in question. However, readers are advised to check the most current information available on procedures included and check information from the manufacturer of each product to be administered, to verify the recommended dose, formula, method and duration of administration, adverse effects and contraindications. It is the responsibility of the practitioner to take all appropriate safety precautions. Neither the publisher nor the author(s)/editor(s) assume any liability for any injury and/or damage to persons or property arising from or related to use of material in this book.

This book is sold on the understanding that the publisher is not engaged in providing professional medical services. If such advice or services are required, the services of a competent medical professional should be sought.

Every effort has been made where necessary to contact holders of copyright to obtain permission to reproduce copyright material. If any have been inadvertently overlooked, the publisher will be pleased to make the necessary arrangements at the first opportunity.

**Inquiries for bulk sales may be solicited at:** jaypee@jaypeebrothers.com

**Textbook of Critical Care Nursing**

First Edition: **2024**

ISBN: 978-93-5696-988-9

*Printed at: Sterling Graphics Pvt. Ltd. India*

# Contributors List

**Anu Baby** MSc(N)
Senior Critical Care Nurse, IQP Lead
Critical Care Unit, Manchester Royal
Infirmary, Manchester University NHS
Foundation Trust, UK

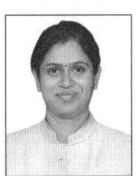

**Neethu Maria Joseph** MSc(N)
Clinical Nurse Tutor with Professional
Education Development Team
Lancashire Teaching Hospital
NHS Trust, UK

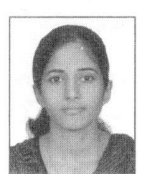

**Bishnupriya Mohapatra** Msc(N)
Tutor
Department of Medical and Surgical
Nursing
SUM Nursing College
SOA (DTU), Bhubaneswar, Odisha, India

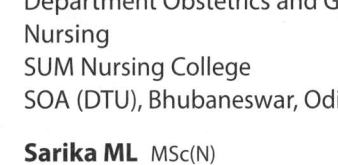

**Pratibha Khosla** MSc(N)
Associate Professor
Department Obstetrics and Gynecology
Nursing
SUM Nursing College
SOA (DTU), Bhubaneswar, Odisha, India

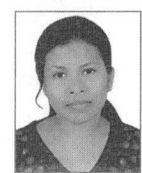

**Debajani Nayak** MSc(N)
Associate Professor
Department of Obstetrics and Gynecology
Nursing
SUM Nursing College
SOA (DTU), Bhubaneswar, Odisha, India

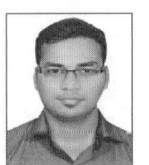

**Sarika ML** MSc(N)
Tutor
Department of Medical and Surgical
Nursing
AIMS Nursing College
Bhubaneswar, Odisha, India

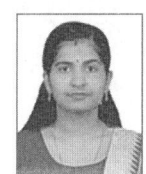

**Dinabandhu Barad** MSc(N)
Tutor
Department of Pediatric Nursing
SUM Nursing College
SOA (DTU), Bhubaneswar, Odisha, India

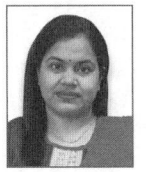

**Sasmita Das** PhD
Associate Dean
Department of Medical and Surgical
Nursing
SUM Nursing College
SOA (DTU), Bhubaneswar, Odisha, India

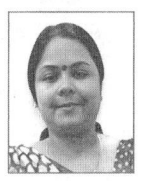

**Jhunilata Pradhan** MSc(N)
Associate Professor
Department of Medical and Surgical
Nursing
SUM Nursing College
SOA (DTU), Bhubaneswar, Odisha, India

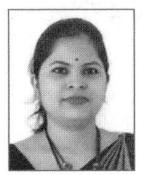

**Suchismita Phantasingh** MSc(N)
Associate Professor
Department of Psychiatric Nursing
SUM Nursing College
SOA (DTU), Bhubaneswar, Odisha, India

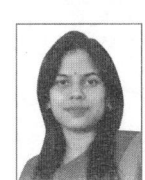

**Madhusmita Nayak** MSc(N)
Assistant Professor
Department of Obstetrics and Gynecology
Nursing
SUM Nursing College
SOA (DTU), Bhubaneswar, Odisha, India

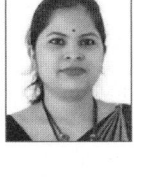

**Susan Konda** MSc(N)
Assistant Professor
Department of Medical and Surgical
Nursing
SUM Nursing College
SOA (DTU), Bhubaneswar, Odisha, India

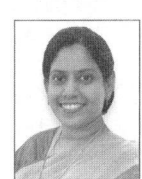

**Mamata Swain** MSc(N)
Assistant Professor
Department of Medical and Surgical
Nursing
SUM Nursing College
SOA (DTU), Bhubaneswar, Odisha, India

**Vasudevan NJ** PhD
Associate Professor
Department of Medical and Surgical
Nursing
SUM Nursing College
SOA (DTU), Bhubaneswar, Odisha, India

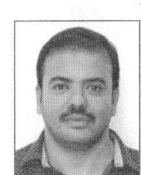

# Preface

Presently, critical care nurse is expected to care for critically ill patients in a variety of setting. Advances in nursing, medicine and technology—the rapidly changing healthcare climate, shortage of nursing staff and faculty are various factors which bring great changes in the practice of healthcare setting.

Today's critical care nurse more than ever before must possess a unique body of knowledge in order to provide competent and compassionate care to critically ill patients and their near and dear ones. Some of the knowledge can be gained through formal education and textbooks. The rest can only be gained through experience. It is our goal, with first edition of *Textbook of Critical Care Nursing,* to assist readers on their journey by providing a comprehensive and up-to-date resource and reference. Our goal with this edition is to continue a tradition of excellence in critical care publishing that has spanned over 50 years. I offer the next generation of critical care practitioners up-to-date information on a holistic perspective.

The entire contents are prepared in very understandable language with adequate tables and figures. This book has 18 chapters along with various subsections drafted as per the requirement prescribed by the nursing syllabus. This book can be utilized by different nursing courses like BSc, MSc and PB BSc nursing, diploma and certificate courses in critical care nursing. It can be used as a reference book for exploring different critical care issues.

With great pleasure, I introduce this resource to promote critical care excellence, so the nurses can help patients and their family to cope with the consequence of illness.

I welcome and wish all the best to all readers.

**Sasmita Das**

# Acknowledgments

First and foremost, I would like to thank our supreme deity "Lord Sri Jagannath", who strengthens our team with his abundant Kripa through innumerable means and giving me the knowledge, ability and opportunity to undertake this project and complete it satisfactorily. Without his blessings, this achievement would not have been possible.

This project was completed with the help and cooperation of many people. First, I want to thank our many colleagues who contributed to the text either by authoring a chapter or by sharing their experience as a reviewer.

I would like to thank M/s Jaypee Brothers Medical Publishers (P) Ltd., who has gone through much changes during the publishing of this edition, but has remained committed to producing the best text possible.

Especially want to thank our management, Dean, our faculty of SUM Nursing College (SNC), SOA (DTU) for their support and words of positive encouragement as they applauded us to the finish line with the project.

Another key person is Ms Jitika Royal (Content Strategist—Nursing) who I want to thank for her timeless attention to organize the chapters in detail and for taking up the publishing of this book. I extend my sincere gratitude to the other members of Jaypee Brothers Medical Publishers team who helped me throughout many stages of this edition.

I conclude with lots of appreciation for all those who have directly or indirectly helped me to make this book a reality.

Finally, I wish to express a word of thanks to my family and nursing colleagues who endured the time while I complete this project.

# Contents

1. **Introduction to Critical Care Nursing** .......................... 1
   *Sasmita Das*
   - Historical Development Review of Critical Care Nursing *1*
   - Review of Anatomy and Physiology of Vital Organs *2*
   - Altered Fluid Electrolyte Balance *2*
   - Electrolyte Imbalance *4*
   - Progressive Patient Care *7*
   - Concept of Critical Care Nursing *8*
   - Critical Care Unit Setup *10*
   - Documentation in Critical Care Unit *11*
   - Evidence-based Critical Care Nursing Practice *13*
   - Future of Critical Care Nursing *14*

2. **Concept of Holism Applied to Critical Care Nursing Practices** ........................ 23
   *Sasmita Das*
   - Patients and Family Perception towards Critical Illness *23*
   - Impact of the Critical Care Environment on the Patient *24*
   - Stress and Burnout Syndromes among Healthcare Professionals *35*

3. **Review of Drugs** .................................... 39
   *Sasmita Das*
   - Principles of Pharmacokinetics *40*
   - Analgesics and Anti-inflammatory Drugs *41*
   - Opioid Analgesics and Antagonists *41*
   - Non-narcotic Analgesics and Nonsteroidal Anti-inflammatory Drugs *44*
   - Antibiotics *48*
   - Antiseptics *53*
   - Inotropics *55*
   - Life-saving Drugs *56*

   **Drugs used in Various Body Systems 56**
   - Drugs used in Respiratory System *56*
   - Drugs used in Nervous System *58*
   - Sedative *59*
   - Drugs used in Cardiovascular System *61*
   - Drugs used in Gastrointestinal System *62*
   - Drugs used on Urinary System *64*
   - Drugs used in Endocrine System *66*
   - Drug Therapy for Diabetes Mellitus *66*
   - Intravenous Fluids *67*
   - Blood and Blood Components *69*
   - Electrolytes *70*
   - Drug Overdoses and Poisoning *71*
   - Role of Nurses (in General) *74*

4. **Pain Management in Critical Care Unit** ...................... 78
   *Vasudevan NJ*
   - Theories of Pain *79*
   - Pain Assessment in Critical Care Unit *81*
   - Pharmacological Pain Management in CCU *83*
   - Nonpharmacological Pain Management *83*
   - Placebo Effect *84*

5. **Infection Control in Critical Care Unit** ........................ 89
   *Vasudevan NJ*
   - Risk Factors for Infection *90*
   - Antibiotic Resistant Infections *91*
   - Postoperative Wound Infection in CCU *92*
   - Prevention and Infection Control Measures *92*
   - Nosocomial Infection in Critical Care Unit *93*
   - Methicillin-Resistant Staphylococcus Aureus *94*
   - Standard Safety Measures in CCU *94*
   - Sterilization and Disinfection in CCU *95*

6. **Common Gastrointestinal Emergencies** .................... 98
   *Jhunilata Pradhan*
   - Anatomy of Gastrointestinal System *98*
   - Physiology of Digestive System *100*
   - Assessment of GI System *101*
   - Parenteral and Enteral Nutrition *105*
   - Gastrointestinal Bleeding *109*
   - Abdominal Injuries *114*
   - Mechanism of Injury *115*
   - Fulminant Hepatic Failure *117*
   - Hepatic Encephalopathy *120*
   - Acute Pancreatitis *123*
   - Intestinal Obstruction *128*
   - Perforated Peritonitis *131*

## 7. Renal System Emergencies and Management .................. 138

✍ *Susan Konda*

- Anatomy of Renal System *138*
- Physiology of Renal System *139*
- Assessment of Renal System *140*
- Acute Renal Failure *143*
- Chronic Renal Failure *146*
- Acute Tubular Necrosis *150*
- Bladder Trauma *153*
- Disorders of Fluid Volume *154*
- End-Stage Renal Disease and Renal Transplantation *156*
- Management Modalities for Renal System Disorders *158*

## 8. Nervous System Emergencies and Management .................. 166

✍ *Neethu Maria Joseph, Anu Baby*

- Anatomy of Nervous System *167*
- Physiology of Nervous System *172*
- Assessment of Nervous System *173*
- Increased Intracranial Pressure *179*
- Cerebrovascular Disease *188*
- Stroke *191*
- Seizure Disorder *195*
- Status Epilepticus *199*
- Guillain-Barré Syndrome *201*
- Myasthenia Gravis *203*
- Encephalopathy *207*
- Head Injury *211*
- Spinal Cord Injury *217*
- Problems Associated with Neurological Disorders *222*
- Brain Death *228*
- Herniation Syndrome *229*
- Management Modalities through Neurosurgical Approaches *232*

## 9. Cardiovascular Emergencies and Management .................. 239

✍ *Sarika ML*

- Anatomy of Cardiovascular System *239*
- Physiology of Cardiovascular System *244*
- Principles of Nursing in Caring for Patients with Cardiovascular Disorders *246*
- Assessment of Cardiovascular System *246*
- Hypertensive Crisis *253*
- Coronary Artery Disease *255*
- Acute Myocardial Infarction *259*
- Cardiomyopathy *262*
- Deep Vein Thrombosis *265*
- Valvular Diseases *267*
- Heart Block *270*
- Cardiac Arrhythmias *272*
- Aneurysm *276*
- Infective Endocarditis *277*
- Heart Failure *279*
- Management Modalities for Cardiovascular System Disorders *284*
- Percutaneous Coronary Intervention *288*

## 10. Respiratory Emergency Diseases .................. 297

✍ *Mamata Swain*

- Respiratory System *297*
- Assessment and Diagnostic Evaluation *304*
- Common Respiratory Emergency Disorders *313*

## 11. Endocrine System Emergencies and Management .................. 368

✍ *Pratibha Khosla*

- Anatomy and Physiology of Endocrine System *368*
- Assessment of Endocrine System *369*
- Hypoglycemia *373*
- Hyperglycemia *376*
- Diabetic Ketoacidosis *379*
- Thyroid Storm *383*
- Myxedema *385*
- Adrenal Crisis *388*
- Antidiuretic Hormone Dysfunction *392*

## 12. Obstetrical Emergency and Management .................. 396

✍ *Debajani Nayak*

- Types of Obstetrical Emergency *396*
- Antepartum Hemorrhage *397*
- Pregnancy-induced Hypertension *407*
- Obstructed Labor *418*
- Postpartum Hemorrhage *420*
- Ruptured Uterus *425*
- Puerperal Sepsis *429*
- Obstetrical Shock *432*

13. **Neonatal and Pediatric Emergencies and Management** .................................................. 439
    *Dinabandhu Barad*
    - Neonatal and Pediatric Emergencies *440*
    - Congenital Disorders *474*

14. **Other Emergency Conditions and Management** .................................................. 512
    *Madhusmita Nayak*
    - Assessment and Mechanism of Injury *512*
    - Shock *534*
    - Systemic Inflammatory Response Syndrome *540*
    - Multiple Organ Dysfunction Syndrome *541*
    - Disseminated Intravascular Coagulation *543*
    - Drug Overdose and Poisoning *547*
    - Acquired Immunodeficiency Syndrome *550*
    - Eye Injuries *554*
    - Nose Injuries *557*
    - Throat Injuries *560*

15. **Psychiatric Emergencies and Crisis Intervention** .................................................. 567
    *Suchismita Phantasingh*
    - Prevalence and Incidence *567*
    - Psychiatric Emergencies *567*
    - Crisis Intervention *575*

16. **Burns and Management** .................................................. 582
    *Susan Konda*
    - Classification and Pathophysiology of Burns *582*
    - Burn Assessment *587*
    - Fluid and Electrolyte therapy *589*
    - Pain Management *590*
    - Wound Care *591*
    - Infection Control *592*
    - Prevention and Management of Burn Complication *593*
    - Grafts and Flaps *594*
    - Reconstructive Surgery *595*
    - Rehabilitation *595*

17. **Legal and Ethical Issues in Critical Care** .................. 600
    *Suchismita Phantasingh*
    - Principles of Critical Care *600*
    - Ethical Issues in Critical Care Unit *601*
    - Principles of Bioethics *601*
    - Legal Issues in Critical Care Unit *606*

18. **Quality Assurance in Critical Care** .............................. 610
    *Bishnupriya Mohapatra*
    - Quality Assurance *610*
    - Standards of CCU *614*
    - Design of CCU *616*
    - Protocols and Policies of CCU *620*
    - Nursing Audit *623*
    - Staffing of CCU *627*

*Review Questions* ........................................................................ 637
*Index* ........................................................................................... 645

# Syllabus

## CLINICAL SPECIALITY – II

## Medical Surgical Nursing - Critical Care Nursing

**Placement:** II Year

*Hours of instruction*
**Theory:** 150 hours
**Practical:** 950 hours
**Total:** 1100 hours

## Course Description

This course is designed to assist students in developing expertise and in-depth knowledge in the field of critical care nursing. It will help students to develop advanced skills for nursing intervention in caring for critically ill patients. It will enable the student to function as critical care nurse practitioner/specialist. It will further enable the student to function as educator, manager and researcher in the field of critical care nursing.

## Objectives

At the end of the course, the students will be able to:
- Appreciate trends and issues related to critical care nursing.
- Describe the epidemiology, etiology, pathophysiology and diagnostic assessment of critically ill patients.
- Describe the various drugs used in critical care and nurses responsibility.
- Perform physical, psychosocial and spiritual assessment.
- Demonstrate advance skills/competence in managing critically ill patients including advance cardiac life support.
- Demonstrate skill in handling various equipment/gadgets used for critical care.
- Provide comprehensive care to critically ill patients.
- Appreciate team work and coordinate activities related to patient care.
- Practice infection control measures.
- Assess and manage pain.
- Identify complications and take appropriate measures.
- Discuss the legal and ethical issues in critical care nursing.
- Assist patients and their family to cope with emotional distress, spiritual, grief and anxiety.
- Assist in various diagnostic, therapeutic and surgical procedures.
- Incorporate evidence-based nursing practice and identify the areas of research in the field of critical care nursing
- Identify the sources of stress and manage burnout syndrome among health care providers.
- Teach and supervise nurses and allied health workers.
- Design a layout of ICU and develop standards for critical care nursing practice.

## Course Content

| Unit | Hours | Content |
|------|-------|---------|
| I | 5 | **Introduction to Critical Care Nursing**<br>• Historical review: Progressive patient care (PPC)<br>• Review of anatomy and physiology of vital organs, fluid and electrolyte balance<br>• Concepts of critical care nursing<br>• Principles of critical care nursing<br>• Scope of critical care nursing<br>• Critical care unit set up including equipment supplies, use and care of various type of monitors and ventilators<br>• Flow sheets |
| II | 10 | **Concept of Holistic Care Applied to Critical Care Nursing Practice**<br>• Impact of critical care environment on patients: Risk factors, assessment of patients, critical care psychosis, prevention and nursing care for patients affected with psychophysiological and psychosocial problems of critical care unit, caring for the patient's family, family teaching<br>• The dynamics of healing in critical care unit: Therapeutic touch, relaxation, music therapy, guided imagery, acupressure<br>• Stress and burnout syndrome among health team members |
| III | 14 | **Review**<br>• Pharmacokinetics<br>• Analgesics/anti-inflammatory agents<br>• Antibiotics, antiseptics<br>• Drug reaction and toxicity<br>• Drugs used in critical care unit (inclusive of ionotropic, life saving drugs)<br>• Drugs used in various body systems<br>• IV fluids and electrolytes<br>• Blood and blood components<br>• Principles of drug administration, role of nurses and care of drugs |
| IV | 5 | **Pain Management**<br>• Pain and sedation in critically ill patients<br>• Theories of pain, types of pain, pain assessment, systemic responses to pain<br>• Pain management—pharmacological and non-pharmacological measures<br>• Placebo effect |
| V | 5 | **Infection Control in Intensive Care Unit**<br>Nosocomial infection in intensive care unit; methyl resistant staphylococcus aureus (MRSA), disinfection, sterilization, standard safety measures, prophylaxis for staff |
| VI | 10 | **Gastrointestinal System**<br>Causes, pathophysiology, clinical types, clinical features, diagnosis, prognosis, management—medical, surgical and nursing management of: acute gastrointestinal bleeding, abdominal injury, hepatic disorders: fulminant hepatic failure, hepatic encephalopathy, acute pancreatitis, acute intestinal obstruction, perforative peritonitis |
| VII | 10 | **Renal System**<br>• Causes, pathophysiology, clinical types, clinical features, diagnosis, prognosis, management: medical, surgical and nursing management of: Acute renal failure, chronic renal failure, acute tubular necrosis, bladder trauma<br>• Management modalities: Hemodialysis, peritoneal dialysis, continuous ambulatory peritoneal dialysis, continuous arteriovenous hemodialysis, renal transplant |
| VIII | 10 | **Nervous System**<br>• Causes, pathophysiology, clinical types, clinical features, diagnosis, prognosis, management: medical, surgical and nursing management of: common neurological disorders: cerebrovascular disease, cerebrovascular accident, seizure disorders, Guillein-Barre syndrome, myasthenia gravis, coma, persistent vegetative state, encephalopathy, head injury, spinal cord injury<br>• Management modalities: Assessment of intracranial pressure, management of intracranial hypertension, craniotomy<br>• Problems associated with neurological disorders: Thermoregulation, unconsciousness, herniation syndrome |

| Unit | Hours | Content |
|------|-------|---------|
| IX | 5 | **Endocrine System**<br>Causes, pathophysiology, clinical types, clinical features, diagnosis, prognosis, management: medical, surgical and nursing management of: hypoglycemia, diabetic ketoacidosis, thyroid crisis, myxedema, adrenal crisis, syndrome of inappropriate/hypersecretion of antidiuretic hormone (SIADH) |
| X | 15 | **Management of Other Emergency Conditions**<br>• Mechanism of injury, thoracic injuries, abdominal injuries, pelvic fractures, complications of trauma, head injuries<br>• Shock: Shock syndrome, hypovolemic, cardiogenic, anaphylactic, neurogenic and septic shock<br>• Systemic inflammatory response: The inflammatory response, multiple organ dysfunction syndrome<br>• Disseminated intravascular coagulation<br>• Drug overdose and poisoning<br>• Acquired immunodeficiency syndrome (AIDS)<br>• Ophthalmic: Eye injuries, glaucoma, retinal detachment<br>• Ear nose throat: Foreign bodies, stridor, bleeding, quincy, acute allergic conditions<br>• Psychiatric emergencies, suicide<br>• Crisis intervention |
| XI | 20 | **Cardiovascular Emergencies**<br>• Principles of nursing in caring for patient's with cardiovascular disorders<br>• Assessment: Cardiovascular system: Heart sounds, Diagnostic studies: Cardiac enzymes studies, Electrocardiographic monitoring, Holter monitoring, stress test. Echocardiography, coronary angiography, nuclear medicine studies<br>• Causes, pathophysiology, clinical types, clinical features, diagnostic prognosis, management: medical, surgical and nursing management of: hypertensive crisis, coronary artery disease, acute myocardial infarction, cardiomyopathy, deep vein thrombosis, valvular diseases, heart block, cardiac arrhythmias and conduction disturbances, aneurysms, endocarditis, heart failure cardiopulmonary resuscitation BCLS/ACLS<br>• Management modalities: thrombolytic therapy, pacemaker – temporary and permanent, percutaneous transluminal coronary angioplasty, cardioversion, intra-aortic balloon pump monitoring, defibrillations, cardiac surgeries, coronary artery bypass grafts (CABG/MICAS), valvular surgeries, heart transplantation, autologous blood transfusion, radiofrequency catheter ablation |
| XII | 15 | **Respiratory System**<br>• Acid-base balance and imbalance<br>• Assessment: History and physical examination<br>• Diagnostic tests: Pulse oximetry, end–tidal carbon dioxide monitoring, arterial blood gas studies, chest radiography, pulmonary angiography, bronchoscopy, pulmonary function test, ventilation perfusion scan, lung ventilation scan<br>• Causes: pathophysiology, clinical types, clinical features, prognosis, management: medical, surgical and nursing management of common pulmonary disorders: pneumonia, status asthmaticus, interstitial drug disease, pleural effusion, chronic obstructive pulmonary disease, pulmonary tuberculosis, pulmonary edema, atelectasis, pulmonary embolism, acute respiratory failure, acute respiratory distress syndrome (ARDS), chest trauma hemothorax, pneumothorax<br>• Management modalities: Airway management<br>• Ventilatory management: Invasive, non-invasive, long-term mechanical ventilations<br>• Bronchial hygiene: Nebulization, deep breathing exercise, chest physiotherapy, postural drainage, intercostal drainage, thoracic surgeries |
| XIII | 7 | **Burns**<br>• Clinical types, classification, pathophysiology, clinical features, assessment, diagnosis, prognosis, management: medical, surgical and nursing management of burns<br>• Fluid and electrolyte therapy—calculation of fluids and its administration<br>• Pain management<br>• Wound care<br>• Infection control<br>• Prevention and management of burn complications<br>• Grafts and flaps<br>• Reconstructive surgery<br>• Rehabilitation |

| Unit | Hours | Content |
|---|---|---|
| XIV | 5 | **Obstetrical Emergencies**<br>Causes, pathophysiology, clinical types, clinical features, diagnostic prognosis, management: medical, surgical and nursing management of: antepartum hemorrhage, preeclampsia, eclampsia, obstructed labor and ruptured uterus, postpartum hemorrhage, puerperal sepsis, obstetrical shock |
| XV | 10 | **Neonatal Pediatric Emergencies**<br>Causes, pathophysiology, clinical types, clinical features, diagnostic, prognosis, management: medical, surgical and nursing management of:<br>• Neonatal emergencies: Asphyxia neonatorum, pathological jaundice in neonates, neonatal seizures, metabolic disorders, intracranial hemorrhage, neonatal sepsis, RDS/HMD (respiratory distress syndrome/hyaline membrane disease<br>• Congenital disorders: Cyanotic heart disease, tracheoesophageal fistula, congenital hypertrophic pyloric stenosis, imperforate anus<br>• Pediatric emergencies: Dehydration, acute bronchopneumonia, acute respiratory distress syndrome, poisoning, foreign bodies, seizures, traumas, status asthmaticus |
| XVI | 2 | **Legal and Ethical Issues in Critical Care-Nurse's Role**<br>• Brain death<br>• Organ donation and counselling<br>• Do not resuscitate (DNR)<br>• Euthanasia<br>• Living will |
| XVII | 2 | **Quality Assurance**<br>• Standards, protocols, policies, procedures<br>• Infection control; standard safety measures<br>• Nursing audit<br>• Staffing<br>• Design of ICU/CCU |

# Chapter 1

# Introduction to Critical Care Nursing

 Sasmita Das

## CHAPTER OUTLINE

- ❖ Historical Development Review of Critical Care Nursing
- ❖ Review of Anatomy and Physiology of Vital Organs
- ❖ Altered Fluid and Electrolyte Balance
- ❖ Progressive Patient Care
- ❖ Concept of Critical Care Nursing
  - ◆ Principles of critical care nursing
  - ◆ Scope of critical care nursing
- ❖ Critical Care Unit Setup
  - ◆ Equipment and supplies
  - ◆ Use and care of therapeutic and diagnostic equipment
- ❖ Documentation in Critical Care Unit
  - ◆ Procedure and monitoring a CCU
  - ◆ Flow sheets
  - ◆ Evidence-based critical care nursing practice
- ❖ Future of Critical Care Nursing

### Learning Objectives

At the end of the chapter, the students will be able to:
- Describe the historical development of critical care nursing.
- Discuss the various components of progressive patient care.
- Express the principles and scope of critical care nursing.
- Explain the requirements needed for critical care unit setup.
- Enumerate the monitoring and documentation system in critical care unit (CCU).
- Apply the AACN synergy model for patient care in CCU.

## HISTORICAL DEVELOPMENT REVIEW OF CRITICAL CARE NURSING

Intensive care in the present day consists of critically ill patients care for in one setting that facilitates the support of organs to preserve physiological regularity. Even though we believe of critical care as a current concept, it supports dates back thousands of years. Since 1500 BC Egyptians had recognized events like tracheostomy to manage airway obstruction and one thousand years later, Hippocrates had started the organ support by cannulating the airway to permit air to be drained into the lungs.

Florence Nightingale marked an innovative pace towards present critical care, throughout the Crimean War of 1850s by separating the injured soldiers as per the severity of their injuries. An important part to intensive care patient is the frequency and intensity of observing by a nurse, a structure that Florence documented by watching the sickest soldiers more frequently by additional nurses. She illustrated and initiated the recovery room care system. Her data collection techniques on hospital acquired infections provided a remarkable difference among hospitals and developed the evidence-based practice that we maintain today.

In 1922, first neonatal intensive care unit established at Sarah Morris Hospital, Chicago, USA. In 1923, the first adult critical care unit came out at John Hopkins Hospital, USA.

A revolutionary incident of 1950s, which brought a remarkable change in the care of the acutely ill. At Copenhagen in 1952, when one of the world's worst polio epidemics occurred. Many patients died from respiratory failure due to increasing muscle weakness and paralysis. Dr Bjorn Ibsen, a Danish anesthetist, planned that the patient could be sustained by inserting a tracheostomy and clearing their secretions and ventilating them with an oxygen/nitrogen mix using positive pressure manually. He also documented the need of carbon dioxide clearance and suggested the carbon dioxide absorbers in the circuit. Ibsen planned to open the first intensive care unit (ICU) in 1953, which was adopted by various hospitals around the world.

Intensive care has been considered as specialty since 1950. Various technological advances developed sophisticated ventilators, cardiovascular monitoring and renal replacement therapy. Intensive care units can be managed by tele or remote ICU systems, providing support to various ICUs in far-away or inaccessible places by a centralized multi-disciplinary Intensive care groups.

In 1975, the critical care nursing registered nurse certificate examination started. In 1980, critical care courses started at CMC. Since 50 years, critical care developed for comprehensive, mostly mechanical laboratory measurements and electronic checking to direct intensive therapy of multiorgan failures by critical care groups.

## REVIEW OF ANATOMY AND PHYSIOLOGY OF VITAL ORGANS

Humans consist of five vital organs that are very essential for survival. These are heart, brain, kidneys, liver, and lungs.

To refresh the readers knowledge on anatomy and physiology of vital organs, refer "UNIT VI, VII, VIII, IX and X".

## ALTERED FLUID ELECTROLYTE BALANCE

Human body consists of extracellular and intracellular fluid, which helps to maintain homeostasis. Fluid and electrolytes act like catalysts and also transporters as well as solvents and solutions for different reactions occurred in the human body. Beyond the normal requirement of fluid and electrolyte, less or more in total or independent volume or concentration may cause abnormalities in systemic findings. Certain regulation by renal and pulmonary systems as well as intake and output of water and electrolytes has a greater role in fluid and electrolyte balance. Body fluids are regulated by fluid intake (thirst mechanism), hormonal control (ADH, renin, aldosterone) and fluid output (kidneys, skin, lungs and GI tracts).

### Altered Fluid Balance

#### Extracellular Fluid Volume Deficit (ECFVD)

It is a condition in which less intravascular interstitial fluids and It is very frequent and severe fluid imbalances which leads to vascular fluid volume loss (hypovolemia). Which is very prone for cellular fluid loss due to shifting of fluid from the cells to re-establish the fluid balance.

*Etiology*

- Excess vomiting or diarrhea
- Excessive blood loss due to traumatic injury
- Abnormal accumulation of fluid within body tissue or a body cavity
- Inadequate fluid intake.

*Risk Factors*

In diabetic ketoacidosis

- Excess vomiting or loose stool
- Swallowing trouble
- In elderly persons who are very confused.

*Clinical Manifestations*

- **Mild ECFVD:** Two percent of body weight and 1–2 liter
- **of water will be loosed.**
- **Moderate ECFVD:** Five percent of weight loss and 3–5 liter of water will be loosed.
- **Severe ECFVD:** Eight percent of body weight and 5–10 L of water will be loosed.
- Thirst
- Reduced skin turgor
- Tachycardia
- Dried up mucus membrane
- Eyeballs sunken and soft
- Elevated body temperature
- Weight loss
- Oliguria (<30 mL/hour)
- Restlessness, coma in severe deficit.

*Laboratory Diagnosis*

- Serum sodium level will be increased
- Blood urea nitrogen will be more than 25 mg/dL
- Elevated hematocrit value (>55%)
- Hyperglycemia (>120 mg/dL).

*Medical Management*

- **Pharmacological management:**
  - Five percent dextrose in water of may be prescribed through an intravenous solution.
  - In case of blood losses are less than one liter, ringers lactate and normal saline solution may be advised.
- **Dietary management:** Diarrhea affected patients should avoid oily food and milk-based products.

#### Extracellular Fluid Volume Excess

This condition increases fluid retention in the intravascular space and interstitial space.

*Etiology*

- Total body sodium will be increased
- Heart failure
- Renal disorder
- Cirrhosis of liver
- Using excess intravenous fluid containing sodium
- Food containing high amount of sodium.

*Clinical Manifestations*

- **Cardiovascular:**
  - Pitting edema in lower extremities
  - Neck vein engorgement in semi fowlers
  - Weight gain
  - Sacral edema
  - Elevated blood pressure
- **Respiratory system:**
  - Irritating cough
  - Dyspnea
  - Crackle lungs
  - Cyanosis
- **Neurological:** Changes in level of consciousness.

*Laboratory Findings*

- Serum sodium level (<135 mEq/L)
- Decreased hematocrit level.

*Management*

- **Pharmacological:**
  - Potassium sparing diuretics
  - Digoxin, a digitalis preparation increased the force of myocardial contraction or to slow the heart rate in case of heart failure.
- **Dietary:** Diet containing low sodium is prescribed for fluid retention patient.

### Extracellular Fluid Volume Shift to Third Space Fluid

Fluid volume shifts basically a change in the location of extra cellular fluid between the intravascular and interstitial space. Vascular fluid shift into interstitial space and considered as a as third space of fluid. Generally it is found in case of tissue injury, which results due to altered capillary permeability. In case of inflammation and traumatic injury more vascular fluids volume appears in the abdomen (**Flowchart 1.1**).

*Causes*

- Simple blisters or sprain
- Crushing injury
- Extensive burns
- Perforated peptic ulcer
- Intestinal obstruction
- Large venous thrombosis

*Clinical Manifestations*

- Cold extremities
- Hypotension
- Weak and rapid pulse
- Oliguria
- Pallor in skin
- Level of consciousness will be decreased.

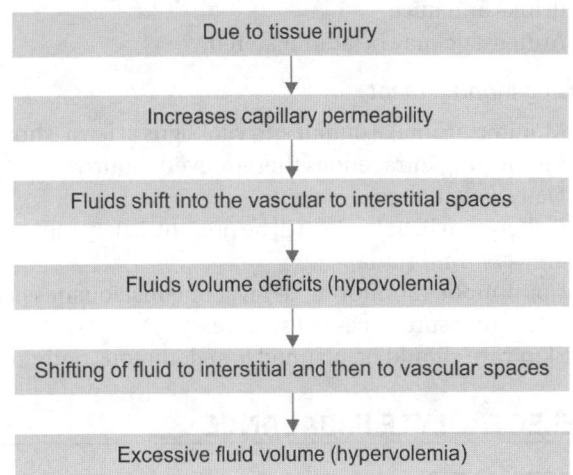

**Flowchart 1.1:** Pathophysiology of extracellular fluid volume shift.

*Laboratory Findings*

- Elevated hematocrit level (fluids returns to blood stream)
- Elevated BUN level (fluids returns to blood stream).

*Management*

Medical management:
- Large volume of fluid administers (tissue injury, burns, i.e., hypervolemia)
- Fluid volume administered limited (hypervolemia).

### Intracellular Fluid Volume Excess (ICFVE)

ICFVE may occur, who receive D 5% IV fluid constantly, patient with brain injury or diseases which enhance production of ADH, which augments water reabsorption from renal tubules.

*Clinical Manifestations*

- Headache
- Nausea, vomiting
- Behavioral changes, irritability
- Weight gain
- Convulsion, confusion
- Increased systolic BP with bradycardia
- Papillary changes

*Laboratory Findings*

- Serum sodium level will be less than 125 mEq/L
- Hematocrit value will be decreased.

*Management*

- If the cause is water excess then 5% dextrose and 0.45% NaCl can be used

- Oral fluids may be administered in the form of soft drinks and juice
- Antiemetic may be administered.

*Nursing Management*

- Monitoring intake output and vital signs at least 8 hourly
- Monitoring intravenous therapy every hourly
- Daily weight measurement
- If alteration in behavior will be present, safety measures are very important
- Continuous monitoring of level of consciousness and safety measure in case of seizure
- Skin care should be planned for edematous patient.

## ELECTROLYTE IMBALANCE

### Hyponatremia

It is the condition where level of serum sodium will be less than 135 mEq/L.

*Causes*

- In case of less total body water
- In case of diuresis
- Using diuretics
- Gastrointestinal suction
- Even if after taking more water excess perspiration.

*Clinical Manifestations*

- Nausea, vomiting, diarrhea, cramps in abdomen
- Diastolic pressure will be decreased, tachycardia, orthostatic hypotension and weak pulse
- Altered rates of respiration
- Headache, lethargy, confusion, weakness, tremors and altered problem solving ability
- Dry skin and pale mucus membrane.

*Management*

*Medical Management*

- Correct body water balance
- Sodium replacement is necessary
- Fluid intake will be reduced for sodium regain.

*Pharmacological Management*

- Administered 0.9% of NaCl or Ringer lactate may be prescribed
- 3% NaCl is advised if serum sodium level is less than 115 mEq/L.

*Dietary Management*

- In case of severe hyponatremia sodium replacement is required
- Fluids can be reduced (800–1,000 mL/day)
- Where hyponatremia will be for excess fluids, in that case fluid restricted diet may be prescribed.

### Hypernatremia

In this case, level of serum sodium will be more than 145 mEq/L.

*Causes*

- Diabetes insipidus
- Renal losses
- Excess NaCl (IV fluids intake)
- Canned vegetables
- Increased salt intake.

*Clinical Manifestations*

- **Gastrointestinal:** Nausea, vomiting and anorexia
- **Cardiovascular:** Tachycardia, hypotension and hypertension
- **Neurologic:** Restlessness, agitation, lethargy, seizures, irritability, and tremors
- **Renal:** Oliguria
- **Integumentary:** Dry and flushed skin, dry mucus membrane and sticky, thirst.

*Laboratory Findings*

Serum sodium level will be more than 145 mEq/L.

*Management*

*Medical Management*

- To balance sodium level, D5w or (0.2 % or 0.45% NaCl) is administered.
- Diuretics like furosemide are administered.

*Dietary Management*

- Restriction of a sodium rich diet is essential in preventing hypernatremia
- In case of renal disorders sodium intake is permissible for 500–2,000 mg/day.

### Hypokalemia

In this condition level of serum potassium will be less than 3.5 mEq/L.

*Causes*

- Diarrhea, vomiting, nasogastric suctioning
- Malnutrition, no potassium in diet, starvation
- Diabetic acidosis
- Diuretics cause in eliminating more potassium in the urine.

### Clinical Manifestations

- Nausea, vomiting, anorexia, and diarrhea
- Dysarrythmia, vertigo, postural hypotension, flattened T-wave
- Shortness breath, shallow respiration
- Decreased tendon reflex, confusion, lethargy, fatigue
- Muscle weakness, leg cramps, paralysis.

### Laboratory Findings

Serum potassium level <3.5 mEq/L.

### Management

*Medical Management*

- In case of severe hypokalemia, cardiac monitoring is very essential.
- Oral potassium replacement therapy is advised if serum potassium is (3.3–3.5) mEq/L.
- IV Potassium may result cardiac arrest and should be administered in doses of 10–20 mEq/hour after diluting with IV fluid and it needs continuous monitoring.
- Potassium chloride must be diluted in IV fluid before administration for moderate to severe hypokalemia.

*Dietary Management*

Administered high rich potassium diet help in correct potassium loss (rich sources of potassium containing foods are cabbage, carrot, mushroom, spinach, tomato and fruits like banana, guava, and orange).

## Hyperkalemia

In this condition level of potassium will be more than 5.0 mEq/L.

### Causes

- In case of potassium retention like renal failure, less urine output, potassium sparing diuretics.
- Excessive release of cellular potassium in case of severe traumatic injury, severe burns, severe infection, metabolic acidosis.
- Excess IV infusion or potassium taking orally.

### Clinical Features

- Tachycardia then bradycardia, abnormal ECG findings like peaked narrow T-wave, wide QRS complex, depressed ST segment, widened PR interval.
- Nausea, vomiting, hyperactive bowel sounds.
- Muscles weakness, muscles cramps and paresthesia.
- Oliguria and anuria.

### Laboratory Findings

- Serum potassium will be more than 5.0 mEq/L.
- Serum creatinine will be more than 1.5 mg/dL.
- Blood urea nitrogen is above 25 mg/dL.

### Management

*Medical Management*

- Restricted potassium riched diet (serum potassium level is 5.0–5.5 mEq/L).
- After enhancing urine output, serum potassium level will be reduced.
- Advice for insulin infusion, glucose or sodium bicarbonate to encourage potassium uptake into cell.
- IV infusions of calcium gluconate to decline the agonist effects of overloaded potassium in the myocardium.

## Hypocalcemia

It is a condition in which level of serum calcium is less than 4.5 mEq/L or 8.5 mg/dL.

### Causes

- Inadequate dietary calcium, vitamin-D deficiency.
- Metabolic alkalosis (less ionized calcium)
- Renal failure with hyperphosphatemia, burns, acute pancreatitis, Cushing's disease, hyperparathyroidism.
- Using medication magnesium sulfate.

### Clinical Manifestations

- Tetany symptoms like twitching around mouth, numbness and tingling finger facial spasm, convulsion.
- Dyspnea, laryngeal spasm
- Increased peristalsis, diarrhea
- Palpitation, dysarrythmias.

### Laboratory Findings

- Facial muscles will be contracted in response to a light tap over the facial nerve in front of the ear (Chvostek's sign)
- By inflating a blood pressure cuff above the systolic pressure for a few minutes, carpal spasm will be induced (Trousseau's sign).

### Management

*Medical Management*

- Calcium supplements should be taken 30 minutes prior to main course food for good absorption and along with a glass of milk because vitamin-D will facilitate absorption of calcium from the intestines.

- For reducing the effect of hypertension and bradycardia, Intravenous calcium chloride and calcium gluconate (10%) should be given very slowly.
- Oral calcium gluconate, calcium lactate or calcium chloride to correct hypocalcemia.

*Dietary Management*

- High rich calcium diet (milk, spinach and fish).
- If hypocalcemia is due to deficiency of parathyroid, the client should not take high phosphate food (milk products, carbonate beverages).

## Hypercalcemia

In this condition level of serum calcium is greater than (5.5 mEq/L to 11 mg/L).

### Causes

- Overactive parathyroid glands (hyperparathyroidism)
- Metastatic malignancy in lung, breast, ovarian, prostatic bladder and kidney
- Diuretic therapy (Thiazide)
- Prolonged immobilization
- More vitamin-D.

### Clinical Manifestations

- Anorexia, vomiting, constipation and decreased peristalsis.
- Mild to moderate hypocalcemia.
- Depression, difficulty to concentration. In severe case extreme lethargy, coma, and confusion.
- Heart block, dysrhythmias.
- Polyuria, kidney stone, renal failure.
- Pain in bone and fractures.

### Laboratory Findings

- Level of serum calcium is more than 5.5 mEq/L.
- Arterial blood gas reading will be PH <7.45, $HCO_3$ >26 mEq/L.

### Management

*Medical Management*

- 0.9% NaCl advised to start rapidly with Furosemide to prevent overload of fluid and enhance excretion of calcium through urine.
- Corticosteroids drugs decrease calcium level.
- A new drug that is etidronate disodium, which reduces serum calcium by reducing both normal and abnormal bone reabsorption of Ca and secondary by reducing bone formation.
- Do not use excess Ca or vitamin-D supplements or Ca containing antacids agent.

*Dietary Management*

- Avoided high rich calcium diet.
- Rapid fluid administration will be needed for hydrating the client and wash out excess calcium through the kidney.

## Hypomagnesemia

Hypomagnesemia in Mg level is less than 1.6 mg/dL.

### Etiology

- Loss of GI fluids, particularly in diarrhea.
- Protein–calorie malnutrition or starvation.
- Administration drugs such as loop or thiazide diuretics.
- Endocrine disorder like diabetic ketoacidosis.

### Clinical Manifestations

- **Neurologic:** Confusion, mood changes, seizures, tremors and muscle weakness.
- **Cardiovascular:** Hypertension, ECG changes prolonged PR interval, widened QRS complex, depression of ST segment with T-wave inversion.

### Laboratory Findings

Serum Mg level less than 1.6 mg/dL.

### Management

*Medical Management*

- Mg is added in IV and TPN solution to prevent hypomagnesemia.
- Treatment is continuing for several days to restore intracellular Mg.

*Dietary Management*

Mild deficiencies are of Mg providing increased intake of Mg rich foods.

## Hypermagnesemia

Hypermagnesemia is serum Mg level is more than 2.6 mg/dL.

### Etiology

Renal failure

### Clinical Manifestations

- **Neuromuscular:** Muscle weakness, depressed deep tendon reflexes.

- **Cardiovascular:** Hypotension, bradycardia, cardiac arrest.
- **GI system:** Nausea, vomiting.

### Management

*Medical Management*

- Administered IV calcium gluconate to reserve neuromuscular and cardiac effects of hypermagnesemia.
- In renal failure cases dialysis or peritoneal dialysis is performed for removing excess Mg.

## Hypophosphatemia

Hypophosphatemia is serum phosphorus level isles than 2.5 mg/dL.

### Etiology

- Refeeding syndrome develop when malnourished clients starts enteral or total parenteral nutrition. Glucose containing solution stimulates insulin secretion and helps the entry of glucose and phosphate into the cell, diminish extracellular phosphate level.
- Medication frequently contributes to hypophosphatemia including IV glucose solution, antacid (magnesium based) and diuretics.
- Alcoholism affects both intake and absorption of phosphate.
- Other causes including diabetic ketoacidosis with extensive phosphate loss in urine.

### Clinical Manifestations

- **CNS:** Irritability, apprehension, weakness, lack of coordination, confusion, seizures, and coma (reduced oxygen and ATP synthesis in the brain).
- **Respiratory:** Chest muscle weakness can interfere with effective ventilation, leading to respiratory failure.
- **GI:** Anorexia, dysphasia, vomiting, nausea, and decreased bowel sounds.
- **Cardiovascular:** Decreased oxygenation of the heart muscle can cause chest pain and dysrhythmia.
- **Musculoskeletal:** Muscle weakness.

### Management

- IV phosphate is given when serum phosphate is less than 1 mg/dL
- Oral phosphate supplements
- Improved dietary pattern.

## Hyperphosphatemia

Hyperphosphatemia is serum phosphate level is greater than 4.5 mg/dL.

### Etiology

- Acute and chronic renal failure is the main reason of impaired phosphate excretion.
- Rapid administration of phosphate containing solution.

### Clinical Manifestations

- Muscle cramps and pain
- Paresthesia
- Tingling around the mouth
- Muscle spasm and tetany.

### Management

- Correct the serum phosphate level by consumption use of phosphate containing drug.
- Intake of phosphate rich diet such as milk, meat, and milk products are avoid.
- IV normal saline should be started to promote renal excretion of phosphate.
- Dialysis can reduce phosphate level in client with renal failure.

## PROGRESSIVE PATIENT CARE

Progressive patient care (PPC) is one of the nursing care concepts. The concept began to take shape in the middle of 1950s, the overall aim of this concept was to organize hospital services so that the client gets optimum care corresponding to his required needs.

### Definition

PPC is described as the group of the hospital services and staff according to the changing medical and nursing need of the clients. Progressive patient care is the area where patients are nursed in different units according to the illness suffered by them.

### Major Concepts of PPC

- It is the improved patient care by the hospital facilities, services and staff around the changing needs of the patient.
- PPC is concerned for the right patient with the correct services at the exact time.
- PPC is organized classification of patients according to their medical needs.
- Critical care nursing is an exciting and challenging field. There are many principles of critical care nurses that contribute to the care that they provide. This lesson describes the principles of critical care nursing.

## Description

Under progressive patient care system, the patient is classified and place in different units of the hospital according to his need and not according to medical diagnosis. The patient may need intensive care or long-term care and accordingly he is admitted to the appropriate unit irrespective of his medical diagnosis. The concept has undergone some changes over the years with the trend towards specialization, a variety of progressive patient care elements have been established under a decentralized setup in major department of large hospitals.

## Principles and Elements of Progressive Patient Care

- **Intensive care:** Critically ill patients who receive intensive care around the clock, who need constant attention are admitted to intensive care unit. The purpose of this unit is lifesaving.
- **Intermediate care:** When the patient no longer needs the close attention by the nurses and they are transferred to the intermediate care unit when condition improves and vital function are stabilized.
- **Self-care:** The ambulatory patient who are mostly self sufficient in terms and need daily care requirement. Self care patient patients require minimal nursing care and are not ready for discharge, as they may need few more days to adjust to activities of daily living, particularly if they have been transferred to this unit from an intensive care unit, e.g., patient recovering from acute poisoning.
- **Long-term care:** Chronically ill patients or disabled patients who require nursing care for a prolonged period. Rehabilitation is occupational therapy and physical therapy may be needed for these patients. Patient teaching is emphasized with a view to helping these patients learn how to adjust to their illness and disabilities, e.g., paraplegia client, cancer client.
- **Home care:** It is a supportive care provided in the home and it is a hospital care-based program provides all the resources for the patient, e.g., short-term and long-term related services.
- **Outpatient care:** For the ambulatory patient requiring simple diagnostic, curative preventive and rehabilitative services.

## Advantages of Progressive Patient Care

- **To the client:** Clients receive specific consideration when they require it. Assistance will be provided to make adjustments of the client to the hospital and later to home and community.
- **To the nursing personnel:** They can be efficient in special abilities and potentials. Placement can be made according to skills and competencies of nursing staff. Team can include semi-skilled staff to extend the nursing services to low risk patients, can be under the guidance of qualified registered nurses. They can deliver increased and improved quality of nursing services.
- **To the hospital:** Can enhance the quality of patient care as a result of effective and efficient use of personnel. Can maintain continuity of care and co-ordinate home care services.

## Disadvantages

There may be discomfort to client who is moved often. It is very difficult to establish long-term nurse client relationships. There is also difficulty in meeting administrative need of the organization like accreditation, staffing and evaluation.

## CONCEPT OF CRITICAL CARE NURSING

As changes in healthcare evolve critical care, nursing continues to expand. Patient desires have become more complex, and nurses need to provide high-quality care with specific competencies like good leadership, participating in health policy, evidence-based practice and research, joint effort and cooperation. Critical illness is a dramatic event for both the individual and their family. Life-threatening physical illness can be coupled with overwhelming psychological responses. As care becomes more complex so are the ethical issues associated with this. The Intensive care nurse as a member of the multidisciplinary team requires education and experience to perform their role competently.

The purpose of critical care is to provide care so that the patient recovers from acute illness or to reduce the complications of the chronic illness.

Since forty years critical care units have been developed. Florence nightingale realized the necessities to think about the impact of sickness in allotment of beds to patients and kept the critically sick patients close to the nurses' location. In 1923, a special care unit for neurosurgical patients developed by John Hopkins University Hospital. After Second World War, modern medicines got its higher ranking. As surgical techniques advanced, the concept of recovery room came out. In 1950, the epidemic of poliomyelitis called for maximum patients depending on intensive nursing care and respiratory assist devices. At that time, also new horizons on cardiothoracic surgery like modification in the techniques of intra operative membrane oxygen came out. A four-bedded unit opened in 1953, at Manchester Memorial Hospital of Philadelphia.

In 1970, the term Intensive care came with various types of special care units along with direct patient care accountability and development of new patterns of care. Pediatric intensive care units and special care unit for babies came out as it was necessary to have separate units with therapeutic and diagnostic equipment and devices for the care of children.

Critical care nursing is a multifaceted and demanding nurse specialty to which various registered nurses desire. Intensive care nurses must be skilled in a variety of sophisticated skills. They must be proficient in administering care, recognizing complications, evaluating intensive care patients and manage with additional members of the intensive care team.

## Principles of Critical Care Nursing

- **Anticipation:** It is the first principle and individual has to distinguish the high-risk clients and predict the necessities, complications and be ready for any emergency. All units should be organized in which all essential supplies and equipment are required for successful management of the unit.
- **Early detection and prompt action:** Accurate prediction of the client depends on the timely recognition of differences, quick and suitable action to check complications is very important. Assessment of cardiac and respiratory functions is most important in first level of management.
- **Collaborative practice:** Critical care practice is a very comprehensive area, which require specific body of knowledge for the nurses and physicians working in the same department, promotes a joint venture to take decision, and make sure about quality and empathetic patient care. Organized teamwork is more reasonable for critical care patients.
- **Communication:** Communication has a considerable significance in the management of all units. Various evidence-based communication models enhance outcome as much as patient, healthcare professionals are concerned. This model gives more importance to the client centered management, promotes clinical decision-making, utilize available medical records and emphasizing on evaluation of client care.
- **Prevention of infection:** Nosocomial infection charges more for healthcare services. Critically sick clients necessitate intensive care are more prone for the risk than other clients because of the less immunity with the stress and antibiotic usage, prolonged stay and severity of illness, invasive lines, mechanical ventilators and surroundings of the critical care department itself.
- **Crisis intervention and stress reduction:** During crisis, partnerships are to be created and bonds are established, becomes stronger during hospitalization between nurses, patients and families. When a client advocates at that time nurses should support the patient to express their fear, recognize their pattern of grieving, and give opportunity for positive coping.

Along with principles of critical care nursing and critical care nurse are very much precious for best nursing practice. Various principles of critical care nurse are:

- **Highly qualified nursing practice:** Bedside practice occurs through quality improvement, being involved at the organizational level, and collection of data. Quality improvements are reviewing care plans of clients, prognosis of prior patients, and using various evidences to enhance the outcomes of the clients.
- **Education is power:** Due to rapid advances in technology healthcare is developing. Critical care nurses should not stop learning and they will have to be very dynamic. As part of their practice and certification, these nurses attend classes and training sessions in order to improve their competency as a critical care nurse.
- **Working with others:** Team spirit is very essential in critical care unit. As part of being in critical care nursing; these nurses share what they know about caring for patients with their co-workers. They provide constructive feedback to help others improve their practice. They also contribute to and support a healthy work environment that is crucial to optimal patient outcomes in the critical care area.
- **Ethics are imperative:** Nurses have a code of ethics they must follow regardless of what area whereever they are working. The ethics guidelines ensure that nurses maintain confidentiality, support their patients physically as well as spiritually, deliver care to any and all patients, and report any illegal or incompetent practices of other healthcare providers.

## Scope of Critical Care Nursing

It presents an outline in which a critical care nurse can provide appropriate services. This scope provides a definition and description of the nursing practice at critical care areas. The scope is very dynamic with the three components.
1. The critically ill patients and their important social relationship.
2. The critical care nurse.
3. The critical care environment where nursing service is practiced.

### Critically Ill Patient

Critical care patients having some essential characteristics like:
- A major health dilemma that brings threat to life.
- Health problem for which client depends upon health-care providers, very frequent need for continuous health maintenance and life support.

**According to the American Association of Critical Care Nurses (AACN):** Critically ill patient described as follows:
- Occurrence of actual and/or potential life-threatening health problems.
- Quick assessment and strategies should be ready to re-establish the health and prevent complications.
- Must include family and significant others during the development of strategy.
- Requirements for critically ill are categorized as physical or non-physical
  - Physical like basic physiological or biological needs.
  - Non-physiological needs may comprise social, spiritual, and psychological needs self-esteem, information and communication communications.

Good social relationship provides the comfort and support, which enhance effective coping. Patient's family need should be considered as first priority. For meeting the needs of critically ill patient, planning the holistic nursing care is very essential.

### Critical Care Nurse

The critical care nurse is a certified professional and accountable for practicing in critical care areas and accountability in making clinical judgments to prevent clinical deterioration in critically ill patients. Anticipation and early prevention of patient problems are vital requirements for critical care nursing practice, and these requirements mandate highly developed assessment and clinical judgment skill.

Patient problems can be predicted through sound understanding of anatomy and physiology and well judged assessment skills. Professional accountability and comprehensive knowledge on biophysical and social sciences is essential for critical care nursing practice.

Knowledge constantly needs revision and development through various research activities and technological novelty. Critical care nursing practice must highlight the need of holistic approach in patient care system.

### Critical Care Environment

Critical care environment is a specific environment that is designed and structured to provide excellent possible patient care and to decline the patient morbidity, and emphasizes safety of both patient and staff as prime concern.

Critical care environment is viewed from three prospective:
1. Direct interaction between the critical care nurse and the critically ill patient.
2. Sufficient resources that always maintain various interactions among patient and healthcare professional.
3. Quality control systems and maintenance of standard of nursing care. Challenging factors of legal, regulatory, social, economic and political factors, which influence the provision of critically ill care.

## CRITICAL CARE UNIT SETUP

The above setup offers a practical and user friendly situation. The central components of an ICU are continuous observation, quick and expert intervention and multi-disciplinary teamwork. Various factors are to be considered like sources of patients, predictable rate of occupancy, economic assets and practicability, admission and discharge criteria, personnel required and technological resources.

### Equipment and Supplies

**Intensive care unit** (ICU) equipment helps in constantly monitoring the patient and providing respiratory and cardiac support, managing intensity of pain, consist of emergency resuscitation devices, and other life support equipment designed to care for patients who are critically ill and life-threatening illness, or have undergone a major surgical procedure, thus necessitate 24-hour care and monitoring.

### Patient Monitoring Equipment

- **Acute care physiologic monitoring system:** It is a complete patient monitoring system that continuously measures and display a number of parameters via electrodes and sensors that are connected to the patient. Each patient bed in an ICU has a physiologic monitor that measures various body parameters (heart rate, BP, $SaO_2$, etc.). All monitors are connected to central nurses' station.
- **Pulse oximeter:** Measures the arterial hemoglobin oxygen saturation with a sensor clipped over the finger or toe.
- **Intracranial pressure monitor:** It measures the pressure of fluid in the brain of patients with head trauma or other conditions affecting the brain such as tumors, edema, or hemorrhage. These devices provide warning for elevated pressure and record various pressure trends.

- **Apnea monitor:** Breathing is monitored continuously via electrodes or sensors positioned on the patient. Incase off risk of respiratory failure, an apnea monitor notice cessation of breathing in infants and adults, show respiration parameters, and activate an alarm in case of absence of breath in patients.

*Life Support and Emergency Resuscitative Equipment*

Critical care equipment for life support and emergency resuscitation includes the following:
- **Ventilator (also called a respirator):** Assists with or controls pulmonary ventilation in patients who cannot breathe on their own. Ventilators check and alarms if any deviation from normal breathing pattern will be in patient. It is connected to a central monitoring system or information system.
- **Infusion pump:** It is a piece of equipment that transports fluids intravenously or epidurally by a catheter. Infusion pumps make use of pumping mechanisms for delivering continuous anesthesia, drugs, and blood infusions.
- **Crash cart:** It is a resuscitation or code cart containing emergency resuscitation equipment for patients. Crash carts are located in the ICU for instant accessibility for the patient during cardiorespiratory failure.
- **Intra-aortic balloon pump:** It is a machine that helps to decrease the heart's workload and assist blood flow in the coronary arteries. The balloon at the last part of a catheter is connected to the pump's console, which exhibit readings of heart rate, pressure, and electrocardiogram (ECG). The patient's ECG shows the inflation and deflation of the balloon.

*Diagnostic Equipment*
- Mobile X-ray for bedside radiography.
- Handheld, portable point-of-care analyzers are used for blood analysis at the bedside.

*Other ICU Equipment*
- Disposable ICU equipment includes urinary (Foley) catheters, catheters used for arterial and central venous lines, Swan-Ganz catheters, chest and endotracheal tubes, gastrointestinal and nasogastric feeding tubes, and monitoring electrodes.
- Some patients may be wearing a posey vest, also called a Houdini jacket for safety; the purpose is to keep the patient stationary.
- Spenco boots are padded support devices made of lamb's wool to position the feet and ankles of the patient.
- Support hose may also be placed on the patient's legs to support the leg muscles and aid circulation.

### Use and Care of Therapeutic and Diagnostic Equipment

Intensive care unit patient monitoring systems are equipped with alarms that sound when the patient's vital signs deteriorate—for instance, when breathing stops, blood pressure is too high or too low, or when heart rate is too fast or too slow.

Disposable items, such as catheters and needles, should be disposed of in a properly labeled container. ICU staff should take out daily check the equipment and when equipment needs maintenance, repair, or replacement, notify biomedical engineering staff. Third-party servicing companies if available, should be kept up-to-date at all times.

All ICU staff must have undergone specialized training on sophisticated ICU equipment and must be trained to act in response to life-threatening circumstances, since ICU patients are in risk for respiratory or cardiac emergencies.

## DOCUMENTATION IN CRITICAL CARE UNIT

A long-ago, mostly clinical data were documented as heart and respiratory rates, blood pressures, and flows, but now a day's integrating various data from monitor and other devices, which measure blood gases, chemistry, as well as combine data from various sources outer to the critical care unit.

Uninterrupted measurement of client's parameters such as heart rate and rhythm, respiratory rate, blood pressure, blood-oxygen saturation, and several other parameters have become vital for critically ill patients. When decision-making is critical for patient care, electronic monitors commonly are used to assemble and display physiological data. Gradually more, such data are collected using non-invasive sensors from less seriously ill patients at medical-surgical units, labor and delivery suites, nursing homes, or patients' own homes to detect unpredicted life-threatening conditions or to record routine data efficiently.

### Procedure and Monitoring at CCU

Patient monitoring is the repeated or continuous observations or measurements of physiological function, and the function of life support equipment, for the purpose of guiding management decisions, therapeutic interventions, and assessment of those interventions.

With the arrival of additional automatic devices, the ICU nurse usually spends less time for assessing the vital signs and more time in caring critically ill patient. Several nursing professionals moved away from the bedside to a central console for monitoring the ECG and vital-sign reports from many patients. Maloney (1968) pointed out that this was an inappropriate use of technology when it deprived the patient of adequate personal attention at the bedside. He also suggested that having the nurse record vital signs every few hours was "only to assure regular nurse–patient contact".

As checking potential expanded, healthcare professionals shortly were dealt with a maze-like number of gadgets; they were threatened by data overload. Several investigators opined that the digital computer may be supportive in problem solving associated with data collection, review, and reporting.

As computer technology has rapidly advanced, the meaning of computer-based monitoring has changed. Systems with database functions, report-generation systems, and some decision-making capabilities are usually called computer-based patient monitors.

**There are at least five categories of patients who need physiological monitoring:**

1. Patients with unstable physiological regulatory systems; for example, a patient whose respiratory system is suppressed by a drug overdose or anesthesia.
2. Patients with a suspected life-threatening condition; for example, a patient who has findings indicating an acute myocardial infarction (heart attack).
3. Patients at high risk of developing a life-threatening condition; for example, patients immediately after open-heart surgery or a premature infant whose heart and lungs are not fully developed.
4. Patients in a critical physiological state; for example, patients with multiple trauma or septic shock.
5. Mother and baby during the labor and delivery process.

**Care of the critically ill patient requires prompt and accurate decisions so that life-protecting and life-saving therapy can be appropriately applied. Computer-based documentation are having following needs:**

- Frequently or continuously assessing physiological data.
- Communicating information to remote locations like radiology departments and various laboratory.
- Reporting, organizing and storing the data.
- Correlating and integrating data of various resources.
- Providing clinical alerts and advisories basing upon various types of data.
- Health professionals can utilize decision-making tool for planning the care.
- Measuring severity of illness, which helps in patient classification.
- Evaluating outcomes of cost effective and clinical effective ICU care.

**Computers assist in the following activities:**

- Monitoring arrhythmia.
- Invasive monitoring events such as the insertion of an arterial catheter.
- Computer checks and verifies reasonable data. Data Calculation and communications errors can be reduced.
- Data can be integrated from various sources and does reliable interpretations and make alerts.
- Assisting physicians in calculating appropriate drug doses.
- Computer networking provides quick access to all laboratory data and can even interpret the results and provide alerts.
- Enteral (tube-feeding) and parenteral (IV) nutritional-support services like estimating the desired volume of dietary supplements.
- Titrated therapeutic interventions with infusion pumps for calculating the administration of intravenous fluids and drugs.

The accessibility of microcomputers has really improved the capability to make the processing of the physiological data used in patient monitoring. Furthermore, exploration is needed by which the computer can be used efficiently to integrate, display and evaluate the results and make simpler the complex data related to critically ill patients.

**Flow Sheets**

The goal of the flow sheet is to effectively and accurately communicate the patient's status and to document nursing care efficiently and accurately have been achieved.

The design of a critical care nursing documentation form in a flow sheet format provides quick access to and makes fast communication about patient information. Flow sheet format is a standardized documentation, which aids in quality assurance and remove duplicate documentation. Healthcare professionals can save time in communicating.

Flow sheet which is a documentation sheet in which graphical representation of various health related parameters, particularly the vital signs, weight, the treatments going on, medications given, and procedures performed.

The flow sheets should be simple and located in one place, so nursing, medicine, and surgery can share the elements.

### *Advantages of using Flowcharts*

- **Communication:** Healthcare professionals can communicate very effectively through flowcharts.
- **Effective analysis:** Analysis of problems can be done very effectively trough flow chart by reducing cost and wastage of time.
- **Proper documentation:** Flowchart is very systematic program documentation, which is essential for making things well-organized.
- **Efficient coding:** It helps as blueprint during the systems analysis and program development phase.

- **Appropriate debugging:** The flowchart facilitates in correcting the process also.
- **Efficient program maintenance:** Operating program can be managed very effectively with the help of flowchart. Programmers can put efforts more competently on that parts and also better the logic of a system can be communicated to all concerned involved.

### Disadvantages of using Flowcharts
- **Complex logic:** Sometimes, the program logic is quite complicated. In that case, flowchart becomes complex and clumsy.
- **Alterations and modifications:** If alterations are required the flowchart may require re-drawing completely. This will usually waste valuable time.
- **Reproduction:** As the flowchart symbols cannot be typed, reproduction of flowchart becomes a problem.

## EVIDENCE-BASED CRITICAL CARE NURSING PRACTICE

The movement of evidence-based practices grounded in the 1980s and 1990s, due in part to the readily available computer databases that prepared accessing healthcare research easier.

The safest care provided by healthcare professionals is evidence-based. It uses current knowledge and best evidence to make decisions about how to care for critically ill patients. This means that research is performed by nursing experts on how to care for patients in ways that ensure the best patient outcomes.

Crystal Bennett, identifies five basic steps in the practice of evidence-based medicine:
1. Formulation of a clinical question.
2. Gathering the best evidence to address the question.
3. Critical evaluation of the best evidence.
4. Merging evidence with the clinician's own experience, the patient's condition, available resources and the patient's preferences and values to come to a clinical decision.
5. Evaluation of evidence implementation, in order to determine practice change.

### Strength of Evidence to Support Practice
- **Level I:** Meta analysis of multiple studies
- **Level II:** Experimental studies
- **Level III:** Well-developed quasi-experimental studies
- **Level IV:** Well-developed non-experimental studies
- **Level V:** Case reports and clinical examples.

In order to implement evidence-based practice we need changes and improve the quality of the care provided within the organization, the group must decide on both the practices for change and the model to guide this process. The best way to integrate this process into practice is through the development of a committee to facilitate evidence-based practice and quality improvement.

### Barriers to Evidence-based Practice
#### Organizational
- Evidence-based practice was a low management priority
- Difficulties with teamwork
- Inadequate systems for managing personal and professional development
- Difficulties in managing innovation
- Inadequate systems for dissemination
- Difficulties in accessing evidence
- Resource constraints.

#### Culture and Practice of Nursing
- Motivation to change practice cannot be assumed.
- Unclear and competing interpretations of nursing roles and practice.
- Cultures emphasize doing and inhibit questioning of practice.

### Benefits of Evidence-based Practice
The final goal of the EBP is to standardize and get better access and quality of care across the healthcare system. Various patient and nurse benefits comprise the following:
- **Improved patient outcomes:** EBP helps nurses to direct patient care as per scientific research, like randomized controlled trials, patient care studies and compiling patient data, based on nursing interventions that have established successful in the past with same type of patient populations.
- **Lower costs of care:** Evidence-based practice across the healthcare spectrum often offers improved patient outcomes, less demands on healthcare resources and in lowering healthcare costs. Patient-centered approach may assist remove needless costs connected to treating serious patients and also lessen expenses for healthier patients.
- **Superior nursing skills:** EBP permits nursing professionals to contribute research to nursing profession and applying the current research and practices while removing untested methods. Incorporating EBP enhances advanced critical thinking and decision-making skills.

## FUTURE OF CRITICAL CARE NURSING

Critical care nursing practice can either serve as the basis for innovative leadership in the continuing evolution of autonomous nursing practice or it can continue on an evolutionary track of critical care medical practice implemented by nurses. If the vision of the future is one in which critical care nurses engage in more than the implementation of pharmaceutical and medical treatment regimens, then the vision is worth making a reality. Each nurse needs to accept responsibility for the current state of nursing. Every nursing personnel should be sure that their part of the future matches their vision for critical care nursing.

A lot of challenges ahead for nurses as far as looking at how:
- We can best integrate palliative care and end-of-life pain management into our critical care environments.
- We can address end-of-life issues best with patients and families.
- Nurses can take good care of themselves because that moral distress can be one of a number of factors that can really cause the nurses to develop compassion fatigue.
- Nurses acquire great skills and knowledge-base working with variety of patients.

In future the expectation of society from the hospital will be:

- The computers that control this can somehow link with the patients around the world who have similar values, expectations, and concerns. if you press the button, a nurse or physician immediately appears on the screen over any other data display, asking the need or want.
- Everything seems to be non-invasive. Video-laser system to evaluate alterations in microcirculation. Also evaluate peripheral cell oxygenation and viability of major organs.
- In severe cases, there will be an intubating robot that can insert an endotracheal tube already connected to the respirator. A machine just scanned the chest for about a minute and then showed these amazing pictures and videos of the lungs on that huge screen. Not only that, but the pictures were in 3D, so one could see lungs from inside and out, and how they altered during breathing, and it is better than, old CT and MRI machines of the past, which provides the interpretation instantly.
- Previously clinical trials taking more time, now done in few weeks along with better individualized result.
- There are still some disciplines, need human contact more, like obstetrics, pediatrics, and intensive care.

*Source:* Vincent, JL, Slutsky, AS and Gattinoni, L. Intensive Care Med (2017) 43: 1401.

Keeping pace with the expectations of society, healthcare professionals should be prepared accordingly.

ICU of the future will be shaped by specifically an aging population and few expert critical care practitioners.

Future healthcare will examine how the hospital of the future will deal with the supply-and-demand dilemma that is previously becoming noticeable in the ICU.

It will also check future potential for staffing structure, critical care guidelines, and innovative technological solutions.

Basically highly developed ICUs are having trained critical care teams for providing best possible care. In the future, all ICUs will follow this model in order to improve patient safety and efficiency of care.

These teams can include "not only physicians and nurses, but also respiratory therapists, nutritional support staff, and pharmacists, who collectively function as a highly integrated team, following protocols," says Dr Buchman. "Jointly this team prepares a patient plan and assess the impact of that plan. This is not restricted to medical care; it will include social and spiritual care also, along with case managers, social workers, and chaplains. These professionals contribute to the integrated care plans.

The future of critical care nursing will be built on the firm foundation of our past: Collaborative relationships with physicians and other healthcare professionals, a commitment to furthering nursing education and certification, and a passion for research and practice that will improve outcomes for our patients. Together with our partners we will create the future of critical care nursing.

### Future Key Message for Critical Care Nursing

- Nurses should give importance upon practice during their education and training tenure.
- Nurses should attain higher levels of education and training through a better system of education.
- Nurses should be full partners, with physicians and other healthcare professionals, in redesigning healthcare in the country.
- Effective workforce planning and policy making require an improved information infrastructure.

 **Summary**

Critical care nursing practice is based on individual professional accountability and a thorough knowledge of biophysical and social sciences. Critical illness is a dramatic event for both the individual and their family. Critical care practice is a very comprehensive area, which requires specific body of knowledge for the nurses and physicians working in the same department, promotes a joint venture to take decisions, and make sure about quality and empathetic patient care. Organized teamwork is more reasonable for critical care patients. Quality improvements are reviewing care plans of clients, prognosis of prior patients, using various evidence to enhance the outcomes of the clients and adopting strong and clear documentation system.

### Points to Ponder

- Intensive care nurses must be skilled in a variety of sophisticated skills and must be proficient in administering care, recognizing complications, evaluating intensive care patients and manage with additional members of the intensive care team.
- Homeostatic is the ability or tendency of an organism or cell to maintain internal equilibrium by adjusting its physiological processes.
- Osmosis is the diffusion of fluid through semi permeable membrane from a low solution with solute concentration to solution with a higher solute concentration until there is an equal concentration of fluid on both side of membrane.
- Diffusion is the process by which solutes move from an area of higher concentration to one area of lower concentration, without any expending extra energy.
- Isotonic relating to a solution having the same osmotic pressure as some other solution, especially one in a cell or a body fluid.
- Osmolality is the concentration of a solution expressed as the total number of solute particles per kilogram.
- Progressive patient care is the improved patient care by the hospital facilities, services and staff around the changing needs of the patient.
- Six important principles of critical care nursing are anticipation, early detection and prompt action, collaborative practice, communication, prevention of infections and crisis intervention and stress reductions.
- The scope is very dynamic with the three components. Those are critically ill patients and their important social relationship, critical care nurse and critical care environment where nursing service is practiced.
- Flow sheet (in a patient record) a graphic summary of several changing factors, especially the patient's vital signs or weight and the treatments and medications given.
- Evidence-based practice (EBP) is a problem-solving approach by which the healthcare provider makes clinical decisions using the best available scientific evidence, one's clinical experiences, and patient preferences in the context of available resources.
- The core concept of the reconceptualized model of certified practice is the AACN synergy model for patient care based upon the needs or characteristics of patients and families influence and drives the characteristics or competencies of nurses.
- Critical care nursing practice can either serve as the basis for innovative leadership in the continuing evolution of autonomous nursing practice or it can continue on an evolutionary track of critical care medical practice implemented by nurses.
- The future of critical care nursing will be built on the firm foundation of our past: Collaborative relationships with physicians and other healthcare professionals, a commitment to furthering nursing education and certification, and a passion for research and practice that will improve outcomes for our patients.

### Abbreviations

- CCU : Critical Care Unit
- AACN : American Association of Critical Care Nurses
- PPC : Progressive Patient Care
- ICU : Intensive Care Unit
- IV : Intravenous
- EBP : Evidenced-based Practice
- DNSc : Diploma in Nursing Sciences
- RN : Registered Nurse

### Short Answer Questions

1. Define critical care nursing.
2. Write down the principles of critical care nursing.
3. Define progressive patient care.
4. Enlist the elements of progressive patient care (PPC).
5. Write down the advantages and disadvantages of PPC.
6. List out the equipment needed for critical care unit setup.
7. Define flow sheets and write its advantages.
8. Define evidence-based practice and mention the barriers to evidence-based practice.
9. Define AACN synergy model for patient care. Describe the patient characteristics of the synergy model.

### Long Answer Questions

1. Discuss the historical development of critical care nursing.
2. Define progressive patient care and explain principles and elements of PPC.
3. Elaborated the scope of critical care nursing in detail.
4. Explain regarding the documentation system of critical care unit with examples.
5. Discuss about AACN Synergy model of patient care with examples.
6. Discuss on the future and various challenges of critical care nursing practice.

### Bibliography

1. Adhikari NK, Fowler RA, Bhagwanjee S, Rubenfeld GD. Critical care and the global burden of critical illness in adults. Lancet. 2010 Oct 16;376(9749):1339-46.
2. Caroline Richmond. Bjørn Ibsen. BMJ 2007; 335:674.

3. Gardner RM, Sittig DF, Clemmer TP (1995). Computers in the intensive care unit: A match meant to be! In WC Shoemaker et al. (Eds.), Textbook of Critical Care (3rd ed., pp. 1757–1770). Philadelphia: WB Saunders.
4. Ginzton LE, Laks MM (1984). Computer aided ECG interpretation. MD Computing, 1:36. This article summarizes the development of computer-based ECG interpretation systems, discusses the advantages and disadvantages of such systems, and describes the process by which atypical systems obtain and processes ECG data.
5. Goran SF. A second set of eyes: An introduction to Tele-ICU. Crit Care Nurse. 2010 Aug;30(4):46-55.
6. Hillman K. Critical care without walls. Curr Opin Crit Care. 2002 Dec;8(6):594-9.
7. Hillman KM, Bristow PJ, Chey T, Daffurn K, Jacques T, Norman SL, Bishop GF, Simmons G. Antecedents to hospital deaths. Intern Med J. 2001 Aug;31(6):343-8.
8. http://www.surgeryencyclopedia.com/Fi-La/Intensive-Care-Unit-Equipment.htmLixzz5CAU9xswl
9. https://www.encyclopedia.com/medicine/encyclopedias-almanacs-transcripts-and-maps/intensive-care-unit-equipment
10. Kause J, Smith G, Prytherch D, Parr M, Flabouris A, Hillman K. A comparison of antecedents to cardiac arrests, deaths, and emergency intensive care admissions.
11. Munro, Cindy L. The 'Lady with the Lamp' Illuminates Critical Care Today. Am J Crit Care 2010;19:315-317.
12. Mushin WW, Lunn JN. The anesthetist and intensive care. Br Med J. 1969 Jun 14;2 (5658):683-4.
13. Savino, Joseph S, C William Hanson III, and Timothy J Gardner. "Cardiothoracic Intensive Care: Operation and Administration." Seminars in Thoracic and Cardiovascular Surgery 12 (October 2000):362–70.
14. Szmuk P, Ezri T, Evron S, Roth Y, Katz J. A brief history of tracheostomy and tracheal intubation, from the Bronze Age to the Space Age. Intensive Care Med. 2008 Feb;34(2): 222-8.

Chapter 1: Introduction to Critical Care Nursing    17

Patient's Name: _____    Date: _____

| | | | | | | | | | | | | | | | | |
|---|---|---|---|---|---|---|---|---|---|---|---|---|---|---|---|---|
| TEMP/HR/RHYTHM | TIME | | | | | | | | | | | | | | | |
| | TEMP C=Celsius, F=Farenheit | | | | | | | | | | | | | | | |
| | HEART RATE | | | | | | | | | | | | | | | |
| | RHYTHM | | | | | | | | | | | | | | | |
| | RESP / SPO | | | | | | | | | | | | | | | |
| BLOOD PRESSURE | ARTERIAL LINE | | | | | | | | | | | | | | | |
| | MEAN / MEAN | | | | | | | | | | | | | | | |
| | NBP | | | | | | | | | | | | | | | |
| SWAN GANZ CATHETER | PAP(S/D) | | | | | | | | | | | | | | | |
| | MEAN | | | | | | | | | | | | | | | |
| | PCWP / CVP | | | | | | | | | | | | | | | |
| | C.O. / C.I. | | | | | | | | | | | | | | | |
| | SVR | | | | | | | | | | | | | | | |
| | PVR / LVSWI | | | | | | | | | | | | | | | |
| IABP | ASSISTED SYS. / DIA | | | | | | | | | | | | | | | |
| | MEAN / AUG | | | | | | | | | | | | | | | |
| | % AUG / FREQ | | | | | | | | | | | | | | | |
| IV FLUIDS (INTAKE) IV GTTS | ENTERAL | | | | | | | | | | | | | | | |
| | | | | | | | | | | | | | | | | |
| | | | | | | | | | | | | | | | | |
| | | | | | | | | | | | | | | | | |
| | | | | | | | | | | | | | | | | |
| | | | | | | | | | | | | | | | | |
| | | | | | | | | | | | | | | | | |
| | | | | | | | | | | | | | | | | |
| | | | | | | | | | | | | | | | | |
| | | | | | | | | | | | | | | | | |
| | | | | | | | | | | | | | | | | |
| MISC. | | | | | | | | | | | | | | | | |
| OUTPUT | URINE | | | | | | | | | | | | | | | |
| | NG | | | | | | | | | | | | | | | |
| | CT #1 | | | | | | | | | | | | | | | |
| | CT #2 | | | | | | | | | | | | | | | |
| | DRAIN | | | | | | | | | | | | | | | |

**24 Hr. Critical Care Flow Record (ICU; CCU & CVS-ICU)**

*Source:* http://www.govthospital-forms.com/114.pdf

# Chapter 1: Introduction to Critical Care Nursing

Date: _____

| | * NARRATIVE NOTE | 00 | 1 | 2 | 3 | 4 | 5 | 6 | 7 | 8 | 9 | 10 | 11 | 12 | 13 | 14 | 15 | 16 | 17 | 18 | 19 | 20 | 21 | 22 | 23 |
|---|---|---|---|---|---|---|---|---|---|---|---|---|---|---|---|---|---|---|---|---|---|---|---|---|---|
| **ACTIVITY** | Up Ad Lib | | | | | | | | | | | | | | | | | | | | | | | | |
| | Bedrest | | | | | | | | | | | | | | | | | | | | | | | | |
| | Turn Self | | | | | | | | | | | | | | | | | | | | | | | | |
| | Turn w/Assist  B=Back  R=Right  L=Left | | | | | | | | | | | | | | | | | | | | | | | | |
| | BSC w/Assist | | | | | | | | | | | | | | | | | | | | | | | | |
| | BRP w/Assist | | | | | | | | | | | | | | | | | | | | | | | | |
| | Dangle w/Assist | | | | | | | | | | | | | | | | | | | | | | | | |
| | Chair  Self  ☐ Cardiac Chair  ☐ High Back Chair | | | | | | | | | | | | | | | | | | | | | | | | |
| | Ambulated Self                Distance | | | | | | | | | | | | | | | | | | | | | | | | |
| | Specialty Bed in Use: (type) _____ | | | | | | | | | | | | | | | | | | | | | | | | |
| **SAFETY** | Bed Low Position | | | | | | | | | | | | | | | | | | | | | | | | |
| | Call Light in Reach | | | | | | | | | | | | | | | | | | | | | | | | |
| | Siderails - x _____ | | | | | | | | | | | | | | | | | | | | | | | | |
| | Bed Exit Alarms on | | | | | | | | | | | | | | | | | | | | | | | | |
| | **C**ontact **D**roplet **A**irborne **N**eutropenic | | | | | | | | | | | | | | | | | | | | | | | | |
| | Monitor Alarms on | | | | | | | | | | | | | | | | | | | | | | | | |
| | Hilrom Bed Mode ☐ Comfort  ☐ Prevention | | | | | | | | | | | | | | | | | | | | | | | | |
| **HYGIENE** | Bath: ☐ Self ☐ Assist ☐ Complete ☐ Refused | | | | | | | | | | | | | | | | | | | | | | | | |
| | Tracheostomy Care Completed | | | | | | | | | | | | | | | | | | | | | | | | |
| | GI Access Care Completed ☐ J-Tube ☐ G-Tube ☐ PEG | | | | | | | | | | | | | | | | | | | | | | | | |
| | Mouth Care | | | | | | | | | | | | | | | | | | | | | | | | |
| | Peri Care | | | | | | | | | | | | | | | | | | | | | | | | |
| | Urinary Cath Care Bag Change Due _____ | | | | | | | | | | | | | | | | | | | | | | | | |
| | Shave | | | | | | | | | | | | | | | | | | | | | | | | |
| | Shampoo | | | | | | | | | | | | | | | | | | | | | | | | |
| **IV SITE** | IV Site(s)  Initials = Intact * Focus (narrative note) | | | | | | | | | | | | | | | | | | | | | | | | |
| | IV Pump Functioning Correctly (assess every shift) | | | | | | | | | | | | | | | | | | | | | | | | |
| | PCA Pump | | | | | | | | | | | | | | | | | | | | | | | | |
| **MISC.** | SCD's  ☐ Knee  ☐ Thigh | | | | | | | | | | | | | | | | | | | | | | | | |
| | Blanket: ☐ Heating ☐ Cooling | | | | | | | | | | | | | | | | | | | | | | | | |
| | Ted Hose ☐ Knee  ☐ Thigh | | | | | | | | | | | | | | | | | | | | | | | | |
| | Dressing Dry & Intact: _____ | | | | | | | | | | | | | | | | | | | | | | | | |

| SIGNATURE | INITIALS |
|---|---|
| | |
| | |
| | |
| | |
| | |

Form 6334 R: 12/01

**24 Hr. Critical Care Flow Record (ICU; CCU & CVS-ICU)**

Date: _____

## 24 HR. CRITICAL CARE FLOW RECORD
### (ICU, CCU, CVS-ICU)

### NEUROLOGICAL

**LOC**
- AL = Alert Wakefulness
- D = Drowsiness
- ST = Stupor
- CO = Coma
- AN = Anesthetized
- C = Confusion

**Orientation To**
- PE = Person
- PL = Place
- X = Time
- 3 = All the above

**Pupil Reaction**
- BR = Brisk
- SL = Sluggish
- NR = Nonreactive

Pupil sizes: 1mm, 2mm, 3mm, 4mm, 5mm, 6mm, 7mm, 8mm, 9mm

**Glasgow Coma Scale**

*Eye Opening*
- 4 = Spontaneous
- 3 = To Speech
- 2 = To Pain
- 1 = No Response

*Verbal Response*
- 5 = Oriented, converses
- 4 = Disoriented, converses
- 3 = Inappropriate words
- 2 = Incomprehensible sounds
- 1 = No Response

*Best Motor Response*
- 6 = Obeys
- 5 = Localizes
- 4 = Flexion (withdrawal)
- 3 = Abnormal Flexion (Decorticate)
- 2 = Extension (Decerebrate)
- 1 = No Response

**HOB**
- FL = Flat
- Degree of elevation 10-45°
- RT = Reverse Trendelenburg
- T = Trendelenburg

**Motor**
- S = Strong
- W = Weak
- A = Absent

**Reflex**
- C = Cough
- G = Gag
- CO = Corneal
- 3 = All the above

### RESPIRATORY

**Respiratory Type**
- R = Regular
- I = Irregular
- S = Shallow
- L = Labored
- H = Hyperventilation
- Ch = Cheyne-Stokes
- T = Trach/ETT

**Breath Sounds**
- Cl = Clear
- Cr = Crackles
- Rh = Rhonchi
- Wz = Wheeze
- E = Expiratory
- I = Inspiratory
- ↓ = Decreased
- O = Absent
- A = Anterior
- P = Posterior
- S = Stridor
- Pr = Pleural Rub

**O₂ Appliance**
- NC = Nasal Cannula
- AFM = Aerosol Face Mask
- VM = Venti Mask
- NR = Nonrebreather Mask
- CPAP = CPAP Mask
- TP = T-Piece / Briggs
- ET = Oral Endotracheal Tube
- NT = Nasotracheal Tube
- TM = Trach Mask
- T = Tracheostomy
- V = Ventilator
- B = Briggs

**CT Type**
- M = Mediastinal
- PL = Pleural

**Leak**
- + = Leak Present
- − = No Leak

**CT Drainage Type**
- B = Bloody
- SS = Serosanguineous
- S = Serous
- P = Purulent

### NEUROLOGICAL / RESPIRATORY

| Time | LOC | Orientation | Glasgow Coma Scale (E/V/M/T/L) | Pupil Size/Reaction (R) | HOB | Reflex | Motor (RUE/LUE / RLE/LLE) | Respiratory Type | Breath Sounds Right | Breath Sounds Left | O₂ Appliance | Ventilator Settings | Secretions Color & Type | Chest Tubes Type | CT Drainage Type | Suction CMH₂O | System Leak | Patient Leak |
|---|---|---|---|---|---|---|---|---|---|---|---|---|---|---|---|---|---|---|
| | | | | | | | | | | | | | | | | | | |

Form 6334  R: 12/01

**24 Hr. Critical Care Flow Record (ICU; CCU & CVS-ICU)**

# Chapter 1: Introduction to Critical Care Nursing

Date: _____
ALLERGIES: _____
ID Band on (location): _____
Allergy Band on: ☐ Yes   Fall Risk Band on: ☐ Yes ☐ N/A

## CIRCULATORY

**Heart Sounds**
A = Absent
P = Present
S = Split
D = Distant

**Murmur**
A = Absent
P = Present
C = Click

**Rub**
A = Absent
P = Present

**Skin**
W = Warm
Cl = Cool
Co = Cold
H = Hot
D = Diaphoretic
Cm = Clammy
Dr = Dry

**Color**
D = Dusky
A = Ashen
CY = Cyanotic
J = Jaundice
F = Flushed
N = Normal / Pink
P = Pale
M = Mottled

**Capillary Refill (hands)**
N = Normal <3 sec.
S = Sluggish >3 sec.
A = Absent

**Edema Location**
Ph = Peripheral
G = General
P = Pedal
S = Sacral
SC = Scleral
B = Bilateral

**Edema Grade**
1+ = Mild
2+ = Moderate
3+ = Pitting
4+ = Profound Pitting

**Pulses**
0 = Absent
D = Doppler
+1 = Weak
+2 = Normal
+3 = Bounding

**Pacemaker**
T = Temporary
P = Permanent
EP = Epicardial
TCP = External

**Sensitivity**
AAI = Atrial Demand
AOO = Atrial Async
VVI = Ventricular Demand
DOO = AV Async
DVI = AV Sequential
DDD = AV Demand
DDI = AV Demand

## GASTROINTESTINAL/NUTRITION/ELIMINATION

**Abdomen**
Fl = Flat
D = Distended
L = Large
T = Tender
S = Soft
F = Firm
R = Rigid

**Bowel Sounds**
P = Present
A = Absent
↓ = Hypoactive
↑ = Hyperactive
(document appropriate quadrants & location)

**GI Tube Placement**
NG = Nasalgastric
OG = Oralgastric
D = Dobhoff
J = Jejunostomy
G = Gastrostomy

**Tube Feeding**
B = Boost
CD = Choice
U = Ultracal
R = Respalor
M = Magnacal Renal
O = Other (specify)

**Amount**
Document rate cc/hr
B = Bolus document amount

**Residual**
Document amount

**Gastro Drainage/Mode**
C = Clamped
G = Gravity
LCS = Low Continuous Suction
LIS = Low Intermittent Suction

**Emesis**
= Emesis occurred and describe

**Stool**
= Bowel Movement and describe

**Urine Color Character**
Describe
F = Foley
N = Nephrotomy
P = Suprapubic

**24 Hr. Critical Care Flow Record (ICU; CCU & CVS-ICU)**

**Chapter 1:** Introduction to Critical Care Nursing

\* = See Notation in Patient Progress Notes  
Blank spaces = Non-applicable to patient's condition

### BRADEN SCALE (score daily)

| | 1 | 2 | 3 | 4 | Score |
|---|---|---|---|---|---|
| Sensory Perception | Completely Limited | Very Limited | Slightly Limited | No Impairment | |
| Moisture | Constantly Moist | Very Moist | Ocassionally Moist | Rarely Moist | |
| Activity | Bedfast | Chairfast | Walks Occasionally | Walks Frequently | |
| Mobility | Completely Immobile | Very Limited | Slightly Limited | No Limitations | |
| Nutrition | Very Poor | Probably Inadequate | Adequate | Excellent | |
| Friction & Shear | Problem | Potential Problem | No Apparent Problem | Braden Total | |

### PAIN
Scale Rating = 0 to 10  
VAS = Visual Analog Scale  
B = Behavioral  

**Location**  
S = Surgical  
C = Chest  
H = Head  
A = Abdomen  
B = Back  
RUE = Right Upper Extremity  
LUE = Left Upper Extremity  
RLE = Right Lower Extremity  
LLE = Left Lower Extremity  
G = Generalized  
Other = Write location  

**Description**  
A = Aching  
S = Stabbing  
B = Burning  
D = Dull  
T = Tingling  
C = Crushing  
P = Pounding  
T = Throbbing  

**Interventions**  
NA = Not Applicable  
M = Medicate  
P = Position Change  
C = Comfort Measures  
Other = Write intervention

### FALL RISK
Document once every shift.  
\* = in any category indicates patient is currently experiencing the assessment criteria and should be considered a Fall Risk  

Risk = Y = Yes - orange wrist band applied  
N = No  
NA = Due to condition  
Yes = Nurse Implements Falls Precautions

### SURGICAL
**Dressing Dry & Intact** = Defines dry & intact (location of dressing)  
**Dressing Change** = Changed at time documented  
**Suture Line Well Approximated** = Well approximated  
**Staples, Sutures, Steri Strips Intact** = Intact  
**Drainage Amount**  
SC = Scant  M = Moderate  
S = Small  L = Large  
N = None  
**Drainage Type**  
S = Serous  
SS = Sero-Sanguinous  
P = Purulent

### SIGNATURES

| Shift 23-07 |
|---|
| SIGNATURE TITLE/INITIALS |
| SIGNATURE TITLE/INITIALS |
| **Shift 07-15** |
| SIGNATURE TITLE/INITIALS |
| SIGNATURE TITLE/INITIALS |
| **Shift 15-23** |
| SIGNATURE TITLE/INITIALS |
| SIGNATURE TITLE/INITIALS |

| PAIN | | | | | FALL RISK (Minimum Every Shift) | | | | | SURGICAL INCISIONS | | | | | MISC. |
|---|---|---|---|---|---|---|---|---|---|---|---|---|---|---|---|
| Pain Scale Rating | Pain Location | Pain Description | Interventions | Pain Reassessment Time/Scale | Unsteady Gait/ Dizziness/ Imbalance | Impaired Memory or Judgement | Incontinence Ongoing Freq./ Diarrhea | New Fall/ Previous Fall/ Hx of Falls | Risk - Y or N | Drsng Dry & Intact | Dressing Change | Suture Line Well Approximated | Staples/Sutures Steri Strips Intact | Drainage Amount | Drainage Type |
| | | | | | | | | | | | | | | | |

**24 Hr. Critical Care Flow Record (ICU; CCU & CVS-ICU)**

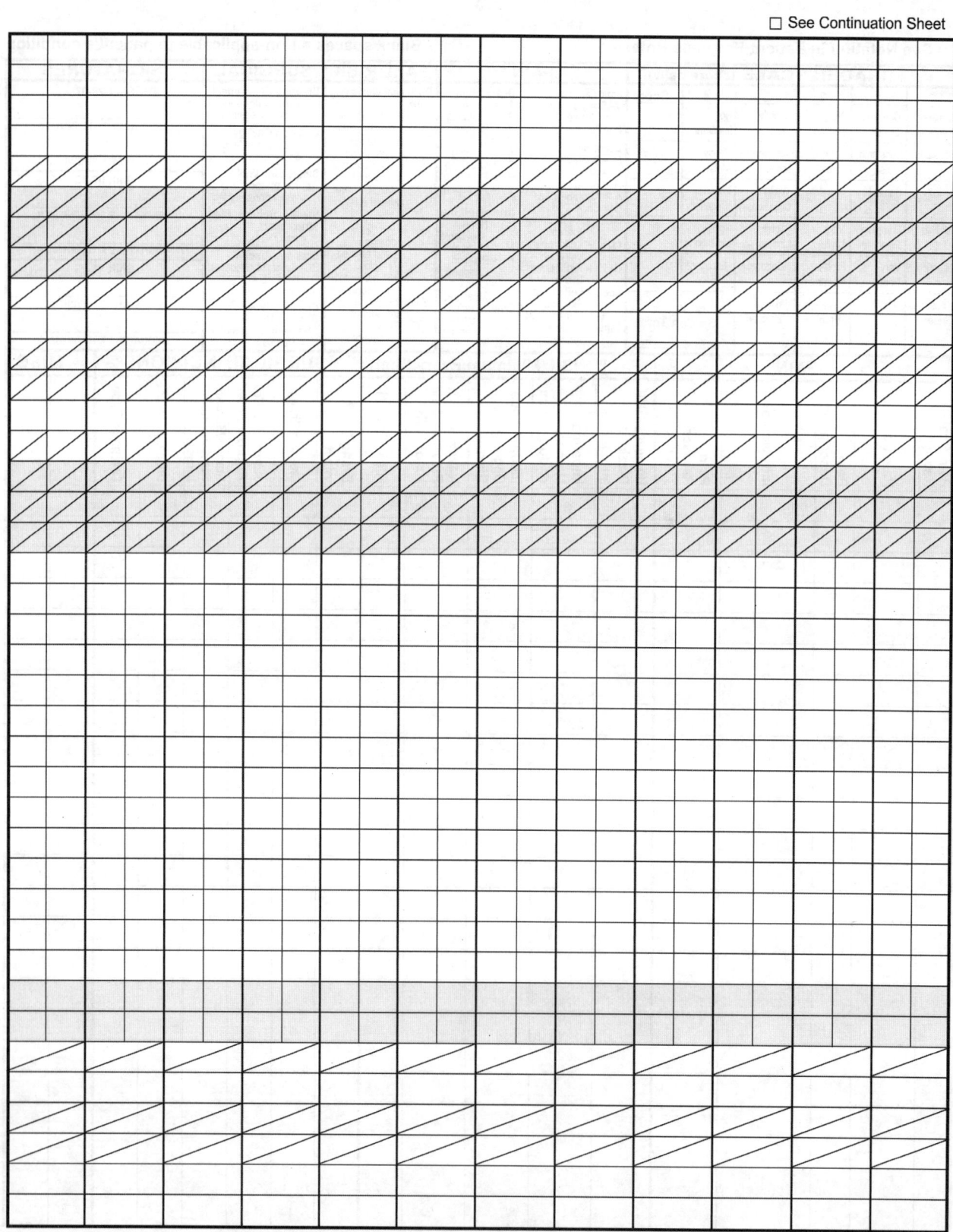

**24 Hr. Critical Care Flow Record (ICU; CCU & CVS-ICU)**

# Chapter 2

# Concept of Holism Applied to Critical Care Nursing Practices

*Sasmita Das*

## CHAPTER OUTLINE

- Patients and Family Perception Towards Critical Illness
- Impact of Critical Care Environment on Patients
  - Environment of critical care unit
  - Assessment of the patient environment interface
  - Critical care psychosis and prevention
  - Psychophysiological and psychosocial problems considerations
- Caring for patient, patient's family and family teaching
- Dynamics of Healing in the Critical Care Unit Environment
  - Healing/therapeutic environment
  - Complementary and alternative therapies in critical care unit
- Stress and Burnout Syndromes among Health Members

### Learning Objectives

At the end of the chapter, the students will be able to:
- Discuss the patients and family perception towards critical illness.
- Describe the impact of critical care environment on the patient.
- Assess patient environment interface.
- Create a healing/therapeutic environment for the patient and caregivers.
- Explain the complementary and alternative therapies used for patient in critical care unit.
- Enumerate various stress and burnout syndromes among health members.

## PATIENTS AND FAMILY PERCEPTION TOWARDS CRITICAL ILLNESS

The intensive care unit (ICU) is a complex clinical setting, where the focus is on the clinical needs of the patient with less attention given to family requirements. Clinical and technical proficiencies are viewed as essential components for nurses working in the critical care, skills that are frequently considered to be of greater importance than caring aspects. Critical illness often occurs without warning, leaving the critically ill relatives feeling vulnerable and help-less with no clear knowledge about the patient's prognosis or outcomes (Eman Ebrahim Fateel, Catherine Sarah O'Neill, 2016).

Holistic caring, the interconnected experience of need and response within a nursing theoretical framework is the nurse's art. It is this art of caring which keeps the balance of technological competency with the art of nursing that promotes adaptations in health crises. Application of holistic caring through established nursing theories such as Watson's theory of nursing and Orem's theory of nursing, enable the critical care nurse to acquire an expert level of nursing ca care.

### Patient Perception

Illness perceptions have a greater impact on outcomes of acute and chronic illnesses. Current evidences show illness perceptions are having strong association with self-management behaviors and quality of life.

Illness perceptions are the prearranged cognitive description or beliefs of the patients regarding their illness. These perceptions have shown effect on treatment adherence and functional recovery. Illness perception components include beliefs about the personal consequences of the condition for the patient and their family, as well as the extent to which the illness is amenable to personal control or to control by treatment.

There are two important aspects:
1. Patients' beliefs about their condition may vary from those treating them. Generally hospital staffs are unaware of patients' view regarding their condition as hospital people rarely asks patients, concerning their own view in clinical meeting.
2. Patients' perceptions varying extensively. Even patients with the same medical condition or injury can have different concepts regarding their illness.

### Family Perception

In India, approximately 18–20% of all deaths in ICU occur in a year and for which family members suffer a lot. When any one in family will be affected by illness, whole family will be suffered. Critical illness frequently happens with no warning and gives no time to get ready. If immediate needs of family members can be met, varieties of problems of family can be resolved. Admitted patients are not capable to talk because of sedation, mechanical ventilation, confusion, and comatose also. Decision making and choosing from treatment options will not be taken by patient and family members, and it leads to increase stress levels and for which various psychological and physical symptoms are manifested.

Various unpredicted stimuli related to therapeutic and diagnostic equipment and unfamiliar sounds frequently bring apprehension and powerlessness and stress among family persons.

As ICU mortality rate is very high that's why patients' family needs physical and emotional support. Nursing professional and other health care professionals should provide clear and right information and empathetic care to family members. Because off they will have to involve in taking decision regarding patients those are unable to communicate.

Nursing care is not only meant for patients but for whole family. In the part of families experiencing severe stress, anxiety, feeling helpless and not able to cope is very common. Assessing their needs is first and foremost steps during ICU patients' and family members care. Many numbers of research work have been carried out to recognize the needs of family in the critical care unit. With the critical care family needs inventory (CCFNI), developed by Molten in 1979 and modified by Leske in 1991, various studies have pointed out some basic needs of family members like information related to health, psychological reassurance, convenience or proximity, and comfort also.

Families having more stress are not capable to sustain the patient related stress and transmit their stress to the patient. Easy access to patient's information and good relationships with health care employees are very important needs for families. Various research studies enumerated that family members of critically ill patient have various needs like needs for assurance and for information, comfort, closeness, support and patient treatment are especially vital for family.

## IMPACT OF THE CRITICAL CARE ENVIRONMENT ON THE PATIENT

The ICU is very tough environment for the vulnerable critically ill patient. Adverse environmental factors can contribute to delirium. Delirium is associated with an increased length of hospital stay and increased mortality. Frequently reported stressful environmental factors are noise, ambient light, restriction of mobility, and social isolation. Improving the ICU environment involves education of critical care staff, modification of equipment, and careful consideration to future ICU design.

### Components of Critical Care Environment

Critical care unit is a specially designed and equipped facility staffed by skilled personnel to provide effective and safe care for dependent patients with a life-threatening problem.

- Certain physical features like wall of ICU with only one color cause sensory' deprivation, sounds of equipments, ventilators, chest tubes, nursing station at foot of ward, unit light only switch and lack of privacy.
- Individual room or walled cubical, room are often either side of hall, central monitoring, open nursing station, some unit without external room windows, Separate switch, calendar and watch in patient room cause increase privacy, better control of lighting, noise, infection. Disadvantage is less patient observation, less control of light and sound if cubical is separated by only glass.
- Individual room, folding glass door arranged in semi-circles. Some unit have decentralize nursing station, patients room have windows with external view control over patient.
- Folding or sliding glass doors with privacy curtains. Circular/pod shaped floor plan. Increased noise reduction designing. Patient windows with a view of outdoors (natural or contrived). Patient controlled lighting— artificial and natural. Planned areas for family in patient rooms. Increased use of color and texture in wall, floor, and ceiling coverings. Nursing access and availability of high-tech care in a more homelike environment.

**Factor of ICU environment that affect patient are noise, odor, light, emotion and color.**

## Noise

The volume of noise in critical care units normally surpasses the suggested limits for hospitals, and need major implications for the psychological and physiological health of patients and healthcare professionals.

Noise affects both caregivers and patients and health care people, not only disturb rest and slow down attention and cognition, but it also impede the communication and augment the risk of accidents.

### Noises Recorded in the Critical Care Unit

Source of noise:
- Items falling onto the floor up to 92 dB (A)
- Equipment movement (e.g., bed) 90 dB (A)
- Connection of gas supply 88 dB (A)
- Door closure 85 dB (A)
- Pager 84 dB (A)
- Talking 75–85 dB (A)
- Ventilator alarm 70–85 dB (A)
- Nebulizer 80 dB (A)
- Telephone 70–80 dB (A)
- Television 79 dB (A)
- Oximeter 60–80 dB (A)
- Monitor Alarm 79 dB (A)
- Ventilator 60–78 dB (A)
- IV infusion alarm 65–77 dB (A)
- Endotracheal aspiration unit 50–75 dB (A)

Sleep deprivation is very common for critically ill patients. Medication effect, physical discomfort, nature of illness has a harmful influence on quality of sleep and environmental factors also. Due to deprivation in sleep, critically ill patient is affected with impaired cognitive and memory formation, lead to confusion also. Less sleep is also linked with cardiovascular stress, less immunity and catabolic metabolism. In case of ICU patients and other healthy people present in ICU, Nearly about 20–25% of EEG-monitored arousals from sleep have been linked with high levels of sound. Noise disrupt sleep is perhaps more significant in recovery phase of patients. Though, noise creates negative effects other than sleep disturbance.

If hearing loss is related to critical illness, it may be aggravated by noise. In hearing impairment noise may hinder communication, which affects understanding of the environment. In case of elderly whose speech-processing capability are more receptive to noise interference. Hearing impairment seen with a greater prevalence of psychotic symptoms in both general and psychiatric populations. Loud unfamiliar noises, which not only brings strangeness in the patient's surroundings but also interrupt sleep, affects recalling capacity and cognition. Later leads to confusion and delirium.

Noise is an important risk factor in developing burnout syndrome among nursing personnel. Noise reduces the performance and mental efficiency of healthcare people. Research work reported for unfavorable staff attitude in noisier situation. An increased level of noise enhances speech amplitude, trying to be more audible (the "Lombard effect"), which affect patient's privacy. Also the communication between staff or among staff and patients may get affected and mistakes can be found also.

## Odors

Exposure to odors could result in health effects ranging from none, to more serious symptoms. Some chemicals with strong odors may cause eye, nose, throat or lung irritation. If an odor lasts a long time or keeps occurring, it also could affect mood, anxiety and stress level.

The perception of smell consists not only of the sensation of the odors themselves but of the experiences and emotions associated with these sensations. Our olfactory receptors are directly connected to the limbic system, the most ancient and primitive part of the brain, which is thought to be the seat of emotion.

One reason this might be has to do with the way your brain processes odors and memories. Smells get routed through your olfactory bulb, which the smell-analyzing region in your brain. It's closely connected to your amygdale and hippocampus, brain regions that handle memory and emotion.

It turns out that your sense of smell is the most powerful of all your five senses. In fact, the deep limbic center (he part of your brain that controls your emotions) is connected to your olfactory system, which means that different scents can affect your mood or evoke certain memories and emotions.

## Light

Light impacts human health and performance by four main mechanisms:
1. **Enabling performance of visual tasks:** The common effect of light is in facilitating vision and performing visual tasks. According to Boyce and colleagues (2003), the nature of the taskas as well as the amount, spectrum, and distribution of the light determines the degree of performance that is accomplished.

    Nurses and physicians are very stressful in ICU work environment. Insufficient light and a disorganized environment are enhancing burden of stress and s main cause of error.
2. **Controlling the body's circadian system:** Light from the retina passes to the hypothalamus control the body's circadian rhythm (biological events that recurs at regular intervals), that is coordinating the body's internal clock

to 24 hours. If the internal rhythms are not matching with workday rhythms, healthcare professionals and other staff can experience lethargic, exhausted, and distracted. In case of individuals, working through the whole night, a 24-hour cycle that make the majority people wakeful and alert in the day and sleep in the night and that leads to fatigue and incapability to carry out their work during the night shift.

Light activation of the pineal gland leads to suppress secretion of melatonin and is accompanied by feelings of depression and sleepiness (Lewy et al., 1985). An increased melatonin level is the cause of drowsiness, whilst less melatonin levels are connected to a state of alertness (Edwards and Torcellini, 2002).

Contact without side daylight is a important cause for the circadian rhythm. By controlling the circadian system, light (both natural and artificial) have a impact on many health outcomes amid patients and health care staff in hospitals such as depression, sleep, circadian rest-activity rhythms, as well as length of stay in the hospital. Eleven research work highlights that bright light is helpful in lessening depression among CCU patients and night-shift health care workers also. Bright morning light exposure has been shown to diminish agitation among aged patients with dementia. Patients, who are exposed to an increased intensity of sunlight experienced less perceived stress, marginally less pain,

3. **Affecting mood and perception:** Alteration in mood affects and brings changes in behavior and performance at work place. On the other hand, mood changes may be different for people with the similar lighting situations.
4. **Facilitating direct absorption for critical chemical reactions within the body:** Skin absorbs the light radiation and which stimulate chemical reactions in the blood and other tissues. It supports Vitamin D metabolism and prevents neonatal hyper bilirubin anemia.

## Risk Factor Assessment and Assessing Patient Environment

### Risk Factors Assessment

Patient safety is one of the nation's most urgent health care challenges, which are in the domain of clinical risk management; in fact, clinical risk management is a principal element of clinical governance.

This is self-assessed and provides an assessment framework to demonstrate how well individual healthcare organizations believe they are performing in key areas including:
- Food
- Cleanliness
- Infection control
- Patient environment (including bathroom areas, lighting, floors and patient areas)
- Privacy and dignity

**Anxiety assessment:** Anxiety is the psycho physiological signal that the stress response has been initiated. Because intense anxiety can create further morbidity in vulnerable patients, the ability to assess anxiety is important. Patients experience anxiety as a result of the interface of the illness with the ICU environment.

Highest priorities of detected potential errors of the ICU Nursing care should be assess very carefully by the health team members:
- Ventilator alarm malfunctions
- DVT formation
- Low position of the head while gavages feeding
- Bede sores
- Patient falls from bed
- Absence of routine disinfectants for washing hand
- Difference in device setting and doctors order
- Absence of washing the suction by nursing professionals
- Failure to identify the type of alarm by the nurse
- Failure to perform hand washing techniques by health care professionals.

ICU potential errors are not due to nursing failure and neglect but there are many factors caused errors such as feeling of patient, patient with complicated disease conditions, malfunctioning of equipment, carelessness and mismanagement of physicians and other personnel, Inadequate training of nursing care professional and weakness due to heavy workload in ICU. Team members have to develop strategies which were categorized in four general categories (https://www.ncbi.nlm.nih.gov)

1. Rigorous training and actions taken for getting better of clinical cares
2. Rescheduling shift duties and motivating healthcare professionals
3. Appointing experienced, energized and skill full people
4. Timely do the maintenance like repairing and calibrating of various therapeutic and diagnostic equipment.

Risk assessment is a logical method to quantitatively and qualitatively assess the risks for persons, materials, used equipments, and the surroundings. It also investigates effectiveness and competence of existing control methods. Through risk assessment various precious information regarding the measures to decrease risks, getting better existing control systems.

For the risk management, first is the detection of errors and their effects and the second is about the analysis of critical points to determine the severity of each error.

### Team to Assess Patient Environment

Healthcare professionals including nurses, matrons, doctors, catering and domestic service managers, executive and nonexecutive directors, dieticians and responsible administrator carries out assessments. Patients, patient representatives and members of the public are also part of this assessment process.

Patient led assessments will provide motivation for improvement by providing a clear message, directly from patients, about how the environment or services can be more effective.

## Critical Care Psychosis and Prevention

CCU psychosis is commonly considered as delirium. It is an acute dysfunction of the brain in which psychiatric manifestations are present with no identified history of mental health history. Even after post recovery of illness, there is a 60% of patient are not recovering from earlier baseline cognitive status (Brummel, 2013).

Data shows that in CCU, 60–80% of ventilated patients and 20–50% of nonventilated patients affected with psychosis. ICU patients too have a more chance on a ventilator for a extensive period an increased risk of self-extubation, and removing urinary catheter by himself. Also having risk for greater mortality after receiving discharge from the hospital (Dembler, 2018).

CCU psychosis is categorized as follows (Yezdani, 2016):
- Hyperactive
- Hypoactive
- Mixed type.

### Contributing Factors Leading to CCU Psychosis

Various contributing factors lead to ICU psychosis:
- Age
- Occurrence of dementia
- Existence of hearing or a visual injury
- Hypertension and renal impairment
- Smoking
- Diagnosis of sepsis
- Taking vasopressors
- Renal replacement therapy
- Acute respiratory distress syndrome
- Irregular bilirubin levels
- Unusual urea levels
- Use of restraints
- Inadequate day light contact
- Inadequate orientation to time place and person.
- Medications may aggravate an episode of ICU psychosis are analgesics and other medications like phenergan, benadryl, cyclobenzaprine, due to its anti cholinergic action, dopamine and steroids.

### Manifestations

Manifestation of ICU psychosis depends on type and it' severity of clinical features. The manifestations are (Welker, 2020):
- Restlessness and hearing of voices
- Clouding of consciousness, hallucinations
- Nightmares, paranoia
- Disorientation, agitation
- Delusions, abnormal behavior

Amid various ICU psychosis, the hypoactive form is very tough to detect because off its inert nature (Farkas, 2020).

### Diagnosis

It is very difficult to detect the severity of ICU psychosis.

Various other conditions have an impact on ICU psychosis, such as metabolic syndromes endocrine related problems, medicine toxicity, brain injury, and cerebral vascular injury, a tumour, and sepsis, etc.

ICU-CAM assessment tool use an algorithm, which is very simple to use and can assess ICU psychosis very fast. Different components of tool were scored categorically.

The first category is based on manifestations, if the beginning is a unexpected and alteration in baseline features or if the mental condition varies over twenty-four hours. In case off unexpected arrival, After going through score nurse move towards phase two. If the beginning is not unexpected, the patient is taken as CAM-Negative.

The second category is for if the patient can give notice by having the patient squeezes the nurse's hand at the time of letter A is heard while the nurse spells out S-A-V-E-A-H-A-A-R-T. If the patient makes two or less errors, the patient is CAM-Negative, but if the patient gets more than two errors, the nurse shifts on to parts three.

The third category measures the patients' level of consciousness, by using the RASS scale. If the patients get besides 0, then the patient is CAM-Positive. If, still, the patient has a 0, then the nurse moves for the assessment and asks basic questions, and the patient reacts with a firm answer. Examples of the questions are:
- "Does a stone float on water?"
- "Does one pound weigh more than two?"
- "Can you use a hammer to pound a nail?"

Subsequent to the questions, the nurse directs the patient to "hold up this two fingers". If the patient carries out the command effectively, the nurse advises the patient to hold the same numbers with the other hand.

If the patient does 0–1 errors, the results are CAM-Negative. If the patient does more than one error, the patient is taken as CAM-Positive (Research Gate, 2012).

### Prevention and Management of ICU Psychosis

Evidences stated that, patient having ICU psychosis may enhance stay in the ICU and hospital, which increase cost of hospitalization by 20%, long-standing anxiety, hopelessness, post-traumatic stress disorder, cognitive impairment, and even death (Vasilevskis et al., 2018).

First aim is to make the patient safe, bring into baseline cognitive functioning, and prevent or alleviate long-term effects.

The first line of treatment may include Haldol, which is a first-generation antipsychotic.

In recent times, second-generation antipsychotics such as olanzapine are used as there are no extrapyramidal complications (Carcella et al., 2019).

The other medication like melatonin and the melatonin receptor agonist ramelteon can lessen the occurrence of ICU psychosis by regulating the sleep-wake cycle in the ICU (Carcella et al., 2019).

Another medication particularly if anticholinergic drugs cause the psychosis, is cholinesterase inhibitors is physostigmine (Arumugam et al., 2017).

### Nonpharmacologic Treatment of ICU Psychosis

Orientation of patients to time place and persons, engaging in diversion activities, supporting with early mobilization, assistance for impaired hearing/vision, providing adequate sleep, adequate hydration and physiotherapy (Arumugam et al., 2017).

The healthcare professionals should remain alert for discharge of patient, the patient may not be aware about the environment of ICU which affects quality of life and the length of that patient's life.

### Post-intensive Care Syndrome

ICU support groups should assist ICU patients improve from the suffering of not only being in an ICU but existing critical illness, PTSD, anxiety, and depression that occur as a consequence (Radigan, 2018).

## Psychophysiological and Psychosocial Problems Considerations

### Challenges of Meeting Psychosocial Needs

- Other conflicting priorities such as addressing the physiologic instability of the patient may preclude or inhibit nurses from meeting the psychosocial needs of the patient and family.
- Psychosocial needs often involve family members due to grief and loss, in most of the cases powerlessness may be relevant to the family members of brain-dead patient.
- Value systems in critical care units in performing nursing tasks for attending the patient and family.
- Emphasizing for a coordinated and multidisciplinary approach to care.
- Handling the barriers in efficiently meeting the psychosocial needs.
- Increasing evidence on association among psychosocial and physiologic problems.

### Patient

- Reassurance and support are needed.
- Psychosocial needs differ as per the patient's status compromised status of patient.
- Psychosocial needs of CCU patients are depend on certain characteristics, like resiliency, vulnerability, stability, complexity, resource availability, participation in care and decision-making, and the predictability of the illness.

### Family

- There is diversity of expected psychosocial needs.
- Family members' psychosocial need may differ basing on patient and family features, status and cultural diversity issues.
- Family members' anticipated needs.

### Critical Care Nurse and Critical Care Environment

- Healthcare professionals in critical care unit are the nursing professional, physician, respiratory therapist, social worker, clergy, physiotherapy, occupational and speech therapist, and other healthcare assistant.
- Through the combined efforts of a multidisciplinary team, psychosocial needs of the patient and family can be fulfilled and each member has a distinctive viewpoint and specific contribution to the nursing care plan and achieving patient goals.
- Stressful environment having high-technology and fast-paced environment brings challenges in meeting psychosocial needs of patient.
- Staff awareness and behaviors also have a deep effect on the patient's environment.
- Developing various approaches in providing healing environment.

### Family Issues

- Family cultural pattern and communication pattern should be analysed in depth by critical care nurse.
- Family systems should be considered like various roles and their power structure, mode of communication, way of problem solving and caregiver's role strain.

## Stress

Selye (1974) categorized two types of stress:
1. **Eustress:** When a person comes in contact with non-threatening stimul.
2. **Distress:** When comes in contact with noxious stimuli Psychological stressors commonly found in critically ill. patients and family members are lack of sleep, hopelessness, loss and grief, sensory overload or deficiency and degrees of pain.

## Caring for the Patient, Patient's Family and Family Teaching

### Psychosocial Assessment of Patient and Family Members

*Nursing History*
- **Patient history:**
  - Pre-existing psychiatric, psychological, and social problems
  - Coping mechanisms
  - Support provided by family, friends, spiritual agency and pet animals
  - Patient is having any power of attorney and living wills
- **Family history:**
  - Family representative and caregivers for the patient
  - Contact person for sending information
  - Culture, language of patient and family
  - Coping strategies
  - Support systems of patient
  - Particular family needs like dependent young children and handicap family members
  - Family concerns regarding patient health
  - Suitable family visit time.

*Assessment of Patient*
- Physical examination
- Cognitive assessment like ability for concentration, intensity of judgment and confusion
- Behavioral assessment like sleeping pattern, agitation, communication with health team and family people
- Analysis of findings from various diagnostic studies.

*Evaluation of Patient*

Critical ill patients may have psychosocial problems and each patient and family carry distinctive characteristics regarding care environment (Hardin and Kaplow, 2005). Nursing personnel can assess as per the followings:
- **Resiliency:**
  - *Level 1—minimally resilient:* Women with previous history of suicide and admitted to emergency ward by self gunshot wound to the head.
  - *Level 3—moderately resilient:* Stable alcohol addicted male patient admitted with automobile accident, preparing for transfer to home town hospital for attending counseling session to stop alcohol addiction.
  - *Level 5—highly resilient:* A healthy adolescent girl admitted in emergency department exhibiting multiple cut and disruptive, aggressive, and delirious behavior at the time of "spring breakout celebration," caused by drinking, some drug experimenting.
- **Vulnerability:**
  - *Level 1—highly vulnerable:* A malnourished 9 years old child who has been a victim of child abuse admitted with "fall down the stairs" and is planning for discharge.
  - *Level 3—moderately vulnerable:* A 37 years old obese woman admitted with depression after unsuccessful suicidal attempt. Treatment endeavour failed and she does not fulfil the criteria of surgical treatment because of morbid obesity.
  - *Level 5—minimally vulnerable:* A 50 years old single father, admitted for monitoring overnight because of an vehicle crash in which he was having habit of aggressive driving,
- **Stability:**
  - *Level 1—minimally stable:* An elderly woman develops sudden respiratory arrest following the ingestion of strong phenyl which is an attempted suicide.
  - *Level 3—moderately stable:* An 60 years woman admitted to the ICU for GI bleeding secondary to a gastric ulcer. He is also on medical management for preventing manifestation of acute alcohol withdrawal.
  - *Level 5—Highly stable:* A 25 years old female admitted in causality, that could not wake up her after heavy drinking. She is now conscious.
- **Complexity:**
  - *Level 1—highly complex:* An 89 years old man is admitted after taking suicidal attempt following the loss of his wife. Patient has multiple medical problems, with stomach cancer.
  - *Level 3—moderately complex:* A 70 years old patient with COPD admitted in ICU and stated that he does not want mechanical ventilation to extend life. Family has also support to the patient's wishes.
  - *Level 5—minimally complex:* A 45 years old man admitted in gastro medicine IPD with GI bleeding secondary to nonsteroidal anti inflammatory use and got delirium after receiving sedatives.

- **Resource availability:**
    - *Level 1—few resources:* A 60 years old destitute man is admitted with a head injury and patient ID is not accessible.
    - *Level 3—moderate resources:* An 60 years old woman is admitted in emergency ward with probable urosepsis. Patient's family is very worried for out of pocket expenses.
    - *Level 5—many resources:* An adult patient is admitted with reconstructive surgery and. Patient has large amount insurance coverage for both inpatient care and outpatient medical care treatment.
- **Participation in care:**
    - *Level 1—no participation:* An adolescent male mitral valvuloplasty repair four days before. Patient has a five year history of dysrhythmia and now is having severe chest pain and respiratory problem. He is intubated and unable to communicate with the staff.
    - *Level 3—moderate level of participation:* A 28 years old man who got head injury after falling out from 3rd story building roof as intoxicated, he is conscious now and need water to drink.
    - *Level 5—full participation:* A 55 years old woman is admitted to the critical care unit following upper abdominal surgery. She wants to do ROM exercises so that she will sit independently and can take her food as per preoperative instructions given.
- **Participation in decision-making:**
    - *Level 1—no participation:* A 50 years old brain-dead patient is on mechanical ventilation. His wife is on severe depression and She asks the patient's doctor to make all the essential decisions for extubation of patient.
    - *Level 3—moderate level of participation:* The mother of a 19 years old boy who requires a tracheostomy after a suicide attempt and desires several consults from other pulmonary specialists.
    - *Level 5—full participation:* An 70 years old patient with end stage of cancer and need to be extubated from the ventilator and be "allowed to die with dignity".
- **Predictability:**
    - *Level 1—not predictable:* A 60 years old lady with breast cancer has been admitted after ingesting one-half of a bottle of acetaminophen to get relieve from pain.
    - *Level 3—moderately predictable:* A 60 years old man admitted for acute respiratory failure and unexpectedly delirium occurred secondary to a hypoxemia and electrolyte imbalances.
    - *Level 5—Highly predictable:* A 19 years old boy came to emergency with altered consciousness after drinking alcohol.

### Diagnostic Studies

- Required, laboratory studies based on manifestations
- EEG
- Cerebral blood flow studies.

### Psychosocial Care Issues

- Interdependence like inefficiently managing degrees of pain.
- Powerlessness of patient and family members in describing problem, communicating goals of care, participating in decision making and in collaborating professionals on health care team.
- Strategies are required like promoting patient-nurse communication, involving family members in decision making and health care system. Counseling on spiritual support and active participation in care delivery and planning system.

### Sleep Deficiency

- **Description of problem:** Sleep deprivation means decline in the quantity, consistency, and/or quality of sleep that arises during 24-hours episode. Sleep breakup takes place if the patient does not have 90-minutes usual sleep cycle that comprises both rapid eye movement and nonrapid eye movement sleep (Gawlinski and Hamwi, 1999).
- **Goals of care:**
    - As a minimum of 90-minutes of sleep in a day
    - Client will state the feeling of rested
    - No signs and symptoms of sleep deprivation.
- **Interventions:**
    - Providing as a minimum of two 90-minutes continuous sleep in a day.
    - Arranging cluster activities for not disturbing patient unnecessarily
    - Control the level of noise to encourage sleep
    - Control room light to promote sleep
    - Advice pain relieve measures if needed
    - Adopt various diversional measures to enhance rest and sleep
    - Advice pharmacologic agents for promoting sleep and should be cautious for use of benzodiazepines for a long period, which may eliminate stage IV sleep.
- **Evaluation of patient care:**
    - No manifestation for sleep deprivation.
    - Patient verbalizes feeling of sufficient sleep

*Grief and Loss*
- **Description of problem**
  - It is response to a loss and experienced by both the patient and family members arises from loss of health, body image.
  - Cause of getting grief in family members related to death of patient or in expectation of possible death
  - Intensity of grief should be analysed on the basis of sense of particular loss to the individual, coping responses, and the accessibility of various support systems
- **Goals of care**
  - Patient and family can articulate feelings of grief and loss
  - Patient and family may tell prognosis and present care plan.
- **Healthcare team can collaborate with each others for fulfilment of goals.**
- **Interventions**
  - Welcome and accept cultural deviation in terms of grief
  - Permit both patient and family for stating their grief how they have perceived?
  - Maintain privacy in the time of providing health care.
  - Always try to provide truthful message to the patient and family concerning the patient's illness and the chances of recovery.
- **Appraisal of patient care:** Patient and family should state grief in a culturally suitable way.

## Therapeutic/Healing Environment

Health care system nowadays are planned not only to sustain the form of the art medicine and technology, patient safety and quality care, but to also to provide psychosocially supportive therapeutic environment. The patient received care in a physical environment may influence patient outcomes, patient and health professional satisfaction and Organizational outcomes.

### Purposes of Therapeutic Environment
- Supports clinical excellence in the treatment of physical body.
- Supports the psychosocial and spiritual needs of the patient, family and staff.
- Produces measurable positive effects on patient's clinical outcomes and staff effectiveness.

### Goal
- Development and maintenance of a situation that will be favorable for the patient (both physical and Psychological well-being and staff).

- The emphasis should be on patient centered care.
- To promote physical welfare, purposeful interaction between the patient and staff that will faster emotional balance and recovery of health within the potential of individual patient.

### Basic Characteristics
The distinguishing elements of such environment include:
- Adequate comfort, food, cleanliness and rest.
- Freedom from injury (mechanical, thermal, chemical, electric, psychology and bacteriologic).
- Individualization of patient care with the opportunity for patient to participate in his or her own plan of care within the limits of patient's capacity and readiness.
- Friendly courteous atmosphere throughout the unit that encourages meaningful communication between patient and nurse.
- A feeling of self worth and security for the nursing personnel.
- Diversional activities available for patient.

### Background of Therapeutic Environment
Therapeutic environment originates from the ground of environmental psychology (the psychology effects of environment), psychoneuroimmunology (the effects of environment on the immune system) and neuroscience (how the brain perceives architecture). In health care organization patients are often apprehensive and unsure about their health, their protection and their separation from usual social affairs. Stress may suppress person's immune system and curb a person's emotional and spiritual status, hinder healing and recovery also.

### Role of Nurses in Maintaining Therapeutic Environment

For creating a therapeutic environment all the members of the team, site and landscape designer, medical planner, architect engineer, nursing officer and interior designer are provided as opportunity to apply design features and make the solutions that will influence the patients and staff in constructive ways all through the facility, from the parking lot, approach and entry, to the public spaces, clinical spaces and eventually the room of patient.

Four key factors which if applied in the design of healthcare environment can measurably improve patient outcome.
1. Reduce or eliminate environmental stressors.
2. Provide positive distractions
3. Facilitate social support
4. Give a sense of control

While application of these factors focused on patient and family, there are also recognized potential benefits for staff and caregivers in terms of satisfaction, effectiveness and staff retention from environmental factors such as:
- Suitable illumination
- Provide 'off stage' region for break
- Nearness to employee
- Suitable use of available technology

*Decrease or Remove Environmental Stressors*
- Acoustical partition from other patients and mechanical noises, staff areas still low noise level (40–58) db can diminish quality of sleep and influence other outcomes negatively.
- Appropriate lighting system "lighting can be a stressor that alters mood increases stress, disrupts daily rhythm and modulates hormone production.
- Providing lighting that supports natural circulation rhythm, providing natural day light where possible or bright white light in the day time. Ensure absolute darkness in the evening; for night time movement only red lights should be present in the room.
- Provide comfortable furnishing.
- Keep up high-quality indoor air.
- Suitable use of color.

*Provide Positive Distractions*
- Views of nature, wherever possible in lobby and other high stress areas.
- Easy to avail the nature and healing gardens.
- Prayer room, meditation room and garden.
- Art work represent nature, as well as back lighted photographs of nature.
- Music should be available in room of patient and public areas.
- Mild physical exercises in corridors and gardens that invite walking when appropriate.
- Pets and other activities that allow a sense of stimulation that helps to nurture a patient's sense of positive well-being.

*Facilitate Social Support*
- Family zone in patient room along with, furniture, Phone, internet connection and reading light with separate control.
- Offer spaces where patients can meet with family members and also kitchen where family members can have food together.
- Give accommodation for family member to be with patient all through the health examination and treatment course.
- Ensure culturally sensitive environments.

*Give a Sense of Control*
- It extends from privacy and lighting to choosing art work beings hangs in patient bed room during hospital stay to arrange meals through room service.
- Patient room privacy.
- Access and control to direct environment, i.e., radio, TV, reading light and night lamp.
- Facility for mini medical library and computer facilities so patients can investigate their conditions.
- Provide choice of art work.
- Room service/menu service.

A safety environment is mainly for maintaining, promoting and restoring health, when a nurse has developed a good relationship with the client the client feel safe and secure in their relationship as well as in the environment, the client will most like demonstrate less anxiety and verbalize satisfaction with surroundings. If the client's expectation has not been met, the nurse must reassess not only the client and environment but also the clients' expressed decisions.

### Nurses in Making Hospital, a Healing Environment

More than 2,000 years ago, the ancient Roman physician Galen has given the idea that environment could provide the healing. Florence nightingale has also emphasized on sanitation and other characteristics of the environment those catalyzes to the health and healing of the patients. She also stated that the environment has a greater impact in patient's healing of body and mind.

Healing environment, for healthcare buildings describes a physical setting and organizational culture that supports patients and families through the stresses imposed by illness, hospitalization, medical visits, the process of healing, and sometimes, bereavement. Wherever professional nursing is practiced; whether this be in a community center or practice, a home, or a hospital ward or unit; a therapeutic environment is created by the presence of nurses. It is a healing culture, rich in therapeutic interpersonal relationships and co-operative attentiveness to patients.

Findings of various research studies have been provided growing concern regarding awareness of the insufficiency of end-of-life care. Intensive care unit nurses have a limited role in end-of-life decision-making and care planning. Cultural issues influencing end-of-life care in intensive care units, explores factors surrounding the limited involvement of critical care nurses in end-of-life decision-making and care planning, and offers recommendations for changing nursing practice. Because improving end-of-life care will require cultural changes, an understanding of the cultural issues involved is needed. Recommendations for changing nursing practice include a model of end-of-life care that incorporates the goals of cure and comfort care, as well as a shared decision-making process. Nurses are essential to improving end-of-life care in today's intensive care units.

Patients in ICU are handled with various strategies; those are perceived to be stressful. Pain during ICU staying, and disturbance related to sudden removal of endotracheal tubes or of intravascular catheters. For which sedatives and analgesics are among the most usually administered drugs in intensive care units. (Michael C Reade, MB, 2014)

*Strategies for Promoting a Healing Environment in the ICU*

Strategies for modifying physical infrastructure, family should involved in various healing actions necessary to the setting of a healing environment. Important elements that diminish stress are enumerated below.

Provide distractions

- Keep artwork, picture of family members, holy items, pet animal photo in the hospital room as the patient desires.
- Use favorite music to which patient likes most comforting.
- Arrange for movies which may distract the patient in a positive way and brings relaxation. Various hospitals have TV and provides story book and newspaper facilities in Intensive care units.
- Arrange for pets, can visit to whom patient like most.
- Patient and family members can move in gardens if provision is there in hospital.
- Outside views through windows also very relaxing for patients.
- Arrange other facilities like provision of exercise, playrooms for children, other entertainment opportunities.

Eliminate environmental stressors

- Arrange nice smells to reduce disinfectant smell which causes anxiety and stress like lavender may induce sleep facilitate healing process also.
- Use ear plugs for outside noise.
- Adjust lights if it is unpleasant for patients.

Work with the staff

- After going through daily schedule, the members who are supporting family can avail break.
- Always give importance to professional care and be sympathetic and humble to all categories of staff.
- Priorly fix the plan of care and plan should be carried out properly.

Try to find out holistic therapies

- Ask if complementary therapies like massage, therapeutic touch, aroma and music therapy, Reiki, acupuncture and other alternative therapies.

Effectively use nutrition for all

- Find out the type of food available in the hospital or any substitute menu choices are there.
- Arrange for family members food in hospital campus try to provide suitable place for food storage options.

Keep up a loving presence

- Do not forget to take care of yourself, be calm and always should have a loving presence. Avail the leisure time whenever you need it and do regular meditation.
- Be optimistic always and also help the patient for the same.
- Always help to create a loving, healing space for patients and family members.

Emotional aspects of recovery

- Staying in a critical care unit for an illness brings a lot of physical and mental stress.
- In case of emergency basis of admissions, patients perceive a range of emotions in a variety of recovery stages, including fear, anger, frustration and hope.
- At the context of sleep, after discharge it is found that, difficult to sleep in the first month, which brings fatigue and alteration in moods. Many patient use sedatives for getting sleep. Some people slept better than previously also.
- In memory and concentration, few patients thought that their short-term memory had been affected and others are unable to retain information when they were having conversations. Some of them told that their concentrations are reduced and loosing their concentration In reading and watching TV.
- Presence of fear is there; when they first came home, some people said that they felt uneasy on thinking up about unsafe environment of hospital because lack of immediate attention if anything went wrong. Other people gets scared for getting ill and going to ICU again, getting panicked even if there is least cough or cold. Ventilating their recovery with medical staff brings better coping ability.
- Feeling depressed for their weakness, late recovery and for depending on other and became weepy when come first outside. Yet others become depressed at different stages of recovery for that cause is not known.
- Some people get paranoia, panic and flashbacks. Sometimes they are not interested to talk with people or to socialize.
- Some people mentioned that, even though they feel weakness and dependent on others, they were easily accepting what had happened previously.
- Anxiety, depression and post-traumatic stress disorder are frequent for people who have affected with

unexpected critical illness to feel shocked and, later, anxious or depressed.
- On the part of Improvement and recovery, people felt confident again because they were more independent.
- Even if in cases of patients having planned admissions and shifted to ICU for surgery, it can be upsetting and the disturbance to normal daily life is very much worried for the family and patient also.

## Complementary and Alternative Therapies in Critical Care Unit

Usually, the stress is not eliminated so easily in critical care unit environment because many other stressors are introduced along with the previous problem. If the coping mechanism is strong, anxiety may be reduced, and energy will be towards rest and healing. Various types of nursing interventions can be helpful in lessening anxiety and encourage coping in seriously ill patients.

### *Therapeutic Sounds/Music Therapy*

Music therapy, which is classified as a noninvasive nursing intervention, is used as an adjunct to medical therapies. Through music, entrainment takes place when two elements coordinate with each other and vibrate with equal sound frequency. Through the soothing music, there will be decrease pulse rate, respiratory rate, metabolic rate, oxygen consumption, and blood pressure. Traditional music acts as a complementary therapy and also psychoacoustic therapy and is considered as an important aspects of nursing intervention. Psychoacoustic therapy encompasses harmonies of therapeutic tones (Stichler, 2001). The sounds of nature like birds, water, rain, and waves incorporated with soft classical music may lessen anxieties in family and caregivers and can keep in waiting area also.

### *Art for Healing*

Basic purpose of artwork in patient room is to provide soothing, peaceful environment for patients and family members. A peaceful nature scene is exceptional in providing calm and safety feelings (Stichler, 2001). Artwork which represents confused impressions, vagueness, and intangible pictures should not be kept, because It will be disturbing the patient and aggravate the illness also.

### *Aromatherapy*

The sense of odor can stimulate a healing ambiance inside the body, mind, and spirit. Aromatherapy and the utilization of necessary oils for healing disease have been experienced since several years. In the 1940s, people started using aromatherapy, after a French chemist used lavender oil to keep away from an unavoidable amputation of his arm due to gangrene found after a severe burn.

### *Guided Imagery and Relaxation Training*

Guided imagery is a method of distracting or focusing the patients' thoughts and has been found to empower patients, improving their happiness and comfort (Tusek DL and Cwynar RE: 2000).

These two useful procedures can be used by the patient to decrease tension. Healthcare professionals can support the patient to imagine that technique as a very pleasant experience. The patient can be trained to concentrate on experiencing the sensation for long time. Guided imagery has a great role in alleviating hopelessness, anxiety, and aggression.

### *Deep Breathing*

Patient's breathing patterns can fluctuate in case of anxiousness, and due to that patient may grasp his breathing pattern. This is harmful both physically and mentally. Instructing for diaphragmatic breathing, which is also called abdominal breathing, which will enhance distraction and coping among patient.

### *Humor*

Belly laugh creates very positive physiological and psychological effects in which the level of endorphins will be increased through laughing; the endorphins are body's natural pain relievers, which are released into the bloodstream. Laughter can alleviate tension and anxiety and helps in relaxing muscles. Critical care nurses can use humor to decrease procedure related anxiety and can provide distraction also. It is also helpful for patients to alleviate their anxiety and make them feel healthier.

### *Meridian Therapy*

Meridian therapy originates from traditional Chinese medicine. Meridian therapy refers to therapies that involve an acupoint, such as acupuncture, acupressure, and the activation of specific sites with electrical stimulation and low-intensity laser. Meridians are complex energy pathways that integrate into complex patterns (Sutherland JA, 2000). These pathways hold sensitive energy points that stimulate to relieve blockages that affect various physiological functions. Research has demonstrated the efficacy of meridian therapy for pain relief, postoperative nausea, and other functions. At present, research is in progress to authenticate acupoint sites. Specialized training is necessary for health professionals to use Meridian therapy.

### Massage and Therapeutic Touch

Massage is the purposeful stroking and kneading of muscles to provide comfort and promote relaxation (Richards KC and Gibson R, 2000). Nurses need different evidenced based massage therapy techniques along with various steps and should add in the care for critically ill patients.

Therapeutic touch is a method where the practitioner's hand should touch over a patient in a methodical technique to rebalance the patient's energy fields (Umbreit AW, 2000). Therapeutic touch is sympathetic intent on part of the healer. The main purpose of therapeutic touch is as a complementary therapy to reduce anxiety and enhance a sense of well-being. Implementation of healing touch therapy involves a formal educational program for healers, and its potential benefits are under active investigation.

### Animal-assisted Therapy

The human–animal bond has been well documented. Pet ownership has been linked to higher levels of self-esteem and physical health. Pet therapy (animal-assisted therapy) has measurable benefits for school children and residents of nursing homes and helps the clients with a multitude of goals such as improving self-esteem and developing social skills, as well as providing help for anxiety and post-traumatic stress disorder.

## STRESS AND BURNOUT SYNDROMES AMONG HEALTHCARE PROFESSIONALS

Nowadays burnout is very common and has a great impact on both individuals and society. Research evidence recommended that burnout and depression are separate, although they may have several common characteristics.

Stress and burnout among nurses are very high as compared to other health care professionals. The prevalence of burnout among nurses is higher incase off oncology, mental health, emergency and critical care. Worldwide statistics highlight that burn out affects 10–70% among nurses 30–50% among physicians, nurse practitioners and physician assistants.

Burnout syndrome is a psychological state resulting from prolonged exposure to job stressors. Because ICUs are characterized by a high level of work-related stress, a factor known to increase the risk of burnout syndrome.

### Definition

"Burnout is a syndrome made up of emotional exhaustion, depersonalization, and reduced personal accomplishment" (Beck, 1995).

An emotional condition marked by tiredness, loss of interest, or frustration that interferes with job performance. Burnout is usually regarded as the result of prolonged stress (Medical Dictionary).

Important factors contribute for burnout syndromes are stress in working environment and coping with job stress is difficult, because usually there are not many things to do in order to modify the job environment. This is similar to the concept of internal versus external control suggested to be a critical factor in the development of coping (Pearlin and Schooler, 1978, Rotter, 1966).

### Healthcare Setting

- Pressure related to time
- No control on process of work
- Role and task related conflict
- Group relationship is weak
- Workload communication
- Inadequate leadership along with personal influence factors.

### Factors in Family

- Family environment
- Responsibilities
- Familial demands.

### Factors in Individual

- Reduced self-esteem
- Competitiveness
- Expectation for higher job and satisfactions also.

### Causes of Burnout

Actually no exact major stressful events cause job stress. Gathering of minor events of everyday life (hassles) may produce considerable stress (Chamberlain and Zika, 1990). Only Job stress may not be a cause of burnout. However, working in highly stressful work environment, like the nursing staff in intensive care units, critical care unit of adults and pediatrics, may marked higher levels of anxiety, anger, behavior disorders along with depression symptoms.

- Providing care around the clock patients
- Constantly changing development of new technologies
- Constant noise
- Work environment
- Work overload (limited time, resources, staff)
- Young age, early in career, high level of education personality
- Low self-esteem
- Need for approval, perfectionism and impatience.

### Preburnout Indicators

- Depressed and changing mood
- Tension and anxiety
- Hopelessness and powerlessness
- Poor self-esteem
- Inability to concentrate
- Fatigue, nausea, sleep disturbances and muscle pain
- Hyperactivity, turnover and absenteeism
- Resignation, disappointment and boredom.

### Manifestations

- Illness and disability exhaustion
- Extinction of passion
- Mental breakdown
- Severe depersonalization
- Other symptom like frustration, depression, fatigue and hypertension.

### Management

Burnout is difficult to prevent. It is vital to put emphasis on team work along with positive psychological feedback which brings satisfaction for working people in their work environment.

Do the changes in shift posting of nurses in work. though, this shift should not be too recurrent and respect the qualification of the person also timely recognition of depression development is very necessary because it will facilitate the early treatment.

### Individual and Organizational Approaches

- Psychotherapy
- Counseling and various skill related training
- Training for enhancing communication skill and social support for relaxation activity
- More training for supervisors and suitable organizational practices
- Strategically planned training to enhance coping and tackle stress
- Modification in shift work structure
- Giving provision for vacations and recreational activities.

### Psychotherapeutic Approaches Group Therapies

- Provide intervention as per manifestations.
- For fatigue, advice physical relaxation techniques
- Behavioral training is very essential for reducing frustration
- Social support is very much needed to recognize interesting areas and motivating
- Cognitive restructuring
- Training for self control and developing active coping skill.

### Coping Strategies

- Cognitive coping like evaluating potential stressful events
- Active behavioral coping like efforts to be taken for handling stressful conditions
- Avoid stressful conditions and problematic situations.

Given the personal, family and social impact of burn-out, and taking into consideration the present situation of change and crisis in the world of work today, it is ever more necessary to apply systematic and continued interventions to promote health in the workplace such as organizational measures, for example workplace training, supportive feedback from supervisors, role clarification, team culture, and coping strategies (Gómez-Gascón et al., 2013, Kristensen, 2000, Martínez García-Olalla, 2004, Ruotsalainen et al., 2008).

 **Summary**

Holism and holistic nursing have taken on a number of forms and been defined in a number of ways, but in recent years it has become an established specialty with a significant impact on both nursing and healthcare. Nursing care should be addressed for patient and the whole family members. Physical and emotional demands of patient should be considered very carefully by healthcare professionals.

 **Points to Ponder**

- Holistic caring, the interconnected experience of need and response within a nursing theoretical framework is the nurse's art.
- Illness perceptions are the organized cognitive representations or beliefs that patients have about their illness.
- Factor of ICU environment that affect patient are noise, odor, light, emotion and color.
- Therapeutic environment stems from the fields of environmental psychology, psychoneuroimmunology and neuroscience.
- Four key factors which if applied in the design of health care environment can measurably improve patient outcome are reduce or eliminate environmental stressors, provide positive distractions, enable social support and Give a sense of control.
- The ICU setting has the potential for providing possible opportunity to heal if therapeutic environment is incorporated into its physical design.
- Healing environment, for healthcare buildings describes a physical setting and organizational culture that supports patients and families through the stresses imposed by illness, hospitalization, medical visits.

- Therapeutic touch is a set of techniques where the practitioner's hands move over a patient in a systematic way to rebalance the patient's energy fields.
- Giving emphasis on team work and providing positive psychological feedback which is vital for the employee for making them feel satisfied from work.

## Abbreviations

- ICU : Intensive Care Unit
- CCFNI : Critical Care Family Needs Inventory
- IV : Intravenous
- EEG : Electroencephalogram
- CCU : Critical Care Unit
- AACN : American Association of Critical Care Nurses
- PPC : Progressive Patient Care
- EBP : Evidenced-based Practice
- DNSc : Diploma in Nursing Sciences
- RN : Registered Nurse

## Short Answer Questions

1. Write down the important factors of ICU environment affect patient care.
2. Enumerate the essential strategies for promoting healing environment.
3. Enlist the team members to assess ICU environment.
4. Prepare one checklist assess emotional aspects of recovery in CCU patient.
5. List out the important factor contribute to the burnout syndrome.
6. Enlist the preburnout indicators.

## Long Answer Questions

1. Describe perceptions of patient and family members toward critical illness.
2. Discuss impact of critical care environment patient and healthcare professionals.
3. Elaborate the role of nurse in maintaining therapeutic environment at CCU.
4. Explain regarding strategies for promoting a healing environment in CCU.
5. Discuss importance of complementary and alternative therapy for the critical unit patient.
6. Describe stress and burnout syndrome among health team members.

## Bibliography

1. Albaqawi HM, Butcon VR, Molina RR. Awareness of holistic care practices by intensive care nurses in north-western Saudi Arabia. Saudi Med J. 2017;38(8):826-31.
2. American Holistic Nurses Association. About us. [Accessed 2017 January 8]. Available from: http://www.ahna.org/About-Us/What-We-Do.
3. Arumugam S, El-Menyar A, Al-Hassani A, et al. Delirium in the Intensive Care Unit. J Emerg Trauma Shock. 2017;10(1):37-46.
4. Boyce WT, Obradović J, Bush NR, Stamperdahl J, Adler NE. Biological sensitivity to context: The interactive effects of stress reactivity and family adversity on socioemotional behavior and school readiness. Child Dev. 2010;81(1):270-89.
5. Brummel NE, Girard TD. Preventing delirium in the intensive care unit. Crit Care Clin. 2013;29(1):51-65.
6. Buckle, J. Aromatherapy and diabetes. Diabetes Spectr. 2001;14(3):124-6.
7. Buxman K, What's so funny about... being a school nurse? Advocacy, access, and achievement through humor and perspective. 2012;27(3):134-5.
8. Cascella M, Fiore M, Leone S, Carbone D, Di Napoli R. Current controversies and future perspectives on treatment of intensive care unit delirium in adults. World J Crit Care Med. 2019;8(3):18-27. Published 2019 June 12.
9. Christina JH, Pratik PP, Christopher GH. Intensive Care Unit Delirium: A Review of Diagnosis, Prevention, and Treatment. Anesthesiology. 2016;125(6):1229-41.
10. Dembler, Tammie. Monitoring for Psychosis in Hospitalized Patients. US Pharm. 2018;43(11):HS-8-HS-12.
11. Dossey BM. The psychophysiology of bodymind healing. In: Dossey BM, et al. (Ed). Holistic Nursing: A Handbook for Practice, Maryland: An Aspen Publication; 1995.
12. Edwards L, Torcellini P. A Literature Review of the Effects of Natural Light on Building Occupants (Technical Report). National Renewable Energy Laboratory, Golde; 2002.
13. Eman EF, Catherine SN. Family members' involvement in the care of critically ill patients in two intensive care units in an acute hospital in Bahrain. The experiences and perspectives of family members' and nurses'—A qualitative study. 2016;4(1).
14. Farkas J. Delirium. Internet Book of Critical Care (IBCC). Published November 3, 2016. Accessed May 24, 2020.
15. Frisch NC. Standard for holistic nursing practice: A way to think about our care that includes complementary and alternative modalities. Diaksestanggal; 2009.
16. Grahl JJ, Stollings JL, Rakhit S, et al. Antimicrobial exposure and the risk of delirium in critically ill patients. Crit Care. 2018;22(1):337. Published 2018 December 12.
17. Hess D, Bark LA, Southard ME. White Paper: Holistic Nurse Coaching. AHNA Holistic Nurse Coach Task Force Members; 2007.
18. https://www.ncbi.nlm.nih.gov/. Int J Prev Med. 2013;4(5):592-8.
19. Hudak CM, Gallo BM. Critical Care Nursing: A Holistic Approach. Philadelphia: JB Lippincott Company; 1994.

20. Leske J. Internal Psychometric Properties of the Critical Care Family Needs Inventory. Heart Lung. 1991;20:236-44..
21. Lewy AJ, Ahmed S, Jackson JM, Sack RL. Melatonin shifts human circadian rhythms according to a phase-response curve. Chronobiol Int. 1992;9(5):380–92. [PubMed]
22. McLaughlin M, Marik PE. Dexmedetomidine and delirium in the ICU. Ann Transl Med. 2016;4(11):224.
23. Michael CR, et al. N Engl J Med. 2014;370(5):444-54.4.
24. Molter NC. Needs of relatives of critically ill patients. Heart Lung. 1979;8(2):332-9.
25. Radigan K. Post-intensive Care Syndrome: What Happens After the ICU? reliasmedia.com. Published; 2018. Accessed May 24, 2020.
26. ResearchGate. Confusion Assessment Method in the ICU. Published January 2012. Accessed on 5/9/20 for CAM-ICU Flowsheet.
27. Stichler J. Creating healing environments in critical care units. Crit Care Nurs Q. 2001;24(3):1-20.
28. Sutherland JA. Meridian therapy: Current research and implications) for critical care. AACN Clin. Issues. 2000;11(1):97-104.
29. Tusek DL, Cwynar RE. Strategies for implementing a guided imagery program enhance patient experience. AACN Clinical Issues. 2000;11:68–76.
30. Umbreit AW. Healing touch: Applications in the acute care setting. AACN Clin Issues. 2000;11(1):105-19.
31. Vasilevskis EE, Chandrasekhar R, Holtze CH, et al. The Cost of ICU Delirium and Coma in the Intensive Care Unit Patient. Med Care. 2018;56(10):890-97.
32. Vyveganathan L, Izaham A, Mat W, Peng S, Rahman R, Manap N. Delirium in critically ill patients: Incidence, risk factors, and outcomes. Crit Care Shock. 2019;22(1):25-40.
33. Wade D, Als N, Bell V, on behalf of the POPPI investigators, et al. Providing psychological support to people in intensive care: Development and feasibility study of a nurse-led intervention to prevent acute stress and long-term morbidity. BMJ Open. 2018;8:e021083.
34. Welker M. ICU Psychosis (Intensive Care Unit Psychosis). MedicineNet. Accessed February 16, 2020.
35. Yezdani, H. ICU Delirium Causes, Symptoms, Diagnosis, Treatment. Med India. Updated December 30, 2016. Accessed 2/16/20.

# Chapter 3

# Review of Drugs

*Sasmita Das*

## CHAPTER OUTLINE

- Principles of Pharmacokinetics
- Analgesics/Anti-inflammatory
- Antibiotics
- Antiseptics
- Inotropics
- Life-saving Drugs
- Drugs uses in Various Body Systems
- Drug Overdoses and Poisoning
- IV fluids, Blood and Blood Components and Electrolytes

### Learning Objectives

At the end of the chapter, the students will be able to:
- Explain the principles of pharmacodynamics and pharmacokinetics.
- Describe the various types of critical care unit drugs and its nursing responsibilities.
- Assess side effects of various drugs on its uses.
- Discuss drug overdoses and poisoning.
- Enumerate various nursing responsibilities pre, intra and post administration of drugs.

## INTRODUCTION

At present most of the drugs are synthetic and produced in large scale. Synthetic drugs are more pure, safer and less expensive. The interactions between a drug and the biologic system are conveniently divided into two classes, i.e., pharmacodynamics and pharmacokinetics.

### Pharmacodynamics

Greek word 'dynamic' means power. Pharmacodynamics is the scientific discipline that studies relationship between the concentration of a drug and the response or effect.

Pharmacodynamics study on how chemicals exert their effects. This includes physiological and biochemical effects of drugs and their mechanism of the action in the body. The practical importance of this knowledge is that it makes possible the plan of new and better drugs to treat disease.

Pharmacokinetics is the scientific discipline that studies the time course of absorption, distribution, metabolism, and excretion of drugs.

### Pharmacokinetics

Greek word 'kinesis' means movement. Pharmacokinetics is about how the body deals with the drugs. This refers to movement of the drug in and alteration of the drug by body: Includes absorption, distribution, binding, localization, storage, biotransformation and excretion. It helps to answer a most important question, i.e., what are the factors that determine the maintenance of a therapeutically useful level of the drug in the bloodstream? Needs exploration of the following questions:

- **Dose:** How much of the chemical (drug) should be used to get the desired effect without getting unwanted effects? (To obtain right dose, the medicine must be carefully measured).
- **Route of administration:** By what route should the drug be administered?
- **Absorption and distribution:** How is the drug absorbed and distributed?
- **Metabolism and excretion:** How long does the drug stay in the body? How can sustained therapeutic effect be achieved?

## PRINCIPLES OF PHARMACOKINETICS

### Drug Transport Across Membranes

For a drug to transfer to its site of action, mechanisms must be available to allow the drug to traverse numerous biological membranes. These include passive diffusion, filtration, active transport, and endocytosis. These mechanisms are also important for the transfer of endogenous substances required for life.

### Drug Administration

Sruges can enter the body from several sites, with the route of administration, having a significant influence on the ability of a drug to accumulate at its site of action.

In principles of administration of drugs some points of terminology need to explain before discussing routes of drug administration.

### *Internal and External Environment*

Physiologists refer about the internal and external environment where the body is concerned. When anything is taken orally, it remains in the external environment until it or one of its breakdown products passes a cell membrane and gets into a cell of the body.

### *Bioavailability*

Bioavailability is defined as the fraction of unchanged drug reaching the systemic circulation following administration by any route. It means that the drug has reached the circulation and is therefore available to all tissues. For an intravenous dose of drug, bioavailability is equal to unity. For a drug given orally, bioavailability may be less than unity for several reasons. The drug may be incompletely absorbed. It may be metabolized in the gut, the gut wall, the portal blood, or in the liver prior to entry into the systemic circulation. The patient may take 600 mg aspirin, but going through the above "passes", less than 600 mg of aspirin is available to the body.

### Drug Absorption

Drugs can be absorbed into the circulation from numerous sites within the body. Absorption is movement of the drug from its site of administration into the circulation (from the external environment to internal environment). Except, when given IV the drug has to cross the biological (cell) membrane. These membranes are designed to control the movement of chemicals across them very strictly.

### Drug Distribution

Once in the circulation, the drug is transferred to the interstitial fluid and to the cells of the body. Once the drug is absorbed into the blood, it may be distributed to different physical compartments of the body. If avidly bound to plasma proteins, it may remain in the vascular compartment until eliminated.

Small water-soluble molecules may be freely distributed in the total body water. Drugs that are highly lipid-soluble are ultimately distributed to fat. Drugs that are not tightly bound to cells or proteins within the blood, leave the vascular compartment.

Blood flow determines how rapidly drug molecules are delivered to a given tissue and how effectively the concentration gradient between blood and tissue is maintained. Once a drug gets into the bloodstream, however it is carried to all parts of the body and therefore will come into close proximity with virtually all its tissues and organs, and that fact explains many cases of drug side effects.

### Drug Biotransformation

There is an increased interest in the chemical changes in a drug once it enters the body. In most cases, these drug biotransformation reactions produce intermediates with less pharmacologic activity than the parent compound; however, some drug metabolites possess significant pharmacologic action. Furthermore, some metabolites are chemically reactive and capable of contributing to toxicity, mutagenesis, carcinogenesis, and birth defects.

### Drug Excretion

The primary sites for drug excretion are the liver and kidney, although the skin, lungs, and bile and intestine may be sites for excretion as well.

Excretion is the passage out of systemically absorbed drugs. The rate of which the body eliminates drugs is the most important determinant of their duration of action. Drugs and their metabolites are excreted in urine, feces, exhaled air, saliva and sweat, breast milk.

Generally, body tries to get rid of drugs through enzymes that chemically change, i.e., metabolized in the liver so that it is eliminated more easily via the lungs, kidneys or the gut. But the liver itself can become damaged and drugs' actions may be prolonged beyond its desired duration. Similarly, excretion of drug may depend on the condition of kidneys.

Clinical pharmacokinetics—each of the above processes affect not only the rate of accumulation of a drug at its site action, but also its rate of removal. Clinical pharmacokinetics provides a quantitative description in humans of the behavior of drugs with different characteristics as well as the differences expected from different routes of drug administration.

An important parameter, i.e., measurement of the drugs duration of stay in the body is the plasma half-life.

## Plasma Half-life

Half-life is an expression of the relationship between volume and clearance. The plasma half-life ($t^{1/2}$) of a drug is the time taken for its plasma concentration to be declined to half of its original value. It can be measured by giving a dose of the drug, sampling blood at intervals.

Half-life is a useful kinetic parameter in that it indicates the time required to attain 50% steady state. Ideally, one should like to give a single dose of a drug that maintains steady levels at therapeutically effective concentration which is called the steady-state. It is required to keep giving doses at intervals to maintain the effective concentrations. After the first dose the blood levels of the drugs start rising, and further doses may be needed to achieve the desired level. From working out the plasma half-life of a drug, it has been observed that the time taken to reach steady-state is approximately five times the half-life of a drug. For example, the drug digoxin has a life of 36 hours, therefore the patient must be given doses regularly for the steady-state.

## Loading Dose

This is a single or few quickly repeated doses administered in the beginning to attain steady-state levels with a drug that has a longer half-life.

## Maintenance Dose

This dose is one that is to be repeated at specified intervals after attainment of steady-state levels, so as to maintain the same by balancing elimination.

# ANALGESICS AND ANTI-INFLAMMATORY DRUGS

**Algesia (pain)** is an ill-defined, unpleasant bodily sensation, usually evoked by an external or internal noxious stimulus (chemical, thermal, electrical, mechanical). Pain is a warning signal and primarily proactive in nature but causes discomfort. Pain receptor organs are distributed throughout the body.

Clinically, pain can be categorized as:
- Superficial or cutaneous pain. It is felt as pricking, and stinging, or burning if prolonged.
- Deep nonvisceral pain from muscles, joints, ligaments and bones usually it has a dull character, and it may be accompanied by a sickening sensation due to an autonomic response. Blood pressure and pulse, however, are not much affected.
- Visceral pain is dull aching in character, diffuse and often accompanied by sweating, nausea, fall in blood pressure and even shock. In addition, muscle rigidity and hyperesthesia are common accompaniments. Examples: Myocardial infarction, renal/biliary colic, appendicitis, pancreatitis.
- Referred pain—deep pain, visceral or somatic in origin, may sometimes be misinterpreted as if it is coming from some part of the body other than the actual site of pathology. This is called referred pain, for example, cardiac pain commonly referred to the left arm, diaphragmatic pain to the shoulder.
- Psychogenic or functional pain is usually a vague pain which follows no definite anatomical pattern of distribution. Such pain is usually continuous from day to day and involves. more than one part of the body.

**Analgesic**—a drug that selectively relieves pain by acting in the CNS or on peripheral pain mechanisms, without significantly altering consciousness.

Pain is a warning signal, primarily protective in nature, but causes discomfort and suffering, may even be unbearable and incapacitating. It is the most important symptom that brings the patient to the physician. Excessive pain may produce other effects-sinking sensation, apprehension, sweating, nausea, palpitation, rise or fall in BP, tachypnoea. Analgesics relieve pain as a symptom, without affecting its cause. They are used when the noxious stimulus (evoking the pain) cannot be removed or as adjuvant to a more etiological approach to pain. Analgesics are divided into two groups:
1. Opioid/narcotic/morphine-like analgesics.
2. Nonopioid/non-narcotic/aspirin-like/antipyretic or anti-inflammatory analgesics.

# OPIOID ANALGESICS AND ANTAGONISTS

**Opioids:** Generic term for drugs with morphine like activity, that reduce pain and induce tolerance and physical dependence, also called as narcotic analgesics.

**The mechanism of action of opioid analgesics and opioid antagonists (Table 3.1).**

| Table 3.1: Opioids and related drugs. | | |
|---|---|---|
| **Agonists** | **Partial agonists** | **Antagonists** |
| • Morphine<br>• Diamorphine<br>• Antagonists<br>• Methadone<br>• Pethidine (Meperidine)<br>• Dihydrocodeine<br>• Dextropropoxyphene | • Buprenorphine<br>• Pentazocine | • Naloxone<br>• Naltrexone |

The body's own types of opioids are endorphins and enkephalins. They interact with several distinct opioid receptors in the nervous system, and they appear to function as endogenous analgesics. When these receptors are stimulated by opioid drugs, transmission of nerve impulses related to pain is inhibited and the pain is suppressed. Among so many opioid receptors, the µ receptors are most important. These are responsible for analgesia, euphoria and respiratory depression.

## Opioid Agonist-Morphine

Morphine is the most important alkaloid of opium and is used as sulfate or hydrochloride **(Table 3.2)**.

### Therapeutic Effects of Morphine

- Effects on central nervous system like depressant Increases threshold for sensation of pain. It relieves all sorts of pain.
- Morphine depresses the emotional component of pain and it depresses respiration as well as cough reflexes.
- Pain tolerance increases as it is mild hypnotic and may produce drowsiness and sleep.
- Decreased GI mobility (propulsive action of gut) and increased anal sphincter tone, Urinary retention occurs due to increased tone and decreased coordinated contracting and bladder.
- Increased tone of smooth muscle and sphincter of Oddi of common bile duct causes increased biliary pressure.
- Morphine causes some histamine release, occasionally leading to bronchoconstriction.

### Contraindications of Administering Morphine

Infants and the elderly are more susceptible to the respiratory depressant action of morphine.

- Morphine is contraindicated in patient with head injury because by retaining carbon dioxide it increases intracranial tension, even therapeutic dose can cause marked depression in the patients.
- Morphine causes histamine release which can cause broncho constriction and can be dangerous in asthmatics.
- It is dangerous in patients with respiratory insufficiency, sudden deaths have occurred.
- Use of morphine during labor can cause hazard. Morphine freely crosses placenta and affect fetus more than the mother; it produces depression of fetal respiration. Due to lack of cough and swallowing reflexes gastric content may choke the bronchial tree of fetus.
- Morphine can aggravate certain conditions, i.e., diverticulitis, biliary colic, pancreatitis. Inflamed appendix may rupture. It can be given after the diagnosis is established. Pethidine, pentazocine, buprenorphine is less likely to aggravate biliary spasm.
- Phenothiazines, tricyclic antidepressants, MAO inhibitors, amphetamine and neostigmine potentiate morphine or other opioids, either by retarding its metabolism or by pharmacodynamic interaction.
- Morphine with antipsychotic and antidepressants is contraindicated as it potentiates sedation.
- Morphine retards absorption of many orally administered drugs by delaying gastric emptying.

| Table 3.2: Routes, uses and doses of morphin. | | |
|---|---|---|
| **Route** | **Use** | **Available formulations and dose** |
| Oral | As an immediate release tablet morphine can be given orally but that must be given every 4 hours<br>♦ Single oral dose of morphine is not effective as liver breaks down about 75% of the dose through first pass metabolism before the drugs reaches the circulation<br>♦ With repeated oral doses, however it is very effective | Morphine tablet (morcontin) 10 mg, 30 mg, 60 mg and 100 mg<br>Adult: 10–30 mg q 3–4 hours as needed<br>Children: 0.2–0.3 mg/kg q 3–4 hours as needed |
| Intramuscular injection | For rapid analgesic effect as is given. morphine injection a action starts within 5–30 mins and usually lasts about 4 hours | Morphine HCI-10 mg/mL in ampule available<br>Dose: Adult: 5–10 mg q 3–4 hour as needed<br>Children: 0.1/kg, 3–4 hourly as needed |
| Intravenous injection | Morphine can also be given intravenously (slow). The analgesic effect starts within 10 minutes. Effect of a parenteral dose lasts for 4–6 hours | IV injection–for 2–10 mg for children (0.1–0.2 mg/kg of body weight as needed). 10–15 mg (for adult). 10–15 mg for adults |
| Subcutaneous injection | Effect starts within 20 minutes and lasts for 3–5 hours | 10–15 mg for adults |
| Continuous-subcutaneous infusion repeatedly | For severe and fluctuating pain small doses of morphine can be continuous-subcutaneous infusion | |

## Nursing Responsibilities in Administering Opioid Analgesics

- The patient who is to receive opioid analgesics must be assessed carefully to determine the degree of risk of such therapy. The history of previous use of these drugs and responses to them to be recorded and to be informed to the physician. Respiratory function must be carefully appraised. Patient with a history of multiple sclerosis, myasthenia gravis other respiratory muscle disorders and obstructive airway disease or myxedema are at high risk for acute respiratory depression when opioids are administered. Obese patients have high-risk of respiratory complications.
- Laboratory data should be explored for indication of conditions that impair tissue perfusion (anomie, poor cardiac function) and liver and renal dysfunction.
- Assess individual response to opioid medication carefully in relation to pain relief, side effects, and signs and symptoms of developing allergy or tolerance.
- Nursing diagnosis may include discomfort due to pain. Potential to impaired gas exchange related to hypopnea due to use of depressant drugs, alteration of bowel function due to central sedation, urinary retention and increased sphincter tone, etc.
- Goals of treatment should be to alleviate pain, maintain respiration and gas exchange, maintain cerebral circulation, prevent or alleviate constipation, prevent urinary to retention and to eliminate knowledge deficit of patients.

### Interventions

- The patient with pain needs proper nursing attention to reduce anxiety and stress in the patient, promote and divert attention from the pain are critical.
- Assess respiration prior to administration of opioids, respiration should be 12 or more per minute in adults. Respiration depth and skin color should be observed. The degree of pupillary constriction is to be observed and recorded report to the physician if respiration becomes less than 12/minute, assisted ventilation may be advised.
- Nursing measures to facilitate fecal elimination is essential by using stool softener or enemas or stimulant laxative hydration, regular exercise and diet containing fiber.
- The patients medicated for pains needs slow in changing positions because they are subject to postural hypotension.
- Request a change of medication if response is undesirable or signs of allergy develop. Teach patients who manage their own opioid regimen monitor their responses to the drugs.
- Provide caution to patients who are under opioid drugs not to engage in potentially hazardous activities like driving, operating machineries.
- Patient and his family should be informed of the purpose of the drug administration. Patient must learn assessment techniques to evaluate their need for the drug and to assess undesirable reactions to the drug like bradycardia and instruct the patient for slow change in position to avoid orthostatic hypotension. Adopting relaxation techniques, the control of other stressors and diversion are helpful, establishing regular bowel habit, storage is to be encouraged to prevent overdose and or theft. Patient must know that prolonged take of opioid may precipitate drug dependence and tolerance. Patient must avoid alcohol and CNS depressants during opioid therapy.

## Pethidine (Meperidine) Hydrochloride

Pethidine is a synthetic substance called phenyl piperidine. It is chemically related to atropine and has some actions like it. Though chemically unrelated to morphine, it has many similar actions and is shown to interact with opioid receptors. Actions of pethidine are blocked by naloxone.

### Important Differences in Comparison to Morphine

With adequate dose its analgesic effect is equated to morphine. Duration of action is shorter three to four hours, but the onset of action is more rapid. It does not effectively suppress cough reflex. Constipation and urinary retention are less as pethidine has less spasmodic action on smooth muscles. This drug can be administered to asthmatics as it releases less histamine.

### Doses and Uses

Available formulations are Tablet 50 mg and 100 mg. Intramuscular or subcutaneous injection can be given to adults. Oral tablet or intravenous injection also can be given. Repeat administration of drug can be done after 3–4 hours. 0.5–2 mg per kilogram of body weight can be given to children. Pethidine can be used as a substitute for morphine.

It is indicated for post operative and moderately acute pain in burns, trauma, fracture, cancer. It can be used to alleviate pain in cholecystitis where morphine is contraindicated. It can be used as obstetric analgesic, although labor may be prolonged, and some neonatal respiratory depression may occur, but to a lesser extent than that with other narcotic analgesics. Used as pre anesthetic agent as well as to control shivering during recovery from anesthesia.

### Contraindication

Respiratory depression due to nonopioid drugs. Adjunctive treatment of alcohol dependence. Acute hepatitis/hepatic failure. Brain injury, allergy, epilepsy, and cardiac arrhythmia.

### Side Effects

Sometimes atropinic side effects may occur, i.e., dryness of mouth, blurring of vision, tachycardia, etc. Overdose of pethidine may cause delirium, convulsion, etc. Prolonged use of pethidine may lead to addiction.

### Nursing Responsibilities

- Take patient's drug history especially opioid intake, and history of past medical conditions like hepatic disorders.
- Assess the duration, location, onset and type of pain. Accordingly recording of vital signs is necessary before administration of the drug.
- Withholding the drug and informing the physician is necessary if the respiratory rate becomes 12 or below in an adult or 20 or less in a child.
- Specific laboratory tests are to be done, to assess hepatic and renal functioning.
- Body weight, vital signs, especially respiratory rate and effort are to be assessed.
- Establish and maintain the airway. Monitor patient's vital signs after administration of pethidine.
- Be alert for BP and change in rate and quality of pulse.
- Place the patient in recumbent position. Administer intravenous push very slowly over two to three minutes to avoid severe apnea, cardiac arrest, and circulatory collapse.
- Degree of pain relief and sedation is to be recorded and reported. The effects of the drug are reduced if a full pain response recurs before the next dose.
- Deep breathing and coughing exercises should be encouraged, particularly in patients with impaired respiratory function.

## Pentazocine

Pentazocine is a prototype of opioids with both agonist and antagonist activity. It has weak antagonists and more marked agonistic actions. It does not come from natural sources like morphine but is prepared synthetically.

It is used for moderate pain relief, less dependence liability than morphine Sedation and respiratory depression is 1/3–1/2 of morphine at lower dose.

Biliary spasm and constipation are less severe. Vomiting is less frequent. Other side effects are sweating and lightheadedness. Occasionally causes dysphoria, hallucinations and depersonalization.

### Indications

Postoperative and chronic or recurrent pain, moderately severe pain, where repeated use of morphine carries a substantial risk of inducing dependence. Special precautions like morphine are needed in administering the drug in pregnancy.

### Contraindications

It is contraindicated in coronary ischemia and myocardial infarction porphyria patients. Pentazocine causes tachycardia and rise in BP due to sympathetic stimulation. As it increases cardiac workload it should be avoided in hypertensive states.

### Opioid Antagonists Naloxone/Naltrexone

Naloxone and naltrexone are called competitive antagonists of opioids. Generally, they resemble morphine in their chemical structure and thus co Naloxone and naltrexone appear to exert little or no agonist action and are considered to be relatively pure antagonists. But their physiologic response to opioid antagonists depends upon a number of factors.

- Degree of potential agonists action of selected drug
- Whether or not opioid drugs are present at receptor site
- Degree of previously physical dependence on opioids
- Concentration of antagonist at receptor site at determined by drug dose.

**Pharmacokinetics:** Naloxone is administered by parenteral route as it is readily absorbed by GI and rapidly deactivated during first pass through liver. Naltrexone is administered orally, and drugs are excreted through kidneys. Onset of therapeutic action is 2–5 minutes and duration is 20–60 minutes and half-life 60–100 minutes.

### Uses of Naloxone

- Use to treat acute morphine poisoning. Especially respiratory depression.
- To precipitate withdrawal symptoms in dependent individuals.

### Uses of Naltrexone

- Used to treat opioid induced toxicity.
- To diagnose physical dependence.

## NON-NARCOTIC ANALGESICS AND NON-STEROIDAL ANTI-INFLAMMATORY DRUGS

Nonopioid analgesics and nonsteroidal anti-inflammatory drugs (NSAIDs) are a large group of drugs. They have varying degree of analgesic, antipyretic and anti-inflammatory effects. These drugs are known as prostaglandin inhibitors. One of the actions of prostaglandins is concerned with the production of painful stimuli, and they are responsible for different features of inflammation (swelling redness). Nonsteroidal anti-inflammatory drugs are most effectively used to relieve pain and inflammation.

## Classification
**Commonly used non-narcotic analgesics are:**
- Propionic acid derivative ibuprofen, naproxen
- Aryl-acetic derivative diclofenac, aceclofenac
- Oxicam derivatives
- Preferential COX-2 inhibitors—nimesulide.

**Nonsteroidal anti-inflammatory substances includes:**
- Salicylates (aspirin)
- Para-aminophenol derivative (paracetamols, acetaminophen)
- Nonselective cox inhibitor NSAIDs
- Selective COX-2 inhibitor NSAIDs.

**Conditions treated with above group of drugs are given below:**
- To treat mild to moderate pain.
- To reduce high body temperature as well as to get some anti-inflammatory effect.
- To prevent and treat diseases associated with hypercoagulability, and thus to reduce the risk of myocardial infarction (MI) and stroke.
- Elevated body temperature.
- Mild to moderate pain.
- Acute painful shoulder.
- Primary dysmenorrhea
- Rheumatoid and osteoarthritis (rheumatic fever and Ankylosing spondylitis).

Many of these agents are nonsuitable for long-term therapy because of toxicity.

## Mode of Actions of NSAIDs

The NSAIDs act by inhibiting prostaglandin biosynthesis as the prostaglandins are closely concerned with the onset and maintenance of inflammatory processes. It was once thought that prostaglandins were secreted by the prostate gland, but the prostaglandins are derivatives of arachidonic acid, a long chain fatty acid, link with phospholipids, is present in cell walls. Cyclooxygenase-1 (COX-1) and cyclooxygenase 2 (COX-2), the two enzymes are concerned with the formation of prostaglandin and subsequently metabolized to the various prostaglandins.

## *Aspirin*
- Generic name and chemical name is acetylsalicylic acid.
- Drug family-analgesics mild anti-inflammatory, antipyretic.

*Available Formulation*
- Tablet (325 and 350/500 mg), enteric coated tablet (75 and 100 mg)
- Rectal suppositories: 65–130 mg.

*Doses*
- **For adult:** 300–900 mg at 4-6 hours interval, but not more than 4 g in a day.
- **For children:** Not safe to use.

*Uses*
- Rheumatoid juvenile disorder.
- Osteoarthritis and other inflammatory disorder.

*Mode Action*
- Aspirin acts on the thermoregulating center by inhibiting prostaglandin production in the hypothalamus and control temperature to normal levels. Salicylates in high doses (4–5 g divided doses for 1–3 days) are particularly useful in the treatment of acute rheumatic fever.
- Relief mild moderate pain and inflammation. Aspirin inhibits cyclooxygenase enzyme of injured body tissue and stops formation of prostaglandins.
- Prevention of blood clots as in phlebitis, heart attack and stroke.

*Possible Adverse Effects*
- Mild adverse effects allergic reactions, skin rash, nasal discharge Gl distress, heart burn, mild nausea. Serious side effects are erosion of stomach lining with silent bleeding.
- Aspirin toxicity may develop in dehydrated and febrile children. Reye's syndrome may occur in case of chickenpox or flu in children and teenagers.
- Hemolytic anemia,
- Headache, dizziness, flushing, tachycardia, diaphoresis and thirst are the symptoms of mile toxicity. Marked toxicity means hyperthermia, restlessness, seizure, respiratory failure and coma.

*Drugs may Decrease the Effects of Aspirin*
- Antacid, urine alkalizer may reduce absorption.
- Phenobarbital may hasten the elimination of aspirin.

*Special Storage Instruction*

Aspirin is to be kept in dry tightly closed container. Suppositories art to be kept in cool place. If the drug has an odor like vinegar, do not administer it. This is due to presence of acetic acid, and indicates the decomposition of aspirin.

*Contraindications*

Aspirin is contraindicated for those who:
- Have had an allergic reaction or an unfavorable response to it before
- Have asthma.
- Have problem in liver and kidney.
- Have any type of bleeding disorder (such as hemophilia)
- Are taking anticoagulant drugs.
- Chickenpox or flu in children and teenagers
- Have an active peptic ulcer (stomach or duodenum).

Aspirin is contraindicated for pregnant woman because it leads to:
- Anemia
- Prolongation of labor (if the drug used in last trimester of pregnancy)
- Death of mother due to postpartum bleeding
- Closure of ductus arteriosus of baby before birth
- It also causes rise of blood pressure of baby, low birth weight, hemorrhage, still
- Jaundice to the neonate.

### Paracetamol

Paracetamol (PCM) is a widely used minor analgesic and antipyretic. Its analgesic action is like aspirin but anti-inflammatory property is weak. It has some cyclooxygenase inhibiting properties, this action is very weak in the peripheral tissues, and it has low anti-inflammatory property. Its main advantage is that unlike other drugs in this group it does not cause gastric complication or gastric bleeding.

PCM can be used as home remedy for pain, fever, menstrual pain, etc. As pain killer, PCM is the safest drug. There is a myth that PCM only reduces fever. But its pain-relieving action is like aspirin only.

**Dose:** Paracetamol is given orally in tablet form.

*For Adult*

500–1000 mg tablet three to four times can be given. But not more than 4 g per day. One should not take more than 4 g of paracetamol continuously. The child should be over 3 months old, except for postimmunization pyrexia is acceptable.

*For Child*

The dose of paracetamol under three months of age is determined body weight of the baby (for other children 100 mg paracetamol/kg of/day (in 4–6 equal doses) can be administered.

*Uses*

As paracetamol does not harm gastric lining it can be administered in empty stomach or preferable for after taking food.

*Therapeutic Use*

Paracetamol is administered orally in tablet form. It is well-absorbed and usually peak plasma concentrations are achieved within 60 minutes. It is partly bound to plasma proteins and inactivated by metabolism in the liver. For the children under 12 years, paracetamol is the preferred mild analgesic and antipyretic, as it does not cause Reye's syndrome.

*Contraindication*

In case of liver disease or the person is alcoholic, paracetamol is to be used cautiously in low dose. Otherwise, it is a safe drug.

### Arylacetic Acid Derivatives Diclofenac (Sodium)

*Available Formulations*
- Tablet: 23 and 50 mg.
- Injection: 25 mg/mL is available.
- 3 mL ampules are available in market. Other form-Ointment and dispersible tablet available.

*Therapeutic Actions*

Diclofenac is nonopioid analgesic group of drugs. It is an effective anti-inflammatory and analgesic drug. In any inflammation the injured cells produce different chemicals like bradykinin, serotonin, histamine, etc. Pain occurs due to stimulation of the nerve endings (pain receptors) by these chemicals. Diclofenac stops production of these endogenous mediators of peripheral nerve stimulation. It also constricts the iris sphincter.

*Dose*

Adult dose

Total 75–150 mg drug can be given in 2–3 divided doses. The drug should be given in full stomach.

Child dose

Child dose is 1–3 mg per kg of body weight. Total drug is to be given in 2–3 divided doses.

*Uses*
- Treatment of chronic inflammatory conditions like rheumatoid arthritis and osteoarthritis.
- Acute musculoskeletal pain, painful dental lesions, sprains and joints pain.
- For reducing pain and inflammation postoperatively.

### Ketorolac

It has analgesic properties to reduce pain postoperatively. It can be used parenterally most of the time and also advices for orally.

### Propionic Acid Derivatives

Ibuprofen is more accepted than aspirin. Acting as analgesic, antipyretic and anti-inflammatory but less than actions of aspirin.

Side effects are same and less severe than aspirin.

*Dose*

Ibuprofen 400–800 mg thrice daily.

*Uses*

- In pain and fever
- Soft tissue injuries, postoperative pain, dysmenorrhea and osteoarthritis
- Gout.

### Anthranilic Acid Derivatives

*Fenamates*

Fenamates are analgesic, antipyretic, anti-inflammatory in action and more toxic, not used in case off children. More than one week should not be permitted.
- **Dose** (250–500) mg TDS
- **Adverse effects**: Diarrhea and less GI bleeding
- **Uses:** Myalgias, dysmenorrhea.

*Oxicams*

Piroxicam is an oxicam derivative. It is long acting, having anti-inflammatory, analgesic and antipyretic activity. Drug interactions are not clinically significant; better tolerated by the patient because of less ulcerogenic.

Dose 20 mg OD. Piroxicam is used for rheumatoid arthritis, osteoarthritis, ankylosing spondylitis, acute musculoskeletal pain and postoperative pain and painful dental lesions.

*Alkanones*

Nabumetone is an anti-inflammatory agent which is beneficial for rheumatoid arthritis and osteoarthritis. Less side effects and less ulcerogenic.

### Selective COX-2 Inhibitors

Celecoxib and rofecoxib are very selective COX-2 inhibitors. Having good anti-inflammatory, analgesic and antipyretic properties and not have an effect on platelet aggregation, better to use because of less gastric irritation. Both celecoxib and rofecoxib can cause salt and water retention that leads to hypertension and edema which is risky for cardiovascular disease patient. They can be used in acute painful conditions like postoperative pain, dysmenorrhea and dental pain as well as in Osteoarthritis and rheumatoid arthritis.

*Dose*

- Celecoxib:100–200 mg OD or BD.
- Rofecoxib analgesic: 50 mg daily.

Nimesulide is a sulfonanilide derivative. It slows down leukocyte function, prevents the release of mediators. It has antihistaminic, anti allergic properties, antipyretic and anti inflammatory actions like other NSAIDs. It can be absorbed orally, and excreted by the kidney,
- **Dose:** 50–100 mg BD
- **Adverse effects**: Mild effects of nausea, epigastric pain, rashes, drowsiness and dizziness. Long-term use can lead to hepatotoxicity which may be severe.
- **Uses:** Nimesulide (NICE, NIMEGISIC) act as analgesic, antipyretic and anti inflammatory agent, but it is now banned in most countries including India because of the risk of hepatotoxicity.

## Nursing Implications in Administering Analgesics

Many NSAIDs have serious or deleterious effects in patients. It is observed that the vast majority of them have common side effects to a greater or lesser degree, i.e., GI and renal system.

### Nursing Process Assessment

History of sensitivity to the prescribed drugs or similar drug to be taken to explore whether the patient has a history of GI or renal complaints, and/or history of bronchial asthma. Prolong drug regimen needs frequent lab test. Patient receiving oral anticoagulants should expect to have frequent prothrombin time assessment as well as renal function test, i.e., urea and creatinine.

### Nursing Diagnosis

Alteration in comfort, pain, restricted activity, sleep pattern disturbance, etc. In using NSAIDs includes potential to adverse effects on GI and renal systems.

### Planning

Plan of care aims to achieve some patient's outcome, i.e., diminished pain improving activity means to take self-care, attaining optimal level of sleep, etc.

### Interventions

- Medicines to be given with food or immediately after meals to avoid adverse effects. Instruct patient to report immediately about GI upset like nausea, vomiting,

diarrhea and evidence of GI bleeding (blood in the stool or tarry stools).
- Progress/deterioration of symptoms are to be recorded.
- Diabetic patients need dose adjustment of insulin or oral hypoglycemic agents. Report serum glucose assessment and any episode of hypoglycemia to be reported.
- Teach the patient about the side effects to watch viz., CNS side effect (drowsiness, dizziness).

## Evaluation

Data which include drug efficacy are relief of pain, relaxed facial expression involvement in activities, etc.

## Patient's Education

- Educate people for proper utilization of NSAIDs especially over the counter preparations. These drugs should be taken after meal or with food. It helps to prevent GI disturbances.
- Proper storage of the drug is necessary to avoid accidental hazards by children.
- Patient should be informed about drug interaction.

# ANTIBIOTICS

The era of antibiotic began with the development of penicillin during World War II. Professor Fleming in 1928 observed that the growth of some cultures of *staphylococci* had been inhibited by the growth of contaminated mould. It was found that a blue-green substance formed by the mould could prevent the growth of certain bacteria and the substance was eventually extracted in quantity and named penicillin, a name derived from the name of contaminated mould. Later, the chemical structure of penicillin was identified and explained.

In the complex molecular structure of penicillin, beta-lactam and thiazolidine ring remain attached to each other. This beta-lactam ring mainly helps to destroy the bacteria. It was observed that so many chemical substances had beta-lactam ring and bactericidal property like penicillin. Invention of different types of penicillin were possible by changing the chemical structure of penicillin.

## Antibacterial Classification

- **Inhibitors of bacterial cell wall biosynthesis**
  - Penicillin
  - Cephalosporins
  - Other transpeptidase inhibitors
    - Azactam: It is a synthetic bactericidal antibiotic.
  - Other inhibitors
    - Imipenem
    - Vancomycin
    - Bacitracin
    - Cycloserine
- **Inhibitors of bacterial protein synthesis**
  - Aminoglycosides
  - Tetracycline
  - Chloramphenicol
  - Erythromycin
  - Clindamycin
- **Inhibitors of bacterial metabolism**
  - Sulfonamides.
- **Inhibitors of bacterial events involving nucleic acids.**
  - *RNA synthesis inhibitor:* Rifampicin
  - *DNA binding agents:* Nalidixic acid, nitrofurantoin norflox, ciprofloxacin, ofloxacin enoxacin.

### Inhibitor of Bacterial Cell Wall Biosynthesis

### Penicillin and Cephalosporins

Penicillin and cephalosporins, the two major antibiotic families, share a common structural component the beta-lactam ring, though their pharmacokinetic properties appear to vary. They exhibit some cross sensitivity, i.e., individuals allergic to penicillin are likely to exhibit allergic sensitivity to some cephalosporins. Drugs from other families are inactivated by an enzyme, beta-lactamase, which is produced by some resistant pathogens.

### Therapeutic Uses

Penicillin derivatives are used in the treatment of many common infections like pneumonia and other respiratory tract infection, UTIs, septicemia, bone and joints infection, syphilis and gonorrhea. This drug acts successfully on penicillin-sensitive organisms as streptococci, staphylococci, pneumococci, clostridium, corynebacterium diphtheria, Bacillus anthracis, Neisseria gonorrhea, etc. This drug only acts on gram-positive organisms, so it is not suitable for all sorts of infections. Some strains of organisms produce an enzyme called penicillinase, which chemically degrades penicillin molecule and develop resistance to it. So, treatment by penicillin will be ineffective if infection caused by pathogens with this type of resistance.

### Adverse reactions

- Hypersensitivity reactions occur in nearly 10% of cases. All types of reactions from simple rash to anaphylaxis can be observed within 2 minutes or up to 3 days following administration of penicillin.
- Direct irritation and pain upon injection site.
- GI upset.
- Cation ($NA^+$ or $K^+$) effects due to large doses of salt form of drugs.

## Nursing Management in Administering Cephalosporin

### Assessment

- Before initiating cephalosporin therapy, a complete drug history is necessary to rule out allergic hypersensitivity to penicillin or cephalosporin.
- Assess the patient for renal dysfunction and history of renal disease.

### Nursing diagnosis

It is concerned with both therapeutic and adverse responses to medication.

### Planning of nursing care

Goals of cephalosporin administration are to resolve the infectious process, to reduce the risk of adverse reaction to the antibiotics and to detect and treat adverse reaction promptly.

### Interventions

- Use fresh solutions for administration by injection. If necessary, solution should be stored in refrigerator.
- Administer intravenous cephalosporin injection slowly, preferably a period of 30 minutes.
- Rapid injection causes pain and irritation of the vein. Pain of intramuscular injection site may be minimized by applying ice packs on the site prior to and following the injection. Teach patient receiving oral cephalosporins to schedule doses at least one hour before and two hours after meals.
- One of the rare side effects of cephalosporin administration is acute allergic reaction. Epinephrine should be available for emergency treatment.
- Evaluate the IM injection site for tenderness. Local irritation can produce severe pain after intramuscular injection.
- Assess the patient's oral cavity for white patches on the mucous membrane and tongue, recommend buttermilk or yogurt with each meal during oral cephalosporin treatment.
- Assess the patient's pattern of daily bowel activity and stool consistency.
- Although mild GI effects may be tolerated, severe symptoms may indicate the onset of antibiotic associated colitis.
- To assess nephrotoxicity monitoring of patient's intake and output and renal function tests are necessary.
- Super infection may be a problem in administering cephalosporin especially due to later generation of drugs administration. Be aware about signs and symptoms of super infection, including abdominal pain or cramping, moderate to severe diarrhea, severe anal or genital pruritus or discharge, severe oral or tongue soreness.
- Consult the physician about the need for antimycotic medication. Give special mouth care and skin care.
- Evaluate the IV site for phlebitis, as evidenced by heat, pain and red streaking over the vein. If cephalosporin are prescribed for reduced dose in case of renal failure patient.
- Cephalosporins should be administered following each dialysis because the drugs are removed from the body by dialysis.

### Evaluation

Evaluation data includes signs and symptoms indicating resolution of the:

- Infection process of adverse reactions to the drug regimen.
- Patients should be monitored for GI upset, vaginitis and renal impairment, neutropenia, impaired clotting or renal dysfunction.
- Patient and family education: Inform the patient that IM injection may cause pain, irritation and discomfort
- Advise the patient or family member to space doses evenly around the clock and to complete full course of treatment.
- Inform the patient, if GI upset occurs the drug can be taken with food or milk.
- Not to take both alcohol and cough syrup. Warn the patient to avoid consuming alcohol and alcohol containing preparations (such as cough syrup) during treatment and 72 hours after drug administration.
- It is to be cautioned not to discontinue medication prematurely, even though the signs and symptoms of infection have resolved completely. Prompt reporting to the physician regarding signs and symptoms of super infection regimen necessary. An alternative antibiotic may be substituted to complete the antibiotic.

### *Inhibitors of Bacterial Protein Synthesis*

#### *Aminoglycosides*

Aminoglycosides is a group of natural and semi synthetic antibiotics, effective against gram-negative bacteria Streptomycin, active against tubercle bacilli was the first member discovered in 1944 by Watman and his colleagues. It was an excellent complement to penicillin and combined therapy with the two drugs was often employed to achieve a broader spectrum of efficacy at present this group includes streptomycin, neomycin, kanamycin, amikacin, gentamicin, tobramycin.

## Mechanism of action

They act as bactericidal agents against susceptible organisms by binding irreversibly to ribosomal subunits within the pathogens, thus preventing protein synthesis, they kill the bacteria rather than preventing them from multiplying.

- **General properties:** Not absorbed orally, parenteral administration is needed. Sometimes used in the site of infection. Do not penetrate cerebrospinal fluid (CSF) the kidneys excrete them all an accumulation occurs with impaired renal function. These drugs are all, to a greater or lesser degree ototoxic (they impair hearing and/or balance) and nephrotoxic.
  Aminoglycosides are valuable therapeutic agents active against most gram-negative aerobic bacteria.
- **Adverse reaction:** Ototoxicity, nephrotoxicity, neuromuscular blockade. It has narrow therapeutic index.

## Nursing management in administering aminoglycosides

- **Assessment of patient:** Before administering the initial dose of aminoglycoside drugs, evaluate the patients for renal dysfunction, hearing loss, allergy to aminoglycosides, and concurrent use of other ototoxic or nephrotoxic drugs.
- **Nursing diagnosis:** Diagnoses relate to both therapeutic and adverse.
- **Intervention:** Verify that the patient has been informed of the risks of therapy, especially the risk of hearing loss. Use only fresh solutions of aminoglycosides because aminoglycoside solutions are relatively unstable solutions that must be stored, should be refrigerated. Before administering each dose, the solutions expired date should be checked from the labeling information.
- **Evaluation:** Monitor patients receiving aminoglycosides for early signs and symptoms of ototoxicity or nephrotoxicity such as ringing or a sense of fullness in the ears and changes in urinary excretion.

## Precautions

- Renal damage may occur if gentamicin is combined with frusemide (Lasix).
- Calculation of dose and maintenance of interval is very important-Gentamicin is ototoxic, causing disorder of balance and hearing, which is dose-related.
- Administration of aminoglycosides just immediately after surgery may precipitate neuromuscular blockade. Gentamicin augments the action of neuromuscular blocking agents. Consult physician before administration of the drug.
- Monitor respiratory status of patients who receive aminoglycosides concurrently with neuromuscular blocking agents.
- It should be avoided during pregnancy as it is ototoxic to the fetus.
- Special precaution is needed in administering the drug to neonates. Respiratory arrest (rarely) may occur if serum magnesium level of the neonate is high.

### Tetracycline

Tetracycline is orally active and affects a wide range of microorganisms hence called broad spectrum antibiotics.

### Mechanism of action

This group of drugs are primarily bacteriostatic. Like the aminoglycosides tetracycline interfere with protein synthesis by microbial ribosomes. These drugs gain access to the interior of the cell by more than one mechanism, including passive diffusion. They affect only multiplying organism but are both bacteriostatic and in high concentrations, bactericidal. All tetracyclines are weakly water-soluble, and all have practically the same microbial activity (with minor differences) The subsequently developed members have high lipid solubility, greater potency and some other differences.

### General properties

Adequately absorbed from the gastrointestinal (GI) tract. Can be administered parenterally. Absorption of older tetracycline in impaired by stomach contents, especially milk and antacids, as a result of complex formation with ions, particularly magnesium, calcium and aluminum.

Minocycline and doxycycline, which are highly lipophilic, completely absorbed irrespective of food and better transported by bacteria. Distributed throughout body fluids and therapeutic concentrations can be achieved in the CSF. Doxycycline is excreted almost entirely via feces hence it is the safest tetracycline to administer to individuals with impaired renal function.

### Adverse effects

Gastrointestinal upset including nausea, vomiting, diarrhea. Hepatic damage can occur at high doses but oxytetracycline and tetracycline are safer in this regard. Tetracyclines are hepatotoxic to pregnant women, as it can precipitate acute hepatic necrosis which may be fatal.

Phototoxicity when exposed to strong sunlight (ultraviolet), dermatological reactions are often observed especially with demeclocycline and doxycycline.

Bones and teeth can complex with bone calcium. Children (6 months to 5 years) receiving tetracycline therapy can develop discoloration of teeth. Can also retard bone growth in neonates. Dry syrups a other liquid oral preparations have been banned and discontinued to discourage use in children.

As tetracycline cause marked suppression of the resident flora, they are liable it superinfection. Superinfection can be life-threatening (especially with impaired immune system).

## Chloramphenicol

Chloramphenicol is a broad-spectrum antibiotic which is now produced synthetically. It is a drug of last resort for the treatment of serious infections that cannot be treated with other antibiotics. The most serious adverse reaction to this drug is bone marrow suppression, which can lead to fatal aplastic anemia.

### Mechanism of action

Inhibits bacterial protein synthesis by ribosome of bacterial cells. Binds to ribosomal subunits that catalyze peptide bond formation. Its action in usually bacteriostatic, but in high concentrations and against highly susceptible organisms it does act as a cidal agent.

### Pharmacokinetics

Absorbed well from the GI tract, following absorption it penetrates to most body compartments including cerebrospinal fluid. It is 50–60% bound to plasma proteins and plasma (t1/2) is 3–5 hours. It readily crosses the placenta and secreted in breast milk.

### Therapeutic uses

This drug in active against most gram-positive and gram-negative bacteria like rickettsia, chlamydia, and mycoplasma but in active against fungi. Because chloramphenicol causes serious and potentially fatal adverse reactions, use of this drug in limited to treatment of infections that cannot be treated with other drugs. These include typhoid fever (although resistance may be a problem), meningitis due to H. Influenzae in patients allergic to penicillin and the newer cephalosporins and some cases of infection caused by ampicillin-resistant strains.

### Available formulation

Chloromycetin, enteromycetin, paraxin 250 mg, 500 mg capsule, 1% eye ointment, 5% eye drops, 5% ear drops and 1% applicaps.

### Adverse effects

- Bone marrow depression (pancytopenia) that may lead to irreversible aplastic anemia.
- Low incidence (1:30,000) but high rate of fatality.
- Reticulocytopenia, perhaps as a result of inhibition of mitochondrial protein synthesis.
- Gray baby syndrome—this is a type of circulatory failure occurs in premature and newborn baby. Symptoms include failure to feed, abdominal distension, vomiting, pallor, cyanosis and vasomotor and respiratory collapse.
- Hypersensitivity reactions.

Checklist of nursing action in administering chloramphenicol before initiating this drug

- History taking and screening to be done about patient's personal or family history of chloramphenicol allergy, impaired liver function, pregnancy and lactation, anemia, etc.
- Verify that the patient has been informed of the risks of their therapy before initiating systemic chloramphenicol treatment.
- During treatment complete blood counts should be carried out at regular interval. Monitor blood counts for decreased levels of blood cells.
- This drug should be used as last resort. So before administering the drug the nurse is supposed to question orders for systemic chloramphenicol that do not appear justified.
- Avoid environmental contamination by chloramphenicol.

## Inhibitors of Bacterial Metabolism

### Sulfonamides

The sulfonamides are an effective nonantibiotic antibacterial agents used systematically to treat infectious diseases, before the penicillins were introduced. At present newer antimicrobial agents have replaced the sulfonamides, but they are still among the most widely used antimicrobial agents in the world, chiefly because of their low cost and effectiveness in treating common bacterial infections. All the sulfonamides used therapeutically are synthetically produced. Systemic use of sulphonamides alone is rare now, for better therapeutic effect trimethoprim or pyrimethamine is combined and administer to the patients.

### Mechanism of action

Primarily sulfonamides are bacteriostatic and structural analogs of para amino benzoic acid (PABA). It interferes with the normal utilization of PABA by the bacteria for the synthesis of folic acid, an essential step in the production of purines. Thus, the bacteria are deprived of folic acid and cease to multiply. Trimethoprim interferes with the next step, conversion of folic acid to folinic acid. These successive steps of inhibition of DNA and RNA synthesis convert two bacteriostatic compounds into one bacteria compound. The organism which is not sensitive to either drug alone may be killed by the combination Man uses preformed folate from leafy vegetable and does not synthesize folic acid inside the bod for this reason metabolic effect of sulfonamides cannot affect human cells.

### Pharmacokinetics

- Well-absorbed from the GI tract (70–100) and readily penetrate the CSF.

- Extensively bound to plasma proteins (20–90%)
- Peak concentration of sulfamethoxazole and trimethoprim combination is 2–4 hours
- Metabolized to various degree in the liver
- Excretion of the sulfonamides occurs through kidney. Where both the free and the acetylated form of the drug are filtered through the glomerulus.

Nursing management

Nursing measures are common to all types of anti-microbial therapy, and following measures should be taken during administration of sulfonamides.

| 1. | Renal toxicity may be a potentially serious problem | Instructed to take large amounts of liquid. To monitor urinary output and assure that it amounts to at least 1,200 mL in 24 hours |
|---|---|---|
| 2. | Careful observation for toxic effects | Observed for toxic effects such as rash, sore throat purpura. Encourage individual or family members to inform these symptoms to the physician and to discontinue taking the drug. In prolonged sulfonamide therapy, blood count should be done to assess the occurrence of hematologic side effects |
| 3. | Cross sensitization | Cross sensitization is not as severe as among penicillin, it is safer to avoid all sulfonamides in patients who develop hypersensitivity to any one agent |
| 4. | Drug administration with antacid | Sulfonamides should not be administered with antacids because the later inhibit their action by decrease absorption |

## Inhibitors of Bacterial Events Involving Nucleic Acids

### RNA Synthesis Inhibitor Rifampicin

Rifampicin

Rifampicin is effective against M tuberculosis.

- **Mechanism of actions:** Rifampin inhibits DNA dependent RNA synthesis.
- **Pharmacokinetics:** Absorbed from the GI tract, widely distributed, including in CSF. It is metabolized in liver to a diacetylated metabolite which is excreted mainly in bile, some in urine also. Rifampin and its diacetyl derivative undergo enterohepatic circulation. The half-life of rifampin is variable, i.e., 2–5 hours.
- **Uses and doses:** Treatment of tuberculosis, in combination with other drugs. Orally INH is given in treatment of leprosy, meningitis. No cross resistance develops with other anti-mycobacterial agents, resistance develops rapidly when used alone.
- **Dose:** Adult and child—10 mg/kg daily or 3 times weekly (maximum, 600 mg daily).
  Rifampin is to be administered 1 hour before or 2 hours after a meal.
- **Drug interactions:** Enhances metabolism of other drugs like anticoagulants, contraceptives and corticosteroids, sulfonylureas, NNRTIs (drug of AIDS) and fluconazole.
- **Precautions:** Dose reduction is necessary in hepatic impairment.
  - Monitoring of liver function and blood count is necessary in liver disorder, elderly, renal impairment and alcohol dependency patients. It is not safe in pregnancy.
  - Advise patients on hormonal contraceptives to use additional means.
- **Adverse effects:** GI disturbances, hepatitis, respiratory symptoms, dermatitis, red orange feces, urines tears, sweat.

### DNA Binding Agents: Nalidixic Acid, Nitrofurantoin Norflox, Ciprofloxacin, Ofloxacin and Enoxacin

Quinolones (DNA-binding agents)

This group of antimicrobial drugs interfere with an enzyme necessary for the cell division of bacteria The first member nalidixic acid was introduced in mid-1960s. Nalidixic acid and other quinolones, oxolinic acid, cinoxacin were useful as urinary antiseptics with little systemic activity. Norfloxacin, ciprofloxacin, pefloxacin, ofloxacin are newer fluoroquinolones, which have much greater antimicrobial activity.

**Mechanism of action:** These drugs cause DNA damage. Quinolones inhibit the enzyme DNA gyrase, the enzyme that maintains helical twists in the DNA. By inhibiting the action of specific enzyme, they prevent the winding of the DNA helix into super coiled form; the precise mechanism of action is not known.

Nalidixic acid

This drug is effective as urinary antiseptics. This is used when the infecting organisms is resistant to the older antimicrobial drug.

It acts against gram-negative bacteria particularly *E. coli*, proteus, klebsiella, Enterobacter, and shigella but not pseudomonas.

- **Pharmacokinetics:** Rapidly absorbed from the GI tract, highly plasma protein bound and partly metabolized in liver, it is excreted by urine.
- **Available drugs:** Gramoneg, wintomylon, urodic and nitrofurantoin.
- **Uses:** Nalidixic acid primarily used as urinary antiseptics. Since therapeutic levels not achieved in blood

at nontoxic levels. Used in gastrointestinal infection caused by proteus, *E. coli*, shigella or salmonella. It is considered as a reserve drug in resistant or recurrent infections especially those caused by proteus.
- **Side effects:** Like other quinolones patient is affected with nauseated tendency, vomiting and loose motion. Occasionally headache, dizziness, tremors, confusion or skin rash develops. Individuals with G, PD deficiency may develop hemolysis. Sometimes super infection, photosensitization are also reported.
- **Contraindication:** This drug should not be administered in children and growing adolescents as it may cause arthropathy.

Ciprofloxacin

Ciprofloxacin in active against both gram-positive and gram-negative bacteria. It is effective against salmonella, shigella, neisseria, campylobacter and pseudomonas. It is also active against chlamydia and some mycobacteria. Most anaerobes are resistant to it. Ciprofloxacin is used with doxycycline and metronidazole to treat pelvic inflammatory disease.
- **Pharmacokinetics:** Bioavailability of ciprofloxacin is about 60%. Antacids reduce the bioavailability of the drug significantly.
- **Uses in disease conditions:**
  - Gastroenteritis (including cholera shigellosis, travelers' diarrhea, campylobacter, salmonella); typhoid, etc., for shigella infection, for cholera
  - Gonorrhea and gonococcal conjunctivitis
  - Chancroid
  - Pelvic inflammatory disease
  - For surgical prophylaxis
  - For prophylaxis of meningococcal meningitis
  - Pseudomonal lower respiratory tract infection in cystic fibrosis
  - Acute uncomplicated cystitis
- **Precautions:**
  - History of epilepsy or conditions that predispose to seizures.
  - GPD deficiency may lead to hemolysis
  - Myasthenia gravis (risk of exacerbation) pregnancy and breastfeeding children and adolescents to avoid arthropathy.
  - Avoid exposure to excessive sunlight to avoid photosensitivity.
- **Adverse effect:** Nausea, vomiting, dyspepsia, abdominal pain, flatulence, diarrhea, rarely drug-induce colitis hyperglycemia, headache, dizziness, sleep disorders, rash, petechiae.
- **Contraindication:** Quinolones are contraindicated in patients who are more prone to tendinitis.

- **Principles of appropriate use of antibiotics:**
  - Cultures should be taken before administering antibiotics.
  - The timing of blood cultures with fever is not critical.
  - Do not delay the administration of antibiotics.
  - Use empirical therapy first; narrow the spectrum later.
  - Ensure initial doses are sufficient—under-doing must be avoided.
  - If the microbiology results suggest decreased susceptibility, consider whether the antibiotics are working clinically. If there is direct bedside evidence that they are working, then continue them in spite of laboratory evidence.
  - A shorter course (e.g., 7 days) is probably as good as a standard 2 week course in most cases.
  - Infectious diseases specialists should be consulted when managing serious infections.
  - Know antimicrobial pharmacokinetics and pharmacodynamics; consider tissue penetration and dose adjustment to correct for altered clearance.
  - Monitor antibiotic levels when available.
  - Limit prophylactic use to appropriate situations
  - Consider noninfective causes of inflammation (sepsis mimics are surprisingly common)
  - Adhere to infection control policies.
  - Have an antimicrobial stewardship program in the ICU.

# ANTISEPTICS

Antiseptic kills the microorganisms and acts upon living tissues.

An ideal antiseptic consists of the following characteristics:
- A wide antibacterial spectrum
- Chemically stable
- Quick in action
- Nonirritating to the tissues
- Does not affect the wound healing process
- Not absorbed into systemic circulation.

## Classification

- Acids
- Alcohols
- Aldehydes
- Surfactants
- Phenol derivatives
- Halogens
- Oxidizing hydrogen peroxide and potassium agents
- Dyes
- Metallic salts.

## Acids
- Boric acid has weak bacteriostatic and fungistatic activity and aqueous solutions of boric acid are used for irrigating eyes, bladder and vagina.
- Benzoic acid is an antibacterial and antifungal agent used as a preservative in laboratory.
- Salicylic acid has bacteriostatic, fungicidal and keratolytic properties. It is used as a dusting powder or 2% ointment for seborrheic dermatitis, warts and corn.

## Alcohols
Ethyl alcohol is having antiseptic activity which rapidly denatures the aerial proteins.

### Disadvantages
- Very slowly works against viruses, fungi and spores.
- Irritant on open wounds
- It is inflammable

### Uses
Used on skin before injections and surgeries.

## Aldehydes
Formaldehyde utilized during fumigation and 40% aqueous solution formalin is noncorrosive. On topical application, it hardens the skin. Formaldehyde has a pungent odor and is highly irritating to respiratory mucous membranes and eyes.

### Uses
- Formaldehyde gas is used for fumigation and sterilizing various instruments
- Formalin in 1 in 200 dilutions is used for disinfection of surgical equipment and preservation of tissues.
- It can also be used (10% solution) for disinfection of excreta.
- Formaldehyde is used in dentistry as a mummifying agent.
- Two percent solution is locally applied in case of more sweating (idiopathic hyperhidrosis) of palms and soles.

## Surfactants
Surfactants are termed as detergents which lower the surface tension of solutions, and they may be anionic, cationic, ampholytic surfactants or polysorbates.

They are:
- Active against gram-positive and gram negative active against spores, viruses and fungi.
- Most effective in neutral solution.
- Incompatible with anionic surfactants-soaps neutralize their action.
- One of the most commonly used germicidal agents.

## Phenol Derivatives
Phenol is one of the oldest antiseptics which is bactericidal and fungicidal but has poor action against spores and viruses.

### Uses
- Phenol is used to disinfect urine, feces and sputum of patients.
- **Cresol** is methyl phenol, which is toxic and used as a disinfectant for utensils and excreta.
- **Lysol** has higher antiseptic activity and is used as a disinfectant for hospital and domestic use.

**Chloroxylenol (DETTOL)** is a less toxic chlorinated phenol, effective against gram positive and gram-negative organisms.

**Hexachlorophene:** This chlorinated phenol is used in surgical scrubbing, for cleaning the skin.

**Chlorhexidine (HIBITANE):** Effective against gram-positive, gram-negative organisms and fungi. It is quick in action and nonirritating and destroys protozoa.

## Oxidizing Agents
Hydrogen peroxide is used for cleansing wounds, abscesses and for irrigation. In dentistry, it is used to clean septic sockets and root canals and also as a mouthwash and deodorant gargle. It is used as ear drops while removing ear wax.

Potassium permanganate is an oxidizing agent and an astringent. The purple crystals are water-soluble. It acts by liberating oxygen which oxidizes bacterial protoplasm. Organic matter reduces its activity, and the solution gets decolorized. The concentrated solution is caustic and causes burns and blistering.

## Dyes

### Gentian Violet (Aniline Dye, Crystal Violet or Medicinal Gentian Violet)
It is effective against gram-positive organisms and fungi. It is a nonirritant and potent antiseptic, 0.5–1% solution is used topically on furunculosis, burns, boils, chronic ulcers, infected eczema, thrush, ringworm and mycotic infections of the skin and mucous membranes.

Various other dyes are also used like brilliant green, methylene blue, acriflavine and proflavine and triple dye lotion.

## INOTROPICS

Inotropes change the contractility of the heart and increase the force of contraction of the heart.

Positive inotropes facilitate the force of contraction and negative inotropes weaken the contraction of heart. Positive inotropes can help when heart cannot get enough blood to the body because it is too weak to pump the amount of blood, body needs.

Negative inotropes like calcium channel blockers reduce the workload of the heart. Negative inotropes keep heart muscles from working too hard by beating with less force. This is helpful when their have high blood pressure, chest pain, an abnormal heart rhythm or a disease like hypertrophic cardiomyopathy.

Positive inotropic agents include:
- Epinephrine
- Norepinephrine
- Dopamine
- Dobutamine
- Levosimendan
- Milrinone
- Digoxin
- Amrinone
- Enoximone

Negative inotropic agents include:
- Flecainide
- Verapamil
- Cibenzoline
- Clonidine
- Atenolol
- Disopyramide
- Sunitinib
- Itraconazole

### Mechanism of Action

The main mechanism of action for most inotropes involves increasing intracellular calcium, either by increasing influx to the cell during the action potential or increasing release from the sarcoplasmic reticulum.

### Catecholamines

Catecholamines are the common inotropes; these can be endogenous like adrenaline and noradrenaline or synthetic like dobutamine and isoprenaline.

These medicines act on the sympathetic nervous system. Most commonly their cardiac effects are attributed to stimulation of alpha and beta-adrenergic receptors (specifically $\alpha 1$, $\beta 1$, and $\beta 2$).

The main receptor in the cardiac muscle that affects the rate and force of contraction is the $\beta 1$ receptor. Binding to $\beta 1$ receptors results in increased calcium entry into the cell via the opening of L-type calcium channels and release of intracellular calcium from the sarcoplasmic reticulum. More calcium is available to bind with troponin C, thereby enhancing myocardial contractility.

Most catecholamines have a short half-life (about two minutes) and steady-state blood concentrations are reached within 10 minutes. They are therefore usually given by continuous infusion.

### *Dobutamine*

Dobutamine is predominantly a $\beta 1$ agonist and therefore increases cardiac contractility and heart rate. It works on $\beta 2$ receptors leads to vasodilatation and reducing afterload. Dobutamine increases heart rate, arrhythmias and increased myocardial oxygen demand and can lead to myocardial ischemia also.

### *Isoprenaline*

Isoprenaline enhances tachycardia. It is sometimes used for patient having bradycardia necessitating inotropic support.

### *Noradrenaline*

Frequently used with other inotropes like dobutamine, for maintaining adequate perfusion.

### *Adrenaline*

Adrenaline acts on all adrenergic receptors, $\beta$ agonist in low doses and $\alpha$ agonist at higher doses. Mostly used in resuscitation after cardiac arrest.

### *Dopamine*

Dopamine is a complex inotrope as pharmacological effects depends upon dose quantity. Low-dose dopamine (2–5 µg/kg/min) exerts mainly dopaminergic effects, at medium doses (5–10 µg/kg/min) the $\beta 1$ inotropic effects predominate and at high doses (10–20 µg/kg/min) vasoconstriction predominates.

### Phosphodiesterase-3 inhibitors

Phosphodiesterase-3 (PDE3) is an enzyme found in cardiac and smooth muscle cells. Inhibition of PDE3 increases intracellular calcium causing vasodilatation and increased myocardial contractility. Commonly used PDE3 inhibitor is Milrinone.

### Levosimendan

Levosimendan is a new inotrope that sensitizes troponin-C to calcium, enhances the force of contraction. In smooth muscle, it acts on potassium channels to cause vasodilatation. It increases cardiac output without increasing myocardial oxygen consumption.

### Monitoring

Hemodynamic can be monitored adequately in case of patient receiving inotropes, like monitoring of MAP, CO and CVP detects various hemodynamic changes very quickly.

It is necessary that pharmacists in critical care should know the pharmacology of inotropes and the hemodynamic monitoring required in ensuring safe practice.

## LIFE-SAVING DRUGS

Life-saving drugs (LSDs) are the drugs that save someone's life, require immediate administration in most of the cases, as they sustain life and prevent complications.

The lists below are the most common drugs that are frequently used in emergency situations. It is very important that to know and understand what these drugs are and when to use it.

## Adenosine

An endogenous nucleoside slows conduction down through the AV node. It has an extremely short half-life, less than 10 seconds and immediately should be used. It is advised in the case of supraventricular and atrial tachycardia patients.

Sublingually this drug may increase physical energy. Through IV, the drug can cause nerve block and surgical pain and also promotes blood circulation.

It may be advised in case of irregular heartbeat, in the prevention of unstable metabolism. This drug is also used effectively for lung cancer, pulmonary hypertension, high blood pressure, herpes, varicose veins, bursitis, neuropathy, nerve pain.

## Amiodarone

Antiarrhythmic that affects the sodium, potassium, and calcium channels. This drug is administered in a hospital setting usually, where their heart rhythm can be monitored by an EKG, EGG or electrocardiograph. This drug is used for patients with irregular heartbeats, congestive heart failure.

## Atropine

Anticholinergic enhances the conduction in the AV nodes. Drug of choice in treating bradycardia. Atropine dries the secretion of saliva. This is used for stomach and intestine spasms intestine. Nurses have to be very careful in checking the patient's history before administering this drug and it may interfere with antidepressants.

## Epinephrine

Potent catecholamine increases heart rate by strengthening contraction of heart, blood pressure, used to treat asystole, ventricular tachycardia, Ventricular bradycardia and bradycardia. It is advised for the patient whose air passages are blocked, asthmatic patients and lung disorders. It augments blood pressure, heart rates and releases glucose from the liver. This is also advised for adrenal glands disorders, various allergic reaction and heart failure patients.

## Lidocaine

It is used as anti-arrhythmic alternatively to Amiodarone treat ventricular fibrillation and tachycardia. It is used as anti-itching drug, treatment of hemorrhoids. Some form of Lidocaine is used as a local anesthetic and also in case of surgery and various invasive procedures.

### Procainamide

**Antiarrhythmic drug:** This is used to treat sustained ventricular tachycardia. This is advised for treatment of ventricular tachycardia or irregular heartbeat. The patient getting procainamide should be monitored very cautiously in case of elderly patient, hypokalemia, hypotension, kidney and liver problems.

## Sotalol

It is a beta blocker which treats arterial fibrillation or arterial flutter. This medicine cause the slow heartbeat at an even pace. It is available in tablet or liquid form. It is having long-term effect on the blood vessels and heart.

## Vasopressin

It is a synthetic ant arrhythmic drug which is used to treat asystole, ventricular tachycardia and ventricular fibrillation. Vasopressin augments the re-absorption of water and advised to treat diabetes insipidus. It is a substitute to epinephrine and is frequently used in the intensive care unit to support the blood pressure of organ donor patients, prevents the buildup of fluid in the abdomen and treats patients with severe kidney problems.

# DRUGS USED IN VARIOUS BODY SYSTEMS

## DRUGS USED IN RESPIRATORY SYSTEM

### Classification

- Bronchodilators
- Anticholinergic

- Mast cell stabilizers
- Corticosteroids
- Antihistamines

## Bronchodilators

It stimulates beta receptors. It expands the airway by relaxing bronchial smooth muscles. It is used in cases of asthma and patients with bronchospasm. It is contraindicated in uncontrolled arrhythmia.

### Drug Examples and Route

- **Salbutamol:** 2–4 mg orally
- **Terbutaline:** 5 mg orally
- **Formoterol:** 80 µg BD orally
- **Albuterol:** 200–400 µg inhaled every six hourly

### Adverse Effects

Nervousness, anxiety, tremor, headache, palpitations, tachycardia and arrhythmias.

### Nursing Responsibilities

- Nurses should monitor the patient's vital signs and breath sounds.
- Explaining and demonstrating regarding use of inhalers.
- Educate to avoid smoke, dust, and strong smell.

## Mast Cell Stabilizers

They restrain mast cell activity, by preventing release of allergic mediators like histamine, serotonin, prostaglandins, and cytokines. It is advised for the patient having asthmatic attack, bronchospasm, rhinitis/conjunctivitis.

### Drug Examples and Doses

- Cromolyn sodium (nebulization solution) 4 times a day, 20 mg
- Ketotifen OD or BD, 1–2 mg

### Contraindications

Hypersensitivity.

### Adverse Effects

Irritations in nose and throat, gain in weight, headache, dry mouth and dizziness.

### Nursing Responsibilities

- Observe continuously for adverse reactions. It should not be used in acute attack.
- Complete instruction should be given to the patient regarding the use of metered-dose inhaler or nebulizer.
- Give two minutes gap If more than one inhalation is advised to patient.

## Anti-inflammatory Drugs (Corticosteroids)

They prevent the release of or counteract the bronchial mediators (kinins, serotonin, histamine) which lead to inflammation of tissue and causes edema and narrowing of airway.

### Drug Example

Prednisolone beclomethasone, budesonide, fluticasone and betamethasone valerate.

### Indication/Uses

It is used in chronic bronchitis, respiratory inflammatory disease, bronchial asthma and allergic rhinitis.

### Contraindications

Acute bronchospasm—use cautiously in patients who are immune suppressed and getting prednisone or other corticosteroids and also in patients with viral respiratory infections.

### Adverse Effects

Hoarseness, candida infections, oropharyngeal irritation and after inhalation of dry powder bronchospasm occurs.

### Nursing Responsibilities

- After using inhaled steroids, the mouth should be washed properly.
- Nurses should demonstrate to patients and their family, regarding the use of and of inhaler.

## Antihistamines

These drugs block the effect of histamine and its receptors and having some sort of sedative action.

### Drug Example and Doses

Highly sedative

- Diphenhydramine
- Promethazine
- Hydroxyzine

Mild sedatives

- Chlorpheniramine
- Cyclizine 50 mg
- Cetirizine 10 mg

### Indications/Uses

Allergic reactions, asthma, anaphylaxis and urticaria, used as antiemetics, mild sedative/anxiolytics and parkinsonism.

### Contraindications/Precautions

In hypersensitivity, during lactation and hypokalemia, particular safety measures in acute asthma, pregnancy, elderly and epilepsy

*Adverse Effects*
- Sleepiness common
- Mouth dryness
- Blurring of vision
- Urinary retention
- Constipation

*Nursing Responsibilities*
- Antihistamines is advisable during evening because antihistamines cause drowsiness
- Avoid to drive vehicle and operating the machinery
- Avoid alcohol and sedative hypnotics

## Mucolytics

It reduces the viscosity of sputum by mucoproteins present, so that sputum will be easily expelled.

*Drug Example*
- Acetylcysteine by inhalation or nebulization
- Bromhexine

*Indications/Uses*
- For thick and hard mucus.
- Act as antidote for acetaminophen overdose (acetylcysteine).

*Precautions*
- Who is having hypersensitivity to this drug.
- In the case of elderly, pregnant or breast-feeding mothers, additional precaution is necessary.

*Nursing Responsibilities*
- Maintaining patency of airway.
- Do the suction as per the need.
- Evaluate bronchial secretions breath sounds and cough.
- Maintain fluid intake of 23 L/day.
- Inform the patient regarding the rotten egg smell of acetylcysteine.

## Decongestants

It is used to relieve nasal congestion. Its effect due to vasoconstriction reduces swelling of mucous formation makes the nasal passage easier.

*Drug Examples*
- Oxymetazoline hydrochloride nasal spray.
- Phenylephrine hydrochloride
- Pseudoephedrine hydrochloride

*Indications*
- Nasal congestion
- Hay fever
- Sinusitis
- Promote nasal and sinus drainage

*Contraindications/Precautions*
- Use carefully in elder patient.
- Nasal congestion not advised for more than three days and oral decongestant not beyond seven days as long-time use may cause rebound congestion.

*Nursing Responsibilities*
- Assessing adverse effect of drugs.
- Check vital sign and ECG.
- The tip of the container should not touch the nasal passage to avoid contamination.

# DRUGS USED IN NERVOUS SYSTEM

- Analgesics are used to reduce pain.
- Antipyretics alleviate temperature.
- Anti-inflammatory is used to reduce inflammation.

## Classification

Analgesics are divided into two:
1. **Narcotic analgesics (opioid analgesics):** Its primary main action on central pain mechanism and on have narcosis as side effects.
2. **Non-narcotic analgesics (opioid analgesics):** Its primary main action on peripheral pain mechanism and does not have narcosis as side effects.
   - Non opioid/non-narcotic analgesics (NSAIDS)
   - These include nonsteroidal anti-inflammatory drugs (NSAIDs)
   - They are effective for mild to moderate headache and pain of musculoskeletal origin, also they lower body temperature.

## Mechanism of Action

**NSAIDs:** They inhibits prostaglandin formation in inflamed tissues by slowing down stimulation of pain receptors, prostaglandins synthesis and stimulating peripheral vasodilatation to reliever fever (antipyretic action).

## Drug Examples

Salicylates, paracetamol, diclofenac sodium, aceclofenac, ibuprofen, naproxen, nimesulide and indomethacin.

## Indications
- Arthritis and osteoarthritis
- Pyrexia
- Inflammatory conditions

- Transient ischemic attacks and myocardial infarction
- Dysmenorrhea

## Contraindications/Precautions
- Pregnancy
- Aspirin hypersensitivity
- Bleeding disorders and GI ulcers
- Used with precaution in patients with asthma or nasal polyps

## Adverse Effects
- GI upset
- Peptic ulcer
- Diarrhea
- Nausea/vomiting
- Heart burn
- Tinnitus
- Headache

## Nursing Responsibilities
- Nursing responsibilities (NSAIDs) drugs should be taken with food to reduce gastric irritation.
- Advise to take liquid aspirin immediately after mixing and educate the patient not to take ibuprofen and naproxen concomitantly.
- Educate the client to report any bleeding, abdominal pain, loss of appetite and heart burn.
- Alert for signs of GI bleeding and immediately report it.
- Observe for hypersensitivity reaction.

# SEDATIVE

A drug that reduces excitement and calms the subject without inducing sleep.

## Benzodiazepine

Benzodiazepines work by binding to a receptor which is located or neurons in the brain called GABA receptors. And GABA is neurotransmitter in the brain.

### Drug Examples

*Long Acting (24–48 Hours)*
- Diazepam
- Chlordiazepoxide
- Clonazepam
- Midazolam
- Triazolam

*Short Acting (12–24 Hours)*
- Lorazepam
- Alprazolam
- Nitrazepam
- Oxazepam

*Indications*
- As sedative
- status epileptics
- Insomnia
- Muscle relaxants
- Used in General Anesthesia

*Adverse Effect*
- Confusion
- Lethargy
- Headache
- Impaired motor co-ordination
- Incontinence
- Drowsiness

*Nursing Responsibilities*
- Drug should be taken as per the dose advised
- It should not be stopped without consultation.
- Educate regarding side effects
- Cautiously monitor vital signs during I/V administration.
- Maintain patients I/O chart for 5 hours if getting parenteral infusion.

## Barbiturates

These drugs are derivative of barbituric acid and depresses the cerebral cortical activity.

### Drug Examples
- Phenobarbitone (long acting)
- Thiopentone
- Hexobarbitone
- Pentobarbitone

### Indications
- As sedative and anticonvalscent
- As anesthesia
- Kernicterus (increase conjugation of bilirubin increase clearance of bilirubin)

### Nursing Responsibilities
- Slowly IV infusion and monitor vital sign carefully
- Instruct to avoid alcohol, sleep inducing drugs
- Avoid becoming pregnant when taking these drugs
- Avoid oral contraceptives

## CNS Stimulants

It enhances the excitability of nervous tissue by blocking in an inhibitory neurotransmitter.

### Drug Example

Amphetamine, dextroamphetamine, doxapram and caffeine.

### Indications

- As sedative, Increase mental alertness and respiratory rate
- Used in case of respiratory failure
- Mental retardation and attention deficit disorder in children
- Memory disturbances

### Contraindication and Precaution

- Severe cardiovascular disorders
- Glaucoma
- Use with caution in patients with psychosis and in pregnant and breast feeding mothers

### Side Effects

- Insomnia
- More irritable
- Low BP
- Exhaustion
- Weight loss

### Nursing Responsibilities

- Check the drug effectiveness
- Assess the patients lung sound, rate and depth of respiration
- Advise for last daily dose, six hours before bedtime

## Antidepressants

It is used to prevent depression.

### Drug Example

- Amitriptyline
- Doxepin
- Phenelzine

### Indications

- Endogenous depression
- School phobia and compulsive phobic states
- Enuresis
- Obsessive compulsive disorder

### Contraindication

- Active liver diseases
- Precautious in aged patient and in hepatic and renal disorders.

### Side Effects

- Orthostatic hypotension, tachycardia, blurred vision, constipation, seizures and dry mouth
- Heart failure
- Anticholinergic effects, restlessness and nauseated
- Overdose can cause CNS stimulation, hallucination and convulsions.

### Nursing Responsibilities

- Slowly discontinue the drug
- Counsel the patient that drug may take more days to produce desired effects
- Avoid alcohol and other noninstructed drugs to prevent adverse drugs reactions
- Tell patient to swallow the whole medicine without crushing it.

## Anticonvulsant

It reduces and also prevents severity and occurrence of seizures in different category of epilepsy by enhancing GABA action and inhibiting sodium channel activity.

### Drug Examples

- Phenytoin
- Phenobarbitone
- Carbamazepine
- Clonazepam

### Indications

- Phenytoin can be used in all epilepsies (except petit mal epilepsy)
- Phenobarbitone used to control grand mal epilepsy, simple partial seizures, febrile convulsions
- Seizures related to drug withdrawal
- Status epilepticus
- Carbamazepine is useful to control psychomotor epilepsy, grand mal epilepsy, and mixed seizures.

### Side Effects

Sedation, drowsiness, drug dependence, dizziness, slurred speech, nausea, vomiting (phenytoin), long use of carbamazepine may cause bone marrow suppression and photophobia.

### Nursing Responsibilities

- Alert for manifestation of toxicity, hypotension and coma
- Educate regarding importance of good oral hygiene and dental check up to avoid gingival hyperplasia
- Advise to avoid alcohol and self medication with over the counter drugs

- Advise for compliance and use of same drug preparation
- Evaluate respiratory condition before and during this therapy
- Monitor for any withdrawal symptoms.

# DRUGS USED IN CARDIOVASCULAR SYSTEM

## Cardiac Drugs

Cardiac drug is a general term used to describe medications that are used to treat various heart conditions and disorders. These drugs can have different mechanisms of action and are prescribed based on the specific cardiac condition and the patient's individual needs. The choice of cardiac drug depends on the specific condition being treated, the patient's medical history and any other medications.

Cardiotonic drugs (inotropic) acts on the intracellular calcium levels in the heart muscle and increase contractility of heart muscle and augment cardiac output, leads to increased renal blood flow and urine production.

### Used

- Hypertension
- Angina pectoris and MI
- Shock
- Arrhythmias
- CHF

### Types

- Cardiac glycosides
- Phosphodiesterase inhibitors

## Cardiac Glycosides

Digoxin is having a positive inotropic effect and increase cardiac output and renal perfusion.

### Indications

- Heart failure (HF)
- Atrial flutter
- Atrial fibrillation
- Paroxysmal atrial tachycardia

### Contraindications

- Hypersensitivity to digitalis preparations
- Ventricular tachycardia or fibrillation
- Heart block or sick sinus syndrome
- Idiopathic hypertrophic subaortic stenosis (IHSS)
- Acute MI
- Renal failure

### Side Effects

- Headache, weakness, drowsiness and vision changes
- Digitalis toxicity

### Nursing Responsibilities

- Do thoroughly the physical assessment and evaluate for any contraindication
- Monitor cardiac parameters and change in quality or rhythm
- Check the apical pulse for one minute before taking the drug
- Stop the medication, If the pulse is <60 beats/min in an adult or <90 beats/min in an infant, take the pulse again in one hour
- Continue intravenous doses very slowly over at least five minutes to check arrhythmias and adverse effects
- Deny the oral drug with food or antacids to avoid delays in absorption
- Monitor the patient for therapeutic digoxin level (0.5–2 ng/mL)
- Maintain emergency equipment on standby if digoxin toxicity develops
- Provide thorough patient teaching regarding the use of drug and it's complication

## Phosphodiesterase Inhibitors

These drugs block the enzyme phosphodiesterase. It is used for short-term treatment of HF that has not responded to digoxin or diuretics alone or that has had a poor response to digoxin, diuretics, and vasodilators.

### Contraindications

- Hypersensitivity to phosphodiesterase inhibitors
- Severe aortic or pulmonic valvular disease
- Acute MI

### Adverse Effects

- Ventricular arrhythmias
- Nausea, vomiting, anorexia and abdominal pain
- Thrombocytopenia

### Nursing Responsibilities

- Check input and output and record daily weight
- Watch platelet counts before and regularly during therapy
- Examine the skin for bruising or petechiae to notice early signs of thrombocytopenia
- Arrange life-support equipment on standby
- Give thorough patient teaching on the details of drug use.

## Antianginals

The nitrates relax and dilate veins, arteries, and capillaries, allowing increased blood flow through the vessels and lowering systemic blood pressure.

Long-acting nitrates taken daily for management of chronic angina and prevention of angina in adults. Short acting nitrates are used for treatment of acute angina attack and prevention of angina attacks also.

### Available Forms

Nitroglycerin can be used as sublingual tablet, translingual spray, intravenous solution, transdermal patch, topical ointment or paste and transmucosal agent.

### Contraindications

- Hypersensitivity
- Severe anemia
- Head trauma or cerebral hemorrhage
- Pregnancy or lactation

### Adverse Effect

- Headache, dizziness, weakness, nausea, vomiting, incontinence and hypotension
- Flushing, pallor and increased perspiration.

### Nursing Responsibilities

- Observe cardiopulmonary status closely
- Instruct the patient, after taking medicine; if pain persists emergency treatment should be started
- Rotate the sites when using topical form of medicine
- Taper the dose gradually after long duration therapy

## Beta Blockers

It is used to block the stimulatory effects of the sympathetic nervous system and decreases the excitability of the heart, less cardiac output, less cardiac oxygen consumption, and reduces blood pressure. Examples of the drug are atenolol propranolol and metoprolol.

It is used in long-term management of angina pectoris and prevent re infarction.

### Nuring Responsibilities

- Do not stop these drugs suddenly and taper the medicine slowly over two weeks and check vital signs cardiac output repeatedly.
- Constantly watch for IV administration of the drugs.

## Calcium Channel Blockers

Calcium channel blockers inhibit the movement of calcium ions across the membranes of myocardial and arterial muscle cells, altering the action potential and blocking muscle cell contraction. Which cause vasodilatation, decreases the preload and afterload, reduces cardiac workload and oxygen consumption.

Examples of drugs are amlodipine, diltiazem, nicardipine, nifedipine and verapamil.

It is used for the patient with chronic angina, effort associated angina and hypertension.

### Nursing Responsibilities

- Observe skin color continuously and maintain skin integrity
- Check blood pressure vigilantly.
- Provide health teaching to patient and their family members on contraindication and uses of drugs.

# DRUGS USED IN GASTROINTESTINAL SYSTEM

## Gastrointestinal Stimulants

Decrease reflux by increasing sphincter tone and enhancing acid clearance and decreasing gastric emptying.

### Drug Example

- Metoclopramide (reglan, plasil and vometa)
- Cisapride (propulsid)

### Indications

- Used to prevent nausea and vomiting related to chemotherapy.
- Used for gastric emptying caused by diabetic gastroparesis, gastroesophageal reflux, postoperative nausea and vomiting.

### Adverse Effects

Drowsiness, diarrhea, fatigue, seizures, agranulocytosis and depression.

### Contraindications

- In the presence of gastrointestinal hemorrhage
- Mechanical obstruction or perforation.

### Nursing Responsibilities

- Watch for potential hypernatremia and hypokalemia, in case of congestive heart failure or cirrhosis of liver.
- Extrapyramidal symptoms may occur in young adults and the elder one if taking high dose of metoclopramide
- Teach client to report signs and symptoms of side effects and sign of acute dystonia without delay.
- Not to drive just after taking metoclopramide.

## Anticholinergics and Antispasmodics

Anticholinergics antagonize the action of acetylcholine at the cholinergic receptor sites. Antispasmodics are similar and they are believed to relax smooth muscle.

### Drug Examples
- Dicyclomine hydrochloride
- Chlordiazepoxide hydrochloride
- Glycopyrrolate

### Indications
- Spasms of the gastrointestinal tract
- Irritable bowel syndrome

### Adverse Effects
- May cause dilated and non reactive pupils
- Tachycardia hyperthermia, hypertension and tachypnoea
- Dysphagia and no bowel sound

### Nursing Considerations
- Administer medications 30–60 minutes prior to meals and at bedtime for better therapeutic action
- Significant loss of potassium prone for the occurrence of paralytic ileus and cardia dysrhythmias
- Alert for metabolic acidosis due to loss of bicarbonate and inadequate renal excretion of acids
- Check vital signs and visual changes
- Check intake and output
- Avoid exposure to high temperatures, hyperthermia may occur
- Teach to report side effects to health professionals
- Advise to take sufficient fluid and dietary modification to reduce constipation
- Advise the patient to inform if any supplementary medications prescribed

## Antidiarrheals

It reduces the GI motility by acting on nerve endings of the intestinal wall and make less volume of stools, increasing viscosity and maintain fluid and electrolyte balance.

### Examples of Drugs
- Attapulgite (donnagel)
- Loperamide (imodium)
- Diphenoxylate HCl (lomotil)

### Nursing Considerations
- Document onset, duration, and frequency of symptoms
- Assess current medications and document, if the allergy is present.
- Assess for evidence of dehydration or electrolyte imbalance and monitor vital signs.
- Check abdomen for tenderness, distention, bowel sounds, or masses
- Advise to take bismuth and tetracycline one hour apart.

### Patient Teaching
- Take sufficient fluid to check dehydration and improve dryness of mouth
- Healthcare provider can advise the client to take BRAT diet: Bananas, rice, apple sauce, tea/toast to reduce dehydration
- Teach client take medicine as per prescribed dose and consult health care professionals if diarrhea persists over 2 days
- Alert for drowsiness.
- Avoid to take dairy products
- Instruct to maintain good personal hygiene and avoid alcohol during medication
- Advise client to inform incase of pregnancy and breast feeding.

## Histamine H2 Antagonists

Diminish gastric acid secretion by blocking histamine 2 in the gastric parietal cells. It is used to treat duodenal ulcer, gastric ulcer, Zollinger–Ellison syndrome, reflux esophagitis and combination therapy to treat Helicobacter pylori.

Common drugs are famotidine, cimetidine and ranitidine.

### Nursing Considerations
- Minimize the dose in case of hepatic or renal impairment.
- Assess for any alteration in nutritional status and dietary interventions.
- Advice the client to quit smoking that enhances gastric stimulation. Teach the patients not to take antacid within one hour of dose
- Only prescribed medicine can be taken
- Take the medicine before meals.

## Proton Pump Inhibitor (PPI)

Block acid production by inhibiting the $H^+$ - $K^+$ ATP as at the secretory surface of the gastric parietal cells, through which block the formation of gastric acid.

It is used for treatment of erosive or ulcerative gastro esophageal reflux disease (GERD) or duodenal ulcers, active benign gastric ulcers and for treatment of pathological hypersecretory conditions such as long term Zollinger Ellison syndrome.

Example of medicines are rabeprazole sodium, Omeprazole, Pantoprazole and esomeprazole.

### Nursing Responsibilities

- Reduce the dose for the patient with severe liver disease
- Document the drug advised and its efficacy in detail
- Check laboratory test results including liver function test, CBC, and BUN and review any other diagnostic findings if patient is having
- Counsel the patient to take prescribed diet and modification in life style to decrease symptoms
- Advise the patient that esomeprazole and omeprazole should be taken before meals
- Inform any difficulty in swallowing because omeprazole, pantoprazole, and rabeprazole must be swallowed as a whole
- Inform the client that lansoprazole and esomeprazole capsules may be opened and sprinkled.

## DRUGS USED ON URINARY SYSTEM

### Diuretics

Diuretics (water pills) are the drugs which increase the urine out put (or) urine volume.

**Diuretic agent:** Any drug when introduce into the body increases the out put of sodium, i.e., loss of sodium in urine.

### Indications

- Cirrhosis of the liver
- Pregnancy associated edema
- Hypertension
- Chronic hepatic diseases
- Nephrotic syndrome
- Chronic heart failure

### Classification of Diuretics

- Loop diuretics (furosemide and torsemide)
- Thiazide diuretics (chlorothiazide, hydrochloride thiazide and benzthiazide)
- Osmotic diuretics (mannitol)
- Carbonic anhydrase inhibitors (acetazolamide)
- Potassium sparing diuretics (spironolactone and amiloride)

### Mechanism of Action (Diuretics)

- **Loop diuretics:** They show their action by reducing absorption of sodium at the level of loop of Henle, e.g., furosemide and torsemide.
- **Potassium sparing:** Drug which antagonized the effect of aldosterone, e.g., spironolactone.
- **Thiazide:** They inhibit reabsorption of sodium and chloride ions from distal convoluted tubules, e.g., chlorothiazide.
- **Osmotic:** It inhibits reabsorption of water and sodium, e.g., mannitol.
- **Carbonic anhydrase inhibitor:** They suppress the activity of carbonic anhydrase, e.g., acetazolamide.

### Indication and Uses

- **Loop diuretics:** Edema, acute pulmonary edema (acute LVF, MI), cerebral edema, hypertension, hypercalcemia and renal calcium stone.
- **Thiazide:** Mild to moderate edema (cardiac failure, nephrotic syndrome), HTN, diabetes insipidus, hypercalciuria/calcium stone and premenstrual tenses.
- **Osmotic:** Acute renal failure during prolonged surgery or trauma to prevent or treat increase ICP, glaucoma.
- **Carbonic anhydrase inhibitor:** Glaucoma, epilepsy, acute motion sickness and periodic paralysis.
- **Potassium sparing:** Hyperaldosteronism, HTN, CHF, edema, combine with furosemide, thiazide to reduce potassium loss produce by these agents.

### Drug Examples and Doses (Diuretics)

- **Furosemide:** 20–80 mg
- **Torsemide:** 5–10 mg orally or IV OD
- **Chlorothiazide:** 500–1000 mg PO or IV OD or Bid
- **Hydrochlorothiazide:** 25–50 mg OD
- **Benzthiazide:** 25 mg
- **Mannitol:** 50–100 g IV
- **Acetazolamide:** 125–250 mg orally IV
- **Spironolactone:** 25–200 mg/day in 1-2 divided doses.
- **Amiloride:** 5–10 mg OD.

### Contraindication and Precautions (Diuretics)

- **Osmotic:** Intracranial bleeding, CHF, urinary tract obstruction, pulmonary congestion and edema.
- **Loop:** Hyponatremia, severe sodium and water depletion, hypokalemia, renal failure and addison's disease.
- **Potassium:** Anuria, hyperkalemia, acute or progressive renal insufficiency.
- **Thiazide:** Severe renal impairment, severe hepatic impairment, hypersensitivity, pregnancy and lactation.
- **Carbonic anhydrase:** Pregnancy and lactation, hepatic insufficiency and severe pulmonary congestion.

### Adverse Effect (Diuretics)

- **Thiazide:** Hypokalemia, metabolic alkalosis, hyponatremia, dehydration, hypotension, hypercholesterolemia, hyperuricemia, azotemia (in renal disease patient)

- **Loop:** Hypokalemia, metabolic alkalosis, hyperuricemia, hypomagnesemia, dehydration (hypovolemia), hypotension, ototoxicity (dose related hearing loss)
- **Osmotic:** Electrolyte imbalance, increase circulatory load and may cause congestive heart failure
- **Potassium:** Hyperkalemia, metabolic acidosis, gynecomastia, (aldosterone antagonist), gastric problems including peptic ulcer.

### Nursing Responsibilities
- Monitor urine output, blood pressure, hourly check for electrolyte imbalance.
- Obtain vital signs.
- Monitor laboratory values like potassium, sodium (diuretics can cause electrolyte imbalance).
- Observe changes in level of consciousness, dizziness, fatigue, and postural hypotension because reduction in blood volume due to diuretic therapy may produce changes in level of consciousness or syncope.
- Observe for sign of hypersensitivity reaction.
- Monitor hearing and vision (loop diuretic are ototoxic).

## Urinary Antiseptics
Drugs used for urinary tract infects which kill or inhibit the growth of microorganism.

### Mechanism of Action
These are bacteriostatic drug. They inhibit the growth of different species of bacteria in urine.

### Indications
- Sulphonamide is used to treat infection causes by susceptible organism in urinary tract.
- Methenamine is used to prevent recurrent urinary tract infection.

### Adverse Effects
Fever, rash, crystalluria, nausea, vomiting, photosensitivity reaction, stevens johnson's syndrome.

### Drug Examples and Doses (Urinary Antiseptics)
- **Sulfadiazine:** 500–1000 mg
- **Sulfamethoxazole:** 1–2 g orally every 6 hourly
- **Ciprofloxacin:** 250–500 mg
- **Levofloxacin:** 250–500 mg
- **Nalidixic acid:** 500 mg
- **Nitrofurantoin:** 50–100 mg orally.

### Contraindication and Precautions
- Contraindicated in pregnant and breast-feeding women, children younger than age 2 years.
- History of Stevens Johnson syndrome.
- Hypersensitive patients with sulphonamides.

Cautiously use in patients with mild to moderate renal or hepatic disorders, severe allergies, blood dyscrasias urinary obstruction.

### Nursing Responsibilities
- Assess the sign and symptoms of urinary tract infections.
- Advice to patient for intake of fluid 2,000–3,000 mL/day to reduce crystalluria.
- Teach the patient proper hygiene measures to reduce the risk of reinfection.
- Monitor the patient urinary elimination patterns Instruct to women who are taking oral conceptive to use an alternative method such as barrier method during the entire course of therapy.

## Antidiuretics
An antidiuretics are the agent that reduce urine volume, and opposing diuresis.

### Mechanism of Action
Reduces urine flow by acting reabsorption of water by kidney tubules.

### Indications
- Cranial diabetes insipidus.
- Primary nocturnal enuresis (bed wetting)
- Nocturia associated with multiple sclerosis.

### Drug Examples and Doses
- Antidiuretic hormone (vasopressin): 5–10 units IM/SC
- Desmopressin: 100–400 µg orally 1–4 µg IV.

### Contraindication and Precautions
- Hypersensitivity
- Impaired renal function with ongoing diuretic treatment.

### Caution
- CV disease edema
- Hypertension
- Cystic fibrosis
- Fluid and electrolyte imbalance
- Pregnancy and lactation

### Adverse Effects
- Nasal irritation
- Rhinitis
- Abdominal cramps
- Urge defecate

- Fluid retention
- Congestion
- Ulceration
- Nausea
- Pallor
- Backache in females (due to uterine contraction)

### Nursing Responsibilities

- Monitor electrolyte imbalance.
- Monitor vital signs and BP regularly.
- Observe for sign of hypersensitivity reactions.
- Monitor laboratory values.
- Stop medication if hypertension exists.

## DRUGS USED IN ENDOCRINE SYSTEM

### Thyroid Medications (Thyroid Hormones)

This medicine is advised for the hypothyroidism and replaces the hormonal deficit also.

### Name of Drugs

- Levothyroxine (synthroid)
- Liothyronine (cytomel)
- Thyroid desiccated
- Liotrix (thyrolar)

### Actions

- Replaces both $T_3$–$T_4$
- Increases metabolic rate
- Increase $O_2$ consumption
- Increase HR, RR and BP

### Indications

- Hypothyroidism
- Diagnostic suppression test

### Adverse Effects

- Nausea and vomiting.
- Signs of increased metabolism, i.e., tachycardia, hypertension, cardiac arrhythmias, anxiety, headache, tremors and palpitations.

### Nursing Responsibilities

- Monitor weight.
- Instruct client to take daily medication the same time each morning without food.
- Monitor blood tests to check the activity of thyroid.
- Advise to report palpitation, tachycardia, and chest pain.
- Instruct to avoid foods that inhibit thyroid secretions like cabbage, spinach and radishes.

### Antithyroid Medications

The thyroid becomes oversaturated with iodine and stop producing thyroid hormone.

- Drugs used to block the thyroid hormones and treat hyperthyroidism.
- Inhibit the synthesis of thyroid hormones.

### Antithyroid Medications

- Methimazole (tapazole)
- Propylthiouracil (PTU) Iodine solution-SSKI
- Lugol's solution.

### Indications

- Grave's disease
- Thyrotoxicosis
- Absorption is good orally

### Adverse Effects

Tiredness, increased heart rate, skin rash, GI disturbances, metallic taste, burning in the mouth, sore teeth and gums, diarrhea and arthralgia.

### Nursing Responsibilities

- Monitor VS, $T_3$ and $T_4$, weight.
- Medications with meals to avoid gastric upset.
- Instruct to report sore throat or unexplained fever.
- Monitor for signs of hypothyroidism.
- Instruct not to stop abrupt medication.
- Lugol's solution: Used to decrease the vascularity and size of the thyroid (in preparation for thyroid surgery)
- $T_3$ and $T_4$ production diminishes.
- Given per oral, can be diluted with juice, administered with foods.
- Use straw to decrease staining.

## DRUG THERAPY FOR DIABETES MELLITUS

Advise the client, if diet modification and exercise cannot control the blood glucose level.

### Uses of Insulin

- Type 1 DM (insulin dependent DM), postpancreatectomy diabetes and gestational diabetes
- Some cases of type 2 DM (noninsulin dependent DM): Not controlled by diet/exercise
- Given as split-mix regimen and Basal Bolus regimen
- For diabetes ketoacidosis
- Regular insulin, in bolus dose followed by 0.1 U/kg/hr infusion as per fall in blood glucose levels
- Hyperglycemic coma

## Adverse Effects

- Hypoglycemia (confusion, nausea, hunger, tiredness, perspiration, headache, blurred vision and muscle weakness)
- Allergic reaction
- Edema

### Pharmacologic Insulin

Onset of action is rapid-acting, short-acting, intermediate-acting, long-acting and very long acting. Only regular insulin may be administered intravenously.

### Rapid Acting Insulin

**Example:** Lispro (humalog) and insulin aspart (novolog), produces a more rapid effect and with a shorter duration than any other insulin preparation.
- **Onset:** 5-15 minutes
- **Peak:** 1 hour
- **Duration:** 3 hours
- Instruct patient to eat within 5-15 minutes after injection.

### Regular Insulin

Also called short-acting insulin. Usually clear solution administered 30 minutes before a meal.
- **Onset:** 30 minutes to 1 hour
- **Peak:** 2-4 hours
- **Duration:** 4-6 hours

### Intermediate Acting Insulin

Called "NPH" or "LENTE"
Appears white and cloudy.
- **Onset:** 2-4 hours
- **Peak:** 4-12 hours
- **Duration:** 16-20 hours

### Long Acting Insulin (Insulin Glargine and Insulin Detemir)

- **Onset:** 6-8 hours
- **Peak:** 12-16 hours
- **Duration:** 20-30 hours.

### Methods of Administration

Cloudy insulin should be thoroughly mixed by gently inverting the vial or rolling between the hands.

Insulin not in use should be stored in the refrigerator, but avoid freezing/extreme temperature.

Insulin in use should be kept at room temperature to reduce local irritation at the injection site.

### Nursing Responsibilities

- Insulin may be kept at room temperature up to one month.
- Select syringes that match the insulin concentration. U-100 means 100 units per mL.
- Instruct the client to draw up the regular (clear) insulin first before drawing the intermediate acting (cloudy) insulin.
- Prefilled syringes can be prepared and should be kept in the refrigerator with the needle in the upright position to avoid clogging the needle.
- The four main areas for insulin injection areabdomen, upper arms, thighs and hips.
- Nurse should keep in mind that quick absorption of insulin is through abdomen and very sluggish through hips.
- Alcohol should not be used as cleaning agent for the skin.
- After each use discard the syringe.

## INTRAVENOUS FLUIDS

Many adult hospital inpatients need intravenous (IV) fluid therapy to prevent or correct problems with their fluid and/or electrolyte status. Deciding on the optimal amount and composition of IV fluids to be administered and the best rate at which to give them can be a difficult and complex task, and decisions must be based on careful assessment of the patient's individual needs.

Disturbances related to fluid and electrolytes are the most common clinical problems encountered in the critical care unit. Critical disorders such as severe burns, trauma, sepsis, brain damage, and heart failure lead to disturbances in fluid and electrolyte homeostasis.

Recent studies have reported that fluid and electrolyte imbalances are associated with increased morbidity and mortality among critically ill patients. To provide optimal care, health care providers should be familiar with the principles and practice of fluid and electrolyte physiology and pathophysiology.

Surveys have shown that many staff who prescribe IV fluids knows neither the likely fluid and electrolyte needs of individual patients, nor the specific composition of the many choices of IV fluids available to them. Standards of recording and monitoring IV fluid and electrolyte therapy may also be poor in these settings. IV fluid management in hospital is often delegated to the most junior medical staff that frequently lacks the relevant experience and may have received little or no specific training on the subject.

## Intravenous IV Therapy

- As many as 75% of patients admitted into hospital receive some type of IV therapy.
- 50–70% of the average human is body fluids.

**Distribution of fluid in the body is:**
- **1/3 extracellular fluid**
  - Interstitial fluid
  - Plasma or intravascular fluid
  - Transcellular fluid
- **2/3 intracellular fluid**
  - Fluid within a cell
  - Red blood cells
  - Other cells

## Uses of IV Therapy

- Establish or maintain fluid and/or electrolyte balance
- Administer medication continuously or intermittently
- Administer bolus medication
- Administer fluid to maintain venous access in case of an emergency
- Administer blood or blood products
- Administer intravenous anesthetics
- Maintain or correct a patient's nutritional status
- Administer diagnostic reagents
- Monitor hemodynamic functions
- Correct acidosis or alkalosis

## Types of IV Fluids

- Crystalloids
- Colloids
- Blood and blood products

### Crystalloids (Table 3.3)

- Crystalloids are water with electrolytes that form a solution that can pass through semi permeable membranes.
- They are lost rapidly from the intravascular space into the interstitial space.
- They can remain in the extracellular compartment for about 45 minutes.

**Table 3.3:** Types, uses and nursing implications for common crystalloids.

| Common crystalloids solution | Type | Uses | Nursing implications |
|---|---|---|---|
| Dextrose 5% in water (D5W) | Isotonic | • Fluid loss<br>• Dehydration<br>• Hypernatremia | • Use cautiously in renal and cardiac patients<br>• Can cause fluid overload<br>• May cause hyperglycemia or osmotic diuresis |
| 0.9% sodium chloride (normal saline-NaCl) | Isotonic | • Shock<br>• Hyponatremia<br>• Blood transfusions<br>• Resuscitation<br>• Fluid challenges<br>• Diabetic ketoacidosis (DKA) | • Can lead to overload<br>• Use with caution in patients with heart failure or edema<br>• Can cause hyponatremia, hypernatremia, hyperchloremia or calorie depletion |
| Lactated Ringer's (Hartmanns) | Isotonic | • Dehydration<br>• Burns<br>• Lower GI fluid loss<br>• Acute blood loss<br>• Hypovolemia due to third spacing | • Contains potassium, do not use with renal failure patients<br>• Do not use with liver disease, cannot metabolize lactate |
| 0.45% sodium chloride (1/2 normal saline) | Hypotonic | • Water replacement<br>• DKA<br>• Gastric fluid loss from NG or vomiting | • Use with caution<br>• May cause cardiovascular collapse or increased intracranial pressure<br>• Do not use with liver disease, trauma or burns |
| Dextrose 5% in 1/2 normal saline | Hypertonic | • Later in DKA | • Use only when blood sugar falls below 250 mg/dL |
| Dextrose 5% in normal saline | Hypertonic | • Temporary treatment from shock if plasma expanders aren't available<br>• Addison's crisis | • Contra-indicated for cardiac or renal patients |
| Dextrose 10% in water | Hypertonic | • Water replacement<br>• Conditions where some nutrition with glucose is required | • Monitor blood sugar levels |

- Because of this, larger volumes than colloids are required for fluid resuscitation.
- Eventually, water from crystalloids diffuses through the intracellular fluid.

### Hypertonic
A hypertonic solution draws fluid into the intravascular compartment from the cells and the interstitial compartments. **Osmolarity is higher than serum osmolarity.**

### Hypotonic
A hypotonic solution shifts fluid out of the intravascular compartment, hydrating the cells and the interstitial compartments. **Osmolarity is lower than serum osmolarity.**

### Isotonic
Because an isotonic solution stays in the intravascular space, it expands the intravascular compartment. **Osmolarity is the same as serum osmolarity.**

### Colloids (Table 3.4)
- Colloids contain solutes in the form of large proteins or other similar sized molecules
- They cannot pass through the walls of capillaries and into cells
- They remain in blood vessels longer and increase intravascular volume
- They attract water from the cells into the blood vessels
- But this is a short-term benefit
- Prolonged movement can cause the cells to lose too much water and become dehydrated.

### Common Colloids
See **Table 3.4**.

## BLOOD AND BLOOD COMPONENTS

Blood is the life-maintaining fluid, which flows through the entire body. It carries electrolytes, hormones, antibodies, vitamins, heat, oxygen and nourishment towards the body tissues. It takes away carbon dioxide and waste matter from the body tissues. Components of human blood are shown **Table 3.5**.

**Table 3.5:** Components of human blood.

| Components | Functions |
|---|---|
| Plasma | ◆ Cryoprecipitate is a concentrated source of certain plasma proteins and is used to treat some bleeding problems |
| Red blood cells | ◆ A transfusion of whole blood or packed red blood cells may be needed to treat acute blood loss or anemia |
| White blood cells | ◆ Fight infection, bacteria and other substances that enter the body. White blood cells include lymphocytes, monocytes, eosinophils, basophils, neutrophils<br>◆ When the WBC becomes very less, it is called neutropenia. G-CSF injections may be needed to treat neutropenia |
| Platelets | ◆ Platelets help blood to clot. Platelet transfusions are given when the platelet count is below normal |

**Table 3.4:** Types, uses and nursing considerations for common colloids.

| Colloid | Action/use | Nursing consideration |
|---|---|---|
| Albumin (plasma protein) 4% or 20% | ◆ Keeps fluids in vessels<br>◆ Maintains volume<br>◆ Primarily used to replace protein and treat stock | May cause anaphylaxis (a severe, often rapidly progressive allergic reaction that is potentially life threatening) watch for/report wheeze, persistent cough, difficulty breathing, throat tightness, swelling of the lips, eyes, tongue, face, loss of consciousness. May cause fluid overload and pulmonary edema |
| Dextran (polysaccharide) 40 or 70 | ◆ Shifts fluids into vessels.<br>◆ Vascular expansion<br>◆ Prolongs hemodynamic response when given with HES | ◆ May cause fluid overdose and hypersensitivity<br>◆ Increased risk of bleeding<br>◆ Contraindicated in bleeding disorder, chronic heart failure and renal failure |
| Hetastarch (HES) (synthetic starch) 6% or 10% | ◆ Shifts fluids into vessels<br>◆ Vascular expansion | ◆ Alert for fluid overload and hypersensitivity<br>◆ Increased risk for bleeding<br>◆ Avoid in case of bleeding disorder, chronic failure and renal failure |
| Mannitol (alcohol sugar) 5% or 10% | ◆ Oliguric diuresis<br>◆ Reduce cerebral edema<br>◆ Eliminates toxins | ◆ May cause fluid overload and electrolyte imbalances<br>◆ Extravasations may cause necrosis |

## Complications of IV Therapy

- Confined complications at the site including extravasations, phlebitis, hematoma and infection.
- Fluid overload cause acute pulmonary edema
- Electrolyte imbalance leads to cardiac arrhythmias.
- Anaphylaxis
- Air embolus

## ELECTROLYTES

Electrolytes are minerals in body fluids that carry an electric charge. Electrolytes affect the amount of water, the acidity of blood (pH), muscle function, and other important processes in the body.

There are six major electrolytes:
1. **Sodium:** $Na^+$ major cation in extracellular fluid (ECF)
2. **Potassium:** $K^+$ major cation in intracellular fluid (ICF)
3. **Calcium:** $Ca^{++}$ major cation found in ECF and teeth and bones
4. **Chloride:** $Cl^-$ major anion found in ECF
5. **Phosphate:** $PO_4^{3-}$ major anion found in ICF
6. **Magnesium:** $Mg^{++}$ major cation found in ICF (closely related to $Ca^{++}$ and $PO_4$).

### Sodium (Na⁺)

**Normal:** Serum level 135–145 mmol/L.

#### Functions

- Keep extracellular function (ECF) osmolarity.
- Affects concentration, excretion and absorption of potassium and chloride.
- Helps in controlling acid-base balance.
- Transmit nerve and muscle fiber impulse.

### Potassium (K⁺)

**Normal:** Serum level 3.5–5.0 mmol/L.

#### Functions

- Keep up cell electro-neutrality and cell osmolarity.
- Helps in conduction of nerve impulses.
- Directly affects cardiac muscle contraction along with re-polarization in the action potential.
- Perform a greater role in acid-base balance.

#### Hypokalemia (Potassium Less Than Normal)

- Decreased peristalsis, skeletal muscle and cardiac muscle function and reflexes
- Muscle weakness or irritability/cramps
- Cardiac arrhythmias and ultimately to cardiac arrest
- Decreased blood pressure and bowel motility
- Paralytic ileus.

#### Hyperkalemia (Potassium More Than Normal)

- Muscle weakness, nausea, diarrhea and oliguria.
- Paresthesia (altered sensation) of the face, tongue, hands and feet.
- Cardiac arrhythmias and cardiac arrest.
- Potassium is a heavy solute that needs to disperse thoroughly in IV fluid care should be taken when administering to avoid fatal consequences.

### Calcium (Ca⁺⁺)

**Normal:** Serum level 2.15–2.55 mmol/L.

#### Functions

- Enhances bone strength and durability, cell-membrane structure.
- Affects activation, excitation and contraction of SA node.
- Participates in neurotransmitter release at synapses.
- Trigger specific steps in blood coagulation.

#### Hypocalcemia (Calcium Less Than Normal)

- Muscle tremor.
- Muscle cramps, tetany, tonic-clonic seizures.
- Paresthesia and bleeding.
- Arrhythmias and hypotension.
- Numbness or tingling in fingers, toes and around the mouth.

#### Hypercalcemia (Calcium More Than Normal)

- Lethargy, fatigue, hypertension, polyuria, headache and muscle flaccidity
- Depression confusion
- Nausea and vomiting
- Anorexia and constipation
- Cardiac arrhythmias and ECG changes (shortened QT interval and widened T-wave.

### Chloride (Cl⁻)

**Normal:** Serum level 95–110 mmol/L.

#### Function

Maintains serum osmolarity.

#### Hypochloremia

- Increased muscle excitability and tetany.
- Decreased respirations.

*Hyperchloremia*
- Headache, trouble in concentrating.
- Drowsiness, stupor and rapid, deep breathing (hypercapnia).
- Muscle weakness.

## Phosphate ($PO_4$)

**Normal:** Serum level 0.8–1.5 mmol/L.

*Functions*
- Keep up bones and teeth and cell integrity.
- Plays a major role in acid-base balance (as a urinary buffer).
- Plays essential role in muscle, red blood cell and neurological function.

*Hypophosphatemia*
- Paresthesia and lethargy.
- Speech defects (such as stuttering).
- Muscle pain and tenderness.

*Hyperphosphatemia*
- Renal failure.
- Vague neuro-excitability to tetany and seizures.
- Arrhythmias and muscle twitching with sudden rise in phosphate ($PO_4$) level.

## Magnesium ($Mg^{++}$)

**Normal:** Serum level 0.70–1.05 mol/L.

*Functions*
- Activates intracellular enzymes; active in carbohydrate and protein metabolism.
- Acts on myo-neural vasodilation.
- Facilitates $Na^+$ and $K^+$ movement across all membranes.
- Influences $Ca^{++}$ levels.

*Hypomagnesemia*
- Dizziness, confusion, seizures and tremor.
- Leg and foot cramps.
- Hyperirritability and arrhythmias.
- Vasomotor changes.
- Anorexia, nausea.

*Hypermagnesemia*
- Drowsiness, lethargy and coma.
- Arrhythmias and hypotension.
- Tremor and nausea.
- Peripheral vasodilation and sense of warmth.
- Weak pulse and facial flushing.

## DRUG OVERDOSES AND POISONING

Any product or substance, including medications, can be harmful if it is used in the wrong way, by the wrong person, or in the wrong amount. A poisoning can occur from that substance by eating it, drinking it, breathing it, injecting it, getting it on the skin, or getting it in the eyes.

A drug overdose is considered a poisoning. In this case, the drug is the product that is used in the wrong way, by the wrong person, or in the wrong amount.

Poisoning may be accidental or intended. Accidental poisoning is generally occurs in children, while intended poisoning is very common in adolescents and young adults. Poisoning can cause from various sources and also affect through ingestion from a infected food or water supply, or through inhalation of toxic gases or sprays.

### Poisoning in Children

Accidental poisoning occurs as a result of natural investigative behavior or of imitating adults unknowingly regarding consequence. This type of poisoning happens during six months to five year, and peak around 18 months to two year.

Some poisoning, which may occur in case of small children are iatrogenic and nonaccident.
- Therapeutic poisoning found in premature infants and neonates with a small error in dose can cause life-threatening toxicity, examples are chloramphenicol, theophylline, and digoxin.
- Intentional poisoning may range from sedating a child in order to make quite to Munchausen's syndrome by proxy.

### Poisoning in Teenagers and Adults

- In teenage children, deliberate self-harm (DSH) and substance misuse are the very frequent causes of poisoning.
- In early adulthood, DSH in the form of parasuicidal gestures is common.
- All through adult life, poisoning can occur in industrial settings.
- Serious suicidal attempts become commoner, in men over 45 years of age. There may be underlying factors such as mental or physical illness, alcohol or substance misuse, unemployment, and relationship problems.

### History Taking

When taking the history, the nurse needs to ask the in the following area:
- Drugs or chemicals have been ingested, injected, or inhaled.

- Patient vomited or not after taking the poison, if vomited, when?
- Any other medications taking.
- Patient is having any known allergies.
- Previous history of depression, mental illness, or attempted suicide.

## Nursing Assessment and Interventions

The overall aim of the nursing assessment is to getting the cause and think for safety of the patient regards to airway, breathing, circulation and reducing further absorption. Not to forget emotional and supportive part of management.

- **Maintain airway, breathing and circulation**
- **Neurological monitoring:** Record the GCS score, neurological status is regularly reassessed. Thorough monitoring and frequent reassessment to find out any deterioration in the level of consciousness.
  Observe pupil size and reaction. Pinpoint pupils due to narcotics. Dilated pupils due to cocaine, amphetamines, atropine, or tricyclic antidepressants. Seizures may appear withdrawal from drugs or alcohol
- **Specific interventions:** Hypothermia may happen after taking barbiturates, cocaine, Ecstasy, monoamine oxidase inhibitors and phenothiazines. Use a warming blanket and warm IV fluids to stable the patient's temperature.
  - If the eyes and/or skin have been contaminated by corrosive agents or pesticides, the eyes must be washed out continuously with water for 10–15 min. Clean the skin with soap and water, with more attention to the thinner areas of the skin (axillae, groins and face).
  - Ingestion of corrosive agents, acids, or alkalis can be immediately treated by giving the water to drink for diluting the substance and so prevent tissue damage.
- **Gastric lavage:** The stomach should only be drained by gastric lavage on the recommendation of the poisons unit. Exceptions include iron, lithium, alcohol, methanol, ethylene glycol, corrosive agents, acids, and alkalis, for which oral antidotes or medication are needed.
- **Whole bowel lavage:** It involves giving isotonic fluid, using solutions that are normally used to prepare the bowel for X-ray procedures. It can be used to clear the gut of sustained-release preparations, iron, lithium, heavy metals, and illicit drug packets.
- **Psychosocial care:** Each purposeful self-poisoning patient should be handled in sympathetic way to make sure that all effort is being made to assist these patients, for preventing further occurrence.

## Poisoning from Therapeutic Drugs

### Paracetamol

Paracetamol is analgesic and safe in therapeutic use, but an overdose of >300 mg/kg can leads to liver failure and sometimes also kidney failure.

### Management of Paracetamol Overdose

Manage with the initial dose of acetylcysteine through infusion over 60 min to reduce the risk of frequent dose-related adverse reactions. Hypersensitivity is no longer a contraindication to treatment with acetylcysteine.

### Salicylates

Toxicity from salicylates includes vomiting, dehydration, tinnitus, deafness, sweating, warm extremities, and hyperventilation. Severe poisoning may brings coma, convulsions, pulmonary oedema, and cardiovascular collapse. Repeated measurements are very essential to know the drug level, because drug concentrations may enhance after ingestion of a large dose.

### Tricyclic Antidepressants

Overdose of tricyclic antidepressants (TCA) includes manifestations like tachycardia, dilated pupils, cardiac arrhythmias and widened QRS complex, hypotension, hot dry skin, dry mouth. Convulsions, respiratory depression, and coma may find. Cardiac monitoring is essential. The patient, if comes to hospital within one hour after ingesting toxic amount then may treat with activated charcoal.

### Benzodiazepines

It can be life-threatening problems, mainly in elder clients with severe chronic obstructive airways disease.

Overdose symptoms are drowsiness, ataxia, and nystagmus to hypotension, respiratory depression, and coma, mostly if benzodiazepines are taken with alcohol or other CNS depressants. Flumazenil can reverse the effect of benzodiazepines.

### Iron Tablets

- Early symptoms of iron overdose include nausea, vomiting, abdominal pain, and diarrhea. The patient's vomit and stools may be grey or black. Hematemesis and rectal bleeding may occur. In severe cases, coma and shock may occur.
- For children it is especially necessary to calculate serum iron levels, possibly gastric lavage, and deferoxamine treatment in spite of symptoms have resolved within a few hours.

## Cardiac Glycosides

In case off digoxin and digitalis toxicity nausea, vomiting, cardiac arrhythmias, hypotension, and death may result. Advise the patient for activated charcoal if they have the ability to swallow with close observation of ABCs.

## Drug Misuse

### Alcohol

Drinking alcohol cause intoxication, by which slurred speech, ataxia, confusion, and aggression occurs. Excess alcohol can be the reason of vomiting, coma, and hypoventilation, and also risk for aspiration of vomit. If a patient becomes unconscious handle like comatose patient.

### Opioids

Opioid poisoning causes progressive depression of the CNS, drowsiness, unconsciousness, respiratory depression, and eventually respiratory arrest.

Initial management depends on the patient's level of consciousness.

- In case of consciousness patient within one hour of ingesting toxic amount of opiate, advise for activated charcoal.
- For inadequate aspiration, consult anesthetist.
- In respiratory depression or impaired consciousness, advise naloxone as prescribed. Patients necessitate very close monitoring and frequent reassessment.

### Illicit Drugs

Illicit drugs consumption is a great challenge for the society. Various types of drugs are available from glue or petrol sniffing to cannabis to hard drugs.

### Heroin

It is vital to keep in mind that 10 mg of heroin IV could be fatal for a nonuser. Sometimes regular dose also brings intolerance to the user.

### Cocaine

High BP and chest pain are the frequent complication which necessitates medical attention. Every patient with immediate problems should be administered IV and patients having chest pain must be administered with aspirin. Long-term users may get accelerated atheroma.

### Hallucinogens

Lysergic acid diethylamide (LSD) some types of mushrooms, and some plant material can lead to a sought-after hallucinatory experience, in which visual images are distorted and pleasant. If possible, talk to patients in a quiet environment. If it does not work, then IV diazepam may be administered to calm down the patient.

### Ecstasy (MDMA)

This is now popular for use as a 'dance drug'. Some people may develop hyperthermic collapse due to dancing for too long without replacing fluid, and the urgent treatment is IV fluid, which should slow the pulse rate and facilitate normal temperature regulation. This drug increases the level of antidiuretic hormone.

### Rohypnol

Rohypnol (flunitrazepam) is a sedative which causes muscle relaxation, confusion, memory loss, dizziness, and impaired coordination.

## Poisoning from Other Substances

### Lead

In adults, lead poisoning may result from contaminated water supplies or occupational causes (e.g., painting, manufacturing). Manifestations are abdominal pain, constipation, muscle weakness and in most severe cases, encephalopathy with convulsions. Children common cause is from pica, usually present with anemia and failure to thrive.

### Caustic Chemicals

Intake of caustic chemicals leads to severe burns and edema of upper GI tract.

If the patient is having swallowing ability, advice to take three cupfuls water or milk instantly to dilute the acid or alkali. Do not advice for neutralizing chemicals.

### Carbon Monoxide

Exposure to carbon monoxide leads to various manifestations like headache, weakness, tachypnea, dizziness, nausea, and agitation. Impaired consciousness, respiratory failure, MI, and cerebral edema may occur in severe cases.

### Nursing Implications

- Taking away of the patient from the CO source.
- Observe the patency of airway and start high-flow $O_2$ (100%).
- Support and reassurance should be provided.

### Organophosphates and Carbamates

Organophosphorus and carbamate insecticides are used to control insects in domestic, garden, and agricultural settings. They can cause serious poisoning, which may be fatal, through inhalation, skin contact, or ingestion. The commencement of symptoms can appear after 12 hour. Features like confusion, exhaustion, nausea, vomiting, diarrhea, wheezing, sweating, salivation, and fasciculation of the muscles. Pulmonary edema and loss of consciousness may occur also First line of treatment is clearing airway secretion; main treatment is to administer atropine in large doses until the mouth is dry. Diazepam may be administered to alleviate anxiety and manage seizures.

## Food Poisoning

Food poisoning is caused by the ingestion of foods that contain bacteria or toxins. *Salmonella* is a bacterium generally appears in poultry, eggs, unprocessed milk, and in meat and water. It affects stomach and intestine and it may affect blood also.

Various manifestations like diarrhea or constipation, abdominal pain, nausea, fever, headache, and exhaustion occur in patients. Mild infections require rest and plenty fluids. In moderate and severe cases stool samples should be advice for investigation, antibiotics may be started.

## Binge Drinking

The NHS definition of binge drinking is the consumption of large amounts of alcohol in a short space of time, or drinking in order to get drunk or to feel the effects of alcohol. As per the marker of National Statistics and the NHS, drinking alcohol more than double the daily unit guidelines in a single session. By which blood alcohol concentration (BAC) increase very rapidly, leads to severe intoxication.

### Nursing Implications

Thorough understanding of the pathophysiological impact of alcoholism is essential for ED nurses.
- Obtain alcohol history and that should be standard, wherever possible.
- Vital signs and a capillary blood glucose level should be obtained.

## Alcohol Withdrawal

Alcohol withdrawal fits are grand mal seizures that take place hours or days after the last alcoholic drink. It is vital to check the patient's capillary blood glucose levels

## Alcoholic Ketoacidosis

This is a metabolic complication of alcohol use and starvation, characterize by hyperketonemia and metabolic acidosis, with no significant hyperglycemia. It may appear in chronic alcohol misusers, and confused with diabetic ketoacidosis.

## Korsakoff's Psychosis

Some alcoholic patients with Wernicke's encephalopathy may also develop Korsakoff's psychosis. This is a chronic, irreversible condition characterized by severe memory loss. These patients may suffer acute confusion and memory loss. Visual disturbance with eyelid drooping and abnormal eye movements may also be apparent.

## Delirium Tremens

This is a severe manifestation of alcohol withdrawal, which is characterized by hallucinations, delusions, disorientation, and confusion. In this condition patient is vulnerable to arrhythmias, and that may be the cause of infection, acidosis, electrolyte imbalance, or cardiomyopathy. Preliminary management consists of IV diazepam to control fits.

## Alcoholic Cirrhosis

This is the most advanced form of alcohol-induced liver disease and affects organs like brain, and kidneys. Various manifestations like portal hypertension, splenomegaly, ascites, renal failure, confusion, and even liver cancer occurs.

### Nursing Implications with Alcohol-related Problems
- Thorough physical assessment and detail history of alcohol consumption.
- Nurses should teach patient when patient is receptive and highlight hazardous drinking effects and counsel patients.
- Screening tools like paddington alcohol test (PAT) and the CAGE screening tool may be used for alcohol addicted patient.

# ROLE OF NURSES (IN GENERAL)

To prevent repetition, the following nursing recommendation should be assumed to apply as appropriate to all drugs, modifications would be appropriate for management of chronic/stable health conditions.

## For Admission
- Monitor level of consciousness.
- Keep side rails up and call bell within patient's reach.
- Monitor scrum electrolytes, BUN, serum creatinine, liver function tests. Reduce most drug dosages in the presence of renal impairment.
- Assess the elderly carefully. Older patients may have an exaggerated response to what would be a normal dose in younger individuals. Usually, doses are reduced in the elderly.

- Monitor intake, output, and weight.
- Assess parameters of system wise functioning on a regular basis: cardiac rhythm and rate, blood pressure and pulse, heart and lung sounds, peripheral pulses, presence of edema especially in dependent areas, jugular venous distension form more detailed guidance
- For titrating intravenous doses based on patient response, use a micro drip intravenous set-up. Use intra venous regulators to control rate of infusion but remember these do not replace vigilant nursing assessment. Use infusion filters as agency policy requires.
- Label all intravenous infusions carefully and keep accurate records of drug additives to prevent inadvertent medication errors.
- Calculate dosages carefully; double-check calculations with a colleague if in doubt.
- Teach patients and families about the desired effects and common side effects of prescribed drugs; even critically ill patients can understand a simple explanation. Encourage patients to report the development of subjective or objective changes.
- Emphasize the importance of all prescribed therapies: all drugs, electrolyte replacements, weight loss, stopping smoking, salt restriction or other dietary changes, exercise program, relaxation techniques, support groups, and so on.

## For Discharge to Home

- Remind patients to keep all medications out of the reach of children.
- Teach patients to keep all health care providers informed of all medications being used; this includes dentists, oral surgeons, podiatrists, nurse practitioners.
- Teach patients with drug allergies or patients taking corticosteroids, anticoagulants, or other serious drugs to wear a medical identification tag or bracelet noting their allergies or chronic medications.
- Emphasize to patients the importance of taking drugs as advised, not discontinuing drugs without consulting with the physician, not sharing drugs with relatives, and not self-medicating with over-the-counter drugs unless approved by the physician. On the other hand, the physician may be able to change drugs or dosages in response to side effects, if the patient will tell the physician about new signs or symptoms.
- Review with patients what to do if a dose is missed. Patients should not double up for missed doses. A common guideline would be to take the missed dose as soon as remembered, unless within 2 hours of the next dose (for a drug ordered every 4 hours). If within 2 hours of the next dose, omit the missed dose and resume dosing with the next scheduled dose. This guideline would be 3 hours for a drug ordered every 6 hours, 4 hours for a drug ordered every 8 hours, or within 6 hours for a drug ordered every 12 hours. Specific guidelines may always be modified based on the specific health problems, drugs and doses ordered, dosing schedule, age of the patient, and ability of the patient to adhere to dosage guidelines.
- Some drugs should be taken on an empty stomach for best effect, but this often contributes to gastric irritation. Taking drugs with meals or snack will lessen gastric irritation, which may improve compliance. Generally, encourage patients to take their drugs consistently, either with or without meals.

## Summary

ICU nurses need to be alert for accidental life and death situation. Their fast response, and timely accurate decision-making skills place them in high demanding position. Nurses should be cautious for patients having various illnesses as their body might not endure some medications. Nurses should be aware that sometimes medications reacting with other medications are not unusual also. Most of the side effects can be prevented through various evidence-based strategies.

## Points to Ponder

- Pharmacodynamics is the scientific discipline that studies relationship between the concentration of a drug and the response or effect.
- Pharmacokinetics is the scientific discipline that studies the time course of absorption, distribution, metabolism, and excretion of drugs.
- The plasma half-life ($t^{1/2}$) of a drug is the time taken for its plasma concentration to be declined to half of its original value.
- Loading dose is a single or few quickly repeated doses administered in the beginning to attain steady-state levels with a drug that has a longer half-life
- Maintenance dose is one that is to be repeated at specified intervals after attainment of steady-state levels, so as to maintain the same by balancing elimination.
- Morphine is contraindicated in patient with head injury because by retaining carbon dioxide it increases intracranial tension, even therapeutic dose can cause marked depression in the patients
- Positive inotropes increase the force of contraction of the heart, whereas negative inotropes weaken it.
- The beta-blockers competitively block beta-adrenergic receptors in the heart and decreasing the influence of the SNS on these tissues.
- Alcohol withdrawal fits may happen hours or days following the last alcoholic drink.

### Abbreviations

- ICU : Intensive Care Unit
- MAO : Monoamine Oxidase
- CNS : Central Nervous System
- NSAID : Nonsteroidal Anti-inflammatory Drugs
- CSF : Cerebrospinal Fluid
- PABA : Para-amino Benzoic Acid
- LVF : Left Ventricular Failure
- CHF : Congestive Heart Failure
- BRAT : Bananas, Rice, Apple Sauce, Tea/Toast
- PPI : Proton Pump Inhibitor
- LSD : Lysergic Acid Diethylamide
- MDMA : Methylenedioxy-methamphetamine
- CBG : Capillary Blood Glucose
- PAT : Paddington Alcohol Test
- CAGE : Cut, Annoyed, Guilty, and Eye.

### Short Answer Questions

1. Define pharmacodynamics and pharmacokinetics.
2. Write down the principles of pharmacodynamics and pharmacokinetics.
3. Enumerate the types of analgesic drugs and its mechanism.
4. Enlist the classification of non-narcotic analgesics and nonsteroidal anti-inflammatory drugs.
5. Prepare one checklist of nursing action in administering chloramphenicol before initiating this drug.
6. List out the nursing measures for all types of antimicrobial therapy.
7. Justify the rationales for inotrope use.
8. Describe briefly various life-saving drugs.
9. Enlist various drugs used in urinary system.

### Long Answer Questions

1. Discuss nurses responsibilities in drug overdoses and poisoning.
2. Describe briefly regarding nurses responsibilities in drugs used for cardiovascular system disorders.
3. Elaborate the inotropics in detail.
4. Explain regarding the emergency drugs used in critical care unit.
5. Discuss about over all nursing responsibilities in drug administration.
6. Discuss on various challenges of critical care nurses during administration of drugs.

### Bibliography

1. Anderson P, Baumberg B. Alcohol in Europe: a public health perspective. A report to the European Commission. London: Institute of Alcohol Studies. Find this resource; 2006.
2. Armitage G, Knapman H. Adverse events in drug administration: a literature review. J Nurs Manag. 2003;11(2):130-40.
3. ASHP. ASHP guidelines on adverse drug reaction monitoring and reporting. American Society of Hospital Pharmacy. Am J Health Syst Pharm. 1995;52(4):417-9.
4. Backes WL. xPharm: The Comprehensive Pharmacology Reference; 2007.
5. Buckley MS, Erstad BL, Kopp BJ, Theodorou AA, Priestley G. Direct observation approach for detecting medication errors and adverse drug events in a pediatric intensive care unit. Pediatr Crit Care Med. 2007;8(2):145-52.
6. Fast bleep. Medical notes – fluid Management. Available from: http://www.fastbleep.com/medical-notes/other/15/31/205.
7. Henry JA, Wiseman H. Management of poisoning: A handbook for healthcare workers. Geneva: World Health Organization; 1997.
8. Hicks RW, Becker SC, Krenzischeck D, Beyea SC. Medication errors in the PACU: A secondary analysis of MEDMARX findings. J Perianesth Nurs. 2004;19(1):18-28.
9. Huether SE. Fluids and electrolytes, acids and bases. In: Huether SE, McCance KL (Eds). Understanding pathophysiology. 5th edition. St. Louis: Mosby; 2012. p. 105-26.
10. I.V. Therapy made Incredibly Easy! 4th ed. Philadelphia: Wolters Kluwer/Lippincott Williams & Wilkins; 2010.
11. Joanna Briggs Institute. Management of peripheral intravenous devices. Best Pract. 2008;12(5):1-4.
12. Leape LL, Cullen DJ, Clapp MD, Burdick E, Demonaco HJ, Erickson JI, et al. Pharmacist participation on physician rounds and adverse drug events in the intensive care unit. JAMA. 1999;282(3):267-70. doi: 10.1001/jama.282.3.267, PMID 10422996.
13. Leape LL. Preventing adverse drug events. Am J Health Syst Pharm. 1995;52(4):379-82.
14. Macklin D, Chernecky C. Real world nursing survival guide: IV therapy. St. Louis: Saunders; 2004.
15. Murphy MD. Individual characteristics of nurses who committed medication administration errors. Cases which resulted in licensure discipline by the Colorado Board of Nursing;13(1992):11-3.
16. National Coordinating Council for Medication Error Reporting and Prevention. What is a medication error? [accessed Oct 1, 2007]. www. Available from: http://nccmerp.org/aboutMedErrors.html.
17. Office for National Statistics. Alcohol-related deaths in the United Kingdom, registered in 2013. London: Office for National Statistics. Available; 2015.
18. Schneider MP, Cotting J, Pannatier A. Evaluation of nurses' errors associated in the preparation and administration of medication in a pediatric intensive care unit. Pharm World Sci. 1998;20(4):178-82.

19. Wakefield DS, Wakefield BJ, Uden-Holman T, Blegen MA. Perceived barriers in reporting medications administration errors. Best Pract Benchmarking Healthc. 1996;1(4):191-7.
20. Walsh KE, Kaushal R, Chessare JB. How to avoid paediatric medication errors: A user's guide to the literature. Arch Dis Child. 2005;90(7):698-702. (PMC Free article).
21. Walters JA. Nurses' perceptions of reportable medication errors and factors that contribute to their occurrence. Appl Nurs Res. 1992;5(2):86-8.
22. Wirtz V, Taxis K, Barber ND. An observational study of intravenous medication errors in the United Kingdom and in Germany. Pharm World Sci. 2003;25(3):104-11.

# Chapter 4

# Pain Management in Critical Care Unit

*Vasudevan NJ*

## CHAPTER OUTLINE

- Definitions and Types of Pain
- Theories of Pain
- Pain Assessment in Critical Care Unit
- Pharmacological Pain Management in Critical Care Unit
- Nonpharmacological Pain Management in Critical Care Unit
- Placebo Effect
- Key Steps of Nursing Management

### Learning Objectives

At the end of the chapter, the students will be able to:
- Define pain.
- Enlist the types of pain.
- Explain the theories of pain.
- Enumerate the pain assessment in critical care unit.
- Discuss the pharmacological management in critical care unit.
- Describe the nonpharmacological management in critical care unit.
- Explain in detail about placebo effect.
- Enumerate the nursing management.

## INTRODUCTION

Pain is the most common symptom of a disease which occurs in an early age. It acts an protective mechanism to which the body react to the situation. Pain clearly states that it is a subjective sensory and an emotional experience. Pain is related to the stimulus that provides an observation of the psychological facts pain always refers to a not a good sensation. The sense of pain can be felt in the skin, joints and other internal organs. The etiology of the pain may also cause problems in the brain and the nervous system. The process of pain is a complex phenomenon **(E Arnaudo, Journal of Pain Research, 2017)**.

Pain receptors are sensitive to mechanical, thermal, and clinical stimuli. This process is mainly conducted by nerve fiber which starts from spinal cord and brain. The physiological process of pain is subjective perception, and it is also consisting of emotional an aspect which suffers towards pain and pain expression. A complete review on pain physiology is essential to understand the concepts on pain management.

Pain is a complex process that constitutes of a physiological and also a psychological response to an opioid stimulus. Pain is also a warning mechanism which covers an organism by control it to handle from harmful stimuli. **(E Arnaudo, Journal of Pain Research, 2017).**

## DEFINITIONS

**Pain** is "an unpleasant sensory and emotional experience associated with actual or potential tissue damage or described in terms of such damage". —**WHO**

It is an uncomfortable feeling that comes from injury, disease or damage to the body.

Pain is defined as whatever the person experiencing says it is, exiting it is whenever he says it is. Pain is subjective, protective, and it is modified by developmental, behavioral, personality and cultural factors. —**Margo Mccaffery**

### Types of Pain (Cleveland Clinic, 2020)

Pain can be classified into different types based on various criteria, including its origin, duration, and underlying causes. Here are some common types of pain:
- **Nociceptive pain:** Pain results which generally starts from the activation of nociceptors, which are specialized nerve endings that detect potentially harmful stimuli

such as heat, cold, pressure, and chemicals. Nociceptive pain can be further divided into two subtypes:
1. *Somatic pain:* Starts from the skin, muscles, bones, and joints. They has been described as a sharp, localized pain.
2. *Visceral pain:* Originates from internal organs and is often described as a deep, dull ache. It can be challenging to pinpoint the exact source of visceral pain.

- **Neuropathic pain:** Neuropathic pain is caused by damage or dysfunction of the nervous system, including nerves themselves. It is often described as shooting, burning, or tingling sensations.
- **Inflammatory pain:** Inflammation in tissues or joints can lead to this type of pain. Conditions like arthritis, inflammatory bowel disease, and other autoimmune disorders can cause inflammatory pain.
- **Acute pain:** Acute pain is typically short-lived and occurs suddenly in response to an injury or trauma. It serves as a warning signal to protect the body from further harm. Once the underlying cause is treated, acute pain usually subsides.
- **Chronic pain:** Chronic pain persists over an extended period, often lasting beyond the expected healing time of an injury. It can have a significant impact on a person's quality of life and may be caused by conditions such as fibromyalgia, chronic migraines, or persistent back pain.
- **Referred pain:** Referred pain starts when pain arouse in an area of the body that is not the actual source of the problem. It mainly caused because the nerve pathways from different areas of the body can overlap and share the same nerve pathways to the brain.
- **Psychogenic pain:** It can be also called as psychosomatic pain, this type of pain is primarily influenced by psychological factors such as stress, anxiety, and emotional distress. The pain experienced is real, but its origin is not solely due to physical damage or dysfunction.
- **Cancer pain:** It results from the tumor itself pressing on nerves, bones, or organs, or as a side effect of cancer treatments. The nature of cancer pain can vary widely based on the type and stage of cancer.
- **Phantom pain:** Phantom pain occurs in a body part that has been amputated or is no longer present. Despite the absence of the actual body part, individuals may still experience sensations of pain or discomfort.
- **Central sensitization:** This type of pain is characterized by an increased sensitivity of the nervous system to pain signals. It often accompanies conditions like fibromyalgia and involves an amplified response to stimuli that would not typically be perceived as painful.

# THEORIES OF PAIN

There are several theories that made an effort to describe how pain is perceived and processed by the body. While our understanding of pain is continually evolving, here are various prominent theories of pain which has been mainly explains about the theories of pain.

### Gate Control Theory (Moyaedi M et al, 2013)

Ronald Melzack and Patrick Wall originally put forth this hypothesis of pain in 1965. According to the hypothesis, there are other influences on pain perception in addition to tissue damage severity, including emotions, beliefs, and the surrounding environment. The spinal cord is thought to include a "gate" that regulates how pain impulses are sent from the body to the brain, according to the gate control hypothesis. Several sources of input, such as sensory data from nonpainful stimuli and impulses from the brain and spinal cord, can open or close this gate. According to the hypothesis, when the gate is open, pain signals are sent from the body to the brain, which causes a person to feel pain.

Facts proving that certain nonpainful stimuli, such massage or acupuncture, can lessen the feeling of pain have been used to support the gate control hypothesis. Transcutaneous electrical nerve stimulation (TENS), a treatment that uses electrical impulses to activate nerve fibers and close the pain gate, is one example of a treatment that has been made possible by the hypothesis.

Gate control theory contends that the sensation of pain is dynamic and complicated, impacted by a variety of circumstances, and that different types of input can affect how painful something feels.

### Specificity Theory (Apkarian et al, 2011)

The theory was framed by Charles Sherrington in the late 19th century. The theory suggests that there are specific nerve fibers in the body that are dedicated to detecting and transmitting pain signals to the brain. These fibers are known as nociceptors and are activated by harmful stimuli such as tissue damage, extreme temperatures, or chemicals.

According to the specificity idea, a person's level of pain is directly correlated with how much tissue damage has been done. Thus, an individual will feel more pain the more damage there is. In consonance to the hypothesis, there are several nociceptors that react to various kinds of pain, such as intense or dull pain. Despite the specificity theory's significance in the development of our understanding of pain, it has been criticized for oversimplifying the complexity of pain perception. It ignores the notion that psychological elements like feelings, expectations, and prior experiences have an impact on pain. For instance, anxiety or dread may cause someone to feel a lot of pain even if there is only modest tissue injury. However, it is now understood that pain perception is a complex process involving a number of components, including sensory input, cognitive processes, and emotional considerations. Overall, specificity theory still serves as a crucial foundation for our knowledge of pain.

## Pattern Theory (Trachsel et al, 2021)

Pattern theory is a theory of pain that was propounded by Ronald Melzack in the 1980s. The theory urges pain is not simply the result of the activation of pointwise pain receptors, but rather is the result of the brain's interpretation of patterns of nerve impulses.

The pattern theory contends that rather than individual pain signals from the body, the brain instead gets a complicated pattern of nerve impulses that it interprets as pain. Many elements, such as prior encounters, feelings, and cultural background, have an impact on this interpretation. For instance, even if there is not any actual tissue damage, the brain may interpret fresh nerve impulses from a particular place of the body as pain if the person has previously experienced pain there. Similar to this, cultural and societal influences may have an impact on how pain is perceived. For exemplar, people might be less likely to report pain or seek treatment if they believe it to be a signature of weakness in particular cultures.

Pattern theory has been supported by research explaining brain processes in pain is a highly complex manner, involving multiple areas of the brain and neural networks. It put forth that pain is a subjective experience that is influenced by many different factors, and influencing the subjective experience of pain which is essential for effective pain management. On balance, the pattern theory of pain suggests that the brain plays a key role in the perception of pain, and that pain is a highly complex and subjective experience that is influenced by a wide range of factors.

## Neuromatrix Theory (Trout et al, 2004)

Ronald Melzack advanced his earlier work on the gate control theory and the pattern theory of pain by putting out the neuromatrix theory of pain in 1999. The hypothesis contends that an intricate web of neuronal connections found throughout the brain and spinal cord is what causes the sensation of pain.

In the manner to the neuromatrix hypothesis, the brain's "pain center" is actually a diffuse network of neurons that work together to create the sensation of pain. The sensory, emotional, and cognitive components of this network, referred to as the "neuromatrix," are influenced by a range of variables, including prior experiences, emotions, beliefs, and cultural background. In keeping with the neuromatrix theory, pain is a subjective experience that results from the interaction of several neuronal circuits rather than being exclusively the result of tissue damage. It also proposes that the brain has the ability to generate pain in the absence of tissue damage, as in the case of phantom limb pain. Theory has important implications for the treatment of pain, as it suggests that pain management should be approached from a multidisciplinary perspective that addresses not only the physical symptoms of pain but also the emotional and cognitive components. Treatment approaches may include medications, physical therapy, psychotherapy, and other interventions aimed at modulating the neural pathways involved in the perception of pain.

Comprehensively, the neuromatrix theory of pain emphasizes the complexity of the pain experience and underscores the importance of a multidisciplinary approach to pain management.

## Evolutionary Theory (MacDonald et al, 2005)

According to the evolutionary view of pain, pain is a significant adaptive mechanism that has developed to keep us safe from damage and to aid in our survival. In accordance with this view, discomfort is a reaction to noxious or possibly hazardous stimuli and acts as a cue for the person to take appropriate action to prevent additional injury or at least lessen it.

Pain has been an important survival mechanism throughout human evolution. It has allowed us to quickly respond to danger by withdrawing from a source of pain or injury, and to adapt our behavior to avoid future harm. For example, if we touch a hot stove, the pain we experience prompts us to quickly withdraw our hand, minimizing further damage. Stint pain can be unpleasant, it serves an important function in promoting our survival. The evolutionary theory of pain suggests that the ability to experience pain has been a critical factor in the survival and evolution of species. Animals that are unable to experience pain are at a significant disadvantage in their ability to avoid harm and to survive. It is also suggesting that pain perception is not solely determined by the severity of tissue damage, but is also influenced by a variety of factors, including the individual's emotional state, cognitive processes, and social context. For example, an individual who is experiencing intense emotions such as fear or anxiety may perceive pain more acutely than someone who is in a calm state.

In general context, the evolutionary theory of pain accentuation how adaptive pain is and how it helps people survive. It also emphasizes how crucial it is to comprehend the intricate variables that affect how people perceive pain in order to create efficient pain management plans.

# PAIN ASSESSMENT IN CRITICAL CARE UNIT (JACKSON M, 2012)

To effectively manage pain, pain evaluation is essential. Due to their extensive interactions with patients and their families while they are in the hospital, nurses are in a unique position to evaluate pain. The most typical symptom that affects kids in hospitals is pain. Acute pain (nociception) does not involve neural tissue and is self-limiting, short-lived, and connected with tissue damage and an inflammatory reaction. Due to the complex nature of pain, an assessment must take into account the phenomenon's biological, psychological, and sociological aspects as well as its impact on activity. Social history/issues, cultural and religious beliefs, prior painful experiences, and the first painful experience are some of the elements that may change how pain is seen and how one copes with it.

## ABCDE for Pain Management (Trachsel et al, 2023)

The acronym "ABCDE" refers to the five crucial processes of providing emergency medical care to seriously ill or injured patients. The characteristics of the initialism has been focused and explained as below:
- **A**sk about pain periodically, assess pain systematically.
- **B**elieve the patient and family in their reports of pain and what makes comfort.
- **C**hoose the pain and control the options appropriate for the patient, family setting.
- **D**eliver measures in correct event, sensible and coordinated on trends.
- **E**mpowering the patients and their families.

Pain assessment in critical care units is crucial to ensuring that patients receive appropriate pain management and optimal care. Patients in critical care often experience a range of painful conditions due to surgeries, injuries, medical procedures, and underlying illnesses. Here are some key aspects of pain assessment in critical care units:
- **Regular assessment:** Pain assessment should be carried out regularly, ideally on a scheduled basis and whenever there is a change in the patient's condition. Assessments can be scheduled along with other routine checks such as vital signs monitoring.
- **Valid and reliable tools:** Making use of validated pain assessment tools is suitable for critically ill patients. These tools help quantify pain and provide a consistent way to measure pain intensity and assess its impact. The most common used tools are described with the pictorial part as below:
  – Visual analog scale
  – Numeric rating scale
  – Nonverbal rating scale

### Visual Analog Scale

The Wong-Baker FACES pain rating scale is a tool designed to be of service to people in expressing how severe their pain is. It consists of a sequence of faces, with various facial expressions signifying various degrees of pain, ranging from a joyful smile (zero) to a crying face (ten).

To help patients communicate their level of pain to healthcare professionals, the scale is frequently used with kids or people with limited speech skills. It is a straightforward and useful technique that is frequently used in clinical settings.

Since its creation in 1983 by Donna Wong and Connie Baker, the Wong-Baker FACES pain rating scale (**Fig. 4.1**) has been applied in a number of healthcare settings.

### Numerical Rating Scales

A measurement instrument for determining the degree or intensity of a specific trait or characteristic is a numerical rating scale. For example, a common numerical rating scale used in research and surveys is a Likert Scale, which asks respondents to rate their agreement or disagreement with a statement on a scale ranging from 1 to 5, where 1 is strongly disagree and 5 is strongly agree. Other numerical rating scales can be used to rate other attributes such as pain intensity, anxiety levels, or quality of life, among others (**Dawes J, 2016**).

Numerical rating scales (**Fig. 4.2**) are facile to administer, also providing a quantitative measure of the degree or intensity of the attribute being unfiltered. They are habitually used in healthcare, psychology, education, marketing, over and above that other fields correct measurement of subjective experiences or suggestion is important.

### Nonverbal Pain Scale

The adult nonverbal pain scale (NVPS) is a tool used to assess pain in individuals who are unable to communicate their pain verbally, such as those with dementia, cognitive impairment, or who are intubated and sedated.

The NVPS consists of five categories of pain behaviors; each assigned a score from 0 to 2. The categories are:
1. **Facial expression:** The presence of a frown, grimace, or other expression of pain on the face.
2. **Activity level:** The level of movement or agitation like restlessness or guarding of a body part.
3. **Body language:** The intensity of tension or rigidity on the body, comparable as clenching of fists or a rigid posture.
4. **Vocalization:** The existence of groans, moans, or other sounds indicating pain.
5. **Consolability:** The ease in the company in which the individual can be comforted.

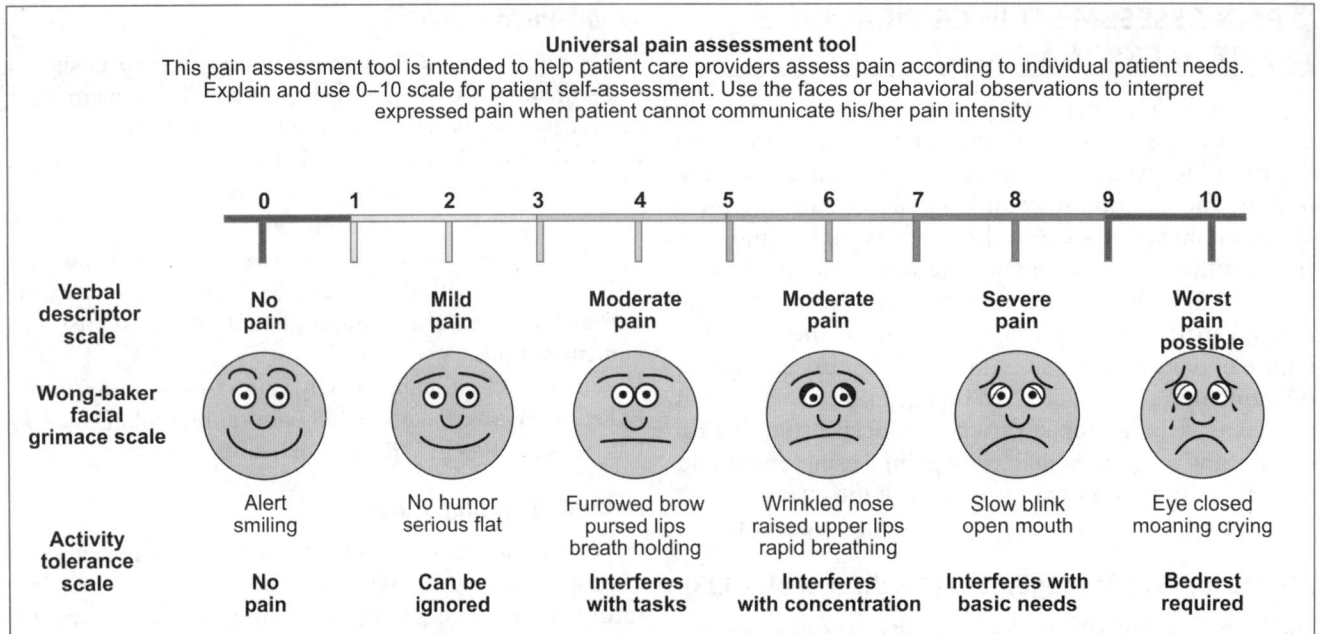

**Fig. 4.1:** Adorn about the universal pain assessment tool (WHO).

| Numerical rating scale | | | | | | | | | |
|---|---|---|---|---|---|---|---|---|---|
| 1 | 2 | 3 | 4 | 5 | 6 | 7 | 8 | 9 | 10 |
| No pain | | Mild pain | | Moderate pain | | Severe pain | | Very severe pain | Worst pain |

**Fig. 4.2:** Illustrates about the numerical rating scale.

The total score ranges from 0 to 10, with higher scores indicating more severe pain. The NVPS can be used in a variety of settings, including hospitals, long-term care facilities, and it is important to note, however, that the NVPS is not a substitute for careful observation and assessment by trained healthcare professionals.

- **Self-reporting:** At any time encourage the patients who are able to verbalize the self-report regarding their pain levels. This direct input from the patient is valuable for tailoring about the pain management strategies.
- **Observational assessment:** For patients who are unable to self-report due to sedation, intubation, or altered consciousness, healthcare providers must rely on observational cues. These cues include facial expressions, body movements, muscle tension, and changes in vital signs.
- **Sedation assessment:** In critical care, patients might be sedated to manage pain and agitation. However, it is important to assess both pain and sedation levels to strike a balance between pain relief and the need for sedation.
- **Communication barriers:** Recognize the various factors, such as language barriers, cultural differences, and cognitive impairments which can hinder effective pain communication.
- **Multi-dimensional assessment:** Pain assessment should consider not only the intensity of pain but also its location, quality (such as sharp, dull, throbbing), and duration. Assess how pain affects the patient's physical and psychological well-being.
- **Documenting findings:** Documentation plays a crucial role in assessing the pain and to mention that accurate and consistent documentation of pain assessment findings is essential. Using the standardized forms or electronic medical records to record pain scores, assessment methods used, patient responses, and any interventions administered which will be a evidence for an patient centered care.
- **Patient context:** Focus on the patient's medical history, current diagnoses, surgical procedures, and the potential sources of pain. These contexts will generally helps determine the main etiology of pain and guides appropriate interventions.

- **Collaborative approach:** Pain assessment is a collaborative effort involving nurses, physicians, and other members of the healthcare team. Regular communication and information sharing are essential for effective pain management.

Pain assessment and management are happening processes that require attention, compassion, and expertise. Individual patient circumstances and critical care unit practices may influence how pain assessment is conducted; hence it's important to adapt approaches as needed while adhering to established guidelines and best practices.

## PHARMACOLOGICAL PAIN MANAGEMENT IN CCU

Pharmacological management in critical care units (CCUs) involves the use of medications to treat various medical conditions and support critically ill patients. The medications used in CCUs aim to stabilize patients, manage symptoms, and improve outcomes.

According to who, there are various pharmacological techniques to relieve pain which has been presented in the below diagram as follows:

### Nonopioid Analgesics

The nonopioid analgesics are increasingly emphasized in a variety of clinics and hospitals as this will be considered as the first line therapy for mild to moderate pain. This analgesics are mainly to be used in the mild pain and the intensity will be based on the drugs given.

### Weak Opioids

Weak opioids, also known as mild opioids or partial agonist opioids, are medications that have a lower affinity for opioid receptors and produce less potent effects compared to strong opioids.
- **Codeine:** This is commonly used for mild to moderate pain relief and is often combined with other medications like acetaminophen (Tylenol) or ibuprofen.
- **Tramadol:** A unique opioid medication that has both opioid and nonopioid mechanisms of action. It's often used for moderate pain and is thought to have a lower potential for abuse compared to strong opioids.
- **Tapentadol:** Another opioid medication which has both opioid and nonopioid mechanisms of action. It's used for moderate to severe pain and is also believed to have a lower risk of abuse.

### Strong Opioids

Narcotics will control the pain and provide a sense of euphoria largely binding to opiate receptors and activating endogenous pain suppression (**Fig. 4.3**) in the central nervous system. There are five primary types of opioids.
1. **Full agonists:** The classification of drugs is generally pure opioid drugs bind together which are tightly to 'M' receptor site producing maximum pain inhalation, an agonist effect, e.g., morphine and codeine.
2. **Mixed agonists:** Antagonists—it can behave as like opioids and relieve the pain. They close the 'M' receptor and activate the receptor site.
3. **Copartial agonists:** It has a covered surface effect in contrast to a full agonist. These are the drugs which are mainly enact in the central block the 'M' receptors which are neutral at that receptor but stuck at a Kappa receptor site common opioids side effects which mainly include constipation, nausea, vomiting, sedation, respiratory depression, pruritis and urinary retention.
4. **Nonopioids/NSAIDS:** Nonopioids include nonsteroidal anti-inflammatory drugs such as aspirin also ibuprofen. They reduce pain by playing a major role on peripheral nerve endings at the injury site and reduce the level of inflammatory mediators generated on the site of injury. They may also increase prostaglandin release at the injury site.

   The most common side effects of nonopioid analgesic is indigestion, stomach ulcers, gastric bleeding.
5. **Adjuvant analgesics:** These are medicines which are developed for uses other than reducing pain but have been started a new basis on pain which is to reduce certain types of chronic pain in addition to their primary action, e.g., diazepam.

## NONPHARMACOLOGICAL PAIN MANAGEMENT (JOHNSON M, 2007)

Nonpharmacological pain management refers to approaches and techniques for managing the various conditions and symptoms without the use of medications. These approaches can be used as standalone treatments or in combination with pharmacological interventions to enhance overall care.

### Cutaneous Stimulation

It changes the client and focuses attention on the tactile reflex, away from painful sensations, thus reducing pain perception. It is believed to:
- Form the release of endorphins that block stimuli transmission.
- Stimulate beta sensory nerve fibers, which creates the transmission of pain impulses through A delta and C fibers.

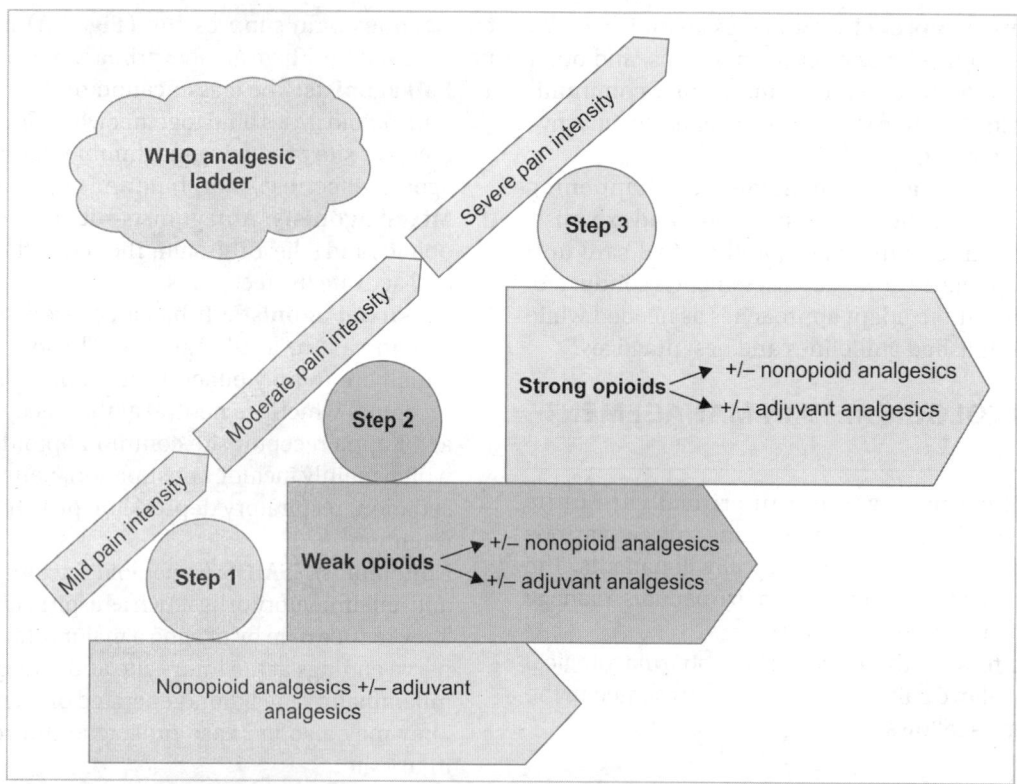

**Fig. 4.3:** Exemplify about the pharmacological pain management.
*Source:* WHO.

There are various cutaneous stimulation technique which mainly include:
- **Massage:** It clearly notes that the relief in affliction on measure that can aid relaxation and change downward in muscle tension, and may promote anxiety as the physical contact communicates caring. It can also extent in small number on pain severity by increasing superficial circulation to the area.
- **Heat and cold applications:** A hot or a warm bath, heating pads, ice bags, ice massage, or cold compress and warm or cold sitz baths in general which is to reduce pain and promote healing of harmed tissues.
- **Acupuncture:** It is a form of an alternative medicine in which small or thin needles are inserted into the body.
- **Contralateral stimulation:** It is a procedure in which it can be accomplished by stimulating the skin in an area opposite to the painful area. It is particularly useful when the painful area cannot be touched because it is hypersensitive, inaccessible by a bandage.
- **Immobilization:** The procedure is mainly to control the episodes of acute pain. Splints or supportive devices also be used in hold joints in the optimal function and can be omitted regularly in accordance with the protocol to provide range of motion exercises.

## Transcutaneous Electrical Nerve Stimulation (TENS)

It is a way of applying electric current to reduce the pain and it mainly involves the benefit of use of low voltage electric power. It is a procedure where it deals with the electrodes which can be placed over the painful area. This is mainly used to treat an effective pain by direct blocking transmission of pain.

There are various nonpharmacological measures used in managing the pain and various therapies is supporting to minimizing the pain and control. **Table 4.1**, explains about the various nonpharmacological therapies and it has been explained.

## PLACEBO EFFECT (MARGO CE, 1999)

Traditional views of placebos as deceptive treatments have prevented them from being comprehended in the context of social symbols and interpersonal aspects that surround the healing process itself. Although the ability of inert drugs to

**Table 4.1:** Explains about the various nonpharmacological measures.

| Therapy | How does it work |
|---|---|
| Music | Reduces pain intensity, fatigue, anxiety as adjunct to pharmacological pain-relieving methods |
| TENS | It consists of a battery-powered device that delivers electrical impulses (low voltage current) through electrodes placed on skin |
| Biofeedback | It is formulated by a special devices to learn how to relax specific muscles in the body to reduce tension |
| Reiki | It generates the energy focus through healing touch |
| Osteopathic manipulation | Helps the body's naturally to heal |
| Heat | Heat can reduce the pain which is mainly caused by sore muscles and muscle spasms |
| ICE | Ice cubes will generally reduce the pain that comes from joint problems or irritated nerves |

heal is widely acknowledged, the placebo effect also has an impact on the effectiveness of traditional treatments. Due to the lack of a shared understanding of the placebo effect and the negative connotations attached to its use, the role of the placebo in contemporary medicine is little understood.

Placebo-controlled experiments are used in research to reduce the placebo effect's therapeutic noise. Few studies are intended to examine the placebo response rate directly. Placebos serve as a reminder of how little is understood about how the mind and body interact. One of the most adaptable and underutilized treatment options at doctors' disposal may be the placebo effect.

## Quick Information About Placebo

- Thousands of medical studies have studied the placebo effect, and many physicians freely acknowledge frequently administering fake medications.
- Before new medications are approved, pharmaceutical companies must demonstrate that they are more effective than a placebo.
- A tablet's color can affect how strong the placebo effect is, and larger tablets have a stronger effect than smaller ones.
- Some people think evolutionary biology can explain how the placebo effect has the ability to cure itself.
- Placebos have been found to have an impact on a number of medical disorders.

## Advantages of Placebo

The premier benefit of employing a placebo spell testing a novel medication is that it reduces or even completely removes the influence that expectations may have on the results.

Researchers may unintentionally provide participants with cues on how they should act if they are hoping for a specific outcome. The study's findings may be impacted by this.

## Nursing Management

### Nursing Diagnoses

- **Acute pain related to tissue damage as evidenced by verbal reports of pain, guarding, grimacing, and increased heart rate (Herr K, Titler MG et al, 2004).**
  Nursing goal for the diagnoses is to provide effective pain management for the patient, to alleviate the discomfort and promote the patient's well-being. The following nursing interventions can be implemented:
  - Assess the patient's pain level and location, using a pain scale and noting the characteristics of the pain (e.g., dull, sharp, throbbing, etc.).
  - Administer pain medication as ordered by the healthcare provider, such as nonopioid analgesics (e.g., acetaminophen, ibuprofen) or opioid analgesics (e.g., morphine, oxycodone) if the pain is not tolerable.
  - Exploit the nonpharmacological pain management techniques, such as positioning the patient in a comfortable position, providing warm or cold compresses, or offering distraction techniques like music or relaxation exercises.
  - Praepostor the patient's vital signs and assess the effectiveness of pain management interventions.
  - Educate the patient about pain management strategies and encourage them to report.
- **Chronic pain related to a medical condition as evidenced by reports of pain lasting longer than 3 months, decreased activity level, and changes in sleep patterns (Becker WC, Dorflinger L, 2017).**
  - *Assessment:* Initiate for patient's pain intensity, location, and any triggers or relieving factors. A thorough assessment is crucial to develop a personalized treatment plan.
  - *Medication management:* Administer analgesics as prescribed by the healthcare provider, monitor for side effects, and adjust doses accordingly. Educate

the patient on the proper use of medications, including potential adverse effects.
- *Nonpharmacological interventions:* Encourage the use of nonpharmacological interventions, such as heat or cold therapy, massage, relaxation techniques, and physical therapy. These interventions can provide relief and improve the patient's quality of life.
- *Patient education:* Educate the patient about the importance of self-management of chronic pain, including adhering to medication regimens, incorporating physical activity into daily routines, and developing coping strategies.
- *Monitor for adverse effects:* Monitor the patient for adverse effects related to medication use, such as dizziness, nausea, constipation, or sedation. Collaborate with the healthcare team to adjust the medication regimen as necessary.
- *Emotional support:* Provide emotional support and counseling to the patient to manage the psychological and emotional impact of chronic pain.
- *Referral:* Collaborate with other healthcare providers to provide multidisciplinary care.

- **Impaired physical mobility related to pain as evidenced by decreased range of motion, difficulty ambulating, and reluctance to move (Carpenito-Moyet LJ, 2006).**
  - Being a nurse there are some nursing responsibilities to manage the impaired physical mobility.
  - To make up one's mind about maintain a thorough assessment on physical mobility status such as extent of the pain.
  - When focusing on the management of pain emboldens the patient in new areas of discomfort.
  - Maintain a therapeutic exercise which helps the patient in range of motion to improve the joint flexibility and credibility.
  - Ensure the patient in a comfortable position such as cushion and pillows.
  - Collaborate with the health team that addresses the patient physical mobility.

- **Anxiety related to pain as evidenced by restlessness, increased heart rate, and verbal reports of anxiety or fear (Doenges ME, Moorhouse MF, 2019).**
  - Conduct a thorough assessment on the patient anxiety level including the intensity, duration and severity of the pain.
  - Educate the patient between the difference of pain and anxiety and teach about the alternative techniques such as guided imagery or relaxation techniques.
  - Provide emotional support to the patient and include active listening validation of their feelings.
  - Reassure the patient that pain is being managed effectively to make sure about the comfort and well being of the client.

### Key Steps of Nursing Management for Pain (Wells et al, 2008)

Pain embraces a extensive approach to identifying, assessing, and treating pain. Presently few available on some key steps nurses can take to manage pain in their patients:

- **Assessment:** Nurses should provide a complete assessment of the patient's pain, taking into account its nature, location, intensity, and duration. Besides, nurses should evaluate how the patient's discomfort affects their everyday activities and emotional health.
- **Communication:** Nurses should encourage open ended phrases with patients about their pain. This includes asking patients to describe their pain in their own words and actively listening to their concerns and preferences.
- **Education:** Nurses should taught patients about pain management strategies, in addition to nonpharmacological techniques such as relaxation exercises, distraction, and guided imagery.
- **Medication:** The healthcare team should collaborate with nurses to choose the best painkiller. Also, they should keep a close watch on the patient for any negative drug side effects and change the dosage as necessary.
- **Evaluation:** Nurses should routinely evaluate the effectiveness of pain management interventions and adjust the plan of care as needed.
- **Collaboration:** Nurses should collaborate with other members of the healthcare team, including physicians, physical therapists, and social workers, to provide comprehensive pain management care.

Overall, nursing management for pain requires a holistic approach that addresses the physical, emotional, and psychological aspects of pain. By providing effective pain management, nurses can help improve the quality of life for their patients.

## Summary

Pain management is a multifaceted approach that encompasses a range of strategies aimed at alleviating or reducing pain, enhancing quality of life, and promoting overall well-being. It involves a combination of pharmacological and nonpharmacological interventions, modified as per individual's condition, pain severity, and specific needs. The goal of pain management is not only to alleviate physical discomfort but also to address emotional, psychological, and social aspects of pain. By implementing a combination of pharmaceutical and nonpharmaceutical interventions, healthcare providers and patients collaborate to achieve the optimal balance between pain relief, functional improvement, and well-being.

### Points to Ponder

- Pain is the most common symptom of a disease which occurs in an early age. It acts as an protective mechanism to which the body react to situation.
- Pain receptors are sensitive to mechanical, thermal and clinical stimuli. This process is mainly conducted by nerve fiber which starts from spinal cord and brain.
- Pain is a complex process that constitutes of a physiological and also a psychological response to a opioid's stimulus.
- **Noncancerous pain** is usually not life threatening but an injured part may have healed long ago.
- Specificity theory is a direct relationship exists between the stimulus and perception of pain.
- Pain is the fifth vital sign.
- Narcotics will control the pain and provide a sense of euphoria.
- Cutaneous simulation form the release of endorphins that block stimuli transmission.
- Massage can clearly notes that the relief in affliction on measure that can aid relaxation and change downward in muscle tension.
- TENS is a way of applying electric current to reduce the pain.

### Abbreviations

- SG : Substantia Gelatinosa
- T Cells : Trigger Cells
- TENS : Transcutaneous Electrical Nerve Stimulation

### Short Answer Questions

1. Define pain and its types.
2. Explain the theories of pain.
3. What are the assessments of pain and explain in detail.
4. Explain the key components of pain assessment.
5. Enumerate the flowchart used in assessment in critical care unit.
6. Write about the WHO analgesic ladder for pain management.
7. Enumerate the common drugs for pain management.
8. What are the ways to reduce pain in nonpharmacological way and brief about it?

### Long Answer Questions

1. Explain theories of pain along with examples.
2. Enumerate the pain assessment in the critical care unit by using various standardized scales.
3. Describe the pharmacological management in CCU in detail.
4. Discuss the nonpharmacological management in CCU.
5. Give a brief explanation on holistic nursing management of pain.

### Bibliography

1. Ahmed El Geziry. et al. Non pharmacological pain management. 2018.
2. Alorfi NM. Pharmacological methods of pain management: narrative review of medication used. Int J Gen Med. 2023;16:3247-56.
3. Apkarian VA, Hashmi JA, Baliki MN. Pain and the brain: Specificity and plasticity of the brain in clinical chronic pain. Pain. 2011;152(3);Suppl:S49-64.
4. Available from: https://my.clevelandclinic.org/health/articles/12051-acute-vs-chronic-pain.
5. Available from: https://www.healthline.com/health/types-of-pain.
6. Becker WC, Dorflinger L, Edmond SN, Islam L, Heapy AA, Fraenkel L. Barriers and facilitators to use of non-pharmacological treatments in chronic pain. BMC Fam Pract. 2017;18(1):41.
7. Carpenito-Moyet LJ, editor. Nursing diagnosis: application to clinical practice. Lippincott Williams & Wilkins; 2006.
8. Cunningham S. Pain assessment and management. In Clinical skills for nursing practice, Routledge; 2016. pp.132-59.
9. Curley MA, Wypij D, Watson RS, Grant MJ, Asaro LA, Cheifetz IM, et al. Protocolized Sedation vs. usual Care in Pediatric Patients Mechanically Ventilated for Acute Respiratory Failure: A Randomized Clinical Trial. JAMA. 2015;313(4):379-89.
10. Dawes J. Do data characteristics change according to the number of scale points used? An experiment using 5-point, 7-point and 10-point scales. Int J Mark Res. 2008;50(1):61-104.
11. Dhaliwal A, Gupta M. Physiology, opioid receptor.
12. Doenges ME, Moorhouse MF, Murr AC. Nursing care plans: guidelines for individualizing client care across the life span. FA Davis; 2019.
13. Gauchan S. Pain assessment in emergency department of teaching hospital in Lalitpur. J Karnali Acad. 2019;2(3):209-13.
14. Herr K, Titler MG, Schilling ML, Marsh JL, Xie X, Ardery G, et al. Evidence-based assessment of acute pain in older adults: Current nursing practices and perceived barriers. Clin J Pain. 2004;20(5):331-40.
15. Hughes CG, McGrane S, Pandharipande PP. Sedation in the intensive care setting. Clin Pharmacol. 2012;4:53-63.
16. Johnson M. Transcutaneous electrical nerve stimulation: mechanisms, clinical application and evidence. Rev Pain. 2007;1(1):7-11.

17. Margo CE. The placebo effect. Surv Ophthalmol. 1999;44(1):31-44.
18. Moayedi M, Davis KD. Theories of pain: From specificity to gate control. J Neurophysiol. 2013;109(1):5-12.
19. Moayedi M. Moayedi M, Davis KD. Theories of pain: from specificity to gate control. J Neuro physiol. 2013;109(1):5-12.
20. Osterweis M, Kleinman A, Mechanic D. The anatomy and physiology of pain. In: Pain and disability: Clinical, behavioral, and public policy perspectives. National Academies Press; 1987.
21. Pain JM. The fifth vital sign. A&C Black; 2012.
22. Raffaeli W, Arnaudo E. Pain as a disease: An overview. J Pain Res;2017(10):2003-8.
23. Trachsel LA, Cascella M. Pain theory. InStatPearls. StatPearls Publishing; 2021.
24. Trachsel LA, Munakomi S, Cascella M. Pain theory. StatPearls. Updated 2022 Apr 20[Internet]; 2023.
25. Trout KK. The neuromatrix theory of pain: Implications for selected nonpharmacologic methods of pain relief for labor. J Midwifery Womens Health. 2004;49(6):482-8.
26. Waxenbaum JA, Reddy V, Varacallo M. Anatomy, autonomic nervous system; 2022.

# Chapter 5

# Infection Control in Critical Care Unit

*Vasudevan NJ*

## CHAPTER OUTLINE

- Risk Factors of Infection
- Common Infections
- Antibiotic Resistant Infections
- Postoperative Wound Infection
- Prevention and Infection Control Measures
- Nosocomial Infection in CCU
- Methicillin-resistant Staphylococcus Aureus (MRSA)
- Standard Safety Measures, Prophylaxis in CCU
- Sterilization and Disinfection in CCU

## Learning Objectives

At the end of the chapter, the students will be able to:
- Define infection.
- Enlist the risk factors of infections.
- Explain the antibiotic resistant infections.
- Enumerate the treatment of fungal infections.
- Discuss about the postoperative wound infection.
- Acquire the understanding on prevention and infection control measures.
- Explain about nosocomial infection.
- Enumerate about MRSA.
- Explain the standard safety measures in CCU.
- List out the prophylaxis method in CCU.
- Discuss about the sterilization and disinfection in CCU.

## INTRODUCTION

Pathological changes which is regularly happened in the hospitals, specifically in the "critical care unit" (CCU) settings, widely between 35% and 45%, can residue to complications in >60% in critically serious ill patients. Concern regarding the healthcare associated infection is affecting hundred of clients for every year with the most prevalence in low developing countries. The extent of patients with infections acquired in intensive care unit in low and middle income countries which is majory ranges from 4.3% to 88.7%. (**Zhao, oral hygiene care for critically ill patients to prevent ventilator-associated pneumonia**).

The immune system is a complex network of cells, tissues, and organs that work together to protect the body from harmful invaders such as bacteria, viruses, fungi, and parasites. The immune system can be divided into two main types of immunity: innate immunity and adaptive immunity.

### Acquired Immunity (Rao VU, 2020)

Acquired immunity **(Flowchart 5.1)** is also called as adaptive immunity in which it is a specific response that develops over time as the body is exposed to specific pathogens. This response involves the production of antibodies and the activation of immune cells such as T cells and B cells. Adaptive immunity has a memory, allowing it to recognize and respond more quickly and effectively to pathogens that have been encountered before.

**Flowchart 5.1:** Immune system and its types.

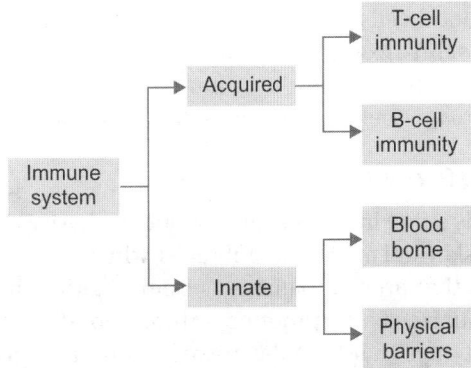

### T-cell Immunity

T-cells, or T lymphocytes, are a type of white blood cell that plays a critical role in the immune system's response to pathogens, infections, and other abnormal cells. It plays a key role in component of adaptive immunity, which allows the immune system to recognize and respond to specific antigens (foreign substances) with precision. T-cell responses are highly specific and are regulated by interactions with other immune cells, including antigen-presenting cells (such as dendritic cells) that capture and present antigens to T-cells. This complex interplay is essential for the immune system's ability to mount targeted and effective responses against infections and diseases.

### B-cell Immunity

B-cells, or B lymphocytes, are a type of white blood cell that plays a central role in the adaptive immune response. They are responsible for producing antibodies, which are proteins that recognize and neutralize specific antigens (foreign substances) such as pathogens, toxins, and other harmful molecules.

## Innate Immunity

Innate immunity (**Flowchart 5.1**) is the first line of defense against invading pathogens. It includes physical and chemical barriers such as skin, mucous membranes, stomach acid, and enzymes in tears and saliva, which help prevent the entry of harmful microorganisms. If a pathogen does manage to enter the body, innate immune cells such as neutrophils, macrophages, and natural killer cells can recognize and destroy it without the need for prior exposure or recognition.

### Blood Borne (Study BS, 2007)

Blood borne are generally plays a vital role in the innate immunity and it mainly focus on phagocytes stays with white blood cells that engulf and digest pathogens and cellular debris. Examples of phagocytes include neutrophils and macrophages. These cells monitor the tissues and the bloodstream, seeking out and destroying invaders.

### Physical Barriers

The body's first line of defense includes physical barriers like the skin and mucous membranes, which act as physical barriers that prevent pathogens from entering the body. These surfaces also produce antimicrobial substances and enzymes that help destroy or inhibit the growth of pathogens.

## RISK FACTORS FOR INFECTION

Patients who are admitted in the critical care unit are at great chance in obtaining nosocomial infections. They include in a positive form of infection because of their underlying diseases and the patients age which is more than 65 years and also patients who are admitted in Intensive care unit. The HCAIs surveys states that widespread surveys provides a exact number of the circumstances or illness or disease in a population at a given time. The increased morbidity and mortality related to health centered acquired infectious state which is transmitted at the critical care setup is an issue of serious difficulty these days. Serious medico legal issues also stand up on part, since the patient or their family sometimes being accusation the healthcare staff for the infection and demand benefits. It has been also mentioned that in healthcare setup with an proper application in hospital acquired infection, contamination might be reduced by using exactly one-third (**Das Gupta, Nosocomial infection in critical care unit, 2015**).

In epidemiology, infections are often analyzed in terms of the interaction between three main components: the agent (pathogen causing the infection), the host (individual susceptible to the infection), and the environment (external factors influencing the transmission). Here are risk factors (**Fig. 5.1**) categorized according to these components are also other categories which is associated with risk factors such as host related which is mainly categorized.

### Host Related

The host related factors play a significant role in which it will mainly encompasses the age in which it mainly focus on the young and old age peoples and they are prone to infect easily. There are also other significant factors such as nutrition, pregnancy and underlying health factors such as diabetes and hypertension.

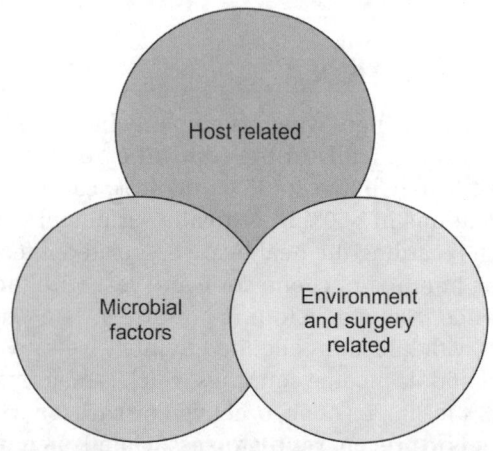

**Fig. 5.1:** Risk factors for infection.

## Environment and Surgery Related

Living conditions plays a vital role in risk factors as an infection is mainly associated with the sanitation and exposure to vectors. In the healthcare setting hospital acquired infections are more likely in environments where hygiene and infection control are measurable. Understanding these factors and their interactions is crucial for preventing and controlling infections at both individual and population levels. Public health interventions often aim to target these risk factors to reduce the burden of infectious diseases.

## Microbial Factors (Kollef MH, 2001)

Infection which is mainly transmitted by vectors (such as mosquitoes which is carrying malaria) are mainly influenced by vector distribution and control measures. These are the factors which are mainly responsible of the infection and microbes will mainly focused on that and leads to form the infection process.

## ANTIBIOTIC RESISTANT INFECTIONS

Antibiotics are commonly drug plot of action which is used to treat and deal with bacterial infections. The resistance happens whilst bacterial changes by situation to the use of these medications. Bacteria, no longer people or mammals, continue to form it's resistant. These medicinal value may also create more microbes on human beings and animals, infections it may reach are cease to treat and deal with the particular because of nonresistant bacteria. It indicates an potential opportunity to higher medical expenses, prolonged healthcare medical institution, and extended mortality.

The global attention has to be different in essence on seeing the method in administering and practice of antibiotic drug. In spite of new medicine are developed, Inspite the behavior change, antibiotic resistance will remain a first rate hazard. Behavior changes additionally encompasses moves to lessen disperse of infections via vaccines, hand wash-up, practicing secured intercourse, and good proper food hygiene (**World Health organization, July 2010**).

## Measures

The measures are extended by the intended intake of antibiotics, in addition to terrible incidence is transmitted and prevention on contamination in action. Steps should be taken to lessen the impact and restrict the spread of resistance.

## Individuals

It is a matter of concern for widely spread antibiotic resistance, administer drug through licensed physician.
- At no time forcefully ask antibiotics.
- Always comply healthcare worker's advice whilst the use of antibiotics.
- Never share or use leftover antibiotics.

Follow the food hygiene techniques by **WHO five keys to safer food:**
1. Keep clean
2. Separate raw and cooked
3. Cook thoroughly
4. Keep food at safe temperatures
5. Use safe water and raw materials

## Healthcare Specialist

To reduce antibiotic resistance, health professionals can:
- Control the suffering via by make sure palm, apparatus, and climate is easy and neat.
- Only prescribe and dispense antibiotics in lying with the current guidelines and recommendations.

### WHO Reaction (With Effect on Antibiotic Resistance)

To block and tackle the infectious resistance is at excessive priority for WHO. A global action plan has been recommended at the World Health Assembly in May 2020. The international focus of action ideas to makes in a certain way to stave off and administration of hazardous diseases with safe and effective medical care and treatment.

"**Global movement plan on antimicrobial resistance**" involves five strategic goals:
1. Improve attention and knowledge of antimicrobial resisting actions.
2. Fortify the ensuring part and research.
3. Downscale the occurrence contamination.
4. Enhance in handling antimicrobial drugs.
5. Clinch on constant funding in chipping the antimicrobial superbugs.

### Treatment of Fungal Infection

Fungi are accountable exactly 20% of biological science recorded at critical care unit (CCU) infections. Originating at a closing years, the degree of invasive fungal infections (IFI), has steadily expanded as a result of the increase numbers of both immunocompromised and critically ailing patients. Invasive fungal infections makes a contribution substantially to nosocomial infections in important gadgets on critical care unit current exercise on guidelines recommends echinocandins, such as micafungin, for the treatment of invasive candidiasis **(Dhingara S, Microbial resistance movements: an overview of global public health threats)**.

The drug classification **(Table 5.1)** has been broadly used and the common pills are indexed underneath as follows.

## POSTOPERATIVE WOUND INFECTION IN CCU

Frequently, surgical wounds exhibit within the first thirty days following the surgical treatment as a routine.

**Unpredictable phenomenon of surgical wound contamination:**
- Poorly managed diabetes
- Problems in immune system
- Obesity
- Smoking
- Intake of corticosteroids (for instance prednisone).

There are specific tiers of wound contamination:
- **Ostensible:** Condition inside pores and on the skin vicinity
- **Profound:** Germs is goes deeper than the pores and skin into the muscle tissue
- **Organ:** The surgery which is deep and includes the organ and space where surgery has been carried out.

### Management

Drugs are used to deal with most of the wound infections. The period of time and instance may vary with the antibiotics based on the disease condition.

### Wound Care

Wound has to be scrubbed together with the dressing to be changed on everyday foundation.

Dispose the vintage bandage and packing. After proper cleansing to moisture the wound, this permits the dressing to return without any difficulties.
- Cleanse out gash area.
- Situate a new, there of packing material and put on a brand new ligature.
- Vacuum-assisted closure (VAC).

It develops gore pattern in the wound and helps with reducing.
- A negative pressure (vacuum) dressing.
- It consists of vacuum pump, a foam piece cut to suit the wound, and a vacuum tube.
- A clean dressing is taped on pinnacle.
- The dressing and the froth piece are changed into each for 2–3 days.

It may take days, weeks, or perhaps even months for the wound to be tidy, clean of infection, and at remaining the contamination to be healed.

Considering approximately the wound inflammation which is not continually very deep and the gap within the wound are tiny, domestic care remedial measures has to be followed.

Based at the wound infection which may be penetrating or there is a bigger opening in the wound, there is a special attention need to focus for a few days in the healthcare setup and the treatment remedy prescribed by the physician **(Majno G, Healing Hands, Harvard University)**.

## PREVENTION AND INFECTION CONTROL MEASURES

Prevention and control measures in critical care units are essential to reduce the risk of healthcare-associated infections (HAIs) and improve patient outcomes. These measures aim to minimize the spread of pathogens, enhance infection control practices, and ensure patient

**Table 5.1:** Explains the common medicine and pills on antifungal drugs.

| S. No. | Name of the drug | Dosage |
|---|---|---|
| 1. | Amphotericin | 0.3 mg/kg |
| 2. | Liposomal amphotericin | 3–4 mg/kg per day |
| 3. | Fluconazole | IV loading dose: 12 mg/kg<br>Maintenance dose: 6 mg/kg |
| 4. | Voriconazole | IV loading dose: 6 mg/kg |
| 5. | Isavuconazole | IV loading dose: 200 mg day 1 day 2<br>Maintenance dose: 200 mg per 24 hour |
| 6. | Caspofungin | IV loading dose: 70 mg/kg<br>Maintenance dose: 50 mg (70 mg if body weight >80 kg) |
| 7. | Anidulafungin | Loading dose: 200 mg |
| 8. | Micafungin | 50 mg for prophylaxis, 100 mg for candidiasis, 150 mg for esophageal candidiasis |

safety. Here are some key prevention and control measures for critical care units:
- **Hand hygiene:** Encourage rigorous hand hygiene practices among healthcare workers. Hand washing with soap and water or using alcohol-based hand sanitizers before and after patient contact is crucial in preventing the spread of infections.
- **Infection control protocols:** Introduce and adhere to infection control protocols for the insertion, maintenance, and removal of invasive devices such as central lines, ventilators, and urinary catheters. Follow strict aseptic techniques to minimize the risk of introducing pathogens.
- **Isolation precautions:** Implement appropriate isolation precautions based on the type of infection and its mode of transmission. This might include contact precautions, droplet precautions, and airborne precautions.
- **Environmental cleaning:** Ensure regular and thorough cleaning and disinfection of patient care areas, surfaces, and equipment. Pay special attention to high-touch surfaces.
- **Patient screening:** Screen patients for potential drug-resistant organisms upon admission and during their stay. This can help identify carriers and prevent transmission.
- **Vaccination:** Ensure that both patients and healthcare workers are up-to-date on vaccinations, especially those recommended for preventing vaccine-preventable diseases.
- **Education and training:** Educate healthcare workers about infection prevention practices, including hand hygiene, proper use of personal protective equipment (PPE), and the importance of adherence to protocols.
- **Personal protective equipment:** Ensure that healthcare workers have access to appropriate PPE such as gloves, gowns, masks, and eye protection when dealing with potentially infectious patients **(Jeong YJ, Kanj, 2019)**.
- **Respiratory hygiene and cough etiquette:** Educate patients and visitors about proper respiratory hygiene, such as covering their mouth and nose when coughing or sneezing, and providing tissues and hand sanitizers.
- **Patient placement:** Assign patients to appropriate rooms based on their infection status and the mode of transmission of the infection. Ensure proper ventilation in rooms if required.

## NOSOCOMIAL INFECTION IN CRITICAL CARE UNIT

Nosocomial infections, which is also known as HAIs infections that patients acquire while receiving treatment in hospitals or critical care units. Critical care units, including intensive care units (ICUs), are particularly prone to nosocomial infections due to the severity of patients' illnesses, invasive procedures, and prolonged hospital stays.

There are various types in nosocomial infection which is seen in critical care unit such as:

### Ventilator-Associated Pneumonia

Hospital acquired pneumonia is defined as pneumonia occurring more than 48 hours after admission to hospital or in the case of ventilator associated pneumonia occurring within 48–72 hours of intubation. The peril of VAP is roughly calculated to be 3–7% during days of 16 of ventilation, decreasing days to 3% during days 4–10% and then 1% day thereafter.

#### Prevention of VAP

- Ensure the hand washing recommendations.
- Front line employee must wear a proper PPE.
- Apposite post operative pain relief to ease the respiratory exercises.
- Chest physiotherapy to be done by the nurse.
- Off the beaten track nursing patients familiar to be colonized transmitted to the microorganism.
- Practice noninvasive ventilation for every occasion possible.
- Carry out each day assessments of readiness to wean and use weaning recommendations.
- Use single use spirometer mouth pieces.
- Keep out the gastric over distension.
- Ensure that all the respiratory instruments and equipment is decontaminated properly and appropriately in between patients according to the manufacturer instructions **(Jeong YJ, Kanj, 2019)**.

### Catheter Related Urinary Tract Infection

Urinary tract incident accounts for 2–6% overall practical consultation and turned out to be identifies as 2nd most similar clinical signal for antibiotic scheduled in primary and secondary care. Ninety seven percentages of healthcare urinary tract infections are connected with instruments like catheterization whilst in approved common place healthcare intervention **(Harrisons, Principles of Internal Medicine)**.

#### Indications

Pointing out reason for catheterization are:
- Spinal/lumbar surgeries
- Traumatic injuries
- Pelvic fracture
- Incontinence.

### Prevention of Catheter-associated Urinary Tract Infection

- **Personnel:** Without human being who is familiar with the perfect method of aseptic insertion and maintenance of the catheter will have to focus on catheter.
- **Practicing silver catheter:** Catheter which is mainly formed of pattern of gold and palladium from a relatively thin of silver reduce microbial adherence to the catheter which minimizes the bio film formation and impede the migration of bacteria along the catheter surface in to the bladder.
- **Hand hygiene:** It is ought which has to be finished right away earlier than and to reduce the infection
- **Catheter insertion:** The catheters has to be inserted properly to avoid the further complications and make sure it has been indicated properly by various measures and techniques used.
- **Closed sterile drainage:** The catheter system forms a group together and it must stay ceased and now not be opened unless surely for vital diagnostic or healing process in irrigation
- **Irrigation:** Continuous irrigation ought to be prevented expect indicated (e.g., after prostatic or bladder surgery).

### Surgical Site Infections

**Lesions** are a common excluding a potentially unsustained complication following any procedure during which the skin is opportunistic resident or transient microorganism. It is significantly casual connection with extreme to the patient and occasionally connected as marker of poor standards of care particularly in related to standards of practice particularly in operation theaters.

### Prevention of Surgical Site Infection (Brunner and Suddarth's, 2008)

- Forbearing must be provided information and explained how to take care of their wound after discharge.
- Stoical need to advised clearly in what way to recognize.
- Convalescent need to be televise for MRSA, if positive decolonize prior to surgery.
- Advice patients to shower or have a hot bath using soap either the day before or on the day of the surgery.
- Staffs maintain their entry and exit of the operation theatre to minimum.
- Do not use nasal decontamination.
- Operating team should wear sterile gowns in the operation theatre during surgery.
- The use of reusable or disposable drapes and gowns does not influence the risk of SSI.
- Maintain adequate perfusion during surgery.
- Do not use the wound irrigation to reduce the risk of SSIs.

## METHICILLIN-RESISTANT STAPHYLOCOCCUS AUREUS

MRSA mainly stands for methicillin-resistant staphylococcus aureus (MRSA). It is a common classification of bacteria that has developed resistance to major antibiotics, including methicillin and other commonly used antibiotics like penicillin and amoxicillin. The treatment can be difficult to provide since the germs are less responsive to the medications that would typically be successful against Staphylococcus aureus. Healthcare-associated MRSA, also known as HA-MRSA, and community-associated MRSA, also known as CA-MRSA, are two different contexts in which MRSA infections can develop.

**Transmission:** It is mainly spread through direct skin-to-skin contact or contact with contaminated surfaces. It can be present on the skin and in the nose of healthy individuals without causing any symptoms.

### Types of MRSA Infections

- **Skin infections:** MRSA frequently causes skin infections like boils, abscesses, and cellulitis. These infections can be red, swollen, and painful.
- **Pneumonia:** In most of the cases, MRSA can lead to pneumonia, especially in people with weakened immune systems or underlying lung conditions.
- **Bloodstream infections:** MRSA can enter the bloodstream through an open wound or invasive medical devices (like central lines or catheters), leading to a bloodstream infection (bacteremia) that can be life-threatening.
- **Surgical site infections:** After surgical procedures, MRSA can infect the surgical site, leading to complications **(CDC, 2019)**.

## STANDARD SAFETY MEASURES IN CCU

In keeping up the standard safety procedures, it plays crucial in a CCU to protect both patients and medical staff. To stop the transmission of illnesses, these precautions include strict hand cleanliness, the appropriate use of personal protective equipment (PPE), and adherence to infection control procedures. To ensure proper treatments, stringent patient identification processes and pharmaceutical safety measures are adhered to. Regular surface and equipment disinfection helps to keep the environment clean. To reduce hazards, careful patient assessment and fall prevention techniques are used, and respiratory hygiene education encourages infection prevention. Priority is placed on effective communication between the medical staff, patients, and families, and emergency readiness training guarantees prompt reactions to life-or-death emergencies. CCUs establish a safe environment for patient care by preserving these safety protocols, minimizing risks **(CDC, 2016)**.

### Prophylaxis in CCU

In a CCU, making sure about on health and safety of healthcare staff is paramount to providing effective patient care. Staff prophylaxis involves a range of preventive strategies aimed at safeguarding the well-being of healthcare workers in this critical environment. Immunization acts as a pivotal role, with periodical updates on recommended vaccinations such as influenza, hepatitis B, and tetanus helping to shield staff from preventable diseases. Regular screening for tuberculosis helps identify potential exposures, and for highly contagious infections like varicella and measles, staff without immunity can receive appropriate vaccines. Respiratory protection measures, particularly in instances of airborne infections like tuberculosis and COVID-19, involve the proper use of N95 respirators. Encouraging safe needle handling practices and providing safety devices minimize needle stick injuries and the risk of blood borne pathogen exposure. In Accordingly as important factor is education and training that empower staff with infection prevention knowledge, ensuring the correct utilization of personal protective equipment and the effective response to exposures. The implementation of standard precautions, stress and fatigue management, and accessible health surveillance programs collectively contribute to the comprehensive approach to staff prophylaxis, promoting a resilient and infection-resistant healthcare workforce within the CCU **(Ray B, 2009)**.

## STERILIZATION AND DISINFECTION IN CCU

Due to the increased susceptibility of critically ill patients to infections, maintaining a sterile environment in a CCU is of utmost importance. To reduce the risk of healthcare-associated infections and ensure the safety of both patients and healthcare workers, prompt sterilization and disinfection measures are strictly implemented.

One of the major key components is hand hygiene, where healthcare professionals diligently wash their hands using soap and water or alcohol-based sanitizers before and after any patient based interaction. This essential procedure stops the spread of dangerous germs. In order to prevent cross-contamination during patient care activities, it is also required that PPE, which includes gloves, gowns, masks, and eye protection, be used.

Aseptic or sterile techniques are painstakingly used during invasive treatments that compromise the body's natural defenses to prevent the introduction of germs. All tools and equipment must be thoroughly cleaned, sterilized, and disinfected in order to stop the spread of illnesses. This procedure, which includes both routine and intensive cleaning steps, closely follows predetermined rules. An essential component of infection control in the CCU is environmental cleanliness. In addition to thoroughly disinfecting patient rooms, common areas and high-touch surfaces also go through routine cleaning and disinfection procedures. Together, these actions support maintaining a sterile and clean atmosphere.

Based on the materials to be sterilized and the particular requirements of the CCU, different sterilization techniques are used, such as autoclaving, chemical disinfection, and ethylene oxide gas sterilization. These procedures are actively monitored by infection control teams, who also carry out surveillance, contain outbreaks, and give healthcare workers continual education. When infectious conditions are found, isolation measures are immediately put in place. The spread of illnesses within the CCU and outside of it is stopped by these measures, which can include contact precautions and airborne precautions **(Blot, S, 2022)**.

Overall, healthcare workers strictly follow these protocols in the safe and tightly supervised environment of the CCU. By doing this, they guarantee the highest levels of infection prevention and patient safety, reducing risks and fostering the best possible patient outcomes.

### Nursing Management in Critical Care Unit

Nursing management in the critical care unit is an essential aspect of care for patients who require intensive and specialized care due to their critical condition. Critical care nurses play a crucial role in ensuring the provision of safe, efficient, and quality care to critically ill patients. The nursing management in a critical care unit involves a wide range of responsibilities and interventions aimed at promoting patient recovery, preventing complications, and ensuring patient safety. Here are some of the key areas of nursing management in the critical care unit.

- **Assessment and monitoring:** Critical care nurses continuously assess and monitor the patient's vital signs, neurological status, and other clinical parameters such as oxygen saturation, urine output, and laboratory values. This enables them to detect changes in the patient's condition promptly and initiate appropriate interventions.

- **Management of invasive devices:** Patients in the critical care unit require several invasive devices such as arterial lines, central venous catheters, mechanical ventilators, and urinary catheters. Critical care nurses are responsible for the proper placement, monitoring, and care of these devices to prevent complications such as infection, bleeding, and obstruction.
- **Medication management:** Patients in the critical care unit require multiple medications, including high-risk drugs such as sedatives, vasopressors, and antibiotics. Critical care nurses are responsible for administering and monitoring these medications to ensure their safety and efficacy.
- **Infection prevention and control:** Critical care nurses follow strict infection prevention and control protocols to prevent the spread of infectious diseases in the critical care unit. This includes regular hand hygiene, proper use of personal protective equipment, and adherence to sterile techniques during procedures.
- **Nutrition and hydration management:** Critically ill patients may have altered nutritional and hydration needs. Critical care nurses are responsible for assessing and monitoring the patient's nutritional and hydration status and implementing appropriate interventions such as enteral or parenteral feeding.
- **Pain and symptom management:** Critical care nurses are responsible for managing the patient's pain and other symptoms such as dyspnea, anxiety, and nausea. They use various interventions such as medication administration, positioning, and nonpharmacological measures to manage these symptoms.
- **Patient and family education:** Critical care nurses provide education to patients and their families on the patient's condition, treatment options, and potential complications. They also provide emotional support and help patients and their families cope with the stress of critical illness.

In conclusion, nursing management in the critical care unit involves a wide range of interventions aimed at promoting patient recovery, preventing complications, and ensuring patient safety. Critical care nurses play a crucial role in the interdisciplinary team, providing comprehensive and vigilant care to critically ill patients **(Ageel M, Shbeer A, 2022)**.

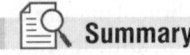

## Summary

Every year, hundreds of patients are concerned about healthcare-associated infections, which are especially common in low-income developing nations. The NAO report concludes that there have been numerous changes, including a shift in culture, and that there are still many areas that need to be improved, most notably the capability of the surveillance system to report HCAI to significant deaths, disabilities, or injuries, as well as the need to increase practice compliance. Because of their underlying conditions, advanced age and admission to an intensive care unit, they are easily evidence to include in a positive type of infection. These days, a major challenge is the rise in morbidity and death from health-related acquired infectious diseases that are spread in critical care settings. Additionally, it has been stated that contamination can be decreased by precisely one-third in a healthcare setting with effective application in hospital acquired infections.

 **Points to Ponder**

- Infection is the invasion of an organism from the body tissues.
- Patients who are admitted in the critical care unit are at great chance in obtaining nosocomial infections.
- Antibiotics are commonly drug plot of action which is used to treat and deal with bacterial infections.
- In spite of new medicine are developed, In spite the behavior change, antibiotic resistance will remain a first rate hazard.
- The period of time and instance may vary with the antibiotics based on the disease condition.
- Ninety seven percentages of healthcare urinary tract infections are connected with instruments like catheterization whilst in approved common place healthcare intervention.
- It is significantly casual connection with extreme to the patient and occasionally connected as marker of poor standards of care particularly in related to standards of practice particularly in operation theatres.
- Hospital acquired pneumonia Is defined as pneumonia occurring more than 48 hours after admission to hospital or in the case of ventilator associated pneumonia occurring within 48–72 hours of intubation.
- 75% people are infected with urinary tract infections
- Respiratory instruments and equipment's is decontaminated properly and appropriately in between patients according to the manufacturer instructions.

 **Abbreviations**

- WHO : World Health Organization
- HAI : Healthcare Associated Infection
- CCU : Critical Care Unit
- NAO : National Audit Office
- PPE : Personal Protective Equipment
- VAC : Vacuum-assisted Closure
- SSI : Surgical Site Infection
- VAP : Ventilator-associated Pneumonia

### Short Answer Questions

1. Define infection and explain its types.
2. Enumerate the risk factors in infection.
3. Explain the role of a nurse in critical care unit.
4. Antibiotic resistant infection.
5. List out the common drugs used in antifungal infection.
6. Explain about VAC in detail.
7. What are the prevention and control measures in CCU by a nurse and explain in detail.
8. Role of a nurse in surgical site infection.
9. List out the common indication for ventilator-associated pneumonia.
10. Explain about WHO recommendations in infection control.

### Long Answer Questions

1. Define nosocomial infection and provide a detailed explanation of the risk factors for infection.
2. What forms of infections are there, and what is a nurse's job in a critical care unit?
3. Describe the typical infections that affect critical care units in detail.
4. What is antibiotic resistance according to who and what does it mean in detail?
5. Detail the management of infection control.
6. Give a brief explanation of the preventative and control strategies used in the critical care unit.

### Bibliography

1. Ageel M, Shbeer A. Assessment of the critical care work environment of Intensive Care Unit nurses in Saudi Arabia. Risk Manag Healthc Policy. 2022;15:2413-20.
2. Blot S, Ruppé E, Harbarth S, Asehnoune K, Poulakou G, Luyt CE, et al. Healthcare-associated infections in adult intensive care unit patients: changes in epidemiology, diagnosis, prevention and contributions of new technologies. Intensive Crit Care Nurs. 2022;70:103227.
3. Center for disease control and prevention. National center for emerging and zoonotic infectious disease; 2019.
4. Center for disease control and prevention. National center for emerging and zoonotic infectious disease, Division of health care promotion; 2016.
5. Dasgupta S, Das S, Chawan NS, Hazra A. Nosocomial infections in the intensive care unit: Incidence, risk factors, outcome and associated pathogens in a public tertiary teaching hospital of Eastern India. Indian J Crit Care Med. 2015;19(1):14-20.
6. Dhingra S, Rahman NAA, Peile E, Rahman M, Sartelli M, Hassali MA, et al. Microbial resistance movements: an overview of global public health threats posed by antimicrobial resistance, and how best to counter. Front Public Health. 2020;4(8):535668.
7. Geneva: World Health Organization; 2010.
8. Harrison's Principles of internal medicine. 16th ed. New York: McGraw-Hill Medical Publishing Division; 2008.
9. Jeong YJ, Kang J. Development and validation of a questionnaire to measure post-intensive care syndrome. Intensive Crit Care Nurs. 2019;1(55):102756.
10. Kollef MH, Fraser VJ. Antibiotic resistance in the intensive care unit. Ann Intern Med. 2001;134(4):298-314.
11. Majno G. The healing hand: Man and wound in the ancient world. Harvard University Press; 1991.
12. Rao VU, Arakeri G, Subash A, Rao J, Jadhav S, Sayeed MS, et al. COVID-19: Loss of bridging between innate and adaptive immunity? Med Hypotheses. 2020;144:109861.
13. Ray B, Samaddar DP, Todi SK, Ramakrishnan N, John G, Ramasubban S. Quality indicators for ICU: ISCCM guidelines for ICUs in India. Indian J Crit Care Med. Peer Reviewed Official publication of Indian Society of Critical Care Medicine. 2009;13(4):173-206.
14. Study BS, National Institutes of Health. Information about mental illness and the brain. National Institutes of Health; 2007. In NIH Curriculum Supplement Series [internet].
15. Suddarths B. Medical surgical nursing. 12th edition. Philadelphia: Lippincott company; 2008.
16. Zhao T, Wu X, Zhang Q, Li C, Worthington HV, Hua F. Oral hygiene care for critically ill patients to prevent ventilator-associated pneumonia. Cochrane Database Syst Rev. 2020;12(12):CD008367.

# Chapter 6

# Common Gastrointestinal Emergencies

*Jhunilata Pradhan*

## CHAPTER OUTLINE

- Anatomy of GI System
- Physiology of GI System
- Assessment of GI System
- Parenteral and Enteral Nutrition
- Gastrointestinal Bleeding
- Abdominal Injuries
- Fulminant Hepatic Failure
- Hepatic Encephalopathy
- Acute Pancreatitis
- Intestinal Obstruction
- Perforated Peritonitis

## Learning Objectives

At the end of the chapter, the students will be able to:
- Describe the basic anatomy and physiology of gastrointestinal system.
- Perform the assessment of a patient with gastrointestine disorder with history collection and physical examination.
- Describe the purposes of different diagnostic procedures involved to study gastrointestinal system disorders.
- Explain enteral and parenteral nutrition methods and nursing responsibility.
- Describe the etiology, clinical manifestations, assessment and management of gastrointestinal bleeding.
- Describe the etiology, pathophysiology mechanisms, clinical manifestations, diagnosis, and management of abdominal trauma.
- Describe the classification, etiology, risk factors, pathophysiology, clinical manifestations, diagnosis, and emergency management of fulminant hepatic failure.
- Describe the causes, types, pathophysiology, diagnosis, complications and management of hepatic encephalopathy.
- Describe the types, etiology, pathophysiology, clinical manifestations, diagnosis, and management of acute pancreatitis.
- Describe the etiology, pathophysiology, clinical features, diagnosis, complications and management of intestinal obstruction.
- Describe the etiology, classification, pathophysiology, clinical manifestations, diagnosis and management of peritonitis.

## ANATOMY OF GASTROINTESTINAL SYSTEM

The digestive system consists of gastrointestinal tract along with the accessory organs. The gastrointestinal tract also known as digestive tract, alimentary tract (**Fig. 6.1**).

The GI tract (digestive system) is seen in abdominopelvic cavity which is covered by serous membrane known as peritoneum.

Organs of digestive tract are as follows:
- Oral cavity
- Pharynx
- Esophagus
- Stomach
- Small intestine (duodenum, jejunum and ileum)
- Large intestine (cecum, colon, rectum and anal canal)
- Anus

Accessory organs of digestive system are:
- Salivary glands
- Liver

- Gallbladder
- Pancreas (Nash, 2005).

## Histology of the Digestive Tract

The GI tract has four major layers like:
1. Innermost mucosa
2. Submucosa
3. Muscularis
4. Outer most serosa or adventitia showing in **(Fig. 6.2)**.

### Basic Functions of Digestive System

- Ingestion
- Mastication
- Propulsion
- Mixing
- Secretion
- Digestion
- Absorption
- Elimination

## Oral Cavity

Oral cavity is the starting of the digestive tract which consists of mouth, tongue, salivary gland and teeth. It helps in mastication, deglutition and speech taste. Specially saliva helps in digestion of food and maintains hygiene of the oral cavity, lubrication and maintains pH level of the cavity.

## Pharynx

It is the part that carries food from the mouth to the esophagus. It is divided into three parts: Naso, oro and laryngopharynx. Only the oropharynx is the part of the digestive system.

## Esophagus

The esophagus lies in the thoracic cavity with 25 cm length and 2 cm wide. It has mucosa, submucosa, muscularis, and adventitia layers. The movement of food particle is controlled by two sphincters at the top and at the bottom. It helps in formation of bolus, swallowing, reduce gastric reflux.

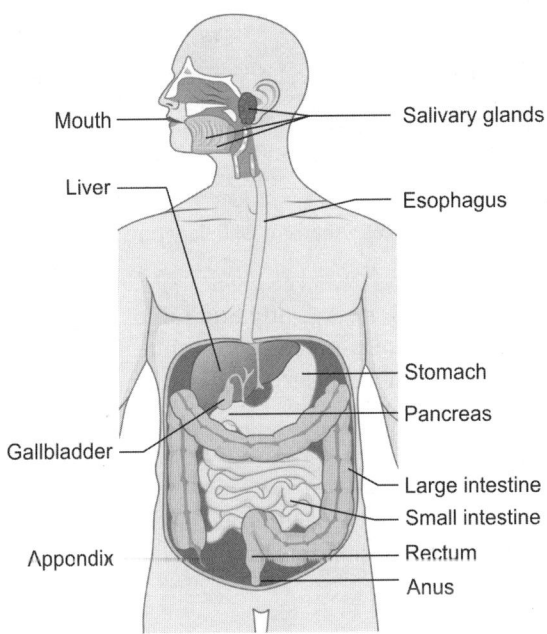

**Fig. 6.1:** Anatomy of digestive system.

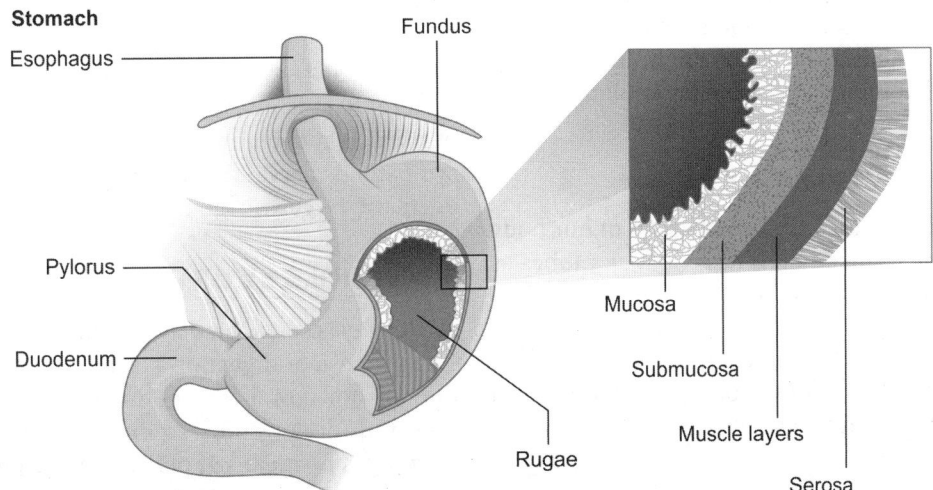

**Fig. 6.2:** Anatomy of liver.

## Stomach

The stomach located left side of the upper abdomen, which receives foods from the esophagus controlled by lower esophagus sphincter or cardiac sphincter. It has four parts cardia, fundus, body and pylorus.

### Gastric Secretory Cells

- **Chief cells:** Helps to secrete pepsinogen (an inactive enzyme).
- **Mucous cells:** Secrete mucus and alkaline substances to help neutralize HCl in the gastric juice.
- **Parietal cells:** Production of "intrinsic factor" and hydrochloric (HCl).
- **G cells:** Secretion of a hormone called gastrin, which stimulates the parietal cells and overall gastric secretion.
- Gastric juice special composed of HCl, pepsinogen, and intrinsic factor which helps in digestion.

## Small Intestine

It lies in between stomach and connects to large intestine. It has three parts, duodenum, jejunum and ileum. It almost 3–5 m length with 2.5–3 cm wide. The small intestine consists of three parts: the duodenum. This part of digestive system is responsible for maximum amount of chemical digestion and absorption. It also helps in to support the immune system. Gallbladder, liver and pancreas supply their secretions to the small intestine to help in chemical digestion of food.

## Large Intestine

It is the last part of the system, with 2–3 inch width. It consists of 5 parts cecum, ascending colon, transverse colon, descending colon, sigmoid colon, rectum, anal canal, and anus. It helps in absorption of water and any remaining absorbable food. Along with bacterial fermentation takes place.

## Liver

It is considered as the largest internal organ of our body placed in right upper quadrant. It has two major lobes as right and left and two minor lobes quadrate and caudate (**Fig. 6.3**). It has a wide range of function like metabolism of carbohydrate protein and fat, secretion of bile, breakdown of insulin and other hormones, storage of vitamins and detoxify the chemical and drugs.

## Pancreas

It is a common organ in digestive and endocrine system which lies behind the stomach in abdominal cavity. It

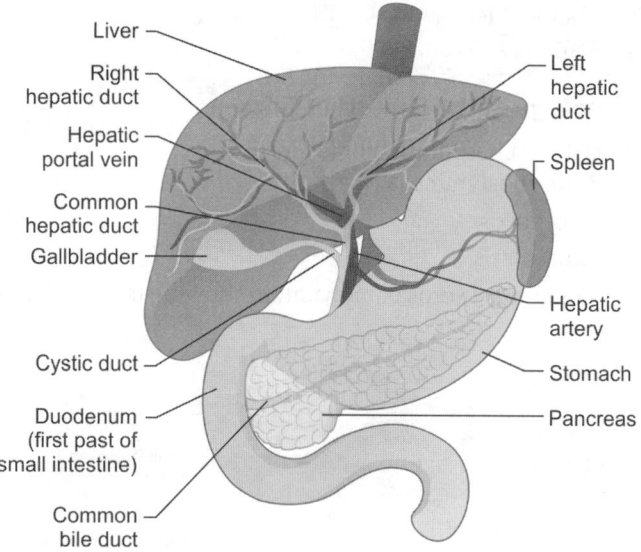

**Fig. 6.3:** Anatomy of biliary tract.

divided into head, neck, body and tail of pancreas. The exocrine function of pancreas is to secrete pancreatic juice and endocrine function is to secrete hormones to control blood glucose level.

## Gallbladder

It is a sac-like structure which is used to store the bile (**Fig. 6.3**). It lies to posterior to liver. Bile is used for digestion of fats.

## Blood and Nerve Supply

The digestive system receives blood from thoracic and abdominal aorta. Maximum portion of the tract supplied by gastric and mesenteric arteries. Both parasympathetic and sympathetic nerve stimulus are supplied to the digestive system. Parasympathetic stimulation helps to increase peristalsis movement and increase secretion where as sympathetic nerve stimulation decreases the secretion and decrease the gastric motility.

# PHYSIOLOGY OF DIGESTIVE SYSTEM

Oral cavity is considered as the entrance of digestive tract. The process of digestion starts from chewing. It helps in breakdown of foods and mixing with saliva. Then the digested food swallowed and go to stomach through esophagus by means of peristalsis movement. At the end the LES opens, and the food bolus enter to stomach, it also prevents from regurgitation of food from stomach to esophagus.

The bolus stores and mixes with secretions in stomach. The gastric juice is acidic in nature due to presence of HCL, it also contains pepsin which helps for protein digestion. Again, the food content travel to pylorus with peristalsis movement. During this time the food content may be paste or liquid.

From stomach the food goes to small intestine through pyloric antrum. Again the digestion continues by mixing the pancreatic juice and bile. Bile helps to digest the fat and removes waste products from blood. The maximum amount of food will be absorbed to blood stream in duodenum and ileum area. After 4 hour of eating waste product of the digestive process passes to the colon through the ileocecal valve. There are two types of colonic secretions: Mucus solution and electrolyte solution. The primary function of colon is reabsorption of electrolyte and water. The waste product stored in the sigmoid colon and with peristalsis movement it empties with act of defecation.

## ASSESSMENT OF GI SYSTEM

Detailed assessment of a patient with gastrointestinal complaints includes history collection and gastrointestinal examination.

### Collection of Health History

History must be collected from the patient if patient is conscious and oriented or can be collected from patient's relatives in case patient will not able to give reliable information.

### Biographical Data

Biographical information such as age, gender, marital status, area of residence, occupation, spiritual beliefs should be collected. All these information might give us an understanding of the exposure of the patient to risk factors of certain diseases.

### Present History of Illness

Present history of illness refers to the detailed course of events leading up to the current admission to hospital. For this, patient's chief complaints should be asked. Some of the common gastrointestinal complaints include: Nausea, vomiting, abdominal pain, weight loss, anorexia, heart burn, etc.

### Past History of Illness

History should be collected regarding any past disorders or diseases. History must be collected any surgery or any invasive procedure related to abdomen or any other system. Past history of medical illness like diabetes mellitus, hypertension, chronic renal failure, hepatitis should be asked. History of immunization is also important.

### Family History

Family history regarding hepatitis, peptic ulcer, liver failure, hypertension, stroke, autoimmune diseases, cancer, degenerating diseases should be collected. Any history of psychiatric disorder or substance abuse among family members should be mentioned.

### Dietary History

Dietary history should include dietary pattern and dietary habits. Information should be gathered related to type of diet, presence of appetite, nausea vomiting and difficulty in swallowing. Body mass index is to be evaluated to check the body built of the patient.

### Exercise History

Patient should be asked for type, pattern and duration of exercise per day, muscular strength, fatigue or weakness experienced. Assess the extent of household or self care activities patient is able to perform.

### Medication History

Use of certain medication like NSAIDs may lead to have different gastro problems. So it is also one aspect to have the detail information regarding the medication patient is taking and the allergy history of medication.

### Personal Habits

This includes activities such as smoking, alcoholism, or substance abuse. These are risk factors for various disease like liver failure, pancreatitis.

### Occupational History

Information regarding the type of work and activities involved during worktime should be collected. Activities such as sedentary work may leads to obesity. Exposure to radiations, toxins, or carcinogens in the workplace can increase the susceptibility of gastrointestinal problems.

It is also required to have the information regarding the social, psychological, spiritual and cultural factors of the patient.

### Pain

The abdominal pain is the most common and important complain of the patient with gastrointestinal disorder. For this all the information regarding pain should be taken very carefully and in detailed.

### Characteristic of Pain (SOCRATES)

- **S:** Site of pain.
- **O:** Onset of pain.
- **C:** Characteristic features of pain (dull/sharp/stabbing/burning/tingling/crushing).
- **R:** Radiation of pain from one place to another place.
- **A:** Associated symptoms with pain (headache and nausea).
- **T:** Timing (episodic, continuous).
- **E:** Exacerbation and reliving factors of pain (medication, food, activity and posture).
- **S:** Severity.

### Nausea, Vomiting and Anorexia

These complains may reflects various gastrointestinal problems. Information to be taken regarding the frequency and duration of symptoms, color and consistency of vomits.

### Bowel Habits

Bowel movements is to be assessed for frequency, consistency and color. Any medication use for bowel movement should be evaluated. Changes in bowel movements and changes in color of stool may be present with variety of disease like intestinal bleeding, colon cancer, hemorrhoids, etc.

### Weight Pattern

Any change in weight like weight loss or weight gain within a specified time period is to be collected. The information related to weight loss may be associated with some disease as well as weight gain may be related to accumulation of fluid or presence of any mass inside the body.

## Physical Examination

Physical examination of gastrointestinal system includes assessment of oral cavity, abdomen and rectum. For physical examination the patient will be in relaxed and supine position with knees flexed slightly. The room must have good source of light with well maintained privacy. Patient must have empty bladder with complete visualization of the abdomen and hands to be kept across the chest.

### Mouth

Complete oral cavity including teeth, tongue, mucus membrane is to be inspected and palpated thoroughly. It will be examined for presence of any inflammation, sores, congenital anomaly, bleeding, mass or swelling. Lips and tongue should be evaluated for dryness, symmetry, sore and crack. Teeth is to be checked for discoloration, loose and missing teeth. Including all patient's breath orders to be checked.

### Abdomen

The order for abdominal examination is inspection, auscultation, percussion and palpation. This sequence is to be followed to avoid the false interpretation of bowel sound due to palpation methods.

#### Inspection

Abdomen is inspected for skin discoloration, presence of sinuses, scars and lesions, striae, stomas, hair distribution and fistula. Along with abdomen must be checked for symmetry and contour. Umbilicus is to be inspected for hernia, position (inverted/everted) and color of umbilicus. Abdominal distension which is caused by 9F (fat, fluids, feces, flatus, fetus, fibroid, false pregnancy, full bladder and fatal tumor) is also assessed. Dilated and distended veins and peristalsis movements can be evaluated in certain disease conditions.

#### Auscultation

Auscultation should be done before percussion and palpation. It will be start from right lower quadrant (RLQ) to right upper quadrant (RUQ), left upper quadrant (LUQ) and left lower quadrant (LLQ) **(Fig. 6.4)**. The diaphragm of stethoscope is to be used for at least 5 min in each quadrant. The average bowel sound present at a rate of 5–30 clicks/min in each quadrant is known as normoactive bowel sound. Bowel sounds more than 30 clicks/min and less than 5 clicks/min is known as hyperactive and hypoactive bowel sound respectively. During certain disease condition like paralytic ileus, intestinal obstruction there may be absences of bowel sound. Special types of bowel sounds are "Borborygmi" (hyper peristalsis movement/characterized by gurgling and audible without stethoscope) and

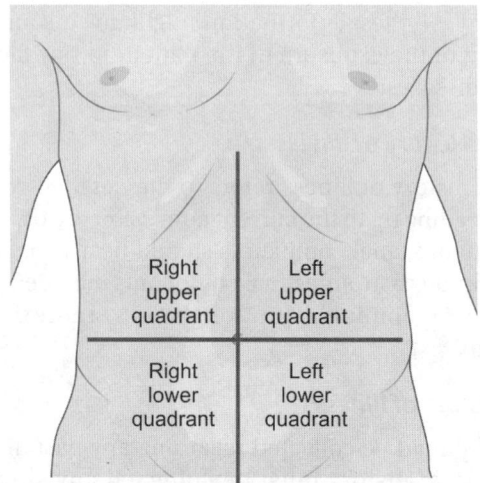

**Fig. 6.4:** Four abdomen quadrant.

"succession splash" (a loud sound like splashing water). The arterial and venous vascular sound (Bruits) must be differentiate from peristalsis movement. If indicated listen for venous hums and friction rub.

*Percussion*

Percussion helps to assess density of abdominal content and identify for abnormal collection of fluids and gases. Percussion must be performed in all four quadrant starting from right lower quadrant. Identify the area of dullness, tympany, and hyperresonance. Special attention given to liver, spleen and bladder. In case of ascites fluid wave is to be assessed.

*Palpation*

Palpation is used to assess the size, location and consistency of abdominal organs and identify abnormal masses and tenderness. Palpation may be light palpation, deep palpation and bimanual palpation. In light palpation use four fingers and depress ½ inch (1 cm) and in deep palpation depress 2–3 inch (5–8 cm) and move clockwise. Bimanual palpation will be carried out by using two hands specially in case of obese and large abdomen. Light palpation will help to assess the involuntary muscle rigidity, guarding, crepitus of abdominal wall and tenderness, deep palpation helps to identify deep mass, enlargement of liver, spleen, kidney and tenderness point. Rebound tenderness/Blumberg's sign can be assessed by palpation. Palpate all the four quadrants:

Liver palpation

Place left hand right side posterior to the patient at the level of lower two ribs with upward movement. Place right hand on right upper quadrant with fingers directed to patient's head or left shoulder. Ask the patient to take deep breath and press gently in and upward direction. The liver edge can be felt when it comes down and touches the finger tips. It should be soft, regular, sharp and smooth surface. For this hooking technique can also be adopted.

Spleen palpation

Place the right hand below the left costal margin and press it towards the spleen. Place left hand to support lower rib cage. instruct the patient for deep breathing. Normally spleen is not palpable. If the size becomes more than 3 times then only it can be palpable.

Kidney palpation

For right side kidney place right hand at the costovertebral area (CVA) and left hand below right costal margin. Instruct the patient for deep breath and try to capture between hands. Repeat the same process for left side. Normal kidneys are not palpable.

Inguinal lymph nodes palpation

Palpate horizontal lymph node in the groin and vertical lymph nodes at the inner aspect of thigh. If it is palpable, it should be smooth, moveable and less than 1 cm.

Bladder palpation

Palpate above the symphysis pubis at the level of midline. An empty bladder usually not palpable.

- **Kehr's sign:** In supine position move the patient's arm to upward direction. Assess for referred pain to left shoulder. It may be positive in case of splenic injury, renal calculi and ectopic pregnancy.
- **Murphy's sign:** Instruct the patient for deep breathing, palpate the mid clavicular line below the costal angel. Observe for pain and breathing restriction. It may be positive in cholecystitis or cancer in gallbladder.
- **McBurney's sign:** McBurney's point is present at the level of two third away from umbilicus to anterior superior iliac spine. Deeply and slowly palpate over the point and assess for the presence of pain. It may be positive in case of appendicitis **(Fig. 6.5)**.
- **Obturator's sign:** Place the patient in supine position and flex right leg at knee and hip. Place one hand above the knee and others at the ankle, then rotate externally and internally. Note the pain at hypo gastric region. Positive sign may indicate pelvic abscess or ruptured appendix.
- **Rovsing's sign:** Rovsing's sign is positive when patient complains pain in right lower quadrant while applying pressure on patient's left lower quadrant. It seen in case of peritonitis or appendicitis.
- **Psoas's sign:** In supine position of patient, place one hand over right lower thigh and instruct the patient to raise right leg by flexing hip while examiner will push

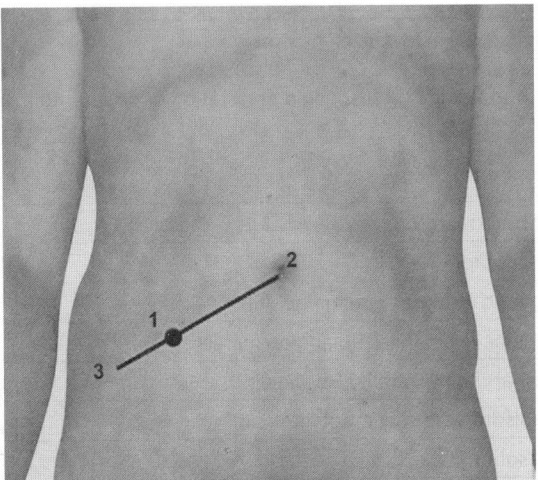

**Fig. 6.5:** Point 1 shows the McBurney's point.

downward. Evaluate pain in right lower quadrant. It is useful in case of appendicitis.

The last part of assessment is the anal and perineal area. Inspection and palpation to be done to find out any fissure, bleeding, fistula or presence of hemorrhoids. If needed digital rectal examination to be done for more detail investigation.

## Diagnostic Evaluation of Gastrointestinal System

All the investigations of gastrointestinal tract system are based on laboratory investigation (**Table 6.1**), imaging investigation (**Table 6.2**), endoscopic procedure, (**Table 6.3**) and other common diagnostic investigations (**Table 6.4**).

**Table 6.1:** Laboratory investigation.

| Name of investigation | Purpose |
|---|---|
| Complete blood count (CBC) | Helps to evaluate the RBC pernicious anemia (b12 absorption), and WBC. Platelets (liver) internal organ (bleeding) |
| Carbon urea breath test | For Helicobacter Pylori |
| PT/PTT | Liver disease/clotting factor |
| Amylase, lipase | Increased with pancreatitis |
| Complete metabolic panel | Albumin (protein made by liver) |
| CEA (carcinoembryonic antigen) and CA 19-9 | Cancer |
| Liver function test | ALT (breakdown protein)/AST (amino acids) ALP, bilirubin |
| D-xylose absorption test | Separate mucosal disease from pancreatic insufficiency |
| Hydrogen breath test | For lactose intolerance |
| Fecal occult blood test | Checks for hidden (occult) blood in the stool |

**Table 6.2:** Imaging investigation.

| Name of investigation | Purpose |
|---|---|
| Plain X-ray | Identify the collection of fluids and gases |
| Barium X-ray in upper GI:<br>• Esophagus<br>• Stomach<br>• Duodenum | Helps in diagnosis of:<br>• Ulcers<br>• Enteritis<br>• Tumors<br>• Obstruction<br>• Malabsorption syndromes<br>• Anatomical structure of organs |
| Barium X-ray in lower GI:<br>• Large intestine<br>• Contraindicated suspected perforation or obstruction | Helps in diagnosis of:<br>• Polyps<br>• Lesions<br>• Tumors<br>• Malfunction of bowel<br>• Anatomic abnormalities |
| Computed tomography scan (CT or CAT scan) | Shows detail picture of organ. Gives more information than X-ray |
| Defecography | X-ray of the anorectal area to evaluate the abnormal findings of the area |
| Magnetic resonance imaging (MRI) | Evaluate the soft tissue, blood vessel, bleeding, neoplasms, fistulas |
| Magnetic resonance cholangiopancreatography (MRCP) | View the biliary tract in detail |
| Oropharyngeal motility (swallowing) study | Useful for gastric motility and gastric emptying |
| Radioisotope gastric emptying scan | Useful for gastric motility and gastric emptying |
| Ultrasound | Evaluate blood vessels tissues and organ |
| Endoscopic ultrasonography | Provide direct imaging of target area |

**Table 6.3:** Endoscopic procedure.

| Name of investigation | Purpose |
|---|---|
| Esophagogastroduodenoscopy (EGD or upper endoscopy) | Complete visualization of inside of the cavity and allows of obtaining tissue sample for other diagnosis<br>Therapeutic procedures:<br>• Remove bile duct stones<br>• Treat gastric bleeding and esophageal varices<br>• Dilate strictures<br>• Laser therapy for neoplasms |
| Anoscope, proctoscopy, and sigmoidoscopy | • Visualization of the large colon<br>• Used for screening<br>   – Cancer<br>   – Polyps<br>   – Unknown diarrhea, occult blood or anemia<br>   – Tissue biopsies and removal of polyps<br>   – Extent of inflammatory disease |
| Endoscopic retrograde cholangiopancreatography (ERCP) | Both diagnose and treat the condition of ductal structures of biliary tract, pancreatic duct, common bile duct and hepatic ducts |

**Table 6.4:** Other common investigations.

| Name of investigation | Purpose |
|---|---|
| Anorectal manometry | Evaluate muscle strength of rectum and anus |
| Esophageal manometry | Identify the esophageal muscle strength |
| Esophageal pH monitoring | Record pH of the esophagus |
| Capsule endoscopy | Useful for small intestine examination |
| Gastric manometry | Record electrical and muscular action of stomach |
| Magnetic resonance cholangiopancreatography (MRCP) | Helpful to scan the internal organs and tissue |
| Laparoscopy (peritoneoscopy) | Useful for the visualization of peritoneal cavity |

# PARENTERAL AND ENTERAL NUTRITION

## Enteral Nutrition

Enteral nutritional support helps to provide carbohydrate, protein, vitamins, electrolytes, minerals, trace elements, and fluids via the gastrointestinal route **(Hospital, Nutrition, and Unit, 2019)**.

It is widely used to deliver feeding into a patient when indicated. The feeding is also given to duodenum, stomach and jejunum.

According to time duration it is of two types:
1. Short-term feeding.
2. Long-term feeding.

### Short-term Feeding

In this type of the time duration is up to 4 weeks. There are different types of feeding are used:

### Nasogastric Tube Feeding (NG)

A nasogastric tube is given through the nose to the stomach. Bolus, intermittent and pump feeding can be given with an nasogastric tube. The tube must be changed in every 4–6 weeks with swapping the nostril. The NG tube must be supervised to avoid the risk of displacement and aspiration.

### Oro-gastric Feeding

A feeding tube is given through the oral cavity into the stomach. The feeding tube must be checked for displacement and changed in every 4–6 weeks.

### Naso-jejunal Feeding

A thin fine feeding tube (FG 6-10) is given through the nose to the jejunum. There is presence of lumen where the distal end may permit for the deflation of the stomach. This type of feeding is evident for patients with gastroesophageal reflux disease or gastroparesis.

### Long-term Feeding

In this type of the time duration of feeding is more than 4 weeks. The different types of feeding used for long term feedings are:

#### Percutaneous Endoscopic Gastrostomy (PEG)

A feeding tube is given to the stomach under endoscopic procedure with local anesthesia. It is fixed by two bumpers both internally and externally, regulated by tubing clam and adapter.

#### Surgically Placed Gastrostomy

If a patient is not able to tolerate an endoscopy procedure, then with general anesthesia surgically a gastrostomy feeding tube is given to stomach. A balloon gastrostomy can replace these feeding tubes once the stoma tract is formed.

#### Radiologically Inserted Gastrostomy (RIG)

A gastrostomy tube given under X-ray (fluoroscopy or ultrasound) guidance and is usually indicated if the patient unable to perform an endoscopic procedure. It can be replaced by balloon gastrostomies once the stoma site has healed.

#### Balloon Gastrostomy

A balloon gastrostomy BGT is a feeding tube (FG10-24) given directly to the stomach through abdomen and held in place by an inflatable balloon. Gastric PH, frequency of tube use and fungal infection may affect the tube.

#### Low Profile Gastrostomy Device

Low profile gastrostomy device (LPGD) also known as button gastrostomy is a small device that fits near to the skin and is usually clenched by a balloon. It has the same function as a PEG but is less cumbersome, easier to conceal, less obtrusive and may be useful for those patients that pull at their gastrostomy. Extension sets are connected onto the "button" part to enable water, feed, or medications to be administered. Once completed, the extension set is removed. LPGDs can be inserted into most patients once a stoma tract is established but are usually used more frequently in children than adults.

#### Jejunostomy

A feeding tube is given directly into the jejunum in surgical method or through endoscopic method.

#### Gastrojejunostomy (PEG–J)

This is an extension of PEG and placed through endoscopic method it passed through the PEG to stomach and passed the pylorus to jejunum. It can be used in case of problem in gastric emptying (*guideline for the care and management of enteral feeding in adults*).

### Nursing Management

#### Meeting Nutritional Needs

All total nutritional requirement of the patient can be fulfilled by this route. After the gastrostomy surgery clear liquid can be given with 10% glucose. On first day only 30–60 mL can be given at one time and the amount can be increased afterward up to 180–240 mL as per the tolerance capacity of the patient and no leakage of fluid around the tube.

#### Providing Tube Care and Preventing Infection

Dressing will be given at the outlet of the gastrostomy tube. Daily observation should be done at the site of tube. Healthcare provider must check about the incision site, tube's placement, and rotates the tube to check the stabilization of the tube.

#### Providing Skin Care

The area near the gastrostomy need special attention as there may be chances of leakage of gastric juice near the tube. So daily cleaning of the area required with soap and water, removes the dead tissue and keep it dry. If there is no drainage and incision site heal completely a dressing may not require. If any skin problem exists, the patient should take an appointment with an enterostomal therapist or wound care specialist.

#### Enhancing Body Image

It may be one challenging issue for the nurses to enhance the body image of the patient who has gastrostomy feeding. Therapist must discuss with the patient and family member regarding the purpose of gastrostomy and daily routine of the feeding. Patient must verbalize his/her feeling towards body image and must be share with the person having the same.

#### Monitoring and Managing Potential Complications

The chances of potential complication may be there during post operative period.

It includes infection at the incision site, cellulitis, wound abscesses. So early identification is very much important to prevent infection and treat the same. If the gastrostomy tube is displaced or removed, the skin around the stoma will be cleaned and a sterile dressing will give, then tube will be placed as soon as possible as the stoma may close within 4–6 hours.

### Complications of Enteral Feeding

There are a number of complications may arise while giving enteral feeding (**Table 6.5**).

**Table 6.5:** Complications of enteral feeding.

| Complication | Causes |
|---|---|
| Diarrhea (most common) | • Hyperosmolar feedings<br>• Lactase deficiency<br>• Rapid infusion/bolus feedings<br>• Bacteria contaminated feedings<br>• Cold formula<br>• Medications/antibiotic therapy<br>• Decreased serum osmolality level<br>• Food allergies |
| Nausea/vomiting | • Change in rate<br>• Inadequate gastric emptying<br>• Hyperosmolar formula |
| Gas/bloating/cramping Dumping syndrome | • Air in tube<br>• Cold formula<br>• Bolus feedings/rapid rate |
| Constipation | • High milk (lactose) content<br>• Inadequate fluid intake/dehydration<br>• Lack of fiber |
| Aspiration pneumonia | • Improper tube placement<br>• Flat in bed<br>• Vomiting and aspirated tube feeding<br>• Use of large tube |
| Tube displacement | • Excessive coughing/vomitus<br>• Tracheal suctioning<br>• Tension on the tube or unsecured tube<br>• Airway Intubation |
| Tube obstruction residue | • Inadequate flushing/formula rate<br>• Flushing after administration<br>• Inadequate crushing of medications |
| Nasopharyngeal irritation | • Tube position/improper taping<br>• Use of large tubes |
| Dehydration and azotemia (excessive urea in the blood) | Hyperosmolar feedings with insufficient fluid intake |
| Tube feeding syndrome | • Excessive urea from high protein mixture and formulas lacking fat<br>• Dehydration |

All the complications must be taken care during the enteral feeding.

## Parenteral Nutrition

It is the method through which nutrition will get inside to human body through vein. The nutrition may include protein, carbohydrate, fat, mineral, electrolyte and trace elements.

### Indications

- Preoperative and postoperative patient
- Nonfunctioning gut (paralytic ileus)
- Any type of abdominal surgery
- Malnourished patient
- Patients with major resections of small intestine
- Critically ill patient
- Systemic inflammatory response syndrome (SIRS)
- Multiple organ failure (MOF)
- Specific conditions like mucositis following systemic chemotherapy
- Upper gastrointestinal fistulae or strictures

### Types

- Peripheral parenteral nutrition
- Central/total parenteral nutrition

Both are different in:
- Composition of feed
- Primary caloric source
- Potential complications
- Method of administration.

### Peripheral Parenteral Nutrition

Given through peripheral vein. it also depends upon the nutritional assessment, baseline weight, venous access evaluation and blood investigation.

Various vascular access devices are used to administer PN solutions in clinical practice. PN may be administered by either peripheral or central IV lines, depending on the patient's condition and the anticipated length of therapy. Through peripheral vein the peripheral parenteral nutrition (PPN) will be supplied. The solutions for PPN are very less hypertonic than PN solution. Through this method the concentration of dextrose will be less than 10% and all nutritional methods cannot be fulfilled by this method of nutrition. The maximum duration for PPN will be 5–7 days **(Hamilton, 2000)**.

### Indications

- Short term use
- Mildly stressed patients
- Needs large amounts of fluid
- Low caloric requirements
- Contraindications to central TPN.

### Central Parenteral Nutrition

The concentration of solution is five or six time more which is very dangerous to the intima of peripheral veins and may cause phlebitis. For this it is to be given through a large blood vessels by which the solution can be quickly diluted to isotonic levels by the blood inside the vessels.

## Types

Four types of **central venous access devices (CVAD)** are available:

1. **Non tunneled central catheters:**
   - It is used for short duration, not more than 30 days.
   - Mostly it is used in long term care, acute care, old age home and home care setting.
   - Percutaneous subclavian, Vas Cath, and Hohn catheters are the example.
   - Most common site is subclavian vein.
   - Other sites are jugular or femoral vein.
2. **Peripherally inserted central catheters (PICC):**
   - It is used for intermediate term, within 3–12 months.
   - Mostly used in hospital, home setting and long-term care.
   - Mostly the cephalic vein or basilica vein is used for PICC.
   - Blood sample and blood pressure will be avoided from the same extremity with PICC.
3. **Tunneled central catheters:**
   - It can remain for many years and used for long term purpose.
   - It will inserted through surgical method to the subclavian vein.
   - The distal part of catheter will remain to superior vena cava and 2–3 cm above the junction of right atrium.
   - Examples are the Hickman, Permacath and Goshong.
4. **Implanted ports:**
   - It is used long term home treatment.
   - Patient will get more freedom in this method.
   - It will be more expensive than others.
   - In this type of the catheter is connected to a chamber which is kept in subcutaneous pocket on the forearm or anterior chest wall.
   - Measurement of blood pressure and taking blood samples from the same extremity should be avoided.

## Nursing Management

- **Maintaining optimal nutrition:** All the nutritional values should be maintained through the parenteral nutrition. The nutritional values must be considered depending upon the condition of the patient, diagnosis, physician and dietician consultation. The pharmacologic requirement must be considered. Daily weight must be checked. Record of intake and output should be maintained carefully.
- **Preventing infection:** The chances of infection will be high if the patient is having long term purpose of parenteral nutrition than the short term purpose. Still daily supervision to be done to check for the sign of infection for every type of catheters. The main origin of the infection is the skin and the hub of the channel. So it must be cleaned everyday and dressing must be done in every alternative day. The site must be checked for redness, tenderness, leakage, kinked catheter, swelling or purulent drainage. The dressing must be done in a sterile technique.
- **Encouraging physical activity:** If the patient is physically active the only nurses can encourage for ambulation and activity. The person must be encouraged for certain type of exercise and physical activity which may not interfere with the existing catheter.

### Complications of Parenteral Feeding

There are a number of complications may arise while giving parenteral feeding **(Table 6.6)**. All the complications should be taken care during parenteral feeding.

**Potential benefits of enteral nutrition over PN include:**
- **Physiologic:**
  - Metabolization and utilization of nutrients will be more effective in enteral more than parenteral route.
  - The gut and liver help maintain the homeostasis of the amino acid pool as well as the skeletal muscle tissue.

**Table 6.6:** Complications of parenteral nutrition.

| Complication | Cause |
|---|---|
| Pneumothorax | Misplacement of the catheter and puncture of the pleura |
| Air embolism | • Tube disconnection<br>• Blocked segment of vascular system<br>• Cap missing from port |
| Clotted catheter line | • Inadequate heparin flushes<br>• Disruption of infusion |
| Sepsis | • Separation of dressings<br>• Infection at insertion site of catheter<br>• Contaminated solution |
| Catheter displacement and contamination | • Excessive movement, possibly with a nonsecured catheter<br>• Separation of tubing and contamination |
| Fluid overload | Fluid infusing rapidly |
| Hyperglycemia | Glucose intolerance |
| Rebound hypoglycemia | Feedings stopped too abruptly |

– The gut and liver process enteral nutrients before their release into systemic circulation."
- **Immunologic:**
  – Gut integrity is maintained by enteral nutrients through the prevention of bacterial translocation from the gut, systemic sepsis, and potential increased risk of multiple organ failure.
  – Lack of GI stimulation may promote bacterial translocation from the gut without concurrent enteral nutrition.
  – Provision of early enteral nutrition may minimize risk of gut related sepsis.
- **Safety (avoid complications related to intravenous access):**
  – Catheter sepsis
  – Pneumothorax
  – Catheter embolism
  – Arterial laceration
- **Cost:**
  – Cost of EN formula is less than PN.
  – Cost of equipment and personnel for preparation and administration is less.

## GASTROINTESTINAL BLEEDING

Gastrointestinal bleeding is one common disorder of gastrointestinal system. The bleeding is not only from the gastroduodenal part, but it can happen with any part of the gastrointestinal tract. It may be occult or overt **(Fig. 6.6)**.

### Definition

Gastrointestinal bleeding is defined as the bleeding originate from any gastrointestinal part includes mouth, esophagus to anus and rectum. It may be occult or overt.

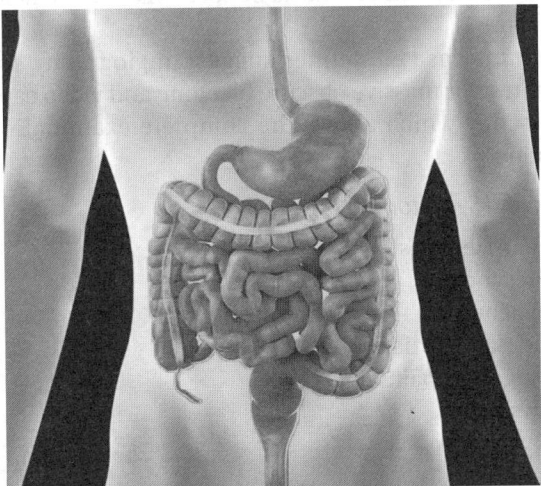

**Fig. 6.6:** Gastrointestinal tract bleeding.

### Classification

According to the location of the bleeding in the gastrointestinal tract it is divided into two types:
1. **Upper GI bleeding:** It is the bleeding from the upper gastrointestinal tract which is starting from mouth to duodenojejunal flexure (DJF) or ligament of treitz.
2. **Lower GI bleeding:** It is the bleeding from the distal part of the gastrointestinal tract, i.e., from duodenojejunal flexure or ligament of treitz to anus or rectum.

### Presentation of Gastrointestinal Bleeding

- **Hematemesis:** It is vomitus associated with red and coffee grounded blood material.
- **Melena:** It is presented as black, tarry and foul-smelling stool.
- **Hematochezia:** It is passage of bright red or maroon blood from rectum. It may be associated with stool.
- **Occult GI bleeding:** It can be diagnosed by absence of overt bleeding, presence of iron deficiency and by obtaining a fecal occult blood test.

### *Upper GI Bleeding*

It is the bleeding from the upper gastrointestinal tract which is starting from mouth to duodenojejunal flexure or ligament of treitz.

The incidence of upper GI bleeding is four times more than the lower GI bleeding.

The cause of upper GI bleeding may be two types:
1. **Variceal bleeding:** It is associated with the complication of liver disease, mostly from the portal hypertension.
2. **Nonvariceal bleeding:** It is mostly associated with peptic ulcer disease and other disease of upper GI tract.

According to anatomical location the causes can be:
- **Esophageal cause:**
  – Esophageal varices
  – Esophagitis
  – Esophageal cancer
  – Esophageal ulcer
  – Mallory-weiss tear
- **Gastric cause:**
  – Gastric ulcer
  – Gastric cancer
  – Gastric varices
  – Gastritis
  – Dieulafoy's lesions
- **Duodenal cause:**
  – Duodenal ulcer
  – Haemobilia
  – Vascular malformation

- Hemosuccus pancreaticus
- Superior mesenteric artery syndrome.
- **Esophageal varices:** It is the enlarged or abnormal dilation of esophageal vein. It is mostly due to portal hypertension.
- **Esophagitis:** It is the inflammation and irritation of esophagus. It is a common medical condition usually caused by gastroesophageal reflux. It may be infectious esophagitis, radiation esophagitis or from direct erosive effect from medication.
- **Esophageal cancer:** It can be defined as any kind of malignant cell found in esophagus.
- **Esophageal ulcer:** It is one type of peptic ulcer disease which can be found at the lining of esophagus mucosa.
- **Mallory-weiss tear:** Mucosal lacerations at the gastro esophageal junction GEJ or in the cardia of the stomach associated with repeated retching or vomiting.
- **Gastric ulcer:** It is one type of peptic ulcer that develop at the lining of the stomach mucosa.
- **Gastric cancer:** It is characterized by the development of cancer/malignant cell at the lining of the stomach.
- **Gastritis:** It is the irritation, inflammation and erosion of gastric mucosa.
- **Gastric varices:** It is the dilated submucosal vein in the stomach usually found in patient with portal hypertension.
- **Dieulafoy's lesions:** It is very uncommon but potentially life-threatening condition characterized by large tortuous arteriole nearly submucosal layer which may that erodes and bleeds. It can present in any part of the gastrointestinal tract.
- **Duodenal ulcer:** It is a sore or ulcer that will be found at the lining of duodenum or first part of abdomen.
- **Vascular malformation:** It may include aortoenteric fistula (AEF) which is the abnormal connection between the aorta and loop of the bowel which remains near to the aorta.
- **Hemobilia:** It defines the bleeding from the biliary tree.
- **Hemosuccus pancreaticus:** It defines the bleeding starts from the pancreatic ducts.
- **Severe superior mesenteric artery syndrome (SMAS):** This condition is very rare. It is characterized by the compression of the duodenum between two arteries (superior mesenteric artery and aorta).

## Lower GI Bleeding

Lower GI bleeding refers to bleeding from distal to ligament treitz to anus.

The majority of lower GI bleeding involves colon/rectum/anus. The bleeding sites from jejunum and ileum is very rare.

*Major Cause of Lower GI Bleeding*
- **Diverticulosis**
- **Colitis**
  - Inflammatory bowel disease
  - Intestinal ischemia
  - Infection
- **Angiodysplasia**
- **Neoplasia**
- **Anorectal**
  - Hemorrhoid
  - Fissure
- **Diverticulosis:** "A condition in which small, bulging pouches develop in the digestive tract."
- **Inflammatory bowel disease:** It is characterized by severe inflammation and ulceration of the colon and rectum. It is associates with two conditions like ulcerative colitis and Crohn's disease.
- **Intestinal ischemia:** It occurs when the blood flow to the intestine will slow down or stop due to blood clots or narrowing of arteries.
- **Angiodysplasia:** It is a small vascular malformation of GI tract, mostly at the caecum or ascending colon with multiple lesions.
- **Hemorrhoid:** It is one of the most common causes of lower GI bleeding. It is defined as the swollen and inflamed vein at the lowest part of rectum and anus.
- **Fissure:** It is also called anal ulcer. It is defined as a small tear in the lining of the anus.

*GI Bleeding of Obscure Origin*

Obscure gastrointestinal bleeding is defined as the continuous or recurrent bleeding with unidentified source by routine endoscopy or contrast X-ray study. It may be overt like melena or hematochezia or occult like iron deficiency anemia.

In this case guidelines suggest angiography as the initial test for massive obscure bleeding and video capsule endoscopy which allows the complete examination of intestine.

*Signs and Symptoms*
- Hematemesis
- Presyncope
- Syncope
- Hematochezia
- Epigastric pain
- Dyspepsia
- Dysphagia
- Jaundice
- Diffuse abdominal pain

- Weight loss
- Orthostatic changes in blood pressure and heart rate.

*Diagnostic Evaluation*

History collection

- A detail history to be collected from the patient regarding abdominal pain with duration of pain, severity, type and radiation of abdominal pain. History of vomiting and stool characteristic is to be evaluated.
- Features of heavy blood loss like shock, anemia and syncope and features of underlying cause like dyspepsia, jaundice and weight loss is to be assessed.
- Drugs history like NSAIDs, aspirin, corticosteroids, anticoagulants to be assessed as these may leads to gastrointestinal bleeding.
- History of epistaxis or hemoptysis to rule out the gastrointestinal bleeding.
- Past history of previous episode of gastrointestinal bleeding or any other chronic diseases like diabetes mellitus, chronic renal failure, coronary artery disease, chronic obstructive pulmonary disease or chronic liver failure is to be checked with any past abdominal surgery history.

Physical examination

- A general and systemic physical examination is to be done to detect any kind of abnormality. Due to heavy blood loss there may be tableplus, hypotension may be orthostatic hypotension may persists.
- Patient may experience signs of shock like cold extremities, tachycardia, hypotension, chest pain, confusion, delirium, oliguria, etc.
- There may be dry mucosa, sunken eyes, reduced skin turgor will present which denotes the signs of dehydration.
- If this condition will be associated with cirrhosis of liver or any bleeding disorder there may be palmar erythema, spider naevi, purpura, ecchymosis, muscle hematoma, etc.
- From digital rectal examination (DRE) there may be fresh blood, occult blood and bloody diarrhea.

Laboratory findings

- Complete blood count (CBC) is to be done to assess the blood loss.
- Blood should be checked for grouping and cross matching for possible blood transfusion as required by the patient.
- The hemoglobin level should be monitored frequently to identify the condition of the patient. Because it will provide the baseline for guiding further treatment also an unbalanced hemoglobin level may signify the ongoing hemorrhage requiring further investigation.
- The initial hematocrit may be normal and may not reflect the loss until 4–6 hours after fluid replacement, since initially the loss of plasma and RBCs is equal.
- Liver functioning test is to be done to determine the underlying cause of liver disease.
- The blood urea nitrogen (BUN) to creatinine ratio which increases with UGIB. A ratio of greater than 36 with a patient without renal disorder is indication of upper gastrointestinal bleeding.
- Prothrombin time (PT) and activated partial thromboplastin time should be checked to identify the presence of coagulopathy.
- All laboratory study to be monitored to estimate the effectiveness of treatment.

Endoscopy

- It is a procedure where a thin tube is inserted inside the body and internal organs can be observed through the camera which is fitted at the top of the tube. It is both diagnostic and therapeutic in nature.
- It is the initial diagnostic examination for all patients having GI bleeding presumed to have upper gastrointestinal bleeding. It should be performed immediately after hemodynamic stabilization and adequate monitoring of the patient.

Imaging

- **Chest X-ray:** Chest radiographs should be done to identify pleural effusion, aspiration pneumonia, and esophageal perforation.
- **Abdominal X-ray:** Erect and supine films should be ordered to exclude perforated viscous and ileus.
- **Computed tomography (CT) scanning and ultrasonography:** May be advisable for the identification of liver disease with cholecystitis, cirrhosis with hemorrhage, aortoenteric fistula pancreatitis with pseudocyst and hemorrhage, and other unusual causes of upper GI hemorrhage.
- **Nuclear medicine scans:** May be useful in determining the area of active hemorrhage.

Angiography

Angiography is used in diagnosing upper GI bleeding when endoscopy cannot be done or when bleeding persists after endoscopic therapy. Angiography is an invasive procedure requiring preparation and setup time and may not be appropriate for a high-risk, unstable patient. In this procedure, a catheter is placed into the left gastric or superior mesenteric artery and advanced until the site of bleeding is discovered.

## Nasogastric lavage

Nasogastric lavage is one important tool for diagnosis. Through this procedure we will be conformed about the recent bleeding, possible active bleeding by observing the gastric content. It must be done with alert and co-operative patient to avoid broncho pulmonary aspiration.

### Assessment of severity of gastrointestinal bleeding

*Interpretation*

Total score is to be calculated by addition:
- A score <3 carries good prognosis
- Total score >8 carries high-risk of mortality **(Table 6.7)**.

### Management of Upper GI Bleeding

Priority of management

- Protect airway, restore circulation and breathing.
- Find out the source of bleeding.
- Active treatment for the cause of bleeding.

Emergency management

- Assess the condition of the patient and protect the airway with required procedure.
- Monitor the vital signs in every 15–30 minutes.
- Two IV lines with 16/18-gauge needle is to be placed for the replacement of fluid and blood products, which can be assessed by physical and laboratory findings.
- Blood sample is to be taken for Hb, PT, PCV and cross match.

**Table 6.7:** Assessment of severity of gastrointestinal bleeding through rochall score.

| Variable | Criteria | Score |
|---|---|---|
| Age | <60 | 0 |
| | 60–79 | 1 |
| | >80 | 2 |
| Shock | No shock | 0 |
| | Pulse >100, SBP>100 | 1 |
| | SBP<100 | 2 |
| Co-morbidity | Nil major | 0 |
| | CHF, IHD, major morbidity | 2 |
| | Kidney failure, liver failure, metastatic cancer | 3 |
| Diagnosis | Mallory-weiss | 0 |
| | All other diagnosis | 1 |
| | GI malignancy | 2 |
| Evidence of bleeding | None | 0 |
| | Blood, adherent clot, spurting vessel | 2 |

- Replacement of circulation – mostly isotonic crystalloid solution will be started (e.g., lactated Ringer's solution). Packed RBCs, Whole blood, and fresh frozen plasma can be used to replace the volume in case of massive hemorrhage.
- When upper GI bleeding is less profuse, infusion of isotonic saline solution followed by packed RBCs permits restoration of the hematocrit more quickly and does not create complications related to fluid volume overload.

**Transfuse blood for:**
- Obvious massive blood loss
- Symptoms due to low hematocrit and hemoglobin
- Hematocrit< 25% with active bleeding supplemental oxygen may be delivered by face mask or nasal cannula will help to increase blood oxygen saturation.
- Patient to be monitored for the response to resuscitation frequently (HR, BP, peripheral temperature, urine output, capillary refill time CRT, level of consciousness)
- Urine output is one of the best measures of vital organ perfusion. Therefore, an indwelling urinary catheter is inserted so that output can be accurately assessed hourly. Watch for signs of fluid overload (raised jugular venous pressure (JVP), pulmonary edema, peripheral edema) NG tube and aspiration (will help differentiate upper from lower GI bleed).
- A central venous pressure line may be inserted for fluid volume status assessment. If the patient has a history of valvular heart disease, coronary artery disease, or heart failure, a pulmonary artery catheter may be necessary to monitor the patient.
- Keep the patient NPO for endoscopic procedure. Organize definitive treatment (endoscopic/ radiological surgical).

### Management of Nonvariceal Bleeding

- Emergency resuscitation to be done.
- Endoscopy is to be done within first 24 hours of bleeding for active treatment. It must be diagnostic and therapeutic in nature.
- Treatment will be administered if there will be active bleeding, adherent blood clots or visible blood vessels. The treatment option includes coagulation, injection and clipping, etc. If re-bleeds then arrange urgent repeat endoscopy.

Medical management

- The aim of drug therapy is to decrease bleeding, reduce and neutralize HCL secretion.
- Empiric IV proton pump inhibiter started before endoscopy which will decrease the amount of re-bleeding and help for endoscopic therapy.

- During endoscopy injection epinephrine (1:10,000 dilution) will be effective for active hemostasis which helps to produce tissue edema and produce pressure on the source of bleeding.
- H2-receptor blocker can be given to reduce acid secretion because acidic environment may impact on platelet function and interfere with clot stabilization.
- Somatostatin or octreotide can be given which helps in reducing blood flow to he gastrointestinal tract along with decrease Hcl secretion and release of gastrin.
- Vasopressin can be given which helps in vasoconstriction and reduce pressure in portal circulation, stops bleeding.
- If H-pyloric is positive, then eradication therapy is to be given.

### Surgical management

Surgical therapy is indicated when the patient not responded to medical and endoscopic management or there is ongoing bleeding despite of two endoscopic treatment. It may necessary when the patient continues to bleed after rapid transfusion of up to 2,000 mL of whole blood or remains in shock after 24 hours.

- Nature of operation depends on cause of bleeding.
- Example, under-running of ulcer (bleeding DU), wedge excision of bleeding lesion (e.g., GU), partial/total gastrectomy (malignancy)
- Peptic ulcer disease: Vagotomy and pyloroplasty to control bleeding.

### Management of Variceal Bleeding

The prime cause of variceal bleeding is liver cirrhosis. "Liver cirrhosis results in portal hypertension and development of porto-systemic anastomosis (opening or dilatation of pre-existing vascular channels connecting portal and systemic circulations)."

Emergency resuscitation to be done as described.

### Drugs

- **Somatostatin/octreotide:** Vasoconstricts splanchnic circulation and reduces pressure in portal system.
- **Terlipressin:** Vasoconstricts splanchnic circulation and reduces pressure in portal system.
- **Propranolol:** Used only in context of primary prevention (in those found to have varices to reduce risk of first bleed).

### Endoscopy

- Band ligation
- Injection sclerotherapy
- **Balloon tamponade:** Sengstaken-blakemore tube
- **Radiological procedure:** Selective catheterization and embolization of vessels.

### Band ligation

Endoscopic variceal ligation (EVL) is one endoscopic procedure where an enlarged vein or a varix in the esophagus will be tied off or ligated with the help a rubber band. It is also called rubber band ligation (RBL).

### Injection sclerotherapy

Endoscopic sclerotherapy procedure involves the passage of an injection of a sclerosing agent into or around esophageal varices with the help of endoscope **(Fig. 6.7)**.

### Balloon tamponade

It is a procedure in which a balloon is inflated within the esophagus or stomach through the endoscopy which help to create pressure on bleeding blood vessels, compress the vessels which causes bleeding and help to stop bleeding.

### Radiological procedure

This can be done if the patient will not respond the medical as well as endoscopic treatment.

"**TIPS procedure:** Transjugular intrahepatic porto-systemic shunt it is a shunt given between hepatic vein and portal vein branch to reduce portal pressure and bleeding from varices."

### Surgical management

- **Surgical portosystemic shunts (splenorenal):** Surgical portosystemic shunting, the formation of a vascular connection within the portal and systemic venous circulation, has been used as a treatment to decrease portal hypertension by decreasing portal venous pressure.
- **Liver transplantation:** It is a surgical procedure which removes the diseased liver which not functioning and replaces by a healthy liver from other person.

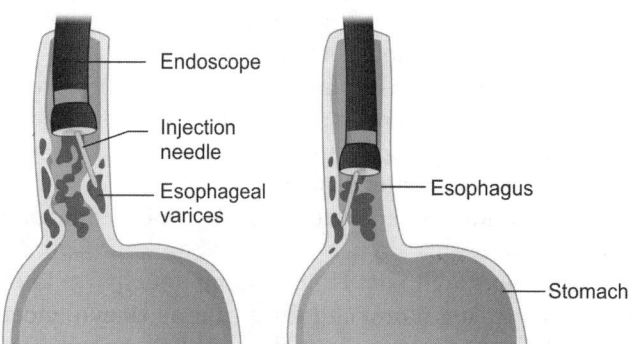

**Fig. 6.7:** Endoscopic sclerotherapy.

### Management of Lower GI Bleeding

- Emergency resuscitation to be done as described above.
- Stop NSAIDS/antiplatelets/anticoagulants as it may worsen the condition.
- First the patient will go through the upper GI endoscopy to evaluate the upper gastrointestinal bleeding.
- Then colonoscopy is to be done. It is both diagnostic and therapeutic in nature.

### Radiological

- **CT angiogram:** It is noninvasive diagnostic in nature. In this procedure X-ray will be used to give detail about heart and blood vessel also it can give the picture of narrowed or blocked blood vessels. It will determine site and causes of bleeding.
- **Mesenteric angiogram:** It is invasive, both diagnostic and therapeutic in nature. It helps to give the detail picture of the blood vessels that supply to small and large intestine. It determines the site of bleeding and allows embolization.

### Surgical

- **Subtotal colectomy:** It is also known as Lane's operation. In this procedure the part of colon will be removed without complete resection of the colon. It can perform where site of bleeding unclear.
- **Segmental colectomy:** It is a surgical procedure where a segment of a colon will be removed. It can be performed where site of bleeding is known.

### Nursing management

- **Nursing diagnosis:** Ineffective tissue perfusion related to GI bleeding/perforation/peptic ulcer disease evidenced by melena, hematemesis, hematochezia, abdominal pain.

  **Expected outcome:** To maintain tissue perfusion.
  **Nursing interventions:**
  - Assess vital signs, oxygen saturation, presence of bleeding and baseline laboratory values.
  - Administer fluid and electrolyte as prescribed to maintain hemodynamic.
  - Obtain the grouping and cross matching and administer blood as prescribed.
  - Monitor the sign of resuscitation.
  - Provide prescribed medication
  - Prepare the patient for indicated endoscopic procedures.

- **Nursing diagnosis:** Fluid volume deficient related to decreased blood and fluid volume as evidenced by hematemesis, melena, tachycardia, hypotension, weakness, nausea/or vomiting.

  **Expected outcome:** To maintain adequate fluid volume.
  **Nursing interventions:**
  - Assess the fluid and electrolyte status along with the nutritional status.
  - Strictly document intake and output chart.
  - Obtain the laboratory values specially the hemoglobin and hematocrit.
  - Provide fluid and electrolyte as need of patient.
  - Provide nutritionally balanced diet for nasogastric tube feeding.
  - Administer the prescribed medications
  - Administer the blood products with safety measures.
  - Close monitoring during blood transfusion
  - Evaluate the condition for shock and dehydration.
  - Prevent further complication.

- **Nursing diagnosis:** Acute pain related to GI perforation as evidenced by restlessness, irritability, report of pain.

  **Expected outcome:** To reduce pain and provide comfort.
  **Nursing interventions:**
  - Assess the level of pain and characteristic of pain.
  - Assess the factor contributing level of pain.
  - Provide comfort measure.
  - Provide nonpharmacologic pain management measures.
  - Plan for sleep and rest time.
  - Administer drugs as prescribed.
  - Evaluate the result of medication.

## ABDOMINAL INJURIES

Abdominal cavity contains so many organs and structures which may be injured, and these conditions may be very difficult to evaluate in clinical setting. The identification of severe chronic abdominal injury is really challenging situation in emergency department. It is of two types of blunt injury and sharp injury. From this, sharp injury or penetrating injury requires immediate medical attention than blunt injury.

### Causes of Abdominal Trauma

- Direct blow to abdomen
- Fall from height
- Child abuse
- Domestic violence
- Motor vehicle injury
- Seat belt injury
- Gunshot injury
- Stab injury
- Bomb blast injury
- Building crash injury

- Endoscopic procedure
- External cardiac compression
- Inadvertent esophageal intubation
- Bag mask ventilation.

Blunt abdominal trauma is more common in young population and also having more mortality and morbidity than other types of abdominal trauma mostly due to delayed in diagnosis, resuscitation and requirement of immediate surgical intervention.

## MECHANISM OF INJURY

### Blunt Injury

#### Deceleration

Rapid deceleration will make different in movement with other organs present in abdominal cavity. Due to which shear force will be created which cause tearing of organs at fixed point of attachment.

#### Crushing Effect

"Intra-abdominal organs will crushed in between anterior abdominal wall and vertebral column or posterior cage. This will create a crushing effect of organ involved mostly liver, spleen, kidney".

#### Compressive Effect

This condition may occur due to direct blow or due to external compression against a fix object like spinal column. it will cause a abrupt rise in intra abdominal pressure and will cause the rupture of hollow organs.

### Sharp Injury

In case of penetrating injury kinetic energy transmit to our body with low velocity, medium velocity and high velocity with different types of injury. The sharp injury severity depends upon the types of object or weapon, velocity of attack to abdomen, and distance between the abdomen and object.

### Clinical Presentation

The patient will show a wide range of clinical manifestation as per the location of the abdominal trauma **(Table 6.8)**.

### Clinical Assessment

- **History collection:** The main aim is to identify the trauma as the exclusive history may not be obtain and the resuscitation procedures to be carried out. However if possible detail history should be taken regarding event of accident and the history of patient's condition.
- **Physical examination:** First responsibility to check the hemodynamic stability by obtaining the vital signs recording. After that the examination to be done to check the abnormality like abdominal tenderness, distension, presence of contusion or abrasion, ecchymosis, rebound tenderness, dullness of abdomen or presence of bowel sound. The patient should be checked for presence of fracture in rib or vertebrae.
- **Diagnostic peritoneal lavage:** It is carried out by aspiration of free peritoneal blood on initial aspiration if it is 10 mL or more frank blood is there then it may be treated as positive.
- **Peritoneal lavage:** If diagnostic peritoneal lavage (DPL) is negative then peritoneal lavage will be carried out to check the condition.
- **X-ray:** Both abdominal and thoracic X-ray to be done to evaluate the site of injury. It can be carried out prior to CT scan.
- **CT scan:** It is necessary to detect the severity and source of injury and also helps in angiography and non operative management. It has more predictive ability of diagnostic peritoneal lavage for operative lesions. It also helps in unnecessary surgery.
- **Ultrasonography:** It is useful both blunt and penetrating type of trauma. It can identify the small amount of hemoperitoneum with good specificity.
- **MRI:** It is helpful for spinal cord injury or diaphragm muscle injury.
  Local wound investigation and laparoscopy can be carried out if necessary.
- **Sigmoidoscopy:** It can be done if the bleeding is present in rectal examination.
- **Magnetic resonance cholangiopancreatography (MRCP):** It is necessary to evaluate the common bile duct injury.

### Management

The main goal of management is to identify and treat the life threating condition.

It includes:
- A: Airway (with cervical spine precaution)
- B: Breathing
- C: Circulation
- D: Disability
- E: Exposure

### Emergency Care

- Initiate IV fluids as soon as possible and as patient's requirement.
- Any external bleeding is present that is to be controlled.
- Provide oxygen therapy with patient's requirement.

**Table 6.8:** Clinical presentation of abdominal trauma.

| Organ involved | Description | Clinical presentation |
|---|---|---|
| Diaphragm muscle | • It is commonly injured by sharp injury<br>• Tear of diaphragm muscle indicates multi organ involvement<br>• May cause due to increase intra abdominal pressure and lead to burst injury | • Acute chest pain<br>• Shortness of breath<br>• Peristalsis sound may be in thorax<br>• Bradypnea<br>• Difficult to diagnosis<br>• Multisystem trauma may be present |
| Esophageal injury | • Mostly due to penetrating injury than blunt injury<br>• May be associated with perforation or cervical spine injury | • Difficulty in swallowing<br>• Cervical tenderness<br>• Severe chest pain<br>• Associated with fever and peritoneal irritation. |
| Stomach injury | • Most common cause is penetrating injury<br>• Both anterior and posterior stomach wall are involved<br>• May happen due to complication of CPR<br>• Associated with gastric dilation | • Epigastric pain and tenderness<br>• Stomach content with bold stain<br>• Peritonitis may occur |
| Liver | • More in incidence of abdominal organ<br>• Common cause is blunt injury than sharp injury<br>• Mostly occur from vehicle crash and involved in gunshot | • Hypovolemic shock<br>• Dull abdomen<br>• Rebound tenderness<br>• Abdominal distension<br>• Peritoneal irritation |
| Spleen | • Involved in blunt abdominal trauma<br>• Involved in case of penetrating trauma to left upper quadrant | • Shortness of breath<br>• Peritoneal irritation<br>• Decreased blood pressure<br>• Abdominal pain and tenderness, more pain at the site of injury<br>• Dullness in percussion in flank region |
| Pancreas | • More common cause is penetrating injury as a result of stabbing and gunshot<br>• Blunt injury may be from steering wheel<br>• Associated with other organ damage inside the abdomen | • Pain at the site of injury<br>• Accompany with paralytic ileus<br>• Associated with nausea and vomiting.<br>• Epigastric pain will radiate to back may show later<br>• Abdominal tenderness |
| Intestinal injury | • Mostly injured by penetrating trauma by means of gunshot<br>• In case of small bowel incidence rate is high in proximal part of jejunum<br>• Sometimes fecal contamination may cause large bowel injury | • Abdominal pain<br>• Pain may radiate to shoulder, back and chest<br>• Peritoneal irritation<br>• Intestinal obstruction<br>• Abdominal tenderness<br>• Blood in rectal examination<br>• Fever |
| Retroperitoneal injury | • It may be the result of both blunt or penetrating trauma to anterior or posterior abdominal wall<br>• May be associated with lumbar vertebral injury and rib fracture<br>• Pancreas, kidney, ureters injury may be present | • Abdominal pain and tenderness<br>• Dull abdomen in percussion<br>• Turner's sign and Cullen's sign may present<br>• Movement restriction due to presence of fracture |

- Exposed organ to be protected with sterile dressing.
- Immobilized the part of fracture if present.
- Provide IV analgesic to reduce pain.
- Provide foley's catheter to record intake and output.
- Nasogastric tube gives for gastric lavage.

*Management as Organ Affected*

- **Diaphragmatic tear:** Surgically it will be repaired to prevent organ herniation in future.
- **Esophageal injury:** GI decompression with nasogastric tube followed by surgical repair of esophageal tear.

- **Gastric injury:** Gastrectomy may be needed as patient's requirement. It may be partial, total or subtotal.
- **Spleen injury:** Splenectomy is the choice when the patient is hemodynamically unstable.
- **Liver injury:** It may be managed surgically or nonsurgically as patient's condition. Other supportive therapy will be given.
- **Small and large bowel injury:** Surgical exploration and repair to be done in case of perforation or laceration is present. If necessary, colostomy is to be done.
- **Pancreatic injury:** Pancreatic drainage is to be done to prevent fistula and damage to other surrounding tissue.

*Supportive Treatment*

- **Nutritional therapy:** It can be provides through total parenteral nutrition and nasogastric feeding. The type and amount of feeding depends upon the patient's prognosis and health condition.
- **Blood and blood component transfusion:** After obtaining the result of blood investigation the necessary amount of blood and blood products is to be provided to meet the patient's demand.
- **Antibiotic therapy:** IV antibiotics may be provided in post operative period and to prevent from other complication.

*Nursing Management*

- **Nursing diagnosis:** Ineffective breathing pattern related to abdominal distention, surgical incision as evidenced by difficulty in breathing.
- **Expected outcome:** To maintain normal breathing pattern.

*Nursing Interventions*

- Assess the vital signs along with the characteristic of respiration.
- Assess the saturation of oxygen level.
- Administer oxygen as prescribed.
- Maintain semi fowler's or upright position.
- Encourage patient for deep breathing exercise.
- Demonstrate and encourage patient for incentive spirometry.
- Evaluate the patient for breathing difficulty.

## Nursing Diagnosis

Risk of hypovolemic shock related to (internal or external) bleeding.

**Expected outcome:** To prevent from hypovolemic shock.

*Nursing Interventions*

- Assess vital signs, check the level of consciousness and oxygen saturation.
- Assess the sign of dehydration through skin and mucous membrane.
- Closely observe for presence of external bleeding.
- Perform the necessary intervention for the cession of the external bleeding.
- Monitor the signs of internal bleeding.
- Administer the IV fluids as per the laboratory blood values and prescription to maintain the hydration status.
- Transfuse blood if it is prescribed.
- Monitor intake and output chart regularly.
- Reassess the condition after intervention.

## FULMINANT HEPATIC FAILURE

Acute liver failure (ALF) or fulminant hepatic failure (FHF) is characterized as rapid onset of hepatocyte dysfunction and associated with coagulopathy and neurologic dysfunction. The incidence rate of Fulminant hepatic failure is more in young individuals than others.

ALF is a clinical syndrome which result from necrosis of hepatocyte leading to hepatic encephalopathy and impaired synthetic function causing coagulopathy (INR >1.5) in individual with previous normal liver or compensated liver disease.

It is again subgroups as three types based on the duration of jaundice and onset of HE

- Hyperacute (less than 7 days)
- Acute (8–28 days)
- Sub-acute (5–26 weeks)

### Etiology

There are several existing causes are there for ALF, but the viral infection and toxin induced hepatitis is the leading cause for this.

### Viral Hepatitis

Hepatitis B virus (HBV) is considered as one of the most important causes for viral hepatitis. Hepatitis C virus (HCV) is very rare cause of acute liver failure and (HDV) hepatitis D virus can be an associated factor with HBV for acute liver failure. Sometimes HEV can lead to ALF in case of endemic areas (mostly seen in antenatal mother). Other viruses which are associated with ALF are herpes simplex virus, cytomegalovirus, Epstein bare virus, hemorrhagic fever virus and paramyxovirus. Autoimmune hepatitis is also one cause of ALF.

### Drug-related Hepatotoxicity

From various study it is cleared that acetaminophen (paracetamol) overdose is one of the common cause for hepatotoxicity. The other medicines are antidepressant, some kinds of antibiotics (doxycycline, erythromycin, isoniazid, tetracycline, ampicilline clavulanate), antiepileptics, NSAIDs, anesthetic agents, etc., also having the hepatotoxicity effect which may lead to ALF.

### Toxin-related Hepatotoxicity

The toxins like *Bacillus cereus* toxin, Yellow phosphorus, cyanobacteria toxin, *Amanita phalloides* mushroom toxin, organic solvents (e.g., carbon tetrachloride) is responsible for ALF.

### Vascular Causes

Vascular reasons are portal vein thrombosis, hepatic arterial thrombosis, hepatic vein thrombosis, ischemic hepatitis and hepatic veno-occlusive disease. These conditions are responsible for ALF.

### Malignancies

Both primary and secondary liver tumor or cancer is one of the cause for ALF.

### Metabolic Conditions

The metabolic conditions are Wilson disease, galactosemia, fructose intolerance, reye syndrome, alpha 1antitrypsin deficiency, etc., may lead to ALF.

### Others

Syndrome hemolysis, elevated liver enzymes, low platelets (HELLP) one conditions seen in case of antenatal mothers with pre-eclampsia and hypertension. Some herbal products may also lead for ALF and some cases it may be idiopathic.

## Pathophysiology

**It has been described in Flowchart 6.1.** In acute liver failure the pathophysiology depends upon the impact of various types of etiological factor. The prime factor for ALF is extensive destruction of hepatocytes which will activate the innate immune system which helps to produce the inflammatory mediators. When the inflammatory mediators go to systemic circulation that results other system disturbances and shows the clinical presentation of ALF. Simultaneously to compensate this condition anti-inflammatory condition develops within the liver cell with an aim to improve the hepatocytes regeneration and control the hepatocytes injury. During this condition the monocyte which is circulating in the systemic circulation may lower the ability to fight against infectious stimuli and the condition known as immune paresis. With a result this

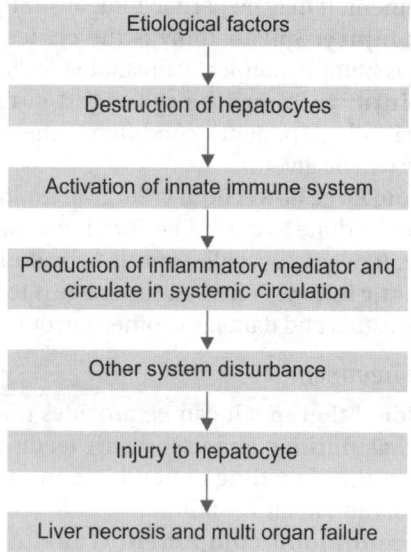

**Flowchart 6.1:** Pathophysiology of fulminant hepatic failure.

condition may refer to multi organ failure and sepsis as clinical presentation (**Flowchart 6.1**).

### Clinical Presentation

The patient primarily develops nausea and malaise, drowsiness, progressive jaundice, ascites, ankle edema, upper right abdominal pain and tenderness. The condition may be worsen with mental confusion, disorientation, muscle tremors, changes in personality, more prone to bleeding and bruising, tachycardia, hematemesis and coma. The person also shows hepatic coma and encephalopathy.

- Fetor hepaticus
  - Sweetish and mild fecal smell of breath
  - May proceed to coma
- Vascular spiders, skin change
- Palmar erythema (liver palms)
  - Hands are warm to touch and palms are bright red in color.
  - Attributed to estrogen excess.
- Symptoms of hormonal imbalances.
  - Reduce libido
  - Loss of hair
  - Failure to ovulation
  - Gynecomastia.

The total clinical presentation of ALF depends upon the degeneration of the hepatocytes and progressive MOF.

### Diagnosis

The patient detail history and physical examination is to be done for accurate diagnosis. The following points are to be assessed during history collection.

- Use of alcohol and medication
- Family history of any liver disease
- Previous history of hepatitis
- Other hepatic toxins
- Presence of jaundice
- History of immunization
- History of bleeding episode
- Features of hepatic encephalopathy

The following conditions to be assessed during physical examination:
- Anemia
- Onset and duration of jaundice
- Vital signs
- Mental status
- Splenomegaly, ascites, spider nevi, spider angioma, contractures, palmar erythema
- Unequal and fixed pupil (increased ICP)
- Hepatic tremor
- Fetor hepaticus
- Papilledema

The other blood investigations are:
- Routine CBC (thrombocytopenia, leukocytosis)
- Blood grouping and cross matching
- Arterial blood gas
- INR, APTT, fibrinogen
- Liver function test must include SGOT, SGPT, serum bilirubin level, ALT, AST, amylase, phosphate, albumin, LDH, alkaline
- Urea, creatinine
- Serum electrolyte (sodium, potassium, magnesium, chloride, calcium, phosphorus, and creatinine kinase)
- Blood sugar levels
- For cupper level (serum free copper, serum ceruloplasmin, 24 hr urinary copper)
- Serological marker (anti HAV IgM, anti HEV IgM, HBsAg, Anti H B Core IgM antibody and the other viruses like CMV (Cytomegalovirus), HSV (herpes simplex virus), VZV (Varicella zoster virus).
- Toxicology, acetaminophen screening
- Intracranial pressure monitoring.
- Autoimmune markers (antinuclear antibody, anti-smooth muscle antibody)
- Immunoglobulin

Other desirable investigations are:
- Trans jugular or percutaneous liver biopsy, electroencephalography (EEG), ultrasonography, CT brain.

## Management

The aim of management is to maintain the hemodynamic stability and to enhance the physiological function of liver.

### Supportive Management

Patient is to be admitted in hospital, if necessary, in ICU to maintain hemodynamic and ventilator support. To prevent volume depletion and hypovolemic syndrome fluid resuscitation has to be done. During the initial phase normal saline with crystalloid is recommended. The resuscitation process must be observed carefully to check the fluid overload.

Hypoglycemia is to be prevent by providing supplementary insulin. If patient develops hepatic encephalopathy (HE), wearly intubation is necessary.

### Pharmacological Therapy

- **Penicillin G:** Intravenous penicillin G is indicated in case of mushroom poisoning.
- **N-Acetylcysteine:** This drug is benefit during paracetamol over dose.
- **Osmotic diuretics:** Mannitol is the drug of choice in case of intracranial hypertension, which helps to reduce the cerebral edema.
- H2 receptor and PPI
- **Benzodiazepine:** It is used in mechanically ventilated patient foe sedation purpose.
- **Anesthetic agents:** Propofol may help to decrease cerebral blood flow.
- Sometimes phenobarbital is used in case of intracranial hypertension.
- Immunosuppressive will be benefit in autoimmune hepatitis.
- TIPS and anticoagulation in case the patient have Budd-Chiari syndrome.
- Antiviral medication for viral hepatitis and other viral infection
- Broad spectrum antibiotics to decrease the bacterial infection.
- Plasmapheresis can be useful in Wilsons disease.

### Liver Transplantation

Orthotopic liver transplantation procedure is one of the definitive therapy for ALF. The patient selection for liver transplantation is based upon King's College criteria which is widely used showing.

*King's College Criteria in ALF*

Acetaminophen-related ALF:
- Single criterion: pH b7.30 or lactate N3.0 mmol/L after adequate fluid resuscitation.
- Three criteria:
  1. Grade III–IV (West-Haven) HE
  2. INR N6.5
  3. Creatinine N3.4 mg/dL

Nonacetaminophen-related ALF:
- Single criterion: INR N6.5
- It is included in five criteria:
  1. Age <10 or >40 years
  2. Time from jaundice to coma >7 days
  3. INR >3.5
  4. Bilirubin >17.5 mg/dL
  5. Unfavorable etiology: Drug-induced, liver injury, Wilson disease, or seronegative liver injury.

### Nursing Management

**Nursing diagnosis:** Excess fluid volume related to excess intake of sodium, decreased plasma protein as evidenced by oliguria, difficulty in breathing, increase weight, edema.

**Expected outcome:** To maintain normal/stable fluid volume.

**Nursing interventions**
- Assess, report and record the patient's condition closely.
- Monitor intake and output strictly.
- Monitor the weight regularly to evaluate the weight gain.
- Assess the sign for dehydration and jaundice.
- Close monitor for oxygen saturation.
- Obtain the record of blood pressure and CVP (if available).
- Observe the sign of tachypnoea and dyspnea.
- Listen the lungs sound for any abnormal breath sounds.
- Observe for peripheral edema.
- Strictly avoid fluid and sodium intake.
- Provide rest and reduce physical activity.
- Provide anti diuretics or other medications as prescribed.

**Nursing diagnosis:** Imbalanced nutrition less than body requirement related to anorexia, indigestion, nausea or vomiting as evidenced by weight loss.

**Expected outcome:** To maintain the desire nutrition status.

**Nursing interventions**
- Assess the patient's nutritional status, weight, height and BMI.
- Evaluate the dietary intake and calory requirement for the patient.
- Involve the patient in meal planning to know the food preferences.
- Encourage the patient to eat and allow the family members to assist in feeding.
- Provide a small and frequent meals with supplementary feeding
- Encourage or assist in mouth care frequently.
- Provide rest period before meals.
- Maintain NPO, NG tube feeding and TPN as indicated.
- Restrict smoking, alcohol strictly to patient
- Obtain the laboratory values as required.
- Consult with doctor and dietitian for special type of diet.

### Complication
- Hepatic encephalopathy
- Cerebral edema
- Increased ICP
- Associated infection
- Hepatic coma
- Multi organ failure
- Metabolic disorder
- Electrolyte imbalance

### Patient Education
- Self-medication to be avoid (paracetamol)
- Make sure for the vaccine of hepatitis
- Avoid taking wild mushrooms.

## HEPATIC ENCEPHALOPATHY

Hepatic encephalopathy is an emergency life threatening neuropsychiatric syndrome usually happens as a complication of chronic liver disease or liver failure. It may be acute or chronic also it can be self-limiting or progressive. The condition may be represented mild confusion to deep coma.

### Definition

Hepatic encephalopathy is defined as brain dysfunction caused by liver insufficiency and/or portosystemic shunting which represents as psychiatric or neurological disturbances may range from confusion to coma.

The advance stage of hepatic encephalopathy shows as hepatic coma. Pathogenesis of this condition includes abnormal neurotransmission, neurotoxic effect of ammonia, inflammatory cytokines and astrocyte swelling.

### Risk Factors

A variety of factors are responsible for hepatic encephalopathy which includes the disorders which effect to the liver tissue. The important factor of hepatic encephalopathy is cirrhosis of liver. Approximately 50% of patient may develop this condition those who are diagnosed as cirrhosis of liver. The other responsible causes are hepatitis, portal hypertension and hepatocellular cancer. In this condition the blood circulation to the liver tissue is compromised by which the function of hepatocyte is restricted.

Other responsible factors are:
- Gastrointestinal bleeding
- Decrease amount of potassium by diuretics medication
- Drug toxicity by narcotics, sedatives, etc.

- Sepsis
- Vascular abnormality (Budd-Chiari syndrome)
- Nonalcoholic fatty liver disease
- Injury/trauma
- Electrolyte abnormalities
- Dehydration
- Intake of more amount of protein
- Renal failure
- Hypoxia
- Alcohol abuse
- Wilson's disease
- Metabolic disease like hemochromatosis, alpha-1 antitrypsin disease
- Autoimmune liver disease

## Pathophysiology

The exact pathogenesis of hepatic encephalopathy is still unclear. But still role of ammonia is considered as a prime factor for hepatic encephalopathy condition. Usually, ammonia is produced by gastrointestinal tract through digestion of protein which will carried out by portal circulation. Inside the liver hepatocyte metabolize the ammonia to urea through urea cycle and excrete from our body through urine.

In case of liver diseases the functioning capability of hepatocyte will be compromised which lead to increase in ammonia level and it will circulate in systemic blood circulation. The increase level of ammonia can cross the blood brain barrier and reaches to brain cell. Astrocytes are the only cell present within the brain cell which can able to metabolize ammonia. Here through astrocytic glutamine synthetase process glutamate and ammonia change to glutamine which is responsible for astrocyte swelling, dysfunction, increased intracranial tension and cerebral edema **(Flowchart 6.2)**.

There are various study proposed that the role neuro-inflammation, sepsis is also responsible for hepatic encephalopathy.

## Grading of Hepatic Encephalopathy

According to West Haven classification system there are total 5 grade of hepatic encephalopathy is described **(Table 6.9)**.

## Clinical Presentation

Hepatic encephalopathy is classified into two broad types, i.e., covert hepatic encephalopathy (CHE) and overt hepatic encephalopathy (OHE). Previously only grade 0 was considered as covert hepatic encephalopathy and grade I to grade IV was considered as overt hepatic encephalopathy.

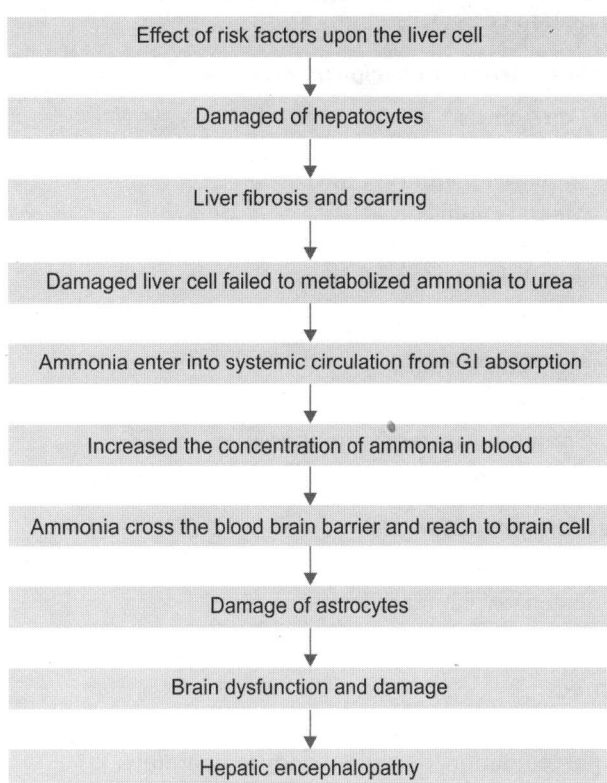

**Flowchart 6.2:** Pathophysiology of hepatic encephalopathy.

**Table 6.9:** West Haven classification system.

| Grade | Description |
|---|---|
| Grade 0 | It shows very minimal hepatic encephalopathy also known as covert hepatic encephalopathy or subclinical HE, very minimal alteration in personality, concentration, memory, behavior |
| Grade I | It can be described by trivial loss of consciousness, reduced attention, mild degree of confusion, depression, insomnia, euphoria, irritability, hypersomnia, not able to perform mental activity |
| Grade II | Apathy, lethargy, slurred speech, disturbed behavior, drowsiness, not able to perform mental activity, obvious asterixis, obvious change in personality, disorientation and somnolence |
| Grade III | It is described by somnolence, amnesia, confusion, disorientation of time and place, incomprehensive speech |
| Grade IV | Characterized by coma |

But now it is redrawn as grade 0 and I taken as CHE and grade II to IV as OHE.

### *Disturbances in Consciousness*
- Drowsiness
- Apathy
- Impaired memory/apraxia
- Mental confusion
- Disturbances in sleep cycle
- Somnolence
- Coma

### *Changes in Personality*
- Euphoric
- Sometime aggressive/outburst
- Fetor hepaticus (foul smelling)

### *Neurological Changes*
- Asterixis (flapping tremor)
- Extensor plantar reflex
- Exaggerated tendon reflex

### *Others*
Tremor, bradykinesia, shuffling gait, hepatic myelopathy, hyperventilation, decreased body temperature.

## Investigation
- History collection and physical examination a complete history to be obtained from patient on present and past illness with medication and previous surgery history. Physical examination along with mental status examination to be carried out to find out the abnormal sign and mental conditions.
- Laboratory investigation routine investigation like CBC, LFT, KFT, urea, creatinine, prothrombin time, albumin and globulin ratio is to be carried out. An increased blood ammonia level is reported in patient with HE. Elevated level of serum bilirubin and prolonged PT may be associated with HE.
- Imaging cerebral edema can be identified through MRI and CT scan may be helpful for to recognize the CVA and subdural hematoma conditions. Chest and abdominal radiograph to be done to assess the chest infection/lungs involvement and bowel obstructions.
- EEG it will show generalized slowing and increased amplitude of brain waves. The findings are not specific for HE but helpful in altered mental status and cirrhosis conditions.
- Different neuropsychological test—it will help to identify the disturbance in memory, attention and motor skill. It is useful in case of minimal HE.

## Differential Diagnosis
- Intracranial lesion (tumor, abscess, subdural hematoma, stroke, intracranial bleeding).
- Metabolic encephalopathy (uremia, electrolyte imbalance, hypoglycemia, anoxia).
- Toxic encephalopathy from alcohol and drugs.
- Organic brain syndrome.

## Management
The main aim of management are to identify and removing the precipitating cause and to reduce level of ammonia absorption.

### *Supportive Treatment*
- Hospitalization with life support procedures to be maintained.
- NG tube feeding and bladder to be catheterized.
- IV fluid initiated to maintain fluid and electrolyte imbalance.
- Diuretic treatment is to be stopped.
- Enema can be given to reduce ammonia absorption from GIT (Gastrointestinal tract).
- Protein restricted and high glucose diet is to be given.

### *Specific Treatment*
- **Decrease of nitrogenous load:** Lactulose given to decrease serum ammonia level by excretion through stool. It helps to reduce the colonic PH and decrease the absorption and synthesis of ammonia. It is known as primary drug choice for HE.
- **Antibiotics (rifaximin):** It is one broad spectrum antibiotics used for HE with minimal systemic absorption. Along with neomycin, metronidazole, and vancomycin can be benefited with the patient with HE. The long-term use of these medication is to avoid as there is having risk for nephrotoxicity and ototoxicity.
- **Maintain amino acid and metabolic imbalance:** For this patient should be given IV or oral administration of BCAA (branched chain amino acid).
- Drugs to be given for the stimulation of metabolic ammonia metabolism. The desired drugs are sodium benzoate, l-ornithine l-aspartate (LOLA), acylcarnitine aspartate and zinc sulphate.
- **Probiotics and prebiotics:** It has the benefit on intestinal flora.
- **Nutrition:** Small and frequent meals to be given to the patients along with late night snacks. The oral BCCA nutrition to be provide the patient with HE. Daily protein intake is to be 1.0–1.5 g/kg as patient's condition. If the person is protein intolerance additional nitrogen supplementation is to be provided.

- **Other treatment:** Large portosystemic shunt embolization help the patient to improve HE with the patient with cirrhosis. Liver transplantation is another option for the patient with chronic or refractory HE.

## Nursing Management

### Nursing Diagnosis

Impaired social interaction related to disorientation, drowsiness as evidenced by mood swing, increase sleeping time.

**Expected outcome:** To improve social interaction.

### Nursing Interventions

- Assessment of neurologic status daily mental status examination is to be assessed to check the condition of the patient.
- Level of consciousness, neurological reflexes, restlessness and agitation to be assessed regularly.
- Observe daily handwriting is to be assessed as it will worsen with the increase in ammonia.
- Involve family members in treatment regimen.
- Reorient the patient frequently and provide a calm and therapeutic environment.

### Nursing Diagnosis

Risk for aspiration related to comatose as evidenced by decreased GCS and not responding to stimuli.

**Expected outcome:** To prevent aspiration

### Nursing Interventions

- Assess the level of consciousness, level of GCS.
- Monitor the laboratory investigation of LFT, BUN, Sr. electrolytes.
- Assess the nutritional status and the nutritional requirement.
- Monitor the deep tendon reflexes along with swallowing reflex.
- Provide NG tube feeding/TPN as indicated to maintain the patients nutritional status.
- Encourage sitting or semi sitting position during NG tube feeding.

### Nursing Diagnosis

Acute confusion related to altered cerebral metabolism as evidenced by cognitive dysfunction.

**Expected outcome:** To reduce agitation and improve cognitive function.

### Nursing Interventions

- Assess the level of consciousness, orientation to time place and person, along with level of confusion.
- Provide the treatment for underlying cause.
- Maintain cerebral tissue perfusion.
- Provide safe and calm environment.
- Monitor the fluid and electrolyte balance.

### Other Nursing Interventions

- Assessment of fluid and electrolyte Intake of lactulose will increase the bowel activity and it may cause the fluid and electrolyte imbalances.
- Intake and output is to be checked with daily weight record. Along with dehydration and hypovolemia is to be assessed.
- Nosocomial infection is to be prevent.
- Monitor other associated infection.
- Monitor serum ammonia value regularly along with diet intake.
- Closely assess the development of coma.
- Administer prescribed dose of medication.
- Care should be taken to prevent bleeding.
- Record vital signs frequently.
- Patient education is to be given regarding diet, and home care management.

## ACUTE PANCREATITIS

Acute pancreatitis is an acute inflammation of the pancreas.

The degree of inflammation ranges from mild edema to severe hemorrhagic necrosis. It is common in middle-aged men and women and affects women and men equally. The rate of pancreatitis in African Americans is three times higher than in whites.

It can be a medical emergency associated with a high risk for life threatening complications and mortality. It is commonly described as autodigestion of pancreas.

In case of mild pancreatitis, the inflammation remains within pancreas and minimal organ dysfunction will present and returns to normal within 6 months. In milder form of pancreatitis there is risk of hypovolemic shock, sepsis, fluid and electrolyte imbalance but in case of severe pancreatitis the pancreatic tissue will become necrosis and it may spread to retroperitoneal tissue.

### Etiology

The most common cause of acute pancreatitis is gall bladder disease mostly in case of women and chronic alcohol consumption in case of men.

### Biliary Tract Disease

The most common cause is presence of gall stone which goes to the bile duct and remain at the sphincter of oddi.

It is assumed that acinar cell destruction occurs leads to increase the pancreatic duct pressure caused by the obstruction at the ampulla of vater.

### Alcohol

It is the major cause of pancreatitis. Due to long term use of alcohol. At the cellular level, ethanol helps to intracellular deposition of digestive enzymes and their premature activation and release. At the ductal level, it help to increases the permeability of ductulus, which permits enzymes to reach the parenchyma and makes pancreatic tissue damage. Ethanol helps to produce more protein content of pancreatic juice and decrease the level of bicarbonate levels and trypsin inhibitor concentrations. It will help to formulate the protein plug and ceases the pancreatic juice outflow.

### Abdominal Trauma

It causes pancreatic injury both in blunt and penetrating injury.

### Endoscopic Retrograde Cholangiopancreatography

Repeated endoscopic retrograde cholangiopancreatography (ERCP) or faulty procedure of ERCP may cause pancreatitis.

### Drugs

Certain kinds of drugs may interfere the pancreatic tissue with their toxic effect. Some drugs may be "azathioprine, sulfonamides, sulindac, tetracycline, valproic acid, didanosine, methyldopa, estrogens, furosemide, 6-mercaptopurine, pentamidine, 5-aminosalicylic acid compounds, corticosteroids, octreotide, etc".

### Infection

Other infectious disease may cause pancreatitis. For example, it may be cytomegalovirus (CMV), Epstein-Barr virus (EBV), varicella-zoster virus (VZV), hepatitis virus and some bacteria may be *mycoplasma pneumoniae, mycobacterium tuberculosis, salmonella, campylobacter*.

### Hypercalcemia

It can cause acute pancreatitis.

#### Developmental Abnormality of Pancreas

- **Pancreas divisum:** It is one type of congenital problem where the dorsal and ventral pancreatic ducts not able to join together to fuse during the time of embryogenesis.
- **Annular pancreas:** It is very rare congenital malformation in which a band of pancreatic tissue surrounds the second part of the duodenum.

### Tumors

The pancreatic duct may have obstruction due to presence of any kind of tumor like solid pseudotumor of the pancreas, pancreatic ductal carcinoma, sarcoma, ampullary carcinoma, lymphoma, islet cell tumor, cholangio-carcinoma, etc. It may cause acute pancreatitis.

### Toxins

Any kind of toxin exposure like organophosphate insecticide, Scorpion and snake bites will cause acute pancreatitis.

### Surgical Procedures

It may occur in post operative surgery of different kinds of surgery mostly in case of abdominal surgery.

### Vascular Abnormalities

Both ischemia and vasculitis may cause acute pancreatitis **(Table 6.10)**.

- **Autoimmune pancreatitis:** Inflammation of pancreas due to autoimmune disease condition.
- **Hypertriglyceridemia:** Serum triglyceride level more than 1,000–2,000 mg/dL is risk factor for acute pancreatitis.
- **Hereditary pancreatitis:** Risk of pancreatitis may pass from generation to generation.

### Pathophysiology

**Premature activation of pancreatic enzyme** within the pancreas leads the autodigestion of pancreas cell. The pancreatic enzyme supposed to activate in the intestine but due to etiology it activates inside the pancreas **(Flowchart 6.3)**. It may be the result of obstruction in the pancreatic duct due to presence of gall stone in common bile duct and blocking the flow of pancreatic juice. it helps to activate the enzymes inside the pancreas rather than intestine. Activation of enzyme within pancreas may lead to increase vascular permeability, vasodilation, necrosis, and hemorrhage.

*Flowchart of Pathophysiology*

See **Flowchart 6.3.**

### Signs and Symptoms

- Severe acute abdominal pain characterized by acute onset, deep, continuous or steady and sharp abdominal pain.
- Pain starts from left upper quadrant of abdomen or may be mid epigastrium and radiates to back due to the retroperitoneal anatomical location of pancreas.

**Table 6.10:** Mnemonic for risk factors of acute pancreatitis. "I get smashed".

| I | Idiopathic |
|---|---|
| G | Gallstones |
| E | Ethanol |
| T | Trauma |
| S | Steroids |
| M | Mumps |
| A | Autoimmune |
| S | Scorpion/snakes |
| H | Hyperlipidemia/hyperglycemia |
| E | ERCP |
| D | Drugs |

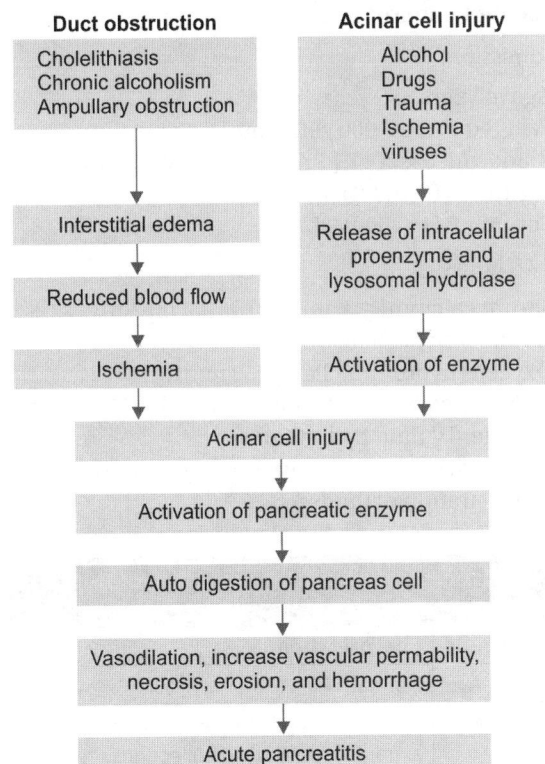

**Flowchart 6.3:** Pathophysiology.

- Abdominal pain may be associated with abdominal tenderness and muscle guarding.
- Pain will be aggravated with meals and alcohol, more often onset in recumbent position and not relived by vomiting and antacid.
- A board like or rigid abdomen may develop
- Nausea and vomiting (mostly gastric origin or bile stained)
- High grade and low grade fever
- Hypotension and shock (due to massive fluid shifts into the retroperitoneal space)
- Tachycardia
- Jaundice
- Decreased or absent bowel sound
- In case of severe abdominal distension paralytic ileus may occur
- Acute renal failure
- Hypoxia and respiratory distress
- Abnormal lungs sound (mostly crackle sound)
- Abnormal ABG
- Hypocalcemia
- Disseminated intravascular coagulopathy (DIC)
- Mental confusion and agitation
- Shallow breathing
- Myocardial depression
- Hyperglycemias
- Patient may do the position of flexion of supine to relieve the abdominal pain.
- Ecchymosis of flank area or bluish flank discoloration known as Gray Turner's sign
- Ecchymosis of periumbilical area or bluish periumbilical discoloration known as cullen's sign. It happens due to leakage of blood stained fluid from pancreas.

### Diagnostic Evaluation

*History Collection*
- A detail history to be collected from the patient regarding abdominal pain with duration of pain, severity, type and radiation of abdominal pain. History of vomiting and hypovolemic shock is to be evaluated.
- Features of shock, difficulty of breathing, mental condition and features of underlying cause like dyspepsia, jaundice and weight loss is to be assessed.
- A full history of alcohol and drugs intake is to be obtained.
- Past history chronic diseases like diabetes mellitus, coronary artery disease, chronic renal failure, chronic liver failure or chronic obstructive pulmonary disease is to be checked with any past abdominal surgery history.

*Physical Examination*
- A general and systemic physical examination is to be done to detect any kind of abnormality. Due to hypovolemic shock there may be feable#pulse, hypotension may be orthostatic hypotension may persists.
- **Abdomen** is to be examined for distension, gray turner's sign and Cullen's sign.
- Patient may experience signs of shock like cold extremities, tachycardia, hypotension, chest pain, confusion, delirium, oliguria, etc.

- Respiratory pattern is to be examined to detect any kind of abnormal respiratory patten.

## Laboratory Findings

- **Plasma amylase:** It is one of the important investigation for acute pancreatitis where it will increased more than four times from the normal level. This condition is known as hyperamylasemia.
- **Isoenzyme:** Helps to differentiate between pancreatic enzyme and nonpancreatic enzyme. In case of acute pancreatitis level of amylase increases in between 2 and 3 hours, peaks at 12–24 hours and come back to normal level after 3–5 days. If the level will not decrease after 5 days then it may be associated with pseudocyst of pancreas.
- **Plasma lipase:** The level of plasma lipase increases between 4–8 hours, highest level at 24 hours, and may continue for 10–14 days.
- **C-reactive protein (CRP):** It is considered as gold standard for assuming the severity of acute pancreatitis. It may be useful to detect the prognosis of the disease.
- **Procalcitonin:** It is also one indicator for pancreatic infection.
- **ABG (arterial blood gases):** It may show hypocapnia, hypoxia and lactic acidosis.
- Hypocalcemia
- Hypomagnesemia
- Hyperglycemia (due to more secretion of glucagon, glucocorticoids and reduce insulin secretion)
- Hyperbilirubinemia,
- Increased plasma enzyme levels (e.g., LDH, AST, ALP)
- Hyperlipidemia
- Hypoalbuminemia
- Increased urinary amylase
- Renal function test
- Liver functioning test
- Increased anion gap
- Complete blood count
- Leukocytosis more than 15,000/mm$^3$.

## Diagnostic Imaging

- **Abdominal X-ray (plain):** It is to be done to differentiate the other cause of abdominal issue.
- **Abdominal CT:** It is considered as gold standard of acute pancreatitis. It will reveal the mild moderate and severe pancreatitis and carried out between 3–10 days of the symptoms.
- **Magnetic resonance cholangiopancreatography (MRCP):** It will help to evaluate pancreaticobiliary tree. It can be performed when ERCP will fail to diagnose the condition.
- **Abdominal ultrasonography:** It will help to detect peritoneal fluid, disease in common bile duct and presence of cyst or abscess.
- **Chest X-ray:** It is helpful to evaluate the ARDS, pleural effusion and other associated lungs disease.
- **Endoscopic ultrasonography (EUS):** It is a mixture of ultrasonography and endoscopy which gives detail picture of internal abdominal organs. This procedure will be helpful when CT scan and MRI is not recommended to the patient (like metallic implantation, antenatal mother, patient not able to mobilize.)
- **Endoscopic retrograde cholangiopancreatography (ERCP):** It is the most important diagnostic and therapeutic tool which help to diagnose the disease as well as treat the condition. The requirement of ERCP is described **(Table 6.11)**.

*Ranson Score for Acute Pancreatitis*

### For alcohol pancreatitis

On admission:

- Age in years >55 years
- WBC count >16,000 cells/mm$^3$
- Blood glucose > 11.11 mmol/L (>200 mg/dL)
- Serum AST >250 IU/L
- Serum LDH >350 IU/L.

After 48 hours:

- Serum calcium <2.0 mmol/L (<8.0 mg/dL)
- Hematocrit fall > 0%
- Oxygen (hypoxemia PaO$_2$ <60 mmHg)
- BUN increased by 1.8 or more mmol/L (5 or more mg/dL) after IV fluid hydration.
- Base deficit (negative base excess) >4 mEq/L
- Sequestration of fluids > 6 L

**Table 6.11:** CT scan grading for interpretation of acute pancreatitis.

| S. No. | Grade | Interpretation |
|---|---|---|
| 1. | A | Normal |
| 2. | B | Focal/diffuse pancreatic edema with small extra-pancreatic fluid collections |
| 3. | C | • Any of the above<br>• Peripancreatic inflammation and <30% pancreatic necrosis |
| 4. | D | • Any of the above<br>• Single extra-pancreatic fluid collection and 30–50% pancreatic necrosis |
| 5. | E | • Any of the above<br>• Extensive extra-pancreatic fluid collection and >50% pancreatic necrosis |

**For gallstone pancreatitis**

On admission:
- Glucose >220 mg/dL
- Age >70 years
- LDH >400 IU/L
- AST >250 IU/L
- WBCs >18,000/mm³.

After 48 hours:
- S Calcium < 8 mg%
- Hematocrit >10%
- Base deficit > 4 mEq/L
- BUN >2 mg%
- Sequestrated fluid >6L.

Interpretation:
- If the score ≥3, severe pancreatitis likely.
- If the score <3, severe pancreatitis is unlikely.

Or:
- Score 0–2: 2% mortality
- Score 3–4: 15% mortality
- Score 5–6: 40% mortality
- Score 7–11: 100% mortality

## Management

Approximately 85–90% of acute pancreatitis may subside within 4–7 days. It will include total collaborative care for the patient. It may include.
- Relief of pain
- Reduction of pancreatic secretion
- Prevention of shock
- Prevention and treatment of other associated infection
- Control of fluid and electrolyte imbalance
- Removal of precipitating factor

### Conservative Therapy

- **Pain management:** IV Pethidine is given with morphine to reduce pain. Patient with severe pain local analgesic or epidural narcotics can be given. Pain medication can be given with antispasmodic agent such as nitroglycerine or papaverine.
- **Supplementary oxygen:** In acute pancreatitis oxygen saturation should be maintain 95%.
- **NPO:** All oral ingestion is to be withheld to reduce the pancreatic activity to reduce pancreatic enzyme secretion.
- **Nasogastric suctions:** Patient should remain NPO and nasogastric suction is to be done to decompress the gastric content. It also helps to reduce nausea and vomiting.
- **Total parenteral nutrition (TPN):** All the nutritional requirement is to fulfilled through parenteral route.
- **Histamine-2 (H2):** Antagonist can be given to reduce pancreatic action by inhibiting HCl acid secretion.
- **Proton pump inhibitor:** It will help to reduce HCl secretion.
- Serum glucose level will be monitored for hyperglycemia.
- Maintain of fluid and electrolyte imbalance with iv fluids like RL and other electrolytes solutions.
- If shock will be present then blood and blood products can be given.
- CVP reading to be taken to be identify the requirement of fluid and electrolyte.
- Vasoactive drugs may be given patient with hypotension.
- Carbonic anhydrase inhibitor helps to neutralize the HCl secretion and reduce production and secretion of pancreatic enzyme and bicarbonate.
- Pancreatic enzyme product can be given to replace the pancreatic enzyme.
- If diabetes is present the insulin therapy can be given.
- In case of chronic illness hemodynamic monitoring and ABG monitoring is to be done.
- **Antibiotics:** Prophylactic antibiotics now recommended with patient to reduce infection.
- **Respiratory care:** Patient may have risk for pulmonary effusion, shifting of diaphragm, etc., for that close observation of the respiratory pattern to be checked. It may range from oxygen supplementation, intubation and mechanical ventilation.
- **Nutritional management:** A small frequent feeding is to be given which will be high in carbohydrates. Supplemental fat-soluble vitamin therapy is to be given. Patient needs abstain from alcohol and smoking.

### Surgical Therapy

If the patient not respond to the conservative therapy, with gallstone, diagnosis is not sure and patient with pseudo cyst or abscess then surgical therapy may be indicated for patient.
- **ERCP with sphincterotomy:** In case of gallstone this procedure can be done through endoscopic method.
- **Percutaneous drainage of pseudocyst:** This procedure can be carried out if the patient has pancreatic abscess or pseudocyst.
- The "**Whipple procedure (pancreaticoduodenectomy)** is an operation to remove the head of the pancreas, the first part of the small intestine (duodenum), the gallbladder and the bile duct. The remaining organs are reattached to allow to digest food normally after surgery".

## Nursing Management

### Nursing Diagnosis

Acute pain related to inflammatory process of pancreas as evidenced by pain scale and verbalization.
**Expected outcome:** To alleviate pain and discomfort.

Nursing interventions

- Periodically pain is to be assessed by pain scale.
- Identify the aggravating and reducing factor of pain.
- Provide bed rest to bedrest during acute pain or provide comfortable position like knee flexed and leaning forward.
- Provide comfort measures and diversional activities with prescribed analgesics is to be provided.
- Reassess the level of pain and comfort.

### Nursing Diagnosis

Ineffective breathing pattern related to ascites, abdominal distention as evidenced by tachypnoea, restlessness.
**Expected outcome:** To maintain normal breathing pattern.

Nursing interventions

- Assess the vital signs, characteristics of breathing pattern.
- Provide semi Fowler's or Fowler's position.
- Assess oxygen saturation level and capillary refill time.
- Provide oxygen supplementation as indicated.
- Oxygen saturation and ABG to be monitored regularly.
- Encourage the patient for deep breathing exercise.
- Arrange for peritoneal lavage if it is indicated to reduce abdominal distention.

### Nursing Diagnosis

**Nutritional alternation:** Less than body requirement related to anorexia, abdominal distention.
**Expected outcome:** To maintain nutritional balance.

Nursing interventions

- Assess the nutritional status and nutritional requirement of the patient.
- Monitor the fluid and electrolyte status of the patient along with laboratory values.
- Parenteral nutritional is to be maintained carefully.
- Offer frequent mouth care. Resume oral intake with a clear liquid diet and if indicated can be provided high protein and high carbohydrate diet.
- Supplemental vitamins A, D, E, and K to be provided with pancreatic replacement enzyme.

### Continuing Care

Monitor the patient for presence of other infection like peritonitis, respiratory tract infection, enteritis. Observe the sign of mental confusion, hyperglycemia, renal failure and intestinal obstruction. During post operative period special attention to be given to minimize infection. Instruct the patient for follow up care.

## INTESTINAL OBSTRUCTION

Acute intestinal obstruction is the most common emergency condition in the world which need emergency management. It occurs approximately 15% of all emergency condition.

### Definition

Intestinal obstruction occurs when there will be interruption or blockage of the normal passage of the bowel content. It may occur partial or complete, may be at small intestine or large intestine, simple or strangulated **(Table 6.12)**.

### Mechanical Obstruction

it is otherwise known as dynamic obstruction. In this type of obstruction, the cause of occlusion in the lumen can be detect **(Table 6.13)**. It is most common in small bowel obstruction and the surgical adhesion is the common one.

### Functional Obstruction

It is otherwise known as adynamic obstruction which occurs mostly due to the vascular or neuromuscular disorder. The common form of this type obstruction is paralytic obstruction where peristalsis sound is absent. It may be in case of:

- Postoperative period of 24–72 hours
- Presence of any infection
- Uremic and hypokalemia condition

### Pseudo-obstruction

The cause of the obstruction cannot be detect by radiological investigation. Mostly idiopathic in nature but neurologic, endocrine and vascular disorders may have greater role for pseudo-obstruction. Vascular obstruction occurs when cessation of blood supply to the part of intestine (emboli and atherosclerosis of mesenteric arteries).

### Pathophysiology

Approximately 6–8 liters of fluids enters in the intestine and absorbs in the colon. Intestinal obstruction is manifested by dilatation of the proximal segment from the site of obstruction and distal part of obstruction will be collapsed. Proximal part contains mostly air, fluid and intestinal content. To maintain homeostasis there will be hyper peristalsis movement to pas the intestinal content downward. This condition may help to develop dehydration as there is fluid loss by means vomiting and bowel edema.

**Table 6.12:** Broad classification of intestinal obstruction.

| According to anatomical position | Small bowel obstruction | • It involves the proximal and distal part of small bowel<br>• It may be acute onset<br>• Vomiting frequent |
|---|---|---|
| | Large bowel obstruction | • It involves all over the large bowel<br>• It may be longer onset<br>• Vomiting is rare or absent |
| According to degree of obstruction | Partial obstruction | • Intestinal lumen constricted<br>• Presence of bowel movement and allows some intestinal content |
| | Complete obstruction | • Intestinal lumen completely obstructed<br>• May occur complete obstipation by means of simple obstruction, strangulation and closed loop |
| According to causes | Mechanical or dynamic | • A detectable obstruction of the intestinal lumen with presence of peristalsis movement |
| | Functional or a dynamic | • Mechanical cause is absent with intestinal atony where peristalsis movement also absent |

**Table 6.13:** Causes of mechanical obstruction.

| Extramural | Intramural | Intraluminal |
|---|---|---|
| • Hernias<br>• Tumor<br>• Volvulus<br>• Congenital deformity<br>• Adhesions | • Inflammatory bowel disease<br>• TB<br>• Tumors<br>• Intussusceptions<br>• Lymphomas | • Presence oh gallstone<br>• Presence of other foreign object<br>• Impacted feces |

Vomiting may cause decrease in potassium, chloride ion, hydrogen of stomach content. Again more dehydration will help to increase renal re absorption bicarbonate and loss of chloride which may lead metabolic alkalosis.

The proximal part of obstruction the intraluminal bowel pressure increases due to persistent of abdominal distension. The increase pressure cause rise in capillary permeability. It will cause retention of fluid in peritoneal cavity. This condition leads to decrease in blood volume circulation results hypotension and hypovolemic shock **(Flowchart 6.4)**.

Decrease amount of blood circulation makes ischemia to bowel tissue, may cause necrosis and perforation. The stasis of intestine leads to overgrowth of intestinal flora and cause more infection.

*Clinical Presentation*
- Colicky abdominal pain, abdominal distention.
- Abdominal pain usually in center in small bowel obstruction and lower abdomen in large bowel obstruction.
- Severe abdominal pain, rigidity and tenderness in case of strangulation and peritonitis.

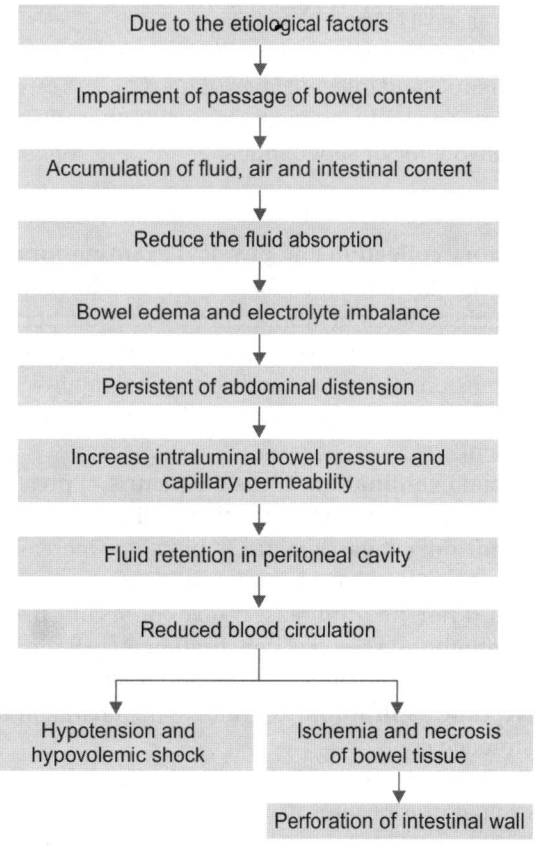

**Flowchart 6.4:** Pathophysiology of intestinal obstruction.

- Nausea and vomiting.
- Small intestine obstruction projectile vomiting occurs with bile.
- If obstruction is proximal vomiting is more frequent than distal obstruction.

- Vomitus with foul smell feculent material denotes chronic obstruction.
- Patient may pass mucus and blood instead of stool or flatus.
- Visible peristalsis in case of proximal loops.
- Acute obstruction increase peristalsis later it will reduces.
- Abdominal bloating due to accumulation of gas and chyme.
- High peach gurgling sound in abdomen.
- Decrease absorption of nutrition and vitamins leads to weakness and fatigue.
- Dizziness and headache may occur.
- Feeling exhaustion and drowsy with normal activity.
- Dehydration due to diarrhea and vomiting.
- Imbalance body fluids and electrolytes.
- Accumulation of fluid in body may leads to decrease urine output.
- Constipation may be absolute or relative.
- Increased TLC or leukopenia.
- Increased body temperature denotes inflammation, ischemia, and intestinal perforation.
- Decreased body temperature or hypothermia denotes hypovolemic or septic shock.

## Investigation

- **History collection and physical examination:** It may indicate the abnormal findings related to obstruction like observation of prominent veins, visible peristalsis, hernial orifice, pervious surgical marks, abdominal distension, tenderness and abdominal rigidity, muscle guarding, bowel sound may be loud and high pitch or absent.
- **Rectal examination:** Gives the picture of presence or absence of fecal material with bleeding.
- **Laboratory investigation:** It may show increase WBC count for infection, electrolyte imbalance for vomiting and ddiarrhea, increased level of serum urea and creatinine as a result of dehydration. Also there may be increased serum amylase, metabolic alkalosis.
- **NG tube aspiration:** To evaluate the characteristic of stomach content.
- **Radiology investigation:** Abdominal and chest X-ray to evaluate the location of obstruction and the collection of fluid or gas. For abdominal X-ray both supine and a erect position X-ay should be taken for adequate diagnosis. There may be ladder like dilation, small diameter and central distension present with small bowel obstruction and large diameter and gross distension and haustral folds present with large bowel obstruction.
- **Contrast study:** Barium enema will help to evaluate intussusception or colon obstruction and oral barium study able to identify ileus.
- **Sigmoidoscopy or colonoscopy:** Help to identify the location of obstruction with presence of tumor or stricture.
- **Abdominal CT scan and ultrasonography:** It may be helpful in patient with history of cancer, previous history of gastro surgery or idiopathic nature.

## Management

Aim of management should be to make stable the patient, manage fluid and electrolyte, prevent the cause and progress of infection, reduce the obstruction and prevent further complication.

### Medical Management

- NG tube suction to decompress the GI tract.
- Maintain the fluid and electrolyte with ringer lactate and potassium as required by the patient.
- If necessary TPN is to be initiated.
- Desired broad-spectrum antibiotic given to treat infection.
- Antiemetic to relive the nausea and vomiting.
- Diuretics provided to reduce fluid retention.
- Analgesic medication to control pain and abdominal discomfort.
- If indicated stool softener can be provided.
- In case of malignance stents can be given through endoscopic method to maintain the patency of intestine. Also colonoscopy method may be helpful to remove tumor, polyps and dilate the stricture.

### Surgical Management

Indication of surgery may be:
- Strangulation
- Irreducible hernia
- Failure of medical management

**Surgical procedures depend upon the site and type of intestinal obstruction**
- Enterotomy indicated in case of foreign body.
- Resection of bowel for obstruction due to lesion or strangulation then end to end anastomosis occurs.
- Temporary ostomy may be provided if it is indicated.
- Other procedures include lysis of adhesions and reduction of hernia, intussusceptions and volvulus.
- If fecal impaction is present, it can be removed digitally with enema but the fecal concretion can be removed with laparotomy as it causes complete obstruction.

*Nursing Management*

Nursing diagnosis

Acute abdominal pain related to inflammation and constipation as evidenced by facial grimacing, pain scale, patient's report.

**Expected outcome:** To provide comfort and reduce pain.

*Nursing interventions*
- Provide NG tube suction to empty the stomach.
- Assess the pain characteristics and level of pain and provide comfortable position.
- Ambulation and mobilization done to relive the gases and improve peristalsis movement.
- Prescribed medication to be administered to relieve pain.

Nursing diagnosis

Ineffective breathing pattern related to abdominal distention.

**Expected outcome:** To maintain normal breathing pattern.

*Nursing interventions*
- Assess the vital signs and oxygen saturation level.
- Monitor respiratory pattern with ABG value.
- Provide Fowler's position to increase ventilation and relieve abdominal distention.
- Oxygen can be given if indicated.

**Other responsibility includes:**
- Maintenance of normal bowel pattern.
- Monitor intake output chart regularly.
- Monitor vital signs with skin condition.
- Monitor the level of electrolytes and other parameters.
- Provide required iv fluids with electrolyte replacement.
- Detect early signs of peritonitis, such as rigidity and tenderness, in an effort to minimize this complication.
- Monitor for signs of shock, pallor, hypotension, tachycardia.
- Monitor for metabolic alkalosis and metabolic acidosis.
- Maintain the nutritional status as required by the patient's condition.
- Take necessary measures to relive fear and anxiety.
- Provide necessary post operative care.

## PERFORATED PERITONITIS

Peritoneum is the largest serous membrane of the body. It consists of two layer: (1) Parietal layer and (2) Visceral layer. Each layer consists of areolar connective tissue covered by mesothelium or simple squamous epithelium. This mesothelium secrets serous fluid which helps the both layer in contraction and relaxation without friction.

### Definition

Peritonitis is defined as the inflammation of peritoneum which may be local or general and may result from infectious and noninfectious agents.

Performative peritonitis occurs due to any perforation in the gastrointestinal tract. This condition is also one common surgical emergency.

### Classification
- Infected or noninfected peritonitis
- Primary or secondary peritonitis

### Infected Peritonitis

It may cause due to any kind of infection to the peritoneum. The main cause will be the perforation of the GI tract. That may include:
- Perforation of lower esophagus
- Perforation of stomach (stomach carcinoma, stomach ulcer)
- Perforation of duodenum (duodenal ulcer)
- Perforation of intestinal tract
- Gallbladder perforation

*Others*
- Septicemia
- Any abdominal surgery
- Abdominal trauma
- Intraperitoneal dialysis
- Peritoneal chemotherapy

### Noninfected Peritonitis

It may occur any kind of chemical or fluid leakage from the organ of GI tract to the peritoneum.

It may include:
- *Bile* extravasated due to trauma or diseases of the gallbladder.
- *Gastric juice* leaked from perforation of stomach.
- *Pancreatic secretions* released from pancreas in acute hemorrhagic pancreatitis.
- *Barium sulfate* from perforation of bowel during radiographic studies.

### Primary Peritonitis

Primary peritonitis is caused by the spread of an infection from the blood and lymph nodes to the peritoneum.

### Secondary Peritonitis

Secondary peritonitis is the more common type of peritonitis, happens when the infection comes into the peritoneum from the gastrointestinal or biliary tract.

## Causative Organism

- E. coli
- Streptococci
- Staphylococci
- Clostridium
- Klebsiella
- Chlamydia
- Gonococcus
- Pneumococcus

## Routes of Inflammation

- **GI perforation:** Any kind of perforation of gastrointestinal tract will cause of infection to the peritoneum as the fluids or juice of the specific organ will come in contact with peritoneum.
- **Exogeneous contamination:** It may include any kind of drain, abdominal trauma, etc.
- **Transmural bacterial translocation:** It means the transmission of the bacteria from the adjacent organ like inflammatory bowel disease, gastritis, etc.
- **Genital tract infection:** Any type of infection to the genital tract may lead to spread of microorganism to peritoneum.
- **Hematogenous spread:** The microorganism may get entry to the peritoneum through infected blood stream, like septicemia.

## Risk Factors

- **Stomach ulcer, perforated colon and ruptured appendix:** These condition may allow the entry of bacteria to the peritoneum.
- **Peritoneal dialysis:** It is considered as the tertiary peritonitis because the equipment used in dialysis and the peritoneal catheter may lead the risk of contamination to the peritoneum.
- **Pancreatitis:** The infection of pancreas may spread to the peritoneum and cause inflammation.
- **Abdominal trauma:** It will allow the direct contact of the microorganism through the trauma.
- **Liver disease:** Due to liver failure there will be accumulation of fluid in the peritoneum known as ascites and that will cause of peritonitis.
- Injury caused by surgery.
- **Diverticulitis:** If one of the infected pouches rupture the infection may transmit to another abdominal organ including peritoneum.
- Weakened immune system.

## Pathophysiology

Peritoneum mostly covers the organs of abdomen and pelvic cavity. The inflammation may cause due to the leakage of fluid from the organ present adjacent to peritoneum as a result of infection process, trauma, perforation, tumor or ischemia. After that the bacterial proliferation will start. Due to bacterial proliferation the involved tissue will became edema and fluid exudation developed. The fluid becomes turbid with more number of protein, cellular debris, blood and white blood cell. For maintaining the balance, the acute response will be hypermobility of intestinal tract which may lead to paralytic ileus gradually due to presence of air and fluid. Further the fluid will become suppurative and pus formation will be there which will create an adhesion, later may form as fibrous tissue or band **(Flowchart 6.5)**.

## Clinical Manifestations

- **Increased temperature:** It is otherwise known as hot belly, as due to the inflammatory response the body temperature remains high.
- **Abdominal pain and tenderness:** Initially a diffuse type of abdominal pain will be there then the pain will be localized, constant and having more intensity around the site of inflammation. The pain may increase with motion, pressure and touch.
- Abdominal rigidity due to accumulation of air and fluid.
- Abdominal distension and bloating.
- Loss of appetite.
- Nausea and vomiting.
- Reduce urine output.

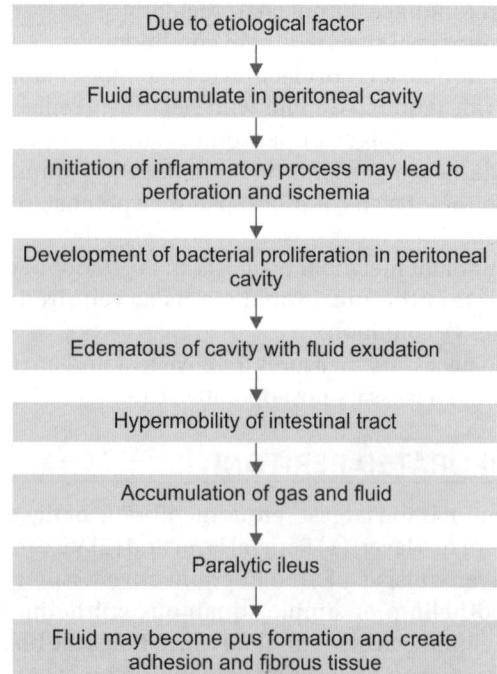

**Flowchart 6.5:** Pathophysiology of peritonitis.

- Sinus tachycardia.
- Increased pulse rate..
- Abdominal guarding
- Board like abdomen.
- Constipation or empty rectum due to intestinal obstruction.
- Unable to pass gas.
- Auscultation results less or absent peristalsis movement due to paralytic ileus.
- In long duration dehydration and the symptoms of shock may present.
- Blumberg sign/rebound tenderness this refers the examiner gently press the abdomen with hand and abruptly release. The person feels worse pain during releasing the pressure from the abdomen than pressing the abdomen.

## Diagnostic Evaluation

- **History taking:** A complete history to be taken regarding the previous disease, ongoing medication, any family disease, nutritional status and other co morbid factor. Special history of peritoneal dialysis should be taken.
- **Physical examination:** Complete head to foot examination is need to identify the sign and symptom related to peritonitis.
- **Blood investigation:** CBC can give the picture of increased WBC
- **Serum electrolyte:** It may result the altered level of sodium, potassium and chloride.
- **Blood culture:** It may be helpful if there is bacterial blood contamination.
- **Radiological findings:** Erect X-ray of abdomen may show the air under the diaphragm and supine X-ray may show the distended bowel loop.
- **Ultrasonography and CECT:** Of abdomen may helpful to localize the infection and perforation. It also helps to identify the abscesses and fluid collection.
- **MRI scan:** Used if necessary.
- **Peritoneal fluid analysis:** This fluid may be examined for increased white blood cell and presence of other bacteria.
- **Urine RE/ME and culture:** To rule out the infection.

## Medical Management

### General Management

- **Bed rest:** The person affected in peritonitis must be advised to hospitalized and take bed rest.
- **NPO:** This is required to minimize the GI activity and reduce the peritoneal irritation.
- **Respiration support:** Mostly patient associated with abdominal distension which may cause respiration difficulty. So the respiration support must be given through oxygen administration and others.
- **IV therapy:** Administration of required amount of IV fluid should be done to correct the fluid and electrolyte alteration. It depends upon the patient's condition and the laboratory values.
- **Urinary catheter:** One urinary catheter must be attached to the patient and monitoring of intake and out put should be done.
- **Intubation and suction:** In this method the abdominal pressure will be released and abdominal distension can be corrected.

### Pharmacologic Management

- **Antibiotics:** Initially this can be given to the patient through intravenous and intra peritoneum route. It may depend upon the result of c/s test of blood and peritoneal fluid sample, e.g., ampicillin.
- **Antipyretics:** Helps to reduce the fever
- **Analgesics:** Helps to reduce the abdominal pain and peritoneal irritation.
- **Antiemetics:** May also indicated.

### Specific Treatment

- **GI decompression:** A tube will be inserted to the stomach and intestine through nasopharynx or oropharynx then removal of the content can be done by suctioning.
- **Peritoneal lavage:** In this procedure a catheter is inserted to the peritoneal cavity to aspirate peritoneal fluid, known as diagnostic peritoneal aspiration (DPA), then with the same catheter fluid can be given to the peritoneal cavity for lavage purpose, known as diagnostic peritoneal lavage (DPL).
- **Paracentesis:** It is a therapeutic and diagnostic procedure where a needle will inserted to the peritoneal cavity and the fluid is to be collected or drained.

### Surgical Management

There is no specific surgery for peritonitis but to treat the cause may need surgical intervention specially in case of secondary peritonitis. It may include removal of etiology and infection. These are may be excision and resection with or without anastomosis and if necessary drainage.

### Nursing Management

*Nursing Diagnosis*

Acute pain related to peritoneal trauma, accumulation of fluid as evidenced by pain scale, patient's report.

**Expected outcome:** To reduce pain and provide comfort.

**Nursing interventions**
- Assess the level of pain, characteristic of pain and factor affecting to pain.
- Monitor the vital signs.
- Provide comfort measures and upright position.
- Administer pain medications as prescription.
- Provide rest and calm environment.
- Engage with other diversional therapy.

*Nursing Diagnosis*

Fluid volume deficiency related to vomiting, fluid accumulation in peritoneal cavity as evidenced by dry skin, oliguria.

**Expected outcome:** To maintain normal fluid volume.

**Nursing interventions**
- Assess the vital signs for hypotension and tachycardia.
- Record patient's intake and output.
- Observe for peripheral edema and abdominal distention due to fluid accumulation.
- Assess the condition of skin to evaluate the level of dehydration.
- Administer fluid and medication as prescribed.
- Plan with physician for GI decompression procedure.

*Nursing Diagnosis*

Risk for infection related to weaken immune system, invasive procedure, recurrent peritoneal dialysis.

**Expected outcome:** To prevent infection.

**Nursing interventions**
- Monitor vital signs to evaluate the sign of sepsis.
- Strictly maintain aseptic procedure during each peritoneal dialysis.
- Assess the dialysis fluid for any abnormality to detect the signs of inflammation.
- Keep the patient and his surroundings clean.
- Monitor the WBC value regularly.
- Administered antibiotics as prescribed.
- Monitor the drainage and tubes attached to the patient.
- Provide necessary health education regarding home management on surgical incision care and self care to prevent infection.

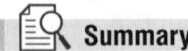
## Summary

This chapter deals with the emergency management of common gastrointestinal disorder. Skill full nursing assessment and correct diagnosis is highly essential for all the nurses to manage these conditions and to provide the desired nursing care to the patient. A detail medical and surgical history is to be taken from the patient which will help to aid in prognosis of the condition. Regular observations is to be done to prevent the complications.

## Points to Ponder

- **Ligament of treitz** is the part where we can divide upper and lower gastrointestinal bleeding.
- **"TIPS procedure:** Transjugular intrahepatic porto-systemic shuntit is a shunt given between hepatic vein and portal vein branch to reduce portal pressure and bleeding from varices."
- **Hematochezia** is the fresh blood in stool.
- **Volvulus:** Volvulus occurs when a loop of intestine twists around itself and the mesentery that supplies it, causing a bowel obstruction.
- **Intussusceptions:** Intussusception is a serious condition in which part of the intestine slides into an adjacent part of the intestine.
- **Grey Turner's sign** refers to bruising of the flanks, the part of the body between the last rib and the top of the hip.
- **Cullen's sign** is described as superficial edema with bruising in the subcutaneous fatty tissue around the periumbilical region.
- **Kehr's sign:** In supine position move the patient's arm to upward direction. Assess for referred pain to left shoulder. It may be positive in case of spleen injury, renal calculi and ectopic pregnancy.
- **Murphy's sign:** Instruct the patient for deep breathing, palpate the mid clavicular line below the costal angel. Observe for pain and breathing restriction. It may be positive in cholecystitis or cancer in gallbladder.
- **McBurney's sign:** McBurney's Point is present at the level of two third away from umbilicus to anterior-superior iliac spine. Deeply and slowly palpate over the point and assess for the presence of pain.
- **Obturator's sign:** Place the patient in supine position and flex right leg at knee and hip. Place one hand above the knee and others at the ankle, then rotate externally and internally. Note the pain at hypogastric region.
- **Rovsing's sign:** The Rovsing's sign is positive when patient complains pain in right lower quadrant while applying pressure on patient's left lower quadrant.
- **Psoas's sign:** In supine position of patient, place one hand over right lower thigh and instruct the patient to raise right leg by flexing hip while examiner will push downward. Evaluate pain in right lower quadrant.

## Abbreviations

- HCL : Hydrochloric Acid
- LES : Lower Esophageal Sphincter
- NSAID : Nonsteroidal Anti-inflammatory Drugs
- RLQ : Right Lower Quadrant
- RUQ : Right Upper Quadrant
- LUQ : Left Upper Quadrant
- LLQ : Left Lower Quadrant

- CVA : Costovertebral Area
- CEA : Carcinoembryonic Antigen
- MRI : Magnetic Resonance Imaging.
- MRCP : Magnetic Resonance Cholangiopancreatography
- EGD : Esophagogastroduodenoscopy
- ERCP : Endoscopic Retrograde Cholangiopancreatography
- MRCP : Magnetic Resonance Cholangiopancreatography
- PEG : Percutaneous Endoscopic Gastrostomy
- BGT : Balloon Gastrostomy
- LPGD : Low Profile Gastrostomy Device
- PPN : Peripheral Parenteral Nutrition
- CVAD : Central Venous Access Devices
- PICC : Peripherally inserted central catheters
- AEF : Aortoenteric Fistula
- SMAS : Severe Superior Mesenteric Artery Syndrome
- CRT : Capillary Refill Time
- JVP : Jugular Venous Pressure
- RBL : Rubber Band Ligation
- EVL : Endoscopic Variceal Ligation
- TIPSS : Transjugular Intrahepatic Portosystemic Shunt
- DPL : Diagnostic Peritoneal Lavage
- FHF : Fulminant Hepatic Failure
- ALF : Acute Liver Failure
- PTT : Partial Thromboplastin Time
- SGOT : Serum Glutamic-oxaloacetic Transaminase
- SGPT : Serum Glutamic Pyruvic Transaminase
- ALT : Alanine Transaminase
- AST : Aspartate Aminotransferase
- LDH : Lactate Dehydrogenase
- CMV : Cytomegalovirus
- HSV : Herpes Simplex Virus
- VZV : Varicella-Zoster Virus
- EEG : Electroencephalography
- HE : Hepatic Encephalopathy
- GIT : Gastrointestinal Tract
- BCAA : Branched Chain Amino Acid
- LOLA : Lornithine–Laspartate
- EBV : Epstein-Barr virus
- DIC : Disseminated Intravascular Coagulopathy
- EUS : Endoscopic Ultrasonography

## Short Answer Questions

1. Explain types of enteral feeding.
2. Describe peritoneal lavage.
3. Enlist the etiology of gastrointestinal bleeding.
4. Describe pathophysiology of fulminant hepatic failure.
5. List out complications of parenteral feeding.
6. Describe different presentation of gastrointestinal bleeding.
7. Classify the abdominal trauma.
8. Describe the risk factor of hepatic encephalopathy.
9. Discuss pathophysiology of acute pancreatitis.
10. Explain nursing responsibility with a patient diagnosed as fulminant liver failure.
11. Enlist the types of peritonitis.
12. List out the types of endoscopic diagnostic studies.
13. Classify the intestinal obstruction.
14. Describe the surgical intervention for intestinal obstruction.
15. Explain the routes of inflammation for peritonitis.
16. Describe Ranson's score for pancreatitis.
17. List out the risk factor for acute pancreatitis.

## Long Answer Questions

1. Mr Saroj admitted in emergency with the diagnosis of acute pancreatitis.
   a. Define acute pancreatitis and describe the pathophysiology.
   b. Explain the diagnostic criteria for acute pancreatitis.
   c. Explain the nursing management of Mr Saroj in the ICU in the first 48 hours with the help of a nursing care plan.
2. a. Define intestinal obstruction and describe the types of intestinal obstruction.
   b. Explain the management in detail with a patient diagnosed as intestinal obstruction.
3. Define hepatic encephalopathy. Write in detail regarding the causes and clinical presentation of hepatic encephalopathy. Explain the management of patient with hepatic encephalopathy.
4. Explain in detail regarding GI bleeding and the management of GI Bleeding.
5. What is peritonitis? What will be the nursing management for a patient with peritonitis?

## Multiple Choice Questions

1. **Which of the following disease is an inflammation of the liver cells?**
   a. GERD
   b. Gastritis
   c. GI bleeding
   d. Hepatitis

2. **Which disorder occurs when motility through the intestine is blocked by a mechanical obstruction?**
   a. Hiatal hernia
   b. Peritonitis
   c. Intestinal obstruction
   d. Paralytic ileus

3. **Peritoneal lavage is the procedure of:**
   a. Aspiration of peritoneal fluid
   b. Aspiration of GI fluid
   c. Administration of medication to stomach
   d. Administration of fluid to peritoneal cavity

4. **An example of an H2 receptor blocker is:**
   a. Pantop
   b. Ornidazole
   c. Ranitidine
   d. Aspirin

5. **Melena is:**
   a. Black tarry stool
   b. Skin pigment
   c. Exocrine hormone
   d. Red color stool

6. **Complication of pancreatitis include the following:**
   a. Pseudocyst
   b. Diabetes mellitus
   c. Deficiency of fat soluble vitamins
   d. All of the above

7. **Stone in bile duct is known as:**
   a. Jaundice
   b. Cholangitis
   c. Choledocholithiasis
   d. Cholelithiasis

8. **Asterix is the:**
   a. Flapping tremor
   b. Severe abdominal pain
   c. Increase PH level
   d. Blood in stool

9. **Nurse is taking vital signs of client admitted with acute pancreatitis. Nurse must aware with the fifth vital sign:**
   a. Anorexia
   b. Pain
   c. Fatigue
   d. Insomnia

10. **An obstruction in bile duct causes _____**
    a. Jaundice
    b. Malaria
    c. Cholera
    d. Acidity

## Answer Key

| 1. | (d) | 2. | (c) | 3. | (a) | 4. | (c) | 5. | (a) |
| 6. | (d) | 7. | (c) | 8. | (a) | 9. | (b) | 10. | (a) |

### Keypoints

Gastrointestinal bleeding, pancreatitis, hepatic encephalopathy, peritonitis, intestinal obstruction, fulminant hepatic failure.

## Bibliography

1. Acharya SK, Panda SK, Saxena A, Gupta SD. Acute hepatic failure in India: A perspective from the East. J Gastroenterol Hepatol. 2000;15(5):473-9.
2. Anders CJ. Abdominal injuries. Postgrad Med J. 1967;43(503):582-6.
3. Berisavac II, Jovanović DR, Padjen VV, Ercegovac MD, Stanarčević PD, Budimkić-Stefanović MS, et al. How to recognize and treat metabolic encephalopathy in Neurology intensive care unit. Neurol India. 2017;65(1):123-8.
4. Boullata JI, Carrera AL, Harvey L, Escuro AA, Hudson L, Mays A, et al. ASPEN safe practices for enteral nutrition therapy. J Parenter Enter Nutr. 2017;41(1):15-103.
5. Brunner LS. Brunner & Suddarth's textbook of medical-surgical nursing. Lippincott Williams & Wilkins; 2010.
6. Cardoso FS, Marcelino P, Bagulho L, Karvellas CJ. Acute liver failure: An up-to-date approach. J Crit Care. 2017;39:25-30.
7. Celiński K, Cichoz-Lach H, Madro A, Słomka M, Kasztelan-Szczerbińska B, Dworzański T. Non-variceal upper gastrointestinal bleeding-guidelines on management. J Physiol Pharmacol. 2008;59;Suppl 2:S215-29.
8. Chowdary KV, Reddy PN. Parenteral nutrition: Revisited. Indian J Anaesth. 2010;54(2):95-103.
9. Estívariz CF, Griffith DP, Luo M, Szeszycki EE, Bazargan N, Dave N, et al. Efficacy of parenteral nutrition supplemented with glutamine dipeptide to decrease hospital infections in critically ill surgical patients. J Parenter Enter Nutr. 2008;32(4):389-402.
10. Ferreira A, Bartelega JA, Urbano HC, de Souza IK. Acute pancreatitis gravity predictive factors: Which and when to use them? Arq Bras Cir Dig. 2015;28(3):207-11.
11. Friedman LS, Martin P. Handbook of liver disease. Elsevier Health Sciences; 2017.
12. Garg PK, Imrie CW. Severity classification of acute pancreatitis: The continuing search for a better system. Pancreatology. 2015;15(2):99-100.
13. Ghishan FK, Kiela PR, Krenitsky J, Coe SG, Wallace MB, Kataria A, et al. Practical gastroenterology. Gastroenterology. 2012;36(9).
14. Heneghan MA, Bernal W. Fulminant hepatic failure. Med Care Liver Transpl Patient. 2012:176-87.
15. https://www.ncbi.nlm.nih.gov/pmc/articles/PMC2131363/table/T0003/?report=objectonly.
16. Jamal A, Fatima N, Monawwar M, Imran M, Mishra S, Bano S. Eval Some Antibiot Manag Hepatic Encephalopathy (He) Overview. 2021:22-39.
17. Johnson-Delaney CA. Anatomy and physiology of the gastrointestinal system of the ferret and selected exotic carnivores. Proceedings of the of the Association of Avian Veterinarians. 2006;2006:29-38.

18. Kattelmann KK, Hise M, Russell M, Charney P, Stokes M, Compher C. Preliminary evidence for a medical nutrition therapy protocol: Enteral feedings for critically ill patients. J Am Diet Assoc. 2006;106(8):1226-41.
19. Koh DC, Luchtefeld MA, Kim DG, Knox MF, Fedeson BC, Vanerp JS, et al. Efficacy of transarterial embolization as definitive treatment in lower gastrointestinal bleeding. Colorectal Dis. 2009;11(1):53-9.
20. Lai WK, Murphy N. Management of acute liver failure. Contin Educ Anaesth Crit Care Pain. 2004;4(2):40-3.
21. Leppäniemi A, Tolonen M, Tarasconi A, Segovia-Lohse H, Gamberini E, Kirkpatrick AW, et al. WSES guidelines for the management of severe acute pancreatitis. World J Emerg Surg. 2019;14(1):1-20.
22. Liao DH, Zhao JB, Gregersen H. Gastrointestinal tract modelling in health and disease. World J Gastroenterol. 2009;15(2):169-76.
23. Lui HF, Jalan R, Hayes PC. Hepatic encephalopathy: Pathogenesis, diagnosis and management. JR Coll Phys Edinb. 1998;28(1):111-8.
24. Marino PL. The ICU book. Lippincott Williams & wilkins; 2007.
25. Mayuga PN. Intestinal obstruction. Philipp J Surg. 1953; 8(3):101-3.
26. McDowell Torres DM, Stevens RD, Gurakar A. Acute liver failure: A management challenge for the practicing gastro-enterologist. Gastroenterol Hepatol (N Y). 2010;6(7):444-50.
27. Nardi GL. Diagnosis and management of acute pancreatitis. Postgrad Med. 1965;37(5):500-3.
28. Pyleris E, Giannikopoulos G, Dabos K. Pathophysiology and management of acute liver failure. Ann Gastroenterol. 2010:257-65.
29. Raghuwanshi S, Gupta R, Vyas MM, Sharma R. CT evaluation of acute pancreatitis and its prognostic correlation with CT severity index. J Clin Diagn Res. 2016;10(6):TC06-11.
30. Sharma S, Kaneria R, Sharma A, Khare A. Perforation peritonitis: A clinical study regarding etiology, clinical presentation and management strategies. Int Surg J. 2019;6(12):4455-9.
31. Volk SW. Peritonitis. Small Anim Crit Care Med. 2015:643-8.
32. Xing TJ. Clinical classification of liver failure: Consensus, contradictions and new recommendations. J Clin Gastroenterol Hepatol. 2017;1(2).

# Chapter 7

# Renal System Emergencies and Management

*Susan Konda*

## CHAPTER OUTLINE

- Anatomy of Renal System
- Physiology of Renal System
- Assessment of Renal System
  - Renal function
  - Electrolyte and acid base balance
  - Fluid balance
- Acute Renal Failure
- Chronic Renal Failure
- Acute Tubular Necrosis
- Bladder Trauma
- Disorders of Fluid Volume
- End-stage Renal Disease and Renal Transplantation
- Management Modalities for Renal System Disorders
  - Renal replacement therapies
  - Hemodialysis
  - Peritoneal dialysis
  - Continuous arteriovenous hemodialysis
  - Management of electrolytic imbalances

### Learning Objectives

At the end of the chapter, the students will be able to:
- Recollect the anatomy and physiology part of the renal system.
- Get knowledge to practice renal assessment.
- Gain knowledge on renal function.
- Manage electrolyte and acid base balance.
- Maintain fluid balance.
- Care of acute renal failure.
- Assess the care of chronic renal failure patients.
- Manage acute tubular necrosis patients.
- Assess the care of bladder trauma.
- Maintain disorders of fluid volume in renal patients.
- Gain knowledge on the emergency nursing care on various renal disorders.
- Acquire the knowledge on different management modalities for pre, post and intradialysis patients.
- Provide care and can prepare the patients for different renal surgeries.

## INTRODUCTION

Genitourinary (GU) problems are a common complaint in the emergency department (ED). In 2015 ED visits in the United States exceeded 2 million for urinary tract infections (UTIs) and 1 million for urinary calculi. The incidence of end-stage renal disease (ESRD) is rising in all industrialized nations, and patients with complications of vascular or peritoneal access for life-sustaining dialysis treatments present to the ED for urgent and emergent intervention. Although they are not as common as UTIs or urinary calculi, the following GU conditions are considered emergent: Testicular torsion with and without epididymitis-orchitis, priapism, rhabdomyolysis, and acute kidney injury.

## ANATOMY OF RENAL SYSTEM

The kidneys, ureters, urinary bladder, and urethra are the major parts of genitourinary system. Fluid volume is regulated by the kidneys and acid-base and electrolyte balance. Ureters transport urine to the bladder for temporary storage. The urine is drained from the bladder to the outside by the urethra (**Fig. 7.1**). External structures of the male GU system have reproductive functions.

The renal artery and renal vein consist of common entry and exit at the medial aspect of either kidney at the hilum. Blood flow to the kidney is supplied by the renal artery, which branches off the abdominal aorta and enters the kidney through the renal sinus. Blood leaves the kidney through the renal vein, which empties into the abdominal inferior vena cava (**Fig. 7.2**).

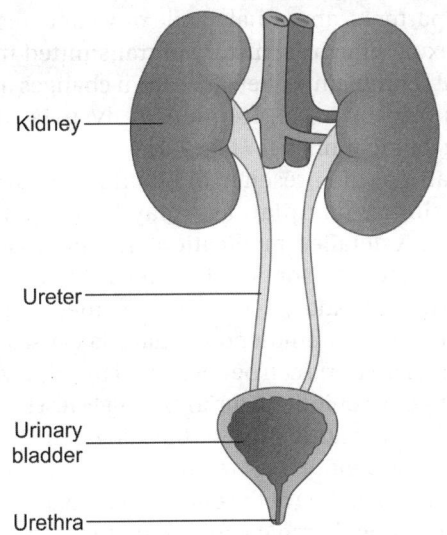

Fig. 7.1: Structure of urinary system.

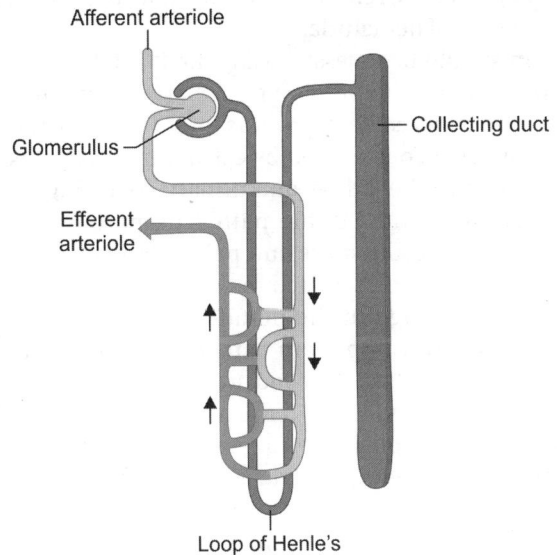

Fig. 7.2: Structure of nephron.

# PHYSIOLOGY OF RENAL SYSTEM

The nephron, the functional unit of the kidney, is composed of the renal corpuscle, proximal convoluted tubule, Henle's loop, distal convoluted tubule, and collecting ducts **(Fig. 7.3)**. Each kidney contains an estimated 1 million nephrons individually capable of producing urine. These nephrons cannot be reproduced once destroyed. The renal corpuscle contains the glomerulus, a web of tightly convoluted capillaries, and Bowman's capsule, which surrounds and supports these structures. Specialized cells called juxtaglomerular cells are located at the entrance to the glomerulus of the afferent arteriole in 15% of

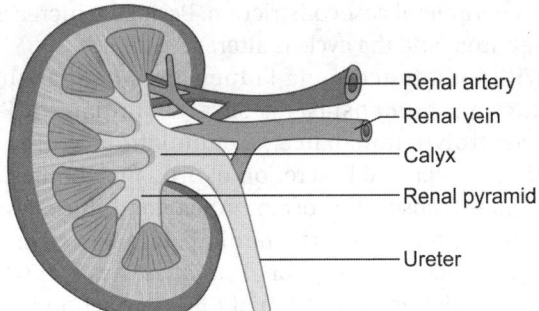

Fig. 7.3: Structure of the kidney with renal arteries.

nephrons. These specialized cells sense changes in pressure and sodium concentration and play a role in the renin-angiotensin-aldosterone (RAA) system.

Filtration of plasma in the renal corpuscle is the first step in urine production and essential solutes. Pressure generated as blood courses through the tight web, oncotic pressure is greater than bowman's capsule pressure so the small solute cross semi-permeable membrane and restricts the flow of red blood cells, proteins and white blood cells to cross. Decreased oncotic pressure, often the result of decreased serum albumin levels, or decreased pressure within the glomerulus produced by systematic hypotension decreases the glomerular filtration rate (GFR) and eventually urine output. GFR in the average adult is 125 mL/min or 180 L/day.

Tubules, Henle's loop, and collecting ducts excrete waste products (e.g., urea, nitrogen, creatinine and drug metabolites), reabsorb water and solutes (potassium, sodium, chloride, hydrogen, glucose, and amino acids) from filtrate, and secrete excess solutes the body does not need into filtrate. Osmosis, diffusion, and active transport occur between the nephron and surrounding capillaries. Hormonal control regulates reabsorption and secretion in the nephron.

The RAA system and antidiuretic hormone (ADH) are feedback loop system within the body maintain homeostasis. Serum osmolarity increases and causes stimulation of the hypothalamus, which release ADH. Pressure changes in the glomerulus are overcome by vasodilation and constriction of the afferent arteriole by a process called auto-regulation. The auto regulation keeps pressure in the glomerulus within a wide range of systolic blood pressures. When the range is exceeded, auto regulation fail and epithelial damage occurs, with eventual scarring and sclerosis followed by decreased permeability, GFR, and urine output. Inadequate nephron perfusion stimulates the juxtaglomerular apparatus to secrete renin that converts angiotensinogen to angiotensin I. Conversion of angiotensin I to angiotensin II by an enzyme in the ling causes peripheral vasoconstriction. Perfusion increases to the nephron, and the cycle is altered.

Without a functioning kidney and adequate urine production, homeostasis is severely impaired. Fluid and electrolyte imbalance, accumulation of urea and creatinine, decreased excretion of drug metabolites, and inadequate reabsorption of amino acids and glucose occur. The kidneys help convert vitamin D into its active form to ensure calcium absorption from intestines and secrete erythropoietin for stimulation of RBC production in bone marrow. Consequently, altered renal function decreases bone mineralization and oxygen-carrying capacity of the blood.

The renal pelvis narrows to enter the ureter, where urine is moved to the bladder by peristaltic contractions. The muscular bladder stores urine until release to the urethra by the micturition reflex.

External genitalia are also part of the GU system. Female genitalia consist of the vestibule, the space into which the urethra and vagina open, and surrounding labia minora and majora. Anatomic position and the short length of the female urethra are responsible for the high frequency of UTIs in female.

Male external genitalia include the penis, scrotum, and scrotal contents. Scrotal contents include the testes, tubules that carry developing sperm cells and secrete testosterone, and the epididymis, which lies along the posterior testes and is the final maturation area for sperm. The prostate is glandular muscle tissue that surrounds the urethra at the base of the bladder. Enlargement of the prostate can cause outlet obstruction and urinary retention. The penis consists of three columns of erectile tissue that become engorged with blood, producing erection. Two columns of corpora cavernosa form the dorsum and sides of the penis, and the corpus spongiosum forms the base and glans. Clinical manifestations of GU disease frequently involve external genitalia.

## ASSESSMENT OF RENAL SYSTEM

Assessment of the GU system should determine history of hypertension, diabetes, previous infections, prostatitis, urethritis, bladder or urethral damage during childbirth, history of renal calculi, and recurrent UTIs. A detailed drug list, including prescription, over-the-counter (OTC), herbal preparations, and illicit drugs, should be obtained. Identification of any history of exposure to occupational chemicals or toxins may identify contact with substances that could cause nephrotoxicity. Sexual history should include discussion of risk factors that can cause GU symptoms (e.g., use of contraceptive jellies or creams, multiple partners, abnormal penile or vaginal discharges, unsafe sexual practices, history of transmitted infections [STIs]). GU complaints often arise from changes in urinary patterns; for example, frequency, dysuria, urgency, dribbling, or incontinence (**Fig. 7.4**).

Hematuria, the presence of blood in the urine, may be the primary complaint or may accompany other symptoms. A detailed medication and diet history may uncover other causes for discoloration of urine-foods such as beets, rhubarb, and blackberries, and medications such as phenytoin are common nonhematuria causes of red or dark urine. Hematuria can be confirmed by urinalysis (UA); however, microscopic hematuria on a single test is common. Early-stream hematuria suggests bleeding from the urethra, hematuria throughout the stream indicates upper GU tract bleeding, and bleeding at the end suggests bladder neck or urethral bleeding. Complete urinalysis and urine cytologic study may indicate the need for further diagnostic testing for urologic cancer, renal disease, infection, or renal calculi as the source of hematuria.

Pain should be assessed using the POSRT mnemonic provocation, quality, region or radiation, severity, and time. The most severe pain associated with the GU system is renal colic caused by calculi. Increase pressure and dilation of the kidney and urinary collecting system cause sudden, unbearable pain. The patient usually presents with restlessness and pallor and complains of flank pain that often radiated to the abdomen and groin. If the stones lodge in the bladder, urinary frequency and urgency develop. Pain can cause tachypnea and tachycardia with elevated blood pressure. Oliguria, defined as urine output less than 75 mL in 24 hours, may be the presenting symptoms. The cause is usually obstruction; however, blood chemistry values should be evaluated for

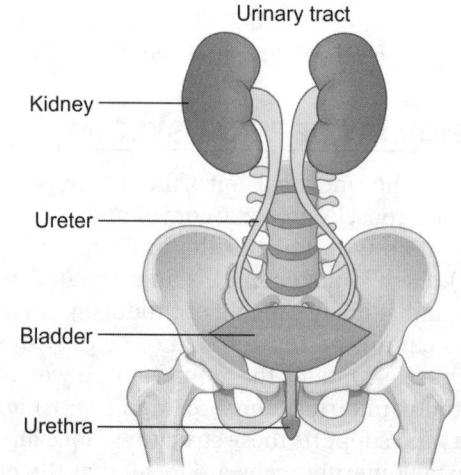

**Fig. 7.4:** Structure of the kidney with renal arteries.

azotemia, which indicates renal failure from prolonged obstruction leading to hydronephrosis or other causes. If the patient has a urinary catheter in place, patency should be assessed. A physical examination can identify urinary retention by palpating the bladder as a firm mass above the symphysis pubis, with an urge to void on palpation; bladder scanning using ultrasonography may also be used to detect bladder distention. History should be obtained to identify drugs that contribute to retention, including OTC nasal decongestants containing anticholinergic ingredients. A neurologic examination or disease that can interfere with the micturition reflex. The prostate is examined for enlargement as the cause of obstruction. After the patient has attempted to void, a urethral catheter may be inserted for residual volume. Bedside bladder ultrasonography may avoid the need for catheterization and allow assessment of prevoid and postvoid volume. If the catheter cannot be inserted without resistance, a Suprapubic bladder tap or assistance from an urologist may be necessary. With a residual volume greater than 500 mL, the catheter may be left in place to allow the bladder to regain muscle tone. If residual volume is minimal, further diagnostic evaluation is aimed at identifying the cause.

## Acid-base Balance

Inadequate tissue perfusion and hypoxia lead to acidosis. The body will attempt to compensate for acidosis in multiple ways. The lungs and the kidney play a key role in acid-base balance for the patient. The major body buffer system are found in the interstitial fluid, the blood, intracellular fluid, urine, and bones.

In early shock, respiratory alkalosis occurs because of tachypnea. This is the body's attempt to increase oxygen levels and decrease carbon dioxide levels in the body's tissue. Increased carbon dioxide and hydrogen ions in chemoreceptors stimulate respiratory centers in the brain and increase the rate and depth of the patient's respirations. Anaerobic metabolism increase serum lactic acid, causing metabolic acidosis. Importantly, lactate level and base deficit can also be influenced by other factors, such as liver and renal diseases. A persistently high base deficit and low pH may be an early indicator of complications. Metabolic acidosis is corrected by providing adequate oxygenation and perfusion through ventilation, fluid, and medications. The cause of the shock state needs to be quickly identified and appropriate management initiated to correct the origin of the anaerobic process. If the pH is less than 7.1, administration of sodium bicarbonate may be needed to correct the pH. However, sodium bicarbonate should not be administered before adequate ventilation and fluid have been established.

## Electrolyte Balance

An electrolyte is a substance capable of carrying an electrical charge. An electrolyte with a positive charge is called a cation, whereas an electrolyte with a negative charge is an anion. Electrolyte are found in varying concentration in ECF and ICF

For the purpose of this chapter, serum electrolyte measurements are equivalent to extracellular electrolyte values. Direct measurement of intracellular electrolyte concentrations in the clinical setting is not yet feasible, so ICF electrolyte concentrations must be inferred from serum electrolyte values.

All fluids outside the cells are collectively referred to as ECF. Electrolytes in ECF, from greatest to least concentration, are sodium, chloride, potassium, bicarbonate, and hydrogen. ECF also contain oxygen, carbon dioxide, protein, and a few miscellaneous anions.

ICF represents fluid found in cell in the body, about 25L. Electrolytes in the ICF, from greatest to least concentration, and potassium, phosphate, and sulfate combined; magnesium; and finally sodium, hydrogen, and bicarbonate in equal concentrations. The ICF also contains several proteins

The delicate balance of water and electrolyte between intracellular and extracellular compartment is an ongoing process of checks and balances easily disturbed by disease or injury. Regulatory processes and the role of each electrolyte are described in the following sections.

### *Sodium*

Sodium, the principal cation in ECF, is primarily responsible for osmotic pressure. Sodium is exchangeable across cell membranes to maintain sodium and water balance and normal arterial pressure. Sodium and chloride play an important role in maintaining body water; movement of glucose, insulin, and amino acids across cell membrane; and maintaining muscle strength, neural function, and urinary output. Sodium is essential for the sodium-potassium pump, which moves sodium and potassium across the cell membrane during repolarization. As sodium diffuses into the cell and potassium out of the cell, an active transport system supplied with energy delivers sodium back to the extracellular compartment and potassium to the intracellular compartment.

Sodium levels are maintained through the renin-angiotensin-aldosterone system, the sympathetic nervous system, and a less well-defined system mediated by atrial natriuretic factor. Decreased fluid volume decreases blood flow and arterial pressure, which stimulate baroreceptors in the kidneys. Baroreceptors stimulate the sympathetic nervous system, which leads to vasoconstriction of renal arterioles, decreased glomerular filtration rate, and retention of sodium and water. The opposite sequence of events occurs when fluid intake (or blood volume) rises above normal.

Atrial natriuretic hormone (ANH), released from the atria in response to increased arterial pressure, produces natriuresis (excretion of abnormal amount of sodium in the urine), diuresis, vasodilation, and antagonistic effects on ADH release, renin, and aldosterone. The resulting increase in sodium excretion eliminates excess volume.

### Chloride

Chloride, the principal anion of blood and ECF, is secreted in various body fluids along with other electrolytes. Sodium and chloride are excreted in sweat, bile, pancreatic fluid, and intestinal fluids. Gastric juice contains chloride and hydrogen. As with sodium, chloride plays a cooperative role in maintaining acid-base balance and take part in the exchange of oxygen and carbon dioxide in red blood cells. Serum chloride levels are passively regulated by serum sodium levels. When serum sodium increases, serum chloride also increases. However, chloride level is inversely related to bicarbonate level because chloride is sacrificed in the kidneys to produce more bicarbonate.

### Potassium

Potassium is the most abundant cation in the body, with 98% in the ICF and 2% in the ECF. Conversely, acute acidosis is the major factor that decreases potassium secretion and increases serum potassium. Acute acidosis increases hydrogen ion concentration in the ECF, causing potassium to move out of the cell in exchange for excess hydrogen ions.

### Calcium

Approximately 99% of the body's calcium is found in bone. However, 1% is found in ICF and 0.1% in ECF. Bone acts as a large reservoir for calcium when ECF calcium levels fall. Calcium is transported in the blood in two forms. Half is bound to plasma protein, usually albumin, and a small amount of nonionized calcium forms complexes with anions such as phosphate, citrate, and sulfate. The rest exists as an ionized form that is free and metabolically active. Most ionized calcium is found in the ECF. Due to the large amount of calcium is found to plasma proteins, assessment of total serum calcium without simultaneous measurement of serum proteins has limited value in determining hypocalcemia or hypercalcemia.

Calcium has many important functions-smooth and skeletal muscle contraction, bone and brain metabolism, blood clotting, and as a primary ingredient in lung surfactant. Calcium is essential for membrane polarization and depolarization, action potential generation, neurotransmission, and muscle contraction. Calcium channels in myocardial cells allow trans membrane calcium transport.

The most important regulatory factors for calcium homeostasis are parathyroid hormone (PTH), calcitonin, and vitamin. When ECF calcium falls below normal levels, parathyroid glands release PTH, which acts directly on bones to stimulate the release of large amount of calcium into ECF. When calcium ion concentration is elevated, PTH secretion decreases, causing excess calcium to deposit in the bones.

Bones rely on proper intake and absorption of calcium stores. Calcium absorption in the kidneys and GI tract is regulated by PTH levels. In hypocalcemia states, PTH activates vitamin D3, the form of vitamin D necessary to increase intestinal calcium reabsorption. PTH also directly stimulates the kidney to increase renal tubular calcium reabsorption, which prevents loss of calcium in the urine.

Another factor influencing calcium reabsorption is plasma concentration of phosphate. Increases in plasma phosphate may indirectly stimulate PTH, which increases calcium reabsorption by renal tubules and reduces calcium loss in the urine.

In response to elevated calcium levels, the thyroid gland secretes a hormone called calcitonin. The effect of calcitonin on plasma calcium level is directly opposite that of PTH. Calcitonin decreases plasma calcium level by increasing calcium deposits in bone and decreasing formation of new osteoclasts, the cell responsible for breakdown and removal of bone. Calcitonin also has minor effects on calcium absorption in the renal tubules and GI tract.

### Phosphate and Phosphorus

Phosphorus, the major anion in the ICF, is essential for metabolism of carbohydrates, lipids, and proteins. Phosphate have active role in hormonal activities and acid-base balance and has a close relationship to calcium in maintaining homeostasis. Renal tubules, maintain a normal phosphate level by an "overflow" mechanism. When the phosphate level in the glomerular filtrate fall below the normal level, essentially all filtered phosphate is reabsorbed.

### Magnesium

Magnesium is the second most important intracellular cation. More than half the body's magnesium is stored in bones, with the rest in cells, particularly muscle. Only a small fraction of the body's magnesium is found in the ECF. Magnesium plays an essential role cellular metabolism.

## Fluid Balance

Water is the most abundant fluid medium in the body, composing 65% of total body weight for the average adult, 75% in a full-term infant, and as little as 45% in an older adults. In a healthy physiologic state, this fluid medium has a constant balance of electrolytes controlled by a unique system of checks and balance. Fluid and electrolyte abnormalities may be caused by gastrointestinal (GI), urologic, cardiac, respiratory, and endocrine disease, as well as many forms of traumatic injury.

Water has many important metabolic functions, including transport of nutrients and other essential substances, removal of metabolic waste product, normal cellular metabolic, and maintenance of normal body temperature, age, weight, body fat, gender, and environmental factors such as ambient temperature determine individual fluid requirements.

Total body water (TBW) is distributed between extracellular and intracellular compartments. Extracellular fluid (ECF) constitutes one-third of TBW, or approximately 15 L. plasma, interstitial fluid, cerebrospinal fluid, intraocular fluid, fluid of the GI tract, and fluid of potential spaces (i.e., pleural space and peritoneal space) are example of ECF. Intracellular fluid (ICF) accounts for two-third of TBW and represents the sum of fluid content for all the cells in the body approximately 25L. Two regulatory mechanism influential in maintaining normal water volume and tonicity, or osmotic pressure, are thirst and renal function. Thirst is the primary regulatory for intake of water. It is triggered by receptors in the anterolateral hypothalamus that respond to increase plasma osmolality (as little as 2%) or decrease body fluid volume. Thirst ensures adequate replacement of fluid losses and is stimulated by ECF hyper tonicity and decrease ICF volume. Similarly thirst is depressed by ECF hyper tonicity and increase ICF volume. Because the thirst mechanism is triggered by increase osmolality, thirst is not effective in hypotonic or hyponatremic dehydration in which water and sodium losses are equal. Hypothalamic dysfunction also decreases the capacity for thirst.

Renal regulation of water balance is twofold, affecting both tonicity and body water. When the glomerular filtrate is hypertonic, osmoreceptors in the hypothalamus are stimulated and antidiuretic hormone (ADH) is resealed by the pituitary gland. ADH makes renal collecting tubules more permeable to water so water is reabsorbed into the body, diluting blood and concentrating urine. The kidneys, through the renin-angiotensin-aldosterone system, regulate the volume of body water. When ECF volume, specifically blood volume, is low, receptors in the kidneys secrete an enzyme called renin. Renin stimulates angiotensinogen (a normal plasma protein) to release angiotensin I, which is then converted to angiotensin II by another enzyme, primarily in the lungs. Angiotensin II stimulates the adrenal cortex to secrete aldosterone, which increase sodium reabsorption from glomerular filtrate in exchange to potassium and hydrogen ions. This exchange increase plasma tonicity, which leads to ADH secretion, water retention, and increased volume. With excessive ECF volume (blood volume), aldosterone secretion is depressed, so tubular reabsorption of sodium and water decrease.

## ACUTE RENAL FAILURE

Renal failure is a reduce or cessation of glomerular filtration. In **acute renal failure**, the kidney abrupt stops working completely. The important characterized of acute renal failure is the suppression of urine flow, usually characterized by oliguria urine output less than 200 mL, or by anuria urine output less than 50 mL.

## Definition

Acute renal failure (ARF) is defined as concept as a quick (over hours to weeks) and generally reversible decline in GFR that may occur either in the setting of preexisting normal renal function or with predetermine renal disease ("acute on chronic" renal failure).

## Etiology

### Prerenal
- Volume loss
- Low effective arterial volume
- Alerted renal vascular auto regulation

### Intrarenal
- Disease of small vessels: vasculitides
- Disease of large vessels: Aortic dissection, vein thrombosis
- Crush injuries

### Postrenal
- Bladder outlet obstruction: Prostatic hypertrophy
- Urothelial malignancy
- Retroperitoneal fibrosis
- Urolithiasis

### Acute Renal Failure Stages
- **Initiation:** Initiation phase period starts with the initial stage and ends with oliguria period
- **Oliguria:** The oliguria period begins when serum concentration level exceed and seen in excretion.

(creatinine, spaceurea, uric acid, organic acids and intracellular caution) metabolic waste produce is 400 mL. In this oliguria period symptoms been observed and it is a life-threatening situation.
- **Diuresis:** Diuresis phase observes slow increase in urine output, laboratory values eventually decrease. The patient must be monitored for dehydration.
- **Recovery:** Recovery phase the kidney function comes to normal condition with normal laboratory values in a period of 3–12 months.

## Pathophysiology

Acute renal failure, also known as acute kidney injury (AKI), is a sudden and rapid decline in kidney function. It is characterized by a sudden decrease in urine output and an increase in serum creatinine and blood urea nitrogen (BUN) levels. The pathophysiology of acute renal failure involves various underlying mechanisms that can be categorized into three main types: Prerenal, intrarenal, and postrenal causes **(Flowchart 7.1)**.

## Clinical Manifestations

- Short-term weight gain or loss
- Nausea and vomiting
- Hematemesis
- Melena
- Dysrhythmias
- Dyspnea
- Stupor or coma
- Compromise or airway, breathing, circulation, and neurologic function require intervention.

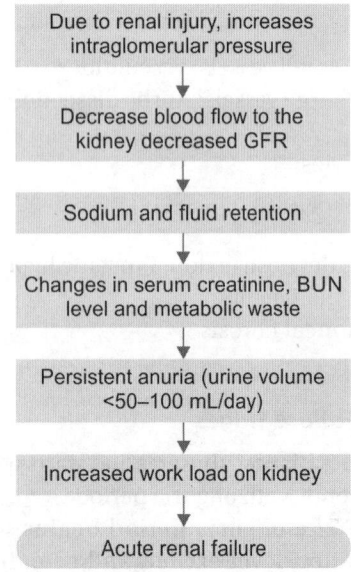

**Flowchart 7.1:** Pathophysiology of ARF.

- Fever may be associated with infection or inflammatory events. Fever reduction measure should be instituted to prevent the continued rise of nitrogenous waste products by catabolic effect of fever.

## Diagnostic Studies

After initial stabilization of the patient, history and diagnostic testing focus on identifying the cause of AKI. Tests include serial blood chemistry values, UA with sodium and potassium concentrations, chest radiograph, renal ultrasonography and Doppler studies, or computed tomography (CT) scan. Imaging procedures are usually done without contrast media because of toxic effects of the media on renal tubules. When contrast is needed, acetyl cysteine or bicarbonate drip may be administered before and after the contrast study to minimize toxic renal effects.

- **Blood test:** Blood studies enumerates elevated blood urea nitrogen, serum creatinine, and potassium levels, and decline in bicarbonate level and hematocrit level.
- **Urine test:** Urine studies reveal proteinuria, hematuria, cellular debris and decreased specific gravity. Urine chemistry reveals decreased amount of sodium (<20 mEq/L) in urine and high potassium level.
- **Kidney biopsy:** Kidney biopsy in which a bit of kidney tissue is removed as a sample to test in a laboratory and grown in artificial culture media.

## Management

The kidneys have remarkable ability to recover. The objective of treatment of ARF is to restore normal chemical balance and prevent complications until repair of renal tissue and restoration of renal function can occur.

- Maintenance of fluid balance is based on daily body weight.
- Proper nutrition is crucial in the management of acute renal failure
- If patient's kidney do not respond to treatment, need to undergo dialysis procedure

### Nursing Diagnosis

- Acute renal failure, also known as acute kidney injury, is a sudden loss of kidney function that can be caused by a variety of factors. Nursing diagnoses for acute renal failure may include:
  - Risk for decreased cardiac output related to fluid and electrolyte imbalances.
  - Excess fluid volume related to decreased urine output and fluid overload.
  - Imbalanced nutrition: Less than body requirements related to anorexia, nausea, and vomiting.

- Risk for infection related to decreased immune function and invasive procedures
- Risk for impaired skin integrity related to edema, skin breakdown, and pressure ulcers
- Risk for injury related to altered mental status, decreased mobility, and seizures
- Anxiety related to the uncertainty of prognosis and treatment
- Risk for impaired urinary elimination related to decreased urine output and/or renal replacement therapy
- Knowledge deficit related to the disease process, treatment options, and self-care management.
• Risk for decreased cardiac output related to fluid and electrolyte imbalances and nursing management includes:
  - Monitor the patient's fluid intake and output, vital signs, and electrolyte levels to identify any changes in their condition.
  - Administer fluids, diuretics, and other medications as prescribed to manage fluid and electrolyte imbalances.
  - Assess the patient's cardiac function, such as heart rate and rhythm, to detect any signs of decreased cardiac output.
  - Educate patients about the importance of maintaining fluid and electrolyte balance to prevent complications.
• Risk for infection related to weakened immune system and invasive procedures and nursing management includes:
  - Monitor the patient's temperature, white blood cell count, and signs of infection to identify any potential infections.
  - Follow proper infection control procedures, such as hand hygiene and proper use of personal protective equipment, to prevent the spread of infection.
  - Administer antibiotics and other medications as prescribed to manage infections.
  - Educate patients about the importance of good hygiene and infection prevention measures.
• Impaired renal function related to damage to the kidneys and nursing management includes:
  - Monitor the patient's urine output, electrolyte levels, and renal function tests to assess the degree of kidney damage.
  - Administer medications and other therapies as prescribed to manage the underlying cause of the ARF and prevent further damage to the kidneys.
  - Provide nutritional support to maintain the patient's energy and protein needs.
  - Educate patients about the importance of managing the underlying cause of the ARF and preventing further damage to the kidneys.
• Anxiety related to the uncertainty of the patient's condition and hospitalization and nursing management includes:
  - Assess the patient's emotional state and provide emotional support as needed.
  - Encourage the patient to express their feelings and concerns.
  - Educate patients and their families about the patient's condition and plan of care to reduce anxiety and promote understanding.
  - Provide a safe and supportive environment to help the patient feel more comfortable and secure.

These nursing diagnoses may vary depending on the cause and severity of the acute renal failure, as well as the individual patient's needs and co-morbidities. It is important for nurses to continually assess and monitor the patient's condition and adjust their care plan as needed.

## General Management

• Administration of intravenous calcium may be needed to antagonize the membrane and improve cardiac conductivity until removal of excess potassium by emergency dialysis can be initiated, IV calcium works within minutes, but duration is short, as evidenced by return ECG changes. Administration of IV sodium bicarbonate ($NaHCO_3$), works within 15–30 minutes, and last approximately 4 hours. Potassium can also be removed by cation exchange resin (e.g., sodium polystyrene sulfonate), but the onset of action is 60 minute when rectally and 120 minute after oral administration. Urine output may be increased or decreased.
• If AKI is nonoliguric, large volume of fluid can be lost, so the patient may be dehydrated and hypotensive. Volume replacement with normal saline is recommended (1–3 L initially at 75–100 mL/h or more unless contraindicated by comorbidities) and is guided by outcome goals such as urine output and tissue oxygenation, jugular vein distention, ling auscultation, and vital signs. Invasive line such as central venous pressure may be used for unstable patients.
• If AKI presents with oliguria, the patient may be volume overloaded and hypertensive, so minimal fluid is given until the volume can be removed by diuretics or through hemodialysis. Metabolic acidosis occurs because renal tubules can no longer regulate concentration of hydrogen ions. IV $NaHCO_3$ may be used unless contraindicated by volume status.

- Indication for emergency dialysis includes stupor, volume overload and pulmonary edema nonresponsive to diuretic therapy, and dangerous hyperkalemia and acidosis unresponsive to medical therapy. Emergency hemodialysis requires vascular access (usually a temporary femoral or subclavian) dual-lumen catheter or internal shunt and an artificial kidney (dialyzer) to act as a semipermeable membrane. The dialysate must be low in ions that the body needs to excrete and high in those to be reabsorbed. Hemodynamically unstable patient may require continuous renal replacement therapy in the intensive care unit.

## CHRONIC RENAL FAILURE

### Definition
Chronic kidney disorder is a permanent decrease in glomerular filtration rate in renal function and it is a long term disease in which patient seeks help of dialysis for entire life and become dependent in hemodialysis.

### Incidence
Millions of people are suffering with chronic kidney disease and seeking dialysis. Heart disease is the major cause of death for all people with chronic kidney disease **(Fig. 7.5)**.

### Classifying Stages CKD
Based on GFR, not based on symptoms:
- **Stage 1:** GFR = 90–120
- **Stage 2:** GFR = 60–89
- **Stage 3:** GFR = 30–59
- **Stage 4:** GFR =15–29 (must be prepared for RRT)
- **Stage 5:** GFR <15 (ESRD–requires transplant or dialysis)

### Etiology
- A strong family history of kidney disorder
- Chronic inflammation of the glomeruli ad renal pelvis
- Diabetes mellitus
- Long-term infections such as tuberculosis and pyelonephritis
- Cysts in the kidney
- Long-term use of nephrotoxic agents
- Immune disorder like systemic lupus erythematous, etc.
- Renal calculi
- Vascular disorders
- Hypertension
- Repeated urinary infections
- Environmental and occupational agents

### Pathophysiology
Chronic renal failure, also known as chronic kidney disease (CKD), is a progressive and irreversible condition characterized by the gradual loss kidney function over time. The pathophysiology of chronic renal failure involves various underlying mechanisms that contribute to the progressive decline in renal function. The key processes involved in the pathophysiology of CKD **(Flowchart 7.2)**:

### Clinical Manifestations
- Acid base abnormalities
- Carbohydrate intolerance
- Fluid and electrolyte imbalance
- Intoxication
- Calcium and phosphate abnormalities and metabolic bone disease
- Hematological abnormalities
- Gastrointestinal abnormalities
- Dermatological abnormalities
- Neuromuscular abnormalities
- Elevated creatinine and BUN levels
- Edema
- Decrease ability to concentrate

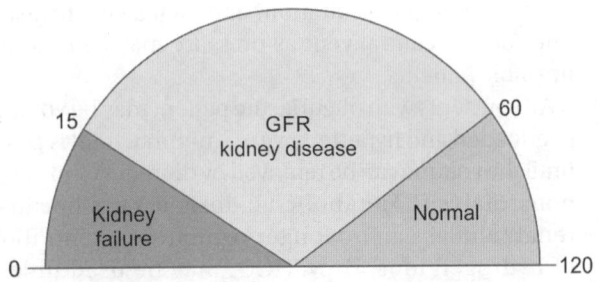

**Fig. 7.5:** Stages of CKD based on GFR.

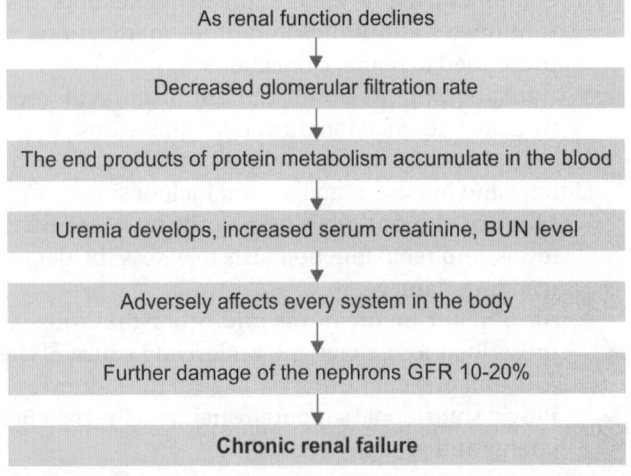

**Flowchart 7.2:** Pathophysiology of CRF.

### Other Symptoms

- Oliguria
- Weakness
- Anemia
- Weight loss
- Nausea and vomiting
- Bone pain
- Muscle twitching
- Amenorrhea
- Sleep problems, such as insomnia, restless leg syndrome

## Diagnostic Findings

- **Renal concentration test:** Evaluates ability of kidney to concentrate solutes in urine.
- **Urine osmolality:** Concentrating ability is lost early in kidney disease; hence these test findings may disclose early defects in renal function.
- **Creatinine clearance:** Detect and evaluate progression of renal disease measured in mL/min/1.7 m$^2$
- Serum creatinine test.
- **Blood urea nitrogen (BUN):** Urea is the nitrogenous end product of protein metabolism. Test values are affected by protein intake, tissue breakdown, and fluid volume changes.
- **Renal biopsy:** Renal biopsy in which a bit of kidney tissue is removed as a sample to test in a laboratory and grown in artificial culture media.

## Management

The main objective in managing chronic renal failure is to maintain sodium and water homeostasis, potassium homeostasis, metabolic acidosis are the common disturbance in advanced CKD. Primary management with medication and dietary therapy. Dialysis is required for maintain fluid and electrolyte balance and remove toxic waste from the body.

### Pharmacologic Therapy

- **Calcium and phosphorus binders:** Such as calcium carbonate these medications binds dietary phosphorous in the intestinal tract.
- **Antihypertensive and cardiovascular agents:** Hypertension is managed by intravascular volume control and a variety of antihypertensive agents. Heart failure is managed by low-sodium diet, diuretic agents such as digoxin.
- Administration of intravenous calcium may be needed to antagonize the membrane and improve cardiac conductivity until removal of excess potassium by emergency dialysis can be initiated, IV calcium works within minutes, but duration is short, as evidenced by return ECG changes.

### Medical Management

- **Diet restriction:** Low potassium, low sodium, and low phosphate.
- **Fluid intake restriction:** 500 mL–1 L/day or that which does not cause volume overload.
- **ACE inhibitor:** Lisinopril, enalapril and captopril.
- **Avoidance of NSAIDs:** Avoid aminoglycosides.

### Nutritional Therapy

- Dietary interventional includes restricted protein intake.
- At the same time, adequate caloric intake and vitamin supplementation must be ensured.
- Potassium is removed through proper dialysis treatment, to prevent hyperkalemia and provide potassium restricted diet.

A kidney transplant is a surgical procedure in which a kidney is removed from one person (donor) and placed into the body of a person suffering from renal failure (recipients).

### Dialysis

Dialysis is the movement of fluid and molecules across a semipermeable membrane from one compartment to another. Technique in which substance move from the blood through semipermeable membrane and into dialysis solution (dialysate).

The two methods of dialysis available are peritoneal dialysis (PD) and hemodialysis (HD).

#### Principles of Dialysis

- **Osmosis:** Through semipermeable water moves from high concentration to low concentration.
- **Diffusion:** Solute from high concentration to low concentration
- **Ultrafiltration:** When there is an osmotic gradient or pressure gradient across the membrane.

#### Hemodialysis

In 1943, Willem Kolff in the Netherlands performed the first successful dialysis on the human. the access blood moves in and out of the body through arteriovenous fistula (AVFs) and grafts (AVGs).

- **Internal arteriovenous fistulas and grafts:** Arteriovenous fistula is created very commonly in the forearm with an end to side anastomosis of the artery (usually radial or ulnar) to a vein (usually cephalic). For hemodialysis of patient the fast flow of blood is required that is arterial blood flow. At least 3 months early AVF initiation should be done for hemodialysis **(Fig. 7.6)**.

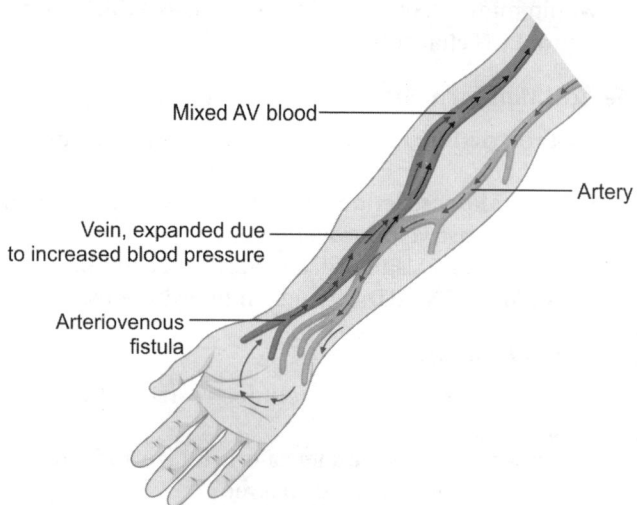

Fig. 7.6: Arteriovenous fistulas.

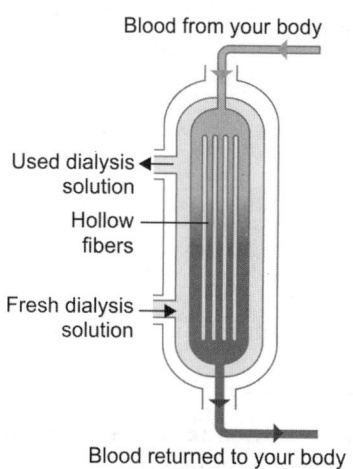

Fig. 7.7: Dialyzer.

- **Arteriovenous graft (AVGs):** Arteriovenous graft is composed of artificial synthetic materials (poltertrafluoroethylene, Teflon) and makes a "bridge" between arterial and venous blood supply. Surgical anastomoses are done between an artery and a vein and it is placed beneath the skin layer known as graft. Allow 2–4 week so that graft should heal. Blood pressure measurement.
  - *Temporary vascular access:* Emergency hemodialysis requires temporary vascular access (usually a temporary femoral or subclavian), dual-lumen catheter or internal shunt and an artificial kidney (dialyzer) to act as a semipermeable membrane. The dialysate must be low in ions that the body needs to excrete and high in those to be reabsorbed. Hemodynamically unstable patient may require continuous renal replacement therapy in the intensive care unit. For maintain the patency of the lumen can give heparin (alteplase) according to doctors order.

### Dialyzers

Dialyzer is a chamber in which, dialysate fluid is pumped on one side of the semipermeable membrane which consist of thousand hollow tubes or fibers. While the patient blood passes through the other side.

- In this dialyzer chamber blood and dialysate flow in either (opposite) direction.
- The composition of dialysis fluid (dialysate) includes sodium, potassium, calcium and bicarbonate which differ with each individual requirements.
- 120 L of water is required during dialysis procedure with flow rate of 250–500 mL/min.
- The process of diffusion, osmosis, and ultrafiltration cleanse the patient blood.
- Then the blood return through a specialized placed vascular access that returns it to the patient **(Fig. 7.7)**.

### Procedure

- The dialyzer and blood lines are usually primed with up to 1,000 mL of saline solution to eliminate air from the system.
- Heparin is added in the dialyzer in order to prevent clot.
- When the blood enters the extracorporeal circuit, it is propelled through the top of the dialyzer by a blood pump at a flow rate of 200–500 mL/min.
- Dialysate circulates in the opposite direction at a rate of 300–900 mL/min.
- Blood is returned from the dialyzer to the patient through the blue catheter lumen.
- Inside the dialyzer the adjustments by ultrafiltration by creating positive pressure on the blood side or negative pressure on the dialysate side or by a combination of both.

### Pre-procedure preparations

- Monitor weight and compare between present and postdialysis, if more than 1–1.5 kg chance of hypotension
- Monitor vital signs hourly.
- Vascular site
- Skin condition.

### Complication of Hemodialysis

Complications occurring early after surgical catheter insertion most commonly include pain, bleeding, obstruction (fluid unable to move in or out of the catheter), and infection and/or leaks. Early complications are generally associated with misplacement of the catheter during insertion.

Significant pain and bleeding are suspicious of perforation of an internal organ during placement. Obstruction may be related to a blockage or kink in the catheter, leaks are associated with weak abdominal wall structure or the need for placement adjustment. If early infection occurs beyond the exit site of the catheter, intraoperative contamination or perforation of the intestines may be the culprit

Late complication includes pain, perforation, peritonitis, catheter obstruction, and herniation at the insertion site. Association symptoms include abdominal pain, nausea and vomiting, fever, bleeding, distention abdominal and cloudy dialysate fluid. Ultrasound, or radiologic dye studies and a CT scan, may be used to further evaluate the exact cause of presenting compliant.

This create high osmotic gradient in brain resulting in the shift of fluid into the brain causing cerebral edema.

## Nursing Management

Chronic renal failure, also known as chronic kidney disease, is a progressive and irreversible loss of kidney function over time. Nursing diagnoses for chronic renal failure may include:

- **Risk for imbalanced nutrition:** Less than body requirements related to anorexia, nausea, vomiting, and malabsorption
- Risk for fluid volume excess related to decreased urine output and fluid overload
- Risk for impaired skin integrity related to edema, skin breakdown, and pressure ulcers
- Risk for decreased cardiac output related to fluid and electrolyte imbalances
- Activity intolerance related to fatigue, weakness, and decreased endurance
- Risk for infection related to decreased immune function and invasive procedures
- Anxiety related to the uncertainty of prognosis and treatment
- Risk for impaired urinary elimination related to decreased urine output and/or renal replacement therapy
- Knowledge deficit related to the disease process, treatment options, and self-care management.

## Nursing Diagnosis

- **Risk for imbalanced nutrition:** Less than body requirements related to decreased appetite and malabsorption and nursing management includes:
  - Monitor the patient's nutritional status and weight regularly to identify any changes.
  - Provide nutritional counseling and education to patients to help them make healthy food choices and maintain their energy and protein needs.
  - Encourage patients to eat small, frequent meals throughout the day and to avoid foods high in salt, potassium, and phosphorus.
  - Administer oral nutritional supplements or parenteral nutrition as prescribed to manage malnutrition.
- Risk for fluid volume excess related to decreased urine output and nursing management includes:
  - Monitor the patient's fluid intake and output, vital signs, and electrolyte levels to identify any changes in their condition.
  - Administer diuretics and other medications as prescribed to manage fluid overload.
  - Educate patients about the importance of maintaining fluid balance to prevent complications.
- Fatigue related to anemia and nursing management includes:
  - Monitor the patient's hemoglobin levels and provide iron supplements and erythropoietin-stimulating agents as prescribed to manage anemia.
  - Encourage patients to take regular breaks and prioritize rest to manage fatigue.
  - Educate patients about the importance of following their medication regimen and lifestyle changes to manage anemia and fatigue.
- Risk for infection related to weakened immune system and invasive procedures and nursing management includes:
  - Monitor the patient's temperature, white blood cell count, and signs of infection to identify any potential infections.
  - Follow proper infection control procedures, such as hand hygiene and proper use of personal protective equipment, to prevent the spread of infection.
  - Administer antibiotics and other medications as prescribed to manage infections.
  - Educate patients about the importance of good hygiene and infection prevention measures.
- Disturbed body image related to changes in physical appearance and nursing management includes:
  - Encourage patients to express their feelings and concerns about their changing physical appearance.
  - Provide emotional support and counseling to help patients cope with the changes in their body image.
  - Educate patients about the available options for managing changes in their physical appearance, such as wigs or other cosmetic treatments.

Overall, nursing management and nursing diagnosis for CRF aim to slow down the progression of the disease, manage symptoms, and prevent complications. Close monitoring of the patient's condition is essential to identify any changes and adjust the plan of care accordingly. It is important for the healthcare team to work together to provide comprehensive care for patients with CRF.

These nursing diagnoses may vary depending on the stage and severity of chronic renal failure, as well as the individual patient's needs and co-morbidities. It is important for nurses to educate patients about their condition, provide support and resources for self-care management, and collaborate with the healthcare team to develop an individualized care plan. Regular monitoring and assessment of the patient's condition and response to treatment is also crucial.

## ACUTE TUBULAR NECROSIS

### Definition

Acute tubular necrosis (ATN) is defined as kidney severe/prolonged hypoperfusion and toxicity that develops ischemia with injury to parenchyma eventually leads to infraction which does not resolve immediately with restoration of renal perfusion.

### Causes of Acute Tubular Necrosis

- Sepsis/cardiac surgery.
- Drugs such as aminoglycosides-gentamycin, neomycin, etc.
- Acute tubular interstitial nephritis.
- Urinary obstruction.

### Pathophysiology

Chronic renal failure, also known as chronic kidney disease (CKD), is a progressive and irreversible condition characterized by the gradual loss of kidney function over time. The pathophysiology of chronic renal failure involves various underlying mechanisms that contribute to the progressive decline in renal function. The key processes involved in the pathophysiology of CKD include:

- **Glomerular injury and loss:** Chronic renal failure often begins with glomerular injury, which can be caused by various factors such as diabetes, hypertension, glomerulonephritis, or autoimmune diseases. The sustained damage to the glomeruli, the filtering units of the kidneys, leads to the progressive loss of functional nephrons.
- **Tubulointerstitial fibrosis:** As chronic renal failure progresses, there is a deposition of excessive extracellular matrix proteins in the tubulointerstitial space. This fibrotic process involves the activation of inflammatory and profibrotic pathways, resulting in the replacement of normal renal tissue with scar tissue. Tubulointerstitial fibrosis further impairs renal function, leading to tubular atrophy and loss of functional nephrons.
- **Renal inflammation and oxidative stress:** Chronic renal failure is associated with chronic low-grade inflammation and increased oxidative stress within the kidneys. The ongoing inflammatory response leads to the production of cytokines and chemokines, which contribute to renal tissue damage and fibrosis. Oxidative stress, caused by an imbalance between reactive oxygen species (ROS) and antioxidant defense mechanisms, also plays a significant role in the pathogenesis of CKD.
- **Renal hypoperfusion and ischemia:** In advanced stages of chronic renal failure, there is often a state of renal hypoperfusion, characterized by reduced blood flow to the kidneys. This can result from progressive narrowing of renal blood vessels, impaired autoregulation, or decreased cardiac output. The reduced perfusion leads to renal ischemia, which further contributes to renal damage and loss of nephrons.
- **Proteinuria and albuminuria:** Proteinuria, the presence of excessive protein in the urine, is a hallmark of chronic renal failure. The damaged glomerular filtration barrier allows the passage of proteins, including albumin, from the bloodstream into the urine. Proteinuria and albuminuria contribute to renal inflammation, oxidative stress, and tubular injury, exacerbating the progression of CKD.
- **Disturbed fluid and electrolyte balance:** As chronic renal failure advances, the kidneys lose their ability to regulate fluid and electrolyte balance. The impaired reabsorption and secretion processes lead to alterations in sodium, potassium, calcium, and phosphate levels in the body. Fluid retention and electrolyte imbalances can cause hypertension, edema, and disturbances in acid-base balance.
- **Endocrine dysfunction:** The kidneys play a vital role in the production and regulation of several hormones, such as erythropoietin (EPO), renin, and active vitamin D. In chronic renal failure, the impaired renal function results in decreased EPO production, leading to anemia. Additionally, the reduced activation of vitamin D can lead to disturbances in calcium and phosphate metabolism, contributing to bone abnormalities.

Overall, the pathophysiology of chronic renal failure involves a complex interplay of glomerular injury, tubulointerstitial fibrosis, inflammation, oxidative stress, renal hypoperfusion, proteinuria, and electrolyte imbalances. These processes contribute to the progressive loss of nephrons and decline in renal function observed in CKD. Timely intervention and management are crucial to slow down the progression of chronic renal failure and preserve renal function **(Flowchart 7.3)**.

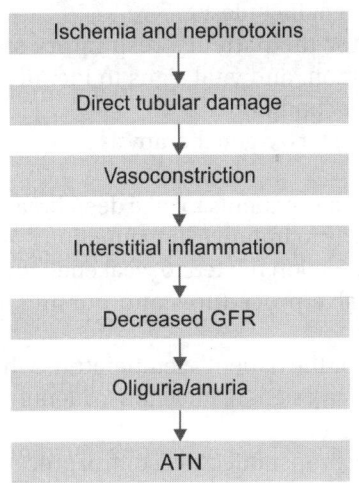

**Flowchart 7.3:** Pathophysiology of ATN.

## Clinical Course of Acute Tubular Necrosis

It is divided into:
- **Initiation stage:** Last for 3 days, with an indications of decreased urinary output sometimes oliguria and decline in GRF rate.
- **Maintenance stage:** Lasting more than 3 weeks, characterized by anuria 100–150 mL urine output, with a risk of hyperkalemia, and increased BUN levels.
- **Recovery phase:** Gradual increase in the urine output. Large amount of potassium, sodium and water are lost through urine outflow by this tubulcs may still damage. This may lead to hypokalemia for hyperkalemia, there is a sudden changes in the renal tubules causes infection. At last renal tubular function is maintained. At the same time, BUN and creatinine levels start to return to normal. Fine tubular functional impairment may persist for months, but most of the patients who reach this phase in due course recover completely.

## Diagnostics Finding

- *Serum chemistries:*
  - BUN and serum creatinine concentrations are increased.
  - Hyperkalemia, hyponatremia, hyperphosphatemia, hypermagnesemia, hypocalcemia, and metabolic acidosis may be present.
- **CBC:** Patient may be anemic. Because erythropoietin production decreased but platelet dysfunction from uremia production decline but platelet dysfunction from uremia also construct bleeding more likely.
- *Urinalysis:* May disclose muddy brown granular casts and epithelial cell casts. In addition, examining urine microscopic–"muddy brown cast".

### Imaging Studies
- Retrograde cystography
- CT scan abdomen
- Ultrasonography
- Renal ultrasound is a simple, relatively inexpensive and noninvasive imaging modality and this procedure should be done in all patients presenting with ATN.

### Renal Biopsy
- Renal biopsy procedure should be performed only when acute renal failure cause is not found. The course is prolonged and knowing the exact cause is perhaps going to change the management.
- Needless to say, pre renal and postrenal causes must be ruled out before subjecting a patient to this invasive procedure.

## Complications

**Intravascular volume overload:** It is characterized by weight gain, raised jugular venous pressure and dependent edema.

## Prevention

Dopamine, mannitol and furosemide, have been tried within 24 hours of ischemic insult to prevent progression to ATN, but have no proven benefit.

## Treatment

- **Fluid intake**
  - Restrict and match the intake of fluid volume to urine output.
  - *Monitor fluid intake:* Treating physician may recommend to monitor the intake of water and other fluids so as to prevent fluid retention. Fluid retention may result in edema feet, liver enlargement and respiratory symptoms.
- **Protein restriction:** In later phase albumin and globulin are reabsorbed by kidney, so to prevent toxic build up of protein in body restrict intake of protein.
- **Restriction of salt:** The kidney retains sodium, potassium and chloride. Salt restriction is advised to prevent excessive build up of salt in the body.
- **Diuretics:** Diuretics are prescribed to remove extra water, which is retained by kidney.
- **Kidney dialysis:** Some individuals need dialysis to clear the body of waste products and excess water.
- Correct underlying problem
- Supportive therapy – maintain fluid balance
- Maintain perfusion of kidneys.

In general, an attempt is made to increase the urine output if oliguria is present, by using loop diuretics, although there is some controversy about this in the literature. One retrospective study showed that diuretics may even increase the risk of death and nonrecovery of renal increase the risk of death and nonrecovery of renal function. The only true indication for diuretic use is volume overload. Furosemide and bumetanide are the commonly used diuretics.

Acute tubular necrosis is a kidney disorder characterized by damage to the renal tubules, which can lead to acute kidney injury. Nursing diagnoses for ATN may include:

- Risk for decreased cardiac output related to fluid and electrolyte imbalances
- Excess fluid volume related to decreased urine output and fluid overload
- Imbalanced nutrition: less than body requirements related to anorexia, nausea, and vomiting
- Risk for infection related to decreased immune function and invasive procedures
- Risk for impaired skin integrity related to edema, skin breakdown, and pressure ulcers
- Risk for injury related to altered mental status, decreased mobility, and seizures
- Anxiety related to the uncertainty of prognosis and treatment
- Risk for impaired urinary elimination related to decreased urine output and/or renal replacement therapy
- Knowledge deficit related to the disease process, treatment options, and self-care management.

These nursing diagnoses may vary depending on the cause and severity of the ATN, as well as the individual patient's needs and co-morbidities. The nursing care for ATN includes careful monitoring of fluid and electrolyte balance, management of nutrition and medications, prevention and management of complications, and support for renal replacement therapy. Nurses should also provide emotional support to the patient and family, and educate them on the management of ATN and the importance of follow-up care.

### Nursing Diagnosis

- Risk for fluid volume deficit related to fluid loss and nursing management includes:
  - Monitor the patient's fluid intake and output, vital signs, and electrolyte levels to identify any changes in their condition.
  - Administer intravenous fluids and electrolytes as prescribed to manage fluid deficit.
  - Educate patients about the importance of maintaining fluid balance to prevent complications.
- Impaired gas exchange related to hypoxia and nursing management includes:
  - Monitor the patient's respiratory status, oxygen saturation, and vital signs to identify any changes in their condition.
  - Administer oxygen therapy as prescribed to manage hypoxia.
  - Encourage patients to take deep breaths and cough regularly to improve lung function.
- Risk for infection related to weakened immune system and invasive procedures and nursing management includes:
  - Monitor the patient's temperature, white blood cell count, and signs of infection to identify any potential infections.
  - Follow proper infection control procedures, such as hand hygiene and proper use of personal protective equipment, to prevent the spread of infection.
  - Administer antibiotics and other medications as prescribed to manage infections.
  - Educate patients about the importance of good hygiene and infection prevention measures.
- Anxiety related to illness and nursing management includes:
  - Provide emotional support and counseling to help patients cope with the anxiety related to their illness.
  - Educate patients about their condition and the treatments they will receive to manage their anxiety.
  - Encourage patients to express their feelings and concerns about their condition.
- Risk for acute pain related to kidney damage and nursing management includes:
  - Monitor the patient's pain level and provide pain medication as prescribed to manage pain.
  - Educate patients about the available pain management options and the importance of managing their pain.
  - Encourage patients to report any new or worsening pain.

### Nursing Management

Gradual increase in the urine output. Large amount of potassium, sodium and water are lost through urine outflow by this tubules may still damage. This may lead to hypokalemia for hyperkalemia, there is a sudden changes in the renal tubules causes infection. At last renal tubular function is maintained. At the same time, BUN and creatinine levels start to return to normal. Fine tubular functional impairment may persist for months, but most of the patients who reach this phase in due course recover completely. Maintain electrolyte balance and prevention of infection. Finally, renal tubular function is restored and tubular concentration ability improves. At the same time, BUN and creatinine levels start to return to normal. Fine tubular functional impairment may persist for months, but most of the patients who reach this phase in due course recover completely

## BLADDER TRAUMA

### Definition

Traumatic injury of the bladder and urethra caused by an outside force. Traumatic injury to the bladder is uncommon. Only 7–10% of pelvic fractures lead to bladder injury. Injury may occur if there is a blow to the pelvis severe break in the bones and cause bone fragments to penetrate the bladder wall leads to bladder trauma.

### Causes of Bladder Injury

- Road traffic accidents
- Blow, kick or fall
- Stabs, gunshot injuries
- Endoscopic trauma
- Diathermy
- Occurs in 20% of bladder rupture cases
- Occurs due to blow, kick or fall
- Instrumentations for example: During hysterectomy, herniotomy, excision of rectum, LSCS, etc.

### Grade Injury

- **Grade Ia:** Hematoma on the wall of bladder.
- **Grade Ib:** Partial laceration found on the wall of bladder.
- **Grade II:** Extraperitoneal less than 2 cm laceration on the wall of bladder.
- **Grade III:** Extraperitoneal and intraperitoneal lesser than 2 cm laceration on the wall of bladder.
- **Grade IV:** Intraperitoneal laceration greater than 2 cm on the wall of bladder.
- **Grade V:** Intraperitoneal or extraperitoneal laceration on wall of the bladder will extend to the urethral orifice.

### Mechanism of Bladder Injury

- Perforation of bladder dome during veress needle/trocar insertion.
- Incidental cystotomy during development of bladder flap and VVS in routine/radical hysterectomy.

### Signs and Symptoms

- Abdominal fullness
- Suprapubic tenderness and pain
- Scrotal swelling
- Strangury and inability to micturate
- Often associated with shock and other injuries
- Abdominal distention
- Lately results in peritonitis, with guarding rigidity, rebound tenderness

### Diagnostic Finding

- Presence of urine is confirmed by peritoneal tap
- Retrograde cystography
- CT scan abdomen
- Ultrasonography

### Complications

- Cystitis and pyelonephritis
- Peritonitis
- Pelvic abscess
- Vesicovaginal or rectovesical fistula
- Paralytic ileus
- Hemorrhage
- Mortality is 100% without surgical intervention

### Management

Urinalysis typically shows gross hematuria. Gunshot wounds to the bladder may result in microscopic hematuria. Rupture of bladder can be seen on routine abdominal CT and more accurately with a CT cystogram. Intraperitonial bladder rupture requires exploratory laparotomy and repair through a layered closure, whereas extraperitoneal injuries can be managed with bladder drainage alone. Urologic follow-up and antibiotics are needed to prevent long-term complications, including strictures, fistulas, infection, and delayed healing.

### Nursing Diagnosis

Bladder trauma is a medical condition that occurs when the bladder is injured, usually as a result of an accident or trauma. Nursing management and nursing diagnosis for bladder trauma aim to manage symptoms, prevent complications, and promote recovery. Here are some nursing management and nursing diagnosis for bladder trauma:

- Acute pain related to bladder trauma and nursing management includes:
  - Assess the patient's pain level and location to determine the best pain management approach.
  - Administer pain medication as prescribed to manage pain.
  - Monitor the patient's response to pain management and adjust the plan of care as needed.

- Encourage the patient to report any new or worsening pain.
- Risk for infection related to bladder trauma and nursing management includes:
  - Monitor the patient's temperature, white blood cell count, and signs of infection to identify any potential infections.
  - Administer antibiotics and other medications as prescribed to manage infections.
  - Encourage the patient to maintain good hygiene and follow infection prevention measures.
  - Provide education to the patient and family about the importance of infection prevention.
- Anxiety related to bladder trauma and nursing management includes:
  - Provide emotional support and counseling to help the patient cope with the anxiety related to their condition.
  - Educate the patient and family about the condition and the treatments they will receive.
  - Encourage the patient to express their feelings and concerns about their condition.
- Impaired urinary elimination related to bladder trauma and nursing management includes:
  - Monitor the patient's urine output, color, and clarity to identify any changes.
  - Administer bladder catheterization as prescribed to help the patient eliminate urine.
  - Educate the patient and family about the catheterization procedure and how to care for the catheter.
  - Monitor the patient for any signs of complications, such as catheter blockage or infection.
- Risk for impaired skin integrity related to bladder trauma and nursing management includes:
  - Monitor the patient's skin condition and identify any signs of breakdown or pressure ulcers.
  - Position the patient appropriately to prevent pressure ulcers.
  - Encourage the patient to maintain good hygiene and follow skin care procedures.
  - Provide education to the patient and family about the importance of skin care and pressure ulcer prevention.

Overall, nursing management and nursing diagnosis for bladder trauma aim to manage the symptoms, prevent complications, and promote recovery. Close monitoring of the patient's condition is essential to identify any changes and adjust the plan of care accordingly. It is important for the healthcare team to work together to provide comprehensive care for patients with bladder trauma.

# DISORDERS OF FLUID VOLUME

Water abnormalities may be due to underlying diseases, iatrogenic causes, environmental factors or psychological abnormalities.

ECF imbalance may be caused by an extra cellular volume deficit, which includes an increase in insensible water loss or perspiration (high fever and heat stroke), diabetes insipidus, osmotic dieresis, hemorrhage, GI loss, inadequate fluid intake and 3rd space fluid shift (burns, intestinal obstruction).

An extra cellular volume excess may be caused by an extreme intake of isotonic or hypotonic IV fluids, heart failure, renal failure, primary polydipsia, syndrome of inappropriate antidiuretic hormone (SIADH), cushing syndrome, and the long term use of corticosteroids.

## Water Depletion

Water depletion may be due to reduced water consumption, diarrhea, vomiting, excessive sweating, excessive respiration, renal disease, ADH deficiency (diabetes insipidus) excessive diuretic use and diabetic ketoacidosis (DKA). Water deficiency is almost always associated with loss of sodium.

Signs and symptoms of water deficiency include thirst, loss of eye ball and skin turgor, dry mucous membrane, flushed skin, decreased urinary output, decreased urine specific gravity, increased temperature, tachycardia, delirium and coma. Most patients with water deficiency are also deficient in sodium and other electrolyte, so oral or parental fluid replacement must be determined on an individual basis. Frequently selected fluids to replenish water and sodium loss include normal saline (0.9%). Serial electrolyte and plasma osmolarity levels are required to determine appropriate fluid replacement.

## Water Excess

Water excess is characterized by weight gain, muscle twitching and cramps, pulmonary or peripheral edema, hyper ventilation, confusion, hallucination, coma and convulsions. Water excess may be due to increased water ingestion, excessive IV therapy, renal disease, excessive ADH and inadequate water transport to the kidney, e.g., shock, heart failure.

The aim of treatment for fluid volume excess is to identify the cause and the treatment goal is to remove fluid volume excess without producing abnormal changes in electrolyte composition. Other possible treatments include restriction of sodium intake, abdominal paracentesis for ascites and thoracentesis for a pleural effusion.

## Nursing Diagnosis

*Disorders of fluid volume refer to conditions in which there is an imbalance between the intake and output of fluids in the body, leading to either excess fluid volume or fluid deficit. Nursing diagnoses for disorders of fluid volume may include:*

- Excess fluid volume related to fluid overload
- Risk for decreased cardiac output related to fluid overload
- Risk for impaired gas exchange related to pulmonary edema
- Risk for impaired skin integrity related to edema, skin breakdown, and pressure ulcers
- Imbalanced nutrition: less than body requirements related to anorexia, nausea, vomiting, and diarrhea
- Risk for injury related to altered mental status, decreased mobility, and seizures
- Risk for infection related to altered immune function and invasive procedures
- Risk for impaired urinary elimination related to fluid overload and/or renal failure
- Knowledge deficit related to the disease process, treatment options, and self-care management.

*Disorders of fluid volume refer to conditions where there is an imbalance in the amount of fluid and electrolytes in the body. Common examples include dehydration, hypovolemia, and fluid overload. Here are some nursing management and nursing diagnosis for disorders of fluid volume:*

- Risk for deficient fluid volume related to excessive fluid loss or inadequate intake, and nursing management includes:
  - Assess the patient's fluid intake and output to determine the extent of the deficit.
  - Administer oral or intravenous fluids as prescribed to restore fluid balance.
  - Monitor the patient's vital signs, skin turgor, and urine output to evaluate the effectiveness of fluid replacement therapy.
  - Educate the patient and family about the importance of maintaining adequate fluid intake and recognizing signs of dehydration.
- Risk for excess fluid volume related to compromised regulatory mechanisms or excessive fluid intake, and nursing management includes:
  - Assess the patient's fluid intake and output to determine the extent of fluid overload.
  - Administer diuretics or other medications as prescribed to remove excess fluid.
  - Monitor the patient's vital signs, lung sounds, and urine output to evaluate the effectiveness of fluid removal therapy.
  - Educate the patient and family about the importance of limiting fluid intake and recognizing signs of fluid overload.
- Risk for electrolyte imbalance related to fluid volume disorders, and nursing management includes:
  - Monitor the patient's electrolyte levels, such as sodium, potassium, and calcium, to identify any imbalances.
  - Administer electrolyte replacement therapy as prescribed to restore electrolyte balance.
  - Educate the patient and family about the importance of maintaining a balanced diet and following medication regimens to prevent electrolyte imbalances.
- Impaired gas exchange related to fluid overload, and nursing management includes:
  - Monitor the patient's respiratory status, such as oxygen saturation and respiratory rate, to identify any signs of impaired gas exchange.
  - Administer oxygen therapy as prescribed to improve oxygenation.
  - Position the patient in a semi-Fowler's position to promote lung expansion.
  - Educate the patient and family about the importance of maintaining good respiratory hygiene and avoiding respiratory irritants.

These nursing diagnoses may vary depending on the cause and severity of the fluid volume disorder, as well as the individual patient's needs and co-morbidities. Nursing care for fluid volume disorders includes monitoring of fluid intake and output, careful management of fluids and electrolytes, administration of diuretics or other medications as needed, and assessment and prevention of complications. Nurses may also educate the patient on self-care management, provide emotional support, and collaborate with the healthcare team to develop an individualized care plan.

## Nursing Implementation

- **Intake output:** 24 hours intake output record gives valuable information. Urine specific gravity measurement can be done.
- **Cardiovascular changes:** Monitor the patient cardio vascular changes to prevent or detect complications.
- **Neurological changes:** Assessment of neurologic functions includes evaluation of level of consciousness, verbal response and painful stimuli. Orientation of time place and person, pupillary response to light and equality of pupil size. Voluntary moment of extremities, degree of muscle strength and reflexes.

# END-STAGE RENAL DISEASE AND RENAL TRANSPLANTATION

First kidney transplantation was performed in 1954 in Boston between identical twins. Kidney transplantation requires taking a donor kidney from the body of one person and implanting it surgically into the recipient body that had lost kidney function. The transplanted kidney then can perform the function of their own kidney. The age range of most suitable kidney donor is 2–70 years.

Kidney transplantation is not a complete cure, even though many people who underwent kidney transplantation are able to have quality of life before their kidneys failed. Client who receive kidney transplantation must be on medication and be monitored by a physician who is specialized in kidney disease for the rest of their live

Patients with a well-functioning transplant have a greater sense of wellbeing and are able to enjoy a lifestyle dialysis free, although they must continue with their transplant medication. Transplant offers freedom from previous dietary and/or fluid restriction and from restriction on time and mobility and have improvement in bone density and anemia.

## Causes of Kidney Transplant

- **Kidney disorder:** The chronic kidney disease also known as chronic renal disease requires the kidney transplant. CKD causes a progressive loss of renal function.
- **Genetic disorder:** Polycystic kidney disease, autoimmune conditions including lupus and good pasture's syndrome and number of inborn errors of metabolism.
- **Other diseases:** Infections, diabetes mellitus and glomerulonephritis and hypertension.

## Recipient Selection

Appropriate recipient selection is important for a successful outcome. The high-risk patients who have co-morbidities such as diabetes mellitus, cardiovascular disease and hypertension should be carefully assessed and monitored appropriately after kidney transplantation.

## Contraindications

- Disseminated malignancies
- Refractory or untreated cardiac disease
- Chronic respiratory failure
- Extensive vascular disease
- Chronic infection
- Unresolved psychosocial disorders
- Hepatitis B or C is not a contraindication

## Donor Sources

Kidney for transplantation may be obtained from compatible blood type deceased donors, blood relatives, emotionally related living donors (e.g., spouse, distant cousin, etc.).

### Live Donor

- Complete history and physical examination
- Compatible blood type deceased donors, blood relatives, emotionally related living donors (e.g., spouse, distant cousin, etc.)
- Live donor must be in good health condition with no co morbidities and no family history of diseases
- One week before transplantation cross matching should do in order to prevent any antibiotics to the donor.

### Advantages

- Live donor kidney includes better patient and graft survival rate.
- Immediate organ availability.
- Immediate function because of minimal cold time.

### Donor Preparation

- The donor will see a nephrologist for a complete history and physical studies.
- Laboratory studies include a 24 hours urine study for creatinine clearance and total protein.
- Complete blood count (CBC) and chemistry and electrolytes profile.
- Cytomegalovirus
- ECG
- Chest X-ray
- CT scan
- Psychologist consultation

### Deceased Donor

Deceased or cadaver kidney donors are brain dead donors have cardiovascular and renal system in a healthy condition and it can be preserve by the help of ventilators.

### Cause for Renal Injury

- Cerebrovascular accident (CVA)
- Sharp or blunt injuries
- Spinal cord injures
- Cardiac arrest
- Brain death: Brain dead donors have cardiovascular system in a good condition and it can be preserve by the help of ventilators.

## Surgical Procedure

### Kidney Transplant Recipient

- Transplanted kidney usually placed extra peritoneally in the iliac fossa.
- Right iliac fossa is preferred to facilitate anastomoses and minimize the occurrence.
- Catheter is inserted in the urinary bladder.
- Peritoneum is left intact.
- Iliac and hypogastric vessels are dissected free.
- The recipient's internal iliac artery or external iliac artery is anastomosed to donor artery.
- The recipient's external iliac artery is anastomosed to donor vein.
- Establish the blood flow to the kidney by removing the clamp, after the completion of anastomoses.
- Immediately after release of clamp urine start flowing from ureter from kidney.
- Mannitol and furosemide may be administered to promote diuresis.
- Transplant surgery takes 3–4 hours.

## Nursing Diagnosis

- End-stage renal disease (ESRD) is a condition in which the kidneys have permanently lost function and require renal replacement therapy, such as dialysis or kidney transplantation. Nursing diagnoses for ESRD and renal transplantation may include:
  - Risk for infection related to invasive procedures and immunosuppressive medications.
  - Risk for imbalanced nutrition: Less than body requirements related to anorexia, nausea, vomiting, and malabsorption.
  - Risk for fluid volume excess or deficit related to fluid and electrolyte imbalances.
  - Risk for impaired skin integrity related to edema, skin breakdown, and pressure ulcers
  - Risk for decreased cardiac output related to fluid and electrolyte imbalances
  - Activity intolerance related to fatigue, weakness, and decreased endurance
  - Anxiety related to the uncertainty of prognosis and treatment
  - Risk for impaired urinary elimination related to decreased urine output and/or renal replacement therapy
  - Knowledge deficit related to the disease process, treatment options, and self-care management.
- Excess fluid volume related to impaired kidney function, and nursing management includes:
  - Monitor the patient's weight, blood pressure, and fluid intake and output to identify any signs of fluid overload.
  - Administer diuretics or other medications as prescribed to remove excess fluid.
  - Educate the patient and family about the importance of following a fluid-restricted diet and limiting sodium intake.
- Risk for infection related to immunosuppressive therapy or chronic disease, and nursing management includes:
  - Monitor the patient's vital signs and laboratory values, such as white blood cell count and culture results, to identify any signs of infection.
  - Administer prophylactic antibiotics or antifungal medications as prescribed.
  - Educate the patient and family about the importance of good hygiene practices and avoiding exposure to infectious agents.
- Risk for impaired skin integrity related to chronic disease or dialysis access, and nursing management includes:
  - Inspect the patient's skin regularly to identify any signs of pressure ulcers or skin breakdown.
  - Provide appropriate wound care and pressure relief interventions as needed.
  - Educate the patient and family about the importance of maintaining good skin hygiene and avoiding prolonged pressure or trauma to the skin.
- Imbalanced nutrition—less than body requirements related to dietary restrictions or anorexia, and nursing management includes:
  - Assess the patient's nutritional status and dietary intake to identify any deficits.
  - Provide nutritional counseling and support to help the patient meet their dietary requirements.
  - Administer appetite stimulants or other medications as prescribed to improve the patient's appetite.
  - Educate the patient and family about the importance of following a nutritious diet and taking medication as prescribed.
- Risk for impaired physical mobility related to chronic disease or dialysis access, and nursing management includes:
  - Assess the patient's mobility status and risk for falls or other complications.
  - Provide assistive devices or physical therapy as needed to improve mobility and prevent falls.
  - Educate the patient and family about the importance of staying active and following a safe exercise program.

These nursing diagnoses may vary depending on the stage and severity of ESRD, the type of renal replacement therapy, and the individual patient's needs and co-morbidities. Nursing care for ESRD and renal transplantation includes careful monitoring of fluid and electrolyte balance, management of nutrition and medications, prevention and management of complications, and support for renal replacement therapy or transplant. Nurses should also provide emotional support to the patient and family, and educate them on the management of ESRD and transplantation, and the importance of follow-up care. Regular monitoring and assessment of the patient's condition and response to treatment is also crucial.

## Nursing Management

### Preoperative Care

- Physical and emotional preparation of patient, because, family and patient waiting for kidney transplantation for a long time.
- Immediate postoperating period will be there.
- There is a chance of kidney may not work immediately after transplantation.
- There is a need for dialysis.
- Need for immunosuppressive drugs.
- Preparation of patient: ECG, XRAY, lab investigation.
- Dialysis if hyperkalemia.
- Vascular access site should be labeled "for dialysis no procedures", for preparation of BP hand area, blood drawing, IV line, etc.

### Postoperation Care

*Live Donor*

- Close monitoring of renal function
- Serum creatinine should be <1.4 mp/dc
- Mostly can discharge 4–5 days, can return to work in 6–8 days.
- Follow up after 1–2 weeks.

*Recipient*

- Fluid, electrolyte balance
- First 12–24 hours in ICU
- Urine output at early hours 1 L/hour.
- Gradual decrease of BUN and serum creatinine to normal
- Urine output replaced by fluid.
- CUP monitoring
- If met acidosis – IV $NaHCO_3$
- Decrease output, increase creatinine, BUN – dialysis.
- Chance of rejection for 1st 3 months

*Immunosuppressive Therapy*

To prevent rejection.

*Complications Transplantation*

- Rejection – may be hyperkalemia.
- Infection:
  - Because suppression of the body's immune system
  - Underlying co-morbidities like DM, systemic lupus earth matters, malnutrition of old age, e.g., pneumonia, wound infection, IV line and drain infection, UTI
  - Prophylactic management.
- Cardiovascular disorders
  - More chance of atherosclerotic vascular disorder
  - *Risk factors:* Hypertension, dyslipidemia, DM, smoking, rejection, infection, ↑ homocysteine level.
- Malignancies: Because of immunosuppressive therapy, because cancer of kidney, skin, lips, hepatobiliary system, vulva, perineum, lymphomas, kaposi sarcoma
- Recurrence of original renal dialysis: Glomerulonephritis, I A nephropathy, diabetic nephropathy, focal segmental sclerosis
- Corticosteroid related complications
  - Aseptic necrosis of hips knees, joints, renal osteodystrophy
  - Peptic ulcer, diabetic mellitus, cataract, hyperlipidemic.

## MANAGEMENT MODALITIES FOR RENAL SYSTEM DISORDERS

### Renal Replacement Therapy

CRRT most commonly uses the venovenous approach of continuous venovenous hemofiltration (CVVH) and continuous venovenous hemodialysis (CVVHD). These approaches are the focus of this discussion of CRRT.

Chronic renal failure requiring dialysis is known as end-stage renal disease, or ESRD. Renal replacement therapy may be provided by peritoneal dialysis or hemodialysis. Peritoneal dialysis involves instilling 1–2 L of dialysate fluid containing varying amount of glucose, magnesium, calcium, chloride, and lactate into abdomen. The peritoneal membrane acts as a semipermeable pathway for exchange of solute and water between the vascular peritoneal space and dialysate by osmosis and diffusion. Access to the peritoneal cavity is achieved through a plastic catheter held in place by a Dacron cuff.

Complications occurring early after surgical catheter insertion most commonly include pain, bleeding, obstruction (fluid unable to move in or out of the catheter), and infection and/or leaks. Early complications are generally associated with misplacement of the catheter during insertion. Significant pain and bleeding are suspicious of perforation of an internal organ during placement. Obstruction may be related to a blockage or kink in the catheter, leaks are associated with weak abdominal wall structure or the need for placement adjustment. If early infection occurs beyond the exit site of the catheter, intra-operative contamination or perforation of the intestines may be the culprit.

Late complication includes pain, perforation, peritonitis, catheter obstruction, and herniation at the insertion site. Association symptoms include abdominal pain, nausea and vomiting, fever, bleeding, distention abdominal and cloudy dialysate fluid. Ultrasound, or radiologic dye studies and a CT scan, may be used to further evaluate the exact cause of presenting compliant.

Depending on the infection, antibiotics may be added to the dialysate fluid or given orally or intravenously. For catheter placement complications, surgical correction may be required. For recurrent peritonitis for which antibiotic therapy is not successful, the catheter should be removed and hemodialysis initiated until peritonitis clears. Unless scarring impairs permeability of the peritoneal membrane, the catheter can be surgically replaced and peritoneal dialysis reinitiated. Care in the ED may include obtaining a sample of peritoneal catheter, carefully adhering to aseptic technique sterile gloves to prevent contamination during access of the peritoneal catheter are extremely important to prevent infection and resultant peritonitis.

Clotted vascular access frequently bring patient with CRF to the ED. Arteriovenous fistulas are surgical connections of a native artery and vein in an extremity or insertion of Gore-Tex graft material to form the connection. Available sites suitable for vascular access may become exhausted, so permanent subclavian dual-lumen catheters are also placed for hemodialysis. Clotting vascular access should be emergently declotted with the use of locally instilled or infused fibrinolytics or surgery. Grafts, fistulas, and insertion sites also become infected and may progress to septicemia. Local symptoms include redness, drainage, or edema. Blood cultures and a complete blood count should be obtained to rile out systemic infection. Access removal may be necessary, so temporary subclavian or femoral access (replaced every 2-3 days) can be used until blood is free of infection. Some type of anticoagulant will reside in the lumens of a dual-lumen dialysis catheter to prevent clotting. When accessing the catheter, failure to withdraw this anticoagulation could cause serious bleeding complications due to alteration of coagulation status **(Fig. 7.8)**.

Bleeding from vascular access sites (fistula, graph) is commonly encountered in the ED. During hemodialysis, the blood is anticoagulated with heparin to avoid clotting and blood loss during the procedure. Direct pressure that does not occlude the fistula or graph should be applied 5-10

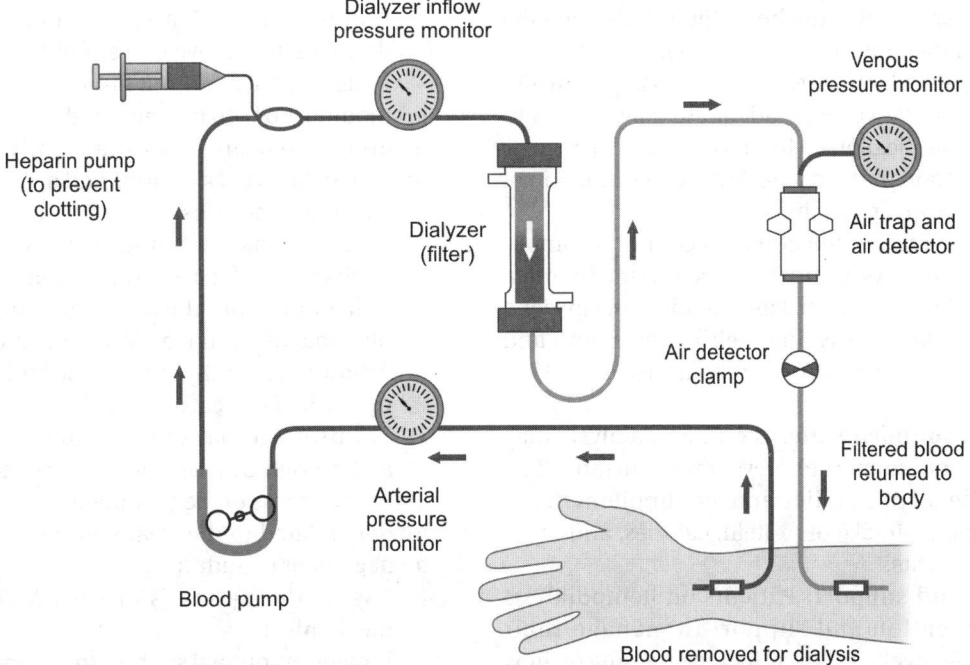

**Fig. 7.8:** Hemodialysis process (renal replacement therapy).

minutes. If direct pressure does not control bleeding, topical hemostatic agent may be used, such as Gelfoam pads (forms a mechanical matrix to enhance clot formation), chitosan (a fibrous complex carbohydrate that promotes adhesion), or thrombin powder. When applying a pressure dressing, avoid excess pressure and circumferential application of tape or other wrap because this may cause clotting of the vascular access. Anticoagulation studies may reveal that reversal of supratherapeutic anticoagulation is needed and protamine administration may be required.

## Hemodialysis

Hemodialysis is a type of renal replacement therapy that removes waste products and excess fluid from the blood using a machine called a dialyzer. The management modalities for hemodialysis include:

- **Access creation:** A vascular access is needed to perform hemodialysis. The most common types of access are fistulas, grafts, and catheters. Fistulas and grafts require surgical creation, while catheters are inserted using a minimally invasive technique.
- **Dialysis prescription:** The dialysis prescription includes the blood flow rate, dialysate flow rate, and the duration of each session. The prescription is based on the patient's needs, and it may be adjusted over time based on the results of regular blood tests.
- **Hemodialysis technique:** Hemodialysis can be performed in a dialysis center or at home. During the treatment, the patient is connected to a dialysis machine that pumps blood out of the body, filters it through the dialyzer, and then returns it to the body.
- **Monitoring:** Regular monitoring is necessary to ensure that the patient is receiving adequate dialysis and to detect any complications. Monitoring includes regular blood tests, blood pressure checks, and examination of the access site for signs of infection.
- **Infection prevention:** Infection is a common complication of hemodialysis, and it can be life-threatening. To prevent infection, patients must follow strict hygiene protocols, including washing their hands before and after each session and keeping the access site clean and dry.
- **Nutritional support:** Patients on hemodialysis may need nutritional support to prevent malnutrition. This may include a special diet and/or supplements to ensure adequate intake of protein, calories, and other essential nutrients.
- **Education and support:** Patients on hemodialysis require education and support to manage their condition effectively. This may include training on how to perform self-care, managing complications, and coping with the emotional and psychological impact of the treatment.

Overall, the management modalities for hemodialysis aim to ensure effective dialysis, prevent complications, and improve the patient's quality of life.

Nursing management and nursing diagnosis for hemodialysis involve a holistic approach to the patient's care, which includes the physical, emotional, and psychosocial aspects of the patient's health. Here are some nursing management and nursing diagnosis for hemodialysis:

### Nursing Diagnosis

- Risk for infection related to the vascular access site, and nursing management includes:
  - Monitor the access site for signs of redness, swelling, warmth, or discharge.
  - Follow strict hygiene protocols, including washing hands before and after touching the access site and wearing gloves during procedures.
  - Educate patients about infection prevention and self-care practices to reduce the risk of infection.
  - Collaborate with the healthcare team to provide appropriate antibiotic therapy for infections.
- Fluid volume excess related to fluid overload and nursing management includes:
  - Monitor the patient's weight before and after each dialysis session to assess fluid balance.
  - Monitor vital signs, such as blood pressure and heart rate, for signs of fluid overload.
  - Administer medications as prescribed, such as diuretics, to remove excess fluid.
  - Educate patients about fluid restriction and dietary modifications to prevent fluid overload.
- Altered nutrition—less than body requirements related to dietary restrictions and anemia, and nursing management includes:
  - Assess the patient's nutritional status and dietary habits to develop a nutrition plan.
  - Collaborate with the dietician to develop a dietary plan that meets the patient's nutritional needs.
  - Administer erythropoietin-stimulating agents as prescribed to treat anemia.
  - Monitor the patient's laboratory values, such as hemoglobin and hematocrit, to evaluate the effectiveness of the treatment.
- Anxiety related to the treatment process and nursing management includes:
  - Assess the patient's anxiety level and coping mechanisms.
  - Provide emotional support to the patient by actively listening and acknowledging their concerns.

- Educate patients about the hemodialysis process and procedures to alleviate their anxiety.
- Provide a comfortable and supportive environment to promote relaxation.

Overall, nursing management and nursing diagnosis for hemodialysis aim to ensure safe and effective dialysis, prevent complications, and improve the patient's quality of life.

## Peritoneal Dialysis

Peritoneal dialysis (PD) is a type of dialysis that uses the peritoneum, a membrane lining the abdomen, to filter waste products and excess fluid from the blood. Management of peritoneal dialysis includes several modalities that aim to ensure effective dialysis and prevent complications. Here are some of the management modalities for peritoneal dialysis:

- **Catheter insertion:** The first step in PD management is the insertion of a catheter into the peritoneal cavity. The catheter is usually inserted under local anesthesia in an outpatient setting.
- **Dialysate prescription:** The dialysate is the solution that is used to remove waste products and excess fluid from the blood. The prescription of the dialysate depends on the patient's needs, and it may be adjusted over time based on the results of regular blood tests **(Fig. 7.9)**.
- **Exchange technique:** There are two main techniques for performing a peritoneal dialysis exchange: continuous ambulatory peritoneal dialysis (CAPD) and automated peritoneal dialysis (APD). In CAPD, the patient manually exchanges the dialysate 4–5 times per day, while in APD, a machine automatically performs the exchanges during the night.
- **Monitoring:** Regular monitoring is necessary to ensure that the patient is receiving adequate dialysis and to detect any complications. Monitoring includes regular blood tests, weight checks, and examination of the catheter exit site for signs of infection.
- **Infection prevention:** Infection is a common complication of peritoneal dialysis, and it can be life-threatening. To prevent infection, patients must follow strict hygiene protocols, including washing their hands before each exchange and keeping the catheter exit site clean and dry.
- **Nutritional support:** Patients on peritoneal dialysis may need nutritional support to prevent malnutrition. This may include a special diet and/or supplements to ensure adequate intake of protein, calories, and other essential nutrients.
- **Education and support:** Patients on peritoneal dialysis require education and support to manage their condition effectively. This may include training on how to perform exchanges, managing complications, and coping with the emotional and psychological impact of the treatment.

Overall, the management modalities for peritoneal dialysis aim to ensure effective dialysis, prevent complications, and improve the patient's quality of life.

## Continuous Arteriovenous Hemodialysis

Continuous arteriovenous hemodialysis (CAVHD) is a type of renal replacement therapy that uses a continuous process to remove waste products, excess fluid, and electrolytes from the blood. CAVHD is typically used for critically ill patients who are hemodynamically unstable and unable to tolerate other forms of hemodialysis.

The CAVHD process involves the placement of two catheters one in an artery and one in a vein which are connected to a hemofiltration machine. Blood is continuously pumped from the arterial catheter to the hemofiltration machine, where it is filtered to remove waste products, excess fluid, and electrolytes. The filtered blood is then returned to the patient through the venous catheter.

Nursing care for patients receiving CAVHD includes monitoring vital signs, fluid status, electrolyte levels, and other laboratory values. The nurse also monitors the function of the catheters, ensuring that they remain patent and free of complications such as infection or dislodgment. The nurse also assesses for potential complications such as hypotension, bleeding, and clotting.

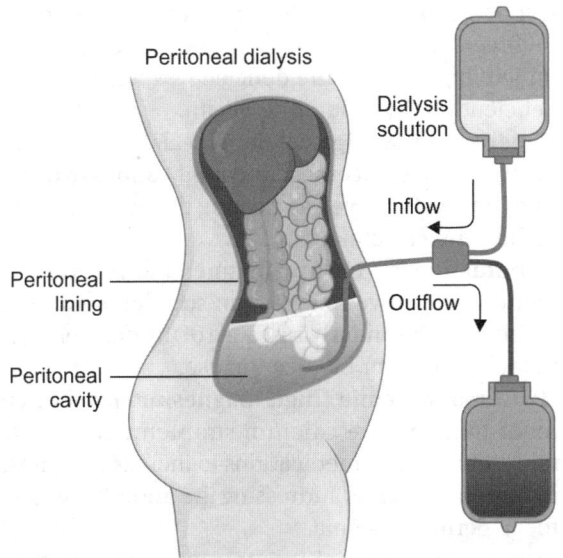

**Fig. 7.9:** Dialyzer.

In addition to monitoring and assessment, nursing care for patients receiving CAVHD includes managing the hemofiltration machine, administering medications and IV fluids as prescribed, and providing education and support to patients and families. Nurses also collaborate with the healthcare team to adjust the treatment plan as needed to optimize patient outcomes.

Overall, the nursing care for patients receiving CAVHD is focused on ensuring the safety and efficacy of the treatment while providing comprehensive care and support to the patient and family.

Some potential nursing diagnoses for patients receiving continuous arteriovenous hemodialysis (CAVHD) may include:
- Risk for infection related to invasive catheter placement and immunocompromised state.
- Risk for bleeding related to anticoagulation therapy and/or coagulopathy.
- Risk for impaired gas exchange related to fluid overload or electrolyte imbalances.
- Risk for electrolyte imbalances related to the removal of fluids and electrolytes during CAVHD.
- Risk for impaired skin integrity related to catheter placement, frequent dressing changes, and immobility.
- Anxiety related to the stress and discomfort of the CAVHD procedure, unfamiliar environment, and uncertainty about the future.
- Deficient knowledge related to the CAVHD procedure, including indications, benefits, risks, and potential complications.

### Nursing Management
- **Continuous monitoring of vital signs, laboratory values, and fluid balance:** The nurse should closely monitor the patient's vital signs, electrolyte levels, and fluid balance to ensure that CAVHD is effectively managing the patient's AKI.
- **Assessment of vascular access site:** The nurse should assess the vascular access site for signs of infection or clotting and ensure that it is functioning properly.
- **Anticoagulation management:** The nurse should monitor the patient's coagulation status and administer anticoagulants as ordered to prevent clotting in the dialysis circuit.
- **Nutrition management:** The nurse should work with a dietitian to ensure that the patient is receiving adequate nutrition during CAVHD.
- **Medication management:** The nurse should ensure that the patient's medications are adjusted appropriately to account for changes in renal function during CAVHD.

These nursing diagnoses serve as a guide for nurses to identify potential problems and develop appropriate nursing interventions to address them. The ultimate goal of nursing care for patients receiving CAVHD is to optimize patient outcomes by ensuring safety, promoting comfort, providing education and support, and collaborating with the healthcare team to individualize the treatment plan for each patient.

### Management of Electrolytic Imbalances

The management of electrolyte imbalances involves identifying the underlying cause and correcting the specific electrolyte abnormalities. The treatment may involve dietary changes, medication adjustments, or medical interventions. The following are some general management strategies for common electrolyte imbalances:
- **Hyponatremia (low sodium levels):** Treatment may involve fluid restriction, increasing dietary sodium intake, or administering medications to increase sodium levels.
- **Hypernatremia (high sodium levels):** Treatment may involve fluid replacement and correcting the underlying cause of dehydration, such as increased water intake or intravenous fluids.
- **Hypokalemia (low potassium levels):** Treatment may involve increasing dietary potassium intake or administering oral or intravenous potassium supplements.
- **Hyperkalemia (high potassium levels):** Treatment may involve dietary restrictions of high potassium foods, administering medications to decrease potassium levels, or medical interventions such as dialysis.
- **Hypocalcemia (low calcium levels):** Treatment may involve calcium supplementation and treating the underlying cause of the deficiency, such as vitamin D deficiency or hypoparathyroidism.
- **Hypercalcemia (high calcium levels):** Treatment may involve fluid replacement and medications to decrease calcium levels, as well as treating the underlying cause of the hypercalcemia.
- **Hypomagnesemia (low magnesium levels):** Treatment may involve magnesium supplementation and addressing the underlying cause of the deficiency, such as malnutrition or medication use.
- **Hypermagnesemia (high magnesium levels):** Treatment may involve calcium supplementation, fluid replacement, and medications to increase magnesium excretion, as well as addressing the underlying cause of the hypermagnesemia.

Nurses play a crucial role in monitoring electrolyte levels, administering medications and supplements, providing education and support to patients and families, and collaborating with the healthcare team to ensure the appropriate management of electrolyte imbalances. Regular monitoring and assessment of electrolyte levels and the patient's response to treatment are crucial to ensure their safety and well-being.

Electrolyte imbalances occur when there is an abnormal level of electrolytes, such as sodium, potassium, calcium, magnesium, and phosphate, in the body. Nursing diagnoses for electrolyte imbalances may include:

- Risk for injury related to cardiac arrhythmias, seizures, and muscle weakness
- Risk for impaired gas exchange related to respiratory muscle weakness and respiratory failure
- Risk for impaired skin integrity related to edema, skin breakdown, and pressure ulcers
- Imbalanced nutrition: less than or greater than body requirements related to anorexia, nausea, vomiting, and diarrhea
- Risk for fluid volume excess or deficit related to fluid and electrolyte imbalances
- Activity intolerance related to fatigue, weakness, and decreased endurance
- Anxiety related to the uncertainty of prognosis and treatment
- Risk for impaired urinary elimination related to electrolyte imbalances and/or renal failure
- Knowledge deficit related to the disease process, treatment options, and self-care management.

Electrolyte imbalances can lead to a variety of complications and symptoms, which can affect various body systems. Nursing management and nursing diagnosis for electrolyte imbalances aim to identify the underlying cause of the imbalance, correct the imbalance, and prevent complications. Here are some nursing management and nursing diagnosis for electrolyte imbalances.

## *Nursing Diagnosis*

- Risk for electrolyte imbalance related to underlying medical conditions, medications, or fluid imbalances and nursing management includes:
  - Monitor electrolyte levels, such as sodium, potassium, calcium, magnesium, and phosphate, to identify imbalances.
  - Review the patient's medical history, medications, and fluid intake to identify potential causes of the electrolyte imbalance.
  - Administer electrolyte replacement therapy as prescribed to correct the imbalance.
  - Educate patients about the importance of maintaining a balanced diet and fluid intake to prevent electrolyte imbalances.
- Fluid volume deficit related to electrolyte imbalances and nursing management includes:
  - Assess the patient's fluid status, including skin turgor, mucous membranes, and urine output, to identify signs of dehydration.
  - Monitor electrolyte levels, such as sodium and potassium, which can be affected by fluid imbalances.
  - Administer fluids, such as IV fluids or oral rehydration solutions, as prescribed to correct the fluid deficit.
  - Educate patients about the importance of fluid intake and signs of dehydration to prevent fluid volume deficits.
- Risk for injury related to muscle weakness or seizures associated with electrolyte imbalances and nursing management includes:
  - Assess the patient's muscle strength and coordination to identify signs of muscle weakness or cramping.
  - Monitor electrolyte levels, such as potassium and calcium, which can affect muscle function.
  - Administer electrolyte replacement therapy as prescribed to correct the imbalance and prevent complications.
  - Educate patients about the signs and symptoms of electrolyte imbalances and potential complications, such as seizures.
- Impaired oral mucous membrane related to electrolyte imbalances and nursing management includes:
  - Assess the patient's oral mucous membranes for signs of dryness or inflammation.
  - Encourage the patient to drink fluids or use oral care products, such as mouthwashes or gels, to hydrate and soothe the mucous membranes.
  - Monitor electrolyte levels, such as sodium and potassium, which can affect the hydration of the mucous membranes.
  - Educate patients about the importance of oral hygiene and fluid intake to prevent dry mouth and oral mucosal irritation.

Overall, nursing management and nursing diagnosis for electrolyte imbalances aim to identify and correct the underlying cause of the imbalance, prevent complications, and educate patients about the importance of electrolyte balance for overall health and well-being. It is essential to work closely with the healthcare team to provide effective and coordinated care for patients with electrolyte imbalances.

These nursing diagnoses may vary depending on the specific electrolyte imbalance and its severity, as well as the individual patient's needs and co-morbidities. Nursing care for electrolyte imbalances includes monitoring of electrolyte levels, administration of electrolyte replacement therapy as needed, and assessment and prevention of complications related to electrolyte imbalances. Nurses may also collaborate with the healthcare team to identify and manage the underlying cause of the electrolyte imbalance, such as renal failure, vomiting, or diarrhea. Education and emotional support for the patient and family are also important aspects of nursing care for electrolyte imbalances.

## Summary

Renal system disorders refer to a variety of conditions that affect the kidneys, ureters, bladder, and urethra. Some common renal system disorders include chronic kidney disease (CKD), acute kidney injury (AKI), urinary tract infections (UTIs), kidney stones, and bladder cancer.

Management modalities for renal system disorders depend on the specific disorder and the patient's individual needs. Treatment options may include medications, dialysis, kidney transplant, and nutrition therapy. Nursing management for patients with renal system disorders involves close monitoring of vital signs, laboratory values, fluid balance, and overall patient status. Nursing diagnosis for these patients may include excess fluid volume, risk for infection, imbalanced nutrition, and impaired physical mobility.

Overall, early detection, prevention, and management of renal system disorders can improve patient outcomes and quality of life. Patients with renal system disorders often require a multidisciplinary approach to care, involving nurses, physicians, dietitians, social workers, and other healthcare professionals. Life is really simple, but we insist on making it complicated. Adequate kidney function is essential to the maintenance of a healthy body. If a person has complete kidney failure and treatment is not provided, death is inevitable. This chapter discusses the structures and functions, assessment, and diagnostic studies of the urinary system.

## Points to Ponder

- The kidneys are located near the twelfth vertebra and extend to the third lumbar vertebra.
- The renal artery and renal vein consist of common entry and exit at the medial aspect of either kidney at the hilum.
- Filtration of plasma in the renal corpuscle is the first step in urine production and essential solutes.
- The RAA system and antidiuretic hormone (ADH) are feedback loop system within the body maintain homeostasis.
- Inadequate tissue perfusion and hypoxia lead to acidosis.
- Metabolic acidosis is corrected by providing adequate oxygenation and perfusion through ventilation, fluid, and medications.
- Renal failure is failure of the kidney to maintain internal homeostasis.
- Acute renal failure is the suppression of urine flow, usually characterized by oliguria urine output less than 200 mL, or by anuria urine output less than 50 mL.
- The main objective in managing chronic renal failure is to maintain sodium and water.
- Homeostasis, potassium homeostasis, metabolic acidosis are the common disturbance in advanced CKD.
- Dialysis is the movement of fluid and molecules across a semipermeable membrane from one compartment to another.
- Arteriovenous fistula is created very commonly in the forearm with an end to side.
- Anastomosis of the artery (usually radial or ulnar) to a vein (usually cephalic).
- The process of diffusion, osmosis, and ultrafiltration cleanse the patient blood.
- Acute tubular necrosis (ATN) is defined as kidney severe/prolonged hypoperfusion and toxicity that develops ischemia with injury to parenchyma.
- Kidney for transplantation may be obtained from compatible blood type deceased donors, blood relatives, emotionally related living donors (e.g., spouse, distant cousin, etc.)
- Transplanted kidney usually placed extra peritoneally in the iliac fossa.
- Arteriovenous graft is composed of artificial synthetic materials (Polytetrafluoroethylene Teflon) and makes a "bridge" between arterial and venous blood supply.
- CRRT most commonly uses the venovenous approach of continuous venovenous hemofiltration (CVVH).
- Renal biopsy in which a bit of kidney tissue is removed as a sample to test in a laboratory and grown in artificial culture media.

## Abbreviations

- UTIs : Urinary Tract Infections
- ADH : Antidiuretic Hormone
- ESRD : End-stage Renal Disease
- RAA : Renin-Angiotensin-Aldosterone
- GFR : Glomerular Filtration Rate
- ADH : Antidiuretic Hormone
- STIs : Sexual Transmitted Infections
- OTC : Over-the-Counter
- ICF : Intracellular Fluid
- ECF : Extracellular Fluid
- ANH : Atrial Natriuretic Hormone
- ARF : Acute Renal Failure
- AKI : Acute Kidney Injury
- PD : Peritoneal Dialysis
- HD : Hemodialysis
- AVGs : Arteriovenous Graft
- AVFs : Arteriovenous Fistula

### Short Answer Questions

1. Renal biopsy.
2. Disorders of fluid volume.
3. Dialysis.
4. Fluid balance.
5. Electrolyte balance.
6. Renal replacement therapy.

### Long Answer Questions

1. a. Define renal failure.
   b. Etiology and categories of acute renal failure.
2. Explain in detail about management modalities for renal system disorders.
3. Define acute tubular necrosis, causes of acute tubular necrosis, pathophysiology and nursing management.
4. Describe about end-stage renal disease and add a note on kidney transplantation.
5. Define bladder trauma, causes of bladder injury, grade injury, complication and management.

### Bibliography

1. Best J, Kitlowski AD, Ou D, Bedolla J. Diagnosis and management of urinary tract infections in the emergency department. Emerg Med Pract. 2014;16(7):1-23. http://www.ebmedicine.net/topic.php?paction=showTopic&topic_id=412. Accessed May 14, 2019.
2. Centers for disease control and prevention. National Hospital ambulatory medical care survey; 2015 ED summary tables.
3. Clement JQ. Management of interstitial cystitis/bladder pain syndrome.
4. Clement JQ. Pathogenesis, clinical features, and diagnosis of interstitial cystitis/bladder pain syndrome.
5. Curhan G, Aronson MD, Preminger GM. Diagnosis and acute management of suspected nephrolithiasis in adults.
6. De Guzman MM, Jung LK, Muscal E. Rhabdomyolysis treatment and management. Medscape website; Updated October 14, 2018. Available from: http://emedicine.medscape.com/article/1007814-treatment. Accessed May 14, 2019.
7. Deveci SP. Available from: http://www.uptodate.com/content/priapism? [updated November 15, 2017, May 14 2019].
8. Fresenius medical care. Complications of PD catheter; updated july 2016. Available from: http://www.advancedrenaleducation.com/content/complications-pd-catheters. [accessed may 14, 2019].
9. Ghanem K, Tuddenham S. Screening for sexually transmitted infections. Available from: http://www.uptodate.com/content/screening –for-sexually-transmitted infections.
10. Han E, Nguyen L, Sirls L, Peters K. Current best practice management of interstitial cystitis/bladder pain syndrome. Ther Adv Urol. 2018;10(7):197-211.
11. Hughes PJ. Classification system for acute kidney injury. Medscape website.
12. Medline plus. Testicular torsion. Medline Plus [website]. Available from: http://medlineplus.gov/ency/article/00517.htm.
13. Okusa M, Rosher MH. Overview of the management of acute kidney injury in adult.
14. Rosner MH, Okusa MD. Acute kidney injury associated with cardiac surgery. Clin J Am Soc Nephrol. 2006;1(1):19-32.
15. Simon E. The dialysis patient: managing fistula complications on the emergency department. Emdocs website. Available from: http://www.endocs.net/diaiysis-patient-managing-fistu.
16. Urology care foundation. What are epididymitis and orchitis? Available from: http://www.urologyhealth.org/urologic-condition/epididymitis-and-orchitis.
17. Workowski KA, Bolan GA, Centers for Disease Control and Prevention. Sexually transmitted disease treatment guidelines, 2015. MMWR Recomm Rep. 2015;64RR-03);64(RR-3):1-137.

# Chapter 8

# Nervous System Emergencies and Management

*Neethu Maria Joseph, Anu Baby*

## CHAPTER OUTLINE

- Anatomy of Nervous System
- Physiology of Nervous System
- Assessment of Nervous System
  - Neurologic examination
  - Invasive brain monitoring and noninvasive brain monitoring
- Increased Intracranial Pressure
- Cerebrovascular Disease
- Stroke
- Seizure Disorder
- Status Epilepticus
- Guillain-Barré Syndrome
- Myasthenia Gravis
- Encephalopathy
- Head Injury
- Spinal Cord Injury
- Problems Associated with Neurological Disorders
  - Thermoregulation
  - Unconsciousness
  - Brain death
  - Herniation syndrome
- Management Modalities through Neurosurgical Approaches
- Assessment of Intracranial Pressure
- Management of Intracranial Hypertension
- Burr hole
- Craniotomy
- Decompressive Craniectomy

## Learning Objectives

At the end of the chapter, the students will be able to:

- Describe the basic anatomy and physiology of nervous system.
- Perform the assessment of a patient with neurologic disorder with history collection and physical examination.
- Describe the purposes and nurses; responsibilities of different diagnostic procedures involved to study nervous system disorders.
- Explain intracranial pressure and its regulation in a normal person.
- Describe the etiology, clinical manifestations, assessment and management of increased intracranial pressure.
- Describe the etiology, pathophysiologic mechanisms, clinical manifestations, diagnosis, and management of subarachnoid hemorrhage.
- Describe the classification, etiology, risk factors, pathophysiology, clinical manifestations, diagnosis, and emergency management of stroke.
- Describe the etiology, classification, diagnosis and management of seizures.
- Describe the causes, types, pathophysiology, diagnosis, complications and management of status epilepticus.
- Describe the types, etiology, pathophysiology, clinical manifestations, diagnosis, and management of Guillain-Barré syndrome.
- Describe the etiology, pathophysiology, clinical features, diagnosis, complications and management of myasthenia gravis.
- Describe the etiology, classification, pathophysiology, clinical manifestations, diagnosis and management of head injury.
- Describe the etiology, pathophysiology, clinical features, diagnosis, complications and management of spinal cord injury.
- Explain the problems associated with neurologic disorders such as thermoregulation, unconsciousness and herniation syndrome.
- Describe the etiopathophysiology, types, clinical manifestations, diagnosis, and treatment of encephalopathy
- Explain the different neurosurgical approaches with perioperative nursing management.

# INTRODUCTION

Out of all the systems in the body, the nervous system can be regarded as one of the most important because it controls the functions of the other systems in the body. An acute neurologic disorder usually calls for emergency management following the basic approach of ABC (airway, breathing, circulation). Neurologic emergencies require immediate management due to the increased dependence of brain tissues on oxygen and glucose supply. An ischemic state makes the tissues nonsalvageable if adequate treatment is not given at the right time. A structured diagnostic system is essential for rapid diagnosis of the underlying disorder. Critical care starts in the emergency department, and it continues in the critical care units, where the patient receives life-saving treatment. This chapter deals with common neurologic emergency conditions and its management in the critical care units.

# ANATOMY OF NERVOUS SYSTEM

The nervous system is divided into two divisions—**central nervous system (CNS)** and **peripheral nervous system (PNS)**.

The central nervous system consists of the **brain** and **spinal cord**. The peripheral nervous system includes all the nervous tissues other that brain and spinal cord, i.e., spinal nerves, cranial nerves, peripheral ganglia, enteric plexuses, and sensory receptors. PNS is further divided into **somatic nervous system (SNS), autonomic nervous system (ANS)** and **enteric nervous system (ENS)**.

## Nervous Tissue

There are two types of cells in the nervous tissue—neurons and neuroglial cells. Neurons are specialized cells which are regarded as the functional units of the nervous system. There are almost 500 billion neurons in the entire nervous sytem. Neuroglial cells are supporting cells in the nervous system and it is 25 times larger than neurons in number. Neuroglia play active role in supporting and protecting neurons, controlling neurotransmitter uptake, recovering neurons from injury, and nourishing neurons. The four main neuroglial cells are—astrocytes, oligodendrocytes, ependymal cells and microglial cells.

A neuron has three basic parts—**cell body, dendrites and axon**. Parts of a neuron are shown in **Figure 8.1**. Cell body is the structure that contains nucleus, cytoplasm with cell organelles like mitochondria, ribosomes, lysosomes, Golgi apparatus and endoplasmic reticulum. Dendrites are the processes that receive electrical impulse from other neurons. Usually, neurons have a single axon, which give out electrical impulses to other neurons, muscle or glands.

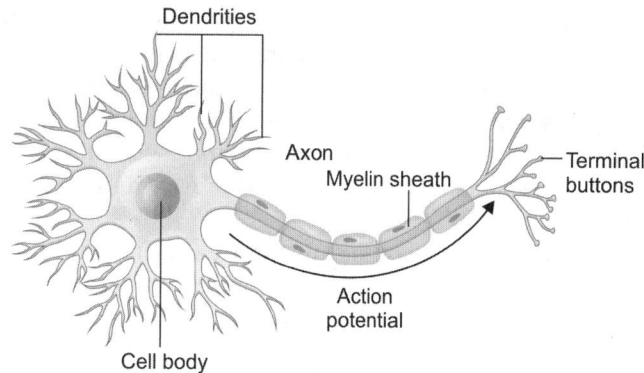

**Fig. 8.1:** Parts of a neuron.

Once the electric impulse reaches at the end of the axon, or the axon terminal, it is transferred to the next cell. This area of communication where a neuron contacts with other cells are called synapse. When the impulse reaches the axon terminal, neurotransmitters such as acetylcholine, gamma-aminobutyric acid, glutamate, epinephrine, norepinephrine, dopamine, serotonin are released from synaptic vesicles. The neurotransmitters cause excitation or inhibition of the cells in the end of synapse.

## Brain

An average adult brain located inside the skull is a soft, complex structure weighing approximately 1,400 g. It accounts for about 2% of the total body weight. Brain contains almost 100 billion neurons (Solomon, 2009; Tortora and Derrickson, 2014).

Brain consists of:
- Cerebrum
- Diencephalon
- Brainstem
- Cerebellum

### Cerebrum

Cerebrum is the largest part of the brain. The outer layer of cerebrum is called cerebral cortex, and the inner layer is called cerebral medulla. Cerebral cortex is made up of cell bodies and dendrites of neurons, thus giving it a gray appearance. Cerebral medulla is made up of axons of neurons giving it a whitish appearance. Thus, cerebral cortex and medulla are known as gray matter and white matter respectively.

Cerebrum is divided into two hemispheres—right and left hemispheres. The two hemispheres are connected to each other with the help of a band made of white matter, corpus callosum. The external surface of cerebrum looks wrinkled with multiple raised and depressed areas. The raised areas or convolutions are called gyri (singular: gyrus) and depressed areas or grooves are called sulci (singular: sulcus). Grooves that are deeper than called fissures.

The sulci and gyri divide cerebrum into four lobes: Frontal, parietal, temporal and occipital. Each of the lobes have specialized functions which are depicted in **Figure 8.2**.

- **Frontal lobe:** Primary motor area in frontal lobe helps in controlling voluntary movement. Prefrontal cortex in the anterior portion of frontal lobe is responsible for personality and executive functions like reasoning, thinking, decision-making, planning and understanding. Broca's area situated in the frontal lobe of the dominant hemisphere helps in the expression of speech.
- **Parietal lobe:** Primary somatosensory cortex in parietal lobe helps in identification of sensations such as touch, vibration and sense of position (proprioception). Somatosensory association area helps in the recognizing objects just by feeling them by touch.
- **Temporal lobe:** Primary auditory cortex in temporal lobe receives information from the ear. Temporal lobe also plays a major part in interpreting taste, smell and hearing sensations. The medial portion of the lobe helps in memory, learning and emotions.
- **Occipital lobe:** Primary visual cortex in occipital lobe is responsible for recognizing, and interpreting visual information. It is also concerned with storage of visual information and visual memory.

### Diencephalon

Diencephalon is the center most portion of the brain. It lies just above the midbrain. Diencephalon is divided into two major parts—thalamus and hypothalamus.

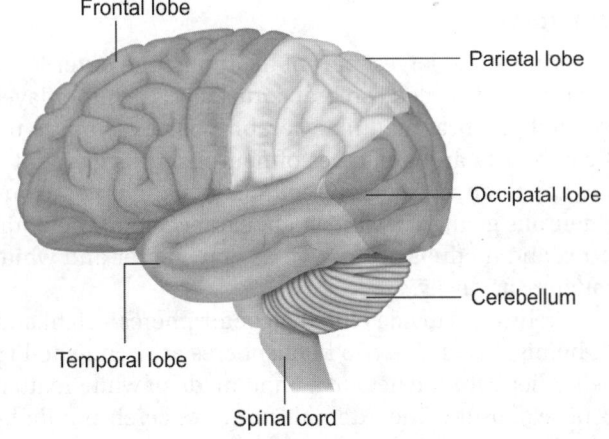

**Fig. 8.2:** Parts of brain.

### Thalamus

Thalamus forms the dorsal portion of the diencephalon and is located on either side of the third ventricle. Thalamus is regarded as the relay station for all the sensory information (except smell) passing from spinal cord to cerebrum. The specific nucleus in thalamus helps in movement by transmitting impulses from cerebellum to primary motor cortex in frontal lobe.

### Hypothalamus

Hypothalamus, as the name implies, is situated below the thalamus. This tiny portion of the brain that accounts for 1% of the brain volume regulates major homeostatic mechanisms in our body like fluid regulation, satiety and thermoregulation. Along with the limbic system, it helps in regulating sexual behavior and emotional behavior. Along with brainstem, hypothalamus helps in regulating circadian rhythms (sleep wake cycle).

Hypothalamus controls and coordinates autonomic nervous system and regulates smooth muscle contraction of visceral organs, heart rate, urinary bladder contraction and movement of gastrointestinal tract.

Oxytocin and antidiuretic hormone (ADH) are hormones produced and secreted from the hypothalamus. Both these hormones are stored in the posterior pituitary for its release into bloodstream. Hypothalamus also produces releasing and inhibiting hormones which act on the anterior pituitary for the secretion or inhibition of hormones produced in the anterior pituitary.

### Brainstem

The midbrain, pons and medulla oblongata are the three parts of the brainstem. The midbrain connects the cerebral hemispheres with pons through huge bundles of neurons. It contains centers for auditory and visual reflexes. Cranial nerves III (oculomotor nerve) and IV (trochlear nerve) originates in the midbrain. Pons is situated anterior to cerebellum and in between midbrain and medulla. Pons acts a bridge between medulla and higher parts of the brain. Centers for regulation of respiration and sleep is located in pons. Cranial nerves V, VI, VII and VIII (trigeminal, abducens, facial and vestibulocochlear nerves respectively) originate in pons. Medulla oblongata contains all the sensory and motor nerve fibers passing through the brain and spinal cord. Most of the motor fibers cross over at the level of medulla. Medulla contain vital centers such as cardiac center, respiratory center and vasomotor centers. Reticular formation, a group of neurons responsible for circadian rhythm and arousal is present in medulla. Cranial nerves IX, X, XI and XII (glossopharyngeal, vagus, spinal accessory and hypoglossal) originates in the medulla.

## Cerebellum

Cerebellum, also called "little brain" is the second largest portion of the brain. Cerebellum is located behind the pons, midbrain and below the occipital lobe. Cerebellum mainly helps in maintaining balance of the body and keeps the movements smooth and coordinated.

## Meninges

Brain and spinal cordis are protected by meninges, which includes three layers namely—dura mater, arachnoid mater and pia mater.

The meningeal layers are shown in **Figure 8.3**. Dura mater is the outermost layer underlying the skull which is tough and inelastic. It provides structural support to the brain tissues. The space between dura mater and skull is known as epidural space. Arachnoid mater lies below dura mater and is thin and delicate. The space between dura mater and arachnoid mater is known as subdural space. The space between arachnoid mater and the underlying pia mater is called subarachnoid space. Subarachnoid space contains cerebrospinal fluid (CSF), which provides buoyancy to the brain tissue. Pia mater is the innermost thin, transparent layer lining the brain closely.

## Cerebrospinal Fluid

Cerebrospinal fluid is a clear, transparent and odorless fluid produced by the ependymal cells in choroid plexus of the ventricles. It circulates through the lateral, third and fourth ventricles, around the brain and spinal cord and in the central canal of spinal cord. CSF is then absorbed through the arachnoid villi (finger-like projections in the arachnoid mater) into the venous sinuses. Thus, CSF enters the bloodstream. Approximately, 400–500 mL of CSF is produced daily and the CSF circulating in the brain and spinal cord is 150–175 mL. Characteristics of normal CSF are as follows:
- **Color:** Colorless
- **Glucose:** 40–80 mg/dL
- **Protein:** 15–45 mg/dL
- **Leukocytes:** 0–5/ μL
- **Red blood cell:** Nil
- **Lactic acid:** <35 mg/dL
- **Specific gravity:** 1.006–1.009.

## Blood Brain Barrier

Blood brain barrier (BBB) is a selective permeable membrane that regulates the movement of ions, cells and molecules between blood and brain. The blood vessels are mainly made up of endothelial cells. It vascularizes the CNS and regulates the homeostasis of the nervous system thereby protecting the neuronal function. When the barrier properties of BBB are destructed, it can lead to varying degrees of neuronal dysfunction and damage.

## Spinal Cord

Spinal cord is a cylindrical structure which begins as a continuation of the medulla oblongata, and it extends through the cervical vertebra to the lumbar vertebra. The spinal cord regions are given in **Figure 8.4**. The spinal cord is surrounded by meninges and vertebra. Conus medullaris is the part where the spinal cord ends. It usually coincides

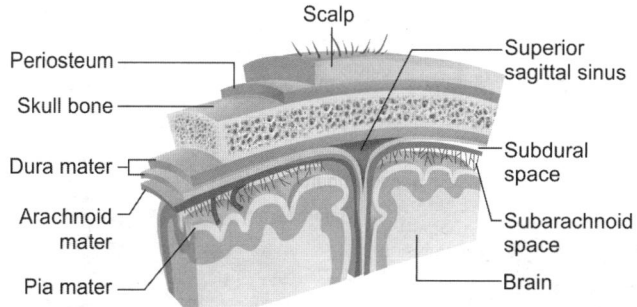

**Fig. 8.3:** Cross-section of head showing scalp, skull, meningeal layers (dura mater, arachnoid mater and pia mater) and brain.

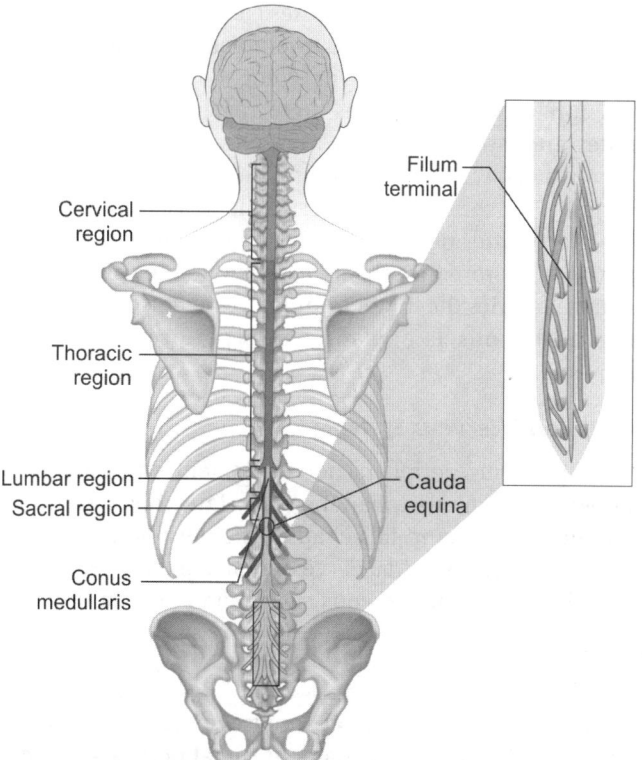

**Fig. 8.4:** Spinal cord regions: Cervical, thoracic, lumbar and sacral regions.

with L1 vertebra of an adult human. Cauda equina is a group of nerves that emerge from the terminal end of spinal cord extending up to L5 vertebral level. Cauda equine has nerves supplying both lower limbs, perineal region, urinary bladder and anal region. Cross-sectionally, the spinal cord has inner gray matter and outer white matter. The spinal cord acts as the link between central nervous system and peripheral nervous system.

Gray matter of the spinal cord contains the ventral and dorsal gray horns. Ventral gray horns are found anteriorly, and it contains cell bodies of motor neurons. The dorsal gray horn is found posteriorly and contains cell bodies of sensory and autonomic neurons. The white matter contains myelinated axons of the sensory and motor neurons that go up and down the brain. This constitutes the ascending and descending tracts. Ascending tracts such as spinothalamic, spinocerebellar tracts carry sensory impulses from spinal cord to cerebrum or cerebellum. Descending tracts such as corticospinal or corticobulbar carry motor impulses from cerebrum to cranial or spinal nerves.

### Reflex Activity

In response to a specific sensory stimulus, an immediate, rapid and involuntary sequence of actions occurs. This is known as reflex, e.g., taking the hand away from the fire, when the hand feels hot. Reflexes can be innate, acquired or learned. Acquired reflex is a complex phenomenon and it includes walking, driving or typing.

In reflex action, there is no involvement of brain. The reflex arc pathway involves the following parts: Sensory receptor (part of the sensory nerve that senses the stimuli), sensory neuron (carries the sensory impulse to the gray matter of the spinal cord), interneuron (carries the impulse from the sensory to the motor neuron), motor neuron (carries the motor impulse to the muscle), effector organ (the muscle or gland which performs the motor movement).

### Peripheral Nervous System

In simple terms, peripheral nervous system is the part of the nervous system other than the central nervous system. As mentioned earlier in this chapter, the peripheral nervous system consists of spinal nerves, cranial nerves, peripheral ganglia, autonomic nervous system and enteric nervous system.

### Spinal Nerves

Spinal nerves carry electrical impulses either to or from the spinal cord. There are 31 pairs of spinal nerves—cervical (8), thoracic (12), lumbar (5), sacral (5) and coccygeal (1). Each of the spinal nerves are a combination of motor and sensory nerve. The motor neurons are located in the anterior (ventral) horn of spinal cord and sensory neurons are located in the posterior (dorsal) horn of spinal cord. Upon exiting the spinal cord, spinal nerves branches into ventral rami, dorsal rami and rami communicants to innervate the trunk, upper limbs and lower limbs.

Sensory neurons in the dorsal gray horn innervate the skin in our whole body. A dermatome is the area of the skin innervated by a sensory neuron from a single dorsal root of a spinal nerve. For example, sensory neurons present in C4 spinal nerve innervate the skin in the upper part of shoulder, upper part of back and lower part of neck. Similarly, motor neurons in the ventral gray horn innervate the muscles in our body. A myotome is the muscle group innervated by a motor neuron from a single ventral root of spinal nerve.

The afferent function of sensory nerves and efferent function of motor nerves are depicted in detail in **Figure 8.5**. Sensory nerves carry sensory impulses from the whole body and transmit them to the brain. In contrast, motor nerves carry motor impulses from the brain and transmit them to the muscles for movement.

### Cranial Nerves

There are 12 pairs of cranial nerves. These are called 'cranial' because it exits from the cranial cavity. Cranial nerves can be sensory, motor or mixed (sensory and motor). The cranial nerves, their origin and functions are given in **Table 8.1**.

### Autonomic Nervous System

Autonomic nervous system (ANS) is divided into sympathetic nervous system and parasympathetic nervous system. Most of the organs are innervated by both sympathetic and parasympathetic nervous system. In autonomic nervous system, the myelinated preganglionic neurons (emerging from brain or spinal cord) extend up to the ganglion and the unmyelinated postganglionic neurons take up the impulse from the ganglion to the target organs.

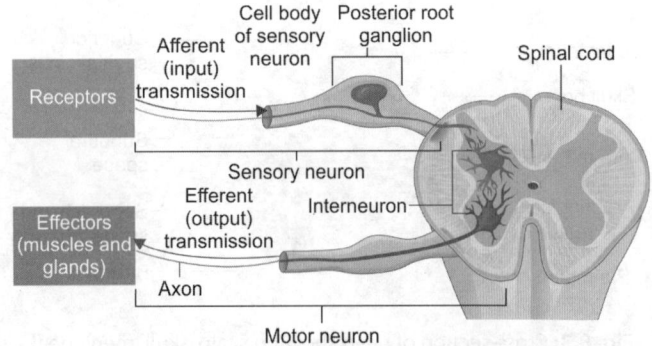

**Fig. 8.5:** Functions of motor and sensory neuron.

Table 8.1: Cranial nerves, its types and functions (Hickey, 1997).

| Cranial nerve | Brain connection | Type | Functions |
|---|---|---|---|
| • Cranial nerve I<br>• Ophthalmic nerve | Anterior cerebrum | Sensory | Smell or olfaction |
| • Cranial nerve II<br>• Optic nerve | Lateral geniculate nucleus | Sensory | Sight |
| • Cranial nerve III<br>• Oculomotor nerve | Midbrain | Motor | Eyelid movement, superior, medial and diagonal movement of eye |
| • Cranial nerve IV<br>• Trochlear nerve | Midbrain | Motor | Inferior and lateral movement of eye |
| • Cranial nerve V<br>• Trigeminal nerve | Pons | • Sensory<br><br>• Motor | • Corneal sensation, and touch, pain, temperature sensation of face (scalp, forehead, cheeks, nose, mouth, teeth, jaw)<br>• Chewing, jaw opening movement, clenching of mouth |
| • Cranial nerve VI<br>• Abducens nerve | Pons | Motor | Lateral movement of eye |
| • Cranial nerve VII<br>• Facial nerve | Pontomedullary junction | • Sensory<br>• Motor | • Taste sensation of anterior 2/3rd portion of tongue<br>• Closing eyelids, closing mouth, movement of facial muscles for facial expression, salivation, lacrimation |
| • Cranial nerve VIII<br>• Vestibulocochlear or auditory nerve | Pontomedullary junction | Sensory | Hearing, balance |
| • Cranial nerve IX<br>• Glossopharyngeal nerve | Medulla | • Sensory<br><br>• Motor | • Taste sensation of posterior 1/3rd portion of tongue<br>• Swallowing, saliva secretion, gag reflex |
| • Cranial nerve X<br>• Vagus nerve | Medulla | • Sensory<br><br><br><br>• Motor | • Sensations in skin behind ear, external auditory meatus, pharynx, larynx, esophagus, thoracic and abdominal viscera<br>• Speaking, swallowing, supply to smooth muscles of thorax and abdomen |
| • Cranial nerve XI<br>• Spinal accessory nerve | Medulla | Motor | Movement of shoulder and neck muscles |
| • Cranial nerve XII<br>• Hypoglossal nerve | Medulla | Motor | Tongue movement: speech, swallowing |

In sympathetic nervous system, the neurotransmitter released by preganglionic fibers is acetylcholine and postganglionic fibers is norepinephrine. In parasympathetic nervous system, the neurotransmitter released by preganglionic and postganglionic fibers is acetylcholine.

### Sympathetic Nervous System

The cell bodies of preganglionic neurons in sympathetic nervous system emerge from T1–L2. Thus, it is called thoracolumbar division. This division of autonomic nervous system is responsible for "flight and fight response". This gets activated in response to any physical or emotional stress. It causes dilation of pupils, increased heart rate, increased blood pressure, bronchodilation, increased blood flow to skeletal muscles, cardiac muscle, glycogenolysis and lipolysis.

### Parasympathetic Nervous System

The cell bodies of postganglionic neurons in parasympathetic nervous system emerge from brainstem and sacral segments (S2,3,4). Thus, it is called craniosacral division. Parasympathetic nervous system helps in "rest and digest response". This enables the body to be in a resting state and helps in conserving the body energy for recovery. It helps in pupillary constriction, decreased heart rate, bronchoconstriction, lacrimation (increased tear secretion), increased salivation, increased gastric motility, and increased urination (contraction of bladder and relaxation of sphincter).

### Enteric Nervous System

Gastrointestinal (GI) system is innervated by two neural plexuses: myenteric plexus and submucous plexus. In response to any changes in the gut wall or the contents in the GI tract, the sensory neurons of the plexus carry the impulse to the spinal cord. The spinal cord contains interneurons processes the impulses and relay the output signal to the motor neurons in the spinal cord. The motor neurons carry the output signals or impulses to the smooth muscle of GI tract and its glands. This mechanism acts like a reflex arc and does not require the intervention of brain.

## PHYSIOLOGY OF NERVOUS SYSTEM

It is well-known that neurons transmit electrical impulses from one neuron to another. The characteristics of neurons which help in this are excitability and conductivity. Excitability refers to the capacity of neurons to generate nerve impulses. Conductivity refers to the capacity of neurons to transmit the impulses from neurons to the next.

### Resting Membrane Potential

The space outside (extracellular fluid) and inside (cytosol) the neuronal cell membrane contains various ions, both positively and negatively charged. But the distribution of ions on either side of the membrane is not equal. In the cytosol, the main cation is $K^+$ and the main anions are proteins, amino acids, sulphates and organic acids. In the extracellular fluid, the main cation is $Na^+$ and main anion is $Cl^-$. There is movement of ions across the cell membrane. However, the number of $K^+$ exiting from the cell is more than the number of $Na^+$ coming inside the cell. Thus, the cytosol is relatively increasingly negatively charged and extracellular fluid is relatively increasingly positively charged. This state is called a "polarized" state. The difference in positive and negative charges (or difference in electrical charge) creates a potential difference across the cell membrane. That is called the resting membrane potential (RMP). It is called "resting" because the neuron is in a resting state, that is, not stimulated. Resting membrane potential is measured in millivolts (mV). The typical value of RMP in a neuron is –70 mV, although it can range from –40 to –90 mV.

### Action Potential—Depolarization

When the neuron is electrically stimulated, there will be changes in the resting membrane potential. The changes can produce either a graded potential or an action potential. Graded potential is generated when the stimulus causes only localized changes and there is only a small deviation from the RMP. In contrast, action potential is generated when the stimulus causes changes in RMP in the entire membrane.

Action potential causes an increase in the membrane potential as shown in **Figure 8.6**. In action potential, when the neuron is stimulated, voltage gated sodium channels in the membrane open. As the number of $Na^+$ ions inside the cell are lower, $Na^+$ ions from the extracellular fluid will go inside the cell following the process of diffusion. As the $Na^+$ ions inside the cell increase, the cytosol becomes more positively charged. As a result, the membrane potential is increased and it rises from -70 mV, crosses zero and reaches upto + 30 mV. This is called depolarization because the polarized state is disturbed. When the potential reaches +30 mV, the voltage gated sodium channels close. This leads to stoppage of movement of $Na^+$ inside the cell.

### Action Potential—Repolarization

As the sodium channels close, voltage gated potassium channels open. As the number of $K^+$ ions outside the cell is lower, $K^+$ ions from the cytosol will go to the extracellular fluid through a process of diffusion. This reduces the membrane potential and it changes from +30 mV to –70 mV (i.e., resting membrane potential). This process is known as repolarization and the membrane polarity is restored.

For a brief period of time after repolarization, the neuron will not be able to generate the next action potential. This period is called the absolute refractory period.

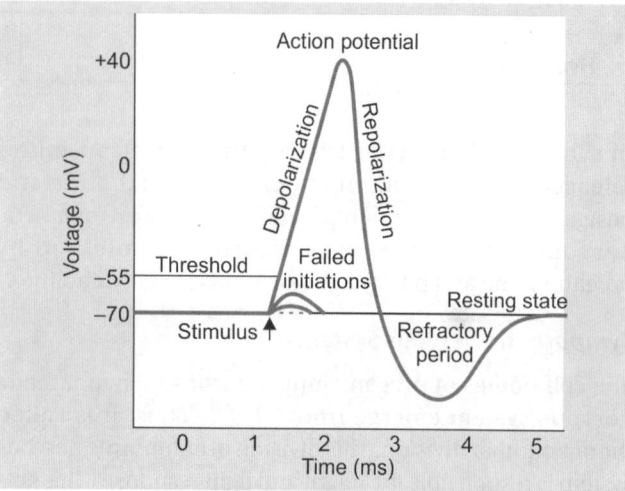

**Fig. 8.6:** Action potential along the neuron: Depolarization and repolarization.

## Threshold Stimulus

For an action potential to generate, the stimulus must raise the membrane potential to a certain value. This is called the threshold value. For a neuron, the typical threshold value is –55 mV. It means that if a stimulus is not strong enough to raise the membrane potential from –70 mV to –55 mV, then action potential will not be generated.

## All-or-none Phenomenon

When the threshold value is crossed, action potential is generated. It will not depend upon the strength or intensity of the stimulus. If an ant bites you or a person pinches you, the same action potential is generated. That means, either an action potential is generated, or it is not generated. That is called the "all-or-none phenomenon".

## ASSESSMENT OF NERVOUS SYSTEM

Detailed assessment of a patient with neurologic complaints includes history collection and neurological examination. In some cases, the patient might be unconscious, semi-conscious, restless or agitated. The assessment of such patients should be tailored as the situation demands.

## History Collection

As mentioned earlier, the patient might be confused, restless or might have aphasia, memory loss, or personality changes. In such cases where the patient information might not be reliable, the primary data should be collected from a patient's close relative or friend.

While collecting history, allow the patient to explain the complaints or the course of events without any interruption. It would be better if probing questions were avoided.

### Biographical Data

Biographical information such as age, gender, marital status, area of residence, occupation, spiritual beliefs should be collected. All this information might give us an understanding of the exposure of the patient to risk factors of certain diseases. For example, we can understand that an elderly person is more at risk for stroke than an adolescent, or males are more at risk for stroke than females.

### Present History of Illness

Present history of illness refers to the detailed course of events leading up to the current admission to hospital. For this, the patient's chief complaints should be asked. Some of the common neurologic complaints include: headache, muscle weakness, confusion, loss of coordination, vertigo, loss of memory, seizures, numbness, problems with vision, hearing, taste or smell and sensation deficits.

While collecting the information regarding each of the complaints, an OLD CARTS format can be used which is given in **Table 8.2**.

It is important to include the patient's description of the symptoms. The specific words as narrated by the patient gives the information in patient's perspective.

**Table 8.2:** Questions to be asked during history collection of a patient with neurological symptoms (Munroe et al., 2015).

| Format | Probing questions |
|---|---|
| **O**–Onset | • When did the symptom start?<br>• What is the frequency of occurrence of the symptoms?<br>• Was it sudden or gradual onset? |
| **L**–Location | • Where is the exact location of the problem?<br>• Is there any radiation pattern noted? (asked mainly for pain) |
| **D**–Duration | • For how long are you suffering from the symptom? |
| **C**–Character | • What is the quality of the symptom? (e.g., stabbing/ dull pain)<br>• Are there any changes in the symptoms from its onset? |
| **A**–Aggravating factors/ associated symptoms | • Aggravating factors: What are the activities that cause the symptom or increase the intensity of the symptom?<br>• Associated symptoms: What are the other symptoms seen along with this symptom? |
| **R**–Relieving factors | • What are the activities that reduce the intensity of the symptom? |
| **T**–Treatment taken | • Have you visited a physician earlier?<br>• What are the medications prescribed earlier for this symptom?<br>• What are the home remedies adopted to relieve the symptom? |
| **S**–Severity | • What is the intensity or severity of the symptom? (e.g., mild/ moderate or severe pain) |

## Past History of Illness

History should be collected regarding any past neurological disorders or diseases. Patients should be asked for any birth injuries, childhood trauma or seizures. Information should be collected regarding any surgery or invasive procedures involving the brain, spinal cord or sense organs. As elderly people are at risk for stroke, history of hypertension, diabetes mellitus, atrial fibrillation or transient ischemic attack (TIA) should be asked.

Immunization history should be noted, especially DPT, Hemophilus influenza or meningococcal vaccine. As the patients might have to undergo imaging studies with contrast, iodine allergy must be ruled out. In addition, any medication allergies should be noted. The patient might be on prescribed or over-the-counter medications for acute or chronic conditions. Assess for anticoagulants, antiplatelets, hormone replacement therapy, sedatives, analgesics, tranquilizers, and mood-elevating drugs (Dillon, 2007).

## Family History

Family history regarding hypertension, stroke, autoimmune diseases, seizures, cancer, demyelinating or degenerating diseases should be collected. Any history of psychiatric disorder or substance abuse among family members should be mentioned.

## Dietary History

Dietary history should include dietary patterns and dietary habits. Patients should be asked for problems related to mastication or swallowing because these problems can cause malnutrition. High cholesterol diet increases the risk of atherosclerosis, thus increasing the risk for ischemic stroke. Vitamin B12, niacin and folic acid deficiencies can lead to peripheral neuropathy. Vitamin deficiencies can also influence the central nervous system and cause irritability, depression, apathy, weakness, and confusion. Use of caffeinated drinks, cheese, chocolate, ice cream, fermented foods can aggravate or trigger headaches in certain individuals.

## Elimination History

The common bowel and bladder elimination pattern problems related to neurological dysfunction include incontinence or retention. Therefore, information should be collected regarding frequency, urgency to pass urine or stools.

## Exercise History

Patients should be asked for type, pattern and duration of exercise per day, muscular strength, fatigue or weakness experienced. Assess the extent of household or selfcare activities patient is able to perform. Also, collect data regarding any history of falls.

## Personal Habits

This includes activities such as smoking, alcoholism or substance abuse. These are risk factors for neurological disorders such as stroke.

## Sleep and Rest

Patients should be enquired the number of uninterrupted hours of sleep per night. Sleep deprivation can be related to pain, and uncomfortable sleeping position due to herniated disc, muscle weakness or paralysis.

## Occupational History

Information regarding the type of work and activities involved during worktime should be noted. Activities such as heavy weightlifting, sedentary work, continuous usage of computers can adversely affect the neurologic system. Exposure to radiation, toxins, or carcinogens in the workplace can increase the susceptibility of neurologic problems.

## Social History

Any change in behavior patterns or communication with the family members should be noted. Any role changes in the family after stroke, paralysis or weakness can affect the person's mental health.

## Sexual History

Sexual activity or sexual desire is affected by hormonal changes or neuronal injury. Any lesions in the cerebrum, pituitary gland, brainstem or spinal cord can affect the sexual life of a patient. Therefore, any problems that influence sexual dysfunction should be assessed.

## Neurological Examination

Neurological examination includes six components:
1. Mental status examination
2. Cranial nerve examination
3. Motor strength assessment
4. Sensory assessment
5. Cerebellar examination
6. Reflexes

## Mental Status Examination

Mental status examination in neurological examination is used to assess a patient's cognitive abilities. Mental status examination involves appearance, level of consciousness, orientation, mood and affect, memory, attention, speech, thought pattern, judgement, reasoning (Newman, 2020).

In an emergency setting, a format of mini mental status examination is used. It includes structured assessment of orientation, registration, attention and calculation, verbal recall, language and copying ability. This test is performed to assess for any cognitive impairment, and the degree of cognitive impairment (Ridha and Rossor, 2005). The patient is asked some questions or assigned to perform certain tasks. Each of these activities are scored. The maximum score of mini mental status examination is 30. A score <24 indicates cognitive impairment.

### Level of Consciousness

In neurological examination, it is essential to assess the level of consciousness of a patient during initial contact and it should be done continued at bedside during regular intervals. One of the common scales used to assess level of consciousness is Glasgow Coma Scale (GCS). This scale is used in the bedside along with other clinical methods to determine the degree of impairment in consciousness. It is also used to assess the prognosis of the patients with acute neurological disorders (Tindall, 1990).

Glasgow Coma Scale was developed in 1974 by Graham Teasdale and Bryan Jennett. It was updated forty years later in his current version which is depicted in **Table 8.3**.

In GCS, three components are observed and assessed: eye opening, verbal response and best motor response. For eye opening, the patient is observed for the responses given in the table. If the patient opens eyes without any stimulus, a score of '4' or 'spontaneous' is assigned. If the patient opens eyes to speech or requests to open eyes in loud voice, a score of '3' or 'to sound' is assigned. If the patient opens the eyes to pressure on fingertips, then a score of '2' or 'to pressure' is assigned. If the patient is not opening the eyes to any stimulus, then a score of '1' or 'none' is assigned. In certain situations, such as head injury, the patient might have both the eyes closed due to periorbital edema. Here, we cannot assess the patient's eye opening. Thus, we chart the eye-opening response as 'NT' denoting 'nontestable'.

For verbal response, we assess whether the patient is oriented by asking for date, time and place. If the patient gives correct response, then a score of '5' or 'orientated' is assigned. If the patient's response is incorrect, but the patient is able to communicate properly, then a score of '4' or 'confused' is assigned. If the patient is unable to verbalize full sentences and gives responses as single words that are incomprehensible, then a score of '3' or 'words' is assigned. If the patient does not even respond with words, but responds verbally as moans or groans, then a score of '2' or 'sounds' is assigned. If the patient gives no verbal response at all, then a score of '1' or 'none' is assigned. In situations where the patient is not capable of giving a verbal response like insertion of endotracheal tube or tracheostomy tube, a score is not assigned. Such a condition is documented as 'NT' or 'nontestable'.

For the best motor response, patient is asked to obey a command for a motor response. For example, raise your hands, put out your tongue, close your eyes, etc. If the patient is obeying the command, a score of '6' or 'obeys commands' is assigned. If the patient is not obeying the command, then a stimulus is provided to elicit a motor response. Stimulus is provided centrally by pinching the trapezius muscle above the shoulder or providing pressure in the supraorbital region. If the stimulus causes the patient to bring hand above and if it crosses the clavicle, then a score of '5' or 'localizing' is assigned. If the hand does not reach above the clavicle, but instead the patient displays a normal bending of the hand at the level of elbow, a score of '4' or 'normal flexion' is assigned. On the contrary, if the patient displays an abnormal bending of the hand at the level of elbow, a score of '3' or 'abnormal flexion' is assigned. If the patient extends arm at the level of elbow, a score of '2' or 'extension' is assigned. If there is no movement in arms or legs, a score of '1' or 'none' is assigned.

The scores of all the three parameters are added. The maximum score of GCS is 15 and the minimum score is 3. A score of 15 is normal and a higher score of GCS indicates good prognosis.

| Table 8.3: Glasgow coma scale (GCS) (Teasdale et al., 2014). | | |
|---|---|---|
| **Eye opening** | **Verbal response** | **Best motor response** |
| 4 – Spontaneous<br>3 – To sound<br>2 – To pressure<br>1 – None | 5 – Orientated<br>4 – Confused<br>3 – Words<br>2 – Sounds<br>1 – None | 6 – Obeys commands<br>5 – Localizing<br>4 – Normal flexion<br>3 – Abnormal flexion<br>2 – Extension<br>1 – None |

## Cranial Nerve Examination

### Olfactory Nerve (CN I)

- Ask patient to close the eyes and close one nostril with his/her finger.
- Place the object (soap/ginger/garlic/lemon/coffee powder/tea powder) in front of the open nostril.
- Ask the patient to sniff and identify the object.
- Repeat the procedure similarly in the other nostril.

### Optic Nerve (CN II)

- **Visual acuity:**
  - Place a snellens chart 20 feet away from the patient
  - Ask the patient to read the numbers or alphabets in the chart.
  - Identify any abnormality, if present.
- **Visual field:**
  - Examiner should stand facing the patient so that eyes of both examiner and patient are at the same level.
  - Ask the patient to close right eye and look directly at the bridge of the examiner's nose.
  - Examiner should close their own left eye.
  - Present an object in the field of vision of the left eye of the patient gradually from the right side of the patient.
  - Ask the patient to notify when the patient is able to start seeing the object.
  - Examiner should validate the response as the examiner is also closing his/her own eyes.
  - Repeat the procedure in the left eye of the patient.

### Oculomotor, Trochlear and Abducens Nerve (CN III, IV, VI)

- **Eye movement:**
  - Place a pointed object or finger in front of the patient's eyes.
  - Move the finger/object horizontally, vertically and diagonally.
  - Ask the patient to follow the movement of the finger.
  - Note any dysconjugate gaze or nystagmus.
- **Pupillary reaction:**
  - Introduce torchlight to the eyes of the patient.
  - Observe for pupillary constriction.
  - Note pupillary size, shape and reaction of both the eyes.

### Trigeminal Nerve (CN V)

- **Corneal reflex:**
  - Take a wisp of cotton.
  - Ask the patient to look towards the left side and bring the cotton tip from the right side and touch the cornea gently.
  - Observe for blinking of the eye.
  - Repeat the procedure in the other eye.
- **Sensory function:**
  - Ask the patient to close the eyes.
  - Inform the patient to notify when the when he/she feels a touch.
  - Brush a piece of cotton over the patient's forehead, cheeks and jaw bilaterally.
  - Note if the patient is responding appropriately. Temperature is assessed using test tubes with warm or cold water.
  - Ask the patient to close eyes.
  - Place the test tube with warm or cold water over the forehead, cheeks and jaw of the patient.
  - Note if the patient is able to identify the warmth or cold temperature.
- **Motor function:**
  - Place the examiner's finger pads over the masseter or temporalis muscles of the patient.
  - Ask the patient to bite down or clench the teeth.
  - Palpate the contraction of the muscles.

### Facial Nerve (CN VII)

- **Motor function:**
  - Ask the patient to smile, frown, puff out cheeks or to bare their teeth.
  - Note for any asymmetry in the facial muscle contraction.
  - Ask the patient to close both eyes tightly
  - The examiner should try to open the eyes.
  - Observe whether the eyes remain closed (which denotes normal eye muscle strength)
- **Taste sensation:**
  - Ask the patient to put out the tongue
  - Place any sweet, sour or salt object in the anterior 2/3rd portion of the tongue
  - Ask the patient to identify the taste.

### Vestibulocochlear Nerve (CN VIII)

- **Watch test:**
  - Ask the patient to close the eyes.
  - Place a ticking watch near the ear.
  - Assess if the patient is able to hear the sound
  - Repeat in the other ear.
- **Rinne's test:**
  - Vibrate the tuning fork and place it over the mastoid bone.
  - Instruct the patient to inform once the vibration stops.
  - Once the vibration stops, place the tuning fork in front of the ear.
  - Ask the patient if the vibration is heard.
  - Repeat the test in the other ear.

- **Weber test:**
  - Vibrate the tuning fork and place it at the center of the head.
  - Ask if the patient is able to hear vibrations equally in both the ears.

*Glossopharyngeal and Vagus Nerve (CN XI, X)*
- **Taste sensation:**
  - Ask the patient to close the eyes and take out the tongue.
  - Place objects such as sugar or salt for taste sensation in the posterior 1/3rd portion of the tongue.
  - Ask the patient to identify the taste.
- **Gag reflex:**
  - Place the tongue depressor inside the mouth of the patient and touch the pharynx.
  - Observe for gag reflex.

*Spinal Accessory Nerve (CN XI)*
- Place the examiner's hands over the shoulders of the patient or the cheek of the patient.
- Ask the patient to exert an opposite force, i.e., to shrug the shoulders or to turn the head to the opposite side.
- Assess the strength of the muscle.

*Hypoglossal Nerve (CN XII)*
Ask the patient to stick out the tongue and observe for asymmetry, deviation or atrophy.

### Motor Strength Assessment

In motor examination, both right and left side of the upper and lower limbs should be assessed and compared. Motor examination includes: Muscle mass, muscle tone, strength, and ability of movement.

*Muscle Mass/Bulk*
Muscle bulk is inspected symmetrically in both upper and lower limbs. Any wasting of muscle, fasciculations or atrophy is noted.

*Muscle Tone*
Muscle tone is checked by inspecting the hanging arms (patient in standing position) or legs (patient in sitting position). The loosely hanging limbs are assessed for ease in movement. If the arms or legs are stiff, it denotes increased muscle tone. There can be two types of abnormal increase in muscle tone: Spasticity and rigidity. The difference between these two can be identified during a passive range of motion. In spasticity, there will be an initial resistance during movement, but the resistance gives way during the remaining movement. It will be easier to move the limbs towards the end of the movement. Spasticity is seen in injuries involving the upper motor neuron. In rigidity, the resistance to movement is present throughout the movement. Rigidity is seen in extrapyramidal diseases such as Parkinson's diseases (cogwheel rigidity). Flaccidity is an abnormal condition seen in lower motor neuron disease with little or no resistance (Cohen, Fadul, Jenkyn, and Ward, 2020).

*Muscle Strength*
While assessing the muscular strength, note any muscle loss or atrophy in upper and lower limbs. Perform motor strength assessment of both right and left upper and lower limbs using power grading (score 0-5)—ask the patient to perform a movement (abduction, adduction, flexion, extension) against gravity or resistance.
- 0: Absent-no contraction detected
- 1: Trace-slight contraction detected
- 2: Weak movement with gravity eliminated (sideways)
- 3: Fair movement against gravity (upward)
- 4: Good movement against gravity with some resistance
- 5: Normal movement against gravity with full resistance.

### Sensory Examination

*Touch Sensation*
- Ask the patient to close the eyes and place the cotton tip at the different parts of the body (except face).
- Ask the patient to notify when the patient feels any touch sensation.

*Pain Sensation*
- Ask the patient to close the eyes.
- Prick the patient's skin with a pointed object over the skin of the body (except face).
- Ask the patient to notify them when the patient feels any pain.

*Temperature Sensation*
- Ask the patient to close the eyes.
- Place test tube with warm or cold water over the patient's skin (except face).
- Ask the patient to identify the temperature (warm or cold).

*Vibration Sensation*
- Vibrate a tuning fork and place it over the bony prominences in the patient's upper and lower limb.
- Instruct the patient to inform when the vibration is no longer felt.

*Proprioception (Position Sense)*
- Ask the patient to close the eyes.
- Move the tip of the finger or tip of toes of the patient either up or down.

- Ask the patient to identify whether the position is up or down.

*Stereognosis*
- Ask the patient to close the eyes and hold out the arms.
- Place any familiar object (coin, key, pen, etc.) on the palm of the patient.
- Ask the patient to identify the object.

*Graphesthesia*
- Ask the patient to close the eyes and hold out the arms.
- Using the blunt end of pencil, write numbers on the palm of the patient.
- Ask the patient to identify the number.

*Two-point Discrimination*
- Ask the patient to close the eyes.
- Gently hold two pins 2–3 mm apart.
- Touch the patient's fingertip.
- Ask the patient to state the number of pins felt.
- Observe whether the patient is able to differentiate the two pins.
- If not, gently increase the distance between the pins and observe the differentiation of stimuli.

## Cerebellar Examination

*Romberg Test*
- Ask the patient to stand up in front of the examiner with feet together.
- Ask the patient to close the eyes and remain in the position for 10–20 sec.
- Observe if the patient begins to sway or has to move the feet for balance.

*Walking Test*
- Ask the patient to walk in a straight line and note for any gait abnormalities.
- If the patient is able to walk properly, instruct the patient to perform tandem walking.

*Finger to Nose Test*
- Examiner has to place the tip of his/her finger in front of the patient.
- Ask the patient to touch examiner's finger with the patient's finger and then to touch the patient's nose.
- Ask the patient to repeat the movement several times quickly.
- Observe for the smoothness of the movement.

*Rapid Alternating Movements*
- Ask the patient to supinate and pronate one hand over the other rapidly.
- Observe for the smoothness of the movement.

*Finger to Finger Test*
- Ask the patient to touch the thumb to each finger as quickly as possible.
- Observe for the smoothness of the movement.

*Heel to Knee Test*
- Ask the patient to lie down on his/her back.
- Instruct the patient to slide the heel of one lower extremity down the shin of the other, starting at the knee.
- Observe for the smoothness of the movement.

## Reflexes

*Superficial Reflexes*
- **Abdominal reflex:**
  - Ask the patient to lie on back.
  - Quickly stroke the abdomen horizontally laterally to medially towards the umbilicus using a stick or tongue blade.
  - Observe contraction of abdominal muscles with the umbilicus deviating towards the stimulus.
- **Cremasteric reflex (in males):**
  - Lightly stroke the inner aspect of the thigh.
  - Observe for rapid elevation of the testicle on the same side.

*Deep Tendon Reflexes*
- **Biceps:**
  - Ask the patient to relax the arm and pronate the forearm midway between flexion and extension.
  - Place the examiner's thumb firmly on the biceps tendon.
  - The reflex hammer is then struck on the examiner's thumb.
  - Observe for contraction of the biceps tendon, followed by flexion at the elbow.
- **Triceps:**
  - Flex the patient's forearm at the elbow and pull the arm towards the chest.
  - Tap the triceps tendon with reflex hammer about 2.5–5 cm above the elbow.
  - Another maneuver is by hanging the patient's arms over the examiner's arms and tapping the tendon.
  - Observe contraction of the triceps tendon with extension at the elbow.
- **Brachioradialis/supinator:**
  - Have the patient's forearm in semiflexion and semipronation.
  - Strike the styloid process of the radius about 2.5–5 cm above the wrist.
  - Observe flexion at the elbow and simultaneous supination of the forearm.

- **Patellar/knee jerk:**
  - Have the patient sit with their legs dangling off the side of the bed.
  - The examiner's hand is placed on the patient's quadriceps muscle.
  - Strike the patellar tendon firmly.
  - Observe contraction of the quadriceps and extension at the knee.
- **Achilles tendon/ankle jerk:**
  - Have the patient sit with the legs dangling off the side of the bed. Leg should be flexed at the hip and the knee.
  - The examiner places a hand under the patient's foot to dorsiflex the ankle.
  - Achilles tendon is struck above its insertion on the posterior aspect of the calcaneus.
  - A patient with a depressed reflex should be asked to kneel on the bed with the feet hanging off the side.
  - Tap the tendon and observe plantar flexion at the ankle.

*Abnormal Reflex*

- **Babinski's reflex:**
  - Stroke the lateral aspect of the sole from the heel to the ball of the foot and curve medially across the heads of the metatarsal bones.
  - Observe for normal response plantar flexion of the big toe (abnormal response dorsiflexion of the big toe, with fanning of the other toes).

## Invasive Brain Monitoring and Noninvasive Brain Monitoring

Once collection of history and physical examination is performed, diagnostic tests are conducted to confirm the disease condition through invasive and noninvasive monitoring. Diagnostic tests can be invasive or noninvasive. Technological advancements have led to the development of newer techniques in diagnosis that adopt a less invasive approach. Nurses are responsible for monitoring and direct care of the patients before, during and after the diagnostic procedure.

The common diagnostic procedures used for neurologic disorders and its nursing responsibilities are given in **Table 8.4**.

## INCREASED INTRACRANIAL PRESSURE

Cranial vault is a closed space with three main components: Brain, Blood, and Cerebrospinal fluid (CSF). The pressure created by the intracranial contents is termed as **intracranial pressure (ICP)**. Normal value of ICP ranges from 5–15 mm Hg. In normal human beings, there can be fluctuations in ICP because of changes in arterial or venous pressure, intrathoracic pressure or intra-abdominal pressure, Valsalva maneuver, postural changes, temperature or blood gas value changes. A measurement of intracranial pressure above 20 mm Hg is considered as increased or raised ICP or intracranial hypertension.

### Regulation of Intracranial Pressure

The volume of each of the contents in the brain that contributes to ICP is approximately as follows: Brain parenchyma—78%, blood—12% and cerebrospinal fluid —10%. Any change in the volume of any one of these contents can thereby cause an increase in ICP. In a healthy person, there are many mechanisms adapted by the body to compensate for the increase in ICP.

*Monro-Kellie Hypothesis*

The Monro-Kellie Hypothesis states that increase in volume of any one of the components of brain can cause a compensatory reduction in the volume of either one or both of the other two components. For example, in a patient with brain tumor, ICP will be increased as the volume of brain is increasing. In order to maintain the normal ICP, either one or both of the other two components, that is, blood or CSF will be reduced. As a result, CSF can be displaced to the spinal cord or CSF absorption can be increased. Also, blood flow to the intracranial cavity can be reduced.

The above compensatory mechanism is effective when there is no skull fracture (that is, the intracranial cavity should remain closed) and if the increase in ICP is gradual. In conditions where the compensation does not occur properly, the ICP increases (Mestecky, 2011a; Zomordi, 2017).

*Cerebral Blood Flow*

As the brain is one of the vital organs of the body, it receives 12–15% of the cardiac output in a resting state. In terms of blood flow, brain receives 750 mL/min and 50–60 mL/100 g/min. Brain receives this huge amount because it requires continuous supply of glucose and oxygen for its functioning. There are certain factors that regulate the constant blood flow to brain: Cerebral perfusion pressure (CPP), autoregulation, chemo regulation and cerebral metabolism.

*Cerebral Perfusion Pressure*

Blood flow to any organ is driven by the pressure difference between the arterial and venous circulation, as arterial pressure is high and venous pressure is low. This pressure difference or the driving force is known as perfusion pressure. In cerebral circulation, arterial pressure pushes

**Table 8.4:** Diagnostic procedures with its purposes, procedure and nurses' responsibilities (Hickey, 1997; Zomordi, 2017).

| Diagnostic procedure | Purpose | Procedure | Nursing responsibilities |
|---|---|---|---|
| Lumbar puncture | To obtain cerebrospinal fluid (CSF) for analysis. Usually used in patients suspected with meningitis or subarachnoid hemorrhage | After cleaning the skin, local anesthetic drug is injected at the site of insertion. Then, a needle is inserted into the L3–L4 space and CSF is aspirated. CSF pressure is monitored. CSF sample is sent for | *Before:* Obtain informed consent, provide lateral recumbent position (lateral position with flexed head and knees), provide privacy, monitor intracranial pressure (ICP) as lumbar puncture is contraindicated in increased ICP. *During:* Ensure the position is maintained, sterile techniques to be followed. *After:* Provide supine position for the patient, monitor for spinal headache, monitor for complications such as hemorrhage, infection, CSF leakage, or difficulty in urination |
| Electroencephalography (EEG) | Used to detect the electrical activity of the brain. It is indicated in patients with seizures. It is also used to confirm brain death. EEG wave patterns produced will help in identifying the activity of brain. EEG also helps in identifying the location of the lesion or abnormality in the cerebrum | 10–20 electrodes are placed on the scalp and then electrical activity is recorded graphically | *Before:* Explain the procedure to the patient, address any fears or anxieties related to the procedure; patient head should be shampooed to clear the scalp of oil or dirt; make sure hair is clean and dry; check if the patient has to avoid anticonvulsants or tranquilizers before procedure *During:* Electrodes should be placed after applying conductive gel *After:* Patients can be instructed to resume any stopped medications; wipe the gel from hair and scalp |
| X-ray | Used to obtain radiographic image of the skull and vertebral column. It helps in identifying fractures or misalignment. It is indicated in road traffic accidents or any trauma | X-rays are passed through the patient's head or trunk and projected onto a photographic plate | *Before:* Patient should be appropriately positioned depending upon the area of injury and view (lateral, anteroposterior, oblique) *During:* Ensure that the patient is not moving during the procedure *After:* Provide a proper position to the patient |
| Computed tomography (CT) | CT scan is used to obtain cross-sectional radiographic images of internal parts of brain or spinal cord. It helps in identifying hemorrhage, tumor, abscess, hydrocephalus, edema, mass shift, infarction, extent of compression in the structures | After the patient lies down on the CT scanner machine table, a series of X-rays cross the body part and multiple coss-sectional images are taken. In some cases, contrast agent can be used to enhance the structures | *Before:* Explain the procedure to the patient, as patients who are claustrophobic might be anxious; If contrast agent is used, check for shellfish or iodine allergy and monitor the renal function of the patient *During:* Ensure that the patient is not moving during the entire procedure; Monitor for any allergic reactions of iodine *After:* Address the needs of the patient |
| Magnetic resonance imaging (MRI) | MRI gives a clearer picture of soft tissues than CT scan. It is also used to obtain cross-sectional images of internal parts of brain and spinal cord. It is indicated in tumors, stroke, traumatic injury, herniation | In MRI, patient is placed inside an MRI machine and body is exposed to powerful magnetic field and then introduced to radiofrequency pulsations. This causes changes in the hydrogen protons in the body and it emits signals that are detected by the machine. | *Before:* Ensure that the patients do not have any metallic objects such as cardiac pacemaker, prosthetic valves, teeth braces, or aneurysm clips. Any metal jewelry or clothing should be removed. In such cases, MRI is contraindicated. While using contrast, monitor renal function. As the procedure takes long time, it is better to sedate the claustrophobic patients. Inform the patient that the machine will be noisy during the procedure. Advise the patient for passing urine before procedure |

*Contd...*

*Contd...*

| Diagnostic procedure | Purpose | Procedure | Nursing responsibilities |
|---|---|---|---|
| | | In some cases, contrast agent (gadolinium) can be used to enhance the structures | *During:* Make sure that the patient is not moving during the procedure<br>*After:* Address the needs of the patient. Instruct the patient that normal activities can be performed after procedure |
| **Cerebral angiography** | Cerebral angiography is used to visualize any abnormalities in the intracranial and extracranial blood vessels. It helps to identify the patency, vasospasm, stenosis, thrombus, blockage of the involved blood vessels. It is indicated in aneurysm, arteriovenous malformations | Just like coronary angiography, a catheter is inserted through femoral artery and then guided to the cerebral arteries. After this, contrast medium is injected through the catheter and serial X-ray images of the head are taken | *Before:* Perform baseline neurological examination, monitor pedal pulses, risk for stroke, allergy to contrast dye; shave the groin region; NPO 4–6 hours before procedure; monitor renal function; sedation provided for some patients<br>*During:* Monitor vital signs; Ensure the patient is not moving during the procedure<br>*After:* Apply pressure on groin region for at least 5 minutes after removing femoral catheter and then apply pressure bandage. Monitor vital signs and neurologic status every 15 minutes in the first two hours, then hourly for next 6 hours and then every 2 hourly for next 24 hours. Advise strict bed rest for up to 2–6 hours with head elevation less than 30 degrees. Restrict movement of punctured leg, as prescribed. Monitor for signs of hematoma in the puncture site in groin. Monitor lower extremities for pulse, change in color, sensations or temperature. Advise patient to increase fluid intake to wash out contrast agent through urine |
| **Myelogram** | It is used to detect compression to nerve root in conditions such as disc herniation, spinal tumor, vertebral fracture or stenosis of intervertebral foramen (contraindicated in pregnancy) | A contrast dye is injected into the subarachnoid space in lumbar region. X-ray table with patient is then tilted in different positions so that contrast dye reaches the whole spinal column. X-ray images of the spinal cord and vertebral column is taken | *Before:* Monitor for NPO for 3–4 hours before procedure. Check for allergy to contrast dye. Instruct patient to void before procedure. Explain about table tilting involved in the procedure<br>*During:* Monitor carefully for nausea as the table is tilted during the procedure<br>*After:* Monitor neurologic signs and vital signs. Observe patient for headache, nausea, vomiting, or seizures. Patient should maintain supine position with head elevation for 24 hours after procedure. Advise the patient to drink fluids in order to wash out contrast dye through urine |
| **Positron emission tomography (PET)** | It is used to detect the metabolic activity of different areas of the brain. It is indicated areas of cell death in stroke, Alzheimer's disease, Parkinson's disease, seizure, and tumors(contraindicated in pregnancy) | At first, patient is administered radioactive glucose or oxygen through injection or inhalation. The areas of the brain with increased metabolism have high blood supply. Therefore, the consumption of radioactive oxygen or glucose in these areas will be high. As the radioactive substance decays, it releases energy. This energy is detected by gamma scanner in PET and it produces colorful images of the active areas of the brain | *Before:* Explain that the procedure is time-consuming. Radio-isotope is administered one hour before PET. Substances that can influence the activity of central nervous system such as caffeine, alcohol or nicotine should be avoided for 24 hours before procedure. Dextrose IV infusion should be stopped for at least 6 hours before procedure. Instruct the patient to void<br>*During:* Ensure the patient is not moving during the procedure. As per the area of the brain being tested, patient will be asked to perform some tasks. Guide and support the patient during these tasks<br>*After:* Advice the patient to drink fluids to wash out the radioisotope |

*Contd...*

*Contd...*

| Diagnostic procedure | Purpose | Procedure | Nursing responsibilities |
|---|---|---|---|
| **Electromyography (EMG)** | It is used to record the electrical activity of a muscle. It is used to distinguish whether the muscle weakness or paralysis is due to muscle, nerve or neuromuscular junction. It is indicated mainly in neuromuscular disease, myasthenia gravis. It is also indicated in disorders involving skeletal muscle or peripheral nerves | Thin needle electrodes are inserted into the muscles. The muscles are stimulated with mild electrical charge. Electrical activity of the muscle is then recorded in a relaxed state and contracted state | *Before:* Inform the patient that insertion of needles can cause pain, pressure or discomfort. Ask patient to avoid caffeine, and nicotine for three hours prior to EMG. Any use of muscle relaxants should be stopped before test<br><br>*During:* Ensure patient is not moving during the procedure as it takes long time<br><br>*After:* Monitor the insertion site for signs of hematoma, bleeding, redness, or swelling. Administer mild analgesics or warm compresses at the insertion site, if it is painful |
| **Nerve conduction studies (NCS)** | It is used to measure the nerve conduction velocity and action potential of motor or sensory neurons in the arm, leg or face. It helps in determining peripheral neuropathy, any disorder of the spinal nerve root or spinal cord | Peripheral nerves (motor or sensory) are electrically stimulated with the help of electrodes. The generated action potential and the velocity of nerve conduction is then measured | *Before:* Monitor the temperature of the patient (lower body temperature can slow the conduction velocity). Explain to the patient that mild electric current will be passed through the body which can create mild discomfort. Ask the patient to remove all jewelery. Ensure whether the patient has no cardiac pacemaker<br><br>*During:* Place the electrodes after applying a special paste and tape them to the skin<br><br>*After:* Monitor for any discomfort or pain at the nerve site |
| **Evoked potentials**<br><br>Types include somatosensory evoked potentials, visual evoked potentials, auditory evoked potentials | It is used to detect any abnormalities in sensory nerve impulse transmission and its pathways. It is used to detect abnormalities in visual or auditory nerve pathways. It is indicated to confirm multiple sclerosis, neuronal damage, optic neuritis, tumors in the eye, retinal damage, auditory nerve lesions | Electrodes are attached to the scalp placed on skin or scalp, depending upon the area to be assessed. Then, a particular stimulus is provided, such as click sound (through headphone) or chequerboard patterns. As a result, an electrical signal is generated in the respective sensory nerve and travels to the cerebral cortex. This electrical signal is detected by the electrodes | *Before:* Explain the procedure to the patient. Instruct the patient regarding the tasks that are given during the procedure. Inform the patient that the test may take long time. Instruct the patient to remove jewelery<br><br>*During:* Ensure the patient is not moving during the procedure. Provide the sensory stimulus to the patient, depending upon the area to be tested |
| **Transcranial doppler sonography** | It is used to measure the velocity of cerebral blood flow and cerebral autoregulation. It is indicated in stroke, subarachnoid hemorrhage, vasospasm, or any blockage in cerebral vasculature | Fiber-optic ultrasonic wave is placed on the bone-windows of the skull – temporal zygoma, transorbital, foramen magnum. (Bone-windows are places where the skull is thin or contains a small gap). The location of placement of probe depends upon the blood vessel to be tested. The probe sends ultrasound waves to the blood vessels and the reflected sound waves are detected by the probe. These reflected sound waves helps in determining blood flow velocity | *Before:* Supine or lateral position is given for the patient. Explain that the procedure is noninvasive.<br><br>*During:* Address the needs of the patient during the procedure<br><br>*After:* Patient can resume normal activities after the procedure |

the blood to the cranium. But there is an additional pressure that opposes blood flow to the cranium. This additional pressure is intracranial pressure. The pressure difference created by the arterial pressure and intracranial pressure drives the blood to enter inside the cranial cavity. This pressure gradient (pressure difference) that drives the blood to flow to the cerebrum is known as cerebral perfusion pressure. Therefore, cerebral pressure is denoted by the following formula:

CPP = MAP − ICP

where CPP is cerebral perfusion pressure
MAP is mean arterial pressure
ICP is intracranial pressure

Mean arterial pressure, in simple terms, is the average value of blood pressure because blood pressure has a systolic and diastolic value. MAP is calculated by the following formula:

$$MAP = \frac{SBP + 2\ DBP}{3}$$

where SBP is systolic blood pressure
DBP is diastolic blood pressure

The normal value of CPP is healthy person ranges between 70–95 mm Hg. We have already seen that CPP is the driving force of blood to the brain. Therefore, theoretically as CPP increases, cerebral blood flow increases and as CPP decreases, cerebral blood flow decreases. But in a healthy body, an increase or decrease in CPP within the range of 50–140 mm Hg will not influence cerebral blood flow. Cerebral blood flow will be maintained constant. This constant cerebral blood flow is being maintained by a mechanism called autoregulation.

### Autoregulation

Based on the formula CPP = MAP − ICP that was seen earlier, any increase in BP will rise MAP. This will cause an increase in CPP, which in turn can increase the cerebral blood flow. In such a situation, in order to maintain the constant cerebral blood flow to brain, cerebral blood vessels, especially microcirculation, constrict to reduce the cerebral blood flow.

In contrast, if there is any decrease in BP, the mean arterial pressure (MAP) will decrease. This will cause a decrease in CPP, which in turn can decrease the cerebral blood flow. In such a situation, in order to maintain the constant cerebral blood flow to brain, cerebral blood vessels, especially microcirculation, dilate to reduce the cerebral blood flow.

This compensatory change in the diameter of cerebral blood vessels to maintain a constant blood flow to brain is termed autoregulation.

But autoregulation has certain limitations and does not happen in all the cases. It does not work properly when the CPP becomes <50 mm Hg and >140 mm Hg. In such cases, cerebral blood flow will depend on mean arterial pressure. Cerebral blood flow will no longer be constant and it will fluctuate depending upon the changes in blood pressure.

### Chemo Regulation

The changes in the cerebral blood vessel diameter with subsequent change in cerebral blood flow depending upon the changes in partial pressure of $CO_2$ ($paCO_2$) and partial pressure of $O_2$ ($paO_2$) is known as chemo regulation.

When there is an increase in $paCO_2$, smooth muscles in the cerebral blood vessels relax and cause vasodilation. This leads to an increase in cerebral blood flow. When there is a decrease in $paCO_2$, the reverse happens. That is, smooth muscles in the cerebral blood vessels contract and cause vasoconstriction. This leads to a decrease in cerebral blood flow.

In hypoxemia, the decrease in $paO_2$ level causes vasodilation in cerebral blood vessels. This results in increased cerebral blood flow to compensate for the reduced oxygen tension. The changes in cerebral blood flow in response to $paO_2$ changes is minimal. There will be a significant increase in cerebral blood flow only when $paO_2$ has decreased to the level of hypoxia.

### Cerebral Metabolism

In the brain, all the areas are not active at the same time. The areas that are metabolically active at a particular time will require more glucose and oxygen delivery than the other areas. As a result, cerebral blood flow is not equal in all the regions of the brain. The metabolically active areas of the brain receive higher blood flow. The cerebral blood flow is mostly dependent upon neuronal activity. Thus, cerebral cortex (gray matter) has higher blood flow than white matter. This is termed as flow-metabolic coupling.

It is suggested that the chemical mediators responsible for vasodilation in the areas with increased metabolic rate are hydrogen ($H^+$) ion, carbon dioxide, potassium ($K^+$) ion, adenosine, nitric oxide. In a patient with hypoxia, the decrease in oxygen results in anaerobic metabolism. This gives rise to lactic acidosis due to lactic acid accumulation. The acidotic state ($H^+$ ion) and hypoxic state further contribute to vasodilation. As it continues, autoregulation will not function and compensatory mechanisms will fail (Tameem and Krovvidi, 2013).

### Pressure-volume Changes

The changes in ICP in relation to the changes in intracranial volume are depicted in the pressure-volume curve

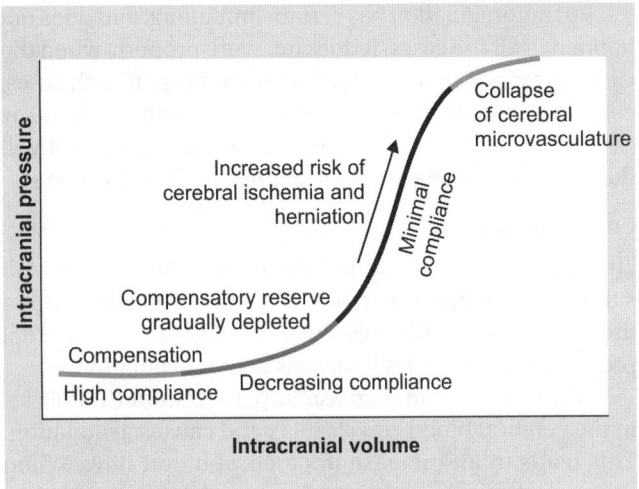

**Fig. 8.7:** Pressure-volume curve in increased ICP.

(**Fig. 8.7**). As the volume inside the cranium increases, blood and CSF helps in maintaining ICP by displacing outside the intracranial space. This is termed as compliance. In other words, compliance is the ability of the brain to expand without changes in ICP.

For example, a patient has an increasing brain tumor. In the initial stages, the brain has high compliance. During this stage, the ICP does not increase as compensatory mechanisms are intact. As the volume increases further, compliance starts to decrease. At this stage, there is a higher risk of increased ICP. Towards the later stages, increase in brain volume causes the compensatory mechanisms to fail and lead to increase in ICP.

### Etiology of Increased ICP

As seen earlier, there will be an increase in ICP when there is increase in any one of the following components in intracranial cavity: Brain, blood and CSF. The causes of increased ICP are given in **Table 8.5**.

### Cerebral Edema

Cerebral or brain edema is the accumulation of fluid in the intracellular and interstitial spaces (that is, extravascular space) in the brain. There are different types of cerebral edema, and these can be seen in combination in certain patients. The different types and causes of cerebral edema are as follows:

- **Vasogenic edema:** The term 'vasogenic' means generated from blood vessels. Vasogenic edema occurs due to the leakage of protein-rich fluid from the blood into the interstitial space of brain. This is the most common type of cerebral edema. Vasogenic edema occurs when the blood-brain barrier is disrupted causing membrane permeability to increase. This allows the movement of fluid from blood vessels to the interstitial space. This edema mainly affects white matter and is mostly associated with brain tumors, cerebral abscesses and toxins.

- **Cytotoxic edema:** Cytotoxic cerebral edema occurs because of the disruption of cell membrane integrity. More specifically, $Na^+$-$K^+$ and $Ca^+$ATP-dependent pumps in the cell membrane are affected. Due to any neurological insult, when the oxygen supply to the brain is reduced, energy dependent pumps fail to function properly. As a result, number of $Na^+$ ions accelerates inside the cell. This causes fluid to flow into the intracellular space through osmosis. Another factor driving $Na^+$ ions inside the cell is the neurotransmitter, glutamate because it opens the $Na^+$ channels. Thus, $Na^+$ ions along with water enter inside the cell. The edema occurs both in gray and white matter and affects neurons and neuroglial cells mainly, astrocytes. Cytotoxic edema is seen mostly in disorders causing reduced oxygen supply, such as stroke, trauma, ischemia, or hypoxia (Ho, et al., 2012, Kimelberg, 1995).

- **Interstitial edema:** Interstitial edema occurs due to hydrocephalus (the accumulation of cerebrospinal fluid inside the ventricles). Due to the rise in CSF volume, the size of ventricles increases. As the pressure inside the ventricles increases, the ventricle wall ruptures and the CSF inside the ventricles will be shifted to the interstitial space of white matter. Interstitial edema is seen mostly in subarachnoid hemorrhage, intraventricular hemorrhage, meningitis, or any tumors compressing the CSF outflow (Ho et al., 2012; Mestecky, 2011).

| Table 8.5: Causes of increased ICP (Mestecky, 2011a, Zomordi, 2017). | | |
|---|---|---|
| **Increase in brain volume** | **Increase in CSF volume** | **Increase in blood volume** |
| • Cerebral edema—vasogenic, cytotoxic, interstitial, hypo-osmolar edema<br>• Space occupying lesions such as tumor, arteriovenous malformation, hematoma (epidural, subdural, subarachnoid, intracerebral), abscess, cysts | • Hydrocephalus—obstruction to flow of CSF<br>• Choroid plexus tumors—increased CSF production<br>• Decreased reabsorption of CSF—meningitis | • Obstruction to venous return—cerebral venous thrombosis, cervical collars, Trendelenburg position<br>• Vasodilation—drugs such as nitrates, severe hypoxia or hypercapnia |

- **Hypo-osmolar edema:** Normally, fluid from the blood vessels crosses the blood brain barrier and shifts to the interstitial space of brain through the process called osmosis. In conditions where the serum osmolality is lowered, the osmotic pressure gradient forces the fluid to pass from the blood vessel to the brain. The swelling thus created in the brain is called hypo-osmolar edema. This is usually seen in water intoxication, syndrome of inappropriate antidiuretic hormone (SIADH), hyponatremia, or diabetic ketoacidosis (Ho et al., 2012).

*Clinical Manifestations of Increased ICP*

Development of signs and symptoms of increased ICP depends on the location, and the rate at which ICP increases. If the rate of increase of ICP is slow (example, slow growing tumors, hydrocephalus), the development of signs and symptoms will be gradual. If the rate of increase of ICP is fast (example, hemorrhage), the signs and symptoms occur suddenly.

*Early signs and symptoms* are commonly seen when a gradual development occurs. They are:

- **Headache:** Compression of cerebral blood vessels and cranial nerves against brain matter leads to headache. The pain is seen to be worse in the morning time and it increases with straining activities like coughing, bending, agitation, etc.
- **Nausea and vomiting:** Vomiting occurs due to pressure changes in the intracranial cavity. Vomiting is usually sudden, not accompanied by nausea and has a projectile nature.
- **Papilledema:** Papilledema is defined as edema in the optic disc. Intracranial compression limits the venous return of retinal vessels. The resulting retinal congestion and vasodilation causes swelling in the optic disc.
- Drowsiness
- Seizures
- **Focal neurologic deficits (FND):** This means signs and symptoms depending upon the location of the affected region of brain. For example, when the primary visual cortex in the occipital lobe is affected, visual problems will ensue, or when the primary motor cortex is affected, hemiplegia will occur. Focal neurologic deficit is most commonly the result of compression of the brain matter due to the mass lesion (Mestecky, 2011; Ropper et., 2019; Zomordi, 2017).

*Late signs and symptoms* are seen when ICP rises rapidly. They are:

- **Changes in level of consciousness:** In patients with increasing ICP, alterations in consciousness can range from unconsciousness to disorientation. These changes occur due to compression and insufficient blood supply to cerebral cortex or reticular activating system (RAS), the area in brainstem responsible for consciousness and alertness.
- Seizures
- **Pupillary changes:** Pupillary dilation occurs due to compression of cranial nerve III or oculomotor nerve. Along with dilation, there can be no reaction or sluggish reaction to light.
- **Cushing's triad:** This is a symptom triad involving the vital signs—BP, heart rate and respiration. Cushing's triad occurs due to compression over thalamus, hypothalamus and brainstem. This includes widening of pulse pressure with increased systolic blood pressure, bradycardia and irregular respirations.
- **Decorticate or decerebrate posturing:** Both these posturing is observed if there is any interruption in the motor pathways. In decorticate posturing, flexion is observed at the level of elbows, wrists and fingers with internal rotation and adduction of arms and extension of legs. In decerebrate posturing, the arms are adducted and extended at the level of elbows, but fingers and wrists are flexed. In addition, the legs are extended with plantar flexion. Among these two posturing, decerebrate posturing has the worse prognosis (Mestecky, 2011a; Zomordi, 2017).

### Assessment of Intracranial Pressure

Although the signs and symptoms denote presence of increased ICP, the health team cannot confirm any increase or decrease in ICP reliably. For this, measurement of ICP is essential in a neurocritical care setting.

*ICP Monitoring*

ICP monitoring is performed to measure the continuous changes in ICP. Clinically, after measuring ICP, cerebral perfusion pressure is calculated as given in the formula earlier in this section. In addition, ICP monitoring also helps in checking the effectiveness of ICU management and thus helps in preventing further complications (EBP, Bradley). There are invasive as well as noninvasive methods of ICP monitoring.

*Techniques*

Invasive ICP monitoring is a procedure which involves introduction of a catheter to the intraventricular, intraparenchymal, subarachnoid, subdural or epidural space as shown in **Figure 8.8**. The specific devices used are fluid-filled devices, and micro transducer devices such as fiber-optic and micro-strain gauge devices. The devices

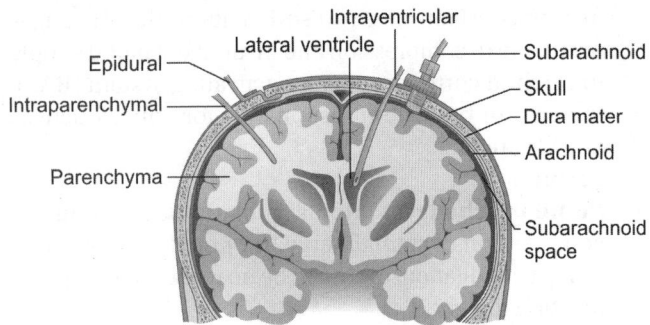

**Fig. 8.8:** Sites for invasive ICP monitoring.

are connected to a pressure transducer which is then connected to the monitor. The ICP value will be displayed on the monitor.

In noninvasive monitoring, the different methods used to determine ICP are: Transcranial ultrasonography, tympanic membrane displacement (TMD), optic nerve sheath diameter (ONSD), MRI and CT scan, fundoscopy and papilledema (Raboel et al., 2012).

*Indications*

Not all the patients with any brain disorder require ICP monitoring. Those who are conscious, alert, and able to follow commands do not require regular monitoring of ICP. The procedure is usually indicated for patients who are at high-risk of developing increased ICP **(Rangel-Castillo et., 2008)**. The indications are:
- **Traumatic conditions:**
  - GCS <8
  - Abnormal head CT scan on admission
  - GCS >8, but if the patients require prolonged anesthesia or prolonged induction of paralysis, high positive end-expiratory pressure (PEEP)
  - A person with normal head CT scan, but if they have two or more of the following risk factors: such as age >40 years, systolic blood pressure <90 mm Hg, and abnormal posture such as decerebrate or decorticate posturing.
- **Nontraumatic conditions:**
  - Presence of mass lesion—tumor, intracerebral hemorrhage with increased chances of deterioration
  - At the end of surgery, involving evacuation of tumor or hematoma **(Rangel-Castillo et al., 2008)**.

*Nursing Responsibility*

Nurses responsibility after catheter insertion for ICP monitoring includes the following:
- The fluid-filled system should be primed with 0.9% normal saline solution.
- The pressure transducer should be at the level of ventricle for accurate readings. For this, the transducer is positioned at the level of external auditory meatus or tragus of ear.
- Rezeroing of the device should be done regularly, that is, at least every 12 hours. This is done to ensure accurate readings.
- ICP value should be recorded every hourly. But if the ICP value is high, then the value should be recorded every half hourly or every 15 minutes.
- CSF is drained when the ICP is elevated. In such cases, CSF drainage, CSF color and clarity should be observed.
- Sterile dressing should be applied at the catheter insertion site.
- Carefully monitor the tubing for any kinks. Observe the drainage tubing for any air bubbles, clots, tissues or debris. In the presence of any debris, flush the tubing away from the patient.
- ICP, CPP, IC3P waveforms, CSF characteristics should be documented **(Salmon et al., 2016; Slazinkski et al., 2011)**.

*Management*

Management is focussed on treating the processes that caused increased intracranial pressure. The goal of the treatment include:
- Maintain cerebral blood flow
- Maintain adequate cerebral oxygenation and perfusion
- Minimize the complications associated with increased ICP.

*Diagnosis*

Ineffective cerebral tissue perfusion related to cerebral edema as evidenced by increase ICP.

*Interventions*
- The head end of the bed should be elevated to 30 degrees to facilitate venous drainage thereby reducing the risk of increasing ICP. The neck should be in a neutral position. Do not flex or hyperextend the neck.
- Avoid restrictive neck taping. Remove or loosen rigid collars to decrease ICP.

*Diagnosis*

Ineffective breathing pattern related to neurologic dysfunction impairment as evidenced by abnormal respiration rate, rhythm/depth.

*Interventions*
- Maintain respiratory pattern.
- Monitor oxygen status.
- Position the patient to maximize the ventilation potential.

## Medical Management and Nursing Care

In the emergency department, airway, breathing and circulation should be paid attention to initially. Increased ICP can lead to cerebral ischemia with decreased cerebral tissue perfusion. Restoring blood and oxygen supply to the brain cells becomes a prioritized need.

### Respiratory Management

Usually, patients with increased ICP manifest hypoxia or respiratory dysfunction with decreased level of consciousness. They are intubated either orally or nasally and connected to the mechanical ventilator to maintain ventilation. Intubation should be done skillfully by an expert because gagging and coughing during the procedure can cause the ICP to increase. Thus, it is recommended to follow rapid sequence induction with intubation, where patient is administered anesthesia inducing agents before intubation.

Increasing positive end-expiratory pressure (PEEP) values in a patient on mechanical ventilator should be done with adequate monitoring. High PEEP can increase the intrathoracic pressure, which can decrease the cerebral venous return. As the venous return decreases, there can be increased ICP (Marik et al., 1999, Rangel-Castillo et al., 2008).

### Positioning

For the patients with increased ICP, a 30° head end elevation is recommended. Head elevation increases the jugular venous return and hence prevents accumulation of blood in the intracranial space. Thus, it helps in lowering the ICP. Head should be kept in a neutral position and certain positions such as Trendelenburg, hip flexion that increase ICP are to be avoided (Dunn, 2002; Tan, Cheng, and Sim, 2015).

### Procedural Precautions

Cervical collar or endotracheal tube ties should not be tied too tightly around the neck. It can cause a reduction in the jugular venous return, which can in turn increase the ICP. Activities that can cause sympathetic nervous system stimulation should be avoided (Godoy et al., 2018).

### Noxious Stimuli

Noxious stimuli specifically auditory stimuli such as noises, monitor alarms that elicit sympathetic response should be minimized or avoided (Godoy et al., 2018).

### Analgesia and Sedation

Propofol, or midazolam is given as sedative and morphine is given as analgesic to depress the activity of central nervous system. Thus, cerebral metabolic activity is reduced, thus decreasing the cerebral blood flow. Sedation also prevents activities that increase ICP such as seizure activity, agitated state, and coughing (Dunn, 2002; Tripathy and Ahmad, 2019).

### Hyperventilation

It is already discussed in this section that decreased $paCO_2$ level causes vasoconstriction, thus decreasing cerebral blood flow. Hyperventilation reduces $paCO_2$ level. Thus, it is helpful in reducing ICP value. But, hyperventilation cannot be continued for a prolonged time as it can rebound the effect with vasodilation, thus resulting in increased ICP (Dunn, 2002; Rangel-Castillo et al., 2008).

### Fever

Fever has certain effects on cerebral physiologic mechanisms. Fever increases the cerebral metabolic rate by 10–13% for every degree Celsius increase in temperature. Fever also can cause vasodilation. Both of these effects can increase cerebral blood flow, thus increasing the ICP. Hence, control of fever is essential in the management of increased ICP. The measures taken to control fever includes: antipyretics and cooling blankets (Rangel-Castillo et al., 2008).

### Prevention of Seizures

Seizure activity can increase the cerebral metabolic rate. Thus, it can result in increased ICP. Seizure prophylaxis is recommended for 7 days after the injury. In order to prevent seizures, anticonvulsants such as phenytoin is used (Marik et al., 1999).

### Hypertension

As patient's cerebral autoregulation is impaired, CPP and cerebral blood flow will be dependent on systemic blood pressure. If the blood pressure is high, it can lead to increased cerebral blood flow. Thus, ICP will be increased. In addition, increased blood pressure can also heighten the risk of intracranial hemorrhage and cerebral edema.

For hypertensive conditions, beta-blockers such as labetalol, esmolol or central acting alpha receptor agonists such as clonidine are preferred. These antihypertensives are specifically used because they do not have any effect on ICP (Rangel-Castillo et al., 2008).

### Hyperosmolar Therapy

Hyperosmolar therapy increases the osmolarity of the blood. Thus, it creates an osmotic effect due to which fluid from the interstitial spaces in the brain is shifted to the intravascular space. This shift is helpful in reducing cerebral edema. The drugs used are mannitol and 3% sodium chloride. Mannitol decreases blood viscosity, which improves blood flow to the brain. The effect of mannitol starts in 15–30 minutes and lasts for 1–6 hours. As mannitol causes diuresis, it is not advised for patients with renal failure. In such situations, hypertonic saline is used. The commonly used 3% sodium chloride increases serum sodium level and serum osmolality without causing diuresis or hypotension (Tan et al., 2015).

### Barbiturate Coma

Administration of high-dose barbiturates such as pentobarbital, thiopentone reduces ICP by reducing cerebral blood flow and cerebral metabolic rate. Barbiturate is not used commonly and is used only for intracranial hypertension that is not responding to treatment. Side-effects of barbiturates includes hypotension, respiratory dysfunction, hypokalemia, hepatic and renal dysfunction. In a patient receiving barbiturate treatment, neurologic functions such as level of consciousness cannot be assessed properly (Dunn, 2002, Tan et al., 2015).

### Steroids

Intravenous dexamethasone 4 mg is preferred for brain tumors as it reduces vasogenic cerebral edema, thus decreasing ICP. But, trials among patients with head injury has shown either no effect or harmful effects, with increased risk of death (Rangel-Castillo et al., 2008).

### Surgical Management

### CSF Drainage

Ventriculostomy is performed to drain the excess cerebrospinal fluid from the ventricles. This can be done intermittently in response to rising ICP. Drainage of the CSF reduces ICP significantly as intracranial volume contributed by CSF is reduced. As a prolonged effect, reduced CSF volume can help in shifting of edematous fluid from brain tissues to the intraventricular space. The complications of this procedure are infection and hemorrhage (Dunn, 2002).

### Resection of Mass Lesions

Mass lesions such as hematoma, tumor, abscess that cause increased ICP is removed. This resection is done through a procedure known as '*craniotomy*' **(Fig. 8.9)**, where a hole is drilled in the skull and the mass lesion is evacuated (Rangel-Castillo et al., 2008).

### Decompressive Craniectomy

'Craniectomy' means removal of skull and 'decompressive' means to relieve compression or pressure. As skull is a rigid structure, it is not able to expand or change its shape in adults. Therefore, when ICP is increased, the brain gets compressed against the skull. In order to relieve the pressure on brain, the portion of the skull above the affected area

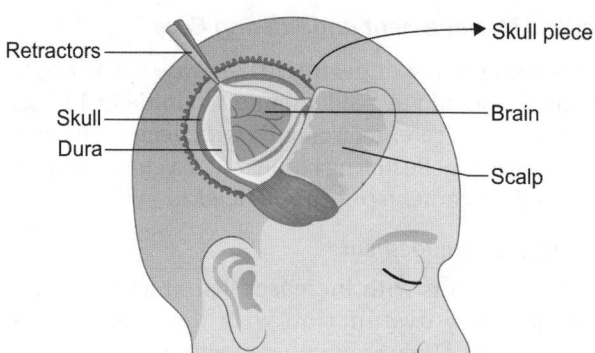

**Fig. 8.9:** Craniotomy: Skull piece removed to expose dura mater and brain.

of brain is removed temporarily. The skull is usually kept in the subcutaneous pocket in the abdomen and replaced later. The surgical procedure where the portion of the skull is replaced is known as '*cranioplasty*'.

Decompressive craniectomy is performed in conditions with uncontrollable intracranial hypertension where the patient is not responding to medical management. This includes intracerebral hemorrhage, subarachnoid hemorrhage or infarction (Rangel-Castillo et al., 2008).

## CEREBROVASCULAR DISEASE

### Subarachnoid Hemorrhage

Subarachnoid hemorrhage (SAH) is bleeding into the subarachnoid space. Aneurysmal rupture is the one of the most common causes of SAH. Aneurysmal SAH is a neurologic emergency that should be treated in a facility with neurologic unit.

### Etiology

The common causes of SAH are:
- **Aneurysmal rupture:** The most common cause of subarachnoid hemorrhage is rupture of cerebral aneurysm. Cerebral aneurysms are protrusion in the arteries of the Circle of Willis. Protrusion occurs due to the thinning of muscular walls of the arteries (Petridis et al., 2017).
- Trauma

Rarely, SAH is caused by the following cerebrovascular abnormalities:
- Arteriovenous malformation
- Vasculitis
- Venous thrombosis
- CNS tumors
- Arterial dissection
- Cocaine abuse

## Pathophysiology

Bleeding after rupture of aneurysm causes an increase in intracranial pressure. There can also be associated intraventricular and cerebral hemorrhage. This can in turn lead to cerebral edema and hydrocephalus.

Bleeding can cause direct damage to the brain and ischemia to the brain tissues which triggers multiple mechanisms in the brain.

SAH can increase the activity of sympathetic nervous system, activate renin angiotensin aldosterone system and inflammatory cytokines. This elicits a systemic response which will then affect multiple organs like lungs, heart and cause fluid electrolyte imbalances **(Macdonald et al., 2017; Petridis et al., 2017)**.

## Clinical Manifestations

The patient mainly manifests severe headaches, which is often described as the worst headache the person has ever experienced. The headache is of sudden onset and maximum severity is reached within 1 minute of onset in half of the patients.

Signs and symptoms of increased intracranial pressure—vomiting, focal neurologic deficit, seizures along with decreased level of consciousness is seen (Macdonald et al., 2017; Petridis et al., 2017).

Signs of meningeal irritation are seen due to presence of blood in CSF. These signs include photophobia, nuchal rigidity, headache and fever.

## Diagnosis

- **CT scan:** Head CT without contrast within the first few hours reveals blood as hyperdense area in the subarachnoid space (basal cisterns, ventricles or brain parenchyma) in majority of the cases.
- **Lumbar puncture (LP):** An LP is done to check for signs of bleeding in the cerebrospinal fluid (CSF)—presence of RBCs or xanthochromia in CSF. Xanthochromia is the yellowish discoloration of the CSF indicative of increased bilirubin due to hemolysis of RBCs. Therefore, xanthochromia is formed about 12 hours after bleeding.
- **Cerebral angiography:** This test is the gold standard for detecting cerebral aneurysm. Digital subtraction angiography (DSA) gives a better visualization of aneurysm along with its relation to the neighboring structures.

## Grading of SAH

Scales are intended to show the severity of patient condition in SAH. The Hunt and Hess classification grades SAH based on the severity of clinical condition of the patient **(Table 8.6)**.

Another grading given by the World Federation of Neurological Surgeons (WFNS) considers level of consciousness and presence or absence of focal neurologic deficit **(Table 8.7)**. It helps in evaluating the severity and patient outcome.

**Table 8.6:** Hunt and Hess grading of SAH (Mestecky, 2011; Macdonald et al., 2017).

| Grades | Description |
|---|---|
| 1. | Asymptomatic, slight headache, nuchal rigidity |
| 2. | Moderate to severe headache, nuchal rigidity, no focal deficit other than cranial nerve palsy |
| 3. | Mild mental status change (drowsy or confused), mild focal neurologic deficit |
| 4. | Stupor, moderate to severe hemiparesis |
| 5. | Comatose, decerebrate rigidity |

**Table 8.7:** WFNS grading of SAH (Mestecky, 2011).

| Grades | Description |
|---|---|
| 1. | GCS score 15, no motor deficit |
| 2. | GCS score 13–14, no motor deficit |
| 3. | GCS score 13–14, motor deficit present |
| 4. | GCS score 7–12, motor deficit may be present or absent |
| 5. | GCS score 3–6, motor deficit may be present or absent |

## Medical and Nursing Management of Aneurysmal SAH

### Nursing Management

**Altered neurological function related to hemorrhage from cerebral aneurysm as evidenced by altered GCS score.**

#### Interventions

- Monitoring of neurological status.
- Monitoring GCS and pupillary reaction to light every hourly

#### Diagnosis

Increased ICP is related to accumulation of blood in the cerebral tissue as evidenced by impaired consciousness.

#### Interventions

- Monitor ICP.
- Elevated the bed 20–30 degrees.

  Patients diagnosed with acute SAH should be immediately transferred to health care facilities with skilled staffs and adequate technology. Aneurysmal SAH can be immediately followed by complications such as rebleeding, delayed cerebral ischemia, hydrocephalus, or increased ICP. Treatment strategies will include management of aneurysm along with its complications.

  Initial management is aimed at maintaining optimal cerebral perfusion pressure, cardiopulmonary resuscitation and delivering adequate oxygen.

- **Neurological assessment:** Close monitoring of neurological status, i.e., GCS and pupillary reaction to light every hourly is essential as there can be sudden change in the neurological status (Mestecky, 2011).
- **Blood pressure control:** Blood pressure management is important to maintain cerebral perfusion pressure and to reduce the risk of rebleeding. It is suggested to maintain systolic blood pressure <160 mm Hg to reduce rebleeding. Recommended antihypertensive drugs include—labetalol, clonidine, calcium channel blockers (Mestecky, 2011; Petridis et al., 2017).
- **Rebleeding:** After ruptured hemorrhage, the peak time for rebleeding is within 24 hours with 5–10% chance within the first 72 hours. Risk factors associated with rebleeding includes increased systolic blood pressure (>160 mm Hg), large size of aneurysm, neurologic status during admission, and initial loss of consciousness (Connolly et al., 2012).

  Blood pressure management is important to prevent rebleeding related to hypertension. Factors that cause stress such as pain, agitation, excess noise should be checked and minimized. Patients should be given a quiet environment and sources of noise such as alarms or ringtones should be avoided. Analgesics such as paracetamol, tramadol, or morphine are prescribed to decrease headache. Antifibrinolytic drugs like tranexamic acid is given to reduce the risk of bleeding. But, studies have shown that there is no significant improvement in using antifibrinolytics (Connolly et al., 2012; Mestecky, 2011).

- **Hydrocephalus:** Presence of blood in the subarachnoid space can cause obstruction to the flow of CSF. This causes hydrocephalus and can result in increased ICP and thus leads to further deterioration of neurological status. External Ventricular Drain (EVD) is inserted to drain out the CSF with bleed.
- **Delayed cerebral vasospasm (DCV):** This is the constriction of the cerebral blood vessels which leads to reduction in blood flow to brain tissue and progresses to cerebral ischemia and infarction. The resulting ischemia can result in symptoms similar to stroke with decreasing level of consciousness and focal neurologic deficits. DCV usually occurs within 3–10 days after the bleeding and is associated with poor prognosis. Treatment measures taken to treat DCV are:

    - *Nimodipine:* Nimodipine is a calcium channel blocker that blocks the influx of calcium into the ischemic neurons, thus providing a neuroprotective effect. It helps in improving cerebral tissue perfusion by dilating small cerebral arteries and improving blood supply. Oral nimodipine 60 mg every four hourly for 21 days or intravenous nimodipine 1 mg/hr via central line is given to reduce the mortality and morbidity related to DCV. Nimodipine is also administered intra-arterially during cerebral angiography or applied on the clips during treatment (Luoma and Reddy, 2013).
    - *Triple-H therapy (hypertension, hypervolemia, hemodilution):* In blood vessels with DCV, autoregulation will be impaired. Thus, blood flow to these vessels will be affected by the changes in BP. In order to maintain adequate blood flow and oxygenation to the cerebral tissues, a state of hypertension is maintained by hypervolemia and hemodilution. Crystalloids and colloids are administered to maintain hypervolemia and this in turn leads to hemodilution. Due to hemodilution, there will be reduction in hematocrit level which improves oxygen delivery to cerebral tissues (Mestecky, 2011). In case of unsecured aneurysm, triple H therapy is not used because this can lead to rebleeding. During treatment, systolic BP and

MAP is targeted above 160 mm Hg and 120 mm Hg respectively. Central venous pressure of 12–16 mm Hg is recommended (Lee et al., 2005).
  - *Magnesium:* Magnesium has vasodilatory effect and thus, studies are being done to establish the effect of magnesium. Intravenous magnesium sulfate is administered to treat vasospasm and delayed cerebral ischemia (T Chen and Carter, 2011).
- **Increased intracranial pressure:** ICP will be increased due to bleeding in the subarachnoid space, hydrocephalus and cerebral edema. Measures taken to reduce ICP are given in the previous section.
- **Seizures:** Seizures are not a common occurrence after SAH. It often occurs due to rebleeding in patients with untreated aneurysm. Prophylactic use of anticonvulsants are not recommended as evidence suggests worsening of seizures after administration of anticonvulsant in SAH (Luoma and Reddy, 2013).
- **Fever:** After SAH, fever is a common occurrence and is associated with high risk of cerebral vasospasm and worse outcome. It can also cause an increase in intracranial pressure and can further deteriorate neurologic function. Antipyretic medications and cooling measures are taken to manage fever.
- **Hyperglycemia:** The severity of blood glucose abnormalities is associated with severity of SAH and hyperglycemia is a predictor of worse outcomes. Therefore, optimum blood glucose level should be maintained with insulin infusions.
- **Cardiac complications:** SAH causes the release of catecholamines into the bloodstream. This causes an increase in myocardial oxygen demand which in turn leads to myocardial ischemia. ECG changes appear in T wave, ST segment and QT interval. Cardiac arrhythmia, ventricular dysfunction and cardiomyopathy can also be seen in patients with SAH.
- **Pulmonary complications:** The complications that affect the lungs include aspiration pneumonitis, neurogenic pulmonary edema, pneumonia, acute lung injury or ARDS.
- **Hyponatremia:** Sodium imbalances in the body occur due to various causes like cerebral salt wasting syndrome, SIADH or due to excessive administration of hypotonic fluids. Therefore, treatment will depend upon the cause of imbalance.

### Surgical Management

- **Clipping of aneurysm:** Clipping requires craniotomy and aneurysmal clips are attached at the neck of an aneurysm. Placement of clip at the base of the aneurysm prevents the entry of blood and subsequent rebleeding (Thompson et al., 2007).
- **Endovascular coiling:** Coiling is a minimally invasive procedure where a catheter is inserted via femoral artery to the location of aneurysm in the cerebral arteries. Platinum detachable coils are attached to the end of the guidewire. This coil is detached into the fundus of the aneurysm when the guidewire reaches the location of aneurysm. The coil placed inside prevents the entry of blood inside the aneurysm and also causes thrombus formation within the aneurysm. Thus, the risk of rebleeding is reduced (Mestecky, 2011; Thompson et al., 2007).

## STROKE

Stroke is a preventable disease, but it has become the second leading cause of death worldwide (Davis, Lees, and Donnan, 2006). Of these, low to middle-income countries contribute to 85% of the global burden of stroke (Kamalakannan et al., 2017).

### Definition

WHO in 1970 defined stroke as "rapidly developing clinical signs of focal (or global in case of coma) disturbance of cerebral function, with symptoms lasting more than 24 hours or longer or leading to death, with no apparent cause other than of vascular origin" (Sacco et al., 2013).

Stroke is an acute cerebrovascular disease which causes disruption to the blood supply to brain due to blockage or hemorrhage in the blood vessel.

### Classification

Depending upon the causes of stroke, it can be classified into ischemic or hemorrhagic stroke (Marino, 2007).
- **Ischemic stroke:** It comprises 80–88% of all strokes. It occurs due to blockage of the cerebral blood vessels and is caused by atherosclerosis, emboli resulting from atrial fibrillation or rheumatic valve disease, hypoxia or hypoperfusion (Bucelli and Ances, 2016; Marino, 2007). Inadequate blood flow to the brain gives rise to reduction in oxygen and nutrients to the brain tissues leads to ischemia, progressing to cerebral infarction (Ekanem, 2018).
- **Hemorrhagic stroke:** It comprises of 12–20% of strokes. It occurs due to intracerebral hemorrhage (bleeding in the cerebral parenchyma) or subarachnoid hemorrhage (bleeding into the subarachnoid space) (Bucelli and Ances, 2016; Marino, 2007).

### Etiology and Risk Factors

The common causes of ischemic and hemorrhagic stroke are highlighted in **Table 8.8**.

| Table 8.8: Causes of ischemic and hemorrhagic stroke (Bucelli and Ances, 2016; Marino, 2007). ||
|---|---|
| **Ischemic stroke** | **Hemorrhagic stroke** |
| • Thrombosis—Atherosclerosis, hypercoagulability<br>• Emboli from atrial fibrillation, or rheumatic valve disease<br>• Hypoxia<br>• Hypoperfusion | Intracerebral hemorrhage<br>• Systemic hypertension<br>• Amyloid angiopathy<br>• Head injury<br>• Anticoagulants<br>• Substance abuse (cocaine, amphetamine)<br>• Arteriovenous malformation<br>• Blood disorders<br>• Vasculitis<br>Subarachnoid hemorrhage<br>• Aneurysmal rupture |

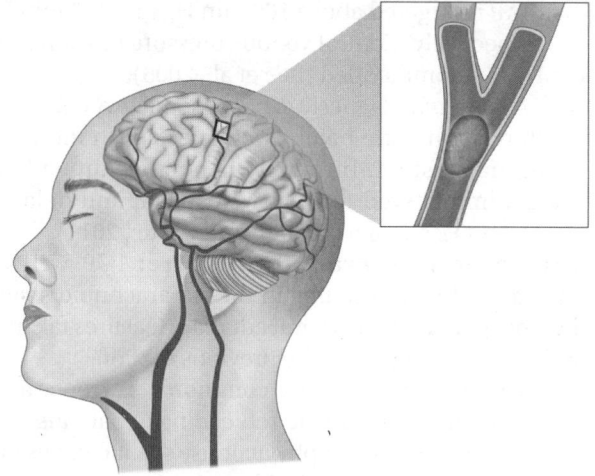

**Fig. 8.10:** Ischemic stroke: Clot in the cerebral blood vessel reduces blood flow to the brain.

### Risk Factors

Risk factors of stroke can be broadly classified into non-modifiable and modifiable risk factors. Nonmodifiable risk factors include age, sex, heredity, race, previous history of stroke, previous history of TIA. Modifiable risk factors are hypertension, diabetes mellitus, current smoking, waist-to-hip ratio, physical inactivity, obesity, diet, hyperlipidemia, alcohol consumption, apolipoprotein, high homocysteine levels (Boehme, Esenwa, and Elkind, 2017; Woodward, Sue, 2011).

### Pathophysiology

#### Ischemic Stroke

Blockage in the cerebral blood vessels results in reduced blood flow to the brain as shown in **Figure 8.10**. Complete occlusion of blood supply causes brain tissue death within 4–10 minutes. When the blood supply per 100 g of brain tissue reduces to <20 mL, it can lead to ischemia and further reduction, that is, <16–18 mL/100 g can cause infarction within 1 hour. The area surrounding the infarcted brain tissue is known as ischemic penumbra, which is salvageable if vascularization is not restored in the right time (Fauci et al., 2018).

When the blood flow to a specific area of brain diminishes, supply of oxygen and glucose to the area reduces. Lack of oxygen leads to reduced production of ATP from mitochondria, which leads to impaired function of ion channels in cell membrane with efflux of potassium to the extracellular space, causing depolarization of neurons. This results in opening of voltage-gated calcium channels which raises intracellular calcium, thus aggravating cellular damage (Fauci et al., 2018; Grotta and Helgason, 1999).

Glutamate is an excitatory neurotransmitter released from synaptic vesicles during neuronal depolarization. This causes neuroexcitability and a further rise in intracellular calcium levels, eventually leading to cell death (Fauci et al., 2018; Frizzell, 2005).

Elevated intracellular calcium levels activate various enzyme systems, in particular, protein kinases, proteases, lipases and nitric oxide synthases. Activation of protein kinases like protein kinase C causes phosphorylation of proteins. Protease activation induces cytoskeletal proteolysis. Activation of lipases such as phospholipase A produces arachidonic acid and free radicals, whereby phospholipase C releases intracellular calcium. Nitric oxide synthase resulting in an increase of nitric oxide. All these ultimately cause damage to neuronal cell membrane, and mitochondrial dysfunction (Grotta and Helgason, 1999).

#### Hemorrhagic Stroke

The hemorrhage in the brain compresses the nearby brain tissues, reducing the blood supply to the area leading to ischemia progressing to necrosis. This initiates an inflammatory response, where macrophages invade the area and engulf or phagocytose the blood and necrosed tissue. Thus, liquefaction of necrosed tissue occurs and a cavity is formed (Frizzell, 2005).

### Clinical Manifestations

Clinical manifestations depend upon the artery affected, location of stroke and the extent of brain damage (Dundas, Bennett, and Slark, 2011). Stroke can affect the following functions in the body—motor, sensory, vision, bladder and bowel elimination, executive functions, personality, swallowing and communication.

- **Motor deficits:** Stroke causes unilateral motor problems like *hemiplegia* (paralysis of one side of the body) or *hemiparesis* (weakness of one side of body). The motor symptoms are contralateral as the upper motor neurons from brain cross over to the opposite side at the level of medulla, i.e., if right side of the brain is affected, left side of the body will be affected causing left sided hemiplegia. Absence or decrease in deep tendon reflexes is seen in the initial stages. Other motor deficits are *ataxia* (unsteady gait), *dysarthria* (difficulty in speech due to paralysis of muscles involved in speech and *dysphagia* (difficulty in swallowing).
- **Sensory deficit:** Loss or decrease in touch sensation, proprioception, difficulty in interpreting visual and auditory stimuli, *paresthesia* (numbness and tingling sensation of extremities) occurs with stroke.
- **Visual deficit:** Temporary or permanent loss of half of visual field (medial half of visual field is called nasal field and lateral part is called temporal field), i.e., *Homonymous hemianopsia*. *Diplopia* or double vision is also a common occurrence among stroke patients (Bowman, 2010).
- **Bladder and bowel:** Continence problems are common following stroke. Due to altered level of consciousness or damage in the areas of brain that control bowel and bladder, patient might have incontinence. Prolonged stay in bed or immobility puts the patient at risk for constipation, fecal impaction, urinary retention and bladder infections. Some medicines that are used in the treatment of stroke such as diuretics (to lower blood pressure) may affect bladder control in the initial phase.
- **Communication problems:** Stroke can affect speech if the areas such as Broca's area and Wernicke's area in the brain are affected. Broca's speech area is located in the lower portion of the frontal lobe is responsible for formation and production of speech. In majority of persons, it is located in the left hemisphere. If Broca's area is affected in stroke, it can cause difficulty in production of speech, where the patients are able to understand, but not able to produce words. This is known as *expressive aphasia* or *Broca's aphasia*. Wernicke's area is an area in temporal and parietal lobes in the left hemisphere. It is responsible for understanding speech. When Wernicke's area is affected, the affected patient will not be able to understand spoken words. The patient might be able to speak by forming sentences, but it will not be an appropriate response. This is known as *receptive aphasia* or *Wernicke's aphasia*. The disorder where both Wernicke's and Broca's area is affected is known as *Global aphasia* (Bowman, 2010; Tortora et al., 2014).
- **Executive functions:** Stroke can cause memory loss, attention deficit, concentration difficulty, with decrease in judgment and reasoning abilities (Bowman, 2010).

### Diagnosis

Immediate assessment of the patient is important. At the scene, FAST test is done to assess the symptoms. F—facial weakness or drooping, A—arm weakness, S—speech problems, T—time to call the ambulance. When the patient is taken to the hospital, CT scanning is done urgently (Dundas et al., 2011). Another tool used in acute setting is National Institutes of Health (NIH) stroke scale which helps in objectively quantifying the impairment caused by stroke and is a guide to predicting clinical outcomes. High stroke scale score indicates more severity and poor prognosis.

### CT (Computerized Tomography) Scan

CT scanning is performed in stroke to identify any intracranial hemorrhage. It also helps to make decisions regarding thrombolytic therapy as intracranial bleeding is a contraindication (Marino, 2007). According to NICE guidelines, the indications to perform nonenhanced CT scan in patients suspected with stroke are to decide thrombolysis, on anticoagulant therapy, with history of bleeding disorders, low GCS score (<13), unexplained progression in symptoms, presence of symptoms of increased ICP. In case of a patient with the above indications, immediate CT scan should be performed within 1 hour of admission to the facility. If patient is suspected of stroke and devoid of any above indications, CT scanning should be done within 24 hours of onset of symptoms (Dundas et al., 2011; National Institute for Health and Clinical Excellence (NICE), 2019).

### Magnetic Resonance Imaging (MRI)

Diffusion weighted MRI images is highly sensitive to detect even small infarcts following ischemic stroke (Dundas et al., 2011; Jauch, 2019).

### Electrocardiogram (ECG) and Echocardiography

ECG is used to identify dysrhythmias such as atrial fibrillation, cardiomyopathy or acute myocardial infarction (MI). Echocardiography is carried out in case of valvular abnormalities or endocarditis (Dundas et al., 2011; Marino, 2007).

### Ultrasound

Doppler of major extracranial arteries are done to identify any stenosis or occlusion especially in the carotid arteries (Dundas et al., 2011).

*Laboratory Studies*

Blood tests that are done for a patient admitted with stroke are:
- Complete blood count
- Blood sugar level
- Serum electrolytes
- Liver and kidney function tests
- Lipid profile
- Coagulation studies—PT-INR, aPTT
- Cardiac biomarkers—CK, CK-MB, Troponin - I, Troponin - T (Ekanem, 2018)

## Emergency Care

### Ischemic Stroke

American Heart Association has recommended time limits from the occurrence of symptoms to provision of care for patients with stroke. Emergency care of patients admitted with acute stroke includes:

- **Airway management:** Maintaining a patent airway is important if the patient's level of consciousness is impaired (Fauci et al., 2018)
- **Breathing:** Supplemental oxygen need to be given only if the $spO_2$ level is <95%. Oxygen therapy is not recommended in a patient with acute stroke without hypoxia National Institute for Health and Clinical Excellence (NICE), 2019.
- **Thrombolysis:** Thrombolytic therapy helps in dissolving the thrombus formed in the cerebral blood vessels. NICE guidelines (2019) recommends use of alteplase, a tissue plasminogen activator for thrombolysis. Therapy should be initiated withing 4.5 hours of onset of symptoms of stroke. It should be administered by staff with specific training in thrombolysis. Monitoring of the patient for any complications during thrombolysis is necessary (NICE), 2019.
- **Antiplatelet drugs:** For patients with acute symptoms of stroke, antiplatelet drugs should be started within 24 hours. Aspirin 300 mg orally is recommended, if the patient has no swallowing difficulty. In case of dysphagia, aspirin is either given through nasogastric tube or aspirin 300 mg is given rectally. Aspirin is continued in the same dosage for 2 weeks (NICE), 2019.
- **Blood pressure management:** Antihypertensives are advised for patients with ischemic stroke only in case of a hypertensive emergency. In patients receiving thrombolysis, blood pressure should be maintained <185/110 mm Hg (NICE), 2019.
- **Blood sugar management:** For a patient with acute stroke, blood sugar should be maintained in the range of 70–200 mg/dL. In case of patients with Type 1 diabetes, intravenous insulin is administered to control sugar levels (NICE), 2019.
- **Swallowing:** Before food or medications are given orally, swallowing function should be assessed in patients. Nasogastric tube should be inserted in those who are diagnosed to have dysphagia and feeding should be started within 24 hours. Measures should be taken to prevent aspiration pneumonia (NICE), 2019.
- **Oral nutrition and hydration:** Patients should be screened for malnutrition, BMI and unexplained weight loss. Oral nutrition supplements can be given orally or through nasogastric tube if the patient is at risk for malnutrition. Hydration should also be assessed regularly (NICE), 2019.
- **Statin treatment:** NICE guidelines 2019 recommends to start statins 48 hours after the onset of symptoms (NICE), 2019.

### Hemorrhagic Stroke

- **Airway management:** As discussed in the management of ischemic stroke, depressed level of consciousness will require airway management (Fauci et al., 2018).
- **Blood pressure management:** Increased blood pressure can cause a further expansion in bleeding. But, there is no clear evidence that shows that reduction in blood pressure reduces the growth of bleed. Non-vasodilating drugs such as labetalol, esmolol, and nicardipine are given intravenously to reduce the blood pressure (Fauci et al., 2018).

## Surgical Management of Stroke

### Carotid Endarterectomy

Carotid endarterectomy is a surgical procedure performed under local anesthesia or general anesthesia where the carotid artery is incised and atherosclerotic plaques are removed. It is indicated in patients with carotid artery stenosis and more than one episode of transient ischemic attack (TIA) **(Howell, 2007)**.

### Decompressive Craniectomy

As discussed earlier under increased ICP, decompressive craniectomy is the removal of a portion of the skull. It is performed to relieve the compression of the brain in the cranial cavity. This surgery is performed in patients with large cerebellar infarction and middle cerebral artery infarction (Pallesen et al., 2019). An early decompressive craniectomy is recommended as it is associated with better prognosis (Dasenbrock et al., 2017).

## Surgery for Intracerebral Hemorrhage

After neurosurgical evaluation, it is decided whether surgery is an option for the patient. Evacuation of the hematoma is commonly done through craniotomy.

## Nursing Management

### Diagnosis

Ineffective tissue perfusion related to decreased cerebral blood flow secondary to thrombus, embolus, hemorrhage or edema as evidenced by ICP 15 mm Hg for 15–30 sec, decreased GCS score and altered respiratory pattern.

### Interventions

- Nurses should undertake regular assessment of the patient with stroke.
- Physiological monitoring of these patients is important to detect early signs of increasing ICP.
- Take actions that will prevent increase in ICP or help in reducing increased ICP

### Diagnosis

Ineffective airway clearance related to inability to raise secretions as evidenced by adventitious breath sounds, diminished breath sounds.

### Interventions

- Assess the breathing pattern of the patient.
- Auscultate the breathing sound and remove the secretions by suctioning.

## Nursing Management of Stroke

Nurses form an integral part of the stroke team. A collaborative approach with various disciplines is essential to manage patients with stroke. Immediate nursing action can improve stroke survival rate.

---

**Nursing management of patient with stroke**

- Nurses should undertake regular assessment of the patient with stroke.
- Physiological monitoring of these patients is important to detect early signs of increasing ICP.
- Monitor blood glucose levels and maintain it within normal limits. High glucose levels can further worsen neuronal damage.
- Temperature monitoring and regulation is imperative since pyrexia can lead to poor stroke outcomes.
- Take actions that will prevent increase in ICP or help in reducing increased ICP.
- Provide change of positions to prevent contracture, pressure ulcer and compression neuropathies.
- A range of motion exercises are encouraged to ensure joint mobility.
- Patients with sensory difficulties should be treated accordingly. For example, a patient who has decreased field of vision following stroke must be approached from the side where visual perception is intact.
- Keep the arm elevated to prevent edema. A pillow should be kept in the axilla of the affected arm to prevent adduction.
- Support the patient in regaining balance.
- Establish an exercise regimen and prepare the patient for early ambulation.
- Do not pull the affected arm of the patient while lifting the patient.
- Elevate the head end of the bed before feeding to prevent aspiration.
- Institute measures for easy bowel movement and prevent bladder infections.

---

## SEIZURE DISORDER

Seizures are defined as sudden, abnormal and excessive electrical discharges from the brain associated with a variety of causes. It can develop at any point in an individual's life and can occur at any time. Seizures can be a single episode or can become recurrent and continue throughout the life. Epilepsy is a brain disorder characterized by recurrent seizures (Linklater, 2011; Ropper et al., 2019).

The mechanism of seizure initiation is characterized by high frequency bursts of action potential due to prolonged depolarization of neuronal membrane and seizure propagation through hyper synchronization of neuronal population (Bromfield et al., 2006).

### Etiological Factors

The major causes of seizure include: (Hickey, 1992; Linklater, 2011):

- **Cerebral causes:** Traumatic brain injury, stroke, expanding brain lesions, infections, hypoxia, vascular diseases, congenital CNS defects, severe birth injury and raised intracranial pressure.
- **Metabolic and other electrolyte imbalances:** Hypoglycemia, acidosis, dehydration, hypokalemia, hyponatremia and hypomagnesemia.
- **Toxins:** Consumption of poison, drugs (prescription/ nonprecription, alcohol and drug abuse.
- Fever associated with any acute infections, septicemia and heat stroke.
- Hypertension and eclampsia (prenatal hypertension).
- **Idiopathic:** Few cases of seizure are of unknown origin.

## Classification

The International League Against Epilepsy (ILAE) classifies seizures into two broad classifications—generalized and partial.

### *Partial Seizure*

Partial seizures, otherwise known as focal seizures, arise from epileptic foci located in any one specific region of the cerebral cortex **(Table 8.9)**.

### *Generalized Seizure*

Generalized seizures involve widespread involvement of both cerebral hemispheres **(Table 8.10)**.

## Diagnosis

The diagnostic tests conducted will depend on whether or not the client has a known seizure disorder.

- **History and physical examination:** Record of events that led to seizure, characteristics of seizure and postseizure events are important aspects in making diagnosis. History must be corroborated with the etiological factors for seizure. Patient should be checked for alterations in level of consciousness, and changes in motor, sensory or autonomic functions (Linklater, 2011; Ropper et al., 2019).
- **Blood tests:** Evaluation is done for electrolyte imbalances, hypoglycemia, infection, and presence of drug or toxins. Function of liver and kidney are also studied to determine possible injury from any drug use, poisoning, drug interaction or alcohol use. Serum levels of antiepileptic drugs should also be assessed (Linklater, 2011).
- **Electroencephalogram (EEG):** It is the most definitive test in locating the area of dysfunction and assessing the brain activity. However, patients should be aware that a normal EEG does not exclude the possibility of seizure. To identify the exact ectopic of seizure, video-EEG and 24 hours EEG can also be conducted.
- **Lumbar puncture:** It detects any cerebral infections, bleeding or abnormal CSF pressure.
- **Radiological studies:** CT and MRI can make it possible in establishing the intracranial causes of seizure. When CT and MRI studies are normal, patients may be sent for single photon emission computed tomography (SPECT) to spot any brain dysfunction. PET scan detects metabolic alterations at the site of lesion (Ropper et al., 2019).

## Management

### *Medical Management*

Antiepileptic drugs (AEDs) are the main choice of treatment in seizure disorders. They treat the symptoms of seizure but do not cure the underlying cause. AEDs have proved to be effective in majority (60-70%) of the patients (Linklater, 2011). NICE guidelines recommend the use of AEDs after second epileptic seizure. It may be considered after a single seizure attack only if there is high risk for more seizure episodes. The first line drug used in the treatment of focal seizure was carbamazepine. However, newer studies have proved lamotrigine to be more effective than carbamazepine in managing seizures. Sodium valproate is the first choice in generalized seizures. Other new AEDS include levetiracetam, pregabalin, zonisamide, and lacosamide. The drugs are commenced at low doses and gradually increased up to therapeutic levels. The patients are managed with one drug if possible. The drug is replaced with an alternative AED when the patient starts experiencing adverse effects of the drug. Drugs are added as adjunct to first line treatment when the first line treatment is not tolerated by the patient or does not prove effective in controlling seizure (NICE guideline, 2012).

### *Surgical Management*

Surgery is considered in patients who are refractory to intensive and prolonged medical management. The most favorable candidates for surgical excision of epileptic foci are those with focal seizures that cause changes in consciousness and antiliteral temporal lobe focus. Though it is estimated that nearly 25% of the patients with

**Table 8.9:** Types of partial seizures (Hickey, 1992b; Linklater, 2011).

| Simple partial seizure | Complex partial seizure |
|---|---|
| • Preservation of full awareness | • Partial or total loss of consciousness as it involves areas of brain responsible for consciousness |
| • May not have notable symptoms | |
| • Can present with motor, somatosensory, autonomic or psychic symptoms (depends on area of origin) | • Forgetfulness on events during seizure |
| • Temporal origin seizure: epigastric rising sensation, déjà or jamais vu, and autonomic changes | • Automatisms such as lip smacking, swallowing, fiddling, chewing, fumbling, fidgeting, undressing, walking, running, or any other repetitive motor actions may be seen |
| • Involvement of motor cortex can present as rhythmic activity contralateral to focal origin | • Period of confusion after seizure (resolves in 10 min) |

| Table 8.10: Types of generalized seizures (Hickey, 1992b; Linklater, 2011). | |
| --- | --- |
| **Types** | **Clinical presentation** |
| Absence seizures | • Sudden onset staring<br>• Momentary impairment of consciousness for few seconds<br>• Mild clonic movements<br>• Commonly seen among children |
| Atypical absence seizures | • Gradual onset and cessation<br>• Momentary impairment of consciousness (longer duration)<br>• Pronounced changes in muscle tone |
| Myoclonic seizures | • Sudden brief jerks<br>• Occurs in arms more often. Patient may even fall when it involves the limbs |
| Clonic seizures | • Rare and most commonly seen in babies<br>• Jerking movements (few seconds to minutes) is more regular and sustained than in myoclonic seizure |
| Tonic seizures | • Sudden onset muscle stiffening<br>• Increased muscle tone<br>• Impaired awareness<br>• High-risk for fall (often backwards) and injuries |
| Tonic-clonic seizures/ Grandmal seziure | • When the tonic-clonic seizure occurs secondary to focal onset, patients may experience simple partial seizure or aura which can be a warning sign to take safety checks<br>• When the tonic-clonic seizure occurs as primary, patient may commence with a tonic phase<br><br>**Aura**<br>It is considered as an early part or warning sign of seizure. It may not be followed by seizure and some seizure attacks may not be preceded by aura. Patients may experience odd smells, dizziness, vision difficulties, nausea, headache, feeling of intense fear, etc.<br><br>**Tonic Phase**<br>• Lasts for 10–20 seconds<br>• Biting of tongue or inside of cheeks<br>• Urinary/fecal incontinence and increased saliva secretion<br>• Cry spell<br>• Apnea due to laryngeal spasm<br>• Elevated heart rate and blood pressure<br><br>**Clonic Phase**<br>• Bilateral rhythmic jerking of limbs<br>• Usually <90 seconds<br><br>**Postictal Phase**<br>• Brief period of unconsciousness (resolves within 10 min to an hour)<br>• Confusion<br>• Headache and muscle ache |
| Atonic seizures | • Sudden loss of muscle tone causes the patient to fall which puts the person at high risk for injury |

epilepsy are suitable for surgery, locating the discharging focus is quite challenging (Ropper et al., 2019). Careful analysis using neuroimaging, video-EEG, EEG monitoring using intraparenchymal depth electrodes, subdural strip electrodes, or subdural grids and specialized EEG analysis will be required. When respective surgery fails, functional surgery is considered. Functional surgery is more of palliative in nature which means the main goal is to provide relief by reducing the frequency or occurrences of seizure (Linklater, 2011).

Vagal nerve stimulation (VNS) is another surgical option for patients who are nonresponsive to AEDs with or without secondarily generalizing seizure. A pacemaker like device is implanted in the anterior chest of the patient and stimulating electrodes are connected to vagus at the bifurcation of left carotid. The effectiveness of VNS in seizure is at an experimental stage though it appears to be a well-tolerated treatment. Patients may complain of hoarseness, cough and discomfort in throat (Linklater, 2011; Ropper et al., 2019).

## Nursing Management

Hickey, 1992b; Linklater, 2011.

### Diagnosis

Ineffective breathing pattern related to neuromuscular impairment secondary to prolong tonic phase of seizure as evidenced by abnormal respiration rate, rhythm/depth.

### Interventions

- Maintain respiratory pattern.
- Monitor oxygen status.
- Position the patient to maximize the ventilation potential.

### Diagnosis

Risk for injury related to seizure activity and subsequent impaired physical mobility secondary to postictal weakness.

### Interventions

- Monitor the compliance in taking antiseizure medications to determine risk of seizure.
- Remove harmful objects from the environment.

The nursing priorities are:
- Prevent/control seizure activity.
- Protect client from injury.
- Maintain airway/respiratory function.

### During Seizure

- Patients experiencing aura must be moved to a safe and private place. Move the patient to the floor and protect the head.
- Maintain strict bed rest if patient experiences aura.
- Place the patient in a lying position on a flat surface. Turn head to side during seizure activity to prevent aspiration of secretions. Suction the patient if required.
- Provide privacy. This protects the dignity of the patient.
- Loosen the constrictive clothing on patient.
- Insert plastic airway as indicated per facility protocol and only if jaw is relaxed.
- Remove any harmful objects from the surroundings that might injure the patient.
- Remove the pillow and raise the side rails, if patient is on bed to avoid the risk of fall.
- Do not restrain the patient as it may cause more injury during movements.
- Stay with the client during and after the seizure.
- Observe for status epilepticus.

### After the Seizure

- Place the patient in a side-lying position to prevent the risk of aspiration.
- Ensure the airway is patented. Provide suctioning in case of increased secretions. It prevents pulmonary aspiration and hypoxia.
- Administer supplemental oxygen or bag ventilation or prepare for intubation as indicated.
- Conduct a neurological and vital signs examination following seizure.
- Patients in the postictal phase might face a period of confusion and drowsiness. Nurses must reorient them to the environment and encourage them to take adequate rest.
- Approach the patient calmly and gently as some of them might feel agitated.
- Maintain seizure precautions (e.g., keeping the side rails up and padded to avoid injury to patient).
- Document the seizure episode. All the events that led to seizure, description of seizure characteristics with duration, complications and treatment measures taken must be recorded.

### Promote Positive Self-esteem

- Encourage the patient to express feelings about diagnosis and evaluate the patient's perception.
- Advice the client to not conceal the problem from the workplace, educational institutions or any other significant persons.
- Encourage supervised activities.
- Reassure the client calmly and help the patient realize the importance of moving away from guilt and blame.
- Explore client's coping ability, strengths and attitude.
- Refer the patients to any support groups known for epilepsy and psychotherapy, if needed.

### Health Teaching

Teaching must be given to both patients and their families:
- Discuss the possible factors triggering seizure in the patient and advice to avoid them.
- Explain the importance of maintaining good general health. This includes having a proper diet, taking adequate rest, moderate exercise, and avoid alcohol, stimulants, smoking and alcohol.
- Ketogenic diet (high-fat, adequate protein and low carbohydrate) and atkins diet (less restrictive than keto diet) are promoted among patients with seizure disorder.
- Practice good oral hygiene and proper dental care.

- Discuss about safety measures related to driving, swimming, use of machinery and any other hobbies.
- Promote acceptance of actual limitations of the patient.
- Inform the patient about local laws or restrictions pertaining to individuals with seizure disorder.
- Include directions on medication regimen, adverse effects potential drug interactions and need for compliance.
- Recommend intake of medicine with meals.
- Encourage to wear identification band or bracelet that also states the diagnosis of seizure.
- Stress the importance of regular follow-up and associated diagnostic tests.

## STATUS EPILEPTICUS

Status Epilepticus is a dangerous complication of epilepsy which can be life-threatening. (Lewis) International League Against Epilepsy (ILAE) task force defined Status Epilepticus as a seizure or repeated seizures lasting more than 5 minutes for generalized tonic-clonic seizures, 10 minutes for focal seizures, and 10–15 minutes for absence seizures (ILAE 2018).

### Causes

Status epilepticus occurs most commonly due to:
- Noncompliance to antiepileptic drugs in chronic epilepsy
- CNS disorders—tumors, infections, cerebrovascular diseases
- Metabolic abnormalities—sepsis, hepatic or uremic encephalopathy, hypoglycemia, hyponatremia, or hypocalcemia.
- Alcohol withdrawal
- Drug toxicity—tricyclic antidepressants
- Refractory epilepsy
- Head injury involving frontal lobe (Fauci et al., 2018; Lindsay et al., 2010; Marino, 2007).

### Types

Status epilepticus has various subtypes. The most commonly found are *generalized convulsive status epilepticus (GCSE), nonconvulsive status epilepticus, refractory status epilepticus,* and *myoclonic status epilepticus.*

*Generalized convulsive status epilepticus* is an emergency condition with higher mortality rates. The patient exhibits tonic-clonic seizures with an altered level of consciousness. But after 30–45 minutes of persistent seizure, the tonic-clonic movements will gradually reduce, and the patient might exhibit subtle signs such as the mild movement of fingers or eyes (Fauci et al., 2018; Marino, 2007).

*Nonconvulsive status* epilepticus is persistent focal or absence seizures, and it exhibits mild motor movements with partial impairment in consciousness. Electroencephalography is used to diagnose these.

*Refractory status epilepticus* is persistent seizure despite the administration of a first-line and second-line medication (benzodiazepine and antiepileptic drug) (Marawar et al., 2018).

*Myoclonic status epilepticus* is characterized by continuous or intermittent myoclonic jerks with or without impairment of consciousness that last for >30 minutes. It occurs due to hypoxic or anoxic state following cardiac arrest (English et al., 2009).

### Pathophysiology

In seizure, during the initiation phase, seizures originate from a specific stimulus. The seizure tends to stop once the stimulus is removed or due to the action of inhibitory neurons. In status epilepticus, there is a second phase called maintenance phase, where a chain of seizures coalesces, and it will continue even after the stimulus is removed. Suppression of inhibitory neurons and excessive neuronal excitation plays a vital role in the initiation and maintenance of status epilepticus (Cherian and Thomas, 2009).

Status epilepticus causes an increase in catecholamine level, which in turn causes a rise in heart rate, blood pressure, and cardiac output. This leads to increased pressure in the left atrium and pulmonary vasculature. The threshold for dysrhythmias decreases resulting in high risk for cardiac arrhythmias. The hypertensive state causes an increase in cerebral perfusion pressure. This along with impaired cerebral autoregulation results in increased cerebral blood flow and thus causes an increase in intracranial pressure. High catecholamine level also leads to hyperglycemia and hyperpyrexia. It is proposed that after a duration of 30 minutes of continuous seizures, neuronal damage occurs (Hawkes and Hocker, 2018).

### Diagnosis

**Electroencephalography (EEG):** EEG is used to identify nonconvulsive status epilepticus. In the case of GCSE, EEG is helpful when the signs of GCSE degenerate, and the patient's level of consciousness is not improving. At this stage, where the patient is in coma and has no visible seizure activity, EEG helps to rule out nonconvulsive status epilepticus **(Cherian and Thomas, 2009; Fauci et al., 2018).**

### Management of Status Epilepticus

Treatment should be initiated immediately as there is a high risk for cardiorespiratory complications and permanent neurologic damage. The efficacy of the therapy is time-dependent; as the duration of seizure increases, the efficacy of drugs reduces.

- **Ongoing monitoring:** ECG, blood pressure, and body temperature should be monitored when the patient is admitted to the facility.
- **Airway support:** Establishing a patent airway should be the first step. Gentle suctioning of the airway is done to prevent aspiration. But, suctioning is done after the seizure is ended because suctioning during a seizure can cause injury to the patient. While performing emergency airway procedures, tongue depressor or oropharyngeal airway should not be inserted forcibly into the oral cavity when the seizure is continuing (Cherian and Thomas, 2009).
- **Breathing:** Supplemental oxygen should be provided through a face mask or nasal cannula. Endotracheal intubation should be considered if the patient is not able to maintain oxygenation (Betjemann and Lowenstein, 2015).
- **Positioning:** Make the patient lie down on a flat surface. Position the patient in such a manner that the least self-injury occurs. Providing a lateral position to the patient during a seizure might cause dislocation of the shoulder. Thereby, it is advised to give a side-lying position after the motor activities are ceased (Cherian and Thomas, 2009).
- **Hyperthermia:** Hyperthermia is associated with the release of cytokines in the brain. This causes further excitation of the neurons, thus aggravating the situation. Passive cooling, administration of antipyretics, ice packs can help to reduce the temperature (Hocker, 2015).
- **Intravenous access:** IV catheters can be inserted to administer fluids and antiepileptic drugs. If possible, a central venous catheter can be placed. Simultaneously, collect blood samples to rule out metabolic abnormalities.
- **Hypoglycemia and hyponatremia:** These metabolic imbalances are the two main causes of status epilepticus which requires immediate correction. The decrease in blood glucose level should be ruled out immediately in patients presenting with seizures. If blood glucose is <60 mg/dL, 50 mL of 50% dextrose in combination with 100 mg thiamine should be administered intravenously.

### Pharmacologic Management

Goal of pharmacologic management is to:
- Stop the seizure immediately.
- Prevent recurrence of seizure.
- Reduce cardiovascular, respiratory and neurologic complications of a seizure.

### Treatment for Generalized Convulsive Status Epilepticus

First line of drugs advised for status epilepticus are benzodiazepines such as diazepam, lorazepam and midazolam.

- **Benzodiazepines:** Benzodiazepines enhances the action of gamma-aminobutyric acid (GABA), which is a CNS inhibitory neurotransmitter. Intravenous lorazepam (0.1 mg/kg) is the initial drug of choice due to its rapid and longer duration of action. Intranasal lorazepam is a noninvasive option with faster absorption. But the intravenous route is widely used. In circumstances where intravenous access is not possible, intramuscular midazolam is administered. Another preferred benzodiazepine is diazepam (0.15 mg/kg), which can be administered intravenously or rectally (Betjemann and Lowenstein, 2015; Trinka et., 2015).
- **Phenytoin/Fosphenytoin:** Phenytoin and fosphenytoin (water-soluble phenytoin prodrug) are the second line of choice for treatment of status epilepticus. These drugs block the sodium channels present in the CNS. Its action mainly occurs in the motor cortex, thus inhibiting the seizure activity. Fosphenytoin is recommended in status epilepticus due to its faster rate of infusion and fewer side effects than phenytoin (Roth, 2018; Trinka et al., 2015).
- **Valproic acid:** Valproic acid exerts antiepileptic action by increasing the levels of GABA and blocking sodium, potassium, and calcium channels in CNS. Valproic acid is given in urgent treatment of status epilepticus and refractory status epilepticus (JWY Chen and Wasterlain, 2006; Hocker, 2015).
- **Levetiracetam:** Levetiracetam binds to protein SV2A present in the synaptic vesicle, thus reducing the rate of release of neurotransmitters from vesicle (Abou-Khalil, 2008).
- **Phenobarbital:** Phenobarbital is a barbiturate, and it causes central nervous system depression by increasing GABA and by blocking sodium and potassium channels.
- **Propofol:** Propofol is a general anesthetic drug with direct stimulation of GABA receptor and inhibition of N-methyl D-aspartate (NMDA) receptor. It is the ideal drug used to treat refractory status epilepticus (Cherian and Thomas, 2009).

### Complications

- **Metabolic:** Muscular contractions during a persistent seizure cause a shift of aerobic to anaerobic respiration. As a result, lactic acid is produced, causing metabolic acidosis. Persistent seizure also causes increased

production of carbon dioxide levels. Alveolar hypoventilation aggravates the condition, and it results in respiratory acidosis.
- **Pulmonary:** Respiratory failure in status epilepticus is associated with apnea, aspiration, airway obstruction, neurocardiogenic pulmonary edema. Neurocardiogenic pulmonary edema develops in status epilepticus due to increased catecholamines causing increased pressure in the pulmonary circulation. Treatment with antiepileptic drugs can cause respiratory depression.
- **Cardiac:** Increased catecholamine level and increased sympathetic stimulation results in subendocardial necrosis and myocyte contraction band necrosis. There is a high-risk for the development of cardiac arrhythmias with abnormalities in conduction.
- **Infections:** Infections commonly affecting patients with status epilepticus are pneumonia (due to aspiration, prolonged mechanical ventilation with weak cough, extended hospital stay or sedative effect of drugs), urinary tract infection (due to presence of indwelling catheter) and sepsis.
- **Renal:** Injury to the muscles in persistent seizures causes rhabdomyolysis leading to reddish colored urine. This ultimately leads to acute kidney injury (AKI).
- **Hematologic:** Peripheral leukocytosis results from either demargination of leukocytes or infections.
- **Musculoskeletal:** Injuries to tongue and tissues of mouth, fractures, shoulder dislocation are commonly seen in patients with seizures (Hawkes and Hocker, 2018).

# GUILLAIN-BARRÉ SYNDROME

Guillain-Barré Syndrome (GBS) is an acute autoimmune disorder affecting the peripheral nervous system characterized by polyradiculopathy. The clinical manifestations ranges from mild muscle weakness to paralysis (quadriplegia) with respiratory failure (Esmail, 2019; Natesan, 2017). Emergency management is required when there is involvement of the respiratory muscles (Winer, 2014).

## Subtypes

GBS has many subtypes or variants on the basis of types of nerve affected and mode of injury **(Dimachkie and Barohn, 2013)**. The commonly seen among these are:
- **Acute inflammatory demyelinating polyneuropathy (AIDP):** This subtype is the predominantly seen form of GBS. In AIDP, segmental demyelination occurs with axonal loss in severe cases. Most common clinical feature is ascending muscle weakness. Some patients may exhibit facial weakness and sensory involvement (Seneviratne, 2000; Woodward, Sue, 2011).
- **Acute motor axonal neuropathy (AMAN):** In AMAN, macrophages are directed at the nodes of Ranvier of motor nerves. This is usually seen among children and young people. Clinical features include sudden progressive muscular weakness, with neck and back stiffness and respiratory failure. Here, disease progresses faster than in AIDP (Dimachkie and Barohn, 2013; Seneviratne, 2000).
- **Acute motor sensory axonal neuropathy (AMSAN):** This is usually seen among adults. Sensory nerves are involved along with motor neurons. AMSAN also exhibits rapid progression of symptoms (Seneviratne, 2000).
- **Miller fisher syndrome:** Clinical features involves ophthalmoplegia, ataxia, and areflexia devoid of any weakness in the body are the classic symptoms of Miller Fisher Syndrome (Dimachkie and Barohn, 2013).

## Etiology

GBS is a postinfectious disorder. The infections can be of bacterial or viral origin. GBS is commonly associated with the following infections (Head and Wakerley, 2016):
- Campylobacter jejuni
- Hemophilus influenza
- Mycoplasma pneumonia
- Epstein-Barr virus
- Cytomegalovirus
- Hepatitis E
- Influenza virus
- Zika virus **(WHO, 2018)**

Usually the onset of symptoms of GBS occurs 2-4 weeks after infection (Meena, Khadilkar, and Murthy, 2011).

## Pathophysiology

Because of the autoimmune response, macrophages act on the myelin sheath of the peripheral nerves and phagocytose the myelin. This causes damage to the myelin sheath, termed as demyelination **(Fig. 8.11)** (Willison, Jacobs, and van Doorn, 2016; Winer, 2014).

It is believed that antibodies attack several target glycolipid antigens present on the nerve terminals and axons. An increase in the levels of antiganglioside antibodies is also seen during the acute phase. These antibodies bind to respective ganglioside antibodies present at unique locations and therefore it can be said that the antibodies determine the distribution of damage in GBS. Multifocal inflammatory demyelination is seen starting at the nerve roots, the earliest changes are observed in the nodes of Ranvier (Meena et al., 2011).

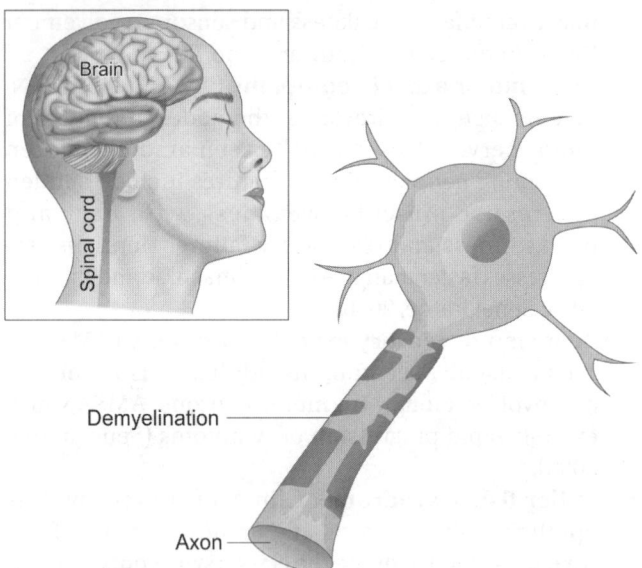

**Fig. 8.11:** Demyelination: damage to myelin sheath along the axon.

## Clinical Manifestations

Classic GBS symptom is acute, bilateral and symmetrical ascending weakness, starting from the distal portion of legs to and continues upwards, which progresses to quadriplegia over a span of days to weeks **(Winer, 2014)**. The progression of symptoms are rapid, with the development of 90% of symptoms within 4 weeks (Meena et al., 2011).

The other symptoms are:
- Hyporeflexia or areflexia
- **Autonomic dysfunction:** Dysrhythmia, fluctuation in blood pressure, excessive sweating, paralytic ileus, or urinary retention
- **Sensory disturbances:** Pain, particularly lumbar pain, numbness, and loss of touch, vibration and proprioception (Seneviratne, 2000)
- **Cranial nerve involvement:** Facial nerve involvement causes facial palsy
- Approximately, 20–30% of patients develop weakness or paralysis of respiratory (diaphragm and intercostal muscles) or oropharyngeal muscles, leading to respiratory failure (Esmail, 2019; Natesan, 2017)

## History Taking and Physical Examination

Since GBS follows infection, history of any infection or fever, abdominal pain with vomiting or diarrhea should be enquired **(Natesan, 2017)**. Neurological examination should include muscle strength and deep tendon reflexes (Steinberg, 2012).

## Diagnosis

Usually clinicians make the diagnosis of GBS just by the patient history of acute progression of weakness (Meena et al., 2011).

### Diagnostic Criteria for GBS

- **Nerve conduction studies:** It helps to not only to diagnose GBS, but also to differentiate between the subtypes of GBS. Nerve conduction studies show deviations after 2 weeks of onset of symptoms. Study findings reveal features of demyelination, such as decreased nerve conduction velocity, conduction block and "sural sparing pattern" (abnormal sensory response in all upper limb nerves excluding sural nerve) (Meena et al., 2011; Willison et al., 2016a).
- **Electromyography:** It is performed to rule out any disorders of the muscle and to assess the extent of damage to axon (Woodward, Sue, 2011).
- **CSF analysis:** Patients with GBS shows increased protein (>45) with low or normal white cell count (Esmail, 2019; Natesan, 2017).
- **Laboratory tests:** Complete blood count (CBC), ESR, kidney function tests, creatine kinase, liver function tests, immunoglobulin levels are tested. Level of antiganglioside antibodies are assessed. These are performed to rule out other diagnoses with similar presentation and to reduce the risk of intravenous immunoglobulin (Esmail, 2019; Head and Wakerley, 2016).
- **Spinal MRI:** It is helpful in excluding other disease conditions with similar symptoms such as disc prolapse, myelitis, cord hematoma or infarction (Esmail, 2019).

## Medical Management

### Plasma Exchange and Intravenous Immunoglobulin (IVIg)

IVIg and plasma exchange is started within 2 weeks of onset of symptoms **(Natesan, 2017)**. Plasma exchange or plasmapheresis is the process of removing patient's plasma containing auto-antibodies and replacing this with fresh frozen plasma (FFP) or albumin. Plasmapheresis is accepted as a first-line treatment for GBS. The effectiveness of plasmapheresis in GBS is usually seen after five to six sessions given over a period of 7–14 days. Complications include hypotension, hypocalcemia, abnormal clotting and septicemia **(Seneviratne, 2000)**.

IVIg is the preferred treatment of choice for most patients. IVIg has an immunomodulatory action by preventing macrophage attack on myelin, upregulation of inhibitory receptors on B-cells and downregulation of activating factors on B-cells (Hughes, Swan, and Van Doorn, 2014). Studies have shown that compared to plasma exchange, IVIg is equally effective and has fewer side-effects (Seneviratne, 2000). The treatment regimen is for 5 days in the dosage 0.4 g/kg body weight or for 2 days at 2 g/kg body weight. Patients should be watched closely during immunoglobulin therapy for reactions such as headache, chills, nausea, back pain, chest pain and muscular pain (Dimachkie and Barohn, 2013; Willison, Jacobs, and van Doorn, 2016).

## Nursing Management

### Diagnosis

Impaired spontaneous ventilation related to progression of disease process resulting in respiratory muscle paralysis.

### Interventions

- Monitor the vital capacity and ABG.
- Maintain the ventilation.

### Diagnosis

**Risk for aspiration related to dysphagia.**

- Bronchial hygiene and chest physiotherapy help clear the secretions.
- Remove the secretions by suctioning.

### Nursing Management in the Intensive Care Unit

Patient with GBS is admitted in the ICU, if the patient displays one or more of the following signs: Rapidly advancing weakness, severe autonomic cardiovascular dysfunction or dysphagia, imminent respiratory distress, or Erasmus GBS Respiratory Insufficiency Score (EGRIS) >4 (Leonhard et al., 2019). The EGRIS tool helps in predicting the probability of respiratory insufficiency in the first week of admission of GBS patients.

Regular monitoring of respiratory function, swallowing ability and muscle strength is carried out. Autonomic dysfunction should be checked with monitoring of blood pressure, heart rate, and bladder or bowel function assessment (Leonhard et al., 2019).

- **Respiratory function:** Patient's Forced Vital Capacity (FVC) should be assessed frequently. FVC <20 mL/kg requires monitoring and should be admitted to the critical care unit. If FVC reduces and is <15 mL/kg, the patient is intubated and connected to the ventilator. $spO_2$ and ABG values are also monitored (Esmail, 2019).
- **Autonomic disturbances:** Since there is a risk of cardiac arrhythmia, postural hypotension, hypertension, heart rate/rhythm, ECG and blood pressure should be monitored. (Esmail, 2019) Antihypertensives such as labetalol, esmolol and nitroprusside are considered for hypertension. For patients with hypotension, management includes intravenous fluids. Paralytic ileus is managed by stopping nasogastric or oral feeds, and nasogastric suctioning.
- **Deep vein thrombosis prophylaxis:** A bedridden state makes the patient at high risk for deep vein thrombosis. Low molecular weight heparin, pneumatic stockings are provided until the patient is capable to ambulate (Esmail, 2019; Meena et al., 2011).
- **Pain:** Pain should be managed with opioid analgesics. Other drugs such as NSAIDs, acetaminophen, gabapentin, carbamazepine, and tricyclic anti-depressants can also be given (Meena et al., 2011).
- **Physiotherapy:** The goal of limb physiotherapy is early mobilization (Esmail, 2019).
- **Nutrition:** Early feeding is initiated to reduce muscle wastage. Diet with high calorie (40–45 kcal excluding protein) and high protein (2–2.5 g/kg) content is recommended. Nasogastric tube is inserted in the patient to avoid aspiration (Meena et al., 2011).
- **Facial palsy:** A patient with facial palsy will find it difficult to close eyes on the affected side. This can lead to dry eyes and corneal damage. Therefore, ointment should be applied to lubricate eyes specifically at night. During nighttime, protective eye shields can also be given to the patients.

## MYASTHENIA GRAVIS

Myasthenia gravis (MG) is an acquired autoimmune disorder which affects the neuromuscular junction. In the neuromuscular junction, acetylcholine is the neurotransmitter that helps in transmission of nerve impulses to muscles. In myasthenia gravis, autoantibodies are directed towards acetylcholine receptors in the post synaptic membrane of motor end plate of voluntary muscles as shown in **Figure 8.12** (Khadilkar 2004; Saini 2017).

### Etiology

- **Autoimmune:** Auto antibodies are targeted against nicotinic acetylcholine receptors or muscle specific kinase (MuSK). MuSK is a tyrosine receptor kinase that helps in the development and maintenance of acetylcholine receptors in the post synaptic membrane (Jacob, 2011; Phillips 2016).
- **Drug induced:** Certain medications such as anti-arrhythmics, D-penicillamine, calcium channel blockers, antimalarials can induce myasthenia gravis (Chaudhuri and Behan, 2009; Thanvi and Lo, 2004).

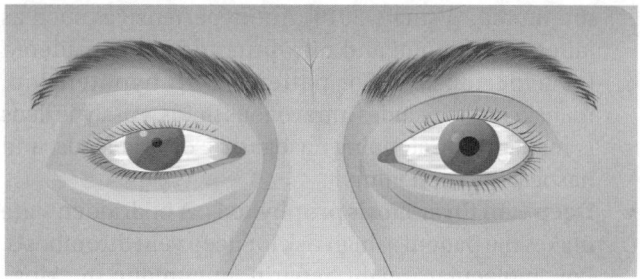

**Fig. 8.12:** Patient with right sided partial ptosis.

- **Thymoma or thymus hyperplasia:** In approximately 65% of patients with MG, thymus hyperplasia is seen. Thymoma is seen in almost 10% of the patients. Thymus gland is hypothesized to be involved in production of autoantigens and thus triggers autoimmune reaction (Fauci et al., 2018).

## Pathophysiology

When the nerve impulse reaches the synapse, acetylcholine in the synaptic vesicles are released into the neuromuscular junction. Acetylcholine binds with the nicotinic acetylcholine receptor (AchR) in the muscle endplate membrane. This causes opening of voltage gated sodium ion channels, thus generating action potential in the muscle and this results in muscular contraction. The remaining acetylcholine present in the neuromuscular junction is hydrolyzed by acetylcholinesterase enzyme (AchE)

In a person with myasthenia gravis, antibodies are attached to the acetylcholine receptors. This limits the number of receptors available for binding of acetylcholine. Thus, amplitude of muscle action potential that is required above the threshold potential reduces and results in weakness of muscles associated with fatigue on exertion (Khadilkar et al., 2004; Saini et al., 2017).

## Clinical Features

The signs and symptoms of the disease is of gradual onset. There will be increasing muscular weakness due to repeated movement of affected group of muscles and it improves with rest (Khadilkar et al., 2004; Kothari, 2004).

The initial symptoms are seen mostly involving the ocular muscles. This leads to:
- **Ptosis (shown in Figure 8.12):** It is drooping of the eyelids (either unilateral or bilateral). Throughout the day, ptosis progresses, and it worsens towards the end of the day.
- **Diplopia:** Double vision, due to weakness of extraocular muscles.

Progressive weakness can be seen in the oropharyngeal muscles or the upper and lower extremities. Generally, upper extremities are affected more than the lower extremities. Bulbar muscle involvement leads to dysphagia, difficulty in chewing, or dysarthria. Weakness of extensor muscles of the neck causes 'dropped head syndrome.'

Respiratory muscle weakness is a complication of myasthenia gravis, but it is a rare occurrence (Khadilkar et al., 2004; Saini et al., 2017).

## Diagnostic Studies

- **Edrophonium chloride (tensilon) test:** Edrophonium chloride is a short-acting acetylcholinesterase inhibitor. This inhibits the acetylcholinesterase enzyme, thus making acetylcholine bind with the accessible acetylcholine receptors (AchR). In a patient with myasthenia gravis, intravenous injection of edrophonium will cause an improvement in muscular weakness temporarily. Initially, 2 mg of edrophonium is given intravenously. If there is improvement in symptoms, then the test is considered positive. If the patient's condition has not changed, then an additional 8 mg is administered intravenously. Side effects of the test include nausea, diarrhea, salivation and bradycardia. Atropine 0.6 mg and emergency trolley should be kept ready beside the patient, in case of bradycardia (Fauci et al., 2018; Kothari, 2004).
- **Acetyl choline receptor antibodies (AchR-Ab):** Assessing the presence of acetyl choline receptor antibodies is the most sensitive and specific test, although all patients affected with myasthenia gravis will not be positive for AchR-Ab (Kothari, 2004).
- **Muscle-specific receptor tyrosine kinase (MuSK):** This test is used for patients who are negative for AchR-Ab.
- **Repetitive nerve stimulation:** The nerves innervating the weak muscles or muscle groups are repetitively stimulated with electric shock at a rate of 2–3 per second and muscle action potentials are recorded. In a normal person, the amplitude of the muscle action potentials will be unchanged after repeated nerve stimulation. But in a patient with myasthenia gravis, amplitude of the muscle action potential will reduce subsequently (Fauci et al., 2018).
- **Single fiber electromyography:** This is the most sensitive test where action potential of muscle fibers innervated by same motor neuron are recorded with a special electrode. Here, "jitter value" is noted, which is the difference in action potential between two muscle fibers. In a normal person, jitter value is <55 microseconds. In a person with MG, jitter is increased and will be >100 microseconds.

- **CT scan:** Computed tomography (CT) scan with contrast of mediastinum is done to rule out thymoma or hyperplasia of thymus gland (Kothari, 2004).

## Management

- **Acetylcholinesterase inhibitors:** Symptomatic relief of symptoms are achieved by long-acting acetylcholinesterase inhibitors such as pyridostigmine or neostigmine. These medications help in improving muscular weakness. These are given in the early phase of disease, as there would be sufficient number of available acetylcholine receptors. Oral pyridostigmine is administered 60 mg three to five times daily (maximum dosage should not exceed 450 mg) (Jacob, 2011; Khadilkar et al., 2004).
- **Immunosuppressive agents:** Since myasthenia gravis is an autoimmune disorder, immunosuppression will benefit the patients in inducing remission (Jacob, 2011; Khadilkar et al., 2004).
  The initial drug of choice for immunosuppression is corticosteroids. Prednisone therapy is given at a dose of 1.5–2 mg/kg/day. Although, worsening of symptoms is commonly seen 2 to 3 weeks after prednisone, there has been improvement in the symptoms 6–8 weeks after therapy. Initially, low dose corticosteroids are given and then the dosage is gradually increased. Side-effects of prednisone include peptic ulcer disease, weight gain, hypertension, hyperglycemia, osteoporosis, electrolyte imbalances, etc.
  To reduce the side-effects of corticosteroids, other immunosuppressant drugs are used. Azathioprine is started at 25–50 mg/day early in the disease as it takes at least 6 weeks to achieve the complete therapeutic benefit of azathioprine. Cyclosporine is also effective in reducing symptoms of myasthenia gravis, but its major side effect is nephrotoxicity. Other immunosuppressants are cyclophosphamide, methotrexate, mycophenolate mofetil and tacrolimus (Jacob, 2011; Kothari, 2004; Thanvi and Lo, 2004).
- **Intravenous immunoglobulins (IVIg):** IVIg is indicated for patients exhibiting severe myasthenia gravis, myasthenic crisis, before or after any surgical procedure. The dosage of administration of intravenous immunoglobulins is 0.4 g/kg/day for five days or 1 g/kg/day for two days. After IVIg, improvement of symptoms are seen after 1–2 weeks and it lasts for 6–12 weeks. (Jacob, 2011; Thanvi and Lo, 2004) IVIg exhibits multiple immunoregulatory actions on macrophages, cytokines, B-cells and antibodies and T-cells. Some of the beneficial actions include blockage of Fc receptors on macrophages, induction of cytokines and cytokine production by regulating T helper cells, reduction in immune complex mediated inflammation, attenuation of complement activation.
- **Plasmapheresis:** It is also indicated for patients with severe myasthenia gravis or in myasthenic crisis. Here, patient blood mixed with anticoagulant is passed through the plasmapheresis machine which then separates the plasma containing AchR antibodies from blood by centrifugation. The separated plasma is then discarded and replaced by fresh frozen plasma. (Jacob, 2011) A total of four to six cycles of plasmapheresis is done on alternate days and in each cycle typically, 2–3 liters of plasma is exchanged. Side-effects of plasmapheresis includes hypotension, infections, bleeding, paresthesia and complications associated with intravenous access. (Jayam Trouth, Dabi, Solieman, Kurukumbi, and Kalyanam, 2012; Thanvi and Lo, 2004)
- **Thymectomy:** In thymoma, removal of thymus gland is helpful in preventing the spread of disease. In nonthymoma MG, thymectomy is recommended for patients with generalized MG positive for AChR antibodies between the age group of 15–60 years. In these patients, thymectomy increases remission of the disease. The therapeutic benefits of thymectomy is seen months to years after the surgery (Jacob, 2011; Khadilkar et al., 2004).

## Complications

### Myasthenic Crisis

Myasthenic crisis is an emergency condition with exacerbation of symptoms of myasthenia gravis. This is characterized by severe muscle weakness and respiratory muscle paralysis leading to respiratory failure. The causative factors of myasthenic crisis are ineffective treatment, infections, or high dose steroid therapy in the initial phase.

Patients are presented with signs of respiratory distress such as dyspnea, tachypnea, nasal flaring, and use of accessory muscles for respiration. In the later stages, tachycardia, increased blood pressure, decreased breath sounds and reduced chest expansion will be manifested. Decrease in oxygen saturation and increase in $pCO_2$ will occur only towards the later stage of crisis as the ventilation and perfusion capacity of lungs will be preserved initially (Jacob, 2011; Thanvi and Lo, 2004).

Aggressive treatment is required with immediate respiratory and ventilator support. Along with that, intravenous immunoglobulins or plasmapheresis is started either alone or in combination (Chaudhuri and Behan, 2009).

## Cholinergic Crisis

Cholinergic crisis occur due to excess intake of acetylcholinesterase inhibitor drugs. Signs and symptoms include excess sweating, lacrimation, salivation, urinary incontinence, diarrhea, bronchospasm and bradycardia. This condition requires immediate management with respiratory support (Jacob, 2011).

## Nursing Management

### Diagnosis

Ineffective breathing pattern related to respiratory muscle weakness as evidenced by abnormal breathing sound.

### Interventions

- Monitor the respiratory status.
- Maintain suctioning.

### Diagnosis

Imbalanced nutrition less than body requirement related to dysphagia as evidenced by difficulty in swallowing and chewing.

### Interventions

- Provide a high fiber diet to prevent constipation.
- Assist the patient to a sitting position before eating or feeding to promote swallowing to reduce the risk of aspiration.

## Nursing Management

### Respiratory Muscle Weakness

Early detection of signs of impending respiratory failure is necessary. If the breathing pattern of the patient is affected, then patient should be connected to the ventilator immediately.

Since patients have muscular weakness, classic signs of respiratory failure like labored breathing, use of accessory muscles, anxious facial expression, nasal flaring might not be elicited. Therefore, continuous monitoring of respiratory rate and vital capacity is essential. Ventilator support should be initiated when the vital capacity is <1 liter or 15–20 mL/kg. While assessing vital capacity, the mouthpiece of the equipment should be sealed by patient lips. This seal can be inadequate as the patient has muscular weakness. Thus, vital capacity should be measured three times during each assessment.

Hypoxia causes a reduction in cerebral oxygenation. So, monitoring of level of consciousness to identify confusion or agitative state is necessary.

Chest physiotherapy is advised for patients with MG, as they will not be able to cough out the secretions properly. Deep breathing and coughing exercises can be scheduled after anticholinesterase medication administration (Jacob, 2011).

### Bulbar Muscle Weakness

Dysphagia and difficulty in chewing can cause malnutrition and increase the risk of aspiration. Swallowing and chewing should be assessed before each meal. It is advised to administer anticholinesterase drugs 30–60 minutes before meals. The patients are advised to refrain from any physical activity before meals to conserve muscular strength. Upright position while feeding will reduce the risk of aspiration. Soft and easily chewable foods are provided to the patient.

In case of any signs of dysphagia, feeding should be stopped, and patients should be sent for further investigations. Suctioning equipment should be kept ready to prevent complications of aspiration. Nasogastric feeding should be initiated for patients showing signs of swallowing difficulty (Jacob, 2011).

### Upper and Lower Limb Weakness

Muscle strength or power should be assessed regularly to identify any worsening of the condition. The patient should be assisted in ambulation and in performing activities of daily living such as bathing, toileting or dressing. After each activity, adequate period of rest should be provided to the patient (Jacob, 2011).

### Fatigue

Patient's ability to perform physical activities should be assessed. Patient's condition should be discussed with the physiotherapist and an activity schedule should be made (Kołtuniuk, 2017).

### Ocular Muscle Weakness

Ocular muscles are frequently assessed for any increase in weakness. For patients with ptosis, 'Lundie loop' can be attached to the eyeglasses. Also, special adhesives are available for lifting eyelids. As patients may not be able to blink their eyes, risk of dry eye, corneal abrasions and infection increase. Carboxymethyl cellulose eyedrops are artificial tears used to moisten the eye. At night, eye ointment is used to lubricate the eye or eyes are shielded with pads (Jacob, 2011; Kołtuniuk et al., 2017).

### Nutritional Support

Assessment of nutritional status and daily dietary intake helps to understand the caloric requirements of the patient.

While considering diet plan, it is important that the chewing and swallowing abilities of the patient are evaluated. The consistency of food can be modified accordingly. Foods rich in potassium must be served as it can be lost during diarrhea episodes and consider a low sodium diet since some medicines (e.g., steroids) used in myasthenia gravis can cause water retention. Diarrhea aggravating foods such as dairy products, high fat and spicy foods should be avoided. However, start including calcium (e.g., milk and other dairy products) and vitamin D in diet when steroids are continued for a longer duration. Steroids can cause bone thinning. Small, frequent feeds are advised to the patient. While placing food in mouth, small portion of should be kept (Kołtuniuk et al., 2017).

## Communication Difficulties

Patient can be referred to a speech and language therapist, in case of speech difficulties. Ask the patient to take deep breaths and pause after each word is spoken. Nonverbal communication methods such as gestures, drawings, communication cards will help the patient in expressing themselves. Nurses and caregivers should show patience and be sensitive towards the patient's effort in communication (Kołtuniuk et al., 2017).

# ENCEPHALOPATHY

Encephalopathy may be defined as a temporary or permanent derangement in the brain function or structure due to varied clinical conditions and physiologic perturbations. Alteration in the mental status is the hallmark of encephalopathy (Ferenci, 2017; Stevens et al., 2010). Emergent management must be initiated to prevent death and neurologic morbidity.

## Types and Etiology-pathophysiology

Encephalopathy can be acute or chronic. Acute encephalopathy, caused by systemic factors, is acute or subacute in onset and can be reversed if the underlying cause is treated promptly. Chronic encephalopathy, on the other hand, results from permanent irreversible brain damage and has gradual progression. Anoxic brain injury, chronic traumatic injury and exposure to heavy metals are some examples that may lead to chronic encephalopathy.

## Metabolic Encephalopathies

Metabolic encephalopathies can develop during the course of illness or as a complication during treatment. It is commonly seen among elderly with chronic illness and those treated in ICUs.

### Hypoxic/Ischemic Encephalopathy

The basic mechanism involved is decreased or lack of blood supply to brain from respiratory or cardiac failure. As neuronal cells begin to die, they release substances that are toxic to other neurons. This can happen in the event of MI, arrhythmia (ventricular), hemorrhage, septic shock, suffocation, paralysis of respiratory muscles (as in GBS, myasthenia gravis) and general anesthesia (when oxygen deficient gas is administered). Prognosis depends on the extent and duration of hypoxia or anoxia of brain tissue. Patients may have permanent neurologic damage (Supanc et al., 2003).

### Hepatic Encephalopathy

Encephalopathy is one of the reversible extra hepatic manifestations and metabolically induced neuropsychiatric condition, mostly due to liver dysfunction. Presence of hepatic encephalopathy is an indicator of severe compromise to liver function. Some of the precipitating factors of acute hepatic encephalopathy are GI bleed, high intake of protein, hypokalemia, hypoxia, infection, excessive diuresis, constipation, and exposure to alcohol, opioids and benzodiazepines. The exact pathophysiology is unknown. Brain edema from metabolic derangemenets in brain following liver dysfunction is believed to be the mechanism. Vasogenic edema from increased BBB permeability and ammonia or neurotoxin driven cytotoxic edema causes cerebral edema. Other noted mechanisms include change in neurotransmitter function, decreased cerebral use of glucose, increase in reactive oxygen molecules, release of inflammatory substances and increase in cerebral blood flow (Stevens et al., 2010; Supanc et al., 2003).

Given below is the West Haven criteria depicting four stages of encephalopathy (Weissenborn, 2019)

- **Grade 1:** Lack of awareness, euphoria or anxiety, shortened attention span, impaired performance of addition or subtraction.
- **Grade 2:** Lethargy or apathy, minimal disorientation for time or place, subtle personality change, inappropriate behavior.
- **Grade 3:** Somnolence to semi stupor but responsive to verbal stimuli, confusion, gross disorientation, bizarre behavior.
- **Grade 4:** Coma (unresponsive to verbal or noxious stimuli).

### Renal Encephalopathy

Uremic encephalopathy is a reversible complication of both acute and chronic renal failure; former being more serious. Diseases of the kidney (e.g., glomerulonephritis, pyelonephritis, etc.), nephrotoxins, shock, immunosuppressive treatment, myoglobinuria, thrombotic thrombocytopenic purpura are other causes. These factors lead to accumulation of uremic neurotoxins in blood. The mechanism of uremic encephalopathy is unknown, but it is clear that cerebral edema does not happen in this type of encephalopathy. Neurotoxin-induced demyelination, endocrine disturbances (increased parathyroid hormone and resultant increase in calcium), increased intracellular sodium and increased neuronal excitability have been implicated as pathologic mechanisms (Supanc et al., 2003).

Complications of dialysis are dialysis disequilibrium syndrome and dialysis encephalopathy. These are also included as renal encephalopathies. Dialysis disequilibrium syndrome is an acute complication of dialysis which leads to swelling of the brain from abrupt changes in serum osmolality. Headache, nausea, vomiting, blurred vision, muscle twitching, hypertension, tremor, asterixis, multifocal myoclonus, disorientation, and in severe cases psychosis, stupor and coma are the symptoms. It usually begins after the third hour of dialysis and is self-limiting. Dialysis encephalopathy or dialysis dementia is a subacute fatal complication that occurs due to aluminum intoxication (aluminum from dialysate) (Supanc et al., 2003).

### Septic Encephalopathy

Sepsis is an excessive inflammatory response to an infection caused by bacteria, virus or fungi. Patients with septic encephalopathy are mostly comatose and are at an increased risk for death. It is estimated that 9–71% of patients with sepsis manifest symptoms of encephalopathy (Ziaja, 2013). Alternation in mental status with diffuse slowing on EEG and normal CSF study are its characteristics. Although the exact pathophysiology is not known, some of the possible mechanism could be disruption of blood brain barrier, effect of leukocytes and inflammatory molecules on brain, infarction and hemorrhage, abscess formation; all of which contributes to cerebral edema and neuronal cell death (Supanc et al., 2003; Ziaja, 2013).

### Hyper or Hypoglycemic Encephalopathy

Hypoglycemia induced encephalopathy is much more common than hyper glgycemia induced encephalopathy. Diabetes mellitus is the most common cause for hypoglycemic coma. Encephalopathy may result from overdose of oral hypoglycemic agents or insulin, insulin secreting tumor, starvation, acute liver disease and chronic renal insufficiency. Patients with hyperglycemia may progress to diabetic ketoacidosis which can result in encephalopathy. It is most commonly seen among young diabetic patients with new onset infection or inadequate insulin therapy (Supanc et al., 2003).

### Wernicke's Encephalopathy

It is an acute onset encephalopathy has classical triad of symptoms: ophthalmoplegia, ataxia and altered mental status. It is caused by thiamine deficiency and is seen among patients with malnutrition, magnesium deficiency, AIDS, alcoholism, cancer or chemotherapy. It is managed with thiamine supplementation. Chronic sequale of wernicke's encephalopathy leads to korsakoff's syndrome, which cannot be reversed and therefore is considered as a form of chronic encephalopathy (Supanc et al., 2003).

### Hypertensive Encephalopathy

It can result from sudden or sustained elevation in blood pressure which includes both primary and secondary hypertension. Long standing hypertension causes adaptive changes in arteries to maintain adequate perfusion and avoids hyper-perfusion. When there is sudden rise in blood pressure more than the regulatory threshold, the vessels are injured (development of fibrinoid necrosis). Resulting ischemia and edema leads to an increase in ICP and severe brain injury. Another mechanism by which brain damage occurs is by vasoconstriction induced increased permeability of BBB. Prompt treatment of hypertension can reverse the condition (Potter and Schaefer, 2020; Sharifian, 2012).

### Encephalopathy Associated with Endocrine Disorders

Encephalopathy associated with endocrine disorders is mostly acute. Hyperthyroidism and hypothyroidism can lead to encephalopathy. Myxedema coma and thyroid storm are extreme forms of thyroid disorders with severe neurological manifestations that can precipitate encephalopathy. A recently described type is Hashimoto encephalopathy of autoimmune origin characterized by high levels of antithyroid antibodies (Stevens et al., 2010).

## Clinical Manifestations

The spectrum of symptoms in encephalopathy can vary slightly based on its cause and severity. Assessment of symptoms combined with appropriate diagnostic test helps in determining the type of encephalopathy **(Table 8.11)**.

## Diagnosis

The diagnosis of encephalopathy can be confusing. A range of diagnostic tests are conducted to arrive at a conclusion.

## Clinical Features

Because encephalopathy is multifactorial in origin, a wide array of symptoms can be present in patients as given in the table above. It requires further testing to diagnose the type and extent of encephalopathy.

**Table 8.11:** Common clinical presentations in encephalopathy (Potter and Schaefer, 2020; Stevens et al., 2010).

| Types | Clinical features |
|---|---|
| Hypertensive encephalopathy | • Altered mental status<br>• Seizure<br>• Headache<br>• Restlessness and confusion<br>• Papilledema (in one-third of patients)<br>• Focal neurological presentations are uncommon (Potter and Schaefer, 2020; Sharifian, 2012) |
| Hypoxic encephalopathy | • Mild hypoxia-inattentiveness, poor judgement and motor incoordination<br>• Profound anoxia (gradual): Patient may tolerate well<br>• Profound anoxia (abrupt): Coma (Supanc et al., 2003) |
| Hepatic encephalopathy | • Mild cognitive impairment to coma<br>• Personality change<br>• Hyperreflexia<br>• Drowsiness, disorientation and forgetfulness<br>• Apraxia<br>• Seizures<br>• Asterixis (Stevens et al., 2010; Supanc et al., 2003) |
| Renal encephalopathy | • Alteration in level of consciousness<br>• Agitation<br>• Hyperpnea<br>• Hyperreflexia<br>• Brainstem signs and nystagmus<br>• Muscle tone abnormalities<br>• Involuntary motor movements-tremor, myoclonus, asterixis, chorea, fasciculations, etc.<br>• Alteration in sensory perceptions (Supanc et al., 2003) |
| Septic encephalopathy | • Alteration in level of consciousness<br>• Impaired cognitive function and inattention<br>• Personality changes and depressive symptoms<br>• Weakness and anorexia (Ziaja, 2013) |
| Hyper or hypoglycemic encephalopathy | Hyperglycemic encephalopathy<br>• Seizure and focal neurologic deficits (e.g., hemiparesis, hypotonia)<br>Hypoglycemic encephalopathy<br>• Blood sugar level at 2.5 mmol/L-anxiety, hunger, sweating, headache, palpitation, vomiting, confusion, drowsiness, occasionally overactivity and bizarre behavior in early stages. Patient may develop motor restlessness, muscular spasms, decerebrate rigidity, convulsions and myoclonus or focal neurologic deficits in the later stages<br>• Blood sugar level at 1 mmol/L deep coma, dilatation of pupils, pale skin, shallow respiration, slow pulse and hypotonia of limb muscles (Supanc et al., 2003) |

### Blood Investigations

- **ABG analysis:** It is used to assess the respiratory, cardiac and metabolic function of the body. This gives a quick review of the oxygenation status, electrolyte balance and bicarbonates level. The findings from ABG report can help in detecting the cause or guide us in ordering further test.
- **Evaluation of blood count:** A complete blood count will provide the hematological indices and an ESR will check for the presence of any infection or auto-immune disorders.
- **Blood chemistry:** Biochemical analysis are mostly helpful in diagnosing metabolic encephalopathy. Evaluation of serum levels of glucose, ammonia, urea, bilirubin, creatinine, electrolytes, C-reactive protein, aspartate aminotransferase (AST), alanine aminotransferase (ALT), gamma-glutamyl transpeptidase (GGT), lactate dehydrogenase (LDH) and creatine phosphokinase (CK) may point towards the underlying etiology. For example, high levels of ammonia with elevated liver enzymes may be due to liver diseases, leukocytosis combined with elevated

CRP indicate septic cause and high BUN values may reveal renal causes for encephalopathy. More tests (test for antibodies, toxins, tumor markers, etc.) are ordered if the above blood investigations remain inconclusive (Berisavac et al., 2017).

### Somatosensory Evoked Potential

It is mainly used in the assessment and prognosis evaluation of coma among patients with encephalopathy of hypoxic or anoxic origin. Changes in conduction velocity, time-frequency distribution, amplitude and latency are noted (Berisavac et al., 2017).

### EEG

It is pivotal in differentiating between the types of encephalopathy. It is reliable indicator of impending coma. Following changes are registered in EEG (Supanc et al., 2003).
- **Hypoxic/anoxic encephalopathy:** Burst suppression pattern or development of alpha-coma in deeply comatose patients
- **Hepatic encephalopathy:** Decreased electrical activity, diffuse slowing of alpha waves, development of delta waves eventually
- **Renal encephalopathy:** Generalized slowing of waves, occasional theta bursts, slowing of predominant posterior alpha
- **Septic encephalopathy:** Slow theta and delta activity
- **Hypoglycemic encephalopathy:** Slowing of EEG pattern.

### Neuroimaging Studies

CT and MRI of the head help in detecting the presence of any organic lesions in brain. Although imaging studies are usually normal in encephalopathy, diffuse or focal cerebral edema can be found. Changes in the signal intensity (hypo or hyper intense) in certain areas of the brain can be registered, which supports differentiation between types of encephalopathy (Berisavac et al., 2017).

### Treatment

The course of treatment is dependent on the neurological symptoms, type and extent of encephalopathy. In cases where the etiology is known, treatment measures are initiated to correct the underlying illness. But patients with unknown etiology undergo various therapeutic procedures in addition to diagnostic testing simultaneously. Management of precipitating factors is the foremost step in the treatment plan of encephalopathy.
- **Hypoxic/anoxic encephalopathy:** The goal is to prevent hypoxic injury to the brain. Restoration of cardiac and respiratory functions improves oxygenation of cerebral tissue. Few evidences support the use of hypothermia and barbiturates in reducing cerebral metabolism (Supanc et al., 2003).
- **Hepatic encephalopathy:** The underlying cause should be treated. For example, if it is GI bleeding associated with hepatic encephalopathy, take measures to stop bleeding and correct related anemia. Other measures include limiting dietary protein intake, reducing intestinal flora using neomycin and kanamycin, and provide lactulose enema. These interventions are targeted towards reducing serum ammonia levels thereby modulating neurotransmission (Stevens et al., 2010).
- **Renal encephalopathy:** Uremic encephalopathy can be reversed with renal transplantation or dialysis.
- **Septic encephalopathy:** Since little is known about the mechanism of septic encephalopathy, management is quite challenging. There does not exist any specific treatment plan for this type of encephalopathy. Supportive treatment is provided to manage the underlying condition.
- **Hypoglycemic/hyperglycemic encephalopathy:** Immediate correction of hypogylcemia is the goal in patients with known and unknown causes of hypoglycemia. Patients with hyperglycemic encephalopathy are treated for diabetic ketoacidosis. Administration of insulin and repletion of intravascular volume are the main management strategy (Supanc et al., 2003).
- **Wernicke's encephalopathy:** Wherever wernicke's encephalopathy is suspected or to prevent its occurrence, a patient presenting with acute encephalopathy is administered intravenous thiamine 100 mg.
- **Hypertensive encephalopathy:** The drug of choice depends on the cause of hypertension. Commonly used antihypertensives are calcium channel blockers, ACE inhibitors, direct vasodilators, and alpha and beta blockers (Sharifian, 2012).
- **Endocrine associated encephalopathy:** Treat the endocrine disorder. For example, encephalopathy due to thyroiditis, treatment with glucocorticoids and plasmapheresis is the standard therapy (Berisavac et al., 2017).

Other neurologic symptoms are also attended concurrently. Benzodiazepines are the first line of choice in seizure due to encephalopathy. In unresponsive cases, the patient is treated with antiepileptic medications (Berisavac et al., 2017). As there is a possibility for increase in ICP, its monitoring and regular neurologic assessment is critical. Osmotic agents are administered to reduce cerebral edema.

## Nursing Management

### Diagnosis

Deficit fluid volume related to bleeding, ascites as evidenced by physical examination.

### Interventions

- Provide IV therapy.
- Maintain input and output chart hourly.

### Diagnosis

Ineffective breathing pattern related to hypoxia as evidenced by abnormal respiration rate, rhythm/depth.

### Interventions

- Maintain respiratory pattern.
- Monitor oxygen status.

# HEAD INJURY

Head injury, or craniocerebral injury is any injury or damage to the scalp, skull or brain. Any brain injury as a result of trauma or external mechanical force is termed as *Traumatic Brain injury* (Pushkarna, Bhatoe, and Sudambrekar, 2010).

## Epidemiology

India has the highest rate of head injury in the world, contributing to almost quarter of the global burden of trauma deaths. Among this, the commonly reported causes of traumatic brain injury are road traffic accidents, followed by falls. Males are affected more than the females with a ratio of 3.8:1 (Massenburg et al., 2017; Traumatic Brain Injury, 2020).

Factors threat influence the disease outcome include age, presence of extracranial injuries, hemodynamic and physiologic status of the patient (Saatman et al., 2008).

## Etiology

The primary causes for head injury are road traffic accidents, falls and violence or assault. Other causes include sports related concussion, injuries occurring at work or at home, blast injury or penetrating injury. Alcohol consumption is a major contributing factor in the occurrence of adult head injuries (Kirankumar et al., 2019; Prins et al., 2013).

## Classification

### Classification Depending on Severity of Injury

Glasgow coma scale (GCS) is used to determine the severity of head injuries.

- **Mild TBI:** GCS 13–15
- **Moderate TBI:** GCS 9–12
- **Severe TBI:** GCS 3–8: Persons with GCS ≤8 has the highest rate of mortality and morbidity (Almulhim and Madadin, 2019; McLernon, 2011).

### Classification Depending on Location of Injury

Head injury is classified depending on the different structures and tissues affected—Scalp injury, skull fracture and brain injury as given in **Table 8.12**.

- **Scalp laceration:** Lacerations are tears in the scalp and underlying tissues as result of blunt trauma. Due to high blood supply to the scalp, most lacerations can result in profuse bleeding. In severe cases, it can lead to hemorrhagic shock and infection if not managed adequately (Almulhim and Madadin, 2019).
- **Skull fracture:** The severity of the skull fracture depends upon the intensity of blow, velocity, momentum and location of impact. Skull fractures can result in damage to the underlying brain tissue causing hematoma and cranial nerve injury (Johnson, 2008). Fractures of the skull can be simple or linear, comminuted or depressed. Basilar skull fracture is a break in the base of the skull (Zomordi, 2017).
- **Brain injury:** Injury to the brain can be diffuse or focal depending upon the area of brain involved.

Concussion is a diffuse brain injury and is also termed as *mild traumatic brain injury*. In concussion, there is a transient loss of neurologic function following a forceful impact. Loss of consciousness, if it occurs, might be followed by a period of amnesia. Patient can also complain of headache, dizziness, disorientation or visual disturbances (McLernon, 2011; Zomordi, 2017). Post-concussion syndrome are a group of somatic (headache, dizziness, nausea, photophobia, tinnitus, anosmia, fatigue), cognitive (mental clouding, memory deficits, difficulty in concentration) and behavioral (irritable

**Table 8.12:** Types of injury based on structure and tissues ffected (Prins et al., 2013; Almulhim and Madadin, 2019)

| Scalp injury | Skull fracture | Brain injury |
|---|---|---|
| • Laceration<br>• Contusion | • Simple fracture<br>• Comminuted fracture<br>• Depressed skull fracture<br>• Basilar skull fracture | • Concussion<br>• Laceration<br>• Contusion<br>• Epidural/extradural hematoma<br>• Subdural hematoma<br>• Subarachnoid hemorrhage<br>• Intracerebral hemorrhage<br>• Intraventricular hemorrhage<br>• Diffuse axonal injury |

behavior, insomnia, hypersomnia, anxiety, depression, changes in personality, labile mood) symptoms that occur after concussive episode (Mullally, 2017). These symptoms usually resolve within a week, but can even persist up to several months (Zomordi, 2017).

Contusion is focal bruising of the brain tissue with areas of hemorrhage, edema, ischemia and necrosis. A contusion occurs when the brain hits the skull due to acceleration and deceleration forces and causes a *coup-contrecoup injury* shown in **Figure 8.13**. When the brain hits the skull at the point of impact, it is known as *coup injury*. Because of the force of the direct impact, the brain moves to the opposite side and hits the skull. This is known as a *contrecoup injury*. So, eventually contusions will appear on opposite sides of the brain. Manifestations will depend upon the location or extent of damage (Zomordi, 2017).

Laceration of the brain is tearing of the brain tissue. It is usually associated with skull fracture or penetrating injuries. The presence of bleeding into the brain tissues can cause focal neurologic deficits.

### Types of Brain Hemorrhage (Fig. 8.14)

- **Epidural hematoma (EDH):** Epidural hematoma is bleeding in the epidural space, that is, between the dura mater and the skull. It is usually associated with skull fracture, tearing of middle meningeal artery or large venous sinuses. In head CT, it appears as a hyperdense biconvex lesion. On admission, patients can present with pupillary abnormalities, limb weakness, decerebrate posturing and seizures (McLernon, 2011).
- **Subdural hematoma (SDH):** Involves bleeding in the subdural space, that is, between the dura mater and the arachnoid mater due to tearing of cortical veins. It is usually accompanied by contusion of the underlying brain. CT findings shows acute SDH as a hyperdense concave area (McLernon, 2011).
- **Subarachnoid hemorrhage (SAH):** Subarachnoid hemorrhage is bleeding in the subarachnoid space, that is, between the arachnoid mater and the pia mater. It occurs due to tearing of cortical veins, arteries or capillaries (McLernon, 2011).
- **Intracerebral hemorrhage (ICH):** Involves bleeding into the cerebral parenchyma, commonly producing mass lesions. It is caused by penetrating injuries like bullet wounds, or tearing of cerebral blood vessels with acceleration deceleration forces (McLernon, 2011). Intraventricular hemorrhage involves extension of bleeding in the intraventricular space. This can cause hydrocephalus.
- **Diffuse axonal injury (DAI):** Occurs in high-speed motor vehicle accidents. Because of the resulting rotational forces within the skull, the brain twists and leads to shearing and tearing of axons. Here, the injury occurs at the cellular level. In severe DAI, there can be complete tearing of the axons, thus affecting the neurotransmission of impulses (McLernon, 2011).

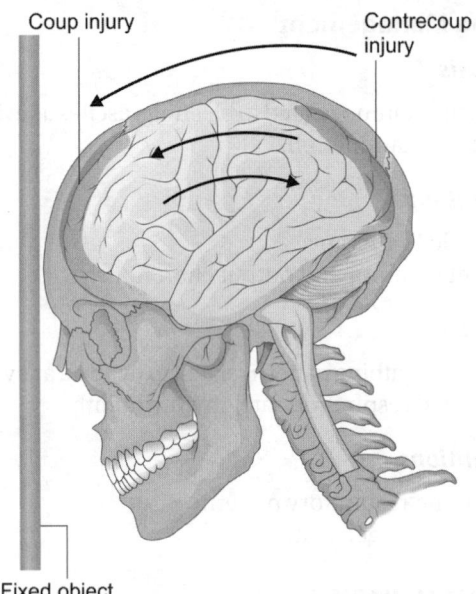

**Fig. 8.13:** Coup-contrecoup injury.

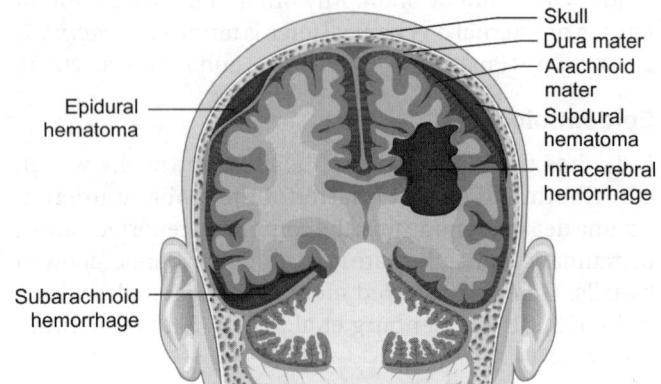

**Fig. 8.14:** Types of brain hemorrhage.

### Depending upon the timing of occurrence of injuries, injuries associated with head injury has been classified into:

*Primary Injury*

Injuries in the intracranial region that occur immediately due to the impact are known as primary injuries. They start to develop in the first few hours to days after injury. It includes contusions, hemorrhage, hematoma or cerebral edema. These events may progress to brain damage due to ischemia (Daniel Agustin Godoy, Khan, and Rubiano, 2020).

## Secondary Injury

The appearance of secondary insults ranges from minutes to days after injury. They can be systemic or intracranial in origin. Systemic secondary insults include: Hypotension, hypoxemia, acidosis, hypercapnia or hypocapnia, agitation, fever, pain, hypo and hypernatremia, hypo and hyperglycemia, severe anemia, disseminated intravascular coagulation and inflammatory systemic response. Intracranial secondary insults include: intracranial hypertension, cerebral edema, vasospasm, hematomas, seizures, hydrocephalus, cerebral hyperthermia (Daniel Agustin Godoy et al., 2020).

## Pathophysiology

In the initial stages after head injury, direct tissue damage and impaired cerebral blood flow and metabolism results in ischemia. This ensues anaerobic respiration leading to lactic acid accumulation and depletion of ATP. Thus, membrane ion pumps that are ATP dependent fail to function. In addition, ischemia increases cell membrane permeability causing cellular fluid accumulation (Prins et al., 2013).

### Cerebral Ischemia

Cerebral blood flow will be decreased to 18 mL/100 g/ min in the initial 48 hours after head injury. Autoregulation mechanism that maintains the cerebral blood flow is failed. Thus, blood flow to the brain becomes dependent on systemic blood pressure. So a hypotensive state can cause cerebral ischemia and hypertensive states can cause injury to the brain cells (McLernon, 2011).

### Excitotoxicity

As a result of the changes in the brain due to injury, there is an excess release of excitatory neurotransmitters like glutamate, aspartate. Such an excessive release activates the NMDA (N-methyl-D-aspartate) receptors which causes excitatory transmission of impulses between neurons. This can lead to nerve cell injury or cell death.

Also, increased release of glutamate causes excess depolarization of neurons. This causes an increased influx of sodium, potassium and calcium ions. The presence of excess intracellular calcium affects the functioning of the mitochondria and endoplasmic reticulum. Thus, excess glutamate further results in neuronal cell damage (Madikians and Giza, 2006; McLernon, 2011).

### Cerebral Metabolism

Initially after severe head injury, cerebral metabolic rate of oxygen consumption and cerebral metabolic rate of glucose increases. This increased demand for energy is not met due to insufficient blood supply. This leads to glycolysis resulting in production of increased lactate. This state can contribute to development of acidosis, cerebral edema, decreased nerve impulse transmission, nerve cell membrane disruption, and interruption in blood brain barrier (Madikians and Giza, 2006).

### Increased ICP

After head injury, there might be intracranial hematoma or hemorrhage, cerebral edema, or inflammatory reactions. All these may lead to increased ICP, which can cause further progression of injury and heighten mortality or morbidity rate.

## Clinical Manifestations

### Signs of Increased ICP

Signs of increased ICP is given earlier in the chapter in the section increased intracranial pressure.

### Focal Neurologic Deficits

Depending upon the location of brain affected, there will be specific neurologic deficits (Greenwood, 2002).

- **Trunk and limb weakness:** Limb weakness is uncommon among patients with head injury. Contralateral (opposite side) limb weakness may be seen in patients with contusion, or large hematomas or lesions. Brain stem injury might result in quadriparesis.
- **Hydrocephalus:** Intraventricular bleeding or subarachnoid hemorrhage can contribute to hydrocephalus. This can result in neurologic deterioration in the subacute phase.
- **Cranial neuropathies:** Injury to the frontal lobe, basal skull fracture and increased ICP account for most of the cranial neuropathies. Cranial nerve involvement can cause anosmia (complete or partial absence of smell), visual field loss, blurred vision, diplopia, and facial nerve palsy. Fractures involving the middle ear resulting in damage to the cochlea or vestibulocochlear nerve can usually cause profound hearing loss (Greenwood, 2002).

***CSF leakage:*** CSF rhinorrhea (leakage of CSF through nostrils) and CSF otorrhea (leakage of CSF through ears) are commonly observed in basilar skull fracture (Greenwood, 2002).

***Raccoons eyes and battle's sign:*** These are the signs of basilar skull fracture. Periorbital ecchymosis or hematoma (tarsal plate is spared) is raccoons eye and postauricular ecchymosis or bruising over the mastoid process is known as the battle's sign. It can be unilateral or bilateral.

***Post-traumatic amnesia:*** Loss of continuous memory of the period following head injury is called post-traumatic amnesia. During this time, patients are disoriented, confused, or agitated. Loss of memory of events that occurred before injury, that is, *retrograde amnesia*, may range from seconds to even years (Greenwood, 2002).

***Cognitive and behavioral changes:*** Once the post-traumatic amnesia is recovered, patients might experience changes in memory, attention, and executive skills. Pertaining to their behavior, often they might display irritability, aggressive behavior, regression, lethargy, lack of interest and initiation in performing activities. In addition, anxiety, depressed mood, and depression are also common after head injury (Greenwood, 2002).

## Diagnostic Investigations

### Skull X-ray

Skull X-rays cannot be used as a routine screening test as it is not sensitive in identifying risk of intracranial injury. However, it is helpful in identifying skull fractures in the absence of a CT scan. Anteroposterior and lateral view of X-ray images are taken (Turner, 2000).

### Computed Tomography Scan

CT scan is done to identify any brain injuries or hematoma. In adults, head CT scan should be performed within 1 hour of occurrence of the following risk factors: GCS <13 during initial assessment, GCS <15 after 2 hours of injury, clinical signs suggestive of basal skull fracture, suspected open or depressed skull fracture, or presence of seizure, focal neurologic deficits, or vomiting. If a patient is receiving anticoagulants with none of the above risk factors, CT scan should be performed within 8 hours of injury (NICE, 2014).

### ICP/CPP Monitoring

ICP and CPP are monitored to identify intracranial hypertension. But any impairment in brain oxygenation or metabolism cannot be detected with ICP or CPP.

### Magnetic Resonance Imaging

MRI is helpful in providing a more detailed account of the abnormalities in the brain than CT scan (Greenwood, 2002).

### Blood Studies

Complete blood count, serum electrolyte levels, blood glucose, coagulation parameters and level of alcohol in blood are tested.

## Management

The goals of management include:
- Maintain adequate oxygenation and circulation
- Protect the cerebral function and prevent functional damage

### Emergency Management

In the early phase, treatment is prioritized—Airway, Breathing, Circulation, Disability and Exposure (ABCDE) should be considered **(Table 8.13)** (EBP). Other parameters to consider are that immobilization of cervical spine and control of hemorrhage (Liew, 2017).

### Initial Assessment

In emergency department, priority should be given to stabilization of airway, breathing and circulation (Daniel Agustin Godoy et al., 2020). If GCS <8, patient should be provided appropriate airway management (NICE, 2014).
- **Glasgow coma scale:** GCS at the time of incident with total score and score of each of the three components should be recorded. In patients with a history of dementia or any chronic neurologic disorders might have GCS <15 even before the injury. In such situations, the preinjury state should be considered during assessment (NICE, 2014). After the initial assessment, GCS should be examined in the following frequency: every half hour for the first two hours, every one hour for next four hours and two hourly thereafter (McLernon, 2011).

| Table 8.13: ABCDE assessment. | |
|---|---|
| Airway | Patency of airway maintained—suctioning, insertion of oropharyngeal airway or endotracheal tube |
| Breathing | • Adequate oxygen support via facemask or mechanical ventilator<br>• Maintain normocapnia |
| Circulation | Target MAP of 90 mm Hg |
| Disability | • Cervical spine injury—cervical immobilization, rigid cervical collar<br>• Intracranial complications—monitor any change in level of consciousness, pupillary size and reactivity to light, imaging |
| Exposure | Examination of the body systems to rule out extracranial injuries |

- **Neurologic assessment:** It should include vital signs, oxygen saturation, GCS, pupillary reaction to light, and limb movements (NICE, 2014). Unequal pupillary size and reaction might indicate increased ICP (Turner et al., 2000).
- **Neck range of movement:** In a patient with head injury, cervical spine immobilization is initiated. But, if there are no risk factors requiring an immediate CT scan and if the patient fulfills any one of the following criteria, range of movement of neck can be assessed carefully. The criteria include:
  - Patient was involved in a simple road traffic accident.
  - Patient is able to maintain a sitting position comfortably.
  - Patient is able to move on his/her own any time since the accident.
  - Patient is exhibiting no tenderness or pain in the middle cervical spine.
  - Patient is manifesting neck pain which is of late onset (Hodgkinson, 2014).
- **Vital signs:** Attach patient to cardiac monitor. Measure and record vital signs including heart rate, blood pressure, respiratory rate and temperature. In case of hypotension, a source of hemorrhage should be identified. Watch for signs of increased intracranial pressure, such as bradycardia and increased systolic blood pressure (Turner et al., 2000).
- **Blood studies:** Blood sample is sent for complete blood count, electrolytes, urea, blood glucose, blood group, arterial blood gas (Turner et al., 2000).
- **History:** Apart from the above mentioned brief neurologic assessment, information regarding the mechanism of injury and patient's level of consciousness (GCS) along with occurrence of seizure at the scene should be enquired. These are assessed to monitor for signs of increased ICP. In case of loss of consciousness, duration of loss of consciousness is to be noted. In addition, presence of headache and/or vomiting, pupillary response following resuscitation and period of hypotension or hypoxia is to be mentioned (Liew et al., 2017; McLernon, 2011). Consumption of alcohol before the accident should be enquired (Turner et al., 2000).

## Ventilatory Support

Patients with GCS <8 require endotracheal intubation and are connected to the mechanical ventilator. Considering the presence of cervical spinal cord injury and increased intracranial pressure, rapid sequence intubation and spine stabilization is necessary. As hypoxemia can contribute to worsening of condition, $saO_2$, $paO_2$ and $pCO_2$ levels are monitored regularly (Daniel Agustin Godoy et al., 2020). Tracheostomy is preferred for patients with severe head injury after 1-2 weeks following injury (Varghese et al., 2017).

### Hemodynamic Stability

Blood pressure should be controlled to maintain a systolic blood pressure >110 mm Hg or MAP >80 mm Hg. It is recommended to maintain CPP in the range of 60-70 mm Hg. Hypotensive state should be prevented. In case of hypotension, initially isotonic crystalloids are administered (preferably 0.9% sodium chloride). Further, vasopressors or inotropic agents are used (Daniel Agustin Godoy et al., 2020).

### ICP Management

The measures to reduce ICP as given earlier in this unit should be followed.

### Hyperthermia

Fever is generally caused by systemic inflammatory response, activation of sympathetic nervous system, damage to hypothalamus or any infections. Hyperthermia results in an increased rate of cerebral metabolism, thus causing rise in ICP. Further, it reduces the seizure threshold. In patients with head injury, fever is managed by providing thermal blankets, or cooling devices. Medications used to control fever are acetaminophen or ibuprofen. In case of shivering, patient should be immediately managed as it can increase metabolic demands (Daniel Agustin Godoy et al., 2020).

### Sodium imbalance

Hyponatremia is common after head injury. Lowered sodium levels can predispose the patient to seizure and increase cerebral edema. Hypernatremia occurs due to dehydration, administration of osmotic fluids or diabetes insipidus. Serum and urine electrolyte levels must be monitored to determine the cause of sodium level abnormalities (Daniel Agustin Godoy et al., 2020; McLernon, 2011).

### Malnutrition

Any severe physical stress creates a hypercatabolic, hypermetabolic and hyperglycemic state in the body after the injury. Rise in metabolic rate can lead to malnutrition with reduced protein levels. This can result in an immunocompromised state and impairment in wound healing. In order to prevent malnutrition, early feeding within 24 hours is initiated with the help of nasogastric tube (Daniel Agustin Godoy et al., 2020; Varghese et al., 2017)

### Hyperglycemia

Stress response contributes to hyperglycemia, which can worsen cerebral damage. Thus, routine monitoring of blood glucose levels is mandatory. It is recommended to start the treatment when the blood glucose levels are >180 mg/dL. Regular insulin is preferred considering its neuroprotective effect (Daniel Agustin Godoy et al., 2020; McLernon, 2011).

### Deep vein thrombosis

Deep vein thrombosis (DVT) is seen in majorly seen in patients with multiple trauma. To prevent DVT, mechanical and/or pharmacologic measures are adopted. Recommended mechanical devices include sequential compression devices with pneumatic stockings. Low dose unfractionated heparin can is also recommended (McLernon, 2011).

### Post-traumatic seizures

Seizures after head injury can occur in the early (<7 days) or in the late phases (>7 days). Prophylactic management of seizures is preferred in some settings. Phenytoin, fos phenytoin and levetiracetam are preferred as prophylactic anticonvulsants after head injury (McCafferty et al., 2018; McLernon, 2011).

### Gastric ulcer prophylaxis

A heightened stress response can lead to gastric ulcer formation. To prevent this, proton pump inhibitors (pantoprazole, omeprazole) or H2 receptor blockers (ranitidine) are administered (McCafferty et al., 2018).

## Surgical Management of Head Injury

Decision for surgery is made based on the following factors: presence of clinical deterioration, size and location of lesion, midline shift and cistern compression. (EBP) Surgery is not recommended for patients with GCS <5 and diffuse anoxic injury (McCafferty et al., 2018).

### Craniotomy

With craniotomy, any hematoma or hemorrhage in the intracranial space is evacuated in patients with a huge lesion on CT scan and GCS ≤8 (Galgano et al., 2017). Burr hole craniotomy is performed in emergency cases.

### Decompressive Craniectomy

Craniectomy, that is, removal of a part of the skull, is performed to relieve the underlying cerebral edema. It is recommended that decompressive surgery is made available within 4 hours to reduce the extent of injury and improve patient outcome.

## Nursing Management

### Diagnosis

Ineffective airway clearance is related to hypoxia as evidenced by abnormal breathing sounds.

### Interventions

- Ensure adequate ventilation and oxygenation.
- Perform suctioning as required. The patient should be preoxygenated with 100% oxygen before and after the procedure. Keep the airway patent.

### Diagnosis

Ineffective tissue perfusion is related to cerebral edema as evidenced by increase ICP.

### Interventions

- The head end of the bed should be elevated to 30 degrees to facilitate venous drainage thereby reducing the risk of increasing ICP. The neck should be in a neutral position. Do not flex or hyperextend the neck.
- Avoid restrictive neck taping. Remove or loosen rigid collars to decrease ICP.

## Nursing Management of Head Injury

Effective nursing management strategies should be practiced having better patient outcome, and reduce the mortality and morbidity rate. In the immediate phase, prevention of hypoxia and hypotension related damage should be the goal as discussed above. The nursing interventions for a patient with head injury are given in the box below:

---

**Nursing management of patient with head injury**

- Ensure adequate ventilation and oxygenation.
- Perform suctioning as required. The patient should be pre-oxygenated with 100% oxygen before and after the procedure. Keep the airway patent.
- Perform neurologic assessment as per the hospital policy and record the findings
- Monitor for signs of increased ICP
- C-spine motion restriction should be considered in all head injury patients while performing any procedures
- The head end of the bed should be elevated to 30 degrees to facilitate venous drainage thereby reducing the risk of increasing ICP. The neck should be in neutral position. Do not flex or hyperextend the neck.
- Avoid restrictive neck taping. Remove or loosen rigid collars to decrease ICP. It is recommended to maintain normothermia as rise in temperature can accelerate the cerebral oxygen demand. Administer antipyretics and use surface cooling devices to manage the body temperature
- Early initiation of nutrition is recommended. It is advised to start early enteral feeding (within 24 hours postinjury) and from 7th days onwards, patient should receive full caloric replacement (Varghese et al., 2017).

- Euvolemia should be maintained using isotonic fluids. Monitor strict intake output chart. Excess administration of fluids can cause cerebral edema.
- Always ensure extreme caution while transporting the patient
- Provide personal hygienic care and tracheostomy care (if present) to prevent the risk of infection. Ventilator associated pneumonia and urinary tract infections are common among patients with head injury (Varghese et al., 2017).
- Dietary plan should take into consideration the blood sugar levels. Hyperglycemia can potentiate cerebral damage and therefore it should be managed with insulin protocol
- Provide analgesia as required to decrease the probability of rise in ICP
- Position changing and range of motion exercises should be encouraged to reduce the risk of venous stasis and to maintain skin integrity

Perioperative nursing management is discussed later in the chapter.

## SPINAL CORD INJURY

### Definition

Spinal cord injury (SCI) is any temporary or permanent insult to the spinal column or the spinal nerves causing neurological impairment. It can lead to devastating complications such as shock, paraplegia, quadriplegia or respiratory failure.

### Etiology

The causes of spinal cord injury can be due to any trauma or any nontraumatic conditions such as malignancy or infections. More than half of the persons affected with SCI are males. There is an increase in SCI among young adults (15–29 years) and older people (> 60 years).

### Traumatic Spinal Cord Injury

This is the most common cause of spinal injuries. Among younger adults, motor vehicle accidents and assaults are the common reasons for spinal injuries. But, in the elderly population, falls are the major cause (NE, Alejandro). Other causes include sports injuries while diving or horse riding, or penetrating injuries with bullet or knives (Harrison and Ash, 2011).

### Nontraumatic Spinal Cord Injury

Nontraumatic injuries include primary or metastatic spinal cord tumors causing spinal compression, viral or bacterial infections such as Pott's spine, inflammatory conditions such as transverse myelitis, ischemia to the spinal cord related to obstruction to blood supply, any congenital or developmental anomalies of the spinal cord such as spina bifida (Harrison and Ash, 2011; McDonald and Sadowsky, 2002).

### Mechanisms of Spinal Cord Injury

- Hyperextension injuries occur in motor vehicle accidents where extension of the cervical region occurs beyond the normal range. This is usually seen in vehicle collisions and falls at home.
- Hyperflexion or flexion with rotation again occur in motor vehicle accidents.
- Axial loading occurs when there is any vertical compression over the spinal cord such as a diving accident where head hits the bottom of the pool or falls from a height in a sitting position. This causes compression fractures over the cervical, thoracic or lumbar vertebrae.
- Penetration injuries usually occur with any violent incidents such as stabbing injury or gunshot. Degree of injury to spinal cord will depend on the speed of impact. These can usually cause tearing and transection of the cord.
- Compression fractures or crush injuries occur when the vertebrae gets crushed and the vertebral fragments compresses the spinal cord (Harrison and Ash, 2011; Hills, 2015).

### Pathophysiology

#### Primary Injury

The injury to the spinal cord is accompanied by vertebral fractures, disc herniation or ligament tearing or traction (pulling) on the spinal cord. This results in direct compression of the spinal cord or compression against the vertebral structures. In addition, hemorrhage or ensuing inflammatory state of the spinal cord leads to edema of the spinal cord. This causes further compression and blood flow to the spinal cord is affected. Reduced blood flow leads to hypoxia and ischemia of the spinal cord (McDonald and Sadowsky, 2002; Rabinstein, 2020).

#### Secondary Injury

This is the continued damage that occurs in the spinal cord after the primary injury. Continued state of reduced blood flow to the spinal cord causes either delay in or complete stoppage of neurotransmission along axons. Hypoxia causes the release of lactic acid and vasoactive substances such as norepinephrine, dopamine. This causes cell death as a result of vasoconstriction and hypoxia.

**Excitotoxicity:** Injured axons and neurons causes release of excessive amount of glutamate, which in turn causes overexcitation of the adjacent neurons. In reaction to this, increased calcium ions triggers various chemical events in the neurons, including oxidative damage. Apart from neurons, excitotoxicity also causes damage to oligodendrocytes and white-matter (McDonald and Sadowsky, 2002).

## Clinical Manifestations

### Complete Cord Lesion

A complete cord lesion is the complete transection of the spinal cord at any level. This causes complete loss of any voluntary activity, sensation and autonomic nerve function below the level of lesion. The body parts affected will depend on the level of cord injury. For example, if the injury is at the level of C4, it can lead to tetraplegia/quadriplegia (paralysis of both upper and lower limbs). If injury is at the level of T4, it can affect the body parts below chest with paraplegia (paralysis of both the lower limbs) (Harrison and Ash, 2011).

### Incomplete Cord Lesion

Incomplete cord lesion results when injury occurs at a specific portion of the spinal cord. This leads to varying degrees of motor and sensory impairments depending upon the part of spinal cord affected and the extent of injury. These clinical syndromes are: Anterior cord syndrome, posterior cord syndrome, Brown-Séquard syndrome, central cord syndrome, conus medullaris and cauda equine syndrome) (Harrison and Ash, 2011).

Some of the clinical syndromes are shown in **Figure 8.15**.

- **Anterior cord syndrome:** As the name suggests, the anterior portion of the spinal cord is injured here. The tracts passing through this portion are spinothalamic tracts and corticospinal tracts. Spinothalamic tracts are responsible for pain and temperature sensation. Corticospinal tracts help in transmitting motor signals to the body. Thus, in anterior cord syndrome, there is loss of pain and temperature and voluntary movements below the level of lesion.
- **Posterior cord syndrome:** As the name suggests, the posterior portion of the spinal cord is injured here. The tracts passing through this area iare the posterior column, which is responsible for deep touch, position and vibration. Therefore, the patient experiences loss of deep touch, sense of position (proprioception) and vibration below the level of injury. But pain and temperature sensation and voluntary movement functions are preserved here. As the proprioception is lost, patients will have no conscious awareness of position of their limbs. This will result in gait abnormalities.
- **Brown-séquard syndrome:** In this, one half (right or left) of the spinal cord is injured. Here, spinothalamic, corticospinal tracts and posterior column are affected. Since only one half of the spinal cord is affected, ipsilateral paralysis, loss of touch, position and vibration occurs and contralateral loss of pain and temperature sensation.
- **Central cord syndrome:** In this, the central portion of the cord is affected. As the center of the cord contains more neuronal tracts responsible for functions of upper extremities, there will be motor and sensory impairments affecting the upper extremities than the lower extremities. The bowel or bladder dysfunction is partially preserved.
- **Conus medullaris syndrome and cauda equina syndrome:** In conus medullaris syndrome, damage occurs to the conus medullaris, that is, the lowermost portion of the spinal cord. In cauda equine syndrome, damage occurs to the cauda equina, the nerve roots distal to the end of spinal cord. These are characterized by unilateral or bilateral leg pain, lower limb paresthesia, paraplegia, bowel or bladder incontinence, back pain, and perineal anesthesia (Dawodu, 2013; Harrop et al., 2004).

### Respiratory System

In patients with cervical injury (above C5), phrenic nerve (supplying the diaphragm) and intercostal muscles are affected. This results in paradoxical breathing because of diaphragamatic breathing and in-drawing of intercostal muscles during inspiration. The complication of high cervical cord injury is respiratory failure (J Lee and Thumbikat, 2015; Rabinstein, 2020).

### Cardiovascular System

In response to injury, catecholamines are released in a huge amount, causing hypertension and tachycardia. But, in case of involvement of thoracic nerves (above T6) or sympathetic ganglion, there can be inhibition of sympathetic activity. This leads to vasodilation, hypotension and bradycardia (Bonner and Smith, 2013).

### Gastrointestinal System

Reduced gastrointestinal tract motility occurs during spinal cord injury above T5. This results in paralytic ileus and subsequent abdominal distension. Due to the stress response, there will be increased release of hydrochloric acid. This causes the formation of gastric ulcers.

When the injury is above T12, bowel movement is reduced with areflexia, rectum is flaccid and sphincter tone is reduced. These bowel changes can also occur as a result of spinal shock. This is termed as neurogenic bowel (Hills, 2015; J Lee and Thumbikat, 2015).

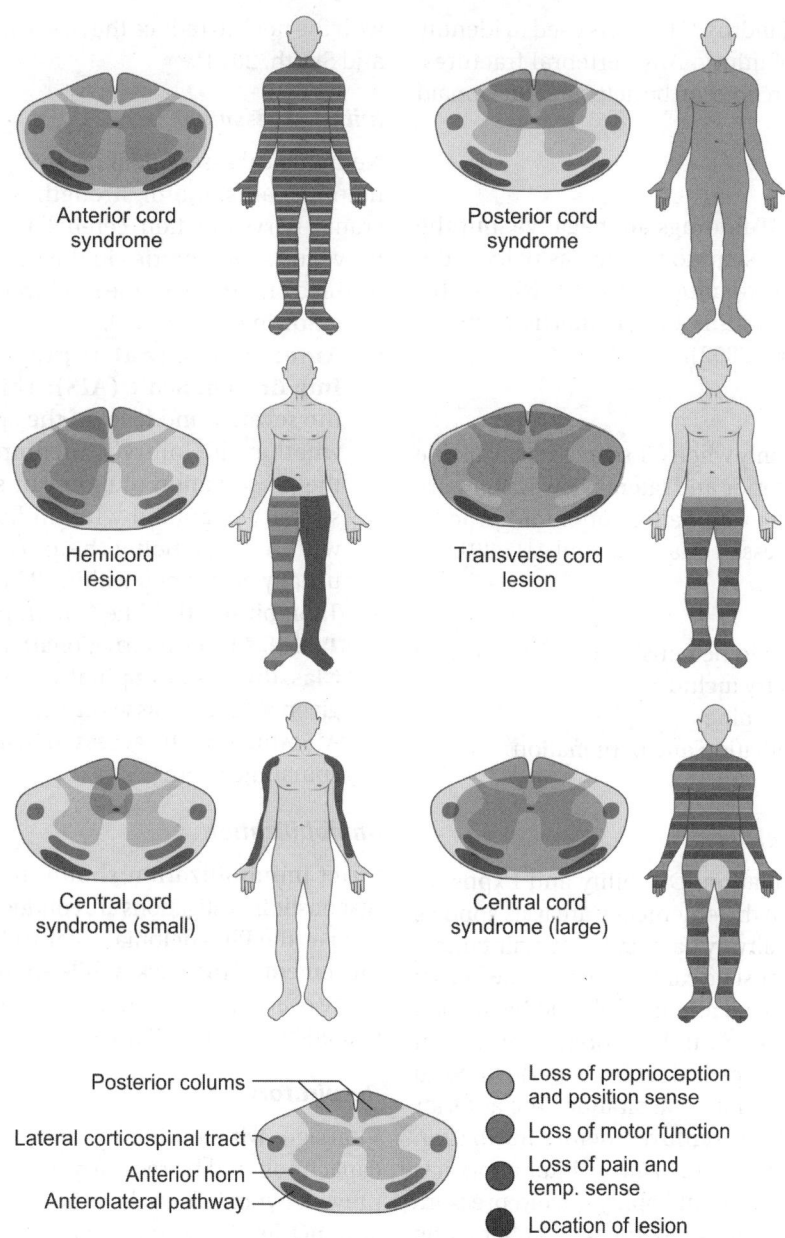

**Fig. 8.15:** Spinal cord syndromes.

### Genitourinary System

The common problem affecting the bladder is urinary retention. In injuries above the sacral level or at the sacral level, the bladder tone is lost (atonic bladder) with detrusor areflexia resulting in bladder distension. This is found in association with spinal injury or spinal shock. Once the reflexes return, there can be loss of inhibitory reflexes from brain. This causes uninhibited bladder emptying or reflex emptying (Linsenmeyer et al., 2006).

### Diagnosis

Radiological examination is important for the diagnosis of acute spinal cord injury. But careful neurologic and physical examination is vital in providing baseline data regarding the involved injury. This helps in evaluating any additional injuries in the head, chest, abdomen or extremities.

### CT Scan

CT scan is done if the patient has signs and symptoms indicative of spinal cord injury with disturbances in level of consciousness (NE – Alejandro). CT scan is used to identify the location and level of injury. Any vertebral fractures, spinal cord edema or infarction can be detected (McDonald and Sadowsky, 2002).

### MRI

MRI is indicated if the CT findings are negative, but the patient exhibits signs and symptoms such as pain in the back or numbness in the extremities (NS fund– Nitin). MRI is indicated to identify any soft-tissue or neural tissue injury (McDonald and Sadowsky, 2002).

### Spinal X-ray

Spinal X-ray is indicated only when CT scan is not available immediately. Anteroposterior and lateral view images are taken. In case of cervical examination, odontoid process and C7-T1 junction is assessed (Harrison and Ash, 2011).

## Management

The therapeutic priorities to be considered after a severe traumatic spinal cord injury include:
- Immobilization of the spine
- Ensure adequate ventilation and oxygenation
- Treat hypotension

### Emergency Management

Airway, Breathing, Circulation, Disability and Exposure should be evaluated in all the emergency areas as soon as the patient is admitted. If airway patency is not maintained, oral or nasal intubation must be carried out with jaw thrust maneuver. In such case, head and neck should be aligned in a neutral position (NS – Anne). Before endotracheal intubation, a rapid sequence induction is performed to reduce the risk of regurgitation or aspiration. The anterior portion of the hard collar is removed before intubation and then replaced after intubation. During intubation, it is recommended that a nurse should apply cricoid pressure and support the posterior portion of the hard collar along with the neck to reduce the risk of neck movement (Bonner and Smith, 2013).

### Initial Assessment

Neurological assessment involving level of consciousness, mental status, motor strength, sensory nerve function, cranial nerve function, cerebellar function and autonomic nerve function. Injuries in the other body systems should be ruled out. To assess the level and severity of spinal injury, the following tool is used:
- **American Spinal Injury Association (ASIA) Impairment Scale (AIS):** This is used to determine the severity and level of the spinal injury. It assesses whether the injury is incomplete or complete, and the preservation of motor or sensory functions. The severity is graded with alphabetical letters A to E, with A grade being the most severe injury. This is usually performed within 72 hours of injury (J Lee and Thumbikat, 2015). The ASIA Impairment Scale is given in **Table 8.14**. The International Standards for Neurological Classification of Spinal Cord Injury (ISNCSCI) has given a detailed assessment of patients with SCI using AIS which can be accessed in the website https://asia-spinalinjury.org/

### Immobilization

Strict immobilization should be maintained until the diagnostic investigations are conducted. Hard cervical collars such as the Philadelphia collar will help in minimizing the movement of the neck. While shifting the patient from the scene of accident, a spinal board and log-rolling movement should be adopted (Bonner and Smith, 2013).

### Respiratory

Vital signs with respiratory rate, oxygen saturation and vital capacity should be regularly monitored in the patients. To prevent hypoxia, $paO_2$ level is maintained above 60 mm Hg and $spO_2$ level above 90%. For those with ventilator support,

| Table 8.14: ASIA impairment scale (Bonner and Smith, 2013; Ahuja et al., 2017). | |
|---|---|
| **Category** | **Description** |
| A | Complete—no motor or sensory function is preserved below the level of injury, including the sacral segments S4–S5 |
| B | Incomplete—sensory function is preserved, but motor function is not preserved below the level of injury including the sacral segments S4–S5 |
| C | Incomplete motor function is preserved below the level of injury; most of the key muscles have a muscle strength grade of <3/5 (5/5 is normal) |
| D | Incomplete—motor function is preserved below the level of injury; most of the key muscles have a muscle strength grade of >3/5 |
| E | Normal—motor function and sensory function are normal |

chest physiotherapy and suctioning should be carried out (Ahuja et al., 2017).

### *Cardiovascular*

Cardiac and hemodynamic monitoring should be carried out in the ICU. Atropine or glycopyrrolate is administered intermittently to increase the heart rate. These medications are also given before any procedures that will stimulate the vagus nerve such as suctioning or laryngoscopy. Intravenous fluids and vasopressor drugs are administered to maintain the systolic blood pressure above 90 mm Hg. Vasopressors will also ensure adequate perfusion of the spinal cord (Ahuja et al., 2017; Bonner and Smith, 2013).

### *Corticosteroid*

Early administration of high dose methylprednisolone is recommended to reduce the level of injury. (Bonner and Smith, 2013)

### *Therapeutic Hypothermia*

The effect of hypothermia in treating spinal cord injury is inconclusive. However, few clinical studies have shown that moderate hypothermia (33°C) using intravascular cooling strategies is safe and has shown certain levels of improvement in long-term recovery following a spinal cord injury (Dietrich, Levi, Wang, and Green, 2011).

### *Thromboprophylaxis*

Patients with spinal cord injury are in a bedridden state for a prolonged period. This puts them at risk for deep vein thrombosis and pulmonary embolus. Use of sequential compression devices or pneumatic compression stockings or anticoagulants to prevent deep vein thrombosis. For anticoagulation, low molecular weight heparin is advised 24 hours after the injury (Bonner and Smith, 2013).

### *Neuropathic Pain*

If a patient is conscious, they complain of severe neuropathic pain in the neck or back. Medications that are given to relieve pain are gabapentin, pregabalin or duloxetine (Rabinstein, 2020).

### *Gastric Ulcer*

Since the patients are at risk for developing peptic ulcer, proton pump inhibitors or H2 receptor antagonists are given prophylactically.

### *Bowel Management*

Lesion in the spinal cord can cause paralytic ileus. In the initial stages, auscultation might reveal normal bowel sounds. Periodic assessment of bowel sounds is essential. Patient should be on nil per oral (NPO) status and a nasogastric tube should be inserted to relieve abdominal distension.

Paralytic ileus and resultant flaccid rectum can lead to constipation. In order to relieve this, suppositories, laxatives or enemas can be administered to soften the stool (J Lee and Thumbikat, 2015).

### *Bladder Management*

An indwelling urinary catheter will be inserted to drain the urine until the patient's condition is stable. Hourly urinary output is monitored. As the patient's condition progresses, intermittent self-catheterization or condom catheterization is a preferred option (J Lee and Thumbikat, 2015).

### *Pressure Sore*

Due to the bedridden stage and loss of sensation, pressure sore is a common complication after spinal cord injury. Patient's position should be changed every 2–3 hours and skin on dependent area should be inspected for any signs of pressure sore. Air mattresses are recommended and patient bed linen should be free of moisture and wrinkles (J Lee and Thumbikat, 2015).

### *Surgery*

Stabilization, open or closed reduction, decompressive laminectomy are recommended to stabilize the spine and relieve the compression of the cord against the vertebral column. Early decompression, that is, within 24 hours, is associated with better prognosis after surgery. Complications after surgery include pain and spinal cord edema that can impair the recovery (Bonner and Smith, 2013; Rabinstein, 2020).

## Complications

- **Spinal shock:** It occurs immediately after spinal cord injury and usually resolves within 2 weeks of injury. The patient will manifest hypotension along with complete loss of voluntary movement, sensation, bowel and bladder control, reflexes and autonomic function below the level of injury (Fund NS – Andrei). As the spinal shock resolves, the symptoms associated with it also resolves. Patient will experience return of muscle tone and deep tendon reflexes (Rabinstein, 2020).
- **Neurogenic shock:** In neurogenic shock, loss of function of sympathetic nervous system is commonly seen in patients where cervical and thoracic cord is involved. This causes hypotension and bradycardia for several days after injury (Rabinstein, 2020).

- **Autonomic dysreflexia:** It is seen in patients where the thoracic cord (T6 or above) is involved. Here, exaggerated sympathetic nervous system stimulation occurs and is characterized by acute headache, hypertension, or tachycardia. This is triggered by any visceral stimulation such as bowel or bladder distension. Therefore, it is essential to avoid situations that can stimulate the triggers (Rabinstein, 2020).

## Nursing Management

### Diagnosis

Impaired physical mobility related to motor and sensory impairment as evidenced by inability to ambulate.

### Interventions

- Ensure proper spine immobilization during any procedures. Use log rolling technique.
- Use of sandbags on either side are advised to limit the cervical movement.

### Diagnosis

Ineffective breathing pattern related to impairment of innervation of diaphragm as evidenced by abnormal respiration rate, rhythm/depth.

### Interventions

- Maintain respiratory pattern.
- Monitor oxygen status.

## Nursing Management

It is vital that nursing actions prevent increasing and permanent damage to the spinal cord. Therefore, we presume that the injuries are unstable until proven otherwise. Early detection and prevention of complications also are part of nursing management. The interventions for a patient with spinal cord injury are discussed above and few additional points are given in the box.

---

**Nursing Actions for a Patient with SCI**

- Preserve life by active resuscitation.
- Ensure proper spine immobilization during any procedures. Use log rolling technique.
- The use of sandbags on either side is advised to limit cervical movement.
- Avoid flexion or hyperextension of the head to prevent further spinal injury. Maintain a head neutral position.
- Clear notice of position must be given to the patient.
- Perform close monitoring of vital signs, cardiac parameters and fluid balance (especially) urine output to identify any complications.
- Serial SCI assessments must be conducted as ordered and any deterioration should be communicated immediately. Document the findings obtained.
- Fluid replacement should be done very cautiously. Excess administration can cause pulmonary edema.
- Ensure hygienic care of the patient to prevent growth of any infection
- Frequent oral care with chlorhexidine is recommended in intubated patients
- Temperature dysregulation being an expected component in SCI patients, body temperature should be monitored, and adequate measures should be taken if any deviations are found
- Institute venous stasis prophylaxis and GI prophylaxis as discussed above
- Range of motion exercises and position changing should be done to prevent DVT, pressure ulcer formation and spasticity. Do not position on bony prominences.
- Conduct regular examination of skin under the splints and braces
- Monitor bowel sounds and check for abdominal distention
- Avoid clustering of nursing interventions to prevent autonomic dysreflexia
- Provide physical and psychological support

---

# PROBLEMS ASSOCIATED WITH NEUROLOGICAL DISORDERS

## Thermoregulation

Body temperature is a critical parameter for cellular functioning and sustenance of life. Thermoregulation is the process by which the human body regulates and maintains the core body temperature. The thermoregulatory strategies support the body in establishing homeostasis and equilibrium despite interaction with the external environment. The elderly and children are at higher risk for disorders of thermoregulation.

The CNS controls and mediates our thermoregulatory behaviors. Temerature-sensitive neurons of hypothalamus are responsible for regulation of body temperature. The temperature center is located at the preoptic area of hypothalamus (Brunker, 2011).

### Mechanism of Thermoregulation

The process of thermoregulation has the following three mechanisms:

1. **Afferent sensing:** Human body consists of afferent receptors that sense both heat and cold throughout the body. Afferent sensing occurs through these receptors when the human body is exposed to varying degrees of external temperature. The hypothalamus also receives the information from the temperature of the blood as it passes through the brain.

2. **Central control:** Thermoregulation is a classic example of an integrative and fully functioning hypothalamus. Hypothalamus is the central controller of body temperature. When a change in temperature is sensed, it sends signals to distinct heat promoting and heat reducing centers.
3. **Efferent sensing:** It includes two responses-behavioral reactions of body to external temperature (e.g., a person using an additional sweater to warm the body in intense cold) and autonomic responses to extremes in temperature (e.g., shivering) (Osilla et al., 2020).

When the body perceives itself as too cold, the hypothalamus acts largely by stimulating the sympathetic activity. It causes vasoconstriction and piloerection thereby preventing loss of heat from skin. At the same time, stimulation of adrenal medulla releases both adrenaline and noradrenaline both of which contribute to thermogenesis by accelerating the basal metabolic rate and production of heat (hormonal thermogenesis). However, when the temperature dips too low the hypothalamus stimulates the motor centers of brainstem. As a result, involuntary responses such as shivering and teeth chattering are initiated which generate heat in the body. Behavioral response includes wearing more clothes, rubbing hands, etc.

The hypothalamus inhibits the sympathetic activity when the body feels too hot. The responses include vasodilation, hair flattening and reduction in the basal metabolic rate; all of which do not allow heat conservation or production in the body. When extreme temperature is felt by the body, the hypothalamus stimulates cholinergic sympathetic response. This induces sweating and increases heat loss from body through evaporation. Removing excess clothing, drinking water, seeking breeze, etc., are few behavioral responses (Brunker, 2011; Osilla et al., 2020).

## Assessment

- **Temperature testing:** We record two body temperatures-peripheral and core. The central or core body temperature is typically higher than the peripheral, but this difference can vary among individuals. The use of pulmonary artery catheters is considered the gold standard technique in recording core body temperature. Rectal and esophageal thermometers are not practical for use in every clinical setting. Oral thermometers pose risk in unconscious patients. Peripheral sites such as the groin and axilla are subject to interference from external factors and are therefore the least reliable (Brunker, 2011).
- **Thermoregulatory sweat test:** This test helps in diagnosing conditions with abnormal temperature regulation and sweat production. The patient is placed in a controlled chamber where the temperature is increased slowly. A special powder is applied on the patient's body before going into the chamber. The color of this powder changes with sweat. Therefore, it helps in detecting the areas where sweat is produced and the nonsweating areas as well. The functioning of the thermoregulatory center is also analyzed. The reliability of tympanic and chemical dot thermometers is criticized and still under debate (Osilla et al., 2020).

## Clinical Significance

- **Brain injury and hyperthermia:** Raised body temperature can exacerbate or cause brain injury. An elevated temperature increases the release of glutamate and free radicals, both of which are responsible for cell damage. The damage to blood brain barrier is also accelerated in pyrexia which leads to cerebral edema and increase in ICP. Increased temperature due to infections such as meningitis, encephalitis, etc., can also lead to severe brain injuries. Alternatively, brain damage can also cause an increase in body temperature. Although the mechanism is not very clear, compression of hypothalamus might be responsible for pyrexia. Hence, brain hemorrhage is thought to be of more risk for pyrexia than any ischemic brain damage.
- **Brain injury and hypothermia:** Although there is lack of firm evidence, it is proposed that lower temperature might protect the brain from further damage. Inducing hypothermia can stop the progress of ischemia. Therapeutic hypothermia or target temperature management (TTM) is now accepted as a neuroprotective strategy (Andersen et al., 2015). It acts by reducing the basal metabolic rate and oxygen consumption by tissues. Other effects include decreasing excitotoxicity and free radical production, prevents intracellular calcium load and ATP depletion. However, the risk of infection, hypovolemia, hypotension and electrolyte imbalance increases with hypothermia. (Osilla et al., 2020)
- **Malignant hyperthermia:** Malignant hyperthermia is a severe reaction to anesthesia most commonly seen among individuals with inherited muscle abnormalities. The clinical presentation may occur within an hour of exposure or may even be delayed up to 12 hours. The body temperature rises abruptly. Unstable vital signs, rigid or painful muscles, sweating, flushed skin, metabolic acidosis and confusion are other symptoms. As calcium release is unregulated in this condition, increased muscle metabolism leads to muscle shortening and rigidity. It can be fatal and therefore rapid management is important. Intravenous

administration of dantrolene sodium controls calcium release. Rapid cooling, 100% oxygen supply and management of metabolic acidosis are other key strategies (Gupta and Hopkins, 2017).
- **Serotonin syndrome and neuroleptic malignant syndrome:** These are also disorders of thermoregulation and may present with clinical hyperthermia (uncommon presentation). Serotonin syndrome develops as an adverse reaction to serotonergic drugs while neuroleptic malignanat syndrome (NMS) develops due to use of antipsychotic medications. Clinical presentation is mostly heterogenous but there are also common features such as fever. As the temperature rises in these conditions, failure to manage immediately can result in serious damages to organs or even organ failure. Both physical (e.g., ice packs, cooling blankets) and pharmacological (e.g., antipyretics, sedatives) measures must be initiated to manage high temperature (Osilla et al., 2020).
- **Hyperthyroidism:** Thyroid hormones regulate both basal metabolic rate and adaptive thermogenesis. An overactive thyroid increases the basal metabolic rate and heat production (adaptive thermogenesis) in the human body resulting in raised core body temperature. The individual often feels warm. The rate of oxygen consumption and ATP turnover are also high. Hyperpyrexia is more likely to occur in severe hyperthyroidism and thyrotoxic crisis (Osilla et al., 2020).

## Management of Raised Temperature

As evidence suggests that high body temperature can accelerate neurological damage, it is vital that body temperature should remain to avoid brain injury. For every 1°C rise in temperature, cerebral oxygen requirement increases by 6–7% (Brunker, 2011).

Pharmacological measures are usually effective in managing hyperthermia, but use of standard antipyretics in managing hyperthermia associated with brain injury has not proven to be much effective. Patients with varied levels of brain insults have been unresponsive to the most commonly used antipyretic acetaminophen (Andersen et al., 2015).

Physical methods of cooling are, therefore, of utmost importance here. This includes cold sponging, air fanning and the use of ice packs. More structured methods of cooling in place are:
- **Surface cooling device:** Examples include air flow blankets and water circulating blankets. The heat from the body is transferred by the mechanism of conduction. Because these devices can cause shivering, warming options must also be included before starting the cooling process.
- **Intravascular cooling device:** Cold saline is passed at a controlled temperature through the small balloons (present at the distal end of catheter) of the specially designed central venous catheter placed in the patient. Chances of shivering are quite less (Andersen et al., 2015; Brunker, 2011).

Neurologic function is closely related to thermoregulation. Effective management against raised temperature is essential to provide safe care and have better clinical outcomes.

## Unconsciousness

In neuro emergency, clinical analysis of unresponsive and comatose patients is a practical and urgent need. Immediate measures should be taken to identify the underlying pathology and its direction of evolution must be determined to prevent any permanent damage to the brain (Ropper et al., 2019).

Consciousness can be defined as a state of awareness of self and the environment, implying arousal in the brain and perceptual processing of an experience (Mashour, 2006). It includes both arousal and cognition. Any damage to the structures responsible for maintaining consciousness and related neural pathways can cause alteration in the level of consciousness (Cook and Woodward, 2011).

### Etiological Factors

Two general categories for cause of altered level of consciousness or unconsciousness are intracranial and extracranial **(Table 8.15)**. The different extracranial and intracranial causes are given in table (Cook and Woodward, 2011).

### Pathophysiology

Consciousness is controlled by reticular activating system (RAS) and its integral components. The ascending reticular activating system, located in the brainstem, is known as the center for arousal. The neurons of ascending RAS, originating from the brainstem structures (dorsal pons and midbrain), are connected to the thalamus and hypothalamus. Neural pathways connect to the cortex via thalamus and to the limbic system via hypothalamus. The cerebral cortex processes the impulses received, integrates it and makes aware of the environment (Ropper et al., 2019).

Neuronal dysfunction resulting from a decrease in cerebral supply of glucose or oxygen can lead to unconsciousness. The arousal center of the brain may get

**Table 8.15:** Intracranial and extracranial causes of unconsciousness (Cook and Woodward, 2011).

| Intracranial causes | Extracranial causes |
|---|---|
| • Intracranial hemorrhages such as SAH<br>• Ischemia and infarction of the brain tissues from vascular diseases or intracerebral hemorrhage<br>• CNS Infections such as meningitis, encephalitis or cerebral abscess<br>• Brain tumors (primary or metastatic)<br>• Brain swelling<br>• Trauma to the contents of central nervous system (e.g., concussion, contusion, EDH, etc.)<br>• Epilepsy | • Hypo/hypertension<br>• Infection and septicemia<br>• Systemic metabolic derangements diabetic ketoacidosis, hypo/hyperglycemia, uremia, hepatic encephalopathy, electrolyte disorders, myxedema<br>• Hypoxia/hypercarbia<br>• Toxicity-heavy metals, carbon monoxide, alcohol, opioids, sedatives, substance abuse<br>• Drug and alcohol withdrawal |

destructed from direct compression caused by structural lesions or by secondary damage from increased ICP, vascular compression or shifting of intracranial contents. Due to various intracranial and extracranial causes, there can be extensive damage to the cortex which also includes neuronal cell death and de-innervation of the cortex (Ganapathy, 2018).

### Alteration in Level of Consciousness

Normal consciousness is characterized by awareness and arousability. Altghough this state may fluctuate during the day, the individual can be brought back to complete alertness and function. **Table 8.16** describes some of the common altered states of consciousness encountered in a clinical setting.

### Diagnostic Tests

***General examination:*** It includes examination of vital signs, skin and odor of breath in the immediate situation (Ropper et al., 2019).

- **Vital signs:** Some of the common variations are given below.
  - *Hypothermia:* Alcohol/barbiturate intoxication, drowning, cold exposure, peripheral circulation failure
  - *Hyperthermia:* Systemic infection, heat stroke, intoxication with drug of anticholinergic properties
  - *Hypertension:* Cerebral hemorrhage, markedly elevated ICP, hypertensive encephalopathy
  - *Hypotension:* Alcohol/barbiturate intoxication, internal hemorrhage, MI, dissecting aortic aneurysm, septicemia, Addison's disease, massive head trauma.
  - *Slow breathing:* Opiate/barbiturate intoxication, hypothyroidism
  - *Rapid breathing:* Pneumonia, diabetic or uremic acidosis, pulmonary edema, intracranial disease that may cause central neurogenic hyperventilation. and Cheyne-stokes respiration related to increased ICP

- **Examination of skin:** Cyanosis indicates inadequate oxygenation. Some abnormalities that can be detected are (Ropper et al., 2019):
  - *Cherry red discoloration:* Carbon monoxide poisoning
  - Multiple bruises in scalp, bleeding, CSF leak, periorbital hemorrhage-suspect for cranial or intracranial injuries or coagulopathy causing hemorrhage
  - Telangiectasis and hyperemia of th face and conjunctiva-suggest alcoholism
  - Facial puffiness-myxedema
  - Sallow complexion-hypopituitarism
  - Marked pallor-internal hemorrhage
  - Macular hemorrhage-meningococcal infection/staphylococcal endocarditis/typhus/rocky mountain spotted fever
  - Excess sweating-hypoglycemia/shock
  - Excessive dry skin-diabetic acidosis/uremia

- **Examination of breath:** The odor of the breath can suggest few causes of coma. The odor of alcohol, spoiled fruit odor (diabetic ketoacidosis coma), uriniferous odor (uremia), musky and fecal fetor odor (hepatic coma), burnt almond odor (cyanide poisoning), etc., are few examples.

***Neurologic examination:*** The GCS scale is the gold standard in assessing the level of consciousness of an individual. Lower score of GCS indicates lower level of consciousness. A GCS score <8 with no eye opening shows that the patient is in coma. Other neurological examination findings will help in diagnosing the cause of altered conscious level. For example, brainstem function can be studied by checking the papillary size and reactivity, ocular movements, vestibulo-ocular reflexes and pattern of breathing. Careful examination of the movements, responses to stimuli, prevailing postures and cranial nerves should be done (Cook and Woodward, 2011).

**Table 8.16:** Common altered states of consciousness (Cook and Woodward, 2011; Ropper et al., 2019).

| State of impaired consciousness | Description | Features |
|---|---|---|
| Confusion | Confusion mostly results from processes that affects the brain globally (e.g., dementia, toxicity), although focal cerebral diseases are also responsible for such state. Patient fails to consider all the elements included in the present environment. Patient may find difficulty in attaching meaning to external or internal stimuli | • Lack of clarity and slowness in thinking<br>• Inattentiveness and disorientation of varying degrees<br>• Imperceptiveness and distractibility<br>• Inconsistent response and inability to stay on a topic<br>• Impersistence and poor planning while movement<br>• Severely confused: difficulty in carrying out simple commands, limited speech to voluble speech<br>• Disoriented/roughly oriented to time and place<br>• Appear to be unaware of what is happening in the environment<br>• May misidentify people or objects which may create fear in patients<br>• Deficit in working memory |
| Drowsiness and stupor | *Drowsiness:* Patient cannot maintain a wakeful state without an external stimuli. They may sustain wakefulness for a brief period of time without external stimulation. A verbal command is sufficient to overcome drowsiness<br><br>*Stupor:* Patient can be aroused only with vigorous and repeated stimuli. For sustaining the arousal also, repeated stimuli will be required. When these patients do not receive stimulation, they go back to a deep sleep like state. A noxious stimuli is required to overcome stupor | *Drowsiness*<br>• Reduced mental, speech and physical activity<br>• Mild confusion and inattentiveness (improves with arousal)<br>• Shifts positions without much prompting<br>• Eyelids droop<br>• Snoring<br>• Muscles of jaws and limbs are slack<br>• Relaxed limbs<br>*Stupor*<br>• Inadequate, slow or absent response to verbal commands<br>• Restless or stereotyped motor activity<br>• Decreased or no natural shifting of body positions<br>• Eyes displaced upward and outward<br>• Diminished or absent tendon and plantar reflexes<br>• Altered breathing pattern |
| Coma | Patient cannot be aroused by external stimuli or inner need.<br>The presentations during this altered state of consciousness should last for more than an hour to be termed as coma. Outcome of coma is dependent mainly on its cause. The prognosis of coma can vary from good recovery to fatality. Cerebral oxygen uptake also decreases during coma | • Absent arousal and conscious awareness<br>• Absent sleep-wake cycle<br>• During deep stages of coma: Absence of any meaningful or purposeful reaction, diminished corneal, pupillary and pharyngeal responses<br>• During light stages of coma: Above mentioned reflexes can be elicited with extensor or flexor plantar reflex |
| Vegetative state | There is total loss of cognitive functioning and absent voluntary response to external stimuli.. They lack the potential for high order activities. Vegetative state for at least a month is termed as persistent vegetative state which may be reversible or irreversible. Vegetative state for more than 6 months is termed permanent vegetative state (PVS) and it is irreversible | • Arousal present (eyes open)<br>• No awareness<br>• Presence of spontaneous movements but purposeless (e.g., facial grimace, verbal sounds)<br>• Circadian rhythms, autonomic responses of hypothalamus and brainstem are preserved<br>• Urinary and fecal incontinence<br>• Conflicting sensory responses (especially to auditory and oculomotor stimuli)<br>• Presence of possible cranial and spinal nerve reflexes |

*Contd...*

*Contd...*

| State of impaired consciousness | Description | Features |
|---|---|---|
| Minimally conscious state | Patient has limited but definite awareness of themselves or environment. Some degree of cognitive processes is present but cannot make complex decisions. They are usually doubly incontinent and may require nutritional support. There is better prognosis than PVS | • Follows simple commands<br>• Gives response with gestures or with a yes/no<br>• Demonstrates intelligible speech<br>• Purposeful behavior but not reflexive<br>  – Response to emotional stimulus (cry, smile, laugh)<br>  – Response to verbal stimulus (vocalization or gestures)<br>  – Trying to reach for an object intentionally<br>  – Accommodates size and shape of object while holding or touching it<br>  – Tracking or fixation of eyes to external stimuli |
| Locked-in syndrome | Patient will be aware of the environment with eye movement as the only mode of communication since limbs movements and facial expressions are absent. It is caused by bilateral injury to the motor pathways in the pons. Functions of RAS and cortex are not affected but patient cannot adequately respond with motor activity and speech. The cognitive ability of the patient is mostly not disturbed | • Awareness is intact<br>• Up-down ocular movements<br>• Eyelid blinking<br>• All other voluntary movements are disrupted<br>• Quadriplegia<br>• Anarthria: Partial or total loss of motor speech control |

***Laboratory tests:*** The tests depend on the findings from initial examination of the patient. Some of the tests that are frequently carried out to establish the possible cause of coma include: (Cook and Woodward, 2011; Ropper et al., 2019)
- Toxic screen of blood and urine sample
- Serum levels of glucose, urea, carbon dioxide, bicarbonate, ammonia, sodium, potassium, chloride, calcium, and aspartate serum transaminase (AST) to detect any extracranial causes of coma
- ABG analysis to assess for acidosis and anoxia
- Blood and urine tests to detect water and electrolyte disorders and infections may help point any cerebral diseases of coma
- Serum levels of ammonia in suspected cases of hepatic failure

***Radio imaging studies:*** Patients with signs of increased ICP or brain herniation are sent for CT or MRI to study the proximate cause for coma.

## Caring for the Unconscious Patient

Nursing care of an unconscious patient can be challenging. Immediate care and long-term care of these patients require good skill and practice. The main goal in the immediate phase is to support and preserve the vital functions of the patient. This includes maintaining adequate airway (A), breathing (B) and circulation (C) and prevent disability (D), and exposure (E). Measures should be taken to prevent rise in ICP and preserve the existing cerebral function. Other management strategies depend on the cause of unconsciousness which is mostly multiple. The damage to the brain is usually severe and irreversible before the treatment begins. Hence, both diagnosis and management should happen concurrently (Cookand Woodward, 2011; Hickey, 1992).

- Establish a clear airway and provide oxygen support. ABG measurements should be taken as indicated.
- Provide lateral position to the patient to allow the secretions and vomitus to come out of the mouth. Perform suctioning as they accumulate. Delay in suctioning can lead to atelectasis and bronchopneumonia. Aspiration pneumonia is one of the common complications of unconscious patients.
- Endotracheal intubation and positive-pressure respirator are usually used in unconscious patients. Regular mouth care should be provided to reduce the risk of ventilator associated pneumonia.
- Treat shock immediately if present.
- Administer 0.5 mg Naloxone IV in cases of narcotic overdose.
- Hypoglycemic coma must be treated with glucose infusion (25–50 mL of 50% solution followed by 5% infusion). Thiamine should also be administered with it.
- When there is evidence to increased ICP from mass lesion, patient is given 20–50 g mannitol in 20%

solution. It should be administered over 10-20 min. Hyperventilation can be performed if there is deterioration in patient condition. Hypertonic saline can also be considered.
- Broad: Spectrum antibiotics are started immediately if meningitis the cause for cerebral dysfunction.
- Treat the convulsions as per the seizure protocol. Intravenous diazepines are usually the choice.
- In instances of drug ingestion, gastric aspiration and lavage is conducted. Patient can recover from the gastric atony caused by the drugs (salicylates, opiates and anticholinergic drugs). Caustic materials can cause GI perforation and therefore they should not be lavaged. Activated charcoal can be used in certain drug poisoning.
- It is vital to maintain normothermia. Hence, measures to regulate temperature must be instituted. Patients may experience hypothermia or hyperthermia depending on the cause of coma.
- Bladder distension can cause further rise in ICP. Patient should be catheterized immediately and fluid balance chart should be maintained strictly.
- Correct fluid and electrolyte imbalances simultaneously. Patients may develop diabetes insipidus, syndrome of inappropriate antidiuretic hormone (SIADH) or cerebral salt wasting syndrome. Water intoxication and severe hyponatremia can further potentiate neuronal damage.
- Insert nasogastric tube in the patient to continue nutrition. In other cases, patient is given nearly 35 mL/kg isotonic fluid every 24 hours (Ropper et al., 2019).
- There is a high risk for deep vein thrombosis among comatose patients. Client is given heparin 5,000 IU subcutaneously every 12 hours or low-molecular-weight heparin can also be considered. Pneumatic compression boots or DVT stockings are applied on the patient (Ropper et al., 2019).
- Regular back care and physical therapy are also provided to maintain the skin integrity.
- Institute measures to prevent the risk of fall.
- Regular eye care and conjunctival lubrication should be done.

## BRAIN DEATH

Brain death refers to permanent cessation of cerebral and brainstem function (Young, 2018). The most common cause of brain death in adults is trauma and subarachnoid hemorrhage. Other causes include ischemic stroke, hypoxic-ischemic encephalopathy and intracerebral hemorrhage.

Several factors that result in extensive neuronal damage can cause cerebral edema and increased ICP. Increased ICP can significantly reduce the cerebral perfusion pressure (CPP) and cerebral blood flow thereby causing aseptic necrosis of neuronal cells. Gradually decreasing CPP and increasing ICP begin to reinforce each other. This continues until the blood flow to the brain stops and trans tentorial herniation occurs along with coning at the foramen magnum. The compression on the brain stem leads to the permanent dysfunction (Ganapathy, 2018).

### Determination of Brain Death

The diagnosis of brain death follows three steps. Neurophysiological and imaging studies are not mandatory to confirm brain death.
- **Establish the etiology:** A clear etiology of brain dysfunction or irreversible coma should be established. Proper history and physical examination, and relevant diagnostic studies including neuroimaging will help in arriving at the cause. Common causes of coma include severe injury to head, intracerebral hemorrhage, aneurysmal SAH, hypoxic brain injury and hepatic failure. (Goila and Pawar, 2009)
- **Exclude potential reversible syndromes that may mimic brain death:** The reversible causes of coma that must be excluded are (Goila and Pawar, 2009):
  - Intoxication
  - Use of drugs including muscle relaxants (they depress the CNS)
  - Primary hypothermia
  - Hypovolemic shock
  - Metabolic and endocrine disorders
- **Demonstrate clinical signs of brain death:** For the determination of brain death three conditions must be present which includes coma, absence of brainstem reflexes and apnea. This is undertaken when the patient satisfies all the above mentioned preconditions.
  The following reflexes must be absent in a patient who is brain dead (Ganapathy, 2018; Goila and Pawar, 2009).
  - *Pupillary reflex:* Pupil is fixed at mid-position when light is shown (unresponsive to light) with a pupil size of 4 mm usually.
  - *Oculocephalic reflex:* The examiner holds the patient's head in middle position and the eyes are kept open. Sudden turns of head are made to either sides. Normally the eyes would move opposite to the direction of head movement.
- **Oculovestibular reflex (cold caloric test):** Position the patient in midline with head elevated to 30 degrees. Slow irrigation of the ear canal using at least 50 mL of iced water is done. Observe the eyes as the irrigation

proceeds and for 1 min after the procedure. Deviation of eyes to the irrigated ear indicates that the test is positive.
- Corneal reflex
- Gag reflex
- Cough reflex
- There is complete absence of facial movements even with noxious stimuli (trigeminal stimulation by applying pressure on supraorbital ridge.

### Apnea Test

If the cause for coma is established and all the brainstem reflexes are absent, apnea test is conducted. It is not indicated in patients with high cervical cord injury and poor respiratory function. Firstly, preoxygenate the patient with 100% $FiO_2$ to a partial pressure of oxygen greater than 200 mm Hg. The ventilator rate must be reduced to 10 breaths per min and positive end expiratory pressure (PEEP) should be reduced to 5 cm of $H_2O$. Check the $SPO_2$ value and if it is more that 95%, sent an ABG. The patient is then disconnected from the ventilator and provided oxygen (100% $FiO_2$) using insufflations tubing at 6L/min through the endotracheal tube. The respiratory movements of the patient are observed for 8–10 min and blood gas is repeated, if no signs of respiratory drive is noticed during the said duration. Carbon dioxide partial pressure reading of more than 60 mm Hg and absence of respiratory movements will confirm positive apnea test (Goila and Pawar, 2009).

### Confirmatory Test

When the clinical diagnosis is doubtful or cannot be completed, confirmatory tests can be done. These tests are not mandatory. Cerebral angiography (4 vessel angiogram) is considered the gold standard test for diagnosing brain death. Other tests include CT angiography, MRI angiography, radionuclide imaging, sensory evoked potentials and EEG (Ganapathy, 2018).

### Caring for the Brain Dead Patient

India considers death equivalent to brainstem death. If the patient is certified brain stem death, then he is legally and medically considered dead. It is mandatory to include the date and time of brain death in patient notes. The legal time of death is the time at which second prescribed clinical tests are carried out. If organ donation is under consideration, then the doctor who diagnosed brain death should not be involved in transplant procedures. Caring for the family is equally important here. The decision on organ donation can be influenced by multiple factors (e.g., religion, culture) and an informed consent should be obtained from the family. The process of organ donation is regulated by the Transplantation of Human Organs Act, 1994 in India (Ganapathy, 2018).

## HERNIATION SYNDROME

When the intracranial pressure rises within the cranial vault, compensatory mechanisms begin as given by the Monro-Kellie doctrine. Overriding of these compensatory mechanisms causes shift of brain tissue from its normal location to the area of least resistance through a rigid opening. Such mechanical forces can compress cerebral blood vessels and cause obstruction to CSF pathways, further rising the ICP. It is a life-threatening event and an urgent attention would prevent any disastrous consequences to the brain (Mestecky, 2011; Munakomi and Das, 2020).

### Etiology

Multiple factors can cause increased intracranial pressure and lead to brain herniation. These include:
- Space occupying lesions-hematoma, contusions, CNS tumors, edema, abscess
- CNS infections
- Stroke
- Hydrocephalous
- Traumatic and postoperative pneumocephalus
- Intracerebral and subarachnoid hemorrhage (diffuse)
- Encephalopathy (metabolic-hepatic) (Munakomi and Das, 2020)

### Types

Herniation syndromes may either happen in isolation or in rapid succession. Types of herniation syndromes is shown in **Table 8.17** and **Figure 8.16**.

### Diagnosis

- **Neurological assessment:** Early detection of salient neurological signs and symptoms are essential to limit progression and any form secondary insult to the brain tissue. Stringent neurological evaluation reveals specific characteristic features of herniation syndromes. The frequency of neurological evaluation is dependent on the status of the patient. (Munakomi and Das, 2020)
- **Radiological imaging:** CT or MRI identifies the reason for displacement of brain tissue and the extent of damage caused. Type of herniation and its possible pathologic consequences can be recognized with imaging studies. Valuable information regarding the location and size of the lesion, CSF obstruction,

decrease in size of ventricles (due to displacement of CSF to lumbar theca as a compensatory mechanism), infarction, signs of raised ICP can be ascertained. CT is the preferred imaging modality to make an accurate diagnosis (Mestecky, 2011).

## Nursing Management

### Diagnosis

Acute pain related to area of compression as evidenced by limited activities.

**Table 8.17:** Types of herniation syndromes and clinical features (Maiese, 2019; Mestecky, 2011; Munakomi and Das, 2020).

| Herniation syndromes | Description | Signs and symptoms |
|---|---|---|
| Subfalcine herniation | When a part of the frontal lobe (cingulated gyrus) shifts under the falx cerebri to the opposite hemisphere, it is called subfalcine herniation. This happens when a mass lesion present in either of the hemispheres compresses the adjacent tissue and pushes the brain tissue from the hemisphere of lesion to the nonaffected one. It is not considered as herniation in the true sense | • Not associated with specific symptoms<br>• Headache<br>• Contralateral leg weakness from compression of anterior cerebral artery<br>• It can progress to transtentorial herniation, if left untreated |
| Central or downward transtentorial | Downward movement of the cerebral hemispheres is referred to as central herniation. The central structures (diencephalon) within the brain are forced downward through the tentorial hiatus either due to a central lesion or diffuse edema of the cerebral hemispheres | Early signs due to compression of diencephalon:<br>• Change in level of consciousness<br>• Small pupils<br>• Difficulty in determining reactivity of pupil to light<br>Midbrain compression presents as:<br>• Unreactive and midsized (about 5 mm) pupils<br>• Loss of consciousness<br>• Cheyne stokes respiration<br>Pons compression can lead to central neurogenic hyperventilation (normal or elevated arterial oxygen tension, decreased arterial carbon dioxide tension, and respiratory alkalosis with hyperventilation)<br>Hyperthermia and diabetes insipidus with compression of the hypothalamus |
| Temporal transtentorial or uncal | Shift of uncus (a part of temporal lobe) through the tentorial notch is uncal herniation. The shift occurs ipsilateral to the supratentorial mass thereby causing compression of midbrain on the same side. The diencephalon is not compressed in uncal herniation and therefore the early signs differ from central herniation | • Early signs include confusion and restlessness<br>• Deterioration in level of consciousness<br>• Dilated and sluggish ipsilateral pupil due to compression of oculomotor nerve of the same side<br>• Typically contralateral hemiparesis. However, there can be ipsilateral hemiparesis if midbrain compression occurs on the opposite side (Kernohan's phenomenon)<br>• Compression of pons and midbrain will result in signs and symptoms similar to central herniation |
| Cerebellar tonsillar herniation | An infratentorial lesion can cause either of the two things downward displacement of brain tissue through foramen magnum or upward shift of the brain tissue into the supratentorial compartment. The former is much more common and serious than the latter. During the downward shift, the cerebellar tonsils are forced through the foramen magnum, and cause compression of other brainstem structures and upper cervical cord | • Loss of consciousness<br>• Erratic breathing<br>• Tetraparesis which leads to cardiac and respiratory arrest |
| Transcalvarial herniation | When there is displacement of brain tissue through calvarial defects or defects in the skull, it is termed as transcalvarial herniation. Such defects may occur following fracture of skull or craniectomy | Compression of cortical vessels can cause hemorrhagic infarction |

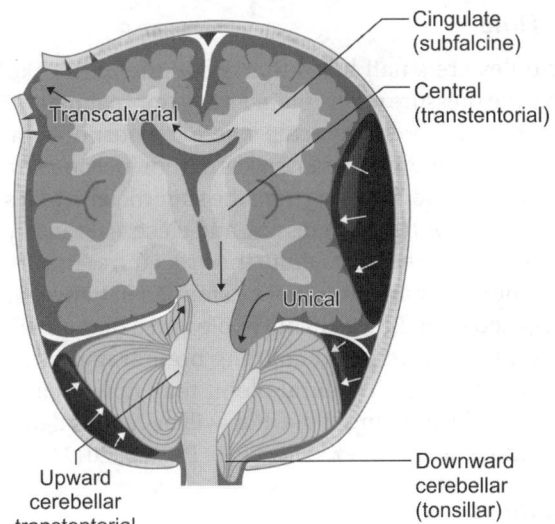

**Fig. 8.16:** Brain herniation types: Cingulate, central (transtentorial), transcalvarial, uncal, upward cerebellar, downward cerebellar (tonsillar).

### Interventions
- Determine the onset, location, and radiation of pain.
- Restricted the movements.

### Diagnosis
Impaired physical mobility related to muscle rigidity as evidenced by inability to ambulate.

### Interventions
- Ensure proper spine immobilization during any procedures. Use log rolling technique.
- Use of sandbags on either side is advised to limit the cervical movement.

## Management of Herniation Syndromes

Treatment measures are dependent on the condition of the patient and the cause of herniation. Delayed treatment can cause irreversible damage to major structures of cerebral hemispheres and brainstem, resulting in permanent neurologic deficits or death. Until a definitive diagnosis and treatment is initiated, the goal is to manage the elevated ICP (≤20 mm Hg) and maintain adequate cerebral perfusion pressure (50–70 mm Hg) (Maiese, 2019).

### Initial Resuscitation and Management

**Managing ABCs:** Adequate resuscitation is the initial step in brain herniation regardless of the cause.
- The first step is to establish a protected and controlled airway. In the field, mask ventilation with 100% oxygen is recommended. Endotracheal intubation must be initiated soon after the patient reaches hospital. Nasotracheal intubation or cricothyroidotomy is considered in suspected cases of basilar skull fracture.
- Controlled ventilation with 100% oxygen should be maintained. The goal is to improve arterial oxygen, reverse hypercarbia and respiratory acidosis. The resultant vasoconstriction from initial hyperventilation helps in lowering ICP. However, excessive vasoconstriction can precipitate cerebral ischemia and therefore, once a mass lesion is detected in the diagnostic studies, $PaCO_2$ must be normalized. In the absence of any mass lesion, $PaCO_2$ is maintained between 30–35 mm Hg, and selective hyperventilation is recommended.
- Prevent or correct systemic hypotension. The most common cause of systemic hypotension among head injury patients is hemorrhagic shock. It is important to support circulation and blood pressure. Treatment modalities include use of volume expanders (crystalloids and blood products) and control of source of hemorrhage. Avoid Overhydration as it can lead to cerebral and pulmonary edema. Administration of hypertonic saline is preferred over mannitol in hemorrhagic shock. If the patient remains unresponsive to volume resuscitation, check other possible causes of hypotension.
- Herniation due to supratentorial lesion: Use of mannitol, hypertonic saline, barbiturates, and hyperventilation is recommended during the initial resuscitation (Andrews, 2016; Mestecky, 2011).

**Administration of mannitol:** Immediate intravenous bolus infusion of mannitol, 1–1.5 g/kg body weight, is recommended (contraindicated in hemorrhagic shock due to its cardiovascular effects). It causes vasoconstriction and improves blood flow to all parts of brain thereby lowering the ICP and improving the intracranial compliance (Andrews, 2016).

### Subsequent Management

After stabilizing the patient, CT scan of the brain is done to study the herniation and its impact. Immediate surgical intervention of the lesion is indicated, if detected. When a preoperative scan is not possible due to unstable client condition, exploratory diagnosis and management is performed (Andrews, 2016).

### Complications

Brain herniation can progress rapidly and therefore any delays to urgent treatment can compromise the vital structures of the brain. Irreversible damage to the brainstem can cause cardiac arrest, respiratory arrest, brain death or death. It can result in global brain infarction due to compression of the cerebral vasculatures' with each type of herniation syndrome.

## MANAGEMENT MODALITIES THROUGH NEUROSURGICAL APPROACHES

Neurosurgery is concerned with the diagnosis and treatment of nervous system disorders. It includes a variety of surgical procedures performed to manage brain, spinal cord and peripheral nerve disorders.

Assessment of Intracranial pressure. *Refer page 185*, increased intracranial pressure.

### Management of Intracranial Hypertension

Effective management of intracranial hypertension involves careful avoidance of factors that precipitate or aggravate increased intracranial pressure.

At the outset, common prophylactic measures such as elevating patient's head, fever control, adequate analgesia and sedation should be applied instantaneously to all patients with suspected intracranial hypertension.

For intracranial hypertension refractory to initial medical management, barbiturate coma, hypothermia, or decompressive craniectomy should be considered. Steroids are not indicated and may be harmful in the treatment of intracranial hypertension resulting from traumatic brain injury. Patients can take a diuretic to reduce fluid retention. In severe cases, patient may need surgery for IIH.

### Common Surgical Procedures in Neuroemergencies

The neurosurgical procedures can be classified into two by the anatomical location.
1. **Supratentorial:** It is the area just above the tentorium and includes cerebral hemispheres. The scalp incision is made within the boundaries of hairline directly above the area that is being considered for surgery. This approach is used to gain access to lesions present in any of the four lobes of the brain (Hickey, 1997).
2. **Infratentorial:** It is the area below the tentorium in the posterior fossa. The incision is made at the nape of the neck usually around the occipital area or posterolaterally in the occipito-temporal region. It gives access to the brainstem and cerebellum. Also, lesions of the temporal or occipital region that are close to the tentorium may be treated using this approach (Hickey, 1997).

### Burr Hole

Burr holes are small holes that are made in the skull to relieve the pressure on the brain tissue. Approximately 5 cm hair is removed from the scalp where the burr holes are to be made. The neurosurgeon makes a 3 cm incision straight down to the bone. Bleeding from the superficial arteries can be controlled with direct pressure and electrical cautery can be used as required throughout the procedure. The drilling should be steady and must not be stopped in between. The drill is used to make a 2 cm burr hole and a blunt hook can be used to remove the remaining bone fragments after removing the drill. Epidural blood may now escape but further careful opening of the dura will be required to drain the subdual blood (Beez et al., 2019; Preece, 2011).

#### Indications

- Extra-axial (epidural and subdural) intracranial hematomas are an indication for emergency burr hole evacuation. Rapidly expanding hematomas with fixed dilated pupil can be fatal.
- Patients with GCS <8 with radio-imaging evidence of extra-dural hematoma causing midline shift and anisocoria. It is also commonly used to insert external ventricular drains, obtain biopsy of brain tissue and for the removal of bone flap during craniotomy (Beez et al., 2019; Preece, 2011).

#### Complications

- Bleeding or re-collection of hematoma which can lead to rising ICP and rapid deterioration
- Infection or injury to the brain tissues
- **Tension pneumocephalus:** It is the entry of air into the subdural, extradural, subarachnoid, intracerebral or intraventricular compartments. If the air trapped is sufficient, it may act as a space occupying lesion and later cause significant neurological deterioration (Beez et al., 2019; Hickey, 1997).

### Craniotomy

During craniotomy the skull is exposed by making an incision on the scalp and small burr holes are created until the underlying dura is revealed. Using a craniotome (special drill), the bone flap is removed from the dura mater. The dura is then incised to expose the brain. Once the lesion is removed, bleeding is stopped and the dura is sutured. The bone flap is replaced using three mini plates while the scalp of the patient is closed using staples. This surgical approach can involve more than one skull bone. Based on the size of the lesion, craniotomy may be small or large. It can vary from burr hole or keyhole craniotomy to complex skull base craniotomies. Awake craniotomy is performed on patients whose lesion are close to speech areas of brain (Preece, 2011).

## Indications

- Closed head injury with expanding lesion such as epidural and subdural hematoma
- Removal of cerebral lobes following traumatic brain injury to reduce intracranial pressure
- Surgical removal of a blood clot, tumor or abscess
- Clipping of an aneurysm
- Removal of vascular malformations such as arterio-venous malformation (AVM) and arterio-venous fistula (AVF)
- Repair meningeal tear or injury and skull fractures
- Implant stimulators such as deep brain stimulator in case of Parkinson's disease
- Perform surgery to treat epilepsy

## Complications

The complex nature of neurosurgery can lead to several life-threatening complications. It also depends on the specific location of the brain being operated.

- Bleeding into tumor site (mainly from large metastatic lesions)
- Seizures occur in approximately 40% cases with tumors in the frontal, temporal and parietal lobes (Preece, 2011)
- Hematoma formation and CSF leak
- Cerebral edema
- Infarction of brain tissue due to inadvertent compression of arteries during surgery
- Infection
- Damage to cranial nerves
- Temporary or permanent neurologic deficit (based on brain tissue involved in surgery).

## Decompressive Craniectomy

It is a surgical procedure used for immediate reduction of intracranial pressure. The procedure involves surgical removal of a portion of skull (bone flap) and expansion of dura mater to accommodate the swollen brain. The bone flap may be temporarily housed in abdominal subcutaneous tissue or ignored until subsequent cranioplasty with acrylic (Wilson et al., 2012). The bone flap should be replaced as soon as the bulging reduces in the craniectomy site to prevent complications (Faleiro and Martins, 2014). Cranioplasty is usually recommended within six months (Preece, 2011).

## Indications

- Intracranial hypertension or brain swelling following traumatic brain injury refractory to medical management
- Malignant infarction of the MCA which can possibly lead to cerebral edema, increased ICP, poor perfusion, hemorrhagic transformation, midline shift or trans-tentorial herniation (Wilson et al., 2012)
- Brain swelling associated with vasospasm (in SAH), hypertensive bleeds, encephalitis and cerebral venous thrombosis (Preece, 2011).

## Complications

- Brain herniation through the craniectomy and subsequent infarct is one of the common complications of decompressive craniectomy.
- **Infection:** It is observed in less than 10% of patients. Infection of surgical site and within CNS are possible.
- **CSF disturbance:** Patients may develop hygroma or internal communicating hydrocephalous. Subdural collections are also common.
- **Seizures:** There is a risk for single or recurrent seizures (6–12%) within 5 years after surgery.
- Syndrome of the trephined or sunken flap syndrome can happen in patients within weeks or months after craniectomy. Patients may present with neurological deterioration after an initial improvement during rehabilitation. The sunken flap overlying the craniectomy defect is evident on clinical and radiological examination (Faleiro and Martins, 2014; Wilson et al., 2012).

## Nursing Management

### Diagnosis

Ineffective tissue perfusion is related to cerebral edema as evidenced by increased ICP.

### Interventions

- The head end of the bed should be elevated to 30 degrees to facilitate venous drainage thereby reducing the risk of increasing ICP. The neck should be in a neutral position. Do not flex or hyperextend the neck.
- Avoid restrictive neck taping. Remove or loosen rigid collars to decrease ICP

### Diagnosis

Disturbed sensory perception related to periorbital edema as evidenced by lack of orientation.

### Interventions

- Assess the vision ability.
- Assess the patients peripheral neuropathy.

## Nursing Management

### Preoperative Management

- Patients must undergo a thorough preoperative
-  assessment before undergoing any neurosurgery
- Obtain informed consent. Ensure that the patient is competent enough to give consent. It is usually obtained by the neurosurgeon doing the procedure. Patients should be given adequate time to make decision and clarify doubts.
- Keep the patient warm in the preoperative phase as hypothermia increases the risk for infections. The patient should be changed to a hospital gown only at the last minute.
- Assess the family support structure of the patient.
- Record the neurological observations and other vital parameters (pulse, blood pressure, respiration, saturation) in the patient notes. It will provide an image of patient status prior to the surgery.
- Chest X-ray and ECG are also recorded to assess for any problems that may affect surgery. Any problems, if detected, must be further evaluated by experts before taking the patient for surgery.
- Conduct all necessary investigations (complete blood count, anticoagulation profile, renal and liver function tests, glucose, blood group, c-reactive protein, calcium) and have a record of all neurodiagnostic procedures related to the patient.
- MRSA screening is mandatory prior to invasive neurosurgical procedure.
- Evaluate all pre-existing conditions. This is to understand the need for extra measures to be taken during and after the surgery. For example, a patient with vascular disease will require more intensive monitoring.
- Check all current medications and note for any allergies. Some medications need to be stopped before surgery (e.g., aspirin, anticoagulants)
- Remove all foreign bodies in the body such as dentures as it may interfere with the intubation. The patient should be examined for any other anatomical oral problems that might make intubation difficult.
- Conducting nutritional assessment as neurosurgery can increase the metabolic rate.
- Maintain NPO status (as recommended) to reduce the risk of perioperative aspiration. Some medications such as oral antiepileptics can be administered with little water 2 hours before the surgery.
- The risk for pressure ulcer should also be checked preoperatively.
- Record the height, weight and BMI of the patient to facilitate calculation of drug dosage.
- Keep the blood sugar under control as hyperglycemia can potentiate brain injury and damage to BBB.
- If there is an opportunity, educate the client on issues related to smoking, alcohol use, weight loss and nutrition.

### Intraoperative Management

- Re-check all the assessments that were made and check for any new developments. This includes verification of patient records including consent.
- Record the neurological findings and vital signs as baseline parameters. Patient should be normothermic before going for surgery.
- Insert a urinary catheter, if not present.
- Consider prophylactic measures for complications associated with immobility and venous stasis such as using antiembolic stockings. Heparin is not administered preoperatively as it can increase the risk of bleeding. Sequential compression boots are generally considered during surgery to prevent pooling of blood in the lower extremities.
- A minimal amount of hair should be removed along the headline. However, sometimes more hair is shaved off in an emergency.
- Provide an optimal position that will allow proper access to lesion. Commonly given positions for neurosurgical procedures include-sitting (posterior fossa surgery), lateral (for access to supratentorial area), prone (for access to infratentorial area).
- Support procedures of ventilation and connect patient to all necessary monitors required for intraoperative monitoring.
- Drugs considered during the intraoperative phase include anesthetics, osmotic diuretics (IV Mannitol), dexamethasone (to control cerebral edema), phenytoin, antibiotics and cardiac drugs (control hypotension or hypertension).
- Ensure adequate cerebral protection during surgery to avoid ICP elevation.

### Postoperative Management

- Regular neurological examination following surgery is recommended. This is to identify any signs of deterioration (e.g., alteration in level of consciousness, unequal pupils) and take appropriate action without delay.
- GCS of the patient is checked concurrently with vital signs, pupillary response and limb movements.
- Neurological examination should be conducted half an hourly until the GCS is 15. When the patient attains a GCS score of 15, neurological observations are then

carried out every half hourly for 2 hours, hourly for next 4 hours and two hourly thereafter.
- Patients pulse and blood pressure must be monitored strictly. Any signs of low circulating volume should be treated with 0.9% sodium chloride as first line management. Avoid dextrose 5% as it can cause cerebral edema. The risk of hypotension is increased if mannitol (osmotic diuretic) was administered during surgery and hypertension can cause bleeding.
- Maintain the oxygen saturation of the patient (≥95%). Hypoxia can lead to decreased cerebral perfusion and cerebral infarction.
- Evaluate the risk for aspiration and other potential respiratory complications. Protect the airway of patients with altered level of consciousness.
- The rate, depth and pattern of respiration of the patient should be monitored and documented.
- Since for every 1°C rise in temperature, the cerebral requirement of oxygen increases by 6–7% it is important to maintain normothermia.
- The head end of the bed is elevated to 30 degrees to facilitate drainage in case of supratentorial procedures. A head end elevation of 30 degrees or lowered flat is preferred in infratentorial cases.
- Increased pain can cause an increase in ICP. Hence, measures for pain relief and antiemetic cover are taken during the intraoperative phase itself (approximately 1 hour before anesthesia reversal). Pain assessment should be performed regularly. Drug choices include: (Preece, 2011).
  - *Codeine phosphate:* Weak opioid for mild to moderate pain, 30–60 mg 4 hourly orally or intra muscularly. Maximum dose: 240 mg/24 hours
  - *Paracetamol:* Nonopioid for mild to moderate pain 1 g 4 hourly oral or IV, maximum dose: 4 g/24 hours
  - *Tramadol:* Synthetic opioid for moderate pain, 50–100 mg IV, 4-6 hourlym maximum dose: 600 mg/24 hours
  - Morphine sulphate opioid with high affinity for μ receptors
    PCA: 100 mg morphine, made up to 50 mL with 0.9% sodium chloride. Initial bolus of 2 mg (1 mL) is given and duration of injection is 1 min with 10 min lockout. Later infusion at the rate of 60 mg/60 mL is titrated to patient requirements (max dose: 30 mg in 4 hours).
- The choice of antiemetics is based on the cause of vomiting. Antiemetic cover is given with:
  - *Cyclizine (50 mg TDS-oral, IM, IV):* It blocks the histamine receptors in the chemoreceptor trigger zone (CTZ) located in the medulla. thereby controlling nausea or vomiting. It is administered to manage anesthesia related nausea/vomiting.
  - *Ondansetron:* It acts by blocking the serotonin receptors in the GI tract and medulla. It is considered in cases where there is risk for surgical manipulation of vomiting center.
- Place observations of drain and drainage in the patient notes regularly, if present. Either a gravity drains or closed suction drain is used. It should not be attached to a wall suction as aggressive suction can cause tears on the brain surfaces.
- Observe the drain sites and wound for any leaks or signs of infection.
- The dressing over the wound site is usually removed after 24 hours and kept open for healing. A turban-style dressing is usually applied initially.
- The scalp sutures/clips are usually removed at 3–5 days (supratentorial sutures) after surgery. The scalp heals quickly due to good blood supply (Preece, 2011).
- Excess straining or irritation can cause a rise in ICP. Therefore, ensure proper functioning of indwelling urethral catheters and provide suppositories for easy bowel movements. Tramadol and codeine can cause constipation.
- Maintain strict fluid balance chart.
- Patient is kept on NPO for first 24 hours; IV fluids are administered slowly.
- Commence oral feed as soon as the patient can tolerate it. Check for swallowing and gag reflexes before starting the feed (especially in infratentorial procedures since cranial nerves IX and X may be manipulated during the procedure).
- Consider GI prophylaxis if the patient is not able to take oral feeds. Omeprazole or ranitidine are the drugs of choice. The BMR may rise up to 60% in the first 48 hours following head injury/major surgery (Preece, 2011).
- Encourage early mobilization to avoid complications associated with immobility (e.g., pneumonia, DVT, pulmonary emboli, pressure ulcer etc.). Ideally patients should be encouraged to wear antiembolic stockings for at least 6 weeks postoperatively.
- Patients who underwent infratentorial procedures are recommended for longer bed rest than those with supratentorial procedures. This is because the frequency of dizziness experienced by them is high.
- There is usually no restriction on turning the patient. However, the patient may not be positioned on the operative side due to risk of shifting of cranial contents (especially in cases of large tumors).

### Postcraniotomy

Patients usually take time to return to their preoperative status after craniotomy. The changes in their mental state after surgery are mostly temporary and resolve gradually. However, nurses should have a clear idea on what is to be expected and when to report to the surgical team.

- Postoperative CT or MRI may be conducted of any significant deviation from baseline recordings are noted.
- Keep the patient adequately hydrated. Overhydration can cause cerebral edema. Generally 2 liters/24 hours is recommended. However, patients who have undergone craniotomy for aneurysm should be given nearly 3 liters of fluids per 24 hours to maintain the circulating volume, prevent vasospasm and ensure adequate cerebral perfusion (Preece, 2011).
- Patients who are on dexamethasone therapy (post-surgery) should undergo daily urinalysis for glucose. Hyperglycemia, if detected, should be managed with insulin since elevated blood sugar levels can disrupt BBB and cause cerebral edema.

### Postcraniectomy

- Provide special attention to the craniectomy site. Observe the site for any leakage, bulging or signs of inflammation. Any deviation in the findings should be immediately reported to the medical staff.
- Tight bandages at the site of bone flap are to be avoided.
- Clear documentation related to bone flap removal should be made on the patient's charts.
- Observe for cranial nerve deficits (infratentorial craniectomy or posterior fossa craniectomy)
- Avoid positioning the patient on the same side of the missing bone flap for the first 48 hours after surgery to prevent compression to the intracranial contents and increase in ICP (Preece, 2011).
- While changing positioning every two hours, ensure that the head of the patient always rests on the solid side of the skull.
- Teach both patient and family the need for extra protection and care for the bony defect. A temporary protective helmet may be given in patients with large craniectomy.

###  Summary

This chapter deals with the emergency management of common gastrointestinal disorder. Neurologic emergencies are one of the common causes for admission in the emergency department. Any downfall in immediate management can lead to fatality or poor functional recovery. Hence, it is imperative that we identify neuroemergencies, make appropriate decisions and manage the neurologic signs.

###  Points to Ponder

- Neuroglial cells are supporting cells in the nervous system and it is 25 times larger than neurons in number and Neuroglia play active role in supporting and protecting neurons, controlling neurotransmitter uptake, recovering neurons from injury, and nourishing neurons.
- Hypothalamus controls and coordinates autonomic nervous system and regulates smooth muscle contraction of visceral organs, heart rate, urinary bladder contraction and movement of gastrointestinal tract.
- Midbrain, pons and medulla oblongata are the three parts of the brainstem. Midbrain connects the cerebral hemispheres with pons through huge bundles of neurons. It contains centers for auditory and visual reflexes.
- Brain and spinal cord are protected by meninges, which includes three layers namely, dura mater, arachnoid mater and pia mater.
- Spinal nerves carry electrical impulses either to or from the spinal cord. There are 31 pairs of spinal nerves— cervical (8), thoracic (12), lumbar (5), sacral (5) and coccygeal (1).
- There are 12 pairs of cranial nerves. These are called 'cranial' because it exits from the cranial cavity. Cranial nerves can be sensory, motor or mixed (sensory and motor).
- According to mental status examination, each of these activities are scored. Maximum score of mini mental status examination is 30. A score <24 indicates cognitive impairment.
- Perform motor strength assessment of both right and left upper and lower limbs using power grading (score 0–5)
- The pressure created by the intracranial contents is termed as intracranial pressure (ICP). Normal value of ICP ranges from 5–15 mm Hg.
- For the patients with increased ICP, a 30° head end elevation is recommended. Head elevation increases the jugular venous return and hence prevents accumulation of blood in the intracranial space.
- Status epilepticus is a seizure or repeated seizures lasting more than 5 minutes for generalized tonic-clonic seizures, 10 minutes for focal seizures, and 10–15 minutes for absence seizures.
- In Guillain-Barré Syndrome (GBS), emergency management is required when there is involvement of the respiratory muscles.
- Myasthenic crisis is an emergency condition with exacerbation of symptoms of myasthenia gravis. This is characterized by severe muscle weakness and respiratory muscle paralysis leading to respiratory failure.
- In case of head injury, the head end of the bed should be elevated to 30 degrees to facilitate venous drainage thereby reducing the risk of increasing ICP. The neck should be in neutral position. Do not flex or hyperextend the neck.

- India considers death equivalent to brainstem death. If the patient is certified brain stem death, then he is legally and medically considered dead. It is mandatory to include the date and time of brain death in patient notes.
- For every 1°C rise in temperature, the cerebral requirement of oxygen increases by 6–7% and it is important to maintain normothermia.

## Abbreviations

- ICU : Intensive Care Unit
- ABC : Airway, Breathing, Circulation
- ADH : Oxytocin and Antidiuretic Hormone
- CSF : Cerebrospinal Fluid
- BBB : Blood Brain Barrier
- ANS : Autonomic Nervous System
- RMP : Resting Membrane Potential
- TIA : Transient Ischemic Attack
- GCS : Glasgow Coma Scale
- CPP : Cerebral Perfusion Pressure
- MAP : Mean Arterial Pressure
- ICP : Intracranial Pressure
- SIADH : Syndrome of Inappropriate Antitdiuretic Hormone
- FND : Focal Neurologic Deficits
- RAS : Reticular Activating System
- PEEP : Positive End-expiratory Pressure
- SAH : Subarachnoid Hemorrhage
- EVD : External Ventricular Drain
- DCV : Delayed Cerebral Vasospasm
- NICE : National Institute for Health and Clinical Excellence
- VNS : Vagal Nerve Stimulation
- GABA : Gamma-Amino Butyric Acid

## Short Answer Questions

1. Briefly explain Monro-Kellie hypothesis.
2. Describe the complications of increased ICP.
3. Describe the management of increased ICP.
4. Discuss the methods of ICP monitoring.
5. Explain the management of cerebral aneurysm.
6. Explain the types of cerebrovascular accident.
7. Explain the types of aphasia.
8. Explain the immediate assessment of a patient with suspected case of stroke.
9. Classify seizure.
10. Elucidate the nurse's role while receiving a patient with generalized tonic-clonic seizure in emergency room.
11. Discuss the emergency management of status epilepticus.
12. Substantiate the pathophysiology in head injury.
13. Enlist the spinal cord syndromes and explain any one in detail.
14. Enlist the levels of consciousness and explain any one.
15. Explain the nursing management of an unconscious patient.
16. Categorize herniation syndromes.

## Long Answer Questions

1. Mr Pramod, 25 years is admitted to ICU after a road accident. He was diagnosed to have head injury with skull fracture and hemorrhage. He is unconscious and connected to mechanical ventilator for support.
   a. What is Monro-Kellie hypothesis?
   b. Clinical manifestations of increased ICP.
   c. Explain the nursing management of Mr Pramod in the ICU in the first 48 hours with the help of a nursing care plan.
2. Ms Anita, 16 years is admitted in ward with the complaints of two episodes of generalized tonic-clonic seizures.
   a. Write the classification of seizures.
   b. Describe in detail the medical management of a patient with seizures.
   c. Explain the nursing management of a patient immediately after seizures.
3. In the emergency department, neurologic examination by a nurse reveals that Mr Chandra, 56 years old has right side weakness, facial droop and impaired speech. CT scan taken within 1 hour of onset of symptoms shows intracerebral bleeding.
   a. Explain the pathophysiological manifestations and discuss the management for Mr Chandra.
   b. Discuss the clinical manifestations and management of a patient with increased ICP.

## Bibliography

1. Abou-Khalil B. Levetiracetam in the treatment of epilepsy. Neuropsychiatr Dis Treat. 2008;4(3):507-23.
2. Ahuja CS, Nori S, Tetreault L, Wilson J, Kwon B, Harrop J, … Fehlings MG. Traumatic spinal cord injury Repair and regeneration. Neurosurg. 2017;80(3):S22-S90.
3. Almulhim AM and Madadin M. Scalp Laceration; 2019; 1–4.
4. Andersen M, Gazmuri JT, Marin A, Regueira T, Rovegno M. Therapeutic hypothermia for acute brain injury. Scand J Trauma Resusc Emerg Med. 2015;23(42).
5. Andrews BT. The Recognition and Management of Cerebral Herniation Syndromes; 2016.
6. Beez T, Munoz-Bendix C, Steiger H-J, Beseoglu K. Decompressive craniectomy for acute ischemic stroke. Crit Care. 2019; 23(209).
7. Berisavac II, Dejana JR, Padjen VV, Ercegovac MD, Stanarčević PDJ, Budimkić-Stefanović MS, … Beslać-BumbaširevićLG. How to recognize and treat metabolic encephalopathy in Neurology intensive care unit. Neurol India. 2017;65(123-8).
8. Betjemann JP, Lowenstein DH. Status epilepticus in adults. Lancet Neurol. 2015;1 (6):615-24.
9. Boehme AK, Esenwa C, Elkind MSV. Stroke Risk Factors, Genetics, and Prevention. Circ Res. 2017;120(3):472-95.
10. Bonner S, Smith C. Initial management of acute spinal cord injury. Continuing Education in Anaesthesia, Crit Care Pain. 2013;13(6):224-31.

11. Chen JWY, Wasterlain CG. Status epilepticus: Pathophysiology and management in adults. Lancet Neurol. 2006;5:246-56.
12. Cook N, Woodward S. Assessment, Interpretation and Management of Altered Consciousness. In: Woodward S Mestecky AM (Eds). Neuroscience Nursing: Evidence-Based Practice, Philadelphia: Wiley-Blackwell. 2011. PP. 107–118.
13. Dasenbrock HH, Robertson FC, Vaitkevicius H, Aziz-Sultan MA, Guttieres D, Dunn IF, ... Gormley WB. Timing of Decompressive Hemicraniectomy for Stroke: A Nationwide Inpatient Sample Analysis. Stroke. 2017;48(3):704-11.
14. Davis S, Lees K, Donnan G. Treating the acute stroke patient as an emergency: Current practices and future opportunities. Int J Clin Pract. 2006;60(4):399-407.
15. Frizzell JP. Acute Stroke: Pathophysiology, Diagnosis, Treatment. AACN Clinical Issues. 2005;16(4):421-40.
16. Galgano M, Toshkezi G, Qiu X, Russell T, Chin L, Zhao LR. Traumatic brain injury: Current treatment strategies and future endeavors. Cell Transplant. 2017;26(7):1118-30.
17. Ganapathy K. Brain death revisited. Neurology India. 2018;66(2):308-15.
18. Godoy, Daniel Agustin, Khan AA, Rubiano AM. Management of Severe Traumatic Brain Injury: A Practical Approach. In: Rabinstein AA (Ed). Neurological Emergencies: A Practical Approach. Switzerland: Springer; 2020. pp. 245-68.
19. Godoy, Daniel Agustín, Lubillo S, Rabinstein AA. Pathophysiology and Management of Intracranial Hypertension and Tissular Brain Hypoxia After Severe Traumatic Brain Injury: An Integrative Approach. Neurosurg. Clin. N. Am. 2018;29:195–212.
20. Goila AK, Pawar M. The diagnosis of brain death. Indian J Crit Care Med. 2009:13(1):7–11.
21. Greenwood R. Head injury for neurologists. J Neurol Neurosurg Psychiatry. 2002;73 (Suppl I):i8–i16.
22. Head VA, Wakerley BR. Guillain-Barré syndrome in general practice: Clinical features suggestive of early diagnosis. Br J Gen Pract. 2016;66:218–9.
23. Head injury: Assessment and early management, 2014.
24. Hickey JV. Management of the Unconscious Patient. In: Hickey JV (Ed). The Clinical Practice of Neurological and Neurosurgical Nursing, 3rd edition. Philadelphia: Lippincott; 1992a.
25. Hickey JV. Seizures and Epilepsy. In: Hickey JV (Ed). The clinical practice of neurological and neurosurgical nursing, 3rd edition. Philadelphia: Lippincott; 1992b.
26. Hickey JV. Management of Patients Undergoing Neurosurgical Procedures. In: Hickey JV (Ed). The clinical practice of neurological and neurosurgical nursing, 3rd edition. Philadelphia: Lippincott; 1997.
27. Hills TE. Nursing Management: Peripheral and Spinal Cord Problems. In: Lewis SL, Dirksen SR, Heitkemper MM, Bucher L, Chintamani, Mani M (Eds). Lewis's Medical-Surgical Nursing, 2nd South; 2017. PP. 1527-37.
28. Ho ML, Rojas R, Eisenberg RL. Cerebral edema. Am J Roentgenol. 2012;199(3):258–73.
29. Munroe B, Curtis K, Murphy M, Strachan L, Buckley T. HIRAID: An evidence-informed emergency nursing assessment framework. Aust Emerg Nurs J. 18(2):83-97.
30. Supanc V, Vargek-Solter V, Demarin V. Metabolic Encephalopathies. Acta Clinica Croatica. 2003;42(4): 351-56.
31. Tameem A, Krovvidi H. Cerebral physiology. Continuing Education in Anaesthesia, Crit Care Pain. 2013;13(4):113-8.
32. Wilson MH, Wise D, Davies G, Lockey D. Emergency burr holes: "How to do it." Scand. J. Trauma, Resusc. Emerg. 2012;20(24):2-4.

# Chapter 9

# Cardiovascular Emergencies and Management

*Sarika ML*

## CHAPTER OUTLINE

- Anatomy of Cardiovascular System
- Physiology of Cardiovascular System
- Principles of Nursing in Caring for Patients with Cardiovascular Disorders
- Assessment of Cardiovascular System
- Hypertensive Crisis
- Coronary Artery Disease
- Acute Myocardial Infarction
- Cardiomyopathy
- Deep Vein Thrombosis
- Valvular Disease
- Heart Block
- Cardiac Arrhythmias
- Aneurysm
- Endocarditis
- Heart Failure
- Management Modalities for Cardiovascular System Disorders
  - Cardiopulmonary resuscitation
  - Pacemaker
  - Percutaneous cronary intervention
  - Cardioversion
  - Intra-aortic ballon pump monitoring
  - Defibrillation
  - Radiofrequency catheter ablation
  - Cardiac surgeries
    – Coronary artery bypass grafting
    – Valvular surgeries
    – Cardiac (heart) transplantation

## Learning Objectives

At the end of this chapter, the students will be able to:
- Recollect the anatomy and physiology part of the cardiovascular system.
- Get knowledge to practice cardiac assessment.
- Gain knowledge on the emergency nursing care on hypertension crisis, coronary artery disease, acute myocardial infarction, cardiomyopathy, deep vein thrombosis, valvular diseases, arrhythmias, heart block, endocarditis and heart failure.
- Acquire the knowledge on different management modalities like CPR, pacemaker, PTCI, cardioversion, defibrillation, intra-aortic balloon pump.
- Provide care and can prepare patients for different cardiac surgeries.

## ANATOMY OF CARDIOVASCULAR SYSTEM

The cardiovascular system (CVS) includes the heart, coronary circulation and the vascular system includes systemic, pulmonary circulation, arterial and venous supply of the body. Knowledge of the cardiovascular system will help to understand about each condition or problems related to this system and to manage or treat the problems easily. The cardiovascular system is the one system that gives blood supply or energy to all other organs. So, the basic knowledge on CVS is very important, then only it is able to understand the clinical manifestation and can correlate with the system.

### Embryology Development

The development of the heart, blood, blood vessels and lymphatic circulation developed fully during the fourth week of gestation from the **mesodermal layer of the embryo**. This development usually starts from the 18–19 days after the fertilization.

The heart developed from the **cardiogenic area** which is near to the head part of the embryo. That is the area in between the base of pericardial cavity and the dorsal wall of yolk sac. After the head fold formation, the developing heart lies on the dorsal to the pericardial cavity and ventral to the foregut.

The cardiogenic area slowly changed to cardiogenic codes due to the chemical signals in the embryo. Immediately a lumen will develop inside the cords and then it is called **endocardial tubes**. These two tubes joined together form **a single primitive heart tube**. Then the heart tube goes to the dorsal side of the pericardial cavity. The dorsal side of the pericardial cavity is lined by the splanchnopleuric mesoderm which multiplying and gives raise to the **myoepicardial mantle**. Later it completely covers the heart tube and form myocardium and epicardium.

This heart tube has five parts including—truncus arteriosus, bulbus cordis, primitive ventricle, primitive atrium and sinus venosus respectively from the head end to the tail end of the heart tube.

The venous blood is flowing into the sinus venosus and the contraction of the heart tube starts from the tail end to the head end of the heart tube.

The primitive heart tubes further elongate and folded within the pericardium and formed a S shape. This process starts from the 4th week onwards (Chaurasia BD, 2019).

### Evolution of Atria

*Evolution of the Right Atrium*

Mainly the right atrium (RA) developed from; right half of the primitive atrium, right horn of the sinus venosus changed into the right half of the primitive atrium, and right half of the AV canal changed into the ventral smooth part. After the formation of the RA, coronary sinus and the vena cava also opens into the RA.

*Evolution of the Left Atrium*

LA developed from left half of the primitive atrial chamber, left half of the AV canal and proximal part of the pulmonary veins and form the rough anterior part and left auricle, anterior smooth part and posterior smooth part between the openings of the pulmonary veins respectively.

*Evolution of the Atrioventricular Canal*

Evolution of the atrioventricular (AV) canal is the connection between the atrium and the ventricle. Initially the AV canal is in the circular in shape later it changed into the transverse shape. The AV endocardial cushions developed at the right and left AV canals. Then it will grow and fuse each other to form septum intermedium **(Figs. 9.1 and 9.2)**.

*Evolution of Interatrial Septum*

The atrium divided into the right and left by the formation of the septum. The sequence includes:
- Appearance of the septum primum.
- Fusion of septum primum with the AV cushion.
- The gap between septum primum and the AV cushion is called foramen primum.
- The foramen secundum formed by the degeneration of the septum primum.
- The septum secundum formed at the right side of the septum primum.
- The free edges of the septum primum covered by the septum secundum.
- The blood flow is from the left to the right via the gap between the two septa.

### Evolution of Ventricle

The right and left ventricles developed from the **primitive ventricle** and **bulbus cordis**. The bulbus cordis at the head end of the heart tube. It is divided into mainly three parts; **proximal** one third, middle one third called **conus** and the distal one third called **truncus arteriosus** (Wong and Whales).

- The proximal part joins with the primitive ventricle and form the bulboventricular chamber subsequently form the trabeculated end of the right ventricle.
- The conus forms the outflow end of the both right and left ventricle. This conus is also associated with the formation of the interventricular septum.
- The truncus arteriosus divide and form the aorto-pulmonary septum between the aorta and the pulmonary artery.

The interatrial septum, interventricular septum and AV septum are formed at the end of the 5th week of gestation (Singh I, 2018).

The AV valves → 5–8 weeks
The Semilunar valve → 5–9 weeks

### Evolution of the Conduction System of the Heart

The two heart tube stage of the cardiac development the sinoatrial node at the caudal end. After the fusion of the two tubes the SA node at the sinus venosus part. Later the sinus venosus changed to form the right ventricle and the SA node will be at the opening area of the superior venacava. The AV node and the AV bundle at the left wall of the sinus venosus. Later stage of development process AV node formed near to the interatrial septum **(Table 9.1)** (Mathew P, 2019).

## Anatomy of the Heart

The heart is a muscular organ situated in the middle of the mediastinum. It is covered by pericardium. The major function of the heart is to pump the blood to the various parts of the body. The heart is situated obliquely back of the sternum body and associated structures of the costal cartilages. That's why the heart is two third deviated to towards the left side and the one third at the right side.

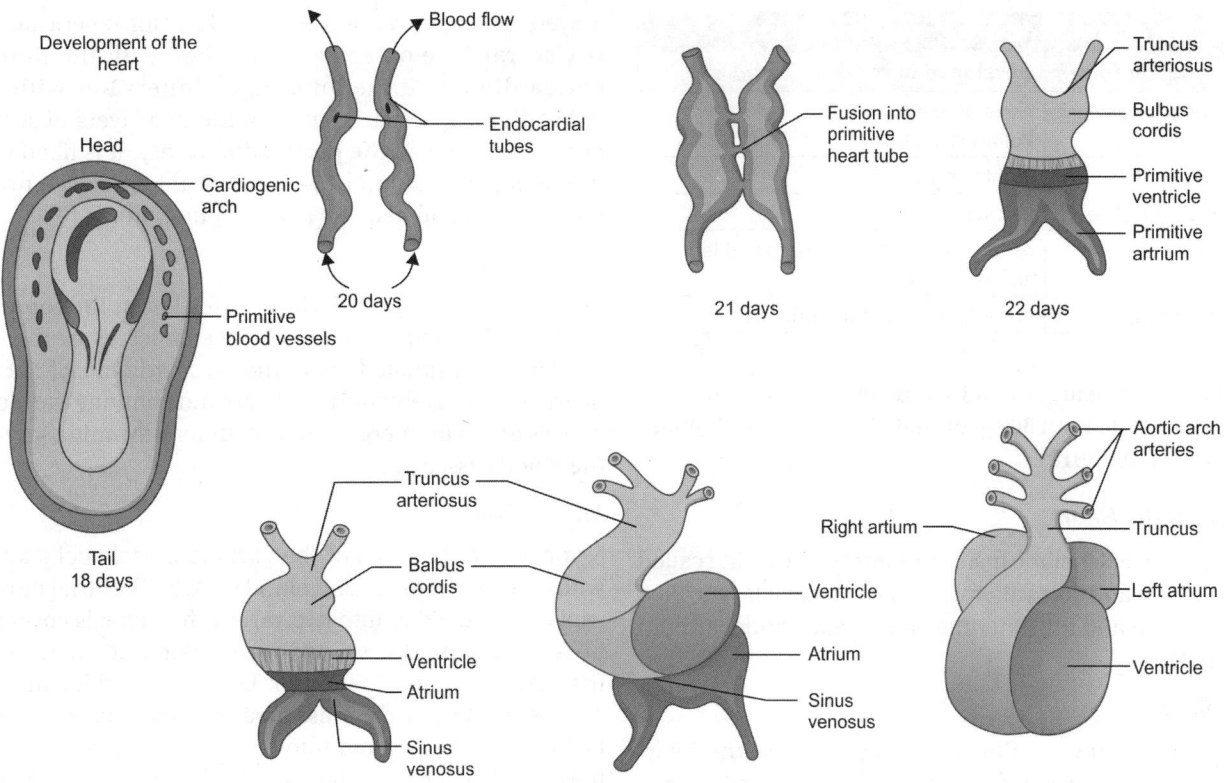

**Fig. 9.1:** Embryology development of heart.

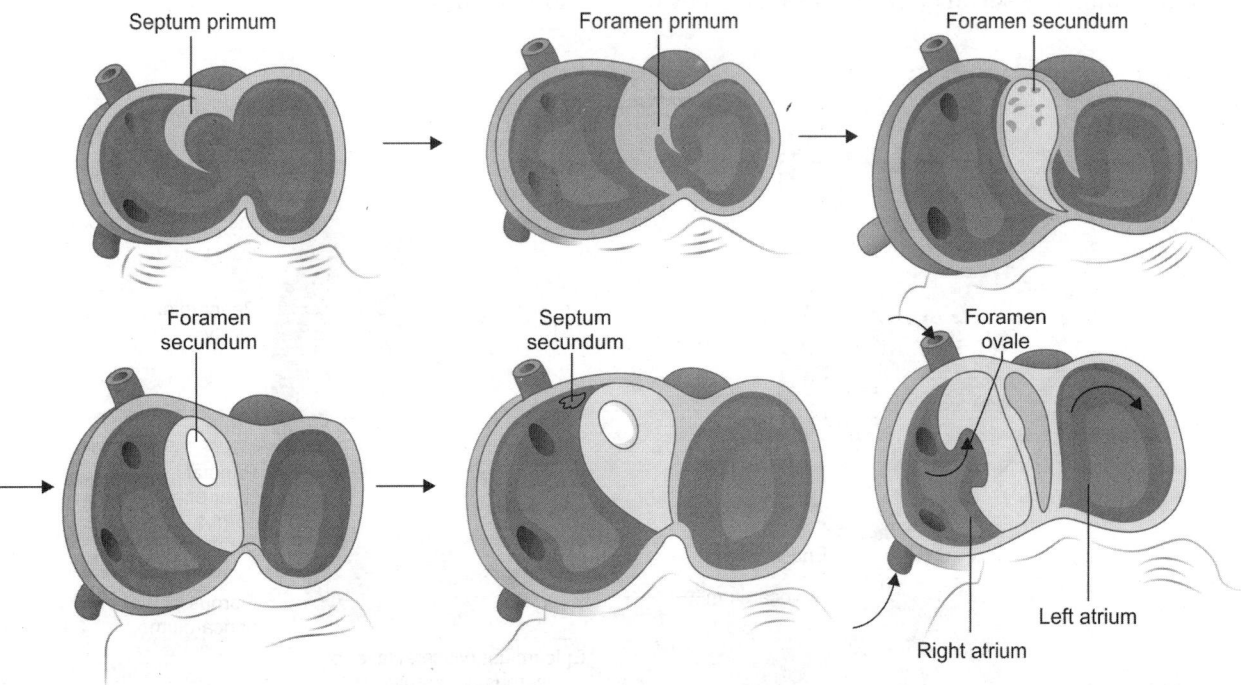

**Fig. 9.2:** Interatrial septum development.

**Table 9.1:** Evolution of different part of the heart.

| Embryogenic form | Developed form |
|---|---|
| Truncus arteriosus | Ascending aorta<br>Pulmonary trunk |
| Bulbous cordis | Right ventricle |
| Primitive ventricle | Left ventricle |
| Primitive atrium | Anterior part of right atrium and left atrium and two auricles |
| Sinus venosus | Posterior part of right atrium, SA |

The size of the heart is about 12 cm length and 9 cm width and the weight about 300 g for males and 250 g for females (Chaurasia BD, 2019).

### Layers of the Heart

The heart layers include mainly; outermost covering called pericardium and epicardium, middle muscular layer called myocardium and the innermost layer called endocardium **(Fig. 9.3)**.

*Pericardium*

The pericardium is a fibroserous covering of the heart and the great vessels; fibrous pericardium and serous pericardium. The **fibrous pericardium** is made up of fibrous tissue and protects the heart from the overfilling. The serous pericardium is a two walled serous membrane by mesothelium. The **serous pericardium** consists of 2 layers; Outer pericardium is parietal and inner pericardium is visceral. The outer layer attached with the fibrous pericardium and the inner layer innervates with the epicardium. The space between the two layers of serous pericardium called **the pericardial cavity**. It is filled with the serous fluid around 10–30 mL, that lubricate between the two layer and help the heart to pump freely.

*Epicardium*

Epicardium is a superficial layer of the heart. The coronary blood vessels, lymphatic vessels, fat and nerves are there in this layer. It is situated above the myocardium layer of the heart. It completely cover the heart and continue the blood vessels and later merge with the tunica adventitia layer of the blood vessels.

*Myocardium*

Myocardium consists of the cardiac muscle cells along with connective tissue and blood vessels. The atrial muscle wall can be divided into two variety; first type is cover the both atrium and the second type is perpendicular to the first layer and it is different for both right and left atrium. The ventricle muscle mass arranged like figure of eight fashion and innervated into the fibrous skeleton. In the horizontal dissection of the muscle it will be like the fan like arrangement (Braunald, 2007).

The myocardial cells divided into:
- **Working myocardial cells:** Generate the contractile force of the heart

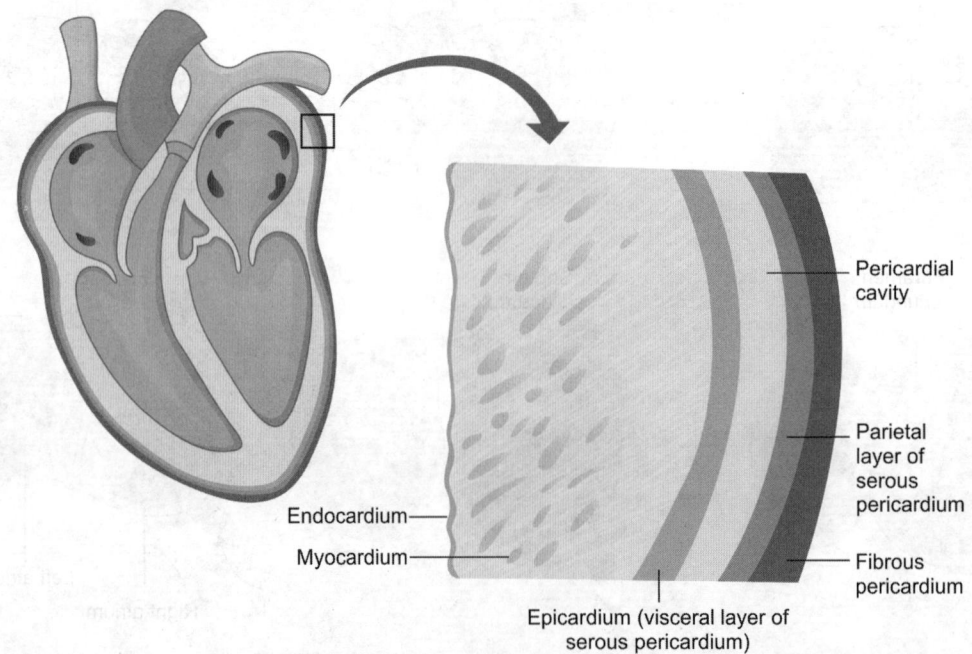

**Fig. 9.3:** Layers of heart.

- **Nodal cells:** For pacemaker function
- **Purkinje cells:** It helps to conduct the electrical signals rapidly through the thick myocardial cells.

*Endocardium*

It is made up of mainly endothelial cells along with few collagen and the elastic fibers. The heart valves are attached to this layer. It continues with the inner layer, tunica intima of the blood vessels.

### Cardiac chambers

#### Right atrium

It is situated at the right upper chamber of the heart. The right atrium (RA) receives the impure or venous blood from the both **superior and inferior vena cava** of the body from upper part of the body and from the lower part of the body respectively. Then it goes to the right ventricle through the **tricuspid valve**, which is present in between the right atrium and ventricle. The upper end of the RA projects towards the left side and form **the right auricle**. **Sulcus terminalis** is a groove that is passes superior vena cava above and the inferior vena cava below. The upper part of sulcus contains the **SinoAtrial Node** (SA node) is the **Pacemaker** of the heart (Chaurasia BD, 2019).

*Tributaries of the RA*
- Superior vena cava
- Inferior vena cava
- Coronary sinus
- Anterior cardiac vein
- Venae cordis minimae
- Right marginal vein

#### Right ventricle

It is a triangular chamber of the heart. It forms the inferior border and it is the large surface of the sternocostal part of the heart. The right ventricle (RV) receives the impure blood from the RA and pumped into the pulmonary artery. The RV consists of mainly 2 surfaces anteriorly sternocostal and inferiorly diaphragmatic. The RV have 2 orifices include; tricuspid guarded by tricuspid valve and the pulmonary trunk by pulmonary or semilunar valve. The wall of the right ventricle is thinner than that of the left ventricle (1:3).

#### Left atrium

It is a posteriorly situated four edged chamber. It occupies the left two third of the base part of the heart. The left atrium (LA) covers the major part of the upper border. It receives the pure or oxygenated blood from the lungs through the pulmonary veins and pumped into the left ventricle trough the mitral or bicuspid valve.

#### Left ventricle

The left ventricle (LV) receives the blood from the LA, and it pumped into the aorta. The LV is the apex of the heart, part of sternocostal surface, left border and the two third part of the left diaphragmatic surface. The LV have two orifices; one is mitral guarded by mitral valve and another one is aortic by aortic or semilunar valve **(Figs. 9.4 and 9.5)**.

#### Coronary circulation

The arterial supply of the heart is by **coronary arteries**. The major branches of the coronary circulation include **right coronary artery** and **left coronary artery**.

#### Right coronary artery

The right coronary artery (RCA) emerging from the right anterior aortic sinus. It is smaller than the left. The RCA goes forward toward the right side between the pulmonary trunk and the right auricle. Then it pass through the right anterior coronary sulcus and reach the right and inferior border of the heart. Then it binds the inferior border of the heart

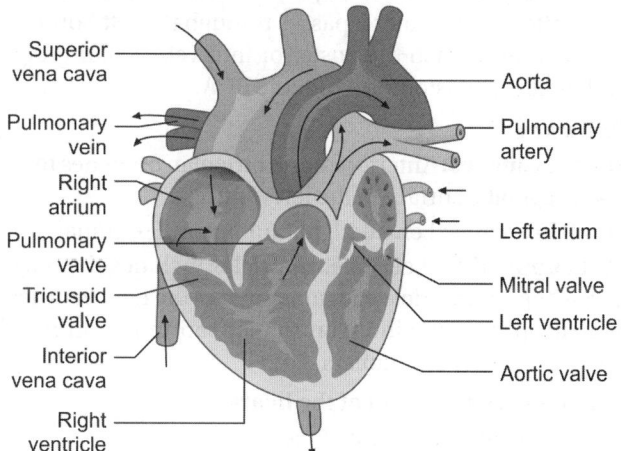

**Fig. 9.4:** Anatomy of heart.

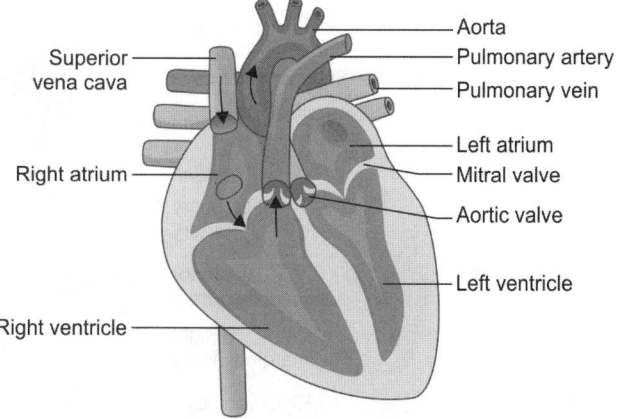

**Fig. 9.5:** Cardiac chambers.

and finally reach the diaphragmatic surface of the heart. Then it progress towards the back and reach the posterior interventricular groove and finally it anastomosis with the left coronary artery.

*Branches*

**Major branches:** Marginal and posterior interventricular.

**Minor branches:** Nodal, right atria, infundibular and terminal.

**RCA supplied to:** Right atrium, ventricles includes; major part of right ventricle, and small part of left ventricle, posterior part of the interventricular septum and the total conducting system of the heart except the left bundle branch.

**Left coronary artery**

The left coronary artery (LCA) emerging from the posterior left aortic sinus. It passes forwards through the left side and passes between the pulmonary trunk and the left auricle. Then the anterior interventricular branch emerging from the major artery then the major branch is named as the left circumflex artery. Later it passes through the left border of the heart and reach the posterior interventricular groove and finally it anastomosis with the RCA.

*Branches*

**Major branches:** Anterior interventricular, branches to the diaphragmatic surface of the left ventricle.

**Small branches:** Left atrial, pulmonary and terminal.

**LCA supplied to:** Left atria, ventricles includes the major part of the left ventricle and minor part of the right ventricle, anterior part of the interventricular septum and the left bundle branch (Chintamani, 2011).

**The venous circulation of the heart**

The major cardiac veins includes:
- Great cardiac vein
- Middle cardiac vein
- Right marginal vein
- Posterior vein of the left ventricle
- Oblique vein of the left atrium
- Right marginal vein
- Anterior cardiac vein
- Venae cordis minimae

The majority of the cardiac veins are drained into the **coronary sinus** except the anterior cardiac vein and the venae cordis minimae, they drain directly into the **right atrium**. The coronary sinus also opens into the right atrium **(Fig. 9.6)**.

**Lymphatic circulation of the heart**

It is mainly divided into two trunks; the **right trunk** that will drain into the brachiocephalic lymph nodes and the **left trunk** into the tracheobronchial lymph nodes at the carina level.

**Nerve supply to the cardiac tissues**

The vagus nerve supply the **parasympathetic** to the heart, it is a cardiac inhibitory type that is if it stimulates then the heart rate will reduce or bradycardia. The **sympathetic** supply is from the thoracic T2–T5 segment of the spinal cord. It is a type of cardiac acceleratory that is when it stimulated then there is tachycardia and coronary artery dilation (Chaurasia BD, 2019).

# PHYSIOLOGY OF CARDIOVASCULAR SYSTEM

## Conduction System of the Heart

The electrical signals initiates from the pacemaker of the heart that is called **SA node**. The SA node is situated at the atrial epicardium. The pacemaker cells having the intrinsic rhythm nature that is the reason without any stimulation of the nerve fibers from the brain, the pacemaker can initiate the cardiac contraction or signals at the regular intervals.

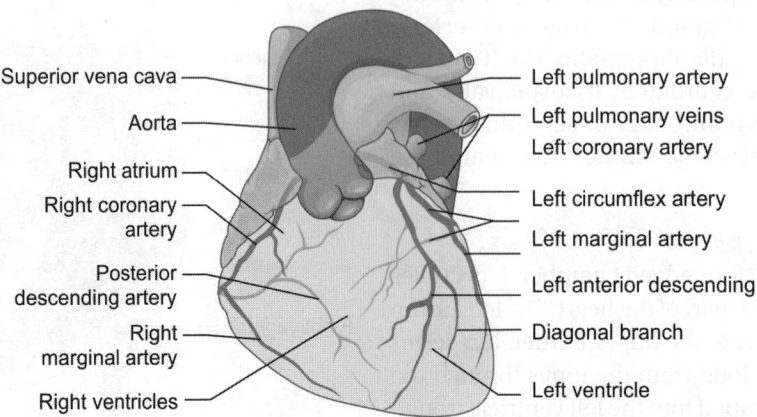

**Fig. 9.6:** Coronary circulation.

When the signal starts from the SA node then it will progress towards the both atria by intermodal pathways through the cell to cell conduction, then the both atria will contract. The specialized pathway between the inter atrial band is called **Bachmann's bundle**. This electrical impulse trigger the cardiac muscle contraction shown as the **P wave** in the ECG as the **atrial depolarization**. The electrical impulse from the atria then it reaches the AV node or atrioventricular node.

The AV node is situated at the inferior part of the right atria in the atrioventricular septum. There is a delay in the impulse transmission before the AV nodal contraction. During this pause the atria completely emptying into the ventricle. The impulses from the AV node then reaches the **Bundle of His**. Further it progressing through the interventricular septum. Then the bundle divided into the **right and left bundle branches**.

The left bundle branch is larger than the right. The left bundle is again branching into **anterosuperior fascicle and posteroinferior fascicle**. Then the electrical impulses passes through the **Purkinje fibers**, the cardiac conductive fibers, followed by the effective contraction of the ventricle as a result the blood is ejecting to the pulmonary trunk and the aorta. The total time duration from the initiation of the impulse from the SA node to the Purkinje fiber will take around 225 ms **(Fig. 9.7)** (Braunald's, 2007).

## Cardiac Cycle

The cardiac cycle is the time interval between the atrial contraction and the ventricular relaxation. The major events during the cardiac cycle are **systole and the diastole**. During the systolic phase the heart contracts and blood pumps into the circulation. During the diastolic phase the heart chambers get relaxed and filled with blood.

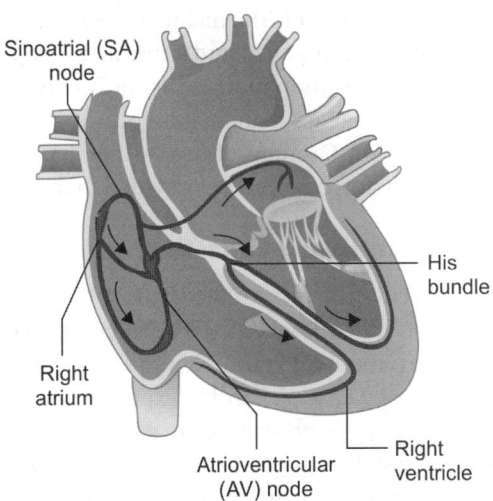

**Fig. 9.7:** Cardiac conduction system.

### Phases

The cardiac cycle starts with the relaxed atria and the ventricles. The impure blood is received in the right atria through the superior and the inferior vena cava and the pure blood is received in the left atria through the pulmonary veins. Then the atria contracts and the blood flows to the ventricles via the tricuspid and the mitral valves called **atrial systole (atrial depolarization or P wave in the ECG)**. At the end before the ventricular systole the atria in the relaxation phase are called **atrial diastole.**

At the end of the atria systole the ventricle contains around 130 mL of blood, called the **end diastolic volume or preload**. Then the heart going to the **ventricular systole (ventricular depolarization or QRS wave in the ECG)**, it has 2 phases, **isovolumic contraction:** The initial phase of the ventricular contraction and **ventricular ejection phase**. Then the ventricles contract and the blood ejected into the aorta and the pulmonary artery through the semilunar valves. The amount of blood ejected from the ventricle in each beat is called the **stroke volume (SV)**, normally around 70–80 mL. The remaining blood in the ventricle is called **end systolic volume**, 50–60 mL.

The last phase is called the **ventricular diastole**, it is the **repolarization of the ventricles** as the **T wave in the ECG**. The early stage of this phase is called **isovolumic ventricular relaxation**. During the second phase, **late ventricular diastole**, the pressure inside the ventricle drops less than that of atria and the next cycle will start again (Woods SL, 2010).

### Cardiac Output

It defines how much volume of blood pumped by each ventricle in one minute.

**CO = SV × HR**

The normal cardiac output (CO) range in a normal adult at rest is 4–8 L/mt.

The cardiac index (CI) is the CO divided by the body mass index. The normal value is between 2.8–4.2 L/mt/m².

### Factors influencing cardiac output

**The factors affecting the stroke volume are:**

- **Preload:** The volume of blood in the ventricle at the end of diastole. According to the Frank Starlings law increasing the stretching of the myocardium the force of contraction also increased. The preload determines the amount of stretching.
- **Contractility:** The contractility increased by the release of the epinephrine and the norepinephrine by the sympathetic system.
- **After load:** It is the resistance against which the ventricle wants to contract. The afterload is determined by the

size of the ventricle, arterial BP and the ventricle wall tension.
- Other factors include heart size, gender and the duration of the contraction.

**Factors affecting the HR are:**
The major factors that increasing the HR and force of contraction:
- Cardioaccelerator–norepinephrine release
- Proprioceptor–during exercise increase the rate of firing
- Chemoreceptor–hypoxia, acidosis, hypercapnia and lactic acid production
- Baroreceptor–decrease the firing rate
- Catecholamines–epinephrine and norepinephrine
- Thyroid hormones–elevated T3-T4
- Calcium–increased $Ca^{2+}$
- Potassium–decreased $K^+$
- Sodium–decreased $Na^+$
- Temperature of the body—elevated
- Nicotine and caffeine—increase the HR

Factors that decreasing the HR and contraction:
- Cardioinhibitory nerve (vagus)—release acetylcholine
- Proprioceptor—decrease firing rate after the exercise
- Chemoreceptors—elevated $O_2$, low $H^+$ ions, and low $CO_2$
- Baroreceptors—increased rate indicating the hypertension
- Catecholamines—decrease epinephrine and norepinephrine
- Thyroid hormones—low T3-T4
- Potassium—elevated $K^+$
- Sodium—elevated $Na^+$
- Temperature of the body—decreased (Chintamani, 2011).

The cardiovascular system is one of the vital system in our body start the activity at the 4 weeks in the fetal life and the last system to cease the activity at the end of the life. The cardiovascular system consists of the systemic circulation and the pulmonary circulation.

## PRINCIPLES OF NURSING IN CARING FOR PATIENTS WITH CARDIOVASCULAR DISORDERS

According to Sidney CS et al. (2004) there are different principles in caring and preventing the cardiovascular diseases.
- Governments, national societies, and foundations should collaborate to develop clinical and public health guidelines for CVD prevention that target risk factors.
- Evidence based guidelines should incorporate professional judgment on the translation of such evidence into effective and efficient care addressing all areas of CVD risk.
- The assessment of total CVD risk should be based on epidemiological risk factor data appropriate to the population to which it is applied.
- Policy recommendations and guidelines should emphasize a total risk approach for CVD prevention.
- The intensity of interventions should be a function of the total risk of CVD, with lower treatment thresholds for higher-risk patients.
- National cardiovascular societies/foundations should promote routine prospective collection of validated national vital statistics on the causes and outcomes of CVD for use in the development of national policies.
- National professional societies should inform policymakers of risk factor targets and drug therapies for prevention of CVD that are culturally and financially appropriate to their nation and ask the government to incorporate prevention of CVD into legislation whenever relevant.
- National professional societies/foundations should facilitate CVD prevention through education and training programs for health professionals.
- National professional societies should assess the achievement of lifestyle, risk factor, and therapeutic targets defined in the national guidelines.
- Health professionals should include prevention of CVD as an integral part of their daily clinical practice.

## ASSESSMENT OF CARDIOVASCULAR SYSTEM

Cardiovascular assessment is an important management part of the cardiac patient. The history collection including the present and past medical and surgical history and the complete physical examination particularly concentrating on the cardiovascular assessment is helpful for the accurate diagnosis and the treatment of the cardiac patient. Then only priority nursing care can be provided to the patient.

### Cardiovascular History Collection

The cardiovascular history collection is the initial step of the assessment part. After getting a detailed history we can categorize the patient into emergency care, acute care and not an emergency case. A cardiac expert nurse or doctor can easily identify the priority of the patient through their experience and skill. Through a thorough history collection help the health care provider to maintain a good and positive therapeutic client relationship.

The important part of the history collection includes:
- Identification data
- Chief complaints
- Present history
- Past history
- System wise review
- Family history of illness
- Personal history
- Socioeconomic history

## Identification Data

Name of the patient, age, gender, address including the contact number of the patient and the relatives, educational status of the patient, income of the family, occupation, and the data should be obtained directly from the patient otherwise from the secondary source that should be mentioned clearly.

## Chief Complaints

This is the important and the key point of the history collection part. The complaints should be state clearly and can write in the quotation mark, e.g., chest pain for 3 hrs. If the patient had more than two complaints then the complaints should be in the priority wise and in the chronologic order.

## Present History

In this step the health care provider should ask about the details of the chief complaints. The complaints should be elaborated as time of onset, frequency and duration, location, quality, quantity, related symptoms, alleviating and aggravating factors, effect of the symptoms on the daily life, etc.

The **time of onset** includes the date and accurate time of starting of the symptoms. The way the symptoms starts also important whether it starts acutely or slowly progressing type. The **duration and frequency** of the symptom also important. It should be specific like, for how long the patient had the problem and the frequency of the symptom, e.g., once in a week or once in a day like that. The duration of the symptom and the time of onset usually determine the type of treatment for that patient.

The next point is the **location** or the site of pain. Usually the pain with the cardiac origin is always sternum or the precordial origin. The pain usually diffuses in nature. If the patient can point the location with a fingertip then it is related to the chest wall abnormality. The **quality** of the symptoms should be asked to the patient to describe on their own words. It includes the type of pain squeezing type/tightening/pressing/strangling/constricting. The quantity of the symptom includes the size, depth and the severity. Sometimes we can measure it with the help of a pain score scale (Woods SL).

The **related symptoms** include palpitation, dizziness, etc., that always along with the actual symptoms. The **alleviating factors** include res, position change, and medication also mention clearly.

The **aggravating** factors include exercise, walking, climbing steps, eating, cold, etc. The recent diagnostic findings, surgery everything should be included in the present history.

## Past History

It includes the past medical problems and the surgical events with details. The major points include childhood illness, accidents, allergy, medicine history like any medication for long term use, etc.

## Family History

The importance of family history is to find out the risk factors in the family. It includes the age and health status of the first-degree family history should made. The history of cardiac diseases, hypertension, diabetes, sudden death, etc., should be confirm with the patient.

## Personal and Socioeconomic History

The important point includes the personal health habits of the patient like smoking, alcohol use, tobacco, drug abuse and the nutritional type, sleep, physical activity, etc., should be covered under the personal history. The socioeconomic history includes the income, the earning member of the family, and the relation with the family members and the neighbors (Chintamani, 2011).

### Causes of the Cardiac Chest Pain and Discomfort

- Coronary artery disease (CAD)
- Acute coronary syndrome
- Stable angina
- Ischemic cardiomyopathy
- Noncoronary artery disease
- Aortic dissection
- Acute pulmonary embolism
- Aortic stenosis
- Aortic regurgitation
- Hypertrophic and restrictive cardiomyopathy
- Pulmonary hypertension

### Causes of the Noncardiac Chest Pain and Discomfort

Pulmonary
- Pleuritis
- Pneumonia

- Tracheobronchitis
- Pneumothorax
- Mediastinitis
- Tumor

Musculoskeletal
- Costochondritis
- Intercostals muscle cramps
- Cervical disc disease

Others
- Herpes zoster
- Emotional
- Chest wall tumor
- Disorder of the breast

### Physical Assessment

The physical examination is an integral part of the cardiovascular assessment. After the completion of the history collection the physician or the assigned nurse can do the physical assessment. The major parts in the physical assessment includes—general appearance, head, skin, musculoskeletal system, arterial pulse, jugular venous pressure, blood pressure, peripheral vascular system and heart assessment. Apart from the cardiovascular assessment the regular head to toe and the system wise assessment also needed.

### General Appearance

The general appearance includes the body build of the patient, dyspnea, skin color, distended neck veins, posture of the patient, appropriateness of weight includes; cachexia, and malnutrition, arachnodactyly, tall stature seen in Marfan's syndrome, others include the conscious level of the patient and orientation status with the time/place/person and along with that the anxiety level of the patient.

### Anthropometric Measurements

It includes height, weight, body mass index (BMI) and the waist circumference of the patient. The weight indicates the nutrition and the fluid status of the patient. The BMI can be calculated by the weight in Kg divided by the height in m$^2$. The BMI more than 25 Kg/m$^2$ is called overweight and the value more than 30 Kg/m$^2$ is called obesity. In overweight people the abdominal waist circumference more than 102 cm for men and 88 cm for females are considered as the cardiovascular risk (Woods SL, 2010).

### Head

It includes the facial features, color, temperature, skin and eyes.

### Facial features

The facial feature examination gives an idea about cardiovascular diseases. The presence of the malar flush, cyanotic lips, jaundice from the hepatic congestion suggesting the rheumatic heart disease with severe mitral stenosis and in aortic regurgitation de Musset's sign or the head bobbing with each heartbeat can be seen. Facial edema can be seen in patients with constrictive pericarditis and tricuspid valve disease. Sever hypertension, tachyarrhythmia and episodic facial flushing can be seen in patients with pheochromocytoma. Butterfly rashes on the face suggestive of systemic lupus erythematosus (SLE) indicating inflammatory heart disease. Dry, sparse hair, loss of lateral eyebrows, dull expression less face and periorbital puffiness can be seen in patients with myxedema due to the reduced cardiac output and heart failure associated with hypothyroidism. Moon face, hirsutism, acne, hypertension and centripetal obesity can be seen in patients with Cushing's syndrome.

### Skin

*Pallor* indicates the anemia and the *jaundice* indicates the hepatic congestion due to right heart failure. Cyanosis is the bluish discoloration of the skin. The *peripheral cyanosis* should be checked at the tip of the nose, earlobe and lips. The *central cyanosis* is more serious than the peripheral cyanosis, for central we should check the buccal mucosa, tongue and oropharyngeal mucosa indicates the right to left shunt in the heart. In the Eisenmenger's syndrome there is clubbing of nails in the fingers and toes and central cyanosis.

The primary and the secondary hemochromatosis patients there will be bronze discoloration of the skin in the unexposed areas. Palmer and plantar keratosis can be seen in patients with arrhythmogenic right ventricular dysplasia. Tendon xanthoma, xanthoma within the palmar creases and subcutaneous lipid nodules indicate the familial hyperlipidemia and suggest coronary artery disease.

### Temperature

The body temperature should be checked for ICU patients every 4 hourly. After the cardiac surgery the temperature should check every 1,530 minutes to verifying the re warmth of the patient body. And also the hyperthermia indicates the infection, that why the temperature should be record regularly (Chatterjee K, 2013).

### Eye

A thin grayish white circle around the iris may be with aging is called senile arcus or corneal arcus. It is due to the hyperlipidemia. Slightly raised yellow colored plaques at the side of the nose in the both eyes called xanthelasma. In case of bacterial endocarditis there will be ophthalmitis, petechial and subconjunctival hemorrhage can see. Red spots in the retina suggestive of the hypertension. In subacute bacterial endocarditis and leukemia case there is roth's spots in the retina with hemorrhages with white center.

## Musculoskeletal System

The patients with Marfan syndrome are tall with kyphoscoliosis, pectus deformities and the head to pubis segment is longer than the pubis to feet segment. Apart from this there is high arched palate, lax joints and arachnodactyly also there. In cases of aortic regurgitation, mitral regurgitation and atrioventricular block, ankylosing spondylitis may be there. Splinter hemorrhage, Osler's node and Janeway lesions are suggestive of bacterial endocarditis.

## Arterial Pulse

The detailed assessment of the arterial pulse is essential to identify the proper evaluation of the peripheral blood supply. The pulse rate/rhythm/amplitude/contour and the blood flow while obstruction of the blood flow is the major characteristics of the pulse. During the initial assessment of the patient the carotid/radial/femoral/tibial dorsal pulses should evaluate and compare with the both sides.

## Rate and Rhythm

The rate and rhythm of the pulse can be check in the radial artery. The normal **rate** is between 60–100 beats/minutes. The pulse rate may change according to the underlying cardiac problems, especially in case of the tachycardia conditions, every heart rate not carried to the periphery. That is the reason the pulse rate should not match with the heart rate monitored in the electronic monitor and the ECG. The pulse rate should count for one minute in case of irregular rhythm and for 15 sec and multiply it by 4 in case of regular rhythm.

The **rhythm** of the pulse is usually regular. The physiologic changes can be seen in respiratory phases. During the inspiration the blood flow to the right heart is increased and the right ventricular output also increased that's why the pulmonary venous capacitance also increased. As a result the left side blood flow decreased that may result in the decreased stroke volume. To compensate to maintain the cardiac output the heart rate may increase slightly during the inspiration phase. During the expiration time the pulmonary blood reaches the left side of the heart and because of the Frank starling's law there is a stretch in the left ventricle and there is an increase in the stroke volume. To maintain the normal cardiac output the heart rate come back to the normal value. This physiological change is called the sinus arrhythmia. Other than the physiological change are not normal (Brunner and Suddarth, 2008).

### Amplitude and Contour

The pulse can be classified into absent, present and bounding pulse or another classification is absent (0), diminished (1+), normal (2+), moderately increased (3+), and markedly increased (4+).

*Small and weak pulse indicates* the diminished pulse because of the reduced cardiac output. Large and bounding pulse indicates the increased stroke volume. The *Corrigan's pulse* can see in case of aortic regurgitation, it is type of bounding pulse seen in carotid artery.

The *contour* of the pulse indicates the rate of rise and the shape of the arterial pulse. The normal contour described as rapid and smooth upstroke. *Pulsus bisferiens* is described as a rapid upstroke and two systolic peak. This can be seen in patients with idiopathic hypertrophic subaortic stenosis, aortic stenosis and aortic insufficiency. Pulsus alternans is the type in which strong pulse and weak pulses alternatively. *Bigeminal pulse* is a type in which there is a bigeminal premature ectopic weak pulse is there. *Pulsus paradoxus* is the pulse with reduced strength during the inspiration.

### Bruit

It is similar to the murmur due to the turbulent blood flow through the arterial blood vessels. If bruit is present on the carotid artery tells that partial obstruction of the blood supply to the brain and in the femoral bruit indicates the partial obstruction of the blood flow towards the lower limbs. During the auscultation for bruit sound tell the patient to withhold the breath during examination to exclude the abnormal breath sounds.

## Jugular Venous Pulse

Jugular venous pulse (JVP) indicates the hemodynamic changes of the right side of the heart. Jugular venous pressure indicates the right ventricular diastolic pressure. The normal value of the JVP is less than 9 cm of $H_2O$ **(Fig. 9.10)**.

*Steps for measuring the JVP include:*

- The right jugular vein reflects the accurate value of the right side hemodynamic value. It lie deeper to the sternocleidomastoid muscle and the pulse is coming to the skin.
- The patient should be in the supine position with the head and neck at the straight line.
- The head end should elevated at 15–30 degrees.
- Turn the neck slightly to the left side to visualize the right internal jugular vein and can see the jugular meniscus properly.

- Place a ruler scale vertically over the angle of Lewis or the sternal angle and place another ruler scale or a tongue blade horizontally at the point of maximum impulse of the jugular vein then it will intersect the vertical scale.
- Measure the vertical distance above the sternal angle. If the value more than 3 cm then the JVP is elevated.

### Blood Pressure

The blood pressure can be measure by either auscultatory method or arterial BP technique. The auscultatory method needs the sphygmomanometer and it should be validated. The normal BP is 120/80 mm Hg. The prehypertension is defined as the systolic BP between 120–139 mm Hg and diastolic BP between 80–90 mm Hg. The pre hypertension people are more prone to progress towards the chronic BP cases. The hypertension can be defined as the systolic BP more than 140 mm Hg and the diastolic BP more than 90 mm Hg (Brunner and Suddarth, 2008).

### Auscultatory Gap

It is a temporary disappearance of the *Korotkoff sound* at the late phase I or in the phase II. It is very common in case of the hypertensive patents. The gap may be around 40 mm Hg. This error can be resolved by the palpatory method of BP technique before going to the auscultatory method.

### Phases of Korotkoff sounds

1. It is the point at which the first faint then continuous tapping sound can hear. The intensity of the sound is increasing during the deflation of the cuff. The first of the at least two sounds called the *systolic BP*.
2. During this phase with the cuff deflation the murmur sound can hear.
3. The more intensity sound.
4. The point at which the sound become soft and muffled in nature, called *diastolic BP*.
5. The pressure level after that the regular sound can hear then no sounds.

### Peripheral Vascular System

In this assessment include both the artery and venous assessment. The assessment should be cross check with the both half of the body **(Figs. 9.8 to 9.11)**.

### Clubbing

It is the enlargement of the nails at the phalanges. There may be change in the angle between the phalanges and the nail bed or floating type of the nails. The normal angle is less than 1,800, in case of clubbing it may be more than 1,950 **(Fig. 9.9)**. Usually the distal phalangeal depth is less than the interphalangeal depth, in case of clubbing the distal phalangeal depth may increase than the interphalangeal depth.

### Capillary Refill

It gives an idea about the peripheral blood supply. The tip of the nail is depressed with pressure, then the nail bed becomes pale and when the pressure released the blood supply is returned back spontaneously, usually less than 3 seconds (Brunner and Suddarth, 2008).

### Edema

It is the extra fluid accumulation at the interstitial spaces. The major causes include right side heart failure, hypoalbuminemia, excessive renal retention of sodium and water, lymph edema. The nature of the edema also should check including the pitting edema score **(Fig. 9.8)**.

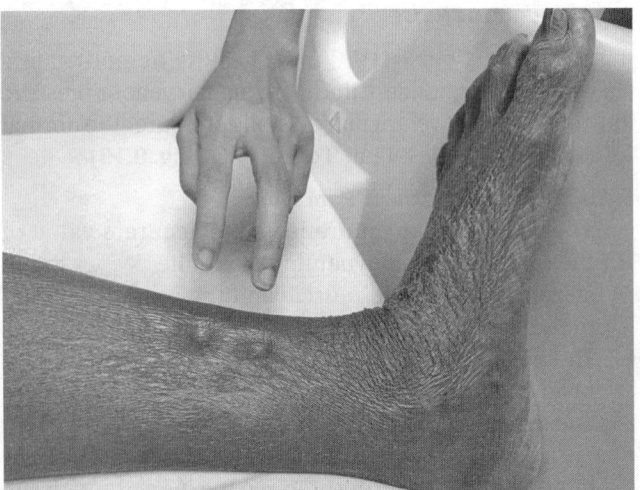

**Fig. 9.8:** Pitting edema.

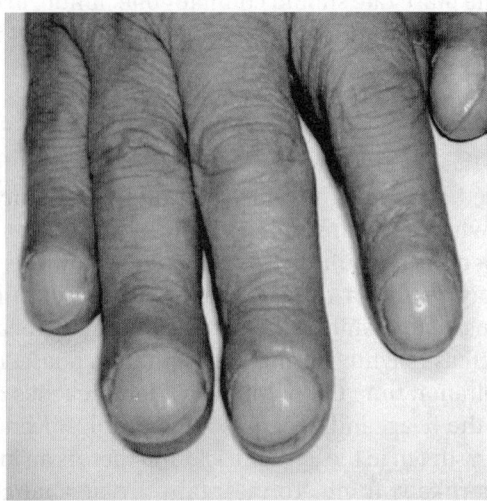

**Fig. 9.9:** Clubbing of nails.

## Thrombophlebitis

It is the inflammation of the vein due to the clot formation. It may be superficial, affecting the superficial veins that may be hard, red, sensitive to pressure, warmth and engorged another type is deep vein thrombosis, there may be pain, edema, and cyanotic in nature. Homan's sign (**Fig. 9.11**) is the pain on the dorsiflexion of the foot.

## Varicose Vein

Varicose veins are the tortuous, dilated superficial veins. It is due to the weakness of the valve of the veins, intrinsic weakness of the vein wall, increased pressure inside the vein and arteriovenous fistulas. During the inspection time should check the presence of varicose veins.

## Cardiac Assessment

The knowledge on the cardiac areas on the chest is very important to assess the heart very easily. The left ventricle or the *mitral area* over the 5th inter costal space (ICS) medial to the mid clavicular line is the apex of the heart, the right ventricle or the *tricuspid area* over the left of the sterna border at the 4–5th ICS, the *pulmonary area* over the left 2nd ICS, *ascending aorta* at the right 2nd ICS (**Fig. 9.12**).

### Inspection

The inspection of the chest is important to assess the visible pulsation. During the inspection phase the patient should be in the supine, propped up position. Check the pulsation and the retraction or the inward movement of the chest. Should note the point where the changes are present. In some patients the apex impulse is visible, but not for all patients. It is visible in the thin patients and not visible in the obese patients, the patients with large breast and barrel chest patients. The visible pulsation over the aortic area indicates the aortic aneurysm, over the pulmonic area indicates the increased filling pressure in the pulmonary artery.

### Palpation

All the cardiac areas should palpate for the pulsation with the fingertip or the base of the fingers. Usually the thrill can elicit with the help of palpation method. Thrill is the turbulence associated with the murmurs. The apex impulse can get easily through the palpation. If the impulse that we felt is diffuse, increased amplitude, laterally or inferiorly displaced indicates that fluid overload or the left ventricular dilation in case of the mitral insufficiency or the left ventricular failure. Palpate the tricuspid area to find the right ventricular enlargement. Then palpate the pulmonary and the aortic area for thrill or any enlargement.

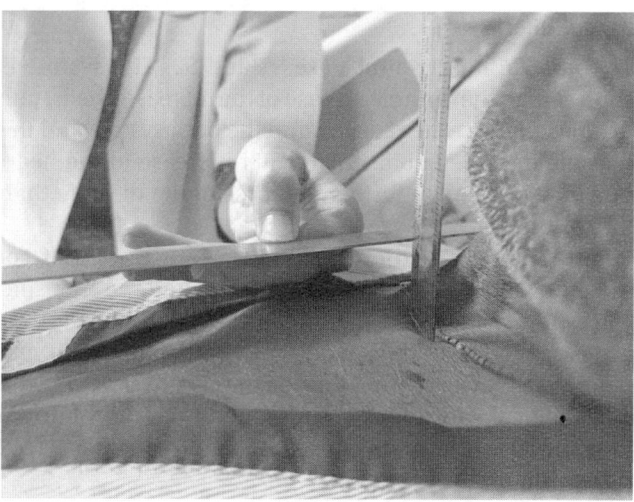

**Fig. 9.10:** JVP monitoring.

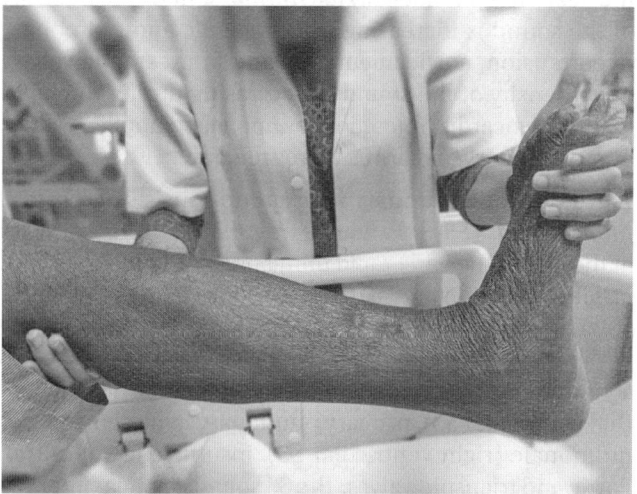

**Fig. 9.11:** Homan's sign.

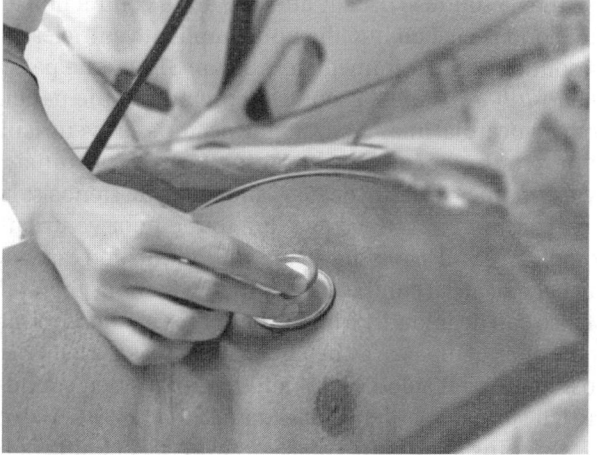

**Fig. 9.12:** Cardiac auscultation.

## Auscultation

The normal heart sounds are S1 and S2. The systole is shorter than the diastole. In case of the increased heart rate the diastole become reduced and the both systole and the diastole become equal. The further increase in the heart rate may lead to the further decrease of the diastole than the systole.

The **first heart sound** or the S1 means the closure of the atrioventricular valves or the mitral and the tricuspid valves. It is the loudest and the apex beat of the heart. S1 is described as the *lub* sound. The splitting of the S1 can hear at the lower sternal border that is physiologic. The pathological splitting is mainly due to the right bundle branch block, tricuspid stenosis and the atrial septal defect. (Chintamani, 2011)

The **second heart sound** or the S2 indicates the closure of the mitral and pulmonary valve; it is loudest at the base of the heart. It is phonetically tell the *dub* sound. The intensity of the sound is increasing with systemic and pulmonary hypertension, aortic aneurysm, and in prosthetic valves. The intensity of the sound is decreasing during the heart failure, myocardial infarction, pulmonary embolism, shock and pulmonary and aortic valve stenosis.

**Extra diastolic sounds:** In this group consists of *diastolic filling sounds (S3–S4)* and *opening snaps*. The S3 sound is at the end of the early rapid filling phase and the S4 is with atrial contraction and at the rapid active filling time.

The *physiologic S3* sound is common in the young athletes and it will disappear at the age of 40 years. The S3 sound after 40 years of age is the indication of left heart failure (left ventricular S3), primary pulmonary hypertension, cor pulmonale (right ventricular S3), insufficiency of mitral, aortic and tricuspid valves. The S3 sound can hear after the S2 sound like *lub-dup-ta*. Usually with help of bell side of the stethoscope can able to differentiate the S3 sound clearly.

The S4 sound is usually after the atrial contraction and the blood is ejected into the noncompliant ventricles. The S4 sound can hear immediately before S1 and the pattern like *ta-lub-dup*. The S4 sound is common in the patients with myocardial infarction, angina pectoris, left ventricular hypertrophy because of the long term hypertension, hypertrophic cardiomyopathy, and in aortic stenosis. It is very common in the old age due to the poor ventricular compliance and it is absent in the atrial fibrillation cases due the need of atrial contraction for the S4. Same as the S3 the S4 also can hear loudly with the bell of the stethoscope and at the apex of the heart when the patient is at the left lateral position for left sided sound and the right sided sound at the left sternal boarder (Chintamani, 2011).

**Opening snaps** are associated with the opening of the stenotic mitral valve. The opening snaps can't hear in the normal valves. The sound is high pitched and is very audible with the diaphragm of the stethoscope. This sound is at the early phase of diastole and medial to the apex.

**Extra systolic sounds:** It consists of mainly early systolic ejection sounds and systolic clicks. Early systolic sounds because of the coincide with the opening of the aortic and pulmonic valves. The aortic ejection sound can better hear at the base or apex of the heart and the pulmonic ejection sound can hear at the 2nd or 3rd left ICS. The major causes for the aortic ejection sound are dilated aorta and aortic stenosis and the causes of pulmonic ejection sounds are pulmonary artery dilation, pulmonary hypertension and pulmonary stenosis. The mid to late systolic clicks are due to the mitral valve prolapsed, and usually they are followed by the murmur (Chintamani, 2011).

### Murmurs

The heart murmur are the extra sounds due to the turbulent blood flow in the heart or great blood vessels. The major causes include:

- Increased flow rate across the normal heart valves, e.g., exercise, pregnancy, anemia
- Blood flow through the partially obstructed valves, e.g., valvular stenosis, pulmonary and systemic hypertension
- Blood flow through the valves with irregularities without obstruction, e.g., bicuspid aortic valves, thickening of the aortic cusps with aging
- Blood flow into the dilated aortic root
- Valvular regurgitation

### Classification of murmurs

- *According to systolic diastolic timing and duration:* Systolic and diastolic, continuous, holosystolic; early systolic, mid systolic or ejection murmur, early or late systolic murmur
- *Intensity:* Grading of murmur **(Table 9.2)**
- *Location:* Where the sound can hear loudly
- *Radiation:* Radiated to back, neck, axilla
- *Configuration:* Crescendo, decrescendo, diamond, plateau and variable

**Table 9.2:** Grading of murmur.

| Grade | Description |
|---|---|
| 1. | Very faint, may not heard in all position |
| 2. | Quiet, but can hear with stethoscope |
| 3. | Moderately loud |
| 4. | Loud with palpable thrill |
| 5. | Very loud with thrill |
| 6. | Very loud with thrill may be with stethoscope completely off the chest |

- *Quality:* Harsh, rough, rumbling, blowing and squeaking, musical.

Pericardial friction rub

- *Timing:* Atrial systole, ventricular systole and ventricular diastole
- *Location:* Variable, best at the 3rd left ICS
- *Radiation:* Little
- *Intensity:* Variable, may increase when the patient bend forward, exhale, and hold breath
- *Quality*: Scratchy and scraping
- *Pitch:* High

# HYPERTENSIVE CRISIS

Hypertensive crisis are the acute, and severe elevation of blood pressure, defines as an elevation of diastolic blood pressure more than 140 mm Hg, with or without target organ damage. Hypertensive emergencies are the type of hypertensive crisis it is characterized by acute, severe elevation of the blood pressure over hours to days usually greater than 180/110 mm Hg or the BP more than 200/120 mm Hg and associated with the presence of target organ damage. Hypertensive urgencies are characterized by similar acute elevation of BP over days to weeks, but no target organ damage. When compare the hypertensive crisis, emergencies and urgency the first two contributes one fourth of the presentations and the last one contributes the major part that is three fourth **(Fig. 9.13)** (Chintamani, 2011).

*Target organ damage includes:*

- **Neurologic:** Cerebral infarction, hypertensive encephalopathy, intracerebral hemorrhage or subarachnoid hemorrhage
- **Cardiovascular:** Acute pulmonary edema, acute congestive heart failure, acute coronary ischemia
- **Renal:** Acute kidney injury/failure
- **Liver:** Liver enzymes elevated (in HELLP syndrome)
- **Ocular:** Retina hemorrhage/exudates
- **Vascular:** Eclampsia, aortic dissection.

## Risk Factors

- Obesity
- Hypertensive patient
- Coronary artery disease
- Higher number of hypertensive medications
- Nonadherence with hypertensive medication
- Intoxications (cocaine, amphetamines, phencyclidine)
- Withdrawal syndrome (clonidine or beta antagonists)
- Drug drug/food interactions (monoamine oxidase inhibitors and tricyclic antidepressants, antihistamines and tyramine)
- Spinal cord disorders
- Pheochromocytoma
- Pregnancy
- Collagen vascular diseases (systemic lupus erythematosus).

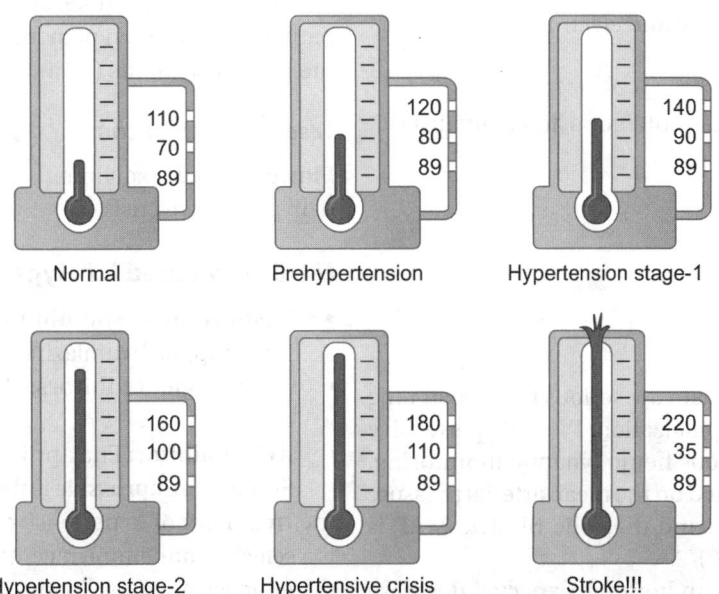

**Fig. 9.13:** Hypertensive crisis.

## Clinical Manifestations

Hypertensive emergencies manifested by *hypertensive encephalopathy*. The clinical manifestations include:
- Sudden rise in BP
- Headache
- Nausea
- Vomiting
- Seizure
- Confusion
- Stupor
- Coma
- Blurred vision
- Transient blindness
- Papilledema
- Retinopathy

*Renal insufficiency:* Minor impairment to complete shutdown of renal function.

*Cardiac decompensation:* Unstable angina to infarction, chest pain, dyspnea (Brunner and Suddarth, 2008).

## Pathophysiological Changes in Patients with Hypertensive Crisis

See **Flowchart 9.1**.

## Diagnostic Evaluations
- History and physical examination; indicates the severe hypertension
- Blood pressure monitoring in both arms
- Urine toxicology screening
- Serum glucose, creatinine and electrolytes
- CBC
- Liver function test
- Urine analysis (to check proteinuria and hematuria)
- Chest radiography
- ECG
- Echocardiography
- Pregnancy screening
- Head and chest CT scan

## Management

Hypertensive emergencies are the serious life-threatening condition. It requires hospitalization, IV antihypertensive medication with continuous hemodynamic monitoring. The major treatment is based on the mean arterial pressure (MAP) instead of systolic and diastolic BP. The MAP is calculated as (SBP + 2 DBP)/3.

In the first minutes to an hour the expected decrease in the MAP in around 25%, not more than that. The next 2–6 hours the target goal of BP is around 160/100–110 mm Hg if the patient is stable. The sudden decrease in the BP may result in the stroke/acute MI or renal failure. If the patient is stable then plan for a gradual reduction of BP in the next 24–48 hours (Chintamani, 2011).

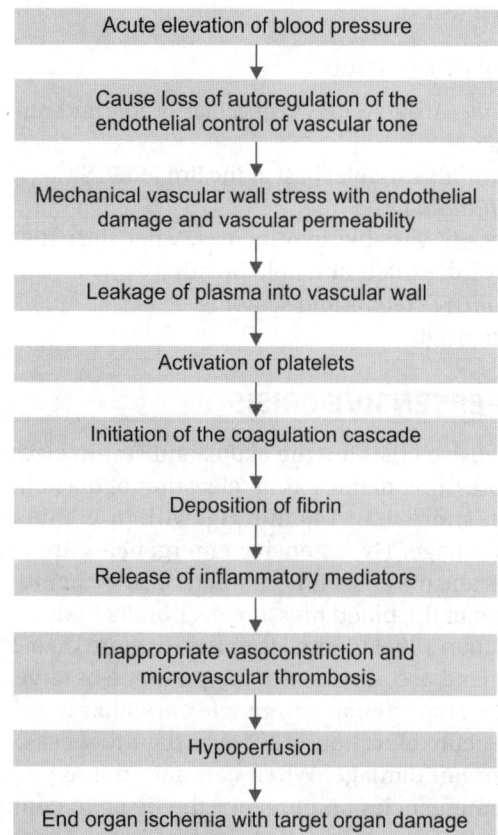

**Flowchart 9.1:** Pathophysiology of hypertensive crisis.

### Treatment Algorithm

**Flowchart 9.2**, explaining about the treatment algorithm of hypertensive crisis.

## Medication used for Hypertensive Emergencies
- **Vasodilators:** Sodium nitroprusside, nitroglycerin, fenoldopam, hydralazine and nicardipine
- **Adrenergic inhibitors:** Phentolamine, labetalol and esmolol
- **ACE inhibitor:** Enalapril

Sodium nitroprusside is the effective drug of choice for the treatment of hypertensive emergencies. Fenoldopam is a selective dopamine receptor activator causes renal and systemic vasodilation (Scott TB) (Brunner and Suddarth, 2008).

**Flowchart 9.2:** Treatment decision algorithm.

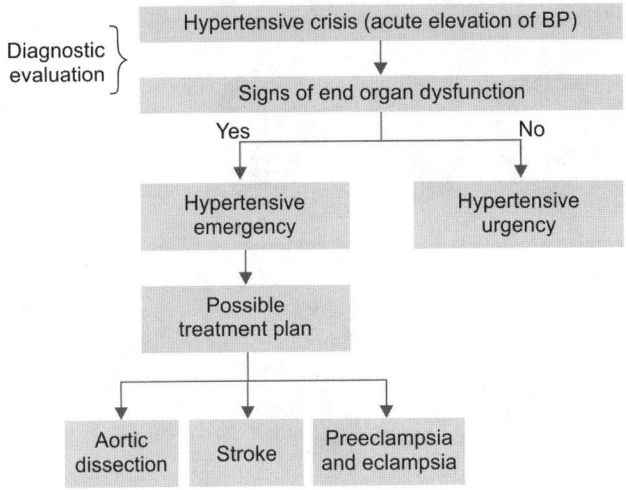

## Nursing Management

### Nursing Diagnosis

Decreased cardiac output related to altered myocardial contractility/inotropic changes as evidenced by increased heart rate (tachycardia), dysrhythmias and ECG changes.

### Nursing Interventions

- Check the BP and pulse rate of the patient every 2–3 minutes after the initiation of the IV antihypertensive medications.
- Regular monitoring of hemodynamic parameters and vital signs.
- Confirm the rate and dose of medication.
- Give oxygen as indicated by the patient's symptoms, oxygen saturation, and ABGs.
- Provide a restful environment and encourage periods of rest and sleep.
- Check for calf tenderness, diminished pedal pulses, swelling, local redness, or pallor of extremity.

### Nursing Diagnosis

Decreased activity tolerance related to abnormal heart rate or BP response to activity.

### Nursing Interventions

- System wise examination
- Patient education for avoid the recurrence
- Instruct patient in energy conserving techniques

Hypertensive crisis are the acute, and severe elevation of blood pressure, defines as an elevation of diastolic blood pressure more than 140 mm Hg, with or without target organ damage. Hypertensive urgencies are characterized by similar acute elevation of BP over days to weeks, but no target organ damage.

# CORONARY ARTERY DISEASE

Cardiovascular diseases are the major cause of death in the world. In which the coronary artery disease plays a vital role to contribute the number of deaths. The CAD mainly divided into asymptomatic or stable angina and acute coronary syndrome (ACS). The acute coronary syndrome refers to a group of conditions that occur due to acute myocardial ischemia and/or infarction as a result of a fast reduction in blood flow through the coronary artery circulation. It includes unstable angina and non-ST segment elevation myocardial infarction (UA/NSTEMI) as a combined phenomenon, as well as STEMI, but it is differentiated from other forms of cardiac ischemia **(Figs. 9.14 and 9.15)** (Brunner and Suddarth, 2008).

## Classification of CAD

**Flowchart 9.3** showing the important classification of coronary artery disease.

## Etiology

Atherosclerosis is the major etiology for the CAD. The intimal layer of the blood vessel wall gets deposited by cholesterol and lipids. The endothelial injury and the inflammatory response of the blood vessel wall make the major contribution to the formation of atherosclerosis **(Flowchart 9.4)** (Harrison, 2005).

## Pathophysiology of CAD

### Atherosclerosis Development—Progressive Stages

The progression of developing the atherosclerosis takes years. Once the patient becomes symptomatic then the individual may reach the advanced stage of the

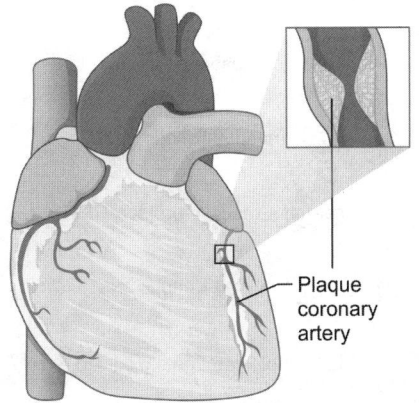

**Fig. 9.14:** Atherosclerosis in the coronary artery.

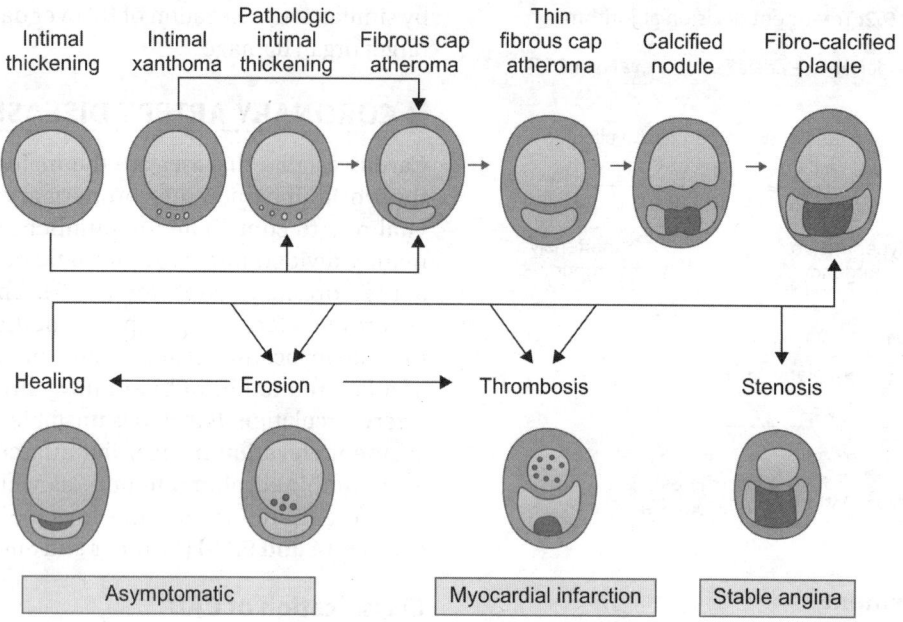

**Fig. 9.15:** Stages of atherosclerosis.

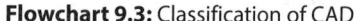

**Flowchart 9.3:** Classification of CAD.

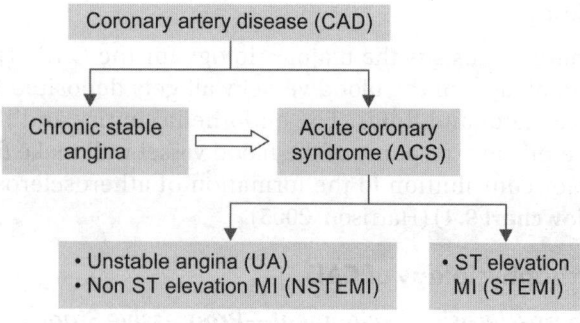

**Flowchart 9.4:** Pathophysiology of CAD.

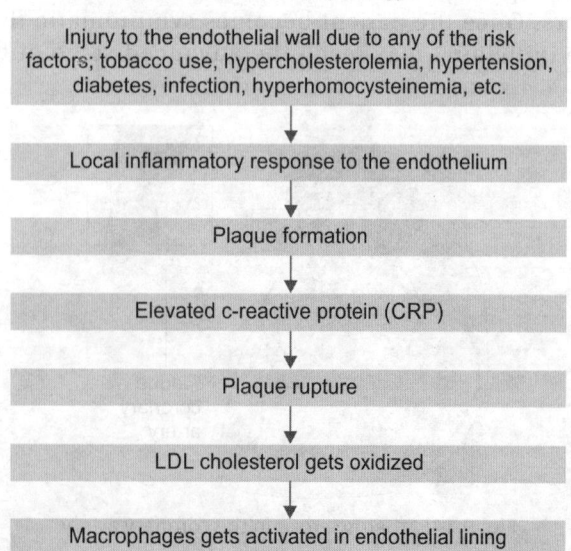

atherosclerosis. The early steps start with the risk factors that lead to the endothelial injury in the intimal layer. It is the important part of the atherosclerosis formation. The macrophages, platelets come ant attach the area near to the endothelial injury. Then there is a progressive stage of development of atherosclerosis takes place (Chintamani, 2011).

The major stages include:
- **Fatty streak:** This is the earliest lesion develop in the intimal layer. The smooth muscle cells emigration from the media to the intima layer and it engulf the fat cells. That is the reason the yellowish discoloration in the intimal layer.
- **Fibrous plaque:** The endothelial layer repairs normally, but the patients at risk for the atherosclerosis the repair takes more time to heal. The smooth muscle proliferation stimulated by the LDL, growth factors, platelets and the thickening of the intimal layer wall. The collagen forming fibrous plaque makes the fatty streak gradually gets thickened and looks grayish and white in color. These plaques either at the one side of the artery or in the entire lumen of the artery. The edges may be smooth/irregular/rough/jagged. Ultimately the size of the lumen decrease and the blood flow to the distal area also decrease.
- **Complicated lesions:** This is the final and fatal stage of atherosclerotic lesion. After the continuous growth and inflammatory process leads to the plaque instability and more chance of ulceration and rupture. There is a loss of integrity of the intimal wall of the artery

leads to the accumulation of the platelets and finally there is formation of thrombus. It adhere the vessel wall and further narrowing of the arterial lumen. The exposed platelets cause binding of the fibrinogen to the glycoprotein IIb/IIIa receptors. That gain leads to the further platelet adhesion and increasing the size of the thrombus and called it as complicated lesion (Chintamani, 2011).

## Risk Factors

### Nonmodifiable Risk Factors

- **Age, gender (male>female):** More common in the middle age men and after the age of 65 years both male and female having the same rate of risk.
- **Ethnicity (Indian > whites)**
- **Family history:** Family history of hyperlipidemia, autosomal dominant disease, diabetes.

### Modifiable Risk Factors

- **Increased serum lipid values:** Total cholesterol more than 200 mg/dL, fasting triglycerides more than 150 mg/dL. Lipoproteins are the proteins that carries the fat in an across the body. There are different types of lipoproteins are there; high density lipoprotein (HDL), low density and very low density lipoproteins (LDL and VLDL). LDL >160 mg/dL is high value, HDL <40 mg/dL also risk factor for CAD.
- **Hypertension:** Patient with BP >140/90 mm Hg.
- **Diabetes mellitus:** Blood sugar level >126 mg/dL in fasting.
- **Smoking and tobacco:** 35–40% of death by smoking people due to CAD. Second hand smoking also may lead to develop CAD. Nicotine in the smoke lead to the release of catecholamine in the body. That leads to the increase HR, peripheral vasoconstriction and hypertension. Also the byproduct carbon monoxide reduces the oxygen carrying capacity of the blood. That may increase the work load of the heart.
- **Obesity and sedentary life style:** Individuals with BMI >30 Kg/m$^2$ is defined as the obese cases are more prone to develop CAD. Physical inactivity is also a major risk factor for CAD.
- **Alcohol use**
- **Psychological states:** Depression, hopelessness, stress, anxiety and anger (Brunner and Suddarth, 2008).

## Signs and Symptoms

**Angina:** Otherwise chest pain or angina is the major clinical manifestation of CAD or reversible myocardial ischemia. The major features of angina including, burning, squeezing or chest tightness. If the patient can point out the chest pain with a finger then it is not related to angina or myocardial ischemia.

### Pathophysiology of Angina

Flowchart 9.5 showing the pathophysiological changes of a patient with angina.

### Types of Angina

- **Stable angina:** It is due to myocardial ischemia/secondary to CAD. The major characteristics include, episodic type of pain lasting 5–15 min, increased by exertion and relieved by rest or nitroglycerin.
- **Unstable angina:** It is due to rupture of the plaque. It a new onset angina with increased frequency, duration and severity. It can occur at rest with less exertion and the pain refractory to nitroglycerin.
- **Prinzmetal's angina/variant angina:** It is due to the coronary vasospasm. It may occur at rest and triggered by smoking. It can present with or without CAD.
- **Nocturnal angina or angina decubitus:** It may occur at night, but no need that the individual in the recumbent position or in the sleeping time. In this type the patient is in the lying down position and the pain relieved by the sting or standing position (Woods SL, 2010).
- Nausea and vomiting
- Cool and clammy extremities
- Pallor
- Sweating
- Xanthelasma
- Dyspnea
- Fatigue

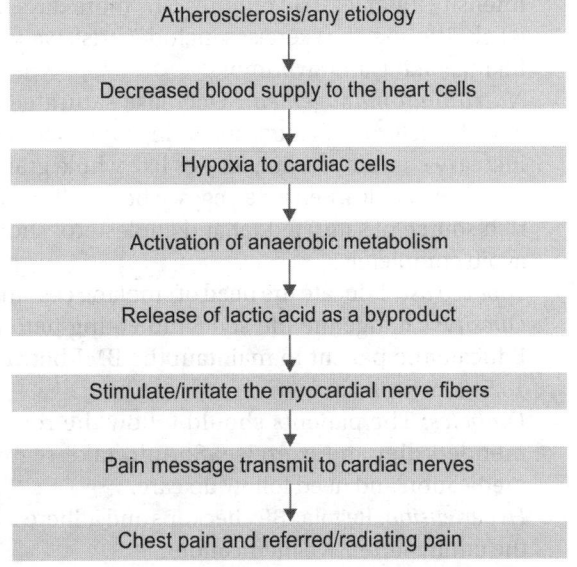

**Flowchart 9.5:** Pathophysiology behind angina.

## Diagnosis

- **Electrocardiography:** Ischemic changes including ST segment depression and T inversion.
- **Exercise stress test:** To detect the ST segment changes during exercise, indicating ischemia.
- **Coronary angiography:** It gives the clear idea about the location and percentage of block.
- **Stress echocardiography:** To find out the abnormal cardiac wall motion.
- **Myocardial perfusion imaging:** With thallium201 used during exercise treadmill test to detect the ischemic areas in the myocardium and it appear as the cold spots.
- **Laboratory studies:** CK MB, CBC, cardiac troponin, myoglobin, lipid profile, CRP, homocysteine (Brunner and Suddarth, 2008).
- Positron emission tomography.
- Electron Beam CT scan.
- Chest X-ray.

## Treatment

### Drug Therapy

- Antiplatelets, e.g., aspirin and clopilet
- Nitroglycerin, e.g., sublingual and IV nitroglycerin
- Beta blockers, e.g., atenolol, metoprolol and carvedilol
- Calcium channel blockers, e.g., nifedipine, verapamil and diltiazem
- ACE inhibitors, e.g., enalapril and captopril
- Lipid lowering agents

### Management of Risk Factors of CAD

- Identification of risk factors
- Management of risk factors:
  - *Physical activity*: Aerobic exercise with moderate intensity for at least 30 minutes 5 or more days in a week. The specific exercises include; brisk walking, hiking, biking and swimming.
  - *Nutritional management:* Decrease saturated fat and cholesterol rich foods including junk foods and increase complex carbohydrates like whole grains/fruits/vegetables. Red meat, eggs, whole milk are the rich source of saturated fat and cholesterol should avoid completely.
  - *Tobacco use:* Educate the need of smoking cessation
  - *Obesity:* Change the life style and eating pattern. Educate the patient to maintain the BMI between 18.5–24.9 Kg/m$^2$.
  - *Diabetes:* The patients should follow the recommended diet and exercise. Should take regular medication and need follow up care.
  - *Hypertension:* Regular BP checkups and adhere with the antihypertensive medications.
  - *Elevated serum lipids:* Reduce fat intake. Follow a strict diet control pattern. Take lipid lowering agents. Include more vegetables and fruits in the diet.
  - *Stress:* Give health education on tips to reduce stress. Consultation with psychiatric department for severe cases (Chintamani, 2011).

### Coronary Revascularization

- Percutaneous coronary intervention (PCI)
- Coronary artery bypass graft.

## Nursing Management

### Nursing Diagnosis

Decreased cardiac output related to CAD as evidenced by ECG changes, cool clammy extremities.

Nursing interventions

- Monitor the cardiovascular status
- Assess the peripheral pulses
- Assess the skin for cyanosis
- Fluid restricted diet
- Instruct the patient to take rest
- Maintain IO chart
- Give medications

Nursing diagnosis

Acute pain related to myocardial ischemia as evidenced by severe chest pain and radiating pain to shoulder.

Nursing interventions

Identify precipitating events, if any, as well as frequency, duration, intensity and location of the pain.

Nursing interventions

- Check the vital signs every five minutes during the initial angina attack.
- Provide complete rest during angina episodes.
- Elevate the head of the bed if the client is short of breath or during nitrates administration
- Administer antianginal medications as per order

Nursing diagnosis

Imbalanced nutrition less than body requirement related to decreased food intake

Nursing interventions

- Check the nutritional status of the patient
- To increase the weight
- To prevent hypertension
- To increase the amount

Nursing diagnosis

Insomnia related to the life-threatening disease condition as evidenced by the verbal statement of the patient.

Nursing interventions
- Assess the sleep pattern of the patient
- Educate the patient regarding the condition of the patient
- Educate the family members to give psychological support

The CAD mainly divided into asymptomatic or stable angina and acute coronary syndrome. The acute coronary syndrome refers to a group of conditions that occur due to acute myocardial ischemia and/or infarction as a result of a fast reduction in blood flow through the coronary artery circulation.

## ACUTE MYOCARDIAL INFARCTION

Myocardial infarction (MI) occurs due to the continuous ischemia and leads to the irreversible damage or infarction of the cardiac cells. When the coronary blood vessels get occlusion that leads to the decreased blood flow and the complete occlusion leads to the halt of blood supply to the particular distal area may lead to myocardial cell death. The acute MI takes time to complete as infarction. The cardiac cells can with stand the ischemia around 20 minutes. Approximately 4–6 hours may take to complete infarction. That is the reason the individual who is getting chest pain and the symptoms of ischemia should attend the hospital casualty as soon as possible. That can save the cardiac cells from infarction (Woods SL, 2010).

**Transmural:** The complete occlusion of the blood vessels causes the transmural type of MI **(Flowchart 9.6)**. As a result the entire myocardium gets infarction. This is otherwise called STEMI.

**Subendocardial:** It is also known as nontransmural or NSTEMI. In this case some parts of the subendocardium gets infarction. It may involve left ventricle/interventricular septum/papillary muscles (Chintamani, 2011).

### Causes
- Family history
- Age: Age advances the risk is increasing
- Gender: More common in males, and postmenopausal women
- Hypertension: >140/90 mm Hg
- Tobacco use
- Alcohol abuse
- Elevated cholesterol values
- Obesity: BMI> 30 Kg/m$^2$
- Sedentary life style
- Stress
- Type A personality
- Cocaine, amphetamine drug abusers.

### Pathophysiology of MI

Described briefly in **Flowchart 9.7**.

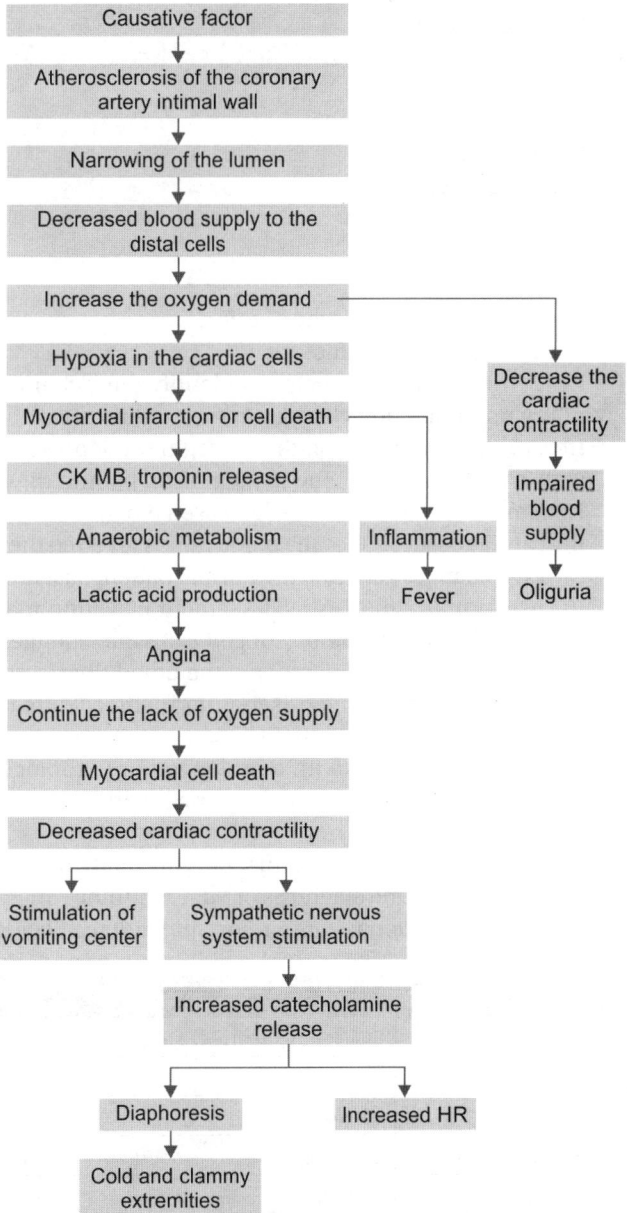

Flowchart 9.7: Pathophysiology of MI.

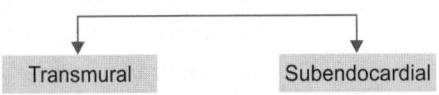

Flowchart 9.6: Classification of acute MI.

## Clinical Manifestations

- Chest pain
- Increased jugular venous pressure
- Elevated BP
- ST segment and T-wave change in ECG
- Tachycardia, Bradycardia and Dysrhythmias (Brunner and Suddarth, 2008)
- Dyspnea
- Pulmonary edema
- Nausea and vomiting
- Oliguria
- Cool and clammy extremities
- Cardiogenic shock
- Dependent edema
- Anxiety
- Restlessness
- Headache
- Blurred vision
- Slurred speech
- Impending doom

## Diagnosis

- **History and physical examination**
- **Identification of risk factors**
- **ECG:** The 12 lead ECG helps to identify the ischemia, injury and infarction changes in the cardiac cells. The *ischemic changes* include the ST segment depression with T wave inversion. The major reason behind these ischemic changes due to the decreased blood supply to the cardiac tissues. Once the blood flow is reverted then the ECG changes get it into the normal patient baseline. In case of *injury* there is a ST segment elevation may present. It is due to the prolonged ischemic changes. That may lead to the *infarction* if the blood flow is not regained. The prolonged ischemia further leads to the stage of infarction. The ECG shows that there is a ST segment elevation with a prolonged or pathologic Q wave (> 0.03 sec) **(Table 9.3)** (Brunner and Suddarth, 2008).
- **Serum cardiac markers:** Cardiac enzymes and troponin are important in the diagnosis of MI. Creatinine Kinase (CK-MB) and troponin are important cardiac specific markers to diagnose the MI. The CK level begins with in 3–12 hours after MI and get normal within 2–3 days. The troponin have more sensitivity and specificity to MI, and the value rise at 3–12 hours of incident and peak at 24–48 hrs and remain in the same for 5–15 days.
- **Coronary angiography:** It gives the clear idea about the location and percentage of block.
- **Stress echocardiography:** To find out the abnormal cardiac wall motion.
- **Myocardial perfusion imaging:** With thallium 201 used during exercise treadmill test to detect the ischemic areas in the myocardium and it appear as the cold spots.
- **Laboratory studies:** CK MB, CBC, cardiac troponin, myoglobin, lipid profile, CRP, homocysteine.
- **Positron emission tomography.**
- **Electron beam CT scan.**
- **Chest X-ray.**

## Management

### For ACS

- Continuous ECG monitoring
- IV access
- Oxygen therapy

*Drug therapy*

- **IV nitroglycerin (Fig. 9.18):** To reduce the angina pain and to increase the coronary blood flow.
- **Morphine Sulphate IV:** To reduce the pain that is not relieved by Nitroglycerin
- **Aspirin:** Loading dose 325 mg
- **Clopilet:** Loading dose 150 mg
- **Atorvastatin:** Cholesterol lowering agent, loading dose 80 mg
- **Heparin**
- **Beta adrenergic blockers:** To decrease the myocardial oxygen demand and to decrease HR, BP and contractility
- **ACE inhibitors:** Recommended for anterior wall MI or decrease the LVEF <40% or pulmonary congestion, e.g., captopril
- **Antidysrhythmic agents:** To reduce the complication of MI

**Table 9.3:** ECG evidence of ACS.

| Area of involvement | ECG leads facing the area | Leads opposite to the area | Related coronary artery |
|---|---|---|---|
| Septal wall | V1, V2 | II, III, aVF | Left anterior descending |
| Anterior wall | V2–V4 | II, III, aVF | Left anterior descending |
| Lateral wall | I, aVL, V5, V6 | II, III, aVF | Left anterior descending or circumflex |
| Inferior wall | II, III, aVF | I, aVL, V5, V6 | Right coronary artery |

- **Stool softeners:** After MI most of the patient suffering with constipation due to the effect of complete bed rest and morphine, e.g., docusate sodium.

## Unstable Angina/NSTEMI

- **Acute drug management:**
  - Nitroglycerin
  - Low molecular weight heparin
  - Clopidogrel
  - Glycoprotein IIb/IIIa inhibitors
- **Coronary angiography:** Percutaneous coronary intervention.
- **Coronary artery bypass graft (CABG)** (Brunner and Suddarth, 2008).

## STEMI

- **Immediate reperfusion therapy:** Percutaneous coronary intervention **(Figs. 9.16 to 9.18)**
- **Fibrinolytic therapy:**
  - Recombinant plasminogen activator
  - Tissue plasminogen activator
  - TNK-tPA

## Nursing Management

### Nursing Diagnosis

Acute pain related to surgical procedure as evidenced by verbalization of pain, facial expression.

### Nursing Interventions

- Immediate assessment and diagnosis
- **Continuous monitoring of the patient:** ECG, vital signs, IV medications
- Pain management
- Medication as per the doctor's order
- Provide adequate rest and comfort
- Provide comfortable position
- Teach distraction techniques

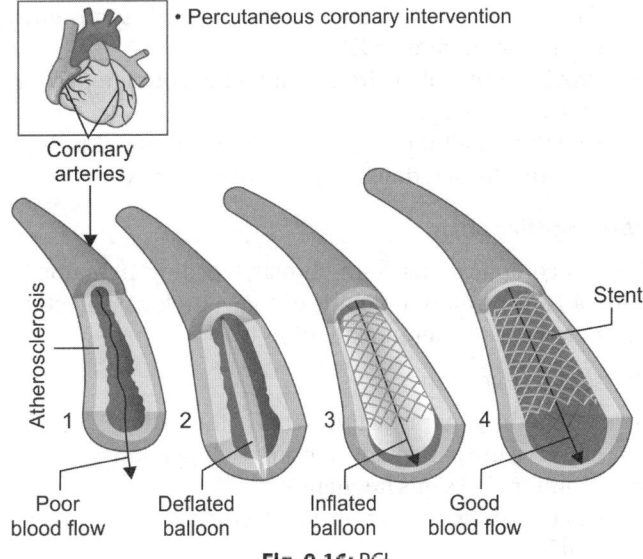

**Fig. 9.16:** PCI.

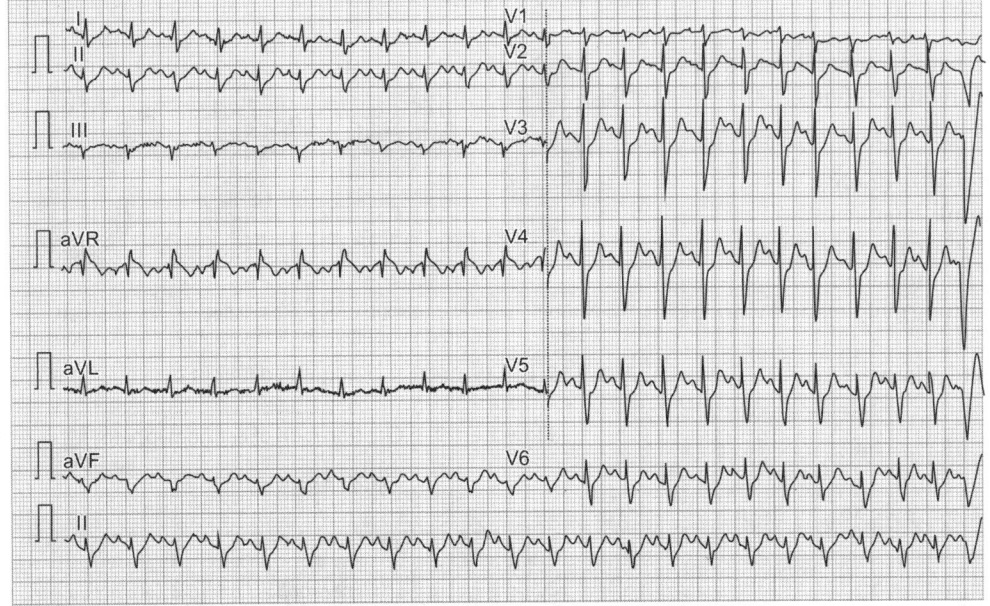

**Fig. 9.17:** ECG changes.

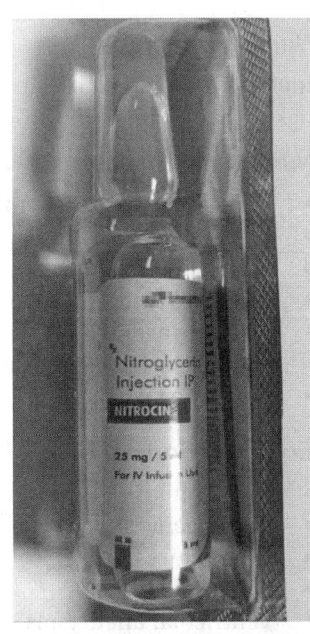

**Fig. 9.18:** Nitroglycerin IV.

## Nursing Diagnosis

Ineffective cardiac tissue perfusion related to myocardial injury as evidenced by dyspnea, dysrhythmias.

*Nursing Interventions*

- Check the BP and Pulse rate of the patient every 2-3 minutes after the initiation of the IV antihypertensive medications.
- Regular monitoring of hemodynamic parameters and vital signs.
- Confirm the rate and dose of medication.
- Give oxygen as indicated by the patient's symptoms, oxygen saturation and ABGs.
- Provide a restful environment and encourage periods of rest and sleep.
- Check for calf tenderness, diminished pedal pulses, swelling, local redness or pallor of extremity.

## Nursing Diagnosis

Risk for complications dysrhythmias, bleeding, hematoma, phlebitis or thrombophlebitis of the vein, local infection related to pacemaker implantation

*Nursing Interventions*

- Assess the general health status of the patient.
- Observe the patient for signs of complications.
- Monitor vital signs frequently.
- Check the pace maker site for bleeding, wound soakage and hematoma.
- Check the venous access site for redness and warmth.
- Administer prophylactic antibiotics as per order.

## Nursing Diagnosis

Ineffective therapeutic regimen management related to lack of knowledge about the procedure undergone.

*Nursing Interventions*

- Encourage the patient to verbalize doubts.
- Explain the condition in simple language.
- Provide health education on the care of pacemaker site.
- Advice to carry the ID card for the pacemaker.
- Advice to avoid exposure to strong magnets and working with powerful electric devices.
- Advice to take medications regularly.

## Complications of MI

- Arrhythmias
- Cardiogenic shock
- Hart failure
- Pericarditis
- Ventricular aneurysms
- Myocardial rupture (Chintamani, 2011)

Myocardial infarction occurs due to the continuous ischemia and leads to the irreversible damage or infarction of the cardiac cells. When the coronary blood vessels get occlusion that leads to the decreased blood flow and the complete occlusion leads to the halt of blood supply to the particular distal area may lead to myocardial cell death. The acute MI takes time to complete as infarction.

## CARDIOMYOPATHY

Cardiomyopathy (CMP) is a group of diseases affects the structural and functional ability of the myocardium. The cardiomyopathy can be diagnosed by patient clinical manifestation and invasive and noninvasive diagnostic methods. CMP can be classified into primary and secondary. The primary CMP refers to the myopathy without known etiology (idiopathic). In this condition some parts of the heart is getting involvement and the cardiac structures are unaffected. The secondary CMP is due to the any related disease conditions (**Fig. 9.19**) (Woods SL, 2010).

### Classification of Cardiomyopathy

The major three types of cardiomyopathies are figured in **Flowchart 9.8**.

### Causes of Cardiomyopathy

#### Dilated Cardiomyopathy

- Cardio toxic agents: Alcohol and cocaine
- Family history: Genetic/autosomal dominant
- Hypertension
- Coronary artery disease

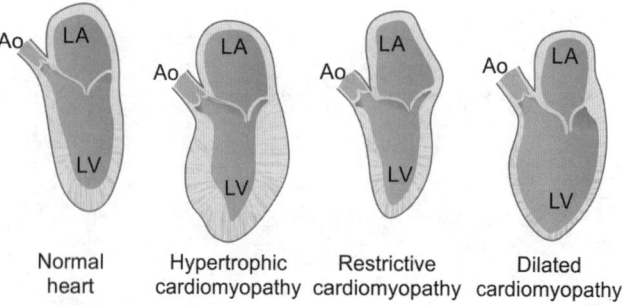

**Fig. 9.19:** Left ventricular changes in different cardiomyopathy.

**Flowchart 9.8:** Classification of cardiomyopathy.

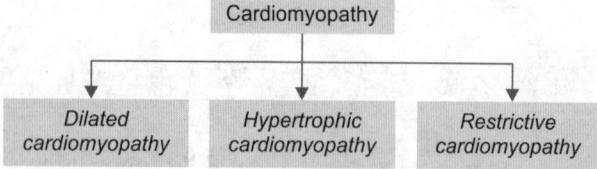

- Metabolic diseases
- Myocarditis
- Pregnancy
- Valvular diseases

### Hypertrophic Cardiomyopathy
- Aortic stenosis
- Family history
- Hypertension

### Restrictive Cardiomyopathy
- Endomyocardial fibrosis
- Amyloidosis
- Neoplastic tumor
- Radiation exposure
- Sarcoidosis
- Ventricular thrombus

### Dilated Cardiomyopathy

Dilated cardiomyopathy common type of cardiomyopathy. It is characterized by inflammation and degeneration of the myocardial fibers resulting into the dilation of ventricles, impaired ventricular function, atrial enlargement, defective systole and finally the pooling of blood inside the ventricles. The dilated CMP is often associated with the infective myocarditis. There may be cardiomegaly due to dilated ventricles but no hypertrophy (Chintamani, 2011).

### Clinical Manifestations
- Left heart failure: Dyspnea and orthopnea
- Right heart failure: Edema, nausea, abdominal pain and nocturia
- Decreased cardiac output
- Fatigue
- Weakness
- Dry cough at night
- Elevated jugular venous pressure
- Weight gain
- Peripheral cyanosis
- Tachycardia
- Murmur
- Arrhythmias
- Chest pain
- Palpitations
- Syncope

### Diagnosis
- *History and physical examination* to find out the etiology and clinical manifestations.
- *Chest X-ray* showing cardiomegaly.
- *ECG*—sinus tachycardia, atrial fibrillation, ventricular arrhythmia.
- *Holter monitoring*—24 hour ambulatory ECG.
- *2D echo.*
- *Cardiac catheterization* to get the pressure changes in the each chamber of the heart (Brunner and Suddarth, 2008).

### Management
- Oxygen therapy
- ACE inhibitors: Decrease the after load by vasodilation
- Diuretics: Decrease the fluid over load
- Beta adrenergic blockers: To reduce the cardiac contractility
- Antiarrhythmic agents
- Pacemaker
- Coronary artery bypass graft
- Heart transplantation
- Life style modification: Smoking cessation, avoid alcohol use, low fat and low sodium diet, increase physical activity according to doctor's order improve the quality of life by reduce stress, anxiety (Woods SL, 2010).

### Hypertrophic Cardiomyopathy

Hypertrophic cardiomyopathy is a type of cardiomyopathy characterized by irregular hypertrophy of the left ventricle without dilation of the ventricle. It is otherwise called as idiopathic subaortic stenosis or hypertrophic obstructive cardiomyopathy or asymmetric septal hypertrophy. It is less common than dilated CMP and more common in the age of 30–40 years.

Major characteristics of HCM are:
- Massive ventricular hypertrophy
- Rapid forceful ventricular contraction
- Impaired diastole
- Obstruction of the aortic out flow

### Clinical Manifestations

Most of the cases asymptomatic, it needs echocardiography to rule out the cases.

Symptomatic cases shows:
- Dyspnea
- Angina
- Fatigue
- Syncope
- Palpitation
- Paroxysmal nocturnal dyspnea
- Heart failure features
- Dizziness
- S4 heart sound
- More than two apical precordial pulse sites

- Systolic murmur
- ECG shows LV hypertrophy and wide deep and broad Q-wave
- Arrhythmias
- Pink frothy sputum
- Crackles
- Orthopnea
- Tachycardia
- Restlessness

*Diagnosis*

- **ECG:** LV hypertrophy, ventricular arrhythmias and atrial fibrillation.
- **Echocardiography:** Asymmetrical thickening of the ventricular wall, increased thickening of the interventricular septum, left ventricular outflow obstruction (Brunner and Suddarth, 2008).
- **Chest X-ray:** Cardiomegaly.
- **Cardiac catheterization:** Increased ventricular end diastolic pressure, left ventricular outflow obstruction
- **Radionuclide studies:** Decreased left ventricular volume, ischemia and increased the myocardial cell mass
- **Thallium scan:** Helps to detect myocardial perfusion defects (Woods SL, 2010).

*Management*

- Atrioventricular pacing
- Surgical management: Ventriculomyotomy and myectomy
- Left ventricular outflow obstruction and the symptoms can manage through alcohol induced percutaneous transluminal septal myocardial ablation.
- Vasodilators: Nitroglycerin
- Lifestyle modification including to avoid strenuous activities, dietary modifications, reduce stress.

### Restrictive Cardiomyopathy

It is a less common type of CMP. In this condition the cardiac muscle cells are restricted to stretch and impair the diastolic function of the heart.

*Clinical Manifestations*

- Fatigue
- Weakness
- Restlessness
- Bradycardia
- Dyspnea
- Dependent edema
- Abdominal ascites
- Hepatomegaly
- S3–S4 sounds
- Increased jugular venous pressure
- Cough
- Crackles
- Pink frothy sputum

*Diagnosis*

- **Chest X-ray:** Cardiomegaly, pericardial effusion and pulmonary congestion.
- **Echocardiography:** Increased ventricular muscle mass, reduced left ventricular size.
- **ECG:** LV hypertrophy, atrioventricular conduction defects.
- **Cardiac catheterization:** Reduced ventricular systolic pressure.
- **Radionuclide studies:** Left ventricular hypertrophy with restricted ventricular filling.

*Management*

No specific treatment, only symptomatic management.

*Nursing Management*

Nursing diagnosis

Decreased cardiac output related to altered myocardial contractility/inotropic changes as evidenced by increased heart rate (tachycardia), dysrhythmias, ECG changes (Brunner and Suddarth, 2008).

*Nursing Interventions*

- Check the BP and pulse rate of the patient every 2–3 minutes after the initiation of the IV antihypertensive medications.
- Regular monitoring of hemodynamic parameters and vital signs.
- Confirm the rate and dose of medication.
- Give oxygen as indicated by the patient's symptoms, oxygen saturation, and ABGs.
- Provide a restful environment and encourage periods of rest and sleep.
- Check for calf tenderness, diminished pedal pulses, swelling, local redness, or pallor of extremity.

*Nursing Diagnosis*

Impaired gas exchange related to increased preload a evidenced by increased respiratory rate, dyspnea.

*Nursing Interventions*

- Position patient in semi-Fowler's position for breathing
- Assist patient to use relaxation techniques
- Monitoring the urine output
- Provide complete bed rest

## Nursing Diagnosis

Decreased activity tolerance related to the imbalance between the supply and demand of the oxygen supply to the body cells.

## Nursing Interventions

- Encourage alternate rest and activity
- Provide adequate medication as per order
- Oxygen if needed
- Maintain the oxygen saturation
- Daily weight monitoring
- Monitor vital signs and hemodynamic parameters
- Provide health education regarding follow up care and need for life style modification
- Psychological support provide propped up position for dyspnea
- Cardiac auscultation
- Continuous physical examination
- Dietary modification
- Ongoing follow up care

Cardiomyopathies a group of diseases affects the structural and functional ability of the myocardium. The cardiomyopathy can be diagnosed by patient clinical manifestation and invasive and noninvasive diagnostic methods. CMP can be classified into primary and secondary.

# DEEP VEIN THROMBOSIS

Venous thrombosis is a common type of disorder of the vein. In venous thrombosis there is a formation of blood clot or thrombus associated with inflammation of the vein. It is mainly classified into superficial thrombosis and deep vein thrombosis (DVT) **(Fig. 9.20)** (Davidson, 2002).

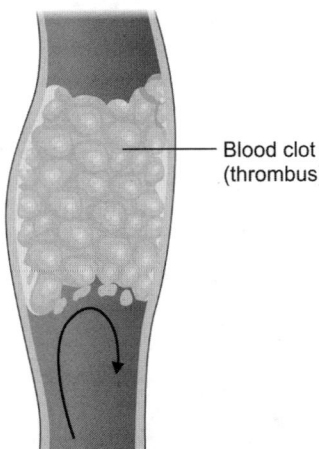

**Fig. 9.20:** Blood flow in DVT.

## Major Types of Venous Thrombosis

There are two different types of venous thrombosis—superficial thrombosis and deep vein thrombosis.

DVT is usually seen in arms include axillary and subclavian veins, legs, e.g., femoral, pelvis, e.g., iliac, inferior and superior vena cava. It is a type of disorder in which the thrombus formation in the deep vein commonly in the iliac and femoral veins. It is very occurs around 5% of all postsurgery cases **(Flowchart 9.9)** (Chintamani, 2011).

## Etiology

The major causes of venous thrombosis are classified into Virchows triad. It include:
- Venous stasis
- Damage of endothelium
- Hypercoagulability of the blood

## Risk Factors of DVT

### Venous Stasis

- Old age
- Atrial fibrillation
- Heart failure
- Obesity
- Postpartum period
- Prolonged bed ridden conditions: Bed rest, hip fracture, spinal cord injury, etc.
- Stroke
- Varicose veins

### Endothelial Damage

- Abdominal surgery
- Pelvic surgery
- IV medications: Hypertonic solutions
- History of DVT
- IV drug abusers
- Indwelling femoral venous catheters
- Trauma

### Hypercoagulability of Blood

- Antiphospholipid antibody syndrome
- Smoking

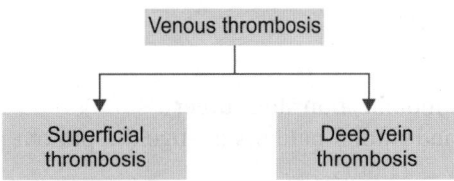

**Flowchart 9.9:** Types of DVT.

- Dehydration
- Malnutrition
- High altitudes
- Hyperhomocysteinemia
- Cancer, e.g., breast, liver, pancreas and gastrointestinal
- Nephritic syndrome
- Oral contraceptives
- Pregnancy
- Sepsis
- Severe anemia

## Pathophysiology

Plate aggregation and fibrin with RBC, WBC and more platelet together forms the thrombus. Usually the thrombus formed at the valve cusp of veins. Gradually the size of the thrombus increases and occludes the vein lumen. Slowly it covered by endothelium and the thrombus formation process gets arrest. Sometimes the thrombus get dislodges and form emboli. This emboli travel throughout the body and get stuck on the pulmonary circulation and causes pulmonary embolus (Harrison, 2005).

## Clinical Manifestations

- Edema on legs
- Extremity pain
- Warm skin
- Skin erythema
- Calf muscle pain
- Positive Homan's sign
- Lower extremity cyanosis

## Diagnosis

- Blood study
- ACT, aPTT, bleeding time and clotting time and platelet count
- **D-dimer test:** D-dimer a fibrin degradation product, raised in the presence of thrombus
- **Venography:** Accurate technique. A radiopaque dye is injecting into the vein and the deep veins can be visualized properly by X-ray imaging
- Ultrasound
- CT Scan
- MRI
- **Duplex ultrasonography:** Highly reliable and non-invasive test and is considered as the gold standard.

## Management

### Prevention

- Early mobilization after surgery
- For bed ridden patients change the patient position every 2–4 hours
- Antiembolism stockings
- Warm compression
- Anticoagulation therapy

### Drug Therapy

- Anticoagulation therapy
- **Vitamin K antagonists:** Warfarin and dicoumarol
- Unfractionated heparin
- **Low molecular weight heparin:** Enoxaparin and dalteparin
- **Direct thrombin inhibitors:** Lepirudin and desirudin
- **Factor Xa inhibitor:** Fondaparinux.

### Surgical Management

- Venous thrombectomy (Brunner and Suddarth, 2008)
- Vena cava interruption devices **(Fig. 9.21)**.

### Nursing Management

**Nursing diagnosis**

Acute pain related to congestion of the veins, improper venous return as evidenced by pain score from the patient.

**Nursing interventions**

- Continuous monitoring of the patient blood coagulation values
- Prevention methods
- Drug therapy
- Health education to prevent the complications

**Nursing diagnosis**

Ineffective tissue perfusion related to interruption of venous blood flow.

**Nursing interventions**

- Check the vital signs and capillary refill
- Provide comfort and rest

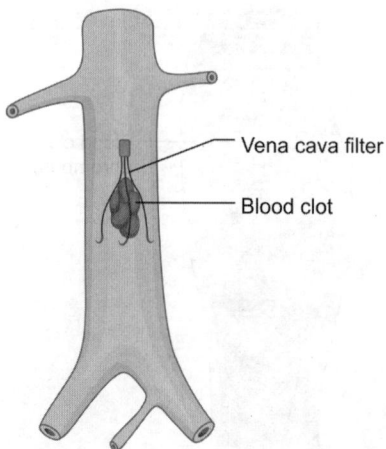

**Fig. 9.21:** Inferior vena cava filter.

- Provide compression devises
- Prevent injuries

**Nursing diagnosis**

Impaired comfort related to vascular inflammation and irritation.

**Nursing interventions**

- Provide bed rest to the patient
- Administer the medication as per the doctors order
- Check for bleeding

*Other possible nursing diagnosis*

- Ineffective health maintenance related to lack of knowledge about the disease.
- Risk for impaired skin integrity related to altered peripheral tissue perfusion.
- Potential complication: bleeding related to anti-coagulation therapy.

Venous thrombosis is a common type of disorder of the vein. In venous thrombosis there is a formation of blood clot or thrombus associated with inflammation of the vein. It is mainly classified into superficial thrombosis and deep vein thrombosis.

## VALVULAR DISEASES

The heart consists of mainly four valves; it includes two atrioventricular valves, mitral and tricuspid valve, and two semilunar valves, aortic and pulmonary valve. The main functions of the valves include controlling the blood flow in the unidirectional way. Mainly the valvular disorders may occur due to the stenosis or regurgitation or the prolapsed of the valves (Chatterjee K, 2013).

In case of stenosis there is narrowing of the valvular opening leads to the increase in the pressure gradient across the valve. If more pressure gradient then more stenosis. In case of regurgitation or the valvular insufficiency there is backflow of the blood is there **(Fig. 9.22)**. Based on the valve involvement and the type of problem in the valve there are different types of valvular disorders are there **(Flowchart 9.10)** (Chintamani, 2011).

### Mitral Valve

*Mitral Valve Stenosis*

It is the stenosis of narrowing of the mitral valve.

*Etiology*

- Rheumatic heart disease
- Congenital mitral stenosis
- Rheumatic arthritis
- Systemic lupus erythematosus
- Rheumatic endocarditis

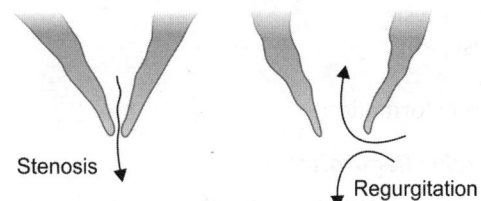

**Fig. 9.22:** Valvular diseases.

**Flowchart 9.10:** Classification of valvular heart diseases.

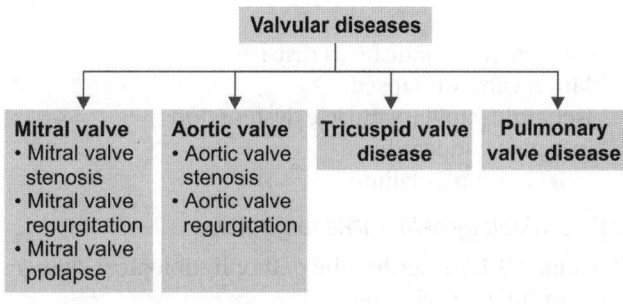

**Flowchart 9.11:** Pathophysiology of mitral valve stenosis.

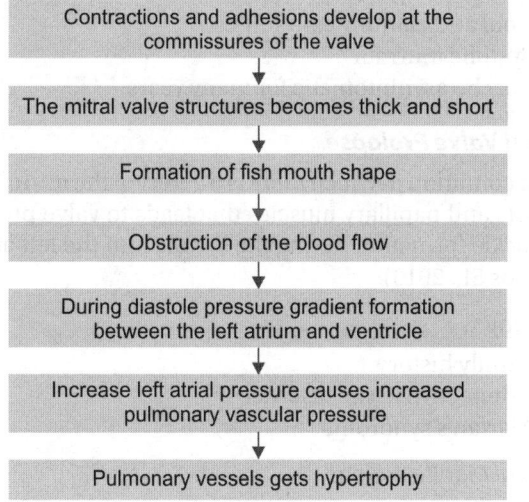

*Pathophysiology of Mitral Valve Stenosis*

The given flowchart describes the pathophysiological changes in the mitral stenosis **(Flowchart 9.11)**.

*Clinical Manifestations*

- Exertional dyspnea
- Fatigue
- Palpitation
- Loud S1
- Diastolic murmur
- Hoarseness

- Hemoptysis
- Chest pain
- Seizure
- Emboli formation

### Mitral Valve Regurgitation

It is due to the damage in one of the mitral leaflets, mitral annulus, chordae tendineae, papillary muscles, left atrium and left ventricle (Woods SL, 2010).

*Etiology*
- MI
- Chronic rheumatic heart disease
- Mitral valve prolapsed
- Ischemic papillary muscle dysfunction
- Infective endocarditis
- Left ventricular failure

*Pathophysiology of Mitral Regurgitation*

**Flowchart 9.12** describes the pathophysiological changes in the mitral regurgitation.

*Clinical Manifestations*
- Thread peripheral pulses
- Cool and clammy extremities
- Systolic murmur
- May be asymptomatic for many years

### Mitral Valve Prolapse

It is a condition in which there is a defect of the mitral valve leaflets and papillary muscles that leads to valve prolapse or buckle formation during the systole into the left atrium (Woods SL, 2010).

*Etiology*
- Family history
- Connective tissue disorder
- Marfan's syndrome

*Clinical Manifestations*
- Asymptomatic in majority of the cases
- Dysrhythmias: Premature ventricular contractions, paroxysmal supraventricular tachycardia and ventricular tachycardia
- Chest pain
- Palpitations
- Lightheadedness
- Dizziness
- Dyspnea

## Aortic Valve

### Aortic Valve Stenosis

It is the stenosis of the aortic valve.

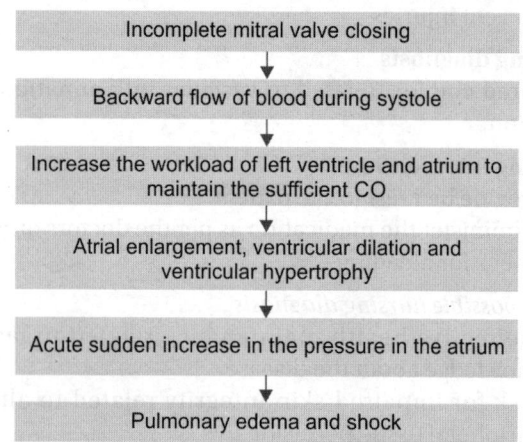

**Flowchart 9.12:** Pathophysiology of mitral valve regurgitation.

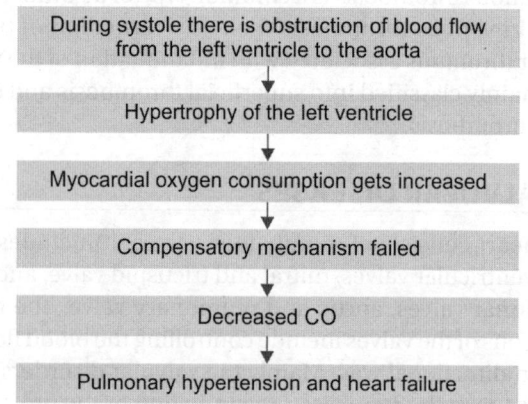

**Flowchart 9.13:** Pathophysiology of aortic valve stenosis.

*Etiology*
- Congenital anomaly
- Rheumatic fever
- Similar etiology of CAD
- Increasing age

*Pathophysiology of Aortic Valve Stenosis*

**Flowchart 9.13** describes the pathophysiological changes in the aortic valve stenosis.

*Clinical Manifestations*
- Angina
- Syncope
- Exertional dyspnea
- Left ventricular failure symptoms

### Aortic Valve Regurgitation

It is the disorder of leaflets of aortic valve, root of aorta or both.

## Etiology

- Infective endocarditis
- Trauma
- Aortic dissection
- Rheumatic heart disease
- Congenital bicuspid aortic valve
- Syphilis
- Ankylosing spondylitis
- Reiter's syndrome

### Pathophysiology of Aortic Valve Regurgitation

**Flowchart 9.14** describes the pathophysiological changes in the aortic valve regurgitation.

### Clinical Manifestations

- Acute aortic regurgitation needs medical emergency and cardiac collapse
- Exertional dyspnea
- Orthopnea
- Paroxysmal nocturnal dyspnea
- Angina

## Tricuspid and Pulmonary Valve

### Tricuspid and Pulmonary Valve Disease

These conditions are very rare. In this type stenosis of the valve is common the regurgitation (Chintamani, 2011).

### Etiology

Tricuspid valve stenosis

- Rheumatic fever
- Drug abusers
- Patients took dopamine agonist treatment (e.g., cabergoline)

Pulmonary stenosis

Congenital cardiac problems.

### Pathophysiology of Tricuspid and Pulmonary Valve Disease

**Flowchart 9.15** describes the pathophysiological changes in the tricuspid and pulmonary valve disease.

### Diagnosis of Valvular Heart Disease

History and physical examination

- **Chest X-ray:** To check the cardiomegaly, alteration in the pulmonary structure
- **ECG:** To rule out the arrhythmias
- **ECHO cardiography:** Shows the valvular structure and functions.
- *Transesophageal echocardiography and color Doppler imaging* helpful for the monitoring and diagnosis of the valvular functions **(Chatterjee K, 2013)**.

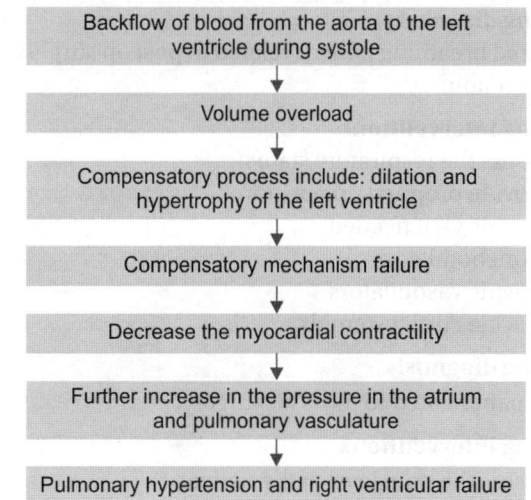

**Flowchart 9.14:** Pathophysiology of aortic valve regurgitation.

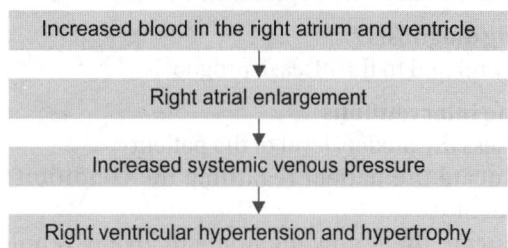

**Flowchart 9.15:** Pathophysiology of tricuspid and pulmonary valve disease.

- **Cardiac catheterization:** Helps to find out the cardiac chambers and the pressure inside the chambers.

### Management

Medical management

- Prophylactic antibiotic therapy for rheumatic fever and infective endocarditis
- Sodium restriction
- Drug therapy
- Vasodilators: Nitrates and ACE inhibitors
- Positive inotropes: Digoxin
- Diuretics
- Beta adrenergic blockers
- Anticoagulation therapy
- Antidysrhythmic agents
- Percutaneous transluminal balloon valvuloplasty

Surgical management

- Commissurotomy
- Valvuloplasty
- Annuloplasty
- Valve replacement

## Nursing management

**Nursing diagnosis**

Impaired breathing pattern related to post op surgery pain and infection

**Nursing interventions**
- Assess the respiratory status
- Provide propped up position
- Provide $O_2$ if needed
- Bronchodilators
- Provide vasodilators
- Provide corticosteroids

**Nursing diagnosis**

Acute pain related to the DVR surgery.

**Nursing interventions**
- Assess the pain level of the patient
- Provide analgesics as per order
- Provide propped up position
- Use spirometry exercise
- Hold the chest with a pillow while coughing.

**Nursing diagnosis**

Anxiety related to the disease prognosis.

**Nursing interventions**
- Assess the anxiety level of the patient
- Educate the patient regarding the condition of the patient
- Educate the family members to give psychological support
- Encourage the patient to follow some distractive techniques

*Other possible nursing diagnosis*
- Activity intolerance related to insufficient oxygenation secondary to decreased cardiac output as evidenced by fatigue, dyspnea and hypotension.
- Excess fluid volume related to heart failure secondary to incompetent valves as evidenced by peripheral edema, weight gain.
- Decreased cardiac output related to valvular incompetence as evidenced by murmurs, dyspnea and dysrhythmias.

**Interventions**
- Monitor the vital signs and hemodynamic parameters
- Provide alternative rest and activity period
- Proper weight chart
- Provide proper medication as per the order
- Health education regarding the home care treatment and follow up care (Brunner and Suddarth, 2008).

The valvular disorders may occur due to the stenosis or regurgitation or the prolapsed of the valves. In case of stenosis there is narrowing of the valvular opening leads to the increase in the pressure gradient across the valve. If more pressure gradient then more stenosis. In case of regurgitation or the valvular insufficiency there is backflow of the blood is there.

## HEART BLOCK

Heart block or atrioventricular block is the delay or failure in the transmission of the electrical signals from the SA node to the AV node or from the atria to the ventricle **(Fig. 9.23)** (Chatterjee K, 2013).

### Etiology
- CAD
- Myocarditis
- Heart failure
- Cardiomyopathy
- Poisoning
- Electrolyte imbalance
- Collagen tissue disorders

### First Degree AV Block

Every impulse conducted to ventricles but the duration of the AV conduction prolonged (Woods SL, 2010).

### ECG Changes
- Regular rhythm
- Depend on the base line rate the heart rate changing
- Prolonged PR interval: >0.20 sec
- Normal QRS

### Etiology

Use of digoxin, beta blockers and calcium channel blockers.

### Clinical Manifestations

Asymptomatic.

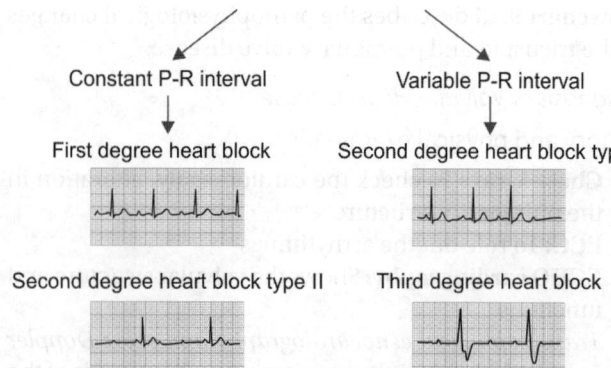

Fig. 9.23: Heart block types.

## Treatment
- Cautious use of medications
- Treatment of etiology.

## Type I or Mobitz I or Wenckebach Heart Block

There is a gradual lengthening of the PR interval. There is prolonged AV conduction time till an atrial impulse cannot conducted and a QRS complex is blocked or missing. **(Flowchart 9.16)** (Chintamani, 2011).

It can be occur at the AV node or the Purkinje system.

### ECG Changes
- Regular atrial rhythm
- Irregular ventricular rhythm
- Atrial rate more than ventricular rate
- PR interval gradual lengthening until drop beat
- PR interval shortens after the drop beat

### Etiology
- Inferior wall MI
- Cardiac surgery
- Acute rheumatic fever
- Vagal stimulation

### Treatment
Temporary pacemaker.

## Type II or Mobitz II

It is a more serious type of heart block. In which the P wave is nonconducted without progressive PR lengthening. In this type the bundle branches is always get block. On the conducted beats the PR interval is same or constant.

Ratio is 2:1 or 3:1 (2P wave and one QRS and 3P wave and one QRS respectively).

### ECG Changes
- Regular atrial rate
- Regular or irregular ventricular rate
- P-P interval constant
- QRS complex absent irregularly

### Etiology
- CAD
- Anterior wall MI
- Acute myocarditis
- Digoxin toxicity

### Clinical Manifestations
- Palpitation
- Fatigue

### Treatment
- Permanent pacemaker
- Discontinue digoxin if needed.

## Third Degree AV Block/Complete Heart Block (CHB)/AV Dissociation

In this type atrial impulses never carried to the ventricles. Atria and ventricle stimulated and contracted independently (Chintamani).

### ECG Changes
- Atrial rate: 60–100 beats per min
- Ventricular rate: 20–40 beats per minute
- Regular rhythm
- Normal P wave
- Varying type of PR interval

### Clinical Manifestations
- Dizziness
- Angina
- Syncope
- Heart failure
- Bradycardia

### Treatment
Permanent pacemaker.

### Nursing Management

**Nursing diagnosis**

Decreased cardiac output related to complete heart block as evidenced by vital sign and ECG changes.

**Nursing interventions**
- Monitor the cardiovascular status
- Assess the peripheral pulses
- Assess the skin for cyanosis
- Fluid restricted diet
- Instruct the patient to take rest
- Maintain IO chart
- Give medications

**Nursing diagnosis**

Imbalanced nutrition less than body requirement related to decreased food intake and BMI.

**Nursing interventions**
- Assess the nutritional status of the patient
- Encourage the patient to take sufficient amount of food

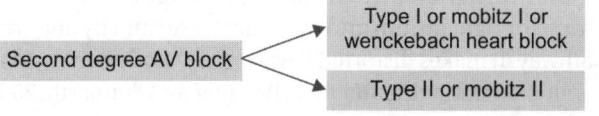

**Flowchart 9.16:** Types of second degree AV block.

- Include high protein, low sodium diet
- Encourage the patient to take small and frequent diet

**Nursing diagnosis**

Insomnia related to the life-threatening disease condition as evidenced by the verbal statement of the patient.

**Nursing interventions**
- Assess the sleep pattern of the patient
- Educate the patient regarding the condition of the patient
- Educate the family members to give psychological support

Heart block or atrioventricular block is the delay or failure in the transmission of the electrical signals from the SA node to the AV node or from the atria to the ventricle (Woods SL, 2010).

## CARDIAC ARRHYTHMIAS

Cardiac arrhythmias are the abnormal conduction system of the heart that may produce the abnormal rate and rhythm changes in the heart.

### Etiology

#### Cardiac Conditions
- Cardiomyopathy
- Conduction defects
- Heart failure
- Myocardial cell degeneration
- MI
- Valvular diseases

#### Others
- Acid base imbalance
- Alcohol, caffeine and tobacco
- Electric shock
- Hypoxia
- Poisoning

### Sinus Bradycardia (Fig. 9.24)

The conduction pathway is normal. The HR <60 beats/min (Woods SL, 2010).

#### ECG
- HR <60 beats/min
- Regular rhythm
- Normal P, QRS and PR interval

#### Clinical Manifestations
- Pale
- Cool skin

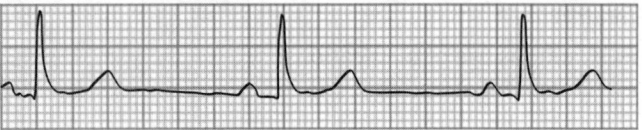

Fig. 9.24: Sinus bradycardia.

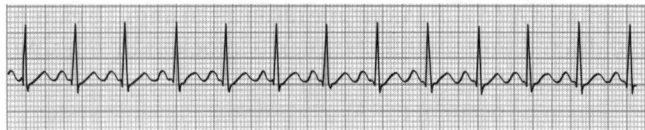

Fig. 9.25: Sinus tachycardia.

- Hypotension
- Angina
- Dizziness
- Syncope
- Shortness of breath

#### Treatment
- Atropine
- Pacemaker

### Sinus Tachycardia (Fig. 9.25)

It is due to the vagal inhibition or sympathetic stimulation. Here there is normal conduction pathway. HR >100 beats/min.

#### ECG
- HR >100 beats/min
- Regular rhythm
- Normal P, QRS and PR interval

#### Clinical Manifestations
- Dizziness
- Dyspnea
- Hypotension
- Angina

#### Treatment
- Adenosine
- Beta blockers

### Premature Atrial Contraction (Fig. 9.26)

In premature atrial contraction (PAC) the electrical impulses starts from the ectopic foci in the atrium other than SA node.

Abnormal electrical impulses originate in the left atrium or right atrium and travel across atrium by abnormal pathway. It makes distorted P wave. At AV node it may stop or conducted normally after that (Brunner and Suddarth, 2008).

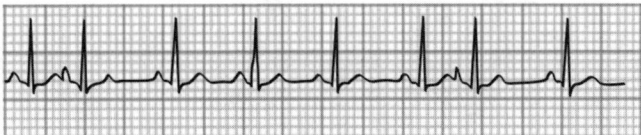

Fig. 9.26: Premature atrial contraction.

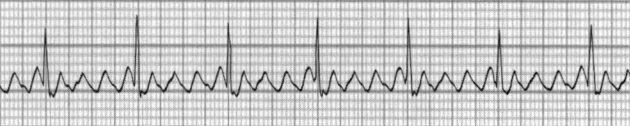

Fig. 9.27: Atrial flutter.

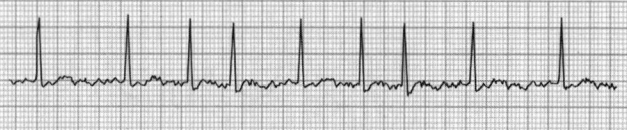

Fig. 9.28: Atrial fibrillation.

HR = 60–100 beats/min

*Rhythm irregular*

It is not much significant if no related heart diseases.

*Treatment*

- Treatment of signs and symptoms
- Beta blockers

## Paroxysmal Supra Ventricular Tachycardia

The dysrhythmias starting from the ectopic focus above the bifurcation of the bundle of His. It is common in the patients with WPW (Wolf Parkinson White) syndrome.

HR = 100–300 beats/min

*Rhythm regular/slightly irregular*

*Clinical Manifestations*

Prolonged HR >180 beats/min leads to decreased blood pressure, breathlessness and angina.

*Treatment*

- Vagal stimulation
- Drug therapy: IV adenosine, beta blockers, calcium channel blockers, digoxin and amiodarone
- If the patient is stable can prefer cardioversion
- Radiofrequency catheter ablation.

## Atrial Flutter (Fig. 9.27)

It is a recurrent; saw toothed shaped ECG waves originated from the ectopic foci in the right atria (Woods SL, 2010).

*ECG*

- Rate: 250–350 beats/min
- A:V = 2:1
- Ventricular rate: 150 beats/min
- P wave: Flutter wave saw toothed shape
- Normal QRS
- Variable PR interval

*Clinical Manifestations*

- Decrease CO
- HF features
- Dizziness
- Dyspnea
- Weakness
- Syncope

*Treatment*

- Calcium channel blockers
- Beta blockers
- Cardioversion
- Antidysrhythmic agents
- Radiofrequency ablation

## Atrial Fibrillation (Fig. 9.28)

It is the total disorganization of the electrical activity due to multiple ectopic foci resulting in loss of electrical activity (Chintamani, 2011).

*ECG*

- Irregular rhythm
- Atrial rate: 350–600 beats/min
- Ventricular rate: 50 or max 180 beats/min
- P wave: No true P wave
- No PR interval
- Normal QRS

Atrial fibrillation with ventricular rate >100 beats/min is called atrial fibrillation with rapid ventricular response.

*Treatment*

- Calcium channel blockers
- Beta blockers
- Digoxin
- Amiodarone
- Cardioversion

## Premature Ventricular Contraction (PVC) (Fig. 9.29)

In this type contractions originating from ectopic focus in the ventricles. Premature occurrence of QRS complex which is wide and distorted type (Woods SL, 2010).

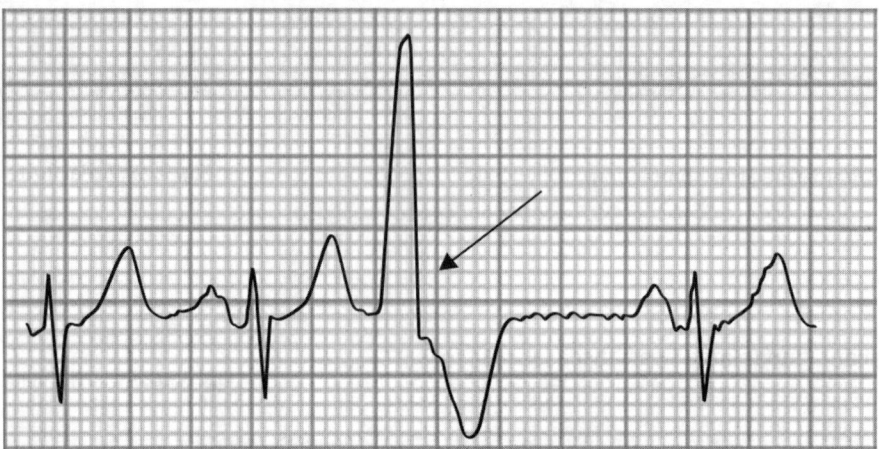

**Fig. 9.29:** Premature ventricular contraction.

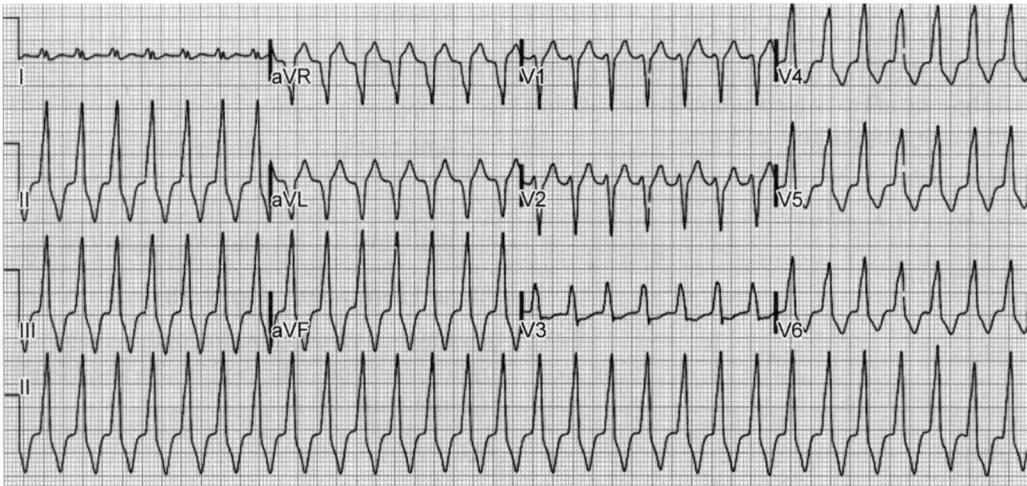

**Fig. 9.30:** Ventricular tachycardia.

## Types

- **Multifocal PVC:** PVCs are initiated from the different foci appear different shapes each other.
- **Unifocal PVC:** Same shape PVC.
- **Ventricular bigeminy:** Every other beat is PVC.
- **Trigeminy:** Every third beat is PVC.
- **Couplet:** Two consecutive PVC.

## Clinical Manifestations

- Palpitations
- Dizziness
- Syncope
- Absence of S2

## Treatment

- Beta blockers
- Amiodarone
- Procainamide

## Ventricular Tachycardia (Fig. 9.30)

It is a run of 3 or more PVCs. Ectopic focus fire repeatedly. Unstable, short paroxysmal burst.

## Types

- **Monomorphic VT:** QRS are same in size, shape, and direction.
- **Polymorphic VT:** QRS gradually change shape, size and direction from series of beats.
- **Torsades de pointes:** Form of polymorphic VT, QRS rotates about the base line, deflecting upward and downward (Woods SL, 2010).

## ECG: Torsades de Pointes

- **Rate:** 150–250 beats/min
- **Rhythm:** Irregular
- **QRS:** Wide and change the amplitude

- **P wave:** Absent
- **Sustained VT:** >30 sec
- **Nonsustained VT:** <30 sec

### ECG

- **Ventricular rate:** 150–250 beats/min
- Rhythm regular/irregular
- QRS-wide and bizarre (>0.12 sec)
- PR interval not measurable
- P wave buried in QRS

### Clinical Significance

- **Stable VT:** With pulse
- **Unstable VT:** Without pulse **(Flowchart 9.17)**

### Treatment

- Precipitating cause management
- **Amiodarone IV dose:**
  - *First dose:* 150 mg over 10 minutes.
  - Follow by maintenance infusion of 1 mg/min for first 6 hours.
- **Sotalol IV dose:**
  - 100 mg (1.5 mg/kg) over 5 minutes. Avoid if prolonged QT.
  - Cardioversion/defibrillation
- **Pulseless VT:** CPR, defibrillation and amiodarone.

## Ventricular Fibrillation (VF) (Fig. 9.31)

- Severe derangement of heart rhythm
- Firing from several ectopic sites
- Mechanically ventricle is quivering—no effective contraction → No CO.

### ECG

Irregular waves of varying shapes and amplitude, HR cannot calculate, no P wave, PR interval and QRS cannot measure.

### Treatment

- Emergency
- CPR
- Defibrillation
- Epinephrine 1 mg every 3–5 min IV
- Vasopressin
- Amiodarone bolus: 300 mg IV
- 2nd dose 150 mg IV

## Asystole (Fig. 9.32)

- Absence of ventricular electrical activity
- Occasionally P wave can see

**Flowchart 9.17:** Changes in sustained VT.

```
Decrease ventricular filling and loss of atrial contraction
                            ↓
                       Decrease CO
                            ↓
Decreased blood pressure, pulmonary edema, decrease
  in cerebral blood flow and cardiorespiratory arrest
```

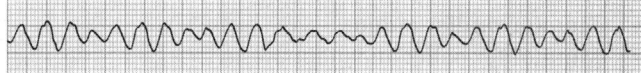

**Fig. 9.31:** Ventricular fibrillation.

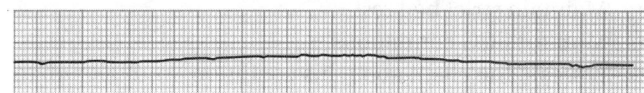

**Fig. 9.32:** Asystole.

- No ventricular contraction
- Patient may be unresponsive, pulseless and apneic.

### Treatment

- CPR
- ACLS

## Pulseless Electrical Activity

There is electrical activity on ECG but no pulse.

### Treatment

- CPR
- IV epinephrine (Chatterjee K, 2013)

## Nursing Management

### Nursing Diagnosis

Deceased cardiac output related to inadequate blood pumped by the heart to meet metabolic demands of the body as evidenced by ventricular tachycardia on ECG.

### Nursing Interventions

- Assess the cardiac function of the patient.
- Assess the heart rate, respiratory rate and blood pressure.
- Monitor cardiac output.
- Monitor for pallor and diaphoresis.
- Administer $O_2$ as required.
- Administer positive inotropic agent.
- Maintain strict bed rest.
- Monitor ECG continuously.
- Educate the client about his condition. And tell to avoid strenuous activities.

### Nursing Diagnosis

Risk for shock related to an inadequate blood flow to the body's tissues which may lead to life-threatening cellular dysfunction.

### Nursing Interventions

- Assess the cardiac function of the patient.
- Assess the heart rate, respiratory rate and blood pressure.
- Monitor cardiac output.
- Monitor for pallor and diaphoresis.
- Administer $O_2$ as required.
- Administer positive inotropic agent.
- Maintain strict bed rest.
- Monitor ECG continuously.
- Educate the client about his condition. And tell him to avoid strenuous activities.

### Nursing Diagnosis

Anxiety related to the disease condition and its complications.

### Nursing Interventions

- Assess the anxiety level of the patient.
- Educate the patient regarding the condition of the patient.
- Educate the family members to give psychological support.
- Encourage the patient to follow some distractive techniques.

## Summary

The abnormal electrical conduction changes the rate and rhythm of the heart is called the cardiac arrhythmias. The severity of the arrhythmia may vary from the mild, asymptomatic and no need of treatment to severe catastrophic ventricular fibrillation which need sudden resuscitation.

## ANEURYSM

Aneurysms are the pathological dilations of normal aortic lumen involve one or several segment of the aorta. Aneurysm is a permanent localized dilation aorta having diameter at least 1.5 times that of expected normal diameter of the aortic segment **(Fig. 9.33)** (Chintamani, 2011).

## Etiology

- CAD
- Hypertension
- Hypercholesterolemia

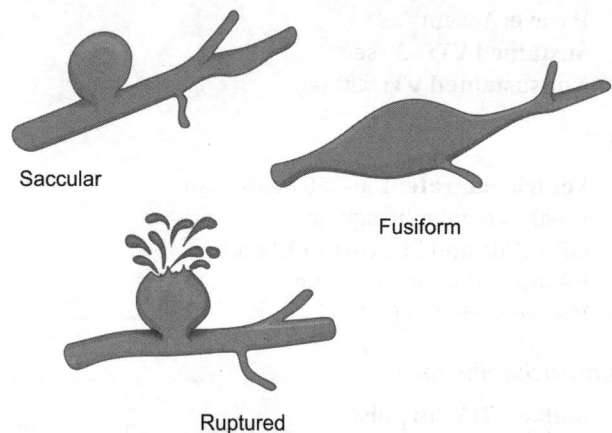

**Fig. 9.33:** Aneurysm.

- Hyperhomocysteinemia
- Elevated CRP
- Tobacco
- Peripheral vascular disease
- Marfan's syndrome
- Bicuspid aortic valve
- Syphilis
- Malignancy
- Inflammatory diseases
- Trauma
- Bacterial infection

## Classification

### According to Location

- Aortic root aneurysm: At the sinus of Valsalva.
- Thoracic aortic aneurysm: At the chest include ascending, aortic arch, descending aortic aneurysm.
- Abdominal aortic aneurysm: Common type.

### Others

- **True aneurysm:** All the three layers of aortic wall involved; intima, media and adventitia.
  - *Saccular:* A bulge at the segment of the aortic wall and it is more localized.
  - *Fusiform:* It is spindle shaped aneurysm. In this type of the dilation of whole circumference of aortic wall and in uniform shape.
- **False/pseudo aneurysm:** The entire wall is injured, and the blood is retained in the surrounding tissue and form a sac communicating with the artery is eventually formed. These blood-filled cavities will eventually either thrombus enough to seal the leak or rupture out of the surrounding tissue.

## Clinical Manifestations

- Asymptomatic in 70% cases.
- Abdominal pain, back pain as the size of the aneurysm enlarges.
- Compression of aneurysm to the nerve roots causes leg pain and numbness.
- Dysphagia due to compression of esophagus.
- Compression of arch of aorta leads to laryngeal nerve compression: Hoarseness of voice.
- Compression of bronchus: Cough, wheezing and dyspnea.
- Aneurysm rupture: Pain, bleeding, hypotension, shock and death.
- Clot formation: Stroke, MI and chest pain.
- Embolism formation.

## Diagnosis

- History
- Physical examination: <5 cm cannot detect by examination
- USG
- Contrast CT: Accurate diagnosis
- Magnetic resonance angiography (MRA)
- Plain X-ray: Calcification within the wall of aneurysm
- ECG: MI (Chatterjee K, 2013)

## Management

- Long-term beta blocker therapy: Metoprolol, propranolol, labetalol and esmolol
- Antihypertensive drugs
- Sodium nitroprusside infusion to decrease the systolic pressure
- Calcium channel blockers
- Direct vasodilators: Hydralazine and diazoxide
- Continuous vital sign monitoring, hemodynamic monitoring and urine output

## Surgical Management

- Bentall procedure aneurysm resected and replaced with prosthetic Dacron graft.
- Percutaneous endovascular stent graft through femoral artery.

## Nursing Management

### Nursing Diagnosis

Anxiety related to impending surgery.

### Nursing Interventions

- Assess the client's anxiety level.
- Provide a quiet environment and privacy.
- Briefly explain all procedures as appropriate, using simple, concrete words.
- Encourage the patient to follow some distractive techniques.

### Nursing Diagnosis

Deficient knowledge related to new disease condition.

### Nursing Interventions

- Provide a quiet environment and privacy.
- Briefly explain all procedures as appropriate, using simple, concrete words.
- Educate the family members to give psychological support.

### Prevention

- Smoking cessation
- Lifestyle modification
- Healthy diet
- BP monitoring
- Avoid alcohol
- Exercise
- Avoid heavy weight lifting
- Continuous treatment follow-up.

Aneurysms are the pathological dilations of normal aortic lumen involve one or several segment of the aorta. Aneurysm is a permanent localized dilation aorta having diameter at least 1.5 times that of expected normal diameter of the aortic segment. Aneurysm may cause no symptoms or may cause severe chest pain. Large size aneurysm may cause the compression effect on the nearby structures.

## INFECTIVE ENDOCARDITIS (IE)

It is the endocardial and vascular endothelium infection of the heart. The endocardium is the inner lining of the heart it continues to form the cardiac valves. That is the major cause that the IE affects the cardiac valves **(Fig. 9.34)** (Chatterjee K, 2013).

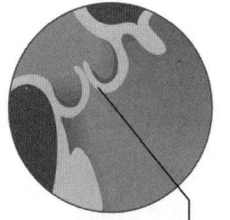
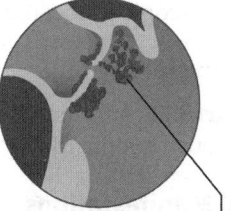

**Fig. 9.34:** Infective endocarditis.

## Classification

- **Subacute:** The individuals with already known case of valvular diseases and it develop over months.
- **Acute:** In this condition the individuals with healthy valves get affected and it is rapidly progressive type.

## Etiology

### Causative Microorganism

*Bacteria*

- Chlamydia
- Staphylococci
- Enterococci
- HACEK group: Hemophilus, Actinobacillus, Cardiobacterium, Eikenella, and Kingella
- Methicillin resistant staphylococcus aureus
- Streptococcus bovis
- Streptococcus group A, B and C.

*Fungus*

Candida albicans.

*Viruses*

Coxsackie B virus.

## Predisposing Factors

- Previous history of endocarditis
- Artificial valves
- Valvular diseases
- Congenital heart diseases
- Rheumatic heart diseases
- Pacemaker
- Marfan's syndrome
- Cardiomyopathy
- IV drug abusers
- Nosocomial infections
- Intravenous devices (invasive arterial line)
- Dental procedures
- Tonsillectomy procedure
- Bronchoscopy, endoscopy, cystoscopy
- Esophageal dilation procedure
- Abdominal surgeries
- Laparoscopic procedure

## Pathophysiology of IE

**Flowchart 9.18** represents the sequential events in a patient with infective endocarditis (IE).

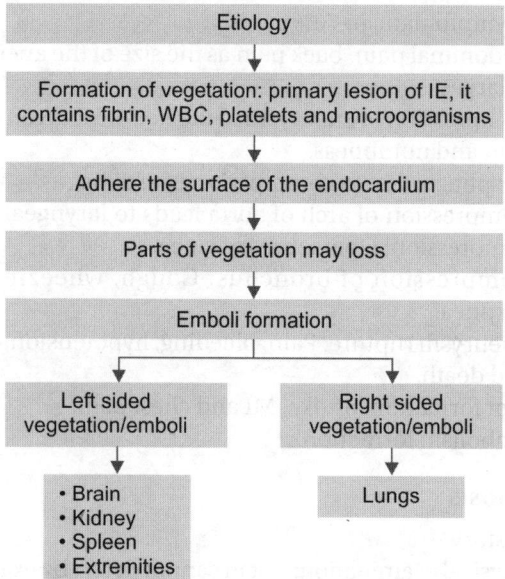

**Flowchart 9.18:** Pathophysiology of IE.

## Clinical Manifestations

- Low grade fever
- Chills
- Weakness
- Malaise
- Fatigue
- Anorexia
- Arthralgia
- Myalgia
- Back pain
- Abdominal discomfort
- Weight loss
- Head ache
- Clubbing of fingers
- Splinter hemorrhage (black longitudinal streaks at the nail beds)
- **Petechiae:** Due to fragmentation of the micro embolism and common in the conjunctiva, lips, buccal mucosa, palate, ankles, feet and popliteal areas
- **Osler's node:** Painful, tender, red, purple, pea shaped lesions at the fingertips and toes
- **Janeway's lesion:** Flat, painless, small, red spots at the palms and soles
- **Roth's spot:** At fundoscopic examination shows hemorrhagic retinal lesions
- Murmur
- Clinical manifestation related to the area of embolization if to brain causes hemiplegia, ataxia, aphasia, visual changes and altered level of consciousness (Chintamani, 2011)

## Diagnosis

- History and physical examination
- Blood culture shows the causative organism.

- Complete blood investigation: Increased WBC, elevated ESR, anemia
- Echocardiography: Vegetation formation and valvular function
- Chest X-ray: Cardiomegaly
- ECG: Atrial fibrillation and atrial flutter

## Management

### Prophylactic Therapy

Antibiotic prophylaxis for all procedure that may lead to IE (Table 9.4).

## Nursing Management

### Nursing Diagnosis

Hyperthermia related to infection of myocardium as evidenced by elevated temperature, tachycardia and malaise.

### Nursing Interventions

- Monitor the patient vital signs and the hemodynamic parameters
- Antipyretic medications
- Antibiotics administration
- Check the patient blood reports
- Encourage to increase the fluid intake according to the output
- Provide rest
- Provide health education to the patient.

### Nursing Diagnosis

Decreased cardiac output related to valvular insufficiency as evidenced by tachycardia, diminished peripheral pulses.

### Nursing Interventions

- Check the BP and pulse rate of the patient every 2–3 minutes after the initiation of the IV antihypertensive medications.
- Regular monitoring of hemodynamic parameters and vital signs.

**Table 9.4:** Drug therapy.

| Causative organism | Antibiotic drug |
|---|---|
| Streptococcus endocarditis | IV penicillin G<br>IM ceftriaxone<br>IM gentamicin<br>IV vancomycin |
| Enterococcal endocarditis | IV ampicillin<br>IV penicillin G |
| Fungal endocarditis | IV amphotericin |

- Confirm the rate and dose of medication.
- Give oxygen as indicated by the patient's symptoms, oxygen saturation and ABGs.
- Provide a restful environment and encourage periods of rest and sleep.
- Check for calf tenderness, diminished pedal pulses, swelling, local redness, or pallor of extremity.

### Nursing Diagnosis

Activity intolerance related to generalized weakness, arthralgia as evidenced by fatigue, dyspnea.

### Nursing Interventions

- Encourage alternate rest and activity
- Provide adequate medication as per order
- Oxygen if needed
- Maintain the oxygen saturation
- Daily weight monitoring
- Monitor vital signs and hemodynamic parameters
- Provide health education regarding follow-up care and need for life style modification
- Psychological support provide propped up position for dyspnea

### Possible Nursing Diagnosis

- Hyperthermia related to infection of myocardium as evidenced by elevated temperature, tachycardia, malaise.
- Decreased cardiac output related to valvular insufficiency as evidenced by tachycardia, diminished peripheral pulses.
- Activity intolerance related to generalized weakness, arthralgia as evidenced by fatigue, dyspnea.
- Knowledge deficit related to lack of information about the disease condition as evidenced by frequent questions.

## Interventions

It is the endocardial and vascular endothelium infection of the heart. The endocardium is the inner lining of the heart it continues to form the cardiac valves. That is the major cause that the IE affects the cardiac valves.

# HEART FAILURE

Heart failure is the disease condition affecting the cardiac pumping action. That results in the vasoconstriction and fluid retention. Heart failure is the major cause of mortality and morbidity in the countries. It is the inability of the heart to maintain adequate cardiac output according to the body demands. It may be right sided or left sided or both biventricular.

## Risk Factors

Heart failure is caused by interference with the normal cardiac mechanisms that regulate the cardiac output including; preload, after load, myocardial contractility, heart rate and metabolic state of the individual (Chintamani, 2011).

## Causes of Heart Failure

Mainly the primary causes of heart failure is divided into acute and chronic (**Flowchart 9.19**).

## Precipitating Causes

- Anemia
- Infection
- Thyrotoxicosis
- Hypothyroidism
- Dysrhythmias
- Bacterial endocarditis
- Pulmonary embolism
- Paget's disease
- Nutritional deficiency
- Hypervolemia

## Pathological Mechanism in Heart Failure

The pathophysiological mechanism of the heart failure is mainly categorized under systolic and diastolic failure (**Flowchart 9.20**).

## Mixed Systolic + Diastolic Failure

- It is seen in the dilated cardiomyopathy
- In this condition the ejection fraction is <35% and high pulmonary pressure and biventricular failure.

## Compensatory Mechanisms in Heart Failure

The sequential compensatory mechanism is given in the **Flowchart 9.21**.

### Counter Regulatory Mechanism

Try to maintain the balance:
- *Natriuretic peptides* (atrial natriuretic peptide and b type natriuretic peptides) are produced by heart myocardium to promote arterial and venous vasodilation leads to decrease the preload and afterload (Chintamani, 2011).
  The major function of the Natriuretic peptides are endothelin and aldosterone antagonists lead to increase dieresis by increase GFR and block RAAS.
  Cardiac hypertrophy, and anti-inflammatory effects may reduce.

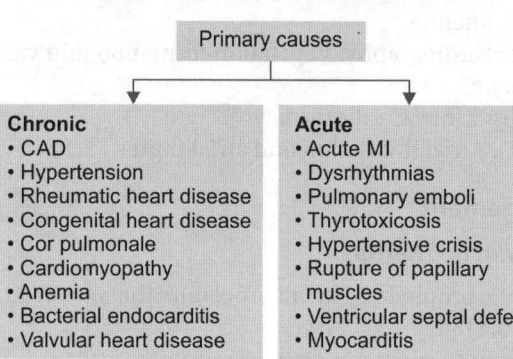

Flowchart 9.19: Causes of heart failure.

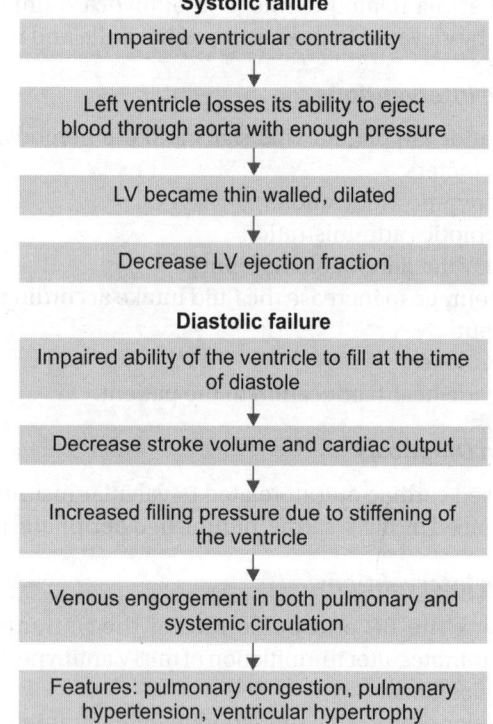

Flowchart 9.20: Pathophysiological changes in systolic and diastolic failure.

ANP primarily triggered by increase in volume and released from the atrium and the BNP triggered by increase in pressure and released from ventricles.
- *Nitric oxide (NO)*

## Change After the Release on Nitric Oxide

The major change after releasing of NO is depicted in **Flowchart 9.22**.

## Types of Heart Failure

The heart failure is mainly divided into systolic and diastolic failure (**Flowchart 9.23**).

**Flowchart 9.21:** Compensatory mechanisms in heart failure.

**Sympathetic nervous system activation**

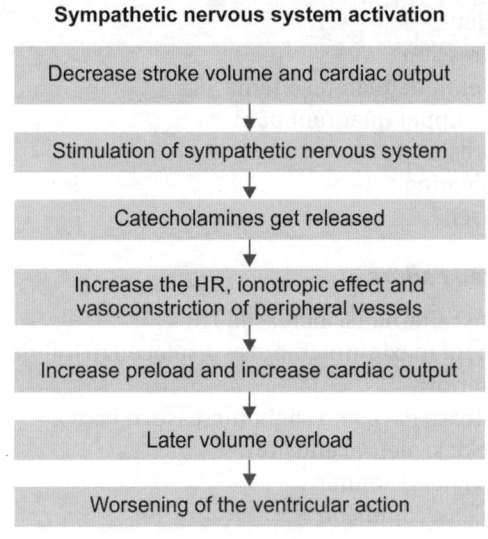

*Angiotensin II effects:*
- Aldosterone released from Adrenal cortex → sodium and water retention
- Peripheral vasoconstriction → increase BP

*Antidiuretic hormone (ADH):*

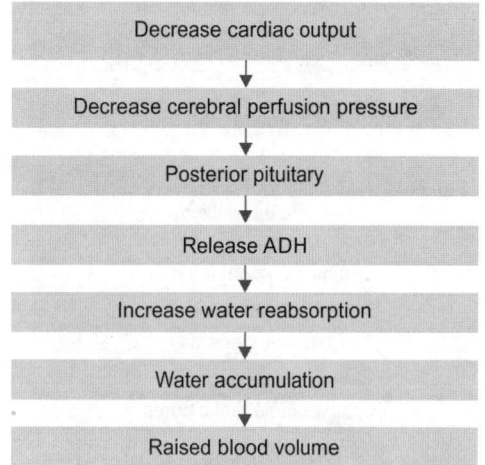

**Neurohormonal performance**
*Renin angiotensin aldosterone system*

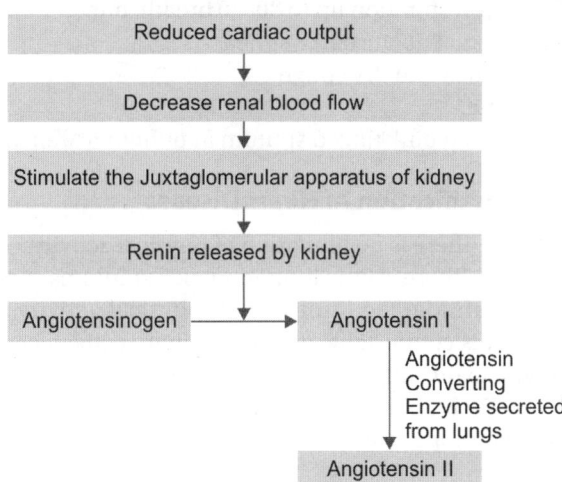

*Endothelin production*

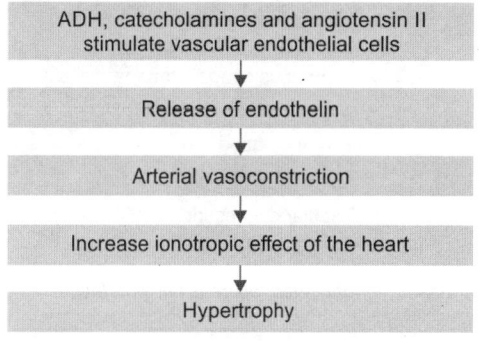

**Flowchart 9.22:** Change after the release on NO.

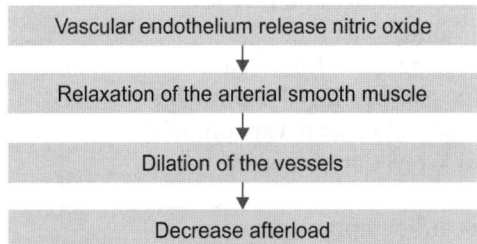

## Clinical Manifestations of Heart Failure

### Right Sided Failure
- Murmur
- Increased JVP
- Edema
- Weight gain
- Increase HR
- Ascites
- Anasarca

**Flowchart 9.23:** Types of heart failure.

*Left sided failure; it is very common*

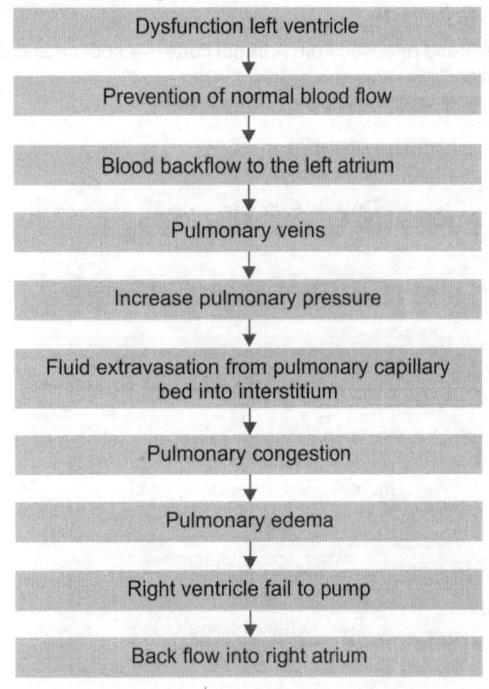

*Right sided failure*

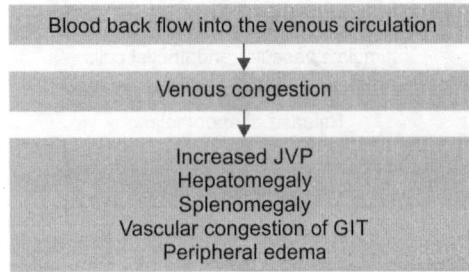

*The major reason of right sided failure is left side failure*

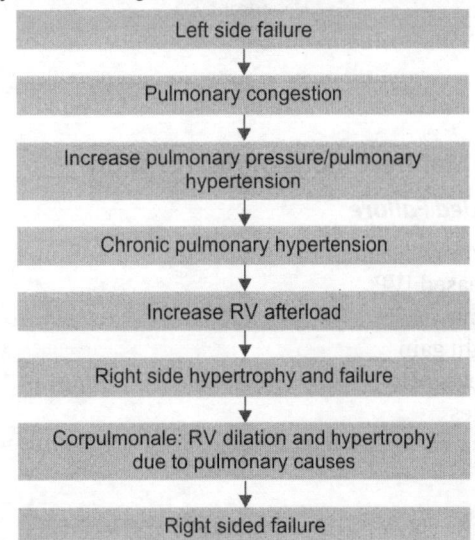

- Hepatomegaly
- Fatigue
- Anxiety
- Depression
- Dependent bilateral edema
- Right upper quadrant pain
- Anorexia
- GI bloating
- Nausea

### Left Sided Failure

- Pulsus alternans, increased HR
- Point of maximum impulse displaced to inferiorly and posteriorly
- Decrease $PaO_2$ and slight increase in $PaCO_2$
- Crackles, pleural effusion
- S3, S4 heart sounds
- Restless, confusion
- Weakness, fatigue
- Anxiety, depression
- Dyspnea
- Shallow respiration up to 30–40 breath/min
- Paroxysmal nocturnal dyspnea
- Orthopnea and dry cough
- Nocturia
- Frothy and pink tinged sputum in pulmonary edema.

## NYHA Classification of Heart Disease

- **Class I:** There is no limitation of physical activity.
- **Class II:** There is little limitation, no symptoms at rest.
- **Class III:** Marked limitation of physical activity and patient is comfortable at rest. Ordinary activity causes angina pain, fatigue and palpitation.
- **Class IV:** Inability to carry out any physical activity and the symptoms present at rest.

### Diagnosis

- History and physical examination
- Find out the etiology
- Cardiac enzymes and BNP level
- BNP value:
  - <100 pg/mL = Heart failure (HF) very improbable
  - 100–500 pg/mL = HF probable
  - >500 pg/mL = HF very probable
- Chest X-ray: Cardiomegaly
- ECG
- Echocardiography
- Exercise stress test
- Hemodynamic monitoring
- Cardiac catheterization

## Management

- **Drugs**
  - Diuretics: Frusemide and torsemide
  - Morphine
  - Vasodilators
  - ACE inhibitors: Captopril and enalapril
  - Nitroprusside
  - Nitroglycerin
  - Beta blockers: Metoprolol and, atenolol
  - Positive inotropes: Digoxin
  - Beta adrenergic agonist: Dopamine and dobutamine
  - Phosphodiesterase inhibitors: Milrinone
  - Angiotensin receptor blockers: Losartan and valsartan
  - Antiarrhythmic agents: Amiodarone
- **Oxygen**
- **Rest and activity period**
- **Daily weight monitoring**
- **Sodium restriction**
- **Ventricular assist device**
- **Cardiac resynchronization therapy**
- **Cardiac transplantation**

## Nursing Management

### Nursing Diagnosis

Decreased cardiac output related to altered myocardial contractility/inotropic changes as evidenced by increased heart rate (tachycardia), dysrhythmias, ECG changes.

### Nursing Interventions

- Check the BP and Pulse rate of the patient every 2–3 minutes after the initiation of the IV antihypertensive medications.
- Regular monitoring of hemodynamic parameters and vital signs.
- Confirm the rate and dose of medication.
- Give oxygen as indicated by the patient's symptoms, oxygen saturation and ABGs.
- Provide a restful environment and encourage periods of rest and sleep.
- Check for calf tenderness, diminished pedal pulses, swelling, local redness or pallor of extremity.

### Nursing Diagnosis

Impaired gas exchange related to increased preload a evidenced by increased respiratory rate, dyspnea.

### Nursing Interventions

- Position patient in semi-Fowler's position for breathing
- Assist patient to use relaxation techniques
- Monitoring the urine output
- Provide complete bed rest

### Nursing Diagnosis

Excess fluid volume related to reduced glomerular filtration rate as evidenced by Oliguria, edema and JVD.

### Nursing Interventions

- Continuous monitoring of ECG to find out the cardiac dysrhythmias.
- Monitoring the urine output.
- Provide complete bed rest.
- Regular neurological assessment; level of consciousness, papillary reaction and size, movement of extremities, etc.
- Follow a low-sodium diet and/or fluid restriction.
- Change position frequently. Elevate feet when sitting. Inspect skin surface, keep dry, and provide padding as indicated.

### Nursing Diagnosis

Decreased activity tolerance related to the imbalance between the supply and demand of the oxygen supply to the body cells.

### Nursing Interventions

- Encourage alternate rest and activity
- Provide adequate medication as per order
- Oxygen if needed
- Maintain the oxygen saturation
- Daily weight monitoring
- Monitor vital signs and hemodynamic parameters
- Provide health education regarding follow up care and need for life style modification
- Psychological support provide propped up position for dyspnea
- Cardiac auscultation
- Continuous physical examination
- Dietary modification
- Ongoing follow-up care

Heart failure is the disease condition affecting the cardiac pumping action. That results in the vasoconstriction and fluid retention. Heart failure is the major cause of mortality and morbidity in the countries. It is the inability of the heart to maintain adequate cardiac output according to the body demands. It may be right sided or left sided or both biventricular.

## MANAGEMENT MODALITIES FOR CARDIOVASCULAR SYSTEM DISORDERS

### Cardiopulmonary Resuscitation

Cardiopulmonary resuscitation (CPR) is an emergency procedure that is used to rescue the patient in cardiac arrest. It may be in the hospital or in the community setting. In CPR the rescuer give chest compression and artificial respiration to the patient after confirming the need of cardiac and pulmonary resuscitation.

#### Chain of Survival

**Flowchart 9.24** shows the chain of survival pattern.

#### Indication

- Cardiac arrest
- Respiratory arrest: Patient has pulse but no respiration.

### CABD (Circulation, Airway, Breathing, Defibrillate)

BLS is a common acronym used to guide providers to use suitable steps to assess and treat patients in respiratory and cardiac arrest. This is in the order; CAB-D (Circulation, Airway, Breathing, Defibrillate) **(Flowchart 9.25)** (AHA, 2020).

CPR is an emergency procedure that is used to rescue the patient in cardiac arrest. It may be in the hospital or in the community setting. In CPR the rescuer give chest compression and artificial respiration to the patient after confirming the need of cardiac and pulmonary resuscitation.

### Pacemaker

A pacemaker is an artificial electrical devise that stimulate the heart muscle to depolarize and causes contraction. The pacemaker can divide into mainly temporary or permanent according to the patient need. The pacemaker works by generating the impulse from the power source and transmitting the impulse to the cardiac myocardium. The major components of a pacemaker are a pulse generator, pacing lead, and electrode tip.

#### Pulse Generator

It contains power source and circuitry. Lithium batteries are there in the permanent pacemakers with a life span of ten years. A microchip is the circuitry of the pacemaker is that guides the heart pacing. In temporary pacemaker a small size radio or telemetry box with alkaline batteries as power source.

#### Stimulus

From the pulse generator an electrical stimulus travel to the electrode chip for the cardiac contraction. If the pacemaker need to stimulate only one chamber of the heart means the leads placed either in the atrium or ventricle it will place, in case of dual chamber then it will be there in the both atrium and ventricle usually on the right side of the heart.

#### Electrodes

It may be one in the unipolar and two in the bipolar lead. It will send the information to the myocardium and give the impulse back to the pulse generator.

### Pacemaker Spikes

The stimulus that travels from the pulse generator to the myocardium can be visible in the ECG as spikes. It is may be large or small appear above or below the isoelectrical line.

### Indication

#### Permanent Pacemaker

- AV block; second or third degree AV block
- Bundle branch block
- Cardiomyopathy; dilated or hypertrophic
- Hear failure
- SA node dysfunction
- Tachydysrhythmias

#### Temporary Pacemaker

- Postcardiac catheterization procedure and coronary angiography
- Before permanent pacemaker implantation
- Prophylactic for cardiac surgeries
- Acute MI
- Second or third degree heart block
- Bradycardia
- Syncope
- Shock myocarditis
- Lyme disease

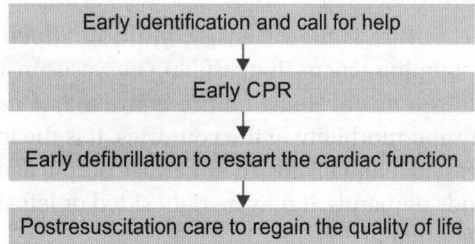

**Flowchart 9.24:** Chain of survival.

**Flowchart 9.25:** BLS algorithm.

### BLS algorithm

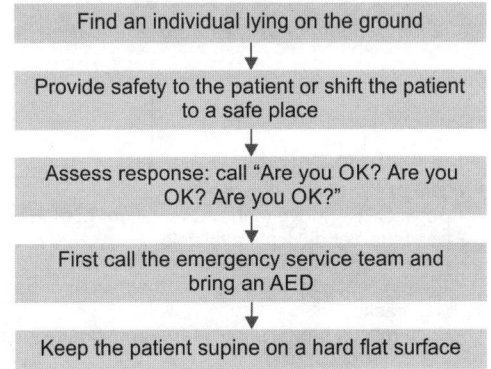

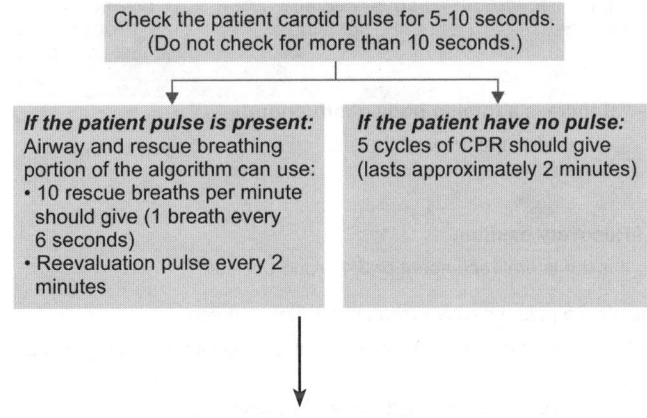

**Start chest compressions**

- Give 100–120 compressions per minute. That is 30 compressions every 15–18 seconds.
- Place the palms in midline position, one over the other, on the lower 1/2 of the patient's sternum between the nipples.
- Lock the arms.
- Using two arms press to a depth of 2–2.4 inches (5–6 cm) or more on the patient's chest.
- Hard and fast compression.
- Allow for full chest recoil with each compression.

*1 cycle of adult CPR is 30:2 is the compression respiration ratio.*
*If two providers are present: change the role between compressor and rescue breather every 5 cycles*

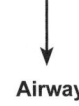

**Airway**

Jaw thrust maneuver can use. This maneuver is used when suspecting a cervical spine injury:
- Place the fingers on the lower rami of the jaw.
- Give pressure anteriorly to advance the jaw forward.

*Use the head Tilt-Chin lift maneuver:*
- Place the palm on the patient's forehead and provide a pressure to tilt the head backward.
- Place the fingers on the other hand under the mental protuberance of the chin and pull the chin forward and cephalic.

*Contd...*

# Chapter 9: Cardiovascular Emergencies and Management

*Contd...*

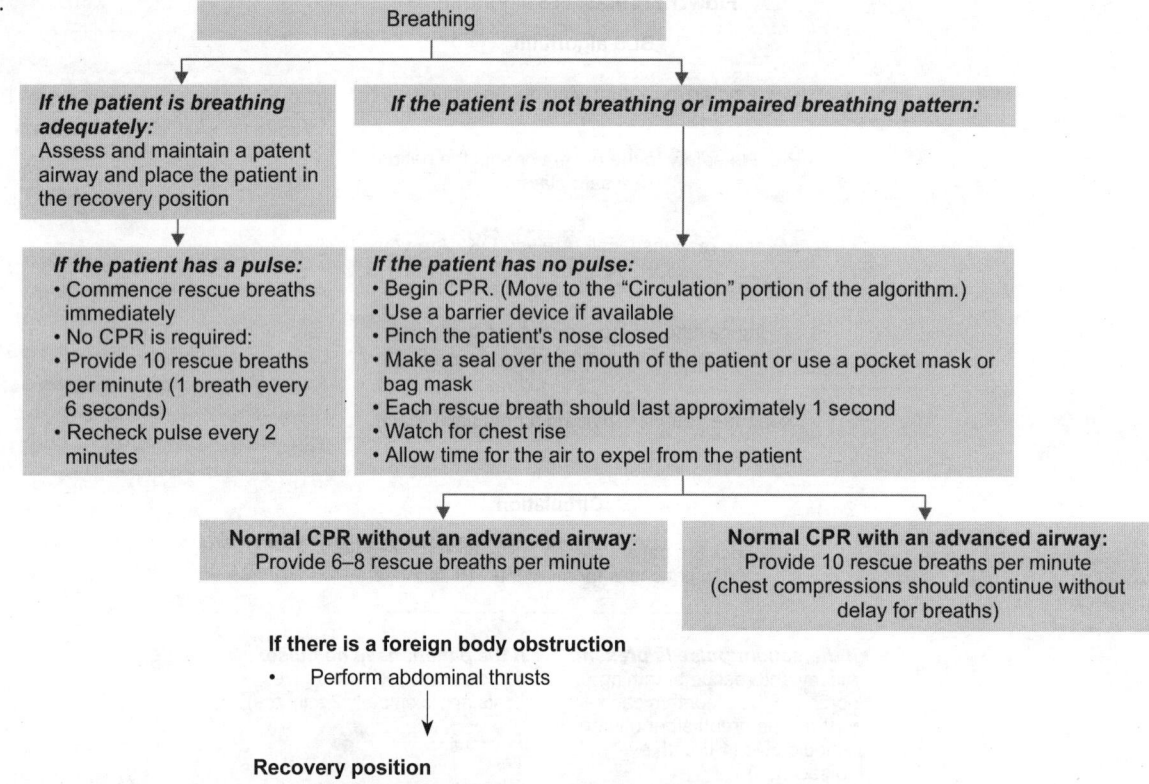

### If there is a foreign body obstruction
- Perform abdominal thrusts

### Recovery position
It is the lateral recumbent or 3/4 prone position:

This position can maintain a patent airway in the unconscious person

- Keep the patient close to a true lateral position with the head dependent to allow fluid to drain
- Maintain stable position
- Don't give pressure on the chest that could impairs breathing
- Position patient in such a way that it allows turning them onto their back easily
- Take precautions to stabilize the neck in case of cervical spine injury

***Assess and maintain access of airway continuously.
Avoid the recovery position if it will cause injury to the patient.***

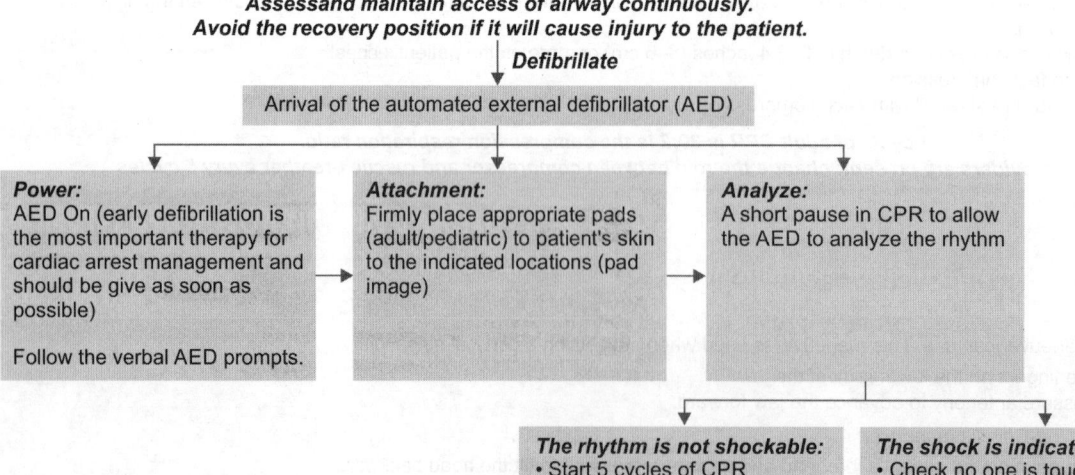

## Types

### Permanent Pacemaker
Under local anesthesia usually this pacemaker may implanted surgically. Through transvenously the leads are placed in the chambers and then fixed into the endocardium. The pulse generator will keep at the pocket made subcutaneously under the clavicle.

### Temporary Pacemaker
It is usually placed at the emergency situation. This can act as a bridge between the temporary to the permanent pacemaker. The temporary can be transvenous, epicardia or transcutaneous.

### Transvenous
It is the insertion of the pacemaker may through the vein like subclavian or internal jugular vein. This procedure can do at the patient bedside or at the procedure room. It is one of the most reliable type of temporary pacemaker. The lead wire inserted into the atrium or ventricle and then it connected to the pulse generator.

### Epicardial
It is commonly using during the cardiac surgeries. The doctors attach the lead wires at the surface of the heart or epicardium and the tip of the wire get out of the patient via the chest wall below the incision area. Then it will attach to the pulse generator. The lead wire will remove after several days of surgery.

### Transcutaneous
It is noninvasive method of temporary pacemaker. In this type the electrode placed on the patient anterior chest wall and one at the back of the chest. The external pulse generator generates the impulse through the skin to the heart. It can be see along with defibrillator for emergency purpose.

## Pacemaker Codes
The pacemaker working can be describes by five letter coding system.

### First Letter
It indicating which chamber the pacemaker paced.
- V-Ventricle
- A-Atrium
- D-Dual (atrium + ventricle)
- O-None

### Second Letter
This letter indicates which chamber pacemaker sensing.
- V-Ventricle
- A-Atrium
- D-Dual (atrium+ventricle)
- O-None

### Third Letter
It indicates the response of the pacemaker to electrical activity it senses the atrium or ventricle.
- T-Triggers pacing (if sensed the atrial activity then the ventricular pacing may be triggered)
- I-Inhibit pacing (if the pacemaker sense the intrinsic activity then the pacemaker didn't fire)
- D-Dual (pacemaker may be trigger or inhibit according to the intrinsic activity of the heart)
- O-None (pacemaker never changes its mode).

### Fourth Letter
It indicates the rate modulation. It is also known as adaptive pacing.
- R-Rate modulation
- O-None (no rate modulation)

### Fifth Letter
It specifies the location and absence of the multisite pacing.
- O-None (no multisite pacing)
- A-Atrium (multisite pacing in the atrium)
- V-Ventricle (multisite pacing in the ventricle)
- D-Dual site.

## Troubleshooting Problems
Malfunction of the pacemaker is a life-threatening problem to the patient and the patient may go the syncope, arrhythmias or hypotension. Common problems include:
- Failure to capture
- Failure to pace
- Under sensing
- Over sensing

## Failure to Capture
It is a pacemaker spike without a complex. This refers that the pacemakers inability to stimulate the chamber.

### Causes
- Hypoxia
- Acidosis
- Electrolyte imbalance
- Fibrosis incorrect lead position
- Broken wire
- Perforation of the lead wire through the myocardium

## Failure to Pace

There is no pacemaker activity in the ECG may indicate failure to pace. It can lead to asystole.

### Causes

- Battery or circuit failure
- Broken leads
- Loose connections
- Oversensing
- Too low voltage

## Failure to Sense

It is otherwise called as under sensing, in which pacemaker spike when there is an intrinsic activity. These spikes can occur at anywhere in the ECG, if it is at the T wave then it is very dangerous and it may lead to ventricular tachycardia and ventricular fibrillation.

### Causes

- High voltage
- Electrolyte imbalance
- Disconnection or dislodgement of the lead
- Improper lead placement
- Increase the sensing threshold from edema or fibrosis
- Drug interactions
- Dead pacemaker battery

## Over Sensing

In this problem the pacemaker is too sensitive and it may misinterpret the muscle involvement or any cardiac events may sense as depolarization. And the pacemaker won't pace when the patient needed and the AV synchronization and heart rate won't be maintained (Woods SL, 2010).

## Nurse's Responsibility

Points should be take care while take care of a patient with a artificial pacemaker:

- Assist the pacemaker implantation procedure
- Regular checkup of patent pacemaker settings, connections and functions
- Monitor the patient vital signs
- Carefully reposition the patient if the patient is on the temporary pacemaker
- Avoid the micro shocks to the patient
- Counter check the pacemaker spies with the patient response
- Monitor the signs of infection
- Check the subcutaneous air around the pacemaker implantation site
- Monitor the hiccups or any pectoral muscle twitching during synchronization with pacemaker
- Check the signs of ventricular perforation and cardiac tamponade
- Check for signs of pneumothorax

## Patient Education

- Explain the pacemaker and its function, need to the patient and the patient family members
- If the patient is on the temporary pacemaker teach them to get the assistance while get out of the bed
- Educate the patient that there will be a muscle twitching for permanent pacemaker implantation
- Instruct the patient that never reposition the pacemaker wires or pulse generator
- The patient should carry the pacemaker identification card all times
- Educate the patient that how to check the troubleshooting problems of the pacemaker like battery problems
- Educate the patient and the relative about hoe to check the pulse rate and incision site care for permanent pacemaker
- Advise the patient do not use tight cloths or direct pressure over the pulse generator
- Avoid MRI and other certain diagnostic evaluation
- Advise the patient to take medical attention if they feel any discomfort like light headedness, palpitation, hiccups, tachycardia

A pacemaker is an artificial electrical devise that stimulate the heart muscle to depolarize and causes contraction. The pacemaker can divide into mainly temporary or permanent according to the patient need. The pacemaker works by generating the impulse from the power source and transmitting the impulse to the cardiac myocardium.

# PERCUTANEOUS CORONARY INTERVENTION

It is a group of procedure performed via percutaneous basis to give any interventional management in the coronary arteries. The PCI initiates with the angiography and can perform the procedures like atherectomy, thrombectomy or drug eluting or without drug eluting stent placement (Chatterjee K, 2013).

## Patient Selection

- Ischemia in the ECG and cardiac biomarkers
- Unstable angina
- ACS

The patient with unstable angina/NSTEMI shows:
- Recurrent angina
- Elevated cardiac biomarkers
- Signs and symptoms of heart failure
- Worsening mitral regurgitation
- Ventricular tachycardia

## Procedure
- Follow aseptic technique
- Access a patent arterial line
- Introduce a guide wire through the artery
- Insert the balloon catheter into the coronary artery via aorta may be into the right or left coronary artery
- The guide wire place across the area of narrowing
- The balloon catheter also place over the lesion
- Inflate the balloon
- The stent will attach over the stenotic area
- Deflate the balloon
- Remove the catheter and the guide wire outside once the planned effect result got, by checking the perfusion by angiogram.

## Types

### Coronary Atherectomy
- It is the removal of the atherosclerotic plaque
- Mainly 2 types.

*Directional Coronary Atherectomy (DCA)*

In this method rotating the cup shaped blade across the plaque and directionally remove the plaque.

*Rotational Coronary Atherectomy*

It is performed by the microscopic diamond chips. It will rotate rapidly by olive shaped atherectomy burr around 160,000 rpm. It is usually used in case of calcified lesions were the stent cannot place.

### Thrombectomy and Aspiration Devices
In this technique the thrombus removed by the dissolution and aspiration. In which the high speed saline jets is there within the tip of the catheter. That will give the local suction effect. Then it may pull the blood, thrombus and the saline into the catheter.

### Emboli Protection Device
There are different types of emboli protection devices:
- Distal occlusion device
- Emboli protection filters
- Proximal occlusion devises

### Coronary Stents
It may be drug eluting or without drug eluting one.

**Drug eluting stent:** In this stent contains anti proliferating agents.
- Example: Sirolimus eluting stent immunosuppressive agent
- Paclitaxel eluting stent anti-inflammatory agents
- Stent material includes stainless steel and cobalt chromium

## Nursing Management of Patient during PCI

### Preprocedure Management
- Informed consent
- History and physical examination documentation
- Laboratory history

*Patient with Diabetes*
- With hold the oral hypoglycemic agents on the day prior to PCI
- Insulin dose change according to physician's order
- Check the blood sugar value on the day prior to the procedure

*Patient with Renal Diseases*
- Check the serum creatinine value, if it is >1.6 mL/dL indicates the renal dysfunction
- Provide adequate hydration before and after the procedure
- Sodium bicarbonate and N-acetylcysteine combination can reduce the risk of renal dysfunction.

### Intraprocedure Management
- Give bolus heparin to maintain the activated clotting time (ACT) around 250–300 sec.
- Radial or brachial arterial access
- Monitor the hemodynamic parameters
- Monitor ECG continuously
- After the procedure prepare the patient for shifting
- Assess the incision site for any bleeding or hematoma
- Sheath may be kept remain for 4–6 hours after the procedure

### Postprocedure Management
- Shift the patient to the intensive coronary care unit
- Monitor the vital signs and hemodynamic parameters continuously
- ECG monitoring
- Lab investigations include hematocrit, platelet, blood urea nitrogen and serum creatinine
- Maintain adequate hydration

- *Removal of the sheath*
  - After 4-6 hours
  - Check the ACT, if it is <180 second can remove the sheath
  - Provide manual pressure at the arterial site for 20 min or more time if needed or once the homeostasis achieved
  - Provide compression bandage at the arterial site
  - Check the arterial site for any complication; bleeding, hematoma

### Anticoagulation Treatment for PCI Patients

#### Oral Antiplatelets

*Before Procedure*

- Aspirin loading dose 75–325 mg at least 2 hours or 24 hours prior to the procedure
- **Clopilet:** 300 mg 6 hours prior to the procedure

*After Procedure*

- **Aspirin:** Daily 150 mg
- **Clopilet:** 75 mg daily

#### Antithrombotic Therapy

- Unfractionated heparin before PCI
- Low molecular weight heparin (LMWH) also can be considered (Woods SL, 2010)

#### Complications Related to PCI

- Angina
- Stent thrombosis
- NSTEMI
- STEMI
- Perforation of the coronary vessel
- Vasospasm
- Arrhythmia
- Contrast related complication
- Acute renal failure
- Cerebrovascular complications

### Cardioversion

It is a synchronized therapy to the patient who is hemodynamically unstable with ventricular or supraventricular tachycardia. A synchronized defibrillator is used to deliver the shock that is programmed to deliver the patient at the R wave in QRS in the ECG. The synchronize button should be on mode for cardioversion.

#### Procedure

- Same as the defibrillator
- Other characteristics or exceptions include
- Cardioversion is under the general anesthesia or sedation (IV midazolam)
- It is an elective procedure
- Turn on the machine
- On the synchronize button
- Attach the adhesive electrodes
- Choose the energy level that will be less than the defibrillator 50J for monophasic and the subsequent energy level can increase by progress to maximum 200 J.
- Get the clear vision of the ECG lead II
- Ensure all clear
- Discharge of the energy; there may be one or two second delay till the machine find out the synchronization
- Check the rhythm of the patient (Woods SL, 2010)

### Intra-aortic Balloon Pump

It is a type of circulatory assist device used to give assistance or support to the ventricle. It is providing a temporary assistance to the compromised ventricle to reduce the afterload by reducing the systolic pressure and improving the aortic diastolic pressure that will result in the improving the coronary circulation **(Fig. 9.35)** (Sheehy, 2017).

#### Indications

- Refractory unstable angina
- Temporary bridge to the cardiac transplantation
- Acute MI
- Acute ventricular septal defect
- Cardiogenic shock
- Pre, post or intraoperative cardiac surgeries
- High risk interventional cardiac procedures
- Left ventricular failure after the cardiopulmonary bypass (CPB)

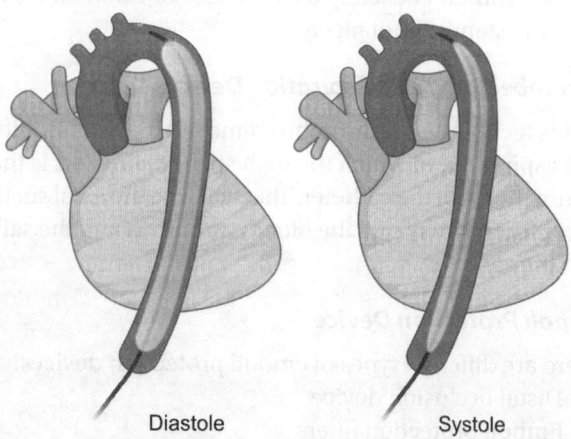

**Fig. 9.35:** Intra-aortic balloon pump.

## Contraindications

- Irreversible brain damage
- Untreatable disease of any major organ system
- Abdominal and thoracic aortic aneurysm
- Moderate to severe aortic insufficiency
- Peripheral vascular diseases

## Procedure and Technique

- Follow aseptic technique
- The balloon (sausage shape) inserted via femoral artery
- Advanced towards heart placed at the descending aorta just above the renal artery and below the subclavian artery
- After the placement confirm the position with chest X-ray
- Helium cyclically fills the balloon at the early phase of diastole that is immediately after the aortic valve closure
- It deflates before the systole helps to eject the blood to the systemic circulation
- The inflation and deflation are triggered by the help of ECG, the balloon will inflate at T wave and deflate at the R wave in the QRS
- The intra-aortic balloon pump (IABP) technique otherwise called as the *counter pulsation* because it is working as opposite of the ventricular contraction
- The ratio of inflation deflation to the heart beat is 1:1

## Mechanism Behind the Counter Pulsation

At the early phase of the diastole the balloon will inflate and give more blood supply to the coronary arteries and peripheral circulation. And at the balloon will deflate just prior to the systole will give a sudden vacuum in the aorta give a pressure drop and the ventricle can easily eject the blood into the aorta. That is the reason the afterload is going to reduce (Woods SL, 2010).

## Complications of IABP

- Infection at the catheter site
- Pneumonia
- Arterial injury
- Thromboembolism
- Platelet aggregation at balloon site
- Hemorrhage from the insertion site
- Balloon leakage or break

## Nursing Management

- Monitoring of vital signs
- Hemodynamic parameter monitoring
- Continuous monitoring of intake and output
- Confirm the position of the IABP by X-ray
- Observe the catheter site for any bleeding or hematoma formation
- Check the CBC
- Maintain the patent airway

## Defibrillation

It is the treatment for life-threatening conditions without pulse including ventricular fibrillation and pulse less ventricular tachycardia. In defibrillation the electrical energy is delivered to the heart to restart the cardiac function as normal. In this the electrical energy may be delivered by mono phasic or biphasic **(Fig. 9.36)** (Woods SL, 2010).

### Monophasic vs Biphasic

- In monophasic the electrical energy passes through one direction that is from one paddle to the other
- In biphasic the current passes in both direction
- Biphasic **(Fig. 9.37)** having less burn and myocardial damage comparing to the monophasic
- In biphasic deliver energy maximum at 150–200 J, but in the monophasic deliver 360 J.
- Nowadays all the defibrillator having biphasic (Sheehy, 2017)

### Mechanism

- Repolarization of the myocardium after the electrical shock.
- Induce asystole temporarily.

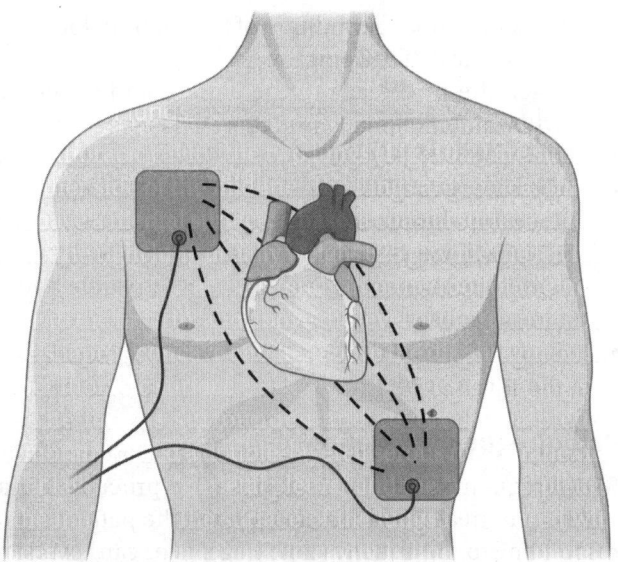

**Fig. 9.36:** Defibrillation.

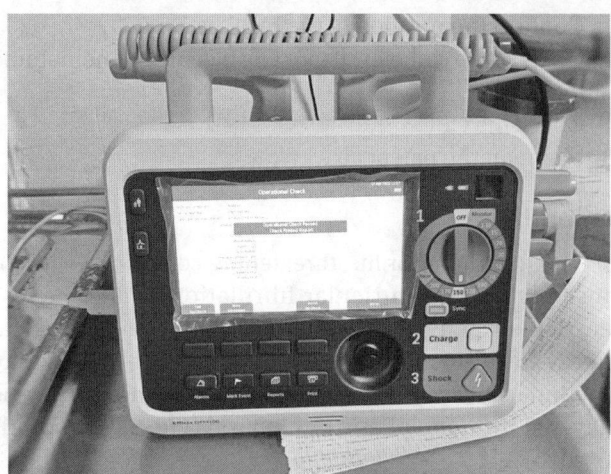

**Fig. 9.37:** Biphasic defibrillator.

## Types of Defibrillators

### Automated External Defibrillator

- It is usually used in the community setting as a part of basic life support.
- There is no need of professional training.
- All instructions are there in the AED.
- Verbal responses are available.
- The machine itself analyze and deliver the shock.

### Standard Defibrillator

- May be monophasic or biphasic.
- It is usually can see in the casualty, ICUs and OT.

### Transvenous/Implanted Type

Procedure

- Check the working condition of the defibrillator.
- Turn on the defibrillator.
- Attach the ECG leads to the patient and check the rhythm.
- Apply conduction gel over the paddles.
- Select the required energy.
- Off the synchronize button.
- Tell I clear, you clear and all clear.
- Deliver the energy by pressing the both paddle button simultaneously.
- Monitor the ECG rhythm.
- Continue if needed.

## Radiofrequency Ablation

Radiofrequency ablation is an invasive procedure that will help to treat the arrhythmias when the patient is not responding to the antiarrhythmic agents or cardioversion therapy. In this procedure, radiofrequency energy delivered through a catheter to the cardiac tissue to destroy or burn the focus of arrhythmia or block the conduction pathway which is responsible for arrhythmia.

### Indications

- Atrial tachycardia
- Atrial fibrillation
- Atrial flutter
- Ventricular tachycardia
- AV nodal reentry tachycardia
- Wolf-Parkinson-White syndrome

### Procedure

First the patient will undergo the electrophysiological study to find out the arrhythmic focus. Then the ablation catheter inserts through the veins usually femoral vein and then advances in to the heart and reaches the selected focus and burst the area. The destroyed focus can't conduct the electrical signals no more (Woods SL, 2010).

Other types includes—microwave, sonar and cryotherapy.

### Nurse's Responsibility

- Continuous cardiac monitoring
- Assess the ECG for any type of arrhythmias
- Provide bed rest for 8 hours
- Keep the affected extremity straight for rest period and maintain the head end elevation at 15–30 degree
- Check the patient vital signs every 15 minutes for the first hour and every 30 minutes for the next 4 hours
- Assess the peripheral pulses, color, sensation, temperature, capillary refill of the affected extremity
- Check the catheter insertion site for any hematoma, bleeding
- Monitor the patient for any complications: Hemorrhage, stroke, cardiac tamponade, arrhythmias, phrenic nerve damage, pulmonary vein stenosis, thrombosis and sudden death.

### Patient Education

- Educate the patient and the family members about the procedure.
- Educate the patient and the family about that it is lengthy procedure may take up to 6 hours.
- Explain the patient that patient may stay in the hospital for 2 days.

## Nursing Management of Patients Undergoing Different Modalities for Cardiovascular System Disorders

Possible priority nursing diagnosis and its interventions.

## Nursing Diagnosis

Ineffective tissue perfusion related to cardiac dysrhythmias, heart blocks, tachydysrhythmias, as evidenced by decreased blood pressure cool, clammy extremities, altered level of consciousness.

## Nursing Interventions

- Assess the ECG for changes in rhythm, rate, and presence of dysrhythmias. Treat as indicated.
- Check the vital signs every 15 minutes
- Identify for muscle twitching or hiccups
- Monitor for sudden complaints of chest pain, and auscultate for pericardial friction rub or muffled heart tones
- Restrict the movement of extremity involved near the insertion site as ordered
- Protect patients from microwave ovens, radar, diathermies, etc.
- Instruct on limitations on activity: avoid excessive bending, stretching, lifting heavy, strenuous exercise, or contact sports.

## Nursing Diagnosis

Impaired skin integrity related to changes in mobility as evidenced by disruption of skin tissue.

## Nursing Interventions

- Change dressing daily, or per hospital protocol, using a sterile technique.
- Instruct on wound care to pacer site and to avoid taking showers for 2 weeks post insertion.
- Instruct the patient and/or family to observe for signs of redness, drainage, fever, pain, tenderness, and swelling at the site.

## Nursing Diagnosis

Risk for injury related to puncture of perforation of heart tissues.

## Nursing Interventions

- Assess the patient for bleeding.
- Check the vital signs: Observe for diaphoresis, dyspnea, and restlessness.
- Instruct the patient on signs and symptoms, such as restlessness, syncope, chest pain, or dyspnea of which to notify the nurse.

# Cardiac Surgeries

## Coronary Artery Bypass Graft

Coronary artery bypass graft (CABG) surgery is defined as the surgical procedure in which the new vascular pathway introduced in between the aorta and the myocardium distal to the obstructed coronary artery. In this procedure the graft may be from the saphenous vein, radial artery, internal mammary artery, gastroepiploic artery or inferior epigastric artery (Woods SL).

### Procedure

- Median sternotomy
- Initiate CPB
- Selection and removal of the graft vessel
- Anastomosis of the graft between the aorta and the myocardium distal to the occluded coronary artery.

### Types

**Minimally invasive direct coronary artery bypass (MIDCAB)**

This technique is used for the patient with single vessel disease in which without the median sternotomy and CPB the surgery can complete.

**Off pump coronary artery bypass**

Without CPB with the help of partial of full sternotomy the bypass surgery can be done.

**Trans myocardial laser revascularization**

It is an indirect technique of revascularization. In this technique the high energy laser create the channels. These channels allow the blood flow to the ischemic areas in the heart.

### Indications

- Significant left main coronary artery stenosis
- 3 vessel coronary artery disease
- Two vessel disease with ejection fraction <50%
- One or two vessel disease with large area of the myocardium at risk
- Failed angioplasty
- Post infarction ventricular septal defect.

### Relative Contraindications

- Severe anatomic abnormalities
- Severe left ventricular failure
- Associated any disease conditions

## Valvular Surgeries

Definition It is the surgical procedure in which the repair of the affected valve according to the disease condition of the patient (Sheehy, 2017).

### Indications

- Mitral stenosis
- Infective endocarditis

- Young age
- No previous valvular surgery

*Types of Surgeries*

**Mitral commissurotomy**

It is indicated for the patient with mitral stenosis. In which the surgical repair of the mitral valve.

**Valvuloplasty**

It is for the treatment of the mitral or tricuspid regurgitation. In which the valvular repair will do.

**Annuloplasty**

In this technique there is repair of the annulus of the valve.

**Prosthetic valvular surgery**

In this technique there is valvular replacement with the prosthetic valves. Types of prosthetic valves:
- **Mechanical caged ball valve:** Starr-Edwards, Sutter, Mcgovern
- **Tilting Disc Valve:** Lillehei-Kaster, Medtronic Hall
- **Leaflet valve:** St Jude, On X, Carbomedic
- **Biologic Porcine Heterograft:** Medtronic
- **Pericardial heterograft:** Edwards
- **Homograft:** Cadaver valve

*Routine Postoperative Care*
- Admit the patient in the ICU for the first 6–24 hour of surgery
- Continuous monitoring of ECG, hemodynamic values, vital signs, $SPO_2$, pulmonary arterial pressure
- Check for any arrhythmias, hypotension, and hypovolemia.
- If any indication of hypovolemia start blood transfusion
- Check the drain output
- Maintain the IO chart

*Nursing Management*
- Long-term anticoagulation therapy
- Monitor for the complications
- Check the vital signs and the hemodynamic parameters
- Regular monitoring of the bleeding time, clotting time, aPTT and PT INR values

*Complications after the Cardiac Surgeries*
- Postoperative bleeding
- Cardiac tamponade
- Myocardial depression
- Myocardial infarction
- Arrhythmias
- Pulmonary embolism
- Renal failure
- Gastroduodenal bleeding
- Cholecystitis
- Brachial and ulnar plexus injury
- Delirium
- Wound infection

### Cardiac (Heart) Transplantation

Cardiac transplantation is the major treatment for the end-stage cardiac disease. The donated heart is placed at the normal anatomical position of the recipient (Woods SL, 2010).

*Selection of Recipients*
- Age <60 years
- End-stage cardiac failure patient with symptoms

*Contraindications*
- Malignancies
- Lung diseases
- Collagen vascular disease
- Autoimmune diseases

*Donor Selection*
- Suitable donor should be <35 years
- Declared as brain death
- No evidence of chest injury
- Check the donor's cardiac history, infection and the duration of CPR
- Check the matching with the donor and recipient blood.

*Procedure*
- After selection of the appropriate donor then surgically open the donor chest.
- Remove the heart from the donor after cooling.
- Prepare the recipient chest.
- After the median sternotomy initiate the cardiopulmonary bypass.
- Remove the heart from the recipient leave the posterior wall of the atria. The blood vessels including the vena cava, and pulmonary vein remain intact. The aorta and the pulmonary artery were transected.
- Then the atria of the donor anastomosed with the recipient atria without harm the SA node. After the anastomosis of the atria, the aorta and pulmonary artery anastomose with the recipient vessels (Braunwald).

*Complications*
- Graft rejection
- Hypertension
- Vasculopathy

## Nursing Management of Patients Undergoing Cardiac Surgeries

### Nursing Diagnosis

Decreased cardiac output related to cardiac ischemia during transplantation as evidenced by bradycardia and hypotension.

Nursing interventions

- Assess the vital signs and the hemodynamic parameters regularly.
- Maintain intake output chart.
- Check for hypotension and shock symptoms.

### Nursing Diagnosis

Risk for ineffective airway clearance.

Nursing interventions

- Positioning the patient upright as tolerated
- Encouraging coughing and deep breathing
- Encouraging and assisting with ambulation as tolerated
- Monitoring oxygen saturation and coordinating with respiratory therapy
- Administering prescribed oxygen and other medications as necessary

### Nursing Diagnosis

Risk for infection related to immunosuppressive therapy as evidenced by elevated temperature, increase WBC.

Nursing interventions

- Maintain aseptic technique
- Monitor laboratory value
- Monitor the signs of rejection

### Nursing Diagnosis

Activity intolerance related to preoperative de-conditioned stage as evidenced by fatigue.

Nursing interventions

- Assess the side effects of immune suppressants
- Monitor the chance of complications

### Nursing Diagnosis

Risk for complications related to cardiac transplantation.

Nursing interventions

- Monitoring the patient's heart rate/rhythm, blood pressure, and respiratory rate
- Assessing extremities for color, temperature, cap refill, edema

## Summary

The cardiovascular system is one of the vital system in our body start the activity at the four weeks in the fetal life and the last system to cease the activity at the end of the life. There are different types of cardiac surgeries are there. When the coronary blood vessels get occlusion that leads to the decreased blood flow and the complete occlusion leads to the halt of blood supply to the particular distal area may lead to myocardial cell death. Reparative surgeries include the closure of PDA, ASD, and VSD, etc. Reconstructive surgeries include the CABG, mitral or aortic valve surgeries, etc.

## Points to Ponder

- The heart is a muscular organ situated in the middle of the mediastinum. It is covered by pericardium.
- Hypertensive crisis are acute, and severe elevation of blood pressure, defines as an elevation of diastolic blood pressure more than 140 mm Hg, with or without target organ damage.
- The cardiac cells can with stand the ischemia around 20 minutes. Approximately 4–6 hours may take to complete infarction.
- Dilated cardiomyopathy common type of cardiomyopathy.
- Mainly the valvular disorders may occur due to the stenosis or regurgitation or the prolapsed of the valves.
- Aneurysm is a permanent localized dilation aorta having diameter at least 1.5 times that of expected normal diameter of the aortic segment.
- A pacemaker is an artificial electrical devise that stimulate the heart muscle to depolarize and causes contraction.
- Heart failure is the major cause of mortality and morbidity in the countries. It is the inability of the heart to maintain adequate cardiac output according to the body demands. It may be right sided or left sided or both biventricular.
- The endocardium is the inner lining of the heart it continues to form the cardiac valves. That is the major cause that the IE affects the cardiac valves.

## Abbreviations

- CVD     : Cardiovascular Disease
- AV      : Atrioventricular
- CAD     : Coronary Artery Disease
- HF      : Heart Failure
- RCA     : Right Coronary Artery
- LCA     : Left Coronary Artery
- MAP     : Mean Arterial Pressure
- MI      : Myocardial Infarction
- STEMI   : ST Elevated MI
- NSTEMI  : Non ST Elevated MI
- PCI     : Percuteneous Coronary Intervention
- CO      : Cardiac Output

- VT : Ventricular Tachycardia
- VF : Ventricular Fibrillation
- $PaO_2$ : Partial Pressure of Oxygen
- $PaCO_2$ : Partial Pressure of Carbon Dioxide
- WPW : Wolf Parkinson White
- HR : Heart Rate
- CRP : C-Reactive Protein
- IE : Infective Endocarditis
- AED : Automated External Defibrillator
- ASD : Atrial Septal Defect
- VSD : Ventricular Septal Defect
- PDA : Patent Ductus Arteriosus

### Short Answer Questions

1. Define hypertension crisis and factors affecting to hypertension.
2. Postoperative nursing care after CABG.
3. Define MI and write its causes, clinical manifestations and management.
4. Describe the coronary circulation with diagram.
5. Describe the heart failure and stages of the heat failure.
6. Describe cardiomyopathy and its management.
7. Write about the vascular disorder.

### Long Answer Questions

1. Mr Arvin, 45 year old admitted in ICU with acute left ventricular failure.
   a. Write the clinical features of the patient.
   b. Mention the diagnostic test done for the same patient.
   c. Draw a nursing care plan for the patient.
2. Describe the etiology, pathophysiology and the management of the patient with infective endocarditis.
3. Write a detailed pre and postoperative nursing management of the patient undergone aortic valve replacement surgery.

### Bibliography

1. American Heart Association (AHA). Instructor manual; 2020.
2. Braunald's textbook of heart disease. London. W B Saunders; 2007.
3. Brunner and Suddarth's textbook of Medical Surgical Nursing. 11th edition. New Delhi: Lippincott and Williams; 2008.
4. Chatterjee K, Anderson M, Heistad D, Kerber RE. Cardiology an illustrated textbook. 1st edition. Jaypee. New Delhi; 2013.
5. Chaurasia BD. Human anatomy; Regional and applied dissection and clinical. 4th edition. Volume I. CBS publisher and distributers. New Delhi; 233-55.
6. Chintamani. Mediacl surgical nursing. New Delhi: Elsevier; 2011.
7. Davidson's principles and practice of medicine. Philadelphia: Churchill Livingstone and Elsevier; 2002.
8. Harrison's Principles of internal medicine. 16th edition. New York: McGraw-Hill Medical Publishing Division; 2005.
9. Mathew P, Bordeni B. Embryology, Heart. Stat Pearl. Treasure Island; 2019.
10. Scott TB. Hypertensive emergencies. CCSAP. Medical issue in ICU. 2018:7-24.
11. Sheehy's emergency Nursing principles and practice. 7th edition. Elsevier; 2017.
12. Smith SC, Jackson R, Pearson TA, Fuster V, Yusuf S, Faergeman O, et al. Principles for national and regional guidelines on cardiovascular disease prevention: A scientific statement from the World Heart and Stroke Forum. Circulation. 2004;109(25):3112-21.
13. Singh I. human embryology. 11th edition. The health science publishers. New Delhi; 2018.
14. Woods SL, Froelicher ESS, Motzer AU, Bridges EJ. Cardiac nursing. 6th edition. Wolter Kluwer. China; 2010.

# Chapter 10

# Respiratory Emergency Diseases

*Mamata Swain*

## CHAPTER OUTLINE

- Respiratory System
  - Anatomy of respiratory system
  - Physiology of respiratory system
- Assessment of Respiratory System
  - History and physical examination
  - Respiratory diagnostic studies
- Common Respiratory Emergency Disorders
  - Pneumonia
  - Status asthmaticus
  - Interstitial drug disease
  - Pleural effusion
  - COPD
  - Pulmonary tuberculosis
- Pulmonary edema
- Atelectasis
- Pulmonary embolism
- Acute respiratory failure
- Acute respiratory distress syndrome
- Chest trauma
- Pneumothorax
- Management Modalities for Respiratory System Disorders
  - Airway management
  - Ventilatory management
  - Bronchial hygiene

## Learning Objectives

At the end of the chapter, the students will be able to:
- Describe the structures and functions of the upper and lower respiratory tracts.
- Describe ventilation, perfusion, diffusion, shunting, and the relationship of pulmonary circulation to these processes.
- Demonstrate the respiratory assessment of a patient and identify the abnormal breathing pattern.
- Discriminate between normal and abnormal breath sounds.
- Use assessment parameters appropriate for determining the characteristics and severity of the major symptoms of respiratory dysfunction.
- Describe the definition, etiology, pathophysiology and diagnostic assessment and management of respiratory emergency conditions.
- Identify the nursing implications of procedures used for diagnostic evaluation of respiratory function.
- Describe the different steps of chest physiotherapy with nursing intervention.
- Identify respiratory emergencies and complications and take appropriate measures.

## RESPIRATORY SYSTEM

### Anatomy of the Respiratory System

The respiratory system of our body is responsible for the exchange of oxygen ($O_2$) and carbon dioxide ($CO_2$) for breathing.

According to the anatomical structure, the respiratory system is divided into two parts:

1. **Upper respiratory tract:** It consists of the nose, pharynx, and nasal cavity.
2. **Lower respiratory tract:** It consists of the larynx, trachea bronchi and bronchioles, lungs, and alveoli (air sacs).

According to the physiological function of the respiratory system is also separated into two divisions:

1. Conducting/dead part
2. Respiratory part

**Conducting/dead part:**
- It consists of the nose, the pharynx, the trachea, the bronchi, and the bronchioles.
- It filters, warms, and conducts air into the lungs.

- The total volume of air in dead space is 150 mL (Waugh Anne GA. 2013).

**Respiratory part:**
- It is the portion of the respiratory system which helps in respiration and perfusion by exchanging gases.
- It includes bronchioles, alveolar duct, alveolar sac and alveoli.
- The total capacity of air in the respiratory portion is 5–6 liters in volume (Waugh Anne GA, 2013).

### Nose and Nasal Cavity

The nose is the first organ of the respiratory tract, by septum, it is divided into two equal passages. The ciliated columnar epithelium is present in the nose lining, and it contains the goblet cells which helps in mucus secretion. Both chronic and acute inflammation of this mucus membrane is called rhinitis. Around the nose, there are four paranasal sinuses (air-filled cavities in the bone) which give resonance to voice and lighten the skull they are—frontal sinuses, maxillary sinuses, ethmoidal sinuses, sphenoidal sinuses. The nasolacrimal duct extends from the nose to the eye, which drains tears from eye to nose. One of the external apertures of the nose is called nostrils or nares. The nose contains an olfactory receptor in the epithelium called the olfactory epithelium. In the olfactory region of the cerebral cortex in the temporal lobe, a sense of smell is perceived.

#### Function of the Nose
- It maintains the warmth of the air for respiration by immense vascularity of the nasal mucosa.
- It helps infiltration and clearance of the inspired air by trapping the dust particles by hairs and lining of the nasal mucosa.
- It helps in the humidification of air that passes over the moist mucosal lining of the nose and saturated with water vapor.
- It helps in the perception of smell with the help of the olfactory nerve.
- It helps in the function of speech by the pronunciation of nasal vowels and consonants, which is called as nasalization (Waugh A, Grant A, 2014).

### Pharynx

It is a 13 cm long funnel-shaped structure. From the nasal cavity to the larynx it acts as a common passageway for air. It also helps in the passage of food from the mouth to the esophagus. It lies behind the nasal and oral cavity and anterior to the cervical vertebra. It is supplied by arteries of "pharyngeal branches of ascending pharyngeal artery, ascending palatine, descending palatine and pharyngeal branches of inferior thyroid artery". The venous drainage by "pharyngeal plexus". The nerve connected to the pharynx is the pharyngeal plexus, maxillary nerve, and mandibular nerve. The pharynx can be divided into three anatomical regions:

#### Nasopharynx
- It lies the oral part of the nose.
- On the lateral wall, there two openings of the auditory tube from both middle ears.
- Posteriorly, the pharyngeal tonsils are present and which consist of lymphoid tissue.

#### Oropharynx
- This is the middle portion of the pharynx locate posteriorly between the epiglottis and the soft palate.
- These portions have both functions of digestive and respiration.
- It lined with stratified squamous epithelium because there is chance of abrasion by food.
- Oropharynx contains two pairs of tonsils called palatine tonsil or faucial tonsil and lingual tonsil.

#### Laryngopharynx
- It lies posteriorly to the esophagus and anteriorly to the larynx and it is otherwise called hypopharynx.
- The lining is made up of stratified squamous epithelium and located between the 4th and 6th cervical vertebrae.
- A mass of lymphoid tissue called the tonsil in the mucus membrane of the pharynx and the tongue base.
- A ring is formed by the palatine tonsils, pharyngeal tonsils, and lingual tonsils which is immunologically active tissue (Patwa A, Shah A, 2015).

### Parts of Respiratory System (Fig. 10.1)

#### Larynx

It is a small passageway that connects the laryngopharynx with the trachea. It is otherwise called a voice box or soundbox. It extended from C4 to C6. The larynx wall, consisting of nine parts of cartilage, is:
- Three cartilages are in pairs such as cuneiform, corniculate and arytenoid.
- Three cartilage are single, such as thyroid, epiglottis, and cricoid cartilage.

The size of the larynx in males larger than females due to larger thyroid cartilage by the influence of the male sex hormone, which causes deep voice in males. The laryngeal prominence formed by two laminae of thyroid cartilage at the top of the trachea in front of the neck is called Adam's apple. Just above Adam's apple a "V" shaped notch known as thyroid notch. The larynx mucus membrane consists of two pairs of folds, upper pairs of false vocal cords, and lower

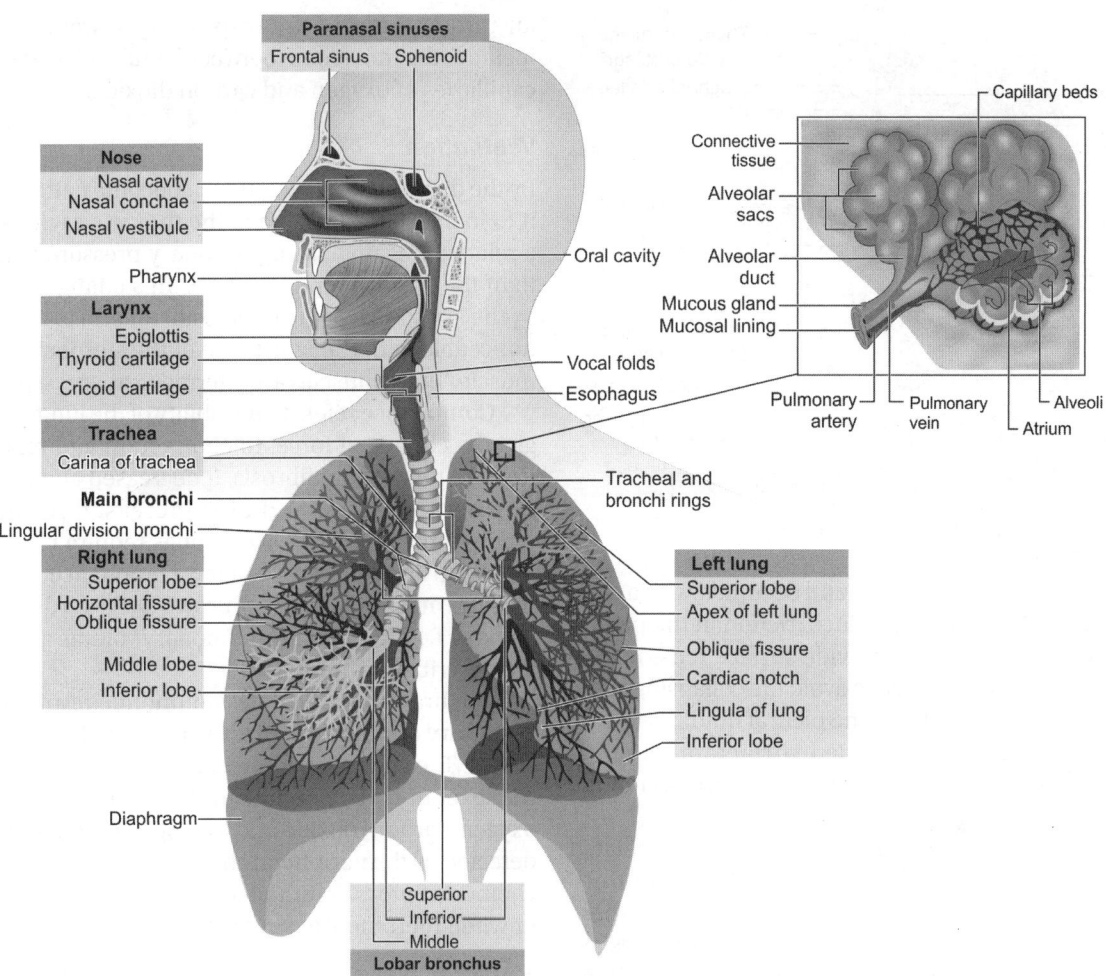

**Fig. 10.1:** Parts of respiratory system.

pairs of false vocal cords called true vocal cords. Sounds derived from the vocal fold vibration. The loudness of voice depended upon the force with which the cord vibrates. (Remington LA, Goodwin D, 2021)

*Trachea*

This is a tubular air passageway. The trachea is 12 cm long with a diameter of 2.5 cm. It lies just in front of the esophagus. The wall of the trachea is composed of 4 layers of tissue; they are the mucosa, submucosa, hyaline cartilage, and adventitia. The mucosa of the trachea consists of ciliated columnar epithelium. Areolar connective tissue consists of submucosa and adventitia. The wall of the trachea is mainly composed of 16 to 20 C shape incomplete rings of 'hyaline cartilage'. It is normal to feel these rings just below the larynx. The open segment of the C-shaped rings is posterior to the esophagus. At T5, the trachea is divided into right and left primary bronchus (Stocks J, Hislop AA, 2002).

*Lungs*

See **Figure 10.2**.

Structure of lungs

In the thoracic cavity, the two lungs (**Fig. 10.2**) are situated on either side of the midline. The lungs are conical shapes and have a medial surface, a base, a coastal surface, and an apex. The right lung usually weighs 625 g, while the left lung weighs 567 g. The apex extends into the root of the neck, close to the first rib, and above the level of the sternum. The base shape is concave and lies above the diaphragm on the upper thoracic surface.

The lung is surrounded and covered by a pleural membrane called a double-layered serous membrane. The outer layer is the "parietal pleura" and the "visceral pleura" is the inner one. The surface of the lungs is enclosed with visceral pleura, the thoracic cavity is lined with parietal pleura. The area between the two pleural membranes is

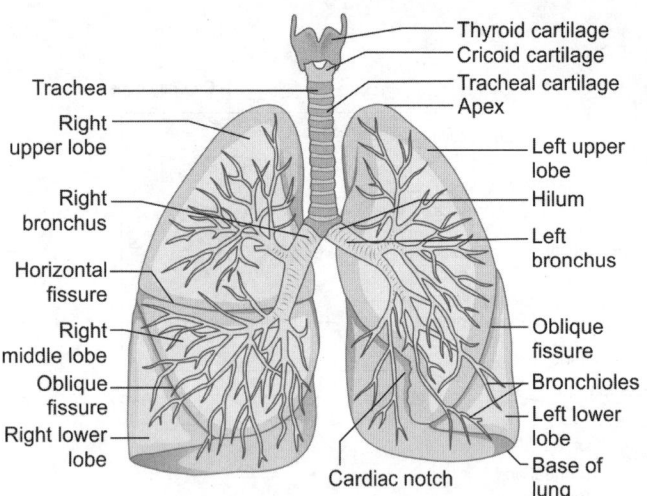

**Fig. 10.2:** Parts of the lungs.

referred to as the "pleural cavity" and occupied with a clear fluid called "pleural fluid" to reduce friction in the pleural cavity between the tissue to provide surface tension. The two pleural membranes attach to avoid the collapsing of the lungs, with water molecules in the pleural fluid.
- A chemical compound called surfactant which is released by the lungs also prevents the friction of the surface.
- The lining of the respiratory tract is made up of ciliated pseudostratified columnar epithelium, smooth muscle and the trachea to the tertiary bronchi there is cartilaginous rings are present. The bronchioles are lined with cuboidal epithelium, and the tract is lined with simple squamous epithelium from the alveolar ducts to the alveoli.
- A layer of skeletal muscle of involuntary control, called the diaphragm, is present lower to the lungs which promotes thoracic volume control (Waugh Anne GA. 2013).

Bronchial tree:
This is the branching tubes of the tree extending from the trachea. The tube diameter is wide and supported by cartilage rings, and majority of the bronchus is surrounded with tissue from primary bronchi to tertiary bronchi.

The diameter of the bronchioles is down to 1 mm and this structure is composed of cuboidal cells. The lining tissue becomes simple squamous epithelium from the alveolar duct to alveoli where gas exchange is possible (Patwa A, Shah A, 2015).

## Physiology of Respiratory System

Ventilation, by the interaction of the musculoskeletal and nervous system, is the mechanical process of transferring air into and out of the respiratory system. Respiration includes the movement between the alveoli and pulmonary capillaries of oxygen and carbon dioxide.

### Ventilation

By the diaphragm contraction, it become flatten and allows it to increase the volume of the thoracic cavity and create a relative negative intrapulmonary pressure which is less than the atmospheric pressure. This change is supported by the assistance of the intercostal muscle to become more noticeable with the assistance of the sternocleidomastoid muscle. These muscles are referred to as accessory muscles.

Compliance refers to the ability of the lungs and thorax, given a chance of force, to contraction and relaxation. In cases of pulmonary fibrosis, it decreased and emphysema fibrosis increased and also increased in the case of emphysema and COPD. The lungs require more pressure for expansion in the case of low compliance, so breathing muscles must work harder (Brown D, Edwards H, Seaton L, Buckley T, 2015). Normal pulmonary volume and capacities are described in **Table 10.1**.

The brainstem regulates autonomic respiration, while voluntary ventilatory effort is regulated by the cerebral cortex. The central chemoreceptor mechanism is to detect the level of hydrogen ions in the blood and the level of oxygen-carbon dioxide and hydrogen ions in the blood are detected by the peripheral chemoreceptors. The function of chemoreceptors to stimulate when changes in acceleration or when there slow in ventilation rate.

### Respiration

Respiration is the process of transportation of oxygen ($O_2$) and carbon dioxide ($CO_2$) within the alveolar-capillary membrane. These transportations occur by the process of diffusion by which the molecules move from higher concentration to lower concentration. Any alteration that occurs in this process harms the process of respiration.

### Ventilation-Perfusion Relationship

Respiration depends on adequate perfusion of alveoli. Trachea and bronchioles usually do not engage in the exchange of gas. Therefore, it is called as anatomical dead space. When an alveolus is not perfused, their alveolar cluster is called alveolar dead space units due to no gas exchange. This occurs in diseases like pulmonary embolism or pulmonary infarct. When alveolus is inadequately ventilated in the presence of perfusion, the clusters are called a shunt unit and here the perfusion exceeds ventilation, which is seen in the diseases like pneumonia and atelectasis. Whenever both ventilation and perfusion are impaired, this condition results in a silent unit and

**Table 10.1:** Normal pulmonary volume and capacities of lungs.

| | Description | Volume | Significance |
|---|---|---|---|
| **Lung volume** | | | |
| Tidal volume (TV) | The volume of air breathed in and out of lungs in a quit respiration | 500 mL | Tidal volume may not vary even with severe disease |
| Inspiratory reserve volume (IRV) | Amount of air inspired forcefully after tidal volume | 3300 mL | |
| Expiratory reserve volume (ERV) | Amount of air that can be expired out forcefully after normal expiration | 1000 mL | Expiratory reserve volume is decreased with restrictive conditions such as obesity, ascites, and pregnancy |
| Residual volume (RV) | The amount of air always remains in the lungs even after forced expiration | 1200 mL | Residual volume may be increased with obstructive diseases |
| **Lung capacity** | | | |
| Total lung capacity (TLC) | The maximum volume of air the lungs can hold. TLC = TV + IRV + ERV + RV  500 + 3300 + 1000 + 1200 | 6000 mL | Total lung capacity may be decreased with restrictive lung diseases like atelectasis and pneumonia and increased in COPD |
| Functional residual capacity (FRC) | The volume of air present in the lungs at the end of the passive expiration. FRC = ERV + RV  1000 + 1200 | 2200 mL | Functional residual capacity may be increased with COPD and decreased in ARDS and obesity |
| Inspiratory capacity (IC) | Amount of air that can be inhaled after the end of a normal expiration IC = TV + IRV  500 + 3300 | 3800 mL | A decreased in inspiratory capacity may indicate restrictive lung diseases and may also be decreased in obesity |
| Vital capacity (VC) | The maximum amount of air can expel from the lungs after a maximum inhalation VC = IRV + ERV + TV  3300 + 1000 + 500 | 4800 mL | A decreased in vital capacity may be found in neuromuscular diseases, generalized fatigue, atelectasis, pulmonary edema, COPD, and obesity |

occurs in severe capital ARDS and pneumothorax (Stocks J, Hislop AA, 2002).

## Breathing Mechanism

The respiratory system of the lungs depends on the law of gas, which explains that the particles of gas molecules always diffuse from an area of higher pressure to a region of lower pressure **(Fig. 10.3)**. Pressure and volume are inversely proportional to each other when the temperature remaining constant. According to Boyle's law, where pressure increases in a smaller volume of gases and pressure decrease in a larger volume of gases.

## Inspiration (Inhalation)

The active mechanism in which the contraction of the diaphragm and external intercostal muscles is triggered by nerve impulses from the medulla oblongata. Thoracic volume increases as the muscles contract, which, according to Boyle's law, reduces the pressure inside the lungs (intra-alveolar pressure). As atmospheric pressure drops below the intra-alveolar pressure (758 mm Hg versus 760 mm Hg respectively), the gas law indicates that gases are now moving into the lungs from the atmosphere (Stocks J, Hislop AA, 2002).

## Expiration (Exhalation)

It is a passive mechanism where the lungs and diaphragm elastic tissues recoil to their original location. Thoracic volume decreases as the diaphragm and external intercostal muscles contract and recoil, which, according to Boyle's law, increases the interalveolar pressure again. Because of the gas law, intra-atmospheric pressure gases travel from the lungs into the atmosphere again.

## Anatomical Dead Space

This refers to the quantity of air remaining in the bronchial tree that is not involved in the exchange of gas due to airflow obstruction or bronchial tree damage.

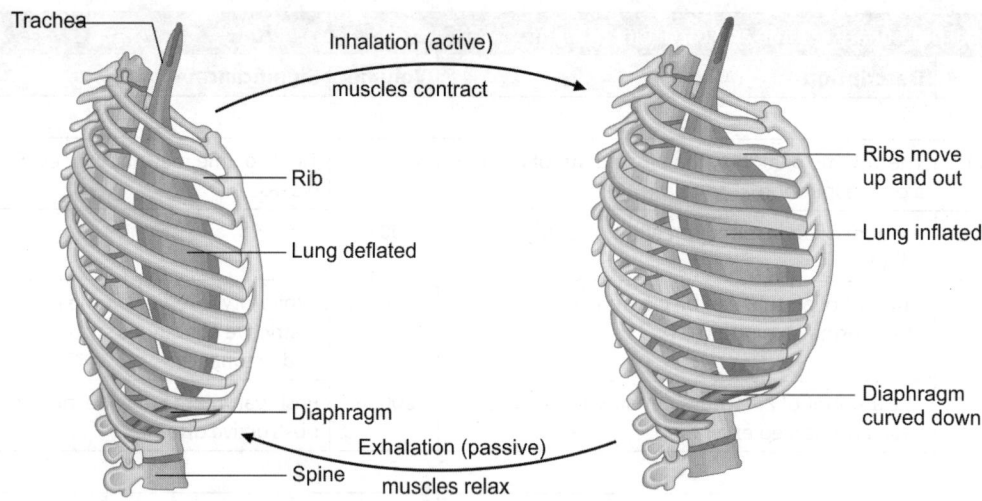

**Fig. 10.3:** Mechanism of breathing of lungs.

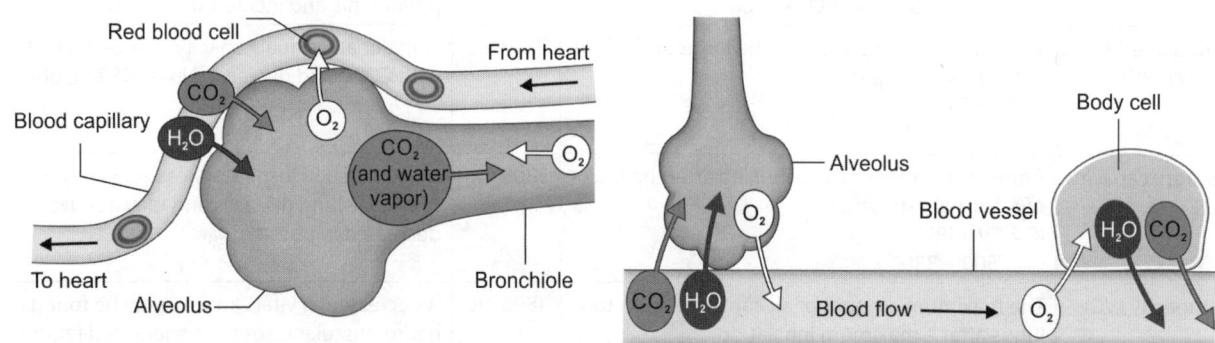

**Fig. 10.4:** Alveolar ventilation.

*Alveolar Dead Space*

This refers to the amount of air in the alveolar ducts or alveolar sacs that, due to poor blood flow or extremely long diffusion distances in the exchange of gases, are not involved in gas exchange.

*Physiology Gas Exchange*

This applies to the total quantity of air in the lungs not involved in gas exchange, (i.e., anatomical dead space + alveolar dead space).

*Breathing Control*

Four key factors that influence normal breathing:
- Stretching of lungs and thoracic wall
- In the blood, the $O_2$ level
- The rate of $CO_2$ in the blood
- In the blood, $H^+$ level

Normal breathing is hindered by lung and thoracic wall stretching, an increase in the level of $O_2$, a decrease in the level of $CO_2$ and $H^+$, whereas normal breathing is induced by relaxation of the lungs and thoracic walls, a decrease in the level of $O_2$ and the levels of $H^+$ ions.
- Chemicals and emotional conditions also impact breathing.
- Lung and thoracic wall tissue stretching prevent inspiration by activating an inflation reflex that limits the duration of inspiratory movements. This also prevents the lungs from being over-inflated during forceful breathing.
- Low blood $PO_2$ improves alveolar ventilation by peripheral chemoreceptors in carotid bodies and low $O_2$ concentrations are detected by aortic bodies.
- High $PCO_2$ in the blood enhances alveolar ventilation.
- High CSF, $H^+$ ion concentration increases breathing rate, and $CO_2$ alveolar ventilation combines to form carbonic acid with water, which in turn releases CSF $H^+$ ions (Stocks J, Hislop AA, 2002) **(Fig. 10.4).**

*Center of Respiration*

In normal breathing the rhythmic, and involuntary activity of respiration is controlled by the respiratory center

(Fig. 10.5) in pons and medulla oblongata of the brainstem. The rhythmic pattern in controlled by medulla on the simple rhythm of inspiration and expiration, which is subdivided into the dorsal respiratory group, which regulates regular breathing. The pneumotaxic region in the pons defines breathing depth, length and rate by influencing the dorsal breath group (Stocks J, Hislop AA, 2002).

## Chemoreceptors

Respiratory centers are associated with primary chemoreceptors. To form carbonic acid, $CO_2$ reacts with water, which in turn releases $H^+$ ion in CSF. Alveolar ventilation is improved by stimulation of these areas.

The carotid and aortic bodies have peripheral chemoreceptors. Such chemoreceptors sense low levels of $O_2$. Alveolar ventilation increases when $O_2$ concentration is low.

### External and Internal Respiration

External respiration takes place in the lungs to oxygenate the blood and remove $CO_2$ from the deoxygenated blood. $O_2$ spreads out in the alveoli into capillaries, while $CO_2$ spreads out into the capillaries.

In body tissue, internal respiration (tissue respiration) occurs to supply the tissue cells with $O_2$ and extract $CO_2$ from the cells. A process known as cell respiration, $O_2$, is necessary for release of the energy molecule ATP while $CO_2$ is a metabolic by-product that can be harmful in significant concentrations to tissue cells. $O_2$ diffuses from the capillaries into tissue cells and $CO_2$ diffuses from the tissue cells into capillaries (Brown D, Edwards H, Seaton L, Buckley T, 2015).

### Oxyhemoglobin Dissociation Curve

Circulation of $O_2$ in blood in two ways about 97% of $O_2$ transported with Hb which is known as $O_2$ saturation ($SaO_2$) and 3% dissolved in serum ($PaO_2$). The oxyhemoglobin dissociation curve (Fig. 10.6) describes the balance of these two-transport methods. Any shift or changes in the cure explains alteration in the respiration process. When it shifts to the right, there is a decrease in the $O_2$ saturation for any given $PaO_2$. This phenomenon is referred to as the Bohr effect, where less Hb saturation occurs, and oxyhemoglobin releases more $O_2$. The factors shift the curve to the right:

- A rise in body temp (fever)
- Reduced pH (acidosis)
- A rise in $CO_2$ (hypercapnia)
- Rise on 2.3 di-phospho-glycerate.

When it shifts to the left, this phenomenon is called the Haldane effect. There is an increased $O_2$ saturation for any $PaO_2$. So, the delivery of $O_2$ to tissue is impaired. The factors shift the curve to the left:

- Low temperature (hypothermia)
- Alkalosis

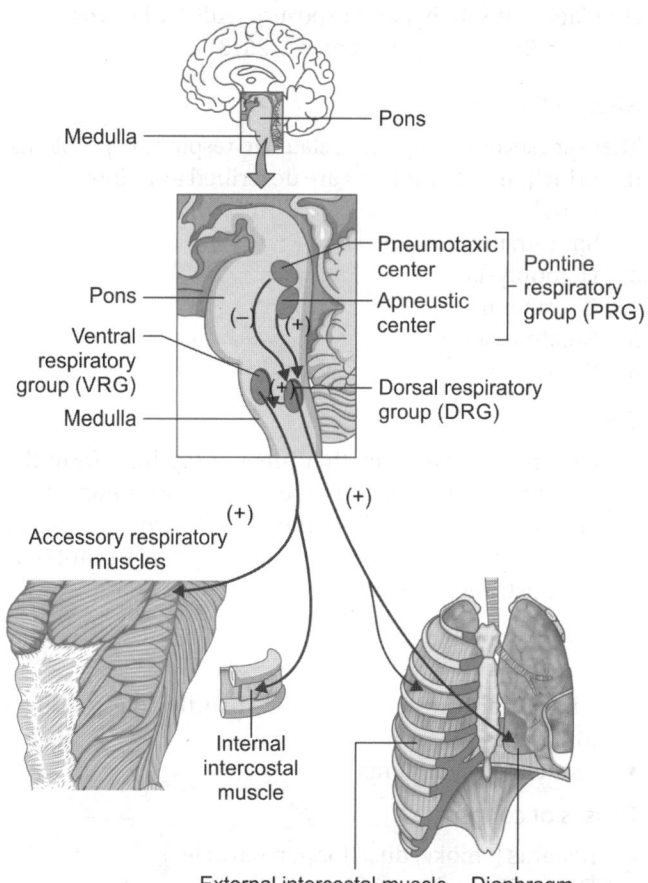

**Fig. 10.5:** Label diagram of respiratory groups in the respiratory center and their influence.

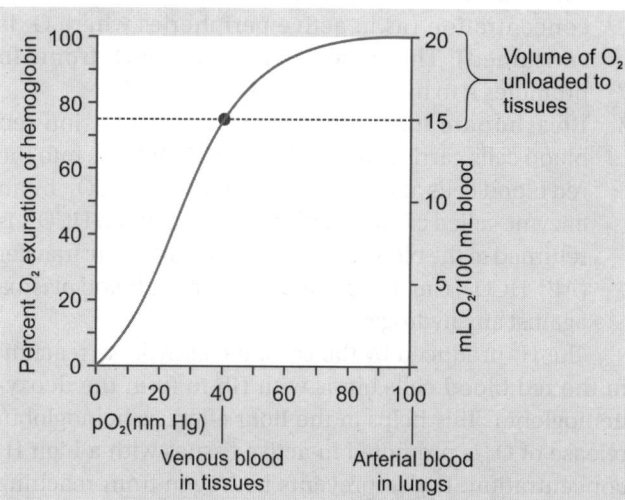

**Fig. 10.6:** Oxyhemoglobin dissociation curve.

- Low $CO_2$ (hypocapnia)
- Low on 2.3 di-phospho-glycerate.

The oxyhemoglobin dissociation curve is significant for the clinician to understand the patient's tissue oxygenation (Suzanne C, Smeltzer, Brenda G Bare, Janice L, 2013).

*Carbon Dioxide Transportation*

The role of $CO_2$ in the blood is very much important. The key function of $CO_2$ is to regulate the pH of the blood—this is significantly more important than carrying $CO_2$ for exhalation to the lungs.

During the resting condition, the 100 mL of deoxygenated blood contains approximately 53 mL of $CO_2$ gases and this is transported in the blood in three ways.

1. **Dissolved $CO_2$:** About 10% of all $CO_2$ in is transported and dissolved in plasma. The amount of gas dissolved in a liquid depends on its solubility and the partial pressure of gas. The water contains high solubility of $CO_2$ and the inspired partial pressure of $CO_2$ is ~40 mm Hg (23 × more soluble than $O_2$). Considering its solubility, plasma carries only a minority of the total $CO_2$ in the blood. This makes the dissolution of more $CO_2$ in the periphery during the gas process in the alveoli where the partial pressure is lower.
2. **Carbamino compound:** Approximately 30% of $CO_2$, as carbamino compounds, are transported. Carbon dioxide bonds specifically to amino acids in high concentrations and the hemoglobin amine groups to form carbaminohemoglobin. In the periphery, where $CO_2$ production is high because of cellular respiration. The influence of Haldane effect also helps to produce carbamino compounds. This indicates the $CO_2$ carriage capacitance of the blood is raised in the lower $O_2$ concentration (as in active peripheries where $O_2$ is consumed). The reason that releasing $O_2$ from Hb promotes it to binding with $CO_2$.
3. **Bicarbonate ions:** The formation of $HCO_3^-$ ion red blood cells carries 60% of all $CO_2$. $CO_2$ diffuses into the red blood cells and is converted to $H^+$ and $HCO_3^-$ by an enzyme called carbonic anhydrase. This anion $HCO_3^-$ is returned to the blood by a chloride-bicarbonate transfer (AE). $HCO_3^-$ can now act as a buffer in the blood plasma against any hydrogen.

The $H^+$ produced by the carbonic anhydrase reaction in the red blood cells binds with Hb to form the deoxyhemoglobin. This helps in the Bohr effect as hemoglobin release of $O_2$ is promoted in active tissues with a high $H^+$ concentration. It also prevents hydrogen from reaching lower pH level in the blood and stabilizes the pH (Suzanne C, Smeltzer, Brenda G. Bare, Janice L, 2013).

# ASSESSMENT AND DIAGNOSTIC EVALUATION

## Assessment

A complete assessment of the respiratory system helps the nurse collect the current baseline status of the patient which helps in the rapid diagnosis of the present health status of the patients.

This is the process of external ventilation assessment which includes observations of breathing rates, depth, and pattern. A detailed breathing assessment is dependent on the normal recognition of movements of the thorax and the abdomen. A detailed respiratory assessment consists of a comprehensive patient history of inspection, palpation, percussion, and auscultation. Using a systematic method to compare results from the left to the right so that the patient can be monitored by himself. The A-E assessment (**Table 10.2**) is a systemic method for rapid assessment and care of seriously diseased or disabled patients, which has been commonly used as a means to track the assessment of respiratory patients. A-E is used as the basis for assessment of airway, breathing, circulation, disability, and exposure (ABCDE) (Suzanne C, Smeltzer, Brenda G. Bare, Janice L, 2013).

### History Collection

There are several symptoms related to respiratory problems. the principle six symptoms are described as follows:
1. Cough
2. Sputum production
3. Hemoptysis
4. Chest pain
5. Breathlessness
6. Wheezing

### Cough

This is a protective reflex that prevent the lung from the entry of any foreign particle or removal of secretion which creates irritation to the mucus membrane of the respiratory tract. The stimulation arises due to any types of irritants like smoke, dust, and chemicals, etc.

#### Assess the cough

- Onset and duration
- Characteristics—dry, moist, productive postural influences
- Associated symptoms

#### Causes of cough

- Irritants (smoke, dust, foreign particles)
- Drugs (B-blockers, ACE inhibitors, etc.)
- Diseases (tumor, asthma, COPD, bronchiolitis, alveolitis, LVF, bronchiectasis, etc.) (Angell ML, 2012).

| | |
|---|---|
| **Table 10.2:** A-E assessment of respiratory status. | |
| **Airways** | • Assess the patency of the airway and the patient's effort for breathing<br>• Check for any obstruction present in the airway which may cause stridor, the hoarseness of voice, orthopnea, drooling, dysphagia, etc.<br>• Assess for self-ventilation of pt. If unable provide mechanical ventilator support<br>• If the patient under mechanical ventilation assess the mode of ventilation, i. e., CPAP, BiPAP |
| **Breathing** | • Assess the respiration rate and rhythm and pattern<br>• Assess the stress of breathing and the use of accessory muscles<br>• Check the saturation ($SPO_2$) level of Pt<br>• Check the ABGs values of $PaO_2$ and $PaCO_2$ level<br>• Assess the report of a chest X-ray<br>• Assess the chest wall movement and chest expansion<br>• In auscultation assess the breath sound and assess for the presence of any abnormal breath sounds like crackles, wheezing, etc.<br>• On palpation assess the body temp. tactile fremitus and edema |
| **Circulation** | • Heart rate<br>• Blood pressure<br>• Skin color<br>• Sweating<br>• Urine output<br>• Blood sugar level |
| **Disability** | • Assess the patient for the level of consciousness and orientation to the environment<br>• Check the patient's alertness, voice pain, and unresponsiveness<br>• Check the patient is sedation not |
| **Exposure** | • Thoroughly assess the patient for any injury like ribs fractures spinal cord fracture which may affect the breathing pattern of the patient<br>• Check for the presence of any surgical wounds<br>• Assess the patients for any presence of drains, catheter, arterial line, HG tubes, etc.<br>• Assess for any swinging or bubbling of the drainage tube |

*Sputum Production*

The thick secretions produced in the respiratory tract and splitting out by coughing is known as sputum or expectoration. During the history collection ensure from the patient about the amount, color, and the nature of the sputum **(Table 10.3)**.

*Hemoptysis*

Hemoptysis is the presence of blood in the sputum. It is generally seen in the case of the cancerous condition of the lungs. It is an essential symptom and must always be properly examined. **Table 10.4** represents the causes of hemoptysis.

Duration and frequency

- Hemoptysis for chronic period suggest bronchiectasis
- Daily for a week in case of lung cancer, tuberculosis, and lung abscess.
- Single episodes of the large amount with associated symptoms suggest thromboembolism and infraction (Booker KJ, 2015).

*Chest Pain*

A valuable tool for identifying, measuring, and recording pain in a condition is the PQRST tool for chest pain assessments mnemonic. The elements of PQRST are "provocative and palliative factors; quality; region or radiation; severity; and time" (Booker KJ, 2015).

Types of pain

- **Pleural pain:**
  - It is usually sharp, stabbing, and perceived during inspiration and coughing.
  - Pain perceived in the upper six ribs by phrenic nerve during irritation of parietal pleura and radiate to neck and shoulder tip.
  - Pain perceived in lower six ribs by intercostal nerve during irritation of outer diaphragm and radiate to the upper part of the abdomen.
- **Chest wall pain:**
  - Pain is perceived in the chest wall in case of respiratory and musculoskeletal diseases.
  - It feels like chest tightness and diffuse type of pain in the case of COPD and asthma.

**Table 10.3:** Sputum analysis.

| Types | Description | Causes |
|---|---|---|
| Saliva | Clear watery fluid | |
| Fetid | Foul-smelling, typical of anaerobic infection | Bronchiectasis, lung abscess or cystic fibrosis |
| Frothy | Pink or white | Pulmonary edema |
| Mucoid | Opalescent or white | Chronic bronchitis without infection, asthma |
| Purulent | • Thick, viscous: Yellow<br>• Dark brown/green<br>• Rusty<br>• Redcurrant jelly | • Hemophilus<br>• Pseudomonas<br>• Pneumococcus, mycoplasma<br>• Klebsiella |
| Mucopurulent | Slightly discolored but not frank pus | Bronchiectasis, cystic fibrosis, pneumonia |
| Rusty | Descriptive of the color of sputum (also called prune juice) | Pneumococcal pneumonia |
| Hemoptysis | From blood specks to frank blood, old blood (dark brown) | Infarction (tuberculosis, bronchiectasis), infarction, carcinoma, vasculitis, trauma also coagulation disorders, cardiac disease |
| Black | Black specks in mucoid secretions | Smoke inhalation (fires, tobacco, heroin), coal dust |

**Table 10.4:** Causes of hemoptysis.

| Tumor | Lung cancer |
|---|---|
| Infection | Endobronchial metastasis, bronchial carcinoid, bronchiectasis, tuberculosis, lung abscess, mycetoma, cystic fibrosis |
| Vascular | Pulmonary infarction, arteriovenous malformation |
| Vasculitis | Wegener's granulomatosis, Goodpasture's syndrome |
| Trauma | Inhaled foreign body, chest trauma, Iatrogenic trauma like bronchoscopic biopsy, transthoracic lung biopsy, bronchoscopic diathermy |
| Cardiac | Mitral valve disease, acute left ventricular failure |
| Hematological | Blood dyscrasias, anticoagulation |

– Sudden onset and localized pain fells in case of rib fracture and intercostal muscle injury.
– Pain which is dull, aching, and gnawing in nature unrelated to respiration perceived in diseases of malignancy of lungs, and ribs.
– Prevesicular herpes zoster and intercostal nerve root compression cause pain which radiates to thoracic distribution.
• **Mediastinal pain:**
– Pain in mediastinum is in the central and retrosternal area unrelated to respiration and cough.
– Tracheobronchial tree irritation and burning pain in case of inhalation of irritant dust and infection which is worsened by cough.

Central chest pain **(Table 10.5)** due to right ventricular pressure produced in the case of myocardial infarction and pulmonary thromboembolism (Booker KJ, 2015).

### Breathlessness

According to the American Thoracic Society (1999), breathlessness is defined as "a subjective experience of breathing discomfort that consists of qualitatively distinct sensations that vary in intensity. The experience is derived from interaction among multiple physiological, psychological, social, and environmental factors and may induce secondary physiological and behavioral responses".

### During history collection

At the time of history collection carefully investigate the breathing pattern of the patient. Assess the "onset, duration, progression, variation, aggravating or relieving factors, severity, and associated symptoms" carefully. There are various factors which causes breathlessness which are described in **Table 10.6**.

**Table 10.5:** Causes of pain.

| Non-central | |
|---|---|
| Pleural | Infection: Pneumonia, bronchiectasis, tuberculosis<br>Malignancy of lungs, pneumothorax, pulmonary infarction, connective tissue diseases like rheumatoid arthritis, systemic lupus erythematous |
| Chest wall | Lung cancer, bony metastasizes, persistent cough/breathlessness, muscle sprains/tear, rib fracture, intercostal nerve compression, thoracic shingles (herpes zoster), Bornholm's disease (Coxsackie B infection), Tietze's syndrome (costochondritis) |
| **Central** | |
| Tracheal | Infection, irritant dust |
| Cardiac | Massive pulmonary thromboembolism, acute myocardial infarction/ischemia |
| Esophageal | Esophagitis, rupture |
| Great vessels | Aortic dissection |
| Mediastinal | Lung cancer, thymoma, lymphadenopathy, metastasis, mediastinitis |

**Table 10.6:** Causes of the breathlessness.

| Causes | Disease condition |
|---|---|
| **Non-respiratory** | |
| Non-cardiorespiratory | Anemia, metabolic acidosis, obesity, psychogenic, neurogenic |
| Cardiac | Left ventricular failure, mitral valve disease, cardiomyopathy, constructive pericarditis, pericardial effusion |
| **Respiratory** | |
| Airways | Laryngeal tumor, foreign body aspiration, asthma, COPD, bronchiectasis, lung cancer, bronchiolitis, cystic fibrosis |
| Parenchyma | Pulmonary fibrosis, alveolitis, sarcoidosis, tuberculosis, pneumonia, metastatic tumor |
| Pulmonary circulation | Pulmonary thromboembolism, pulmonary vasculitis, primary pulmonary hypertension |
| Pleural | Pneumothorax, pleural effusion, diffuse pleural fibrosis |
| Chest wall | Kyphoscoliosis, ankylosis, spondylitis |
| Neuromuscular | Myasthenia gravis, neuropathies, muscular dystrophies, guillain barre syndrome |

**Table 10.7:** Degree of dyspnea according to the modified Medical Research Council Dyspnea Scale (mMRC-Scale).

| Grade | Degree of dyspnea |
|---|---|
| 0 | No dyspnea except with strenuous exercise |
| 1 | Dyspnea when walking up an incline or hurrying on the level |
| 2 | Walks slower than most on the level, or stops after 15 minutes of walking on the level |
| 3 | Stops after a few minutes of walking on the level |
| 4 | With minimal activity such as getting dressed, too dyspneic to leave the house |

**Duration, mode, and progression of breathlessness**

The Medical Research Council Dyspnea Scale (mMRC-Scale) is helpful in the description of systemic dyspnea in patients with respiratory disease and assesses breathless impairment. During assessment collect the history from the patient regarding duration, mode of onset, and progression of breathlessness. According to the modified Medical Research Council Dyspnea Scale (mMRC-Scale) (Hsu KY, Lin JR, Lin MS, Chen W, Chen YJ, Yan YH, 2013) there are various degree of dyspnea (**Table 10.7**).

**Aggravating and relieving factors:**
- Breathlessness when the patient is in laying position (orthopnea) in case of left ventricular failure.
- Breathlessness when waking up of patient from sleep (paroxysmal nocturnal dyspnea) in case of asthma and LVF.
- Breathlessness of a patient and morning awaking in case of COPD, may subside after coughing up sputum.
- Breathlessness due to exposure to irritant and allergens like perfume, dust, cold air, smoke, etc., in case of asthma.
- Breathlessness due to the taking of nonsteroidal anti-inflammatory drugs like aspirin.
- Breathlessness that improves on weekends and holidays in case of occupational asthma and allergic alveolitis. (Hsu KY, Lin JR, Lin MS, Chen W, Chen YJ, Yan YH, 2013)

*Wheezing*

Wheezing is defined as "a high-pitched, coarse whistling sound during breathing." The patient produces noise during respiration. Wheezing, which causes night waking is a feature of asthma, after waking from morning suggest COPD (Suzanne C. Smeltzer, Brenda G. Bare, Janice L, 2013).

General examination

The respiratory examination is incomplete without a general examination of the patient. The four phases of tests should be performed after positioning the patient upright with his or her arms by his or her side with the chest free of clothes. The patient is asked to move his arm forward to listen to the lungs from behind to avoid the scapulae (blades) obstructing the upper lung fields. Both fields need to be correlated with the lungs and are also examined on the front and the back of the chest walls (Malarvizhi S, Gugan R, 2019).

Breathing pattern

The important aspect of the assessment of breathing patterns in the respiration rate and depth (**Table 10.8**). In the case of adults, the normal breathing rate is 16–20 breath per minute. Normal respiration is called as eupnea.

Use of accessory muscle during breathing

The accessory muscles of respiration include sternocleidomastoid, platysma, and pectoral muscle. During breathing the use of accessory muscle suggests COPD. Patient have hyperinflated lungs.

**Stridor**

This is a high-pitched, wheezing airflow sound. Musical breathing or foreign airway obstruction can also be known as Stridor. Airflow is normally interfered with a larynx (voice box) or trachea (wind tube) obstruction. Children more frequently than adults are affected by Stridor. Conditions like abscess (a wretched fluid), swelling, problems of vocal cords such as fracture or paralysis, allergy, tumor-like growths, foreign body inhalation, chest or esophagus surgery, surgery of the thyroid, a tube for respiration (intubation) can causes strider (Malarvizhi S, Gugan R, 2019).

**Hoarseness**

Hoarseness is an abnormal change in the voice that sometimes feel with a dry or scratchy throat. The following conditions can cause hoarseness:

| Table 10.8: Pattern of respiration. | |
|---|---|
| **Pattern** | **Description** |
| Tachypnea | Rapid shallow breathing rate >24 breaths per minute. A normal response to fever, fear or exercise. Also caused by respiratory insufficiency, pneumonia, alkalosis, pleurisy and lesions in the pons |
| Bradypnea | Slow breathing <10 breaths per minute. May be caused by drug induced depression of the respiratory center in the medulla, increased intracranial pressure and diabetic coma |
| Cheyne-stokes respiration | A cycle in which respirations wax and wane in a regular pattern, increasing in rate and depth and then decreasing. Breathing patterns last 30–45 seconds with periods of apnea (20 seconds) alternating the cycle. Causes include severe heart failure, renal failure, meningitis, drug overdose and increased intracranial pressure. May be normal in infants and the elderly in sleep |
| Hyperventilation | An increase in both rate and depth. Normally occurs in extreme exertion, fear or anxiety. Also occurs with diabetic ketoacidosis, hepatic coma, salicylate overdose, lesions of the midbrain and alteration in blood gas concentrations |
| Hypoventilation | An irregular, shallow pattern caused by an overdose of narcotics or anesthetics. May occur with prolonged bed rest or conscious splinting of the chest to avoid respiratory pain |
| Biot's respiration | A pattern with an irregular rate and depth. A series of respirations is followed by periods of apnea. The cycle length lasts between 10 seconds and 1 minute. Can be seen with head trauma, brain abscess, heat stroke, spinal meningitis and encephalitis |

- Reflux of acidic stomach
- Smoking cigarettes
- Alcoholic and caffeinated drinks
- Screaming, singing prolonged or using your vocal cords otherwise
- Allergy
- Toxic substances inhalation
- Coughing heavily
- Polyps on the vocal cords (abnormal growths)
- Thyroid cancer or cancer of the throat
- Intubation
- Male puberty (the deepening of the voice)
- Thyroid gland that functions poorly
- Nerve or muscle disorders that impair the function of the voice box (Angell ML, 2012).

**Cyanosis**

It is defined as "a bluish discoloration, especially of the skin and mucos membranes, due to excessive concentration of deoxyhemoglobin in the blood caused by deoxygenation." It is of two types, i.e., central cyanosis and peripheral cyanosis.
1. Central cyanosis (lip and tongue due to arterial hypoxia) seen in diseases like pneumonia, obstructive sleep apnea, high altitude, COPD, heart failure and valvular diseases, etc.
2. Peripheral cyanosis (figure and toes due to tissue hypoxia) seen in diseases like reduced cardiac output, arterial obstruction, venous obstruction, COPD, etc., (Burns SM, Delgado SA, 2019).

**Blood pressure**

Hypotension due to community acquired pneumonia, septicemia, pneumothorax, and life-threating asthma.

**Skin appearance**

Some respiratory disorder causes changes in skin color and appearance.
- Bluish discoloration of skin due to hypoxia
- Erythema nodosum seen in case of acute sarcoidosis
- Lupus pernio over cheeks and the nose perceived in case of cutaneous sarcoidosis
- Subcutaneous non-tender nodules identify in patient with disseminated cancer
- Aquagenic wrinkling of palm due to higher concentration of electrolyte in blood
- Changes in the nail seen in pleural effusion, lymph-edema, and respiratory distress.

**Tremor**

Tremor is seen in patient of some respiratory disorders.
Flapping tremor (asterixis) seen in case of patients of severe ventilatory failure and retention of $CO_2$.

*Steps in Examination of Thoracic Region*

There are four steps to carry out the respiratory examination. These are inspection, palpation, percussion, and auscultation of respiratory sounds.

Inspection

The inspection of thorax includes skin over the thoracic region, symmetry, anatomical deformity, skin turgor, and any loss of subcutaneous tissue.

By this method, the examiner can find the number of breaths the patient is taking in one minute. The normal breathing rate in adults is 16–20 breaths per minute. But in the case of infants, it may 44 breaths/minute. Along with the respiratory rate, there are some other signs of respiratory distress that can find out during this time. Cyanosis (both peripheral and central also), pursed lip breathing, and use of accessory muscle during breathing (Chulay Marianne, 2010).

Chest configuration

The normal ration of antero-posterior diameter with lateral diameter is 1:2. But some types of deviations are noted in various respiratory diseases. These are explained as follows:
- **Barrel chest:** Due to overinflation of lungs caused by increased antero-posterior diameter of thorax seen in patients with emphysema.
- **Funnel chest (pectus excavatum):** Caused by depressed lower portion on the sternum and may be chances of compression of heart, and great vessels. In case of Marfan syndrome and Rickets Funnel chest has been seen. The compression may results murmurs.
- **Pigeon chest (pectus carinatum):** Results due to displacement of sternum and antero-posterior diameter increased in this case. It has been seen in Rickets, Marfan's syndrome, and severe kyphoscoliosis.
- **Kyphoscoliosis:** This condition limits in expansion of the lungs, results from osteoporosis, and skeletal disorder of spine and thorax. There is the elevation of scapula with S-shaped spine (Booker KJ, 2015).

Thoracic palpation

Palpation is the procedure of physical touch of the test. The doctors check for areas of tenderness, skin abnormalities, respiratory expansion and fremitus during palpation both front and back side of the chest.
- Tenderness between the ribs indicates inflammation of pleura and bluish discoloration seen in case of rib fracture.
- Palpate the front and back of the chest for any abnormal masses or structures. Irregular masses or sinus tracts are the route of the infection.

- Place palms on the patient's back with fingertips parallel to ribs and thumbs on tenth rib to observe the chest wall expansion on the back of the chest. Change positions to raise skin from one side of the spine to another. Teach the patient how to inhale and watch the thumbs move on the back of the patient. Replace the process on the lower edge of the front of the chest for each hand to help observe the expansion of the chest. Chest asymmetry may be caused by lung or pleura disease.
- Put the bony parts of palm on the edges of the patient's scapulae when he or she says "ninety-nine" or "oneoneone" for fremitus examination. Repeat the same procedure on front of the chest.
- A decreased in Fremitus can usually happen while the patient is having soft voices, bronchial obstructions, COPD, pneumothorax, or other infections, or injuries which can restrict larynx vibrations (Booker KJ, 2015).

Thoracic percussion
- Percussion (**Table 10.9**) is the taping act on the surface of the body to assess the structures under the skin.
- Percussion and resonance are used to analyze the lung function and potential problems in the lung. Sound consistency and sensation.
- In fact, the percussion is carried out by putting the middle finger in the field of interest.
- Used to touch the last joint of the finger by the middle finger of the other hand. Percussion takes place from upper to lower ribs in a systematic manner and the resonance from the left to right side of the chest is compared. This is performed from the front to back of the thorax (Booker KJ, 2015).

Auscultation

The areas of the lungs can be heard by a stethoscope are called the lung regions, which are the posterior, lateral and anterior pulmonary areas. The patient needs to take deep breath through mouth during auscultation. The normal lung sounds are vesicular, broncho-vesicular, bronchial, and tracheal. The absent of breath sounds experienced in disease conditions like obstruction of mainstem bronchi, pleural effusion, pneumonectomy, and severe atelectasis. The abnormal lung sounds are described in **Table 10.10**.

## Diagnostic Evaluation

### Pulse Oximetry

Pulse is the fifth vital sign. The pulse oximetry is a continuous, non-invasive procedure of measuring

**Table 10.9:** Percussion over various body tissues leads to five typical types.

| Types | Characteristics |
| --- | --- |
| Resonance | Loud and low pitched. Normal lung sound |
| Dullness | Medium intensity and pitch. Experienced with fluid. A dull, muffled sound may replace resonance in conditions like pneumonia or hemothorax |
| Hyper-resonance | Very loud, very low pitch and longer in duration. Abnormal lung sound. Hyper-resonance can result from asthma or emphysema |
| Tympany | Loud and high pitched. Common for percussion over gas-filled spaces. Tympany may result in pneumothorax |
| Flatness | Soft and high-pitched sound of short duration heard over very dense tissue where air is not present, such as posterior chest below the level of diaphragm |

**Table 10.10:** Types of abnormal sounds of lungs.

| Abnormal breath sound | Description |
| --- | --- |
| Wheezes | Describes a continuous musical sound on expiration or inspiration. A wheeze is the result of narrowed airways. Common causes include asthma and emphysema |
| Rhonchi | Characterized by low pitched, musical bubbly sounds heard on inspiration and expiration. Rhonchi are the result of viscous fluid in the airways |
| Stridor | A high-pitched musical breath sound resulting from turbulent air flow in the larynx or lower in the bronchial tree. It is not to be confused with stertor. Causes are typically obstructive, including foreign bodies, anaphylaxis, croup, epiglottitis, tumors and infection |
| Crackles | Intermittent, non-musical and brief sounds heard during inspiration only. They may be described as fine (soft, high-pitched) or coarse (louder, low-pitched). These are the result of alveoli opening due to increased air pressure during inspiration. Common causes include congestive heart failure |

hemoglobin saturation ($SPO_2$) by using a light signal transmitted through tissue. The normal range for patients without pulmonary pathology ranges from 95–99%. It is used where the patient's oxygen saturation is unstable, including ICU, OT, recovery room, emergency, and hospital ward settings. Due to convenient use, the ability to provide continuous and immediate assessment of oxygen saturation value in blood, pulse oximeters are used in every critical care setting. It is useful for patients with respiratory and cardiac problems, especially COPD, sleep disorders apnea and hypopnea (Civetta JM, Taylor RW, Kirby RR, 1990).

### End-tidal Carbon Dioxide Monitoring

End-tidal carbon dioxide ($ETCO_2$) is the level of carbon dioxide that is released at the end of an exhaled breath. Its level reflects the adequacy with which carbon dioxide ($CO_2$) is carried in the blood back to the lungs and exhaled. Non-invasive methods for $ETCO_2$ measurement include capnometry and capnography. The numerical value of $ETCO_2$ is provided by capnometry along with the graphical waveform of $CO_2$. Due to this reason, capnography is the most widely used method for measuring $ETCO_2$. Capnography procedure is used in patients with pulmonary diseases like COPD, bronchiolitis, pulmonary embolism, heart failure, and other diseases like diabetic ketoacidosis (DKA), metabolic disorders, shock, etc.

### Arterial Blood Gas Studies

Arterial blood gas measures the pH of blood along with $PaO_2$, $PaCO_2$, bicarbonate ion, and saturation of hemoglobin. These values are important in the case of respiratory illness. In case of respiratory problems, these values show abnormal, and the patient needs oxygen administration or ventilatory support. The important of ABGs are as follows:
- Helps in founding a diagnosis and severity of respiratory failure.
- Assess the capability of ventilation and oxygenation.
- Assess the capability of $CO_2$ excretion.
- Measure the variations in acid-base homeostasis.
- Assist to guide the treatment protocol
- Helps in the management of ICU patients.

The followings are some contraindications for ABG:
- Cellulitis or other infections over the puncture site.
- Absence of palpable arterial pulse.
- A negative result of an Allen test.
- Coagulopathies/anticoagulant therapy
- History of arterial spasm following the previous puncture.
- Arterial graft
- Severe peripheral vascular diseases.
- Dialysis shunt—choose another site.

Site selection to collect blood for ABG procedure are as follows:
- Dorsalis pedis artery
- Radial artery –45° insertion angle (ideally)
- Brachial artery –60°–90° insertion angle
- Femoral artery –90° insertion angle
- Posterior tibial artery

The syringe should be flushed with 0.05 mL to 0.10 of 1:1000 heparin solutions and emptied before collection of the blood. Ensure no our bubbles present in the syringe. The syringe must be sealed immediately after withdrawing the sample group of a noninvasive procedure (Nettina SM, Msn AB, Nettina SM, 2013).

Different conditions of acid-base imbalance its causes and sign and symptoms (Malarvizhi S, Gugan R, 2019) are described in **Table 10.11**.

### Pulmonary Function Test

The pulmonary function test is the procedure in which the primary purpose is to assess and recognize the severity of pulmonary impairment. It is a diagnostic and therapeutic test that helps clinicians to detect the lung diseases of patients. PFTs generally done by a respiratory therapist, physiotherapist, pulmonologist, and general practitioner. The indication are as follows:
- Long-term history of shortness of breath
- Asthma, chronic bronchitis, respiratory infection, COPD, lung fibrosis, bronchiectasis
- Restrictive lung disease, etc.

It is based on the measurement of volumes of air breathed in and out in normal and forced breathing. It is carried out by using a spirometer. Spirometry is a procedure for measuring the air capacity of the lung. Spirometry is used to measure airflow, ventilatory regulation, ventilatory mechanics, and lung volume during a forced expiratory maneuver from full inspiration. The purpose of the test is as follows:
- Assessment of various aspect of pulmonary physiology
- Defect and quantify respiratory diseases
- Evaluation of the disease and its response to therapy
- Provide valuable clinical information

Lung volume changes and changes in capacities are generally consistent with the pattern of impartment. TLC, FRC, and RV value rises with obstructive lung diseases and falls with restrictive diseases of the lung (Vincent JL, Abraham E, Kochanek P, Moore FA, Fink MP, 2016).

### Chest Radiography

Chest radiography or imaging studies includes X-ray, CT scan, MRI, contrast studies and radioisotopes diagnostic scan, etc. These tests determine the extent of infection to

**Table 10.11:** Different conditions of acid-base imbalance.

| Disturbance | Frequent causes | Signs and symptoms |
|---|---|---|
| Respiratory acidosis<br>$PaCO_2$ > 45 mm Hg<br>pH < 7.35 | • Central nervous system depression<br>• Hypoventilation<br>• Atelectasis<br>• Bronchial obstruction<br>• Severe pulmonary infections<br>• Heart failure and pulmonary edema<br>• Pulmonary embolism | • Restlessness<br>• Confusion<br>• Lethargy<br>• Decreased responsiveness<br>• Tachycardia<br>• Dysrhythmias<br>• Dyspnea<br>• Respiratory distress |
| Respiratory alkalosis<br>$PaCO_2$ <35 mm Hg<br>pH > 7.45 | • Central nervous system lesions<br>• Hyperventilation<br>• Anxiety, fear or pain<br>• Fever and sepsis | • Lightheadedness<br>• Confusion<br>• Tingling in hands<br>• Dysrhythmias and palpitations |
| Metabolic acidosis<br>$HCO_3$ <22 mEq/L<br>pH <7.35 | **Excess acid**<br>• Anaerobic metabolism (shock)<br>• Renal failure<br>• Ketoacidosis<br>**Base deficit**<br>• Diarrhea<br>• Intestinal fistulas | • Mental status changes<br>• Hyperventilation (possibly Kussmaul respirations)<br>• Dysrhythmias |
| Metabolic alkalosis<br>$HCO_3$ >26 mEq/L<br>pH >7.45 | **Base excess**<br>• Lactate administration<br>• Excessive administration of bicarbonate<br>**Acid deficit**<br>• Vomiting or nasogastric suction<br>• Hypokalemia and hypochloremia | • Mental status changes<br>• Hypoventilation<br>• Muscle cramps and twitching |

the growth of tumors in the thoracic cavity. It also helps to detect the accumulation of fluid, pies any types of secretion, fracture of a bone in the chest cavity (Civetta JM, Taylor RW, Kirby RR, 1990).

### Chest X-ray

This reveals any type of pathological or anatomical changes in the thoracic cavity. It detects the fluid, tumors, foreign bodies, and other pathological conditions. Two types of views seen in routine Chest X-ray. The posteroanterior projection and the lateral projection. After a deep inspiration Chest X-rays always is taken to clear visualization of the lungs (Civetta JM, Taylor RW, Kirby RR, 1990).

### Computed Tomography (CT Scan)

CT scan is the procedure which provides a cross-sectional view of the chest. It provides more detailed information about the nodules present in pulmonary structure and small tumors present adjacent to the pleural surface which is not identified by X-rays. The use of a contrast agent is more useful in clear visualization and assessing the mediastinum and its adjacent parts (Vincent JL, Abraham E, Kochanek P, Moore FA, Fink MP, 2016).

### MRI (Magnetic Resonance Imaging)

In the case of MRI, there is the use of radiofrequency signals in a magnetic fields. It provides a more detailed diagnostic image than the CT scan. MRI procedures provide a clear visualization of soft tissue, which cannot be assessed by CT scan or X-ray. Pulmonary nodules, stage of bronchogenic carcinoma, pulmonary embolism, inflammatory diseases of lungs, etc., are detected early by an MRI study (Vincent JL, Abraham E, Kochanek P, Moore FA, Fink MP, 2016).

### Pulmonary Angiography

This is an invasive procedure usually used to visualize the thromboembolic disease of lungs. These diseases include the pulmonary embolism and congenital abnormalities of the pulmonary vasculature. This procedure is done by the speedy injection of a radiopaque agent into the vasculature of the lungs through the veins of arms or into the femoral vein by the help of a needle or catheter (Civetta JM, Taylor RW, Kirby RR, 1990).

### Bronchoscopy

Bronchoscopy is a procedure which allows direct inspection and observation of internal organ of the respiratory system.

a flexible fiberoptic bronchoscope such as larynx, trachea, and bronchi through. Two types of bronchoscopes are available, i.e., flexible fiberoptic and rigid bronchoscope. Flexible fiberoptic bronchoscope is the most usable scope now a days. In children and endobronchial tumor resection, rigid bronchoscopy is preferable (Vincent JL, Abraham E, Kochanek P, Moore FA, Fink MP, 2016).

*Purposes*

- To examine tissue or collect secretions which obstruct the trachea-bronchial tree
- To examine any pathological changes of tissue and for taking tissue for diagnosis purpose
- To treat any small tumor growth by surgical method
- To visualize bleeding or injury site
- To visualize and removal of any foreign body obstruction
- Treatment of postoperative atelectasis

Possible complication of bronchoscopy

- Infection
- Pneumothorax
- Aspiration
- Bronchospasm
- Hypoxemia
- Bleeding and perforation

*Nursing Care before and After the Procedure*

- Informed permission is obtained from the patient or parent in the case of children
- To reduce the risk of aspiration, food and fluid restriction of patient advised before 6 hours of the procedure
- Administration of postoperative medications such as atropine and sedatives or opioids
- Remove the artificial dentures of the patient before the procedure
- Apply topical anesthesia to minimize cough reflex and discomfort before the procedure
- After the procedure offer ship of water to check the return of cough reflex of patient
- Assess for lethargy, bradycardia, hypoxia, dysrhythmia, hypertension, tachycardia, dyspnea, and hemoptysis. Any abnormality found report promptly to the physician
- Discharge patient after the complete restoration of the cough reflex and respiratory status
- Instruct family members to report in case of shortness of breath or bleeding immediately (Vincent JL, Abraham E, Kochanek P, Moore FA, Fink MP, 2016).

## Ventilation-Perfusion Scan

A ventilation-perfusion scan (V/Q) scan is a type of imaging isotopes to evaluate any blood clot, air present in the circulation of lungs. It also determines the ventilation/perfusion ratio. Their test is done to rule out a pulmonary embolism. It also evaluates lung function in case of pulmonary disease such as COPD and pneumonia, etc., to detect abnormal circulation (shunt) in pulmonary blood vessels (Civetta JM, Taylor RW, Kirby RR, 1990).

## COMMON RESPIRATORY EMERGENCY DISORDERS

### Pneumonia

*Definition*

Pneumonia is defined as "a respiratory disorder caused by inflammation of the lung parenchyma which is caused by various microorganisms including bacteria, mycobacteria, chlamydiae, mycoplasma, fungi, parasites and viruses. In pneumonia, there is an inflammatory process that occurs in lung tissue **(Figs. 10.7A to C)** and due to these patients may have an increased chance to develop microbial invasion." It is the most common cause of death among all respiratory disorders (Suzanne C. Smeltzer, Brenda G. Bare, Janice L, 2013).

*Causes/Risk Factors*

- Conditions that are responsible for increasing the production of mucus and causes bronchial obstructions. (cancer, smoking, COPD)
- Immunosuppressive patients with low neutrophil count (neutropenia, AIDS, chemotherapy heart failure, DM, etc.)
- Prolong immobility and shallow breathing pattern
- Foreign body aspiration
- Patient under NG tube, orogastric tube, prolong antibiotic therapy
- Alcohol intoxication (decrease body reflexes, decrease WBC mobilization, and tracheobronchial ciliary motion)
- Advanced age
- Patient under mechanical ventilation due to the use of improperly cleaned equipment
- Prolonged hospitalization (Suzanne C. Smeltzer, Brenda G. Bare, Janice L, 2013)

*Pathophysiology*

Pneumonia is an inflammatory response. This can be caused by an infection or things like aspiration where fluid gets into the lungs, which causes the alveoli to fill with fluid or pus. When the alveoli are filled with fluid or

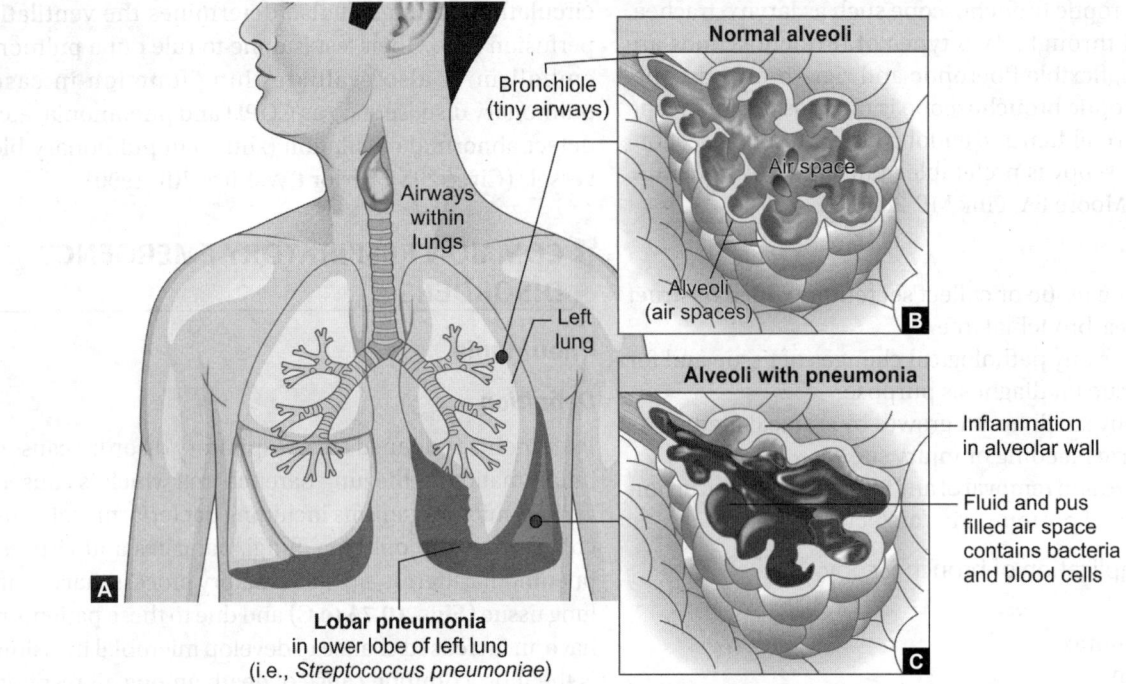

**Figs. 10.7A to C:** Label diagram of pneumonia: (A) Location of the lungs and airways in the body. Pneumonia affecting the lower lobe of the left lung; (B) Normal alveoli; (C) Infected alveoli.

*Courtesy:* Heart, Lung and Blood Institute, 2013.

pus then proper gas exchange does not occur as well. In **Flowchart 10.1**, it is described in detail.

*Classification*

It is classified into four categories as follows:
1. Bacterial or typical
2. Atypical
3. Anaerobic/cavitary
4. Opportunistic

There is another classification of pneumonia according to a different setting if occurs:
- Community-acquired pneumonia.
- Hospital-acquired (nosocomial) pneumonia
- Pneumonia in immune-compromised host
- Aspiration pneumonia (Suzanne C. Smeltzer, Brenda G. Bare, Janice L, 2013).

*Community-acquired Pneumonia*

Community-acquired pneumonia occurs in the community setting or within 48 hours after hospitalization. The causative agent for CAP is *S. pneumoniae, H. influenzae, Legionellae, Pseudomonas aeruginosa*, etc. The most common microorganism which causes CAP is *S. pneumoniae*. It is common in people younger than 60 years. with comorbidity and older than 60 years with comorbidity. *Mycoplasma pneumoniae* is another type of which is caused by *M. pneumoniae*. Its occurrence is mostly seen in older children and younger adults. It spreads through droplets or person to person contact. It affects the entire respiratory tract including bronchioles and causes bronchopneumonia. *H. influenzae* is another microorganism that causes CAP. It affects elderly people having co-morbidities like COPD, alcoholism, DM.

In the case of infants and children, viruses are the most common cause of CAP. The immunosuppressive host is mostly affected by influenza viruses type A and B, adenovirus, parainfluenza viruses, coronavirus, and varicella-zoster viruses. It mostly affects the tracheobronchial tree and extends into the alveolar area clinical sign and symptoms are difficult to identify in case of a viral infection than bacterial pneumonia (Suzanne C. Smeltzer, Brenda G. Bare, Janice L, 2013).

*Hospital-acquired Pneumonia*

HAP, is defined as "the onset of pneumonia symptoms more no evidence of after admission in patients with no evidence of infection at the time of admission". It affects mostly 15% of cases among the total hospital-acquired infection. From estimation; it has been seen that 0.5 to 1% of all admitted patients and 15 to 20% of ICU patients are affected by HAP, (CDC, 2004). Ventilator-associated pneumonia is one type

**Flowchart 10.1:** Pathophysiology of pneumonia.

```
The entry of causative organisms by aspiration/inhalation/pulmonary
circulation and impairs host defenses and trapped in the pulmonary
capillary bed
           ↓
Affect both ventilation and diffusion
           ↓
An inflammatory reaction happens in alveoli and productions of
exudates occurs
           ↓
Interfere with the diffusion process of oxygen and carbon dioxide
cells, mostly neutrophils, and migrate and filled the normally
air-filled spaces
           ↓
Due to secretions and mucosal edema affected area of the lungs in
not adequately ventilated and caused. Partial occlusion of bronchi
or alveoli
           ↓
The resultant decrease in alveoli oxygen tension, bronchospasm
because of hypoventilation
           ↓
Arterial hypoxemia due to the mixing of oxygenated and
deoxygenated/poorly oxygenated blood which travels through the
under the ventilated area of the lungs
           ↓              ↓
Lobar pneumonia involvement    Bronchopneumonia distributed
of substantial portion of      in patchy fashion which originated
one/more lobes                 one or more localized areas
                               within the bronchi and may
                               extends to surrounding adjacent
                               lung parenchyma
```

of HAP, which occurs during endotracheal intubation and mechanical ventilation and develops acute respiratory failure after 48 hours of mechanical ventilation.

HAP, occurs in at least one of these conditions.
- Impaired host defense
- Growth and invasion of microorganism in the lower respiratory system and affect the host defenses
- Presence of highly virulent microorganisms

HAP, causes highly mortality rate because of highly virulence microorganisms presence and their resistance to antibiotics and patient's co-morbid conditions. Common microorganisms responsible for HAP include *E. coli, H. influenzae, Klebsiella* species, *P. aeruginosa, MRSA,* and *S. pneumoniae, S. pneumoniae* causes 30% of cases of HAP, through inhalation or hematogenous route. Overuse or misuse of antibiotics is a major risk factor of *S. pneumoniae*. (Suzanne C. Smeltzer, Brenda G. Bare, Janice L, 2013).

### Pneumonia in the Immunocompromised Host

Pneumonia in an immunocompromised host occurs with overuse of corticosteroid, chemotherapy, use of broad-spectrum antibiotics, HIV infection, malnutrition, genetic immune disorder, and patient under long-term mechanical ventilation. The causative organism is gram-negative bacilli like *Klebsiella, E. coli, pseudomonas, proteus, entero-bacteriae. M. tuberculosis,* etc., (Suzanne C. Smeltzer, Brenda G Bare, Janice L, 2013).

### Aspiration Pneumonia

Aspiration pneumonia the lower respiratory tract causes due to the entry of endogenous or exogenous substances in respiratory system (Suzanne C. Smeltzer, Brenda G Bare, Janice L, 2013).

### Clinical Manifestations (Fig. 10.8)

- High-grade fever (38.5°C to 45.5°C) with sudden onset of chills.
- Pleuritic chest pain which aggravates by coughing and breathing.
- Tachypnea (25 to 45 breaths/min)
- A rapid and bounding pulse
- Bready cardia
- Nasal congestion, sore throat (in case of upper respiratory tract infection)
- Mucoid and mucopurulent sputum production
- Central cyanosis due to hypoxemia
- Shortness of breath
- Orthopnea
- Use of accessory muscles during respiration.

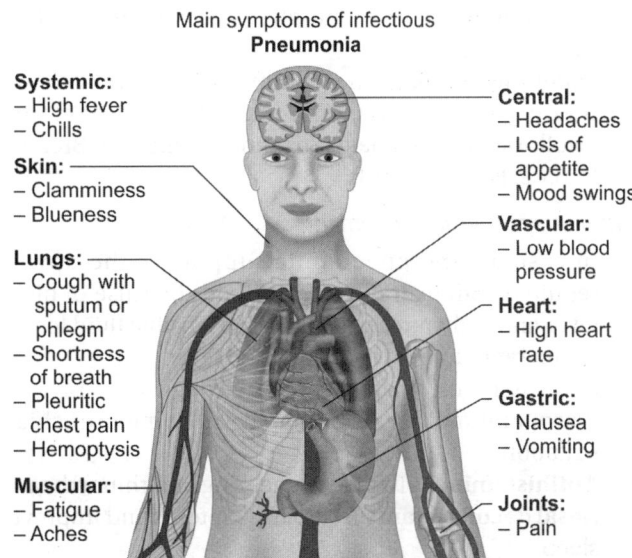

**Fig. 10.8:** Symptoms of pneumonia.
*Source:* Häggström, Mikael, 2014.

## Assessment and Diagnostic Finding

- Recent history of any infection in respiratory tract
- Physical examination
- Chest X-ray
- Blood culture
- Sputum examination
- Bronchoscopy (in case of acute and severe infection, patient under mechanical ventilator) (Suzanne C Smeltzer, Brenda G Bare, Janice L, 2013).

## Medical Management

- Patient with drug-resistant *S. pneumoniae*-macrolide antibiotic (azithromycin, clarithromycin, or erythromycin)
- Patients with risk factors for CAP-Fluoroquinolone (moxifloxacin, gemifloxacin or levofloxacin or beta-lactam agent (cefpodoxime or cefuroxime) plus a macrolide
- Patient under ICU-Broad spectrum antibiotic with septic shock plus vasopressors failure
- For pseudomonas infection-Anti-Pneumococcal antipseudomonal beta-lactam with ciprofloxacin or levofloxacin
- For community-acquired MRSA-Vancomycin/linezolid added with the regimen.
- Patient with suspected HAP, broad-spectrum IV antibiotic
- Patient with multidrug resistance-Three combine therapy may be used-Antipseudomonal cephalosporin or ceftazidime or antipseudomonal carbapenem or piperacillin-tazobactam with antipseudomonal fluoroquinolone or amino-glycoside with linezolid or vancomycin
- Patient with unknown to multidrug resistant-monotherapy with ceftriaxone, ampicillin/sulbactam, levofloxacin/ertapenem (Suzanne C. Smeltzer, Brenda G. Bare, Janice L, 2013).

## Other Supportive Management

- In case of viral pneumonia supportive therapy is required with hydration (by IV fluid) because of high fever and tachypnea with causes insensible fluid loss
- Antipyretics to treat headache and fever
- Anti-tussive medication to reduce cough
- Warm and moist inhalations for relieving bronchial irritation
- **Antihistamines:** To reduce sneezing and rhinorrhea
- **Nasal decongestants:** To treat symptoms and improve sleep
- **For hypoxemia:** Oxygen administration, pulse oximetry and ABG analysis to evaluate the effectiveness (Suzanne C Smeltzer, Brenda G Bare, Janice L, 2013).

## Nursing Management

### Assessment

- Measure body temperature for fever, chills, or night sweats
- Assess for pleuritic pain, fatigue, tachypnea
- Assess for use of accessory muscle during breathing, bradycardia, cough, and purulent sputum
- Assess the pulse, tachypnea, and shortness of breath
- Assess the mental status of patient unusual behavior, hydration, fatigue, etc.

### Nursing diagnosis

- Ineffective airway clearance related to excessive tracheobronchial secretion
- Activity intolerance related to impaired respiratory function
- The risk for deficient fluid volume related to fever and rapid respiratory rate
- Imbalance nutrition less than body requirement related to disease condition as evidence by decrease body weight
- Deficient knowledge of Rt disease condition treatment regimen and preventive health measure

### Goals

- Improve airway patency
- Provide adequate fluid to balance the fluid volume
- Provide adequate nutrition
- Absence of complication

### Nursing interventions

- To improve the patency of the airway
- Promoting rest and conserving energy
- Providing adequate fluid intake
- Providing nutritious food
- Enhancing knowledge of the patient
- Control and management of possible complications
- Promoting treatment both at home and in the community

### Prevention

- Pneumococcal vaccine (patient infected with *S. pneumoniae*)
- Vaccinate to the following group of people:
  - Older adults more than 65 years
  - Immunosuppressive people (heart diseases, DM, respiratory disease, chronic liver disease cases)
  - People with functional/anatomical anemia
  - Population of slum and industrial area
  - Specific strategies for prevention like staff education, case surveillance, prevention of transmission, etc.

*Complications*
- Respiratory failure (in case of gram-negative bacterial disease)
- Pleural effusion
- Atelectasis
- Heart failure
- Cardiac dysrhythmias
- Pericarditis
- Myocarditis
- Hypotension and shock (Suzanne C Smeltzer, Brenda G Bare, Janice L, 2013).

## Status Asthmaticus

### Definition

Status asthmaticus is defined as "a medical emergency, as an extreme form of asthma exacerbation characterized by hypoxemia, hypercarbia, and secondary respiratory failure."

"Status asthmaticus is an acute exacerbation of asthma that does not respond to initial bronchodilator therapy. It is an acute aggravation of asthma that does not respond to initial bronchodilator therapy." Asthmatic symptoms can range from a moderate to an extreme type of bronchospasm, irritation of the airways, and mucus plugging which create breathing problems, $CO_2$ retention, hypoxemia, and respiratory failure (Malarvizhi S, Gugan R, 2019).

*Causes*
- Air pollutants (dust, cigarette smoke, and industrial pollutants)
- Exposure to allergen
- Genetic predisposition
- Environmental factors
- Family history of asthma
- Gastroesophageal reflux disease
- Viral infections
- Certain medications (beta-blockers, aspirin, non-steroidal anti-inflammatory drugs)
- Exposure to cold
- Heavy exercise (Malarvizhi S, Gugan R, 2019)

*Clinical Manifestations*

Respiratory symptoms include:
- Tachypnea
- Wheezing (during expiration in early stage, later in both expiration and inspiration and disappear in severe airflow obstruction)
- Hyper expansion of chest wall and accessory muscle
- Hypoxia

Cardiovascular symptoms include:
- Tachycardia
- Pulsus paradoxus
- Hypercarbia
- Hypotension

Central nervous system symptoms include:
- Lethargy
- Agitation
- Air hunger
- Syncope
- Seizure
- Coma

*Complications*
- Cardiac arrest
- Respiratory failure or arrest
- Hypoxia with hypoxic-ischemic central nervous system injury
- Pneumothorax
- Toxicity from medication

*Diagnostic Evaluation*
- Complete blood cell count
- ABGs analysis
- Serum electrolyte level
- Serum glucose level
- Peak expiratory flow measurements
- Chest X-ray
- ECG
- Blood theophylline level (Malarvizhi S, Gugan R, 2019)

*Management*

Status asthmaticus care priorities include:
- Accelerated healing of airway blocking by effective use and appropriate use of beta-2 agonists
- The monitoring and administration of additional oxygen to reverse hypoxemia
- The prevention or treatment of symptoms such as pneumothorax and respiratory arrest

**Nursing management of the patient with status asthmaticus**

The main objective of the management is as follows:

**Airway management**
- Administer oxygen to maintain the saturation of 90 percent or above. It reduces the ventilation-perfusion mismatching and promotes bronchodilation.
- Closely monitor the patient for avoiding oxygen toxicity.
- Administer bronchodilation as prescribed to relieving bronchoconstriction the short-acting and long-acting B2-agonist are generally used to relieve the bronchial muscle (i.e., salbutamol, albuterol, levalbuterol, etc.).
- Nebulize the patient intermittently or continuously according to disease condition with nebulizing beta-2 agonists.

- Administer systematic corticosteroids as prescribed. It helps to suppress the inflammation of the airway, reduces hypersensitivity and edema. Examples of this group of drugs are prednisone, methylprednisolone, etc.
- In case of severe condition of the patient, it is advised for mechanical ventilation with non-invasive positive pressure ventilation (NPPV). Monitor the patient to reduce the stress of breathing.
- Assist the patient with NPPV to avoid complications like vomiting, gastric distension, aspiration, stress ulcer, and eye irritation.
- Assist the patient in case of endotracheal intubation. Clear the airway by suctioning to avoid respiratory blockage.
- Reduce the anxiety of the patient by administrator sedatives and neuromuscular blockade of prescribed (Malarvizhi S, Gugan R, 2019).

**Nurses role in other supportive therapy procedures are:**
- Monitor the fluid balance of the patient to avoid dehydration.
- Monitor the vital signs and airway breathing and circulation patterns.
- Relax the patient by providing him a comfortable position (high Fowler's or sitting position).
- Providing a calm and quiet environment and ensure the patient's safety avoiding respiratory irritants (tobacco, smoke, perfume, dust, etc.).
- Teach the patient about the prevention and control of asthma at home. Teach him to maintain a healthy lifestyle.
- Educate him regarding follow of rehabilitation program regarding the disease (Malarvizhi S, Gugan R, 2019).

## Interstitial Lung Disease

### Definition
A group of lung disorders caused by scarring of lung tissue. Progressively which affects the breathing pattern. It is the irreversible change of the interstitium by hazardous materials such as various dust particles like asbestos, coal dust grain dust, silica dust, metal dust (Brown D, Edwards H, Seaton L, Buckley T, 2015).

### Causes
Occupational and environmental factors:
- Asbestos
- Silica dust
- Grain dust from farming
- Coal dust from mining
- Talc
- Bird and animal dropping

### Risk Factors
- Age (most likely affect adults than infant and children)
- Exposure to an occupational and environmental toxin (mining, farming, and construction)
- Genetic factors
- GERD
- Smoking
- Radiation and chemotherapy

### Types
- Interstitial pneumonia—it causes by bacteria viruses fungi. The most common bacteria which affect is *Mycoplasma pneumoniae*
- Idiopathic pulmonary fibrosis which causes scar tissue formation
- Nonspecific interstitial pneumonitis caused by auto-immune diseases like rheumatoid arthritis and scleroderma
- Hypersensitivity pneumonitis—occurs by irritation to the lung tissue dust and molds, etc., through inhalation
- Cryptogenic organizing pneumonia—it is otherwise called as bronchiolitis obliterans with organizing pneumonia (BOOP)
- Acute interstitial pneumonitis—it is an acute and severe condition of lung disease which require the mechanical ventilation
- Desquamative interstitial pneumonitis—partially damage of lung tissue by smoking
- Sarcoidosis—which affect the lymph nodes, heart, skin, and eye
- Asbestosis—causes by breathing of asbestos which later produces fibrous tissue production in the lungs (Brown D, Edwards H, Seaton L, Buckley T, 2015).

### Symptoms
- Dry cough
- Weight loss
- Shortness of breath

### Diagnostic Evaluation
- Blood test
- CT scan shows the extent of lung damage
- Chest X-ray
- An echocardiogram determines the function of the heart
- Pulmonary function test
- Spirometry
- Oximetry
- Bronchoscopy to visualize and remove a small tissue sample for examination
- Bronchoalveolar lavage

- Surgical biopsy (Brown D, Edwards H, Seaton L, Buckley T, 2015)

## Management

### Medication

- Chemotherapy drugs (methotrexate, cyclophosphamide)
- Heart medications (amiodarone, propranolol
- Antibiotic (nitrofurantoin, ethambutol)
- Anti-inflammatory drugs (rituximab, sulfasalazine)
- Autoimmune diseases (rheumatoid arthritis, lupus scleroderma, sarcoidosis)
- Antibiotics-effective in case of bacterial infection. Azithromycin and levofloxacin are commonly used. In the case of fungal infection, antifungal drugs are used for viral diseases of the lungs are self-limiting
- Corticosteroids: To reduce inflammation of the tissue. Prednisolone and methylprednisolone are commonly used
- Lung transplantation
- Azathioprine (Imuran)
- N-acetylcysteine (Mucomyst) (Brown D, Edwards H, Seaton L, Buckley T, 2015)

### Nursing Management

- To improve the breathing pattern, administer oxygen therapy
- Assess the $SpO_2$ level of the patient and record it
- Teach the patient about smoking cessation
- Encourage patient for deep breathing coughing exercise
- Administer bronchodilators as prescribed by the physician
- Clear secretion from lungs by adequate hydration
- Advice patient to reduce activities to prevent fatigue
- Clear the excess secretions by suctioning

### Health Education

- Teach patients about the hazardous effect of smoking on health
- Teach the patient about the methods of smoking cessation
- Advice about adequate nutrition and exercise
- Teach the patient about the occupational health hazards of lungs diseases and its preventive methods
- Teach the patient about the use of protective equipment during working environments like mask respiration and hoods, etc. (Brown D, Edwards H, Seaton L, Buckley T, 2015)

### Complications

- Pulmonary hypertension
- Right side threat failure
- Respiratory failure

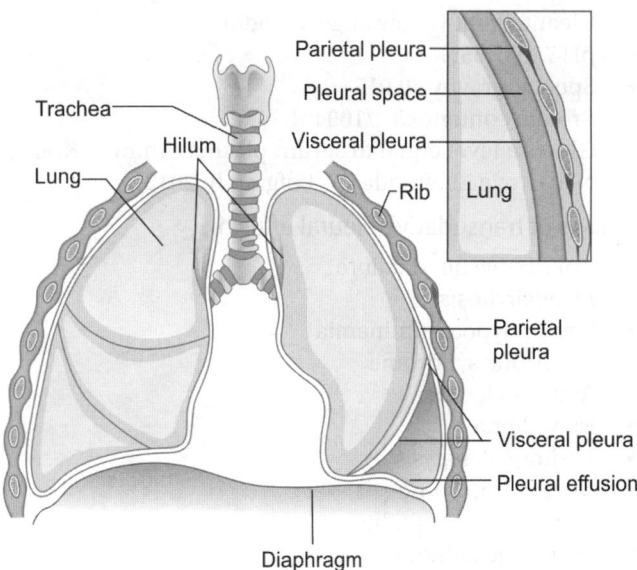

**Fig. 10.9:** Pleural effusion.

## Pleural Effusion

### Definition

Pleural effusion is defined as "the accumulation of the excess amount of fluid in the pleural cavity." It occurs due to an imbalance between the formation and absorption of pleural fluid **(Fig. 10.9)**. An excessive amount of fluid impairs the breathing pattern by limiting the expansion of the lungs during respiration (Thim T, Krarup NH, Grove EL, Rohde CV, Løfgren B, 2012).

### Types

According to the origin of the fluid, it is classified as:
- Hydrothorax (accumulation of serous fluid)
- Hemothorax (blood)
- Chylothorax (chyle which contains lymph and emulsified fat)
- Pyothorax or empyema (pus)
- Urinothorax (urine)

According to pathophysiology, it is divided as:
- Transudative pleural effusion
- Exudative pleural effusion

### Transudative Pleural Effusion

It is also known as hydrothorax. It occurs primarily in noninflammatory conditions by an accumulation of low protein and low cell count.

#### Characteristics

- Occurs primarily in non-inflammatory conditions.
- Low protein, low cell count fluid.

- Clear to faint yellow tinge, no odor
- pH 740–7.55%
- Specific gravity <0.015
- Protein content <3 g/100 mL
- Glucose level equal to serum plasma (Thim T, Krarup NH, Grove EL, Rohde CV, Løfgren B, 2012).

Causes of transudative pleural effusion
- Congestive heart failure
- Liver cirrhosis
- Severe hypoalbuminemia
- Nephrotic syndrome
- Acute atelectasis
- Myxedema
- Peritoneal dialysis
- Meigs's syndrome
- Obstructive uropathy
- End-stage kidney disease

*Exudative Effusions*

It occurs by increased capillary permeability characterized by an inflammatory reaction. It occurs in an area of inflammation by the accumulation of high protein fluid. This type of effusion occurs secondary to conditions like pulmonary malignancies. Pulmonary infections and pulmonary embolization.

Characteristics
- Often turbid or purulent
- pH <7.30
- Specific gravity >1.016
- Protein content >3 g/100 mL
- Glucose level <60 mg/dL
- High protein fluid

Causes of exudative pleural effusion
- Bacterial pneumonia
- Cancer of lungs, breast, and lymphoma
- Viral infection
- Pulmonary embolism
- Incomplete drainage of blood in heart surgery
- Trauma
- Pulmonary infarction
- Autoimmune disorders
- Pancreatitis
- Ruptured esophagus
- Rheumatoid pleurisy
- Drug-induced lupus

Other causes
- Pulmonary tuberculosis
- Autoimmune diseases like systemic lupus erythematosus
- Chylothorax
- Accidental infusion of fluid
- Some fewer common causes include—intra-abdominal abscesses, esophageal rupture, due to surgical interventions like CABG, lung transplantation, insertion of a ventricular shunt, etc. (Thim T, Krarup NH, Grove EL, Rohde CV, Løfgren B, 2012).

*Pathophysiology*
- There is an collection of large volume of fluid in the pleural cavity due to which an imbalance occurs in the formation and malabsorption of the process. The fluid may be clear or bloody or purulent. This condition causes imbalances in hydrostatic or oncotic pressure.
- Transudative pleural effusion is the type of effusion in which there is an increase in hydrostatic pressure and a decrease in oncotic pressure. Due to this, there is unable to remain the fluid within an intravascular space. So, the fluid shift into interstitial space and causes pleural effusion.
- In the case of exudative effusions, there is an invasion of microorganisms, and initiation of inflammatory reactions occurs which results in vasodilation and causes increase capillary permeability. There is leakage of plasma protein which decreases oncotic pressure. So, the fluid shift into interstitial space and causes pleural effusion.

*Clinical Manifestations*
- Dyspnea (most common symptoms when more than 500 mL fluid accumulate in pleural space)
- Pleuritic chest pain
- Decreased or absent breath sounds
- Dullness or flatness to percussion
- Pneumonia which causes fever, chills, and chest pain
- Shortness of breath
- Pleural friction rub

*Diagnostic Evaluation*
- Physical examination: On physical examination, there is
  - Decreased or absent breath sounds
  - Dull, flat sound on percussion
  - Decreased fremitus
  - Tracheal deviation
- Chest X-ray confirms the presence of fluid
- CT of chest
- **Thoracentesis (Fig. 10.10):** Aspiration of pleural fluid to analyze for bacterial growth, presence of RBC and WBC, glucose, amylase, protein, etc.
- Pleural biopsy

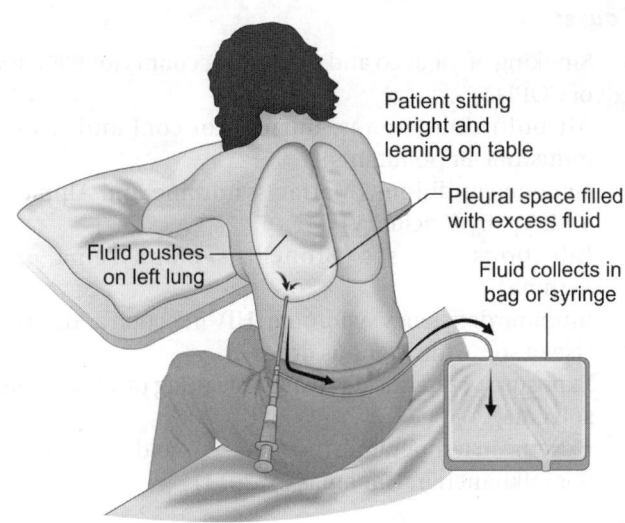

**Fig. 10.10:** Thoracentesis aspiration of pleural fluid. The illustration shows a person having thoracentesis. The person sits upright and leans on a table. Excess fluid from the pleural space is drained into a bag.
*Source:* National Institutes of Health, 2023.

## Medical Management

The objective of management of pleural effusion is to find out the cause of it and to prevent from re-accumulation of fluid.

**Thoracentesis:** By this procedure, the fluid can be removed and send the specimen for analysis.

It also helps to relieve dyspnea and discomfort. It can be done under ultrasound guidance.

- The thoracentesis procedure depends on the size and amount of fluid accumulate in pleural space. If a large amount of fluid present, then a large bone needle is inserted into pleural space and connected with a water seal drainage system. It is called tube thoracotomy. Sometimes suction evacuation is needed for re-expansion of the lung
- Antibiotics to prevent the risk of infection
- Analgesic medication to reduce pain
- Fibrinolytic therapy
- Open thoracostomy
- Decortications (Thim T, Krarup NH, Grove EL, Rohde CV, Løfgren B, 2012)

### Algorithm for the Evaluation of Patients with Pleural Effusion

Algorithm for the evaluation of patients with pleural effusion is shown in **Flowchart 10.2**.

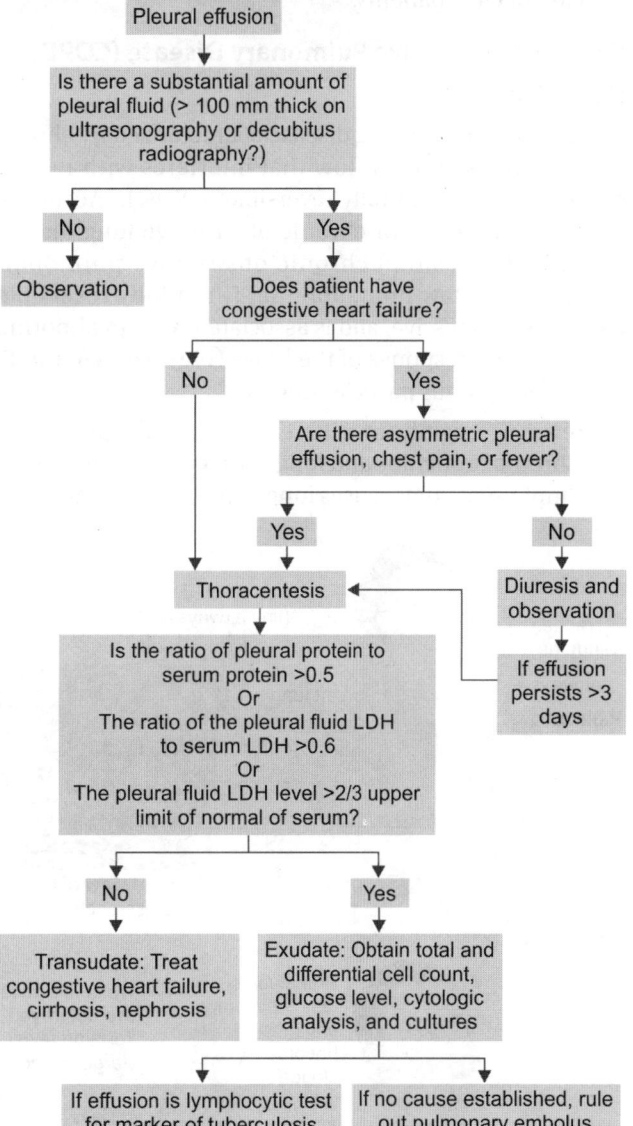

**Flowchart 10.2:** The Algorithm for the evaluation of patients with pleural effusion.

### Nursing Management

- Inform the patient about procedure and take sign in a written consent.
- Send the aspirated pleural fluid for laboratory testing.
- In the case of water seal drainage and tube drainage, the nurse has to monitor the functioning and keep recording for the amount of drainage in advised intervals.
- Provide a comfortable position to minimize pain.
- Provide analgesics to reduce pain as prescribed by the physician.

- Educate the patient and family members regarding the management and care of the chest tube drainage in the case of OPD patients.

## Chronic Obstructive Pulmonary Disease (COPD)

### Definition

This is defined as "a lung disease characterized by chronic obstruction of lung airflow that interferes with normal breathing and is not fully reversible" (WHO). "According to global initiative for chronic obstructive lung disease (GOLD) defines that chronic obstructive pulmonary disease as airflow limitation that is not fully reversible, usually is progressive, and is associated with an abnormal inflammatory response of the lungs **(Figs. 10.11A and B)** to inhaled noxious particles or gases."

There are two significant different features of COPD:
1. Chronic bronchitis and long-term cough with mucus
2. Emphysema that causes lung damage over time.

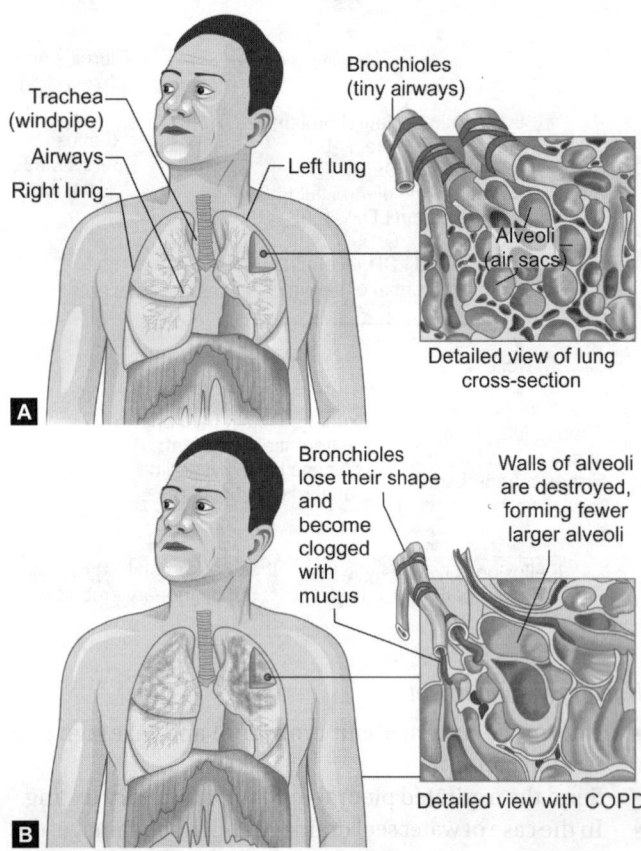

**Figs. 10.11A and B:** (A) Normal lungs: Location of the lungs and airways in the body. The inset image shows a detailed cross-section of the bronchioles and alveoli; (B) Lungs with COPD: Lungs damaged by COPD. The inset image shows a detailed cross-section of the damaged bronchioles and alveolar walls.
*Source:* National Heart Lung and Blood Institute, 2013.

### Causes

- Smoking of tobacco and cigarette accounts for 90% risk of COPD
- Air pollution (fumes, burning of coal and wood, industrial air pollutants)
- Genetic conditions (Marfan syndrome and Alpha -1 antitrypsin deficiency)
- Infectious diseases (Bronchitis, emphysema, and Asthma)
- Immune deficiency syndrome (HIV infection and AIDS)
- Use of some intravenous drugs
- Exposure to chemicals (paints, cleaning products, and solvents)
- Extreme in temperature (extreme hot/cold) (Qureshi H, Sharafkhaneh A, Hanania NA, 2014)

### Pathophysiology

See **Flowchart 10.3**.

### Clinical Manifestations (Fig. 10.12)

*Early Stage*

- Cough with sputum
- Chest pain
- Breathlessness
- Wheezing

*Late Stage*

- Respiratory distress
- Tachypnea
- Cyanosis
- Use of accessory muscle during breathing
- Hyperinflation
- Chronic wheezing
- Prong expiration
- Elevated jugular venous pulse
- Peripheral edema
- Abnormal lung sound (crackle)

### Stages and Treatment Modalities

See **Table 10.12**.

### Diagnosis

- **History and physical examination:** The physical assessment includes the respiratory history of the patient, smoking history and family history of COPD are critical factors of COPD diagnosis.
- **Chest X-ray:** An X-ray can indicate lung enlargement in some COPD (due to hyperinflation) patients. However, X-rays become more helpful if other conditions like COPD, such as pneumonia.

**Flowchart 10.3:** Pathophysiology of COPD.

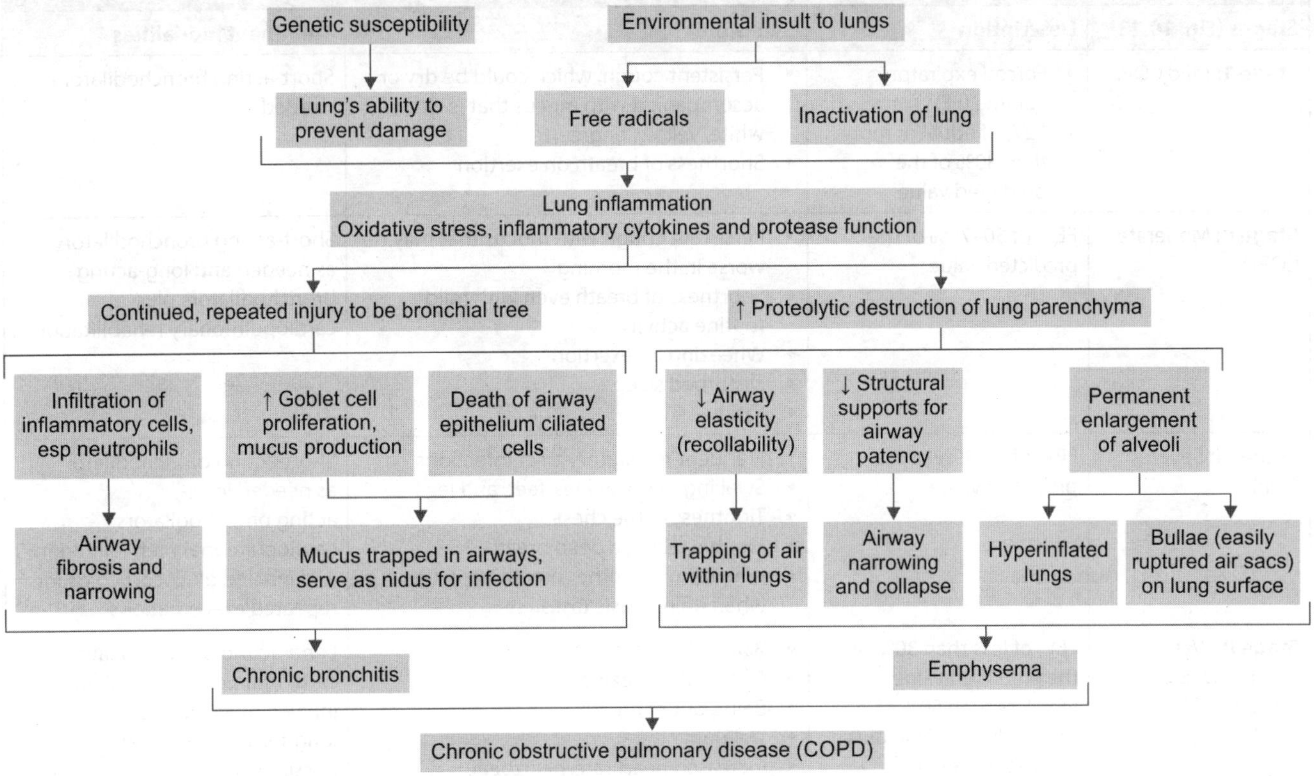

```
Genetic susceptibility          Environmental insult to lungs
        ↓                          ↓           ↓
Lung's ability to           Free radicals    Inactivation of lung
prevent damage
                    ↓
        Lung inflammation
        Oxidative stress, inflammatory cytokines and protease function
            ↓                                       ↓
Continued, repeated injury to be bronchial tree    ↑ Proteolytic destruction of lung parenchyma

Infiltration of      ↑ Goblet cell      Death of airway    ↓ Airway        ↓ Structural    Permanent
inflammatory cells,  proliferation,     epithelium ciliated elasticity     supports for    enlargement
esp neutrophils      mucus production   cells              (recallability) airway patency   of alveoli

Airway              Mucus trapped in airways,            Trapping of air   Airway         Hyperinflated  Bullae (easily
fibrosis and        serve as nidus for infection         within lungs      narrowing      lungs          ruptured air sacs)
narrowing                                                                  and collapse                  on lung surface

        Chronic bronchitis                                      Emphysema

                Chronic obstructive pulmonary disease (COPD)
```

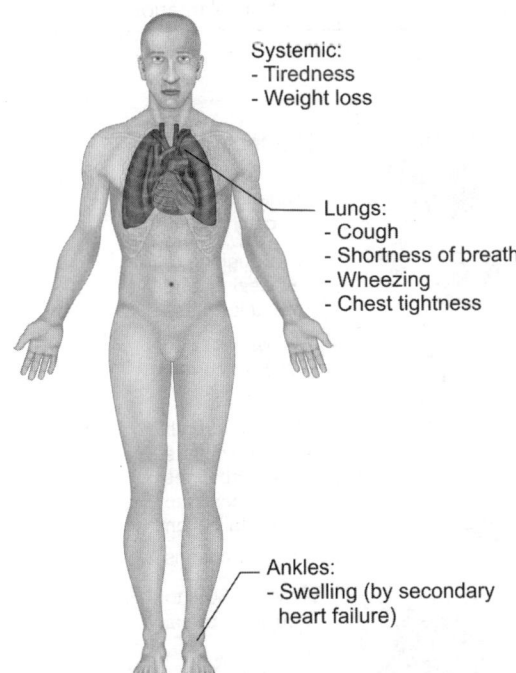

Systemic:
- Tiredness
- Weight loss

Lungs:
- Cough
- Shortness of breath
- Wheezing
- Chest tightness

Ankles:
- Swelling (by secondary heart failure)

**Fig. 10.12:** Symptoms of COPD.
*Source:* National Heart Lung and Blood Institute, 2013.

- CT scan of lungs.
- Pulse oximetry.
- **Spirometry:** Spirometry is a test that measures how much air can pass inside and outside the lungs over a short period and is used for COPD testing. Spirometry involves breathing in a large tubing, called a spirometer, attached to a pump. The test can diagnose early COPD and evaluate the level of COPD. The test also demonstrates how certain medications affect the effects of COPD in a person.
- ABGs analysis.
- Pulmonary function test (PFT)—gold standard test for COPD (Qureshi H, Sharafkhaneh A, Hanania NA, 2014).

## Management

### Medical Management

- **β-2 agonist and bronchodilator (inhaler) in short- and long-term:** Bronchodilators are medicines that are widely used for relaxing bronchial muscles in COPD. The airway is widened and makes airflow into the lungs easier by releasing these muscles. Some are fast-acting (4 to 6 hours), whereas longer-acting bronchodilators are used regularly to relieve more severe COPD

**Table 10.12:** Stages of COPD and its symptoms with treatment modalities.

| Stages (Fig. 10.13) | Description | Symptoms | Treatment modalities |
|---|---|---|---|
| **Stage 1:** Mild COPD | • Forced expiratory volume ($FEV_1$)<br>• $FEV_1$ of equal or more than 80% of the predicted value | • Persistent cough, which could be dry or accompanied with mucus that is clear, white, yellow, or green<br>• Shortness of breath on exertion | Short-acting bronchodilator as needed |
| **Stage II:** Moderate COPD | $FEV_1$ of 50–79% of the predicted value | • Persistent cough with mucus that may be worse in the morning<br>• Shortness of breath even with mild routine activity<br>• Wheezing on exertion<br>• Disturbed sleep<br>• Fatigue | Short-acting bronchodilator as needed and long-acting bronchodilators plus cardiopulmonary rehabilitation |
| **Stage III:** Severe COPD | $FEV_1$ of 30-49% of the predicted value | • Frequent respiratory tract infections<br>• Swelling of the ankles, feet, and legs<br>• Tightness in the chest<br>• Trouble taking a deep breath<br>• Wheezing and other breathing issues when doing basic tasks | Short-acting bronchodilator as needed long-acting bronchodilators cardiopulmonary rehabilitation and inhaled glucocorticoids for repeated exacerbations |
| **Stage IV:** Very severe COPD (end-stage of COPD) | $FEV_1$ of less than 30% of the predicted value or $FEV_1$ less than 50% of the predicted value plus respiratory failure | • Barrel-shaped chest<br>• Constant wheezing<br>• Being out of breath<br>• Delirium<br>• Increased heart rate/heartbeat<br>• Loss of appetite and weight<br>• Increased blood pressure | Long-acting bronchodilators, cardiopulmonary rehabilitation, inhaled glucocorticoids, long-term oxygen therapy, possible lung volume reduction surgery and possible lung transplantation |

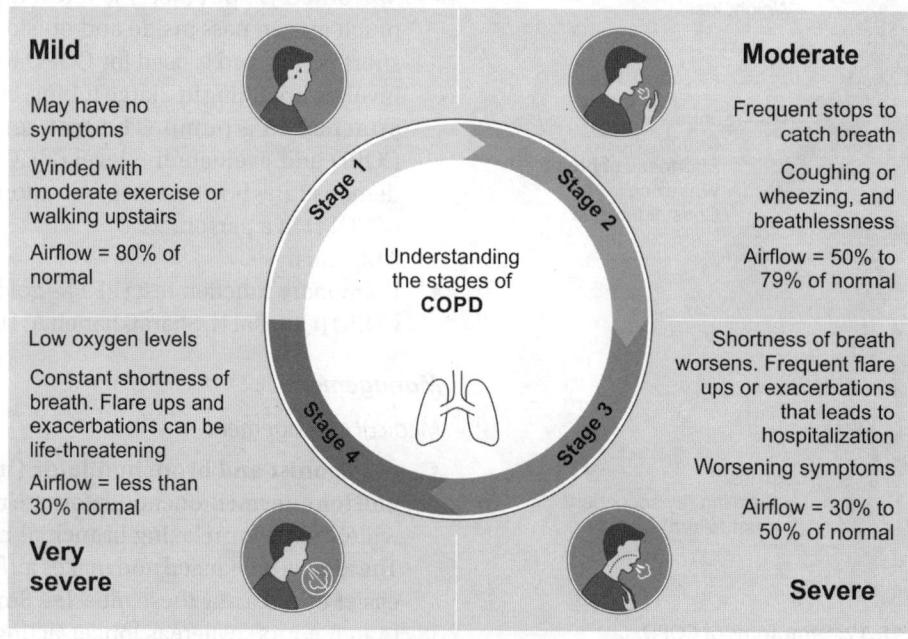

**Fig. 10.13:** Stages of COPD.

symptoms. People with COPD, depending on their symptoms, can use both forms.

Some examples of short-acting bronchodilators are: Albuterol, Metaproterenol, Levalbuterol, Pirbuterol, etc. Some examples of long-acting bronchodilators are Salmeterol, Formoterol, Arformoterol, Indacaterol, etc. Some examples of anti-cholinergic bronchodilators are Ipratropium, Tiotropium, Aclidinium, etc.

- **Inhalation of nasal steroids or oral steroid drugs:** Corticosteroids minimize airway inflammation and thereby free up the airways. The inhaler is sometimes given for this drug, although tablets and/or injectors may also be used. Oral corticosteroids are used to treat COPD when symptoms get rapidly worse. Corticosteroids and bronchodilators are frequently prescribed for COPD patients.

**Mucolytics:** Mucolytics are medicines that reduce the thickness, stickiness of cough. They are used for treating respiratory problems, such as (productive) cough, characterized by excessive or sticky mucus. Some examples are Mucinex, Bromhexine, Hyperosmolar saline, etc.

Antibiotics drugs to remove the mucus and clear the airway infection

**Quit smoking and avoiding other irritants:** Nicotine replacement therapy helps the patient to quit tobacco smoking by reducing the withdrawal symptoms. Nicotine contains chewing gums and nicotine patches are available which is absorbed through mucus membranes and skin. Varenicline is an oral drug that helps to the cessation of smoking. Bupropion is one type of antidepressant which helps to reduce the withdrawal symptoms of nicotine.

**Oxygen therapy:** Oxygen administration can increase life expectancy and quality of life in certain individuals. This is particularly effective for individuals with COPD whose blood levels are consistently poor. It may also lead to developing stamina. Oxygen supply systems are also convenient and lower cost (Qureshi H, Sharafkhaneh A, Hanania NA, 2014).

*Surgical Management*

There are usually three types of surgery to treat some types of COPD patients including:

1. **Bullectomy:** Removal of giant bullae is bullectomy surgery. Air-filled spaces are generally referred to as bullae in the lung periphery which typically occupy lung space in people with emphysema. About 33% of lung tissue will take place in giant bulls, compress adjacent lung tissue, and decrease blood flow and ventilation into healthy tissue. Surgical removal may allow for the expansion of compressed lung tissue.

2. **Lung volume reduction surgery** includes removal of 20% to 30% of the pulmonary tissue most affected by cigarette smoke. This technique is generally done in patients with serious emphysema and significant inflammation of the airways and airways are usually affected. This technique is not used much.

3. **Lung transplantation** is a surgical treatment for advanced pulmonary disease patients. COPD is the main group of individuals seeking lung transplantation. Those other patients with COPD normally have extreme effects at COPD stage III or IV needs lung transplantation and generally have a life expectancy of about 2 years or less without transplantation.

*Nutrition, Vitamins and Complementary Therapy*

- Exercises for breathing—if a person with the chronic obstructive pulmonary disease has moderate to mild symptoms, they will also benefit from exercises to limit the development of COPD. Yoga may be another type of good workout that improves breathing effectiveness and regulation of the breathing muscles.
- Vitamin E improves lung function
- Omega-3 fatty acids (found in tuna, herring, mackerel, sardines, soybeans, canola oil, etc.) to minimize inflammation
- Anti-oxidants to minimize inflammation (found in spinach, peppers, broccoli, green tea, red grapes)
- Acupuncture therapy

*Nursing Management*

- The nurse has to assist the patient in improvement of gas exchange by administering oxygen therapy.
- To assist the patient in the clearance of the airway by coughing and deep breathing exercise. Administer bronchodilators and corticosteroids to avoid potential complications.
- For improving breathing patterns, the nurse has to train the patient about inspiratory muscle training, diaphragmatic and pursed-lip breathing.
- Check the values of pulse oximetry and measure the patient for supplemental $O_2$.
- Prevent the infection by providing vaccines against influenza and *S. pneumonia*.
- Check the vital signs and identify any deviations like fever, hypoxia, breathlessness, etc.
- Document the intervention, treatment plan, and modification of the plan of care.
- Communicate with the respiratory therapist for chest physiotherapy and postural drainage to prevent possible aspiration and avoiding complications.

- Encourage the patient to enroll himself in a pulmonary rehabilitation program.
- Provide a healthy diet and nutrients for early recovery and maintaining good health.
- Advise the patient to quit smoking if the patient is taking and encourage him to join a smoking cessation program (Qureshi H, Sharafkhaneh A, Hanania NA, 2014).

## Pulmonary Tuberculosis

Pulmonary tuberculosis in the infection of lung parenchyma causes by *M. tuberculosis* is an acid-fast aerobic basilica. It is one of the droplet infections (Marty AT, 2016).

- It also affects the other body parts including meninges, kidneys, bones and lymph nodes.
- This disease is closely related with malnutrition, poverty, overpopulation, and the leading cause of death in the world's populous country among infectious diseases (WHO, 2007).

The **Ghon complex**, typical of pulmonary tuberculosis, consists of a parenchymal focus and hilar lymph node lesions. The detailed section of the diagram **(Fig. 10.14)** show's typical features of tuberculous granuloma: Central caseous necrosis surrounded by epithelioid cells, multinucleated giant cells, and lymphocytes.

### Transmission and Risk Factors

- It transmitted through the air by droplet nuclei (1 to 5 mu in diameter) by coughing sneezing and talking, etc.
- Close contact with a patient with active T3.
- Patient with immunocompromised status (HIV infection, transplanted organs, cancer, high dose of corticosteroids for prolong period).
- Alcoholism and substance abuse people.
- Children under 15 years and older adults.
- Poor socioeconomic status (malnutrition, homelessness, inadequate health care).
- Co-morbidity conditions (diabetics mellitus, chronic renal failure, hemodialysis, transplanted organs).
- People migrated from a high prevalence country of TB (Asia, Africa, Latin America, Caribbean).
- Urban and slum area and industrial area.
- Overcrowded and substandard housing.
- Health care workers performing high-risk activities (sputum, induction, procedure, suctioning, coughing procedure, bronchoscopy, caring of immunosuppressed patients) (Marty AT, 2016).

### Pathophysiology

*See* **Flowchart 10.4**.

### Clinical Manifestations (Fig. 10.15)

- Low-grade fever
- Cough (non-productive or mucopurulent sputum)
- Night sweats
- Fatigue
- Weight loss
- Hemoptysis
- Anorexia

### Assessment and Diagnostic Finding

- Assess complete history of the patient regarding socioeconomic status previous medical history (cancer, DM, HTN, cardiac diseases HIV infection)
- Surgical history (previous surgery)
- Medication history (corticosteroid, antibiotics, chemotherapy)
- Family history
- Personal habits (smoking, tobacco)
- Assess the lung sound (crackles, fremitus)

### Diagnostic Evaluation

- Chest X-ray detects the lesions present different in lobes
- Sputum culture
- **Tuberculin test (Mantoux test):** It is a standardized method to detect TB infection. 0.1 mL of PPD (purified protein derivative) injected intradermally by a half-inch 26 or 27-gauge needle. The injected area is marked and evaluated after 72 hours after injection. A reaction of 0 to 4 mm is considered as not significant and 5 mm or greater may be significant for people at risk. 10 mm or greater is considered significant for people who have normal.
- **QuantiFERON-TB Gold test:** It is the enzyme-linked immunosorbent assay (ELISA) that detects the release

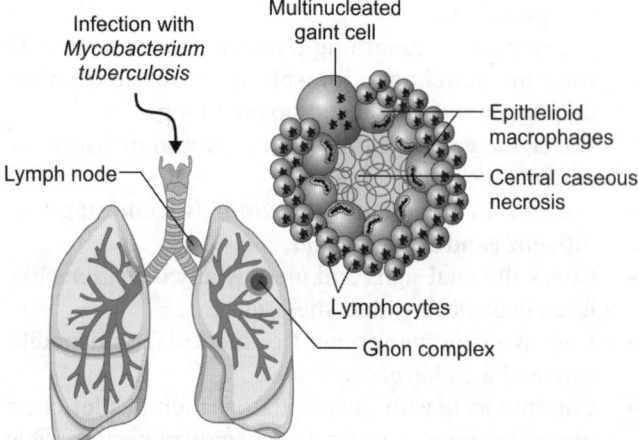

**Fig. 10.14:** Pulmonary tuberculosis.

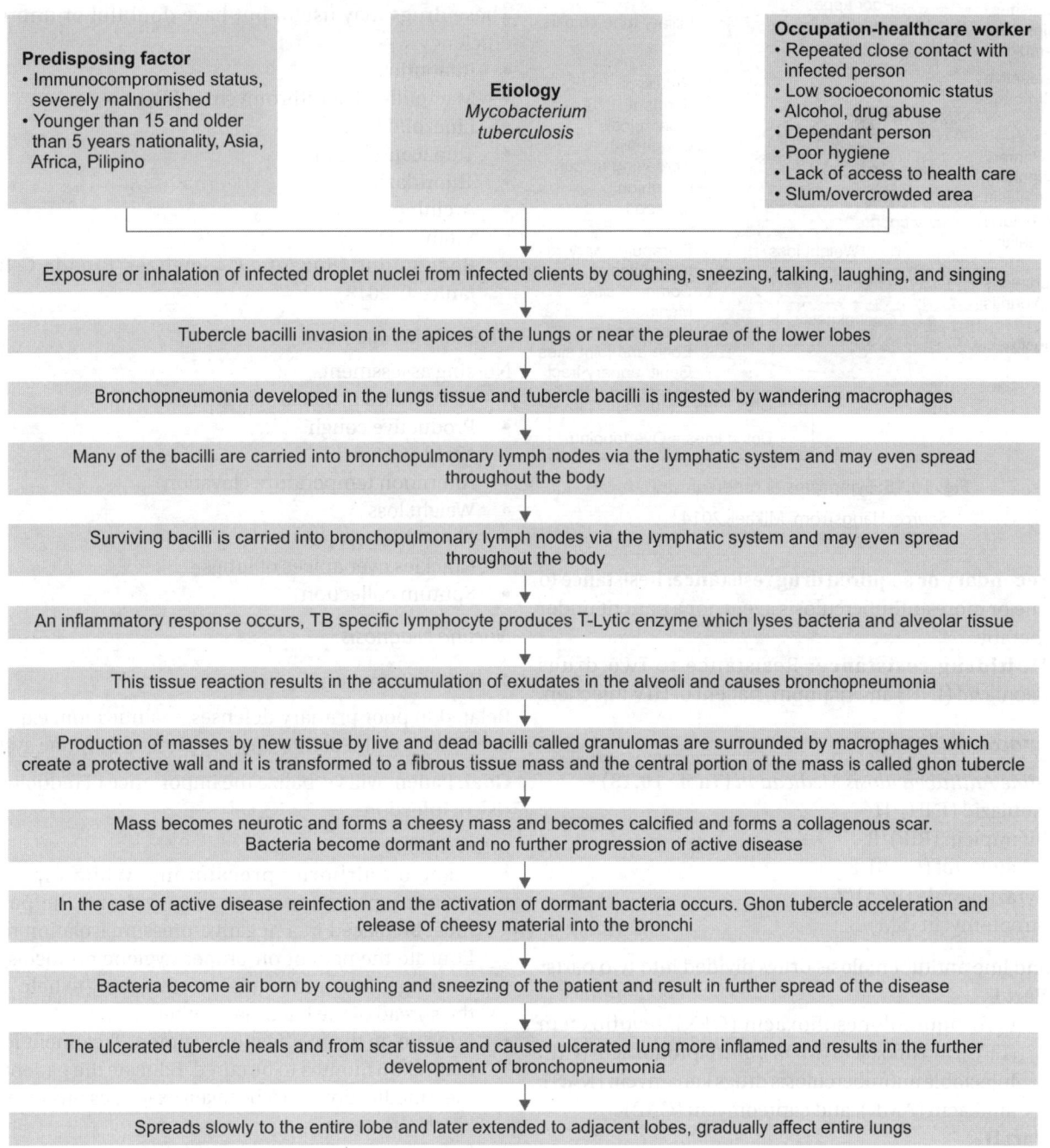

**Flowchart 10.4:** Pathophysiology of pulmonary tuberculosis.

of interferon-gamma by WBC when the blood of the patient with TB is incubated with peptides similar to those in *M. tuberculosis*. The result of the test is available for less than 24 hours. and is not affected by prior vaccination with BCG. A positive QFT-G test only indicates that a person has been infected with TB (Marty AT, 2016).

## Medical Management

Pulmonary TB is primarily treated with antituberculosis agents for 6 to 12 months. Several types of drug therapy available for the treatment of the disease effectively.

- **Primary drug resistance:** Resistance to one drug among first-line antituberculosis agents, those who have not infected before.

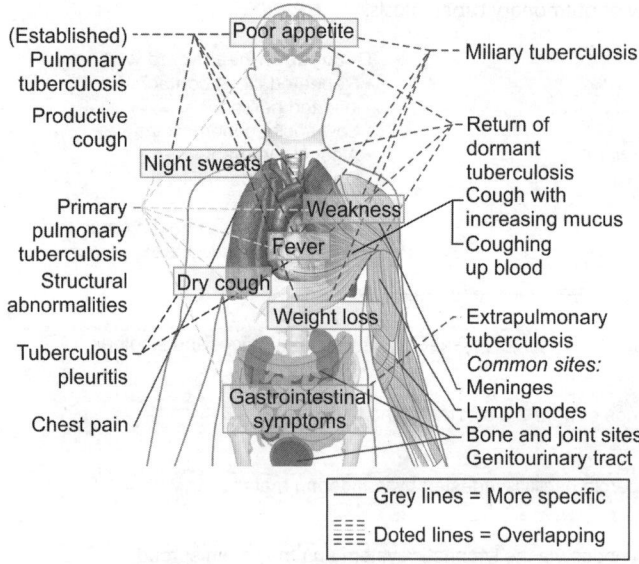

**Fig. 10.15:** Symptoms of tuberculosis.
*Source:* Häggström, Mikael, 2014.

- **Secondary or acquired drug resistance:** Resistance to one or more antituberculosis agent, for a patient under therapy.
- **Multidrug resistance:** Resistance to two drugs (isoniazid (INH) and rifampin) patient of HIV infection.

*Pharmacologic Therapy*

*First-line Antituberculosis Medication* (**Table 10.13**)
- Isoniazid (INH)/H
- Rifampicin (RIF)/R
- Ethambutol (EMB)/E
- Pyrazinamide (PZA)/Z
- Streptomycin (SM)/S

Second line antituberculosis drugs divided into two parts:
1. **Part I**
   - Fluoroquinolonesofloxacin (OFX), levofloxacin (LEV), moxifloxacin (MOX), and ciprofloxacin (CIP)
   - Injectable antituberculosis drugs kanamycin (KAN), amikacin (AMK), and capreomycin (CAP)
2. **Part II**
   - Less effective second-line antituberculosis drugs
   - Ethionamide (ETH)/protionamides (PTH), cycloserine (CS)/terizidone, P-amino salicylic acid (PAS).

The second-line drugs are used only in case of resistance to the first-line therapy (extensively drug-resistant tuberculosis (XDR-TB) or multidrug-resistant tuberculosis (MDR-TB).

**Third-line drugs:**
These drugs may useful but have doubtful or unproven efficiency.
- Rifabutin
- Macrolides [Clarithromycin (CLR)]
- Linezolid (L ZN)
- Thioacetazone (T)
- Thioridazine
- Arginine
- Vitamin D
- Bedaquiline (Suzanne C. Smeltzer, Brenda G Bare, Janice L, 2013)

*Nursing Management*

Nursing assessment
- History and physical symptoms
- Productive cough
- Night sweats
- Afternoon temperature elevation
- Weight loss
- Pleuritic chest pain
- Crackles over apices of lungs
- Sputum collection

*Nursing Diagnosis*

1. Risk for infection

Related to poor primary defenses, malnutrition, exposure to environmental pathogens, suppressed immune system.

**Goal:** Patient will verbalize the importance of reducing the risk of infection.

*Interventions*
- Place on airborne precautions. While inpatient, airborne precautions are required and the patient must be placed in a negative-pressure isolation room. Educate the patient on proper hygiene protocols, like wearing masks and regular handwashing to help avoid the spread of the bacteria to others.
- Educate on the medication regimen. Treatment for TB may take 6 months to be cured. Educate the patient that their medication must be taken exactly as prescribed to kill the bacteria.
- Reiterate the importance of follow-ups and regular retesting of sputum. Monitoring the progression or regression of the disease is important to ensure the effectiveness of treatments.
- Monitor symptoms like fever, tachycardia and changes in sputum production are common symptoms of infection.
- Encourage a well-balanced diet. TB may cause a loss of appetite and weight loss. Teach patients to eat small

**Table 10.13:** First line antituberculosis medications with side effects and drug interactions.

| Commonly used agent | Adult daily use dosage | Most common side effects | Drug interactions | Remarks |
|---|---|---|---|---|
| Isoniazid (INH) | 5 mg/kg (300 mg maximum daily) | Peripheral neuritis, hepatic enzyme elevation, hepatitis, hypersensitivity | Phenytoin-synergistic Antabuse alcohol | • Bactericidal<br>• Pyridoxine is used as prophylaxis for neuritis<br>• Monitor AST and ALT |
| Rifampin (Rifadin) | 10 mg/kg (600 mg maximum daily) | Hepatitis, febrile reaction, purpura (rare), nausea, vomiting | Rifampin increases the metabolism of oral contraceptives, quinidine, corticosteroids, coumarin derivatives and methadone, digoxin, oral hypoglycemic; PAS may interfere with absorption of rifampin | • Bactericidal orange urine and other body secretions<br>• Discoloring of contact lenses<br>• Monitor AST and ALT |
| Rifabutin (Mycobutin) Rifapentine (Priftin) | 5 mg/kg (300 mg maximum daily) 10 mg/kg (600 mg twice weekly) | Hepatotoxicity, thrombocytopenia | Avoid protease inhibitors | • Orange-red coloration ob body secretions, contact lenses, dentures<br>• Use with caution in the elderly or those with renal disease<br>• Bactericidal |
| Pyrazinamide | 15–30 mg/kg (2.0 g maximum daily) | Hyperuricemia, hepatotoxicity, skin rash, arthralgias, GI distress | | • Monitor uric acid, AST, ALT |
| Ethambutol (Myambutol) | 15–25 mg/kg (on maximum daily dose, but base on lean body weight) | Optic neuritis (may lead to blindness; very rare at 15 mg/kg), skin rash | | • Bacteriostatic<br>• Use with caution with renal disease or when feasible. Monitor visual eye testing is not acuity, color discrimination |
| Combinations: INH + rifampin (e.g., Rifamate) | 150 mg and 300 mg caps (2 caps daily) | | | |

frequent snacks if they cannot tolerate larger meals. A nutritious diet will help in preventing malnutrition.
- Check liver function studies (ALT/AST). Since the treatment plan includes a months-long multi-drug regimen, the liver may be affected.
- Report to the appropriate health authorities. TB is a reportable disease. In most states, healthcare workers are required to report cases and potentially exposed persons to the local health department within 24 hours.

2. Ineffective airway clearance

Related to secretions that may be thick, bloody, or viscous, fatigue leading to weaker coughing, inflammation of the airway as evidenced by irregular breathing (abnormal respiratory rate, rhythm, depth), abnormal breath sounds, dyspnea, tightness in the chest, productive, chronic cough.

**Goal:** Patient will display a patent airway as evidenced by unlabored breathing and clear breath sounds.

*Interventions*
- Place the patient in Fowler's position. Semi or high-Fowler's position can increase the lung capacity, therefore allowing the patient to breathe more effectively.
- Instruct on the use of respiratory devices. An incentive spirometer expands the lungs and encourages deep breathing. A flutter valve can mobilize secretions.

- Suction when necessary. If the patient is unable to expectorate secretions, suctioning may be necessary. Clearing the airways helps in preventing obstruction and aspiration.
- Administer oxygen if necessary. Oxygen may be needed if a patient is having extreme dyspnea. Oxygen saturation levels that fall below 95 may require the assistance of oxygen delivered by nasal cannula or oxygen masks.
- Advise the patient to increase their fluid intake unless advised otherwise. Proper hydration helps in thinning secretions, making expectoration easier.

3. Risk for impaired gas exchange

Related to thick, viscous secretions, bronchial edema, destruction of the alveolar-capillary membrane, atelectasis as evidenced by a risk diagnosis is not evidenced by signs and symptoms as the problem has not yet occurred and the goal of nursing interventions is aimed at prevention.

**Goal:** Patient will have improved arterial blood gasses and demonstrate adequate ventilation and oxygenation of the tissues.

*Interventions*
- Demonstrate and encourage pursed-lip breathing during exhalation. This helps in distributing air throughout the lungs by creating resistance against outflowing air to prevent collapse or narrowing of the airways, ultimately relieving shortness of breath.
- Encourage adequate rest and limit activities. Promote a calm and restful environment. Reduce oxygen consumption and demand by promoting plenty of rest.
- Provide supplemental oxygen. Choose the lowest concentration that is indicated by the situation and manifested symptoms. Supplemental oxygen can worsen hypoxemia that may occur due to decreased ventilation from a high concentration of oxygen.
- Consider supportive medications. A corticosteroid inhaler or oral prednisone may assist with dyspnea and chronic coughing.

4. Imbalanced nutrition

Related to fatigue, dyspnea; frequent coughing, disease process, financial or socioeconomic factors as evidenced by aversion to eating, expressed lack of interest in food, body weight 20% or more under ideal, muscle wasting, imbalanced electrolytes.

**Goal:** Patient will demonstrate progressive weight gain toward their individual goal.

*Interventions*
- Monitor intake and output and weigh regularly. Documenting the % of meals consumed along with progress in gaining weight will help determine the effectiveness of nutritional support and interventions.
- Encourage adequate rest and sleep periods. Conserving energy will help in slowing metabolic processes, especially when the patient is febrile.
- Encourage small, frequent meals high in fats and protein. Smaller meals require less effort than forcing larger ones, ultimately leading to maximized nutritional intake.
- Refer to a dietician if necessary. Dieticians will provide accurate adjustments in dietary composition, and in planning a diet with adequate nutrients to meet metabolic requirements, dietary preferences, and financial constraints.
- Monitor BUN, serum protein, iron, and albumin. Abnormal values indicate malnutrition and may point to a need for further intervention or a change in the therapeutic regimen.
- Manage side effects of medications. Nausea, vomiting, GI upset, and anorexia are common side effects of TB medications. Administer closer to bedtime if possible to minimize upset. Antiemetics may be required to allow for adequate food intake.

5. Deficient knowledge

Related to misinterpretation of information, unfamiliarity with information resources, lack of interest in learning, lack of exposure as evidenced by request for information, statement of misconception, inaccurate follow-through of instructions, poor adherence to the treatment plan, development of complications, spread of disease

**Goal:** Patient will initiate necessary lifestyle changes to prevent transmitting the disease to others.

*Interventions*
- Provide written instructions and an after-visit summary. Provide written details including medication schedules, laboratory testing requirements, and follow-up appointment dates to help relieve any burden of remembering specific details in large amounts.
- Encourage questions and clarifications. Correcting misunderstandings with the patient and their family will help in preventing misconceptions. Encourage questions to develop trust and ensure thorough comprehension.
- Explain medication dosages and possible adverse effects. Antibiotic treatment for TB is long; 6 months at the least. Reiterate the importance of not stopping treatment as the bacteria may become resistant, causing multidrug-resistant TB (MDR TB). Serious side effects include liver toxicity, ototoxicity, skin reactions, and more. Explain to contact their doctor if side effects become bothersome.

- Review how TB is transmitted and reactivation. Knowledge of how an illness is transmitted to other persons will help in preventing the further spread of the disease. Reactivation can occur in patients with weak immune systems and chronic conditions such as HIV, diabetes, or cancer.

## Pulmonary Edema

### Definition

"Pulmonary edema **(Fig. 10.16)** is defined as abnormal accumulation of fluid in the lung tissue, alveolar space, or both. It is one of the life-threatening diseases" (Malarvizhi S, Gugan R, 2019).

### Types (Fig. 10.17)

- **Cardiogenic:** Causes that are the failure of the left ventricle to remove adequate blood from the pulmonary circulation, e.g., congestive heart failure, hypertensive crisis, kidney failure, coronary artery diseases, cardiomyopathy, etc.
- **Non-cardiogenic:** Causes injury to the lung tissue or blood vessels that supply to the lung, e.g., general anesthesia, pulmonary embolism, neurogenic causes include seizures, head trauma, strangulation, electrocution, high altitude, etc.

### Causes

- Transfusion related lung injury
- Viral infections
- Smoking
- High altitude
- Exposure to toxins
- Acute respiratory distress syndrome (ARDS)
- Hypovolemia
- Near drowning
- Pulmonary embolism
- A sudden increase in the intravascular pressure in the lungs
- Evacuation of fluid from patient harm pleural effusion
- Rapid inflammation of the lung after removal of air from a pneumothorax
- Adverse drug reaction or drug overdose (Malarvizhi S, Gugan R, 2019)

### Pathophysiology

See **Flowchart 10.5**.

### Clinical Manifestations

Early signs are:
- Dyspnea
- Air hunger

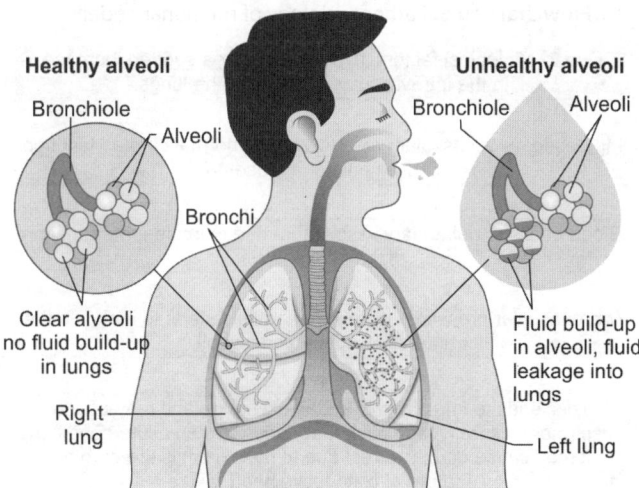

**Fig. 10.16:** Pulmonary edema.

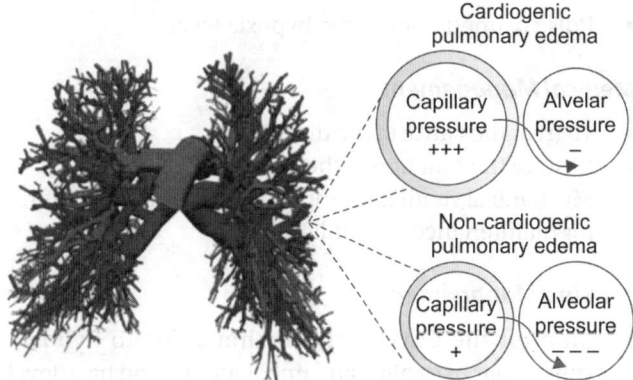

**Fig. 10.17:** Differences between cardiogenic and non-cardiogenic pulmonary edema.

- Restlessness
- Headache
- Fatigue
- Tachycardia
- High blood pressure

Due to the progress of hypoxemia, the signs are as follows:
- Lethargy
- Confusion
- Tachypnea
- Tachycardia
- Diaphoresis
- Central cyanosis
- Finally, respiration arrest (Malarvizhi S, Gugan R, 2019)

### Diagnostic Evaluation

- Chest X-ray
- CT scan of the thoracic cavity

**Flowchart 10.5:** Pathophysiology of pulmonary edema.

```
Due to etiological factors, hypervolemia or a sudden increase
in the intravascular pressure in the lungs
                        ↓
Increased microvascular pressure from abnormal cardiac function
causes pulmonary edema
                        ↓
Blood backs to pulmonary vasculature due to inadequate function
of the left ventricle
                        ↓
Microvascular pressures increases and fluid starts to leak into the
interstitial space and alveoli
                        ↓
This leads to impairments in gas exchange and may cause
respiratory failure. When pulmonary edema is an acute condition,
it may cause cardiac arrest due to hypoxia. It is the cardinal
feature of congestive heart failure
```

- ABGs analysis
- Pulse oximetry detect the hypoxia level

### Medical Management

- To treat the cause of the disease
- Restore the function of the lungs
- Mechanical ventilation and intubation may be required for maintenance of ventilation

### Nursing Management

- Monitor the ECG for dysrhythmia due to hypoxia, ventricular irritability and imbalance of acid base level.
- Hourly document the input and output status and weight the patient regularly.
- Assess the patients heart rate, BP and respiration rate to avoid the complication of cardiopulmonary deterioration.
- Assist the patient in case of mechanical ventilation.
- Assess the reports of ABGs for hypoxia and acidosis.
- Administer diuretics as prescribed by the physician, which will reduce the circulating volume and improve oxygenation.
- To reduce anxiety, administer morphine sulfate and improve the preload and after load reduction (Malarvizhi S, Gugan R, 2019).

## Atelectasis

Atelectasis that affect most of the lung or occurs suddenly is almost often triggered by a life-threatening condition, such as severe airway blockage, or where a significant amount of water or air is compressed (**Fig. 10.18**) with one or both lungs (Civetta JM, Taylor RW, Kirby RR 1990).

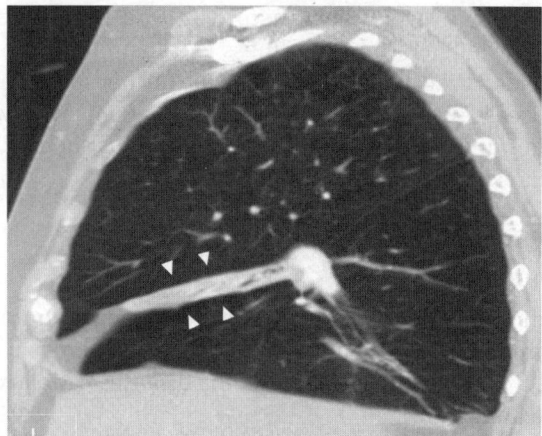

**Fig. 10.18:** Atelectasis of the middle lobe on a sagittal CT reconstruction.

### Definition

Atelectasis is defined as "a complete or partial collapse of the entire lung or lobe of the lung". The alveoli of the lung becomes deflated or may be filled with alveolar fluid. Atelectasis is one of the common postoperative respiratory complications of a patient under general anesthesia (Malarvizhi S, Gugan R, 2019).

### Pathophysiology

The pathophysiology is depending according to the nature of the obstruction. The following are the description of the pathophysiology of both obstructive and non-obstructive types.

### Types

Atelectasis is generally two types:
1. Obstructive atelectasis
2. Non-obstructive atelectasis

### Obstructive Atelectasis

The blood circulating in the alveolar-capillary membrane absorbs the alveolar gas following obstruction of a bronchus. In a few hours, this process will lead to the lung in the airless condition and retraction of air inside the alveoli. Blood then perfuses the unventilated lung in the early stages. This leads to shunting and arterial hypoxemia, potentially. Following a blockage of the bronchus, the alveolar spaces may be filled with cells and secretions, thus preventing complete atelectatic lung failure. The unaffected lung tissue relaxes and displaces the tissues around it. The heart and mediastinum move to the atelectic region, the diaphragm is elevated, and the wall of the chest flattens. When the obstruction of the bronchus is removed and the postoperative infection subsides, the lungs return to normal position. Fibrosis and/or bronchiectasis may occur where the obstruction is chronic, and infection persists.

Obstructive atelectasis occurs when a blockage forms in the airway and prevents the airflow to the alveoli, which results in the collapse of the alveoli. The most frequent form of obstructive atelectasis is the reabsorption of gases by alveoli in the event of blocking of contact between alveoli and trachea. The blockage can occur at the level of a smaller or larger bronchial tube.

The cause of obstructive atelectasis includes:
- Inhalation of foreign particles like peanuts, a small part of toys, small food particles, etc.
- Mucus plug obstruct the airway
- Tumor growth in the small airway
- Tumor in lung tissue (Malarvizhi S, Gugan R, 2019)

### Non-obstructive Atelectasis

The major cause of non-obstructive atelectasis is the lack of contact between the visceral and parietal pleurae. The relaxation of the alveoli or passive atelectasis triggers by pleural effusion and pneumothorax. Pleural effusions more often impact the lower lobes than the upper lobes. The upper lobe is mostly affected by the pneumothorax. A large pleural lung mass can cause compression atelectasis by decreasing lung volumes.

The lack of surfactants is responsible for adhesive atelectasis. The surfactant has phospholipid dipalmitoyl phosphatidylcholine, which inhibits the collapse of the lungs by minimizing alveolar surface tension.

Failure to produce or surfactant inactivation that may occur in the acute respiratory distress syndrome (ARDS), radiation pneumonitis, and blunt trauma to the lungs may cause alveolar instability and collapse. Atelectasis is caused by a tumor-like bronchoalveolar carcinoma, which fills the entire lobe (Vincent JL, Abraham E, Kochanek P, Moore FA, Fink MP, 2016).

Non-obstructive atelectasis refers to the type of atelectasis which doesn't create any obstruction in the airway. It is caused by loss of contact between parietal and visceral pleura, which causes scarring of parenchymal tissue and infiltrative diseases by compression and loss of surfactant.

Common causes of non-obstructive atelectasis include:
- Surgery under general anesthesia (postsurgical atelectasis)
- Pleural effusion (build of fluid in pleural space)
- Pneumothorax (build of air in alveoli)
- Lung scarring/pulmonary fibrosis (due to long-term infection like pulmonary tuberculosis, due to chronic exposure to irritants, cigarette smoking)
- Chest tumor (create pressure on the lung and causes air out from alveoli and deflate them)
- Surfactants deficiency (seen in infants born in prematurely) (Malarvizhi S, Gugan R, 2019).

### Classification

- **Acute atelectasis:** This has been collapsed for a short period due to airlessness.
- **Chronic atelectasis:** In the case of chronic atelectasis lung has been affected by various conditions like chronic infection, bronchiectasis, scar tissue formation, etc.
- **Absorption (resorption) atelectasis:** It happens when the oxygen is exchanged with nitrogen with a large volume and causes a decrease in alveolar volume and collapsed.
- **Compression (relaxation) atelectasis:** It occurs due to the accumulation of blood, body fluid, or air in the pleural cavity, which causes the mechanical collapse of the lung. This happens because of diseases like pleural effusion, congestive heart failure, pneumothorax, and causes compression atelectasis.
- **Patchy atelectasis:** This occurs in newborn babies due to a lack of surfactant in hyaline membrane disease. It is also seen in adults who are suffering from acute respiratory distress syndrome (ARDS).
- **Right middle lobe syndrome:** This is the one form of chronic atelectasis. The contraction of the middle lobe of the right lung occurs, due to pressure on the bronchus from enlarged lymph node glands of by tumor in lungs occasionally. Pneumonia may be developing due to blockage, contraction, and failure to resolve completely which can lead to scarring, chronic inflammation, and bronchiectasis.
- **Rounded atelectasis:** In this condition, the outer portion of the lungs collapses slowly as a result of scarring and shrinkage of the pleura, which is identified by the thickening of the visceral pleura and entrapment of the lung tissue. In the X-ray of the lungs, it shows a rounded appearance. Rounded atelectasis occurs due to complications of asbestos-induced disease of the pleura and also due to scarring or thickening of the pleura for a chronic period (Vincent JL, Abraham E, Kochanek P, Moore FA, Fink MP, 2016).

### Clinical Manifestations

- Difficulty in breathing (fast and shallow)
- Sharp chest pain during breathing and coughing
- Rapid breathing (tachypnea)
- Increased heart rate (tachycardia)
- Cyanosis (skin, lip, fingernails, or toenails)
- Pneumonia with productive fever cough and chest pain

### Diagnostic Evaluation
- Chest X-ray
- CT scan of the thoracic cavity
- ABGs analysis
- Pulse oximetry detect the hypoxia level
- Bronchoscopy to visualize the airway. This procedure also helps to remove foreign particles and surgical intervention of removal of small tissue of tumor or removal of muscle plug which obstructs the airways

### Medical Management
- **Oxygen therapy:** Oxygenation through a face mask and nasal cannula by the mode of continuous positive pressure is beneficial for re-expanding the collapsed lung. By adequate oxygenation, postoperative atelectasis can be prevented. Always ensure the blood saturation is greater than 90 percentages.
- **Fibreoptic bronchoscopy:** It has an important role in the management of atelectasis. It helps to detect the degree of obstruction of the bronchial tree and its causes. Single suction fibreoptic bronchoscopy helps to the removal of foreign particles in case of failure of removal by coughing and normal suctioning.
- **Chest physiotherapy:** Chest physiotherapy along with postural drainage, chest wall vibration, and percussion help the clearance of the airway and assess the characteristics of sputum (i.e., volume, viscosity, and weight)
- **Spirometry:** This procedure helps to reduce postoperative atelectasis. It encourages the patient to deep breathing and early ambulation after surgery.
- **Mechanical ventilation:** In case of severe hypoxia and respiratory distress the patient requires mechanical ventilation. For re-expanding, the collapsed lung's segment positive pressure ventilation and larger tidal volume may helpful.

### Pharmacological Management
- **Bronchodilator:** This increases ventilation by decreasing muscle tone of both larger and smaller airways. These are including drugs like anticholinergic agents, methylxanthines. Examples of some drugs are albuterol, metaproterenol, etc.
- **Antibiotics:** It is used to treat post-obstructive infections and bronchitis. Examples of some drugs are cefuroxime, cefaclor, etc.
- **Mucolytic agents:** The recommended drugs for direct instillation through fibreoptic bronchoscopy or in the case of intubated patients is N-acetylcysteine. It helps to the removal of a thick mucus plug that blocks the airways by liquifying it. Instillation of N-acetylcysteine helps sputum expectoration in patients with mucus plugging (Vincent JL, Abraham E, Kochanek P, Moore FA, Fink MP, 2016).

Surgical management
- **Lobectomy:** A surgical procedure of removal of collapsed lobes of the lung. It has been preferred for a permanently reversible portion of the lung for removal.
- **Segmental resection:** It is the removal of a section of the lobe which is affected and collapsed permanently.

### Complications
The complications of atelectasis may include the following:
- Acute pneumonia
- Bronchiectasis
- Hypoxia and respiratory failure
- Postoperative drowning of the lung
- Sepsis
- Pleural effusion and empyema (Vincent JL, Abraham E, Kochanek P, Moore FA, Fink MP, 2016).

### Nursing Management of the Patient with Atelectasis
- Monitor the vital signs pulse oximetry reading and ABGs values to detect hypoxia or oxygen toxicity.
- Assess the abnormal breath sound and respiratory status frequently.
- Provide oxygen therapy in case of hypoxia.
- Encourage the patient to take adequate fluid to mobilize the secretions and humidify the inspired air.
- Provide a comfortable position to patient to manage pain and breathing difficulties. Give analgesics to reduce pain as prescribed.
- Support patient in daily activity or allow the family members to assist the patient.
- Assist the patient in postural drainage and chest physiotherapy to remove secretions.
- Suction the airway to avoid blocking if the patient is intubated unable to clear the secretion.
- Administer sedatives to relax the patients coughing reflex.
- Provide emotional support and reassurance to the patient and family members. provide comfort measures to which helps in relaxation and conservation of energy.

## Pulmonary Embolism
**Definition:** This is defined as "the obstruction of the pulmonary artery (**Fig. 10.19**) or one of its branches by a thrombus (or thrombi) that originates somewhere in the venous system or the right side of the heart". This condition is associated with trauma, due to surgery, pregnancy, old age, heart failure, hypercoagulable states, and due to long term immobilization (Perrin KO, MacLeod CE, 2009).

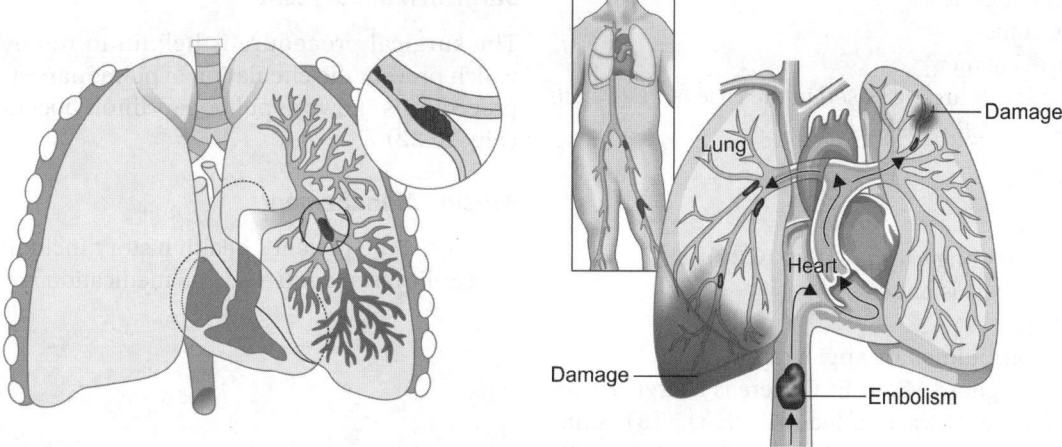

**Fig.10.19:** Pulmonary embolism.

## Causes

- Deep vein thrombosis.
- According to Virchow's tried. These factors are responsible for the formation of a clot. These are:
    - Alteration in blood flow (e.g., postoperative conditions, pregnancy, obesity, cancer)
    - Factors in the vessel wall which causes injury (endothelial injury) (e.g., surgery and catheterization in case of some procedures)
- Factors affect blood properties:
    - Hormonal contraception of estrogen
    - Genetic thrombophilia (e.g., protein C deficiency, antithrombin deficiency, fibrinolysis disorders)
    - Acquired thrombophilia (nephritic syndrome, antiphospholipid syndrome, paroxysmal nocturnal hemoglobinuria). Cancer (Perrin KO, MacLeod CE, 2009)

## Risk Factors

See **Table 10.14**.

## Clinical Manifestations

- Dyspnea (shortness of breath)
- Tachypnea (rapid breathing)
- Pleuritic chest pain
- Cough and hemoptysis
- Cyanosis
- Pleural friction rub
- Raised JVP
- Low-grade fever
- Low blood pressure
- Swelling and warmth of proximal and distal extremity (Perrin KO, MacLeod CE, 2009)

**Table 10.14:** Risk factors of pulmonary embolism.

| | |
|---|---|
| Venous stasis | ♦ Prolonged immobilization<br>♦ Prolong periods of sitting traveling<br>♦ Varicose vein<br>♦ Spinal cord injury |
| Hypercoagulability | ♦ Injury<br>♦ Tumor (pancreatic, gastrointestinal, genitourinary, breast, lung)<br>♦ Increased platelet count (polycythemia, splenectomy) |
| Venous endothelial disease | ♦ Thrombophlebitis<br>♦ Vascular disease<br>♦ Foreign bodies (IV/central venous catheters) |
| Certain disease states (combinations of statis, coagulation alteration, and venous injury) | ♦ Heart disease (especially heart failure)<br>♦ Trauma (factor of help, pelvis, vertebra, lower extremities)<br>♦ Postpartum period<br>♦ Diabetes mellitus<br>♦ COPD |
| Other predisposing conditions | ♦ Advanced age<br>♦ Obesity<br>♦ Pregnancy<br>♦ Oral contraceptive use<br>♦ History of previous thrombophlebitis and pulmonary embolism<br>♦ Constrictive clothing |

## Diagnostic Evaluation

*Blood Test: D-dimer Level*

- Complex blood cell count
- Clotting status (PT, PTT, TT)
- ESR test

- Kidney function test
- Liver enzymes
- Electrolyte balance
- Troponin levels are increased in the case of PE (Perrin KO, MacLeod CE, 2009)

*Imaging Studies*

- Chest X-ray
- CT pulmonary angiography (**Fig. 10.20**)
- Ventilation/perfusion scan
- USG of legs
- Fluoroscopic pulmonary angiography
- **ECG**—To diagnose MI. In ECG there is a large S wave in lead I, large Q wave in lead III (S1 Q3 T3). Sinus tachycardia, right axis deviation, and right bundle branch block are found in ECG
- **Echocardiography:** Dysfunction of Rt side heart which is seen in echocardiography (Perrin KO, MacLeod CE, 2009)

*Medical Management*

- **Anticoagulation therapy:** It reduces the chance of occurrence of thrombus formation and reduces the size of the thrombus the medications the INR (international normalized ratio) value.
- **Thrombolysis:** It is used is to breakage of the clots and contraindicated incase of intracranial hemorrhage, risk of bleeding, etc.
- **Inferior vena cava filter (Fig. 10.21):** It is used in case of contraindication to the administration of anticoagulant therapy. It prevents the existing DVTs to enter into the pulmonary artery (Perrin KO, MacLeod CE, 2009).

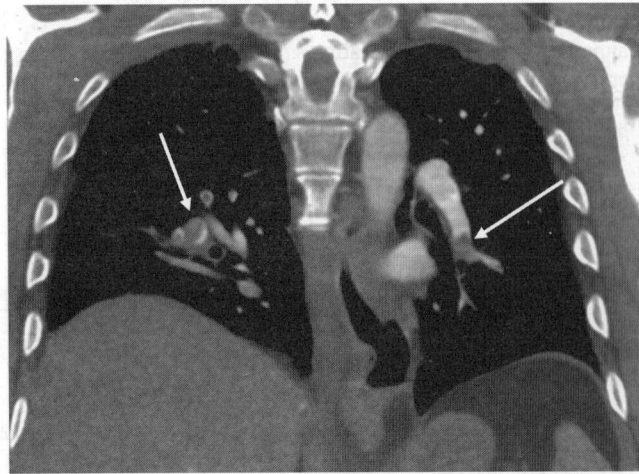

**Fig. 10.20:** Segmental and subsegmental pulmonary emboli on both sides on CT report.

*Surgical Management*

The surgical procedure is helpful to remove the clots which prevent the circulation of pulmonary structure. The procedure is known as pulmonary thromboendarterectomy (**Fig. 10.22**).

*Nursing Management*

- Assess the patient's health history including previous cardiovascular disease and medication records.

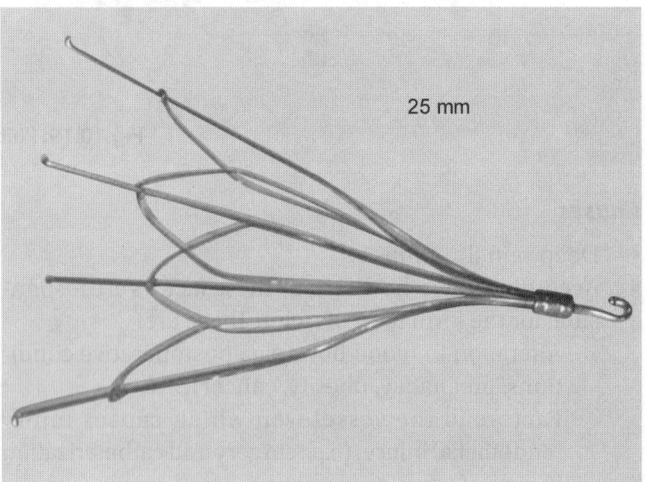

**Fig. 10.21:** Used inferior vena cava filter.

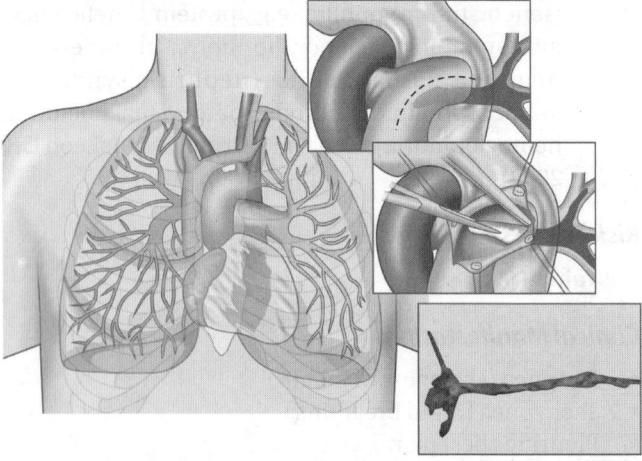

**Fig. 10.22:** Pulmonary thromboendarterectomy for CTEPH involves quick but painstaking removal of thin scarred clot tissue lining the pulmonary arteries. The residual scar is grasped and dissected from the lobar and segmental branches, as shown in the middle inset. The bottom inset shows an operative specimen. The procedure in each lung is ideally completed within 20 minutes to avoid the need for re-perfusion.

*Source:* Heart, Vascular and Thoracic/Research, 2016.

- Assess the family history of the patient may predispose to pulmonary embolism.
- Do physical examination for evaluating warmth, inflammations and redness of the extremities.
- Encourage the patient for ambulation, active and passive exercise of legs to prevent venous stasis.
- Administer thrombolytic therapy and anticoagulant therapy and monitor through INR and PTT (partial thromboplastin time).
- Manage the pain by repositioning the patient which improve the ventilation prefusion ratio.
- Provide oxygen to manage hypoxia and encourage the patient for deep breathing exercise.
- Observe the patient for potential risk of anticoagulant drug therapy such as bleeding or hemorrhage.
- Inspect the wounds of invasive procedure check the oral mucosa and nares for bleeding.
- Assess the patient knowledge regarding treatment regimen and explain the procedure to reduce anxiety.
- Keep record and document each procedure and change in treatment plan for further management (Perrin KO, MacLeod CE, 2009).

## Acute Respiratory Failure

### Definition

"Respiratory failure is a syndrome of inadequate gas exchange due to the dysfunction of one or more essential components of the respiratory system." Acute respiratory failure (ARF) is defined as "a decrease in arterial oxygen tension ($PaO_2$) to less than 50 mm Hg (hypoxemia) and an increase in arterial carbon dioxide tension ($PaCO_2$) to greater than 50 mm Hg (hypercapnia) with an arterial Ph of less than 7.35". It is the condition of an altered gas exchange function that is either in oxygen ($O_2$) or carbon dioxide ($CO_2$) by lung and not able to give adequate oxygenation or ventilation for blood (Loscalzo J, 2013).

### Classification

Acute respiratory failure is classified as two types such as type I or hypoxemic and type II or hypercapnic **(Flowchart 10.6)**.

### Causes

#### Type I: Respiratory Failure (Hypoxemic Failure)

This category of respiratory failure is caused by lack of oxygenation such as:
- Low environmental oxygen (i.e., high altitude)
- Cardiogenic pulmonary edema due to increased hydrostatic pressure
- Non-cardiogenic pulmonary edema caused by increased permeability such as acute lung injury (ALI) and acute respiratory distress syndrome (ARDS), atelectasis, and pneumonia
- Ventilation–perfusion mismatch pulmonary embolism
- Pulmonary fibrosis
- Right to left shunt

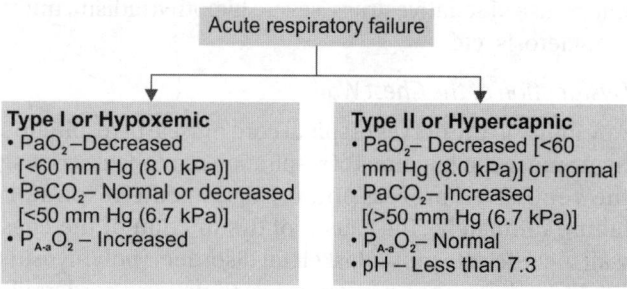

**Flowchart 10.6:** Classification of acute respiratory failure.

#### Type II: Respiratory Failure (Hypercapnic Failure)

Inadequate alveolar ventilation causes type II respiratory failure in which both oxygen and carbon dioxide are affected. Here the accumulation of $CO_2$ occurs in the body, but not disposes. The reasons behind this are:
- Due to increased airway resistance (i.e., COPD, asthma, and suffocation)
- Reduced effort of breathing (i.e., extreme obesity, brain steam lesion, etc.)
- Neuromuscular and chest wall disorder (i.e., myopathies, neuropathies, kyphoscoliosis, myasthenia gravis, ctc.)

Some other causes include:
- Inadequate postoperative analgesia, upper abdominal surgery
- Ascites
- Preoperative tobacco smoking
- Shock (cardiogenic, septic shock, and hypovolemic shock) (Loscalzo J, 2013)

### Pathophysiology

The ventilation or perfusion mechanism is impaired in case of acute respiratory failure. The impairment of respiratory system occurs due to the following conditions:
- Hypoventilation of alveoli
- Diffusion abnormalities
- Mismatching of ventilation-perfusion ratio
- Shunting

The common factors which may cause the ARF includes decreased respiratory drive, chest wall dysfunction, lung parenchyma dysfunction and some other causes.

### Decreased Respiratory Drive

The respiration drive decreases due to decrease response of chemo receptors to normal respiratory stimulation.

This may occur in disease conditions like severe brain injury, use of sedative drugs, severe hypothyroidism, multiple sclerosis, etc.

### Dysfunction of the Chest Wall

Any injury to the nerves of spinal cord muscle of respiration, neuromuscular junctions of respiration may affect seriously the ventilation process and it causes acute respiratory failure ultimately. The causes of dysfunction of the chest wall includes the musculoskeletal disorders (polymyositis, muscular dystrophy), neuromuscular junction disorders like myasthenia gravis, poliomyelitis and some peripheral nerve disorders like cervical injury, Guillain Barre syndrome, etc.

### Dysfunction of Lung Parenchyma

Due to disinfection of lung parenchyma that may lead to ARF. Such diseases include pulmonary embolism, pulmonary edema, pneumonia, lobar atelectasis and status asthmaticus. These diseases cause the obstruction in the ventilation of lungs which may further leads to AFR.

Some other causes include the following:
- Postoperative stage of abdominal and thoracic surgery due to effect of anesthetic drugs, analgesics and sedatives which depresses the respiration and increases the opioids effect and leads to hypoventilation.
- Pain may affect the deep breathing and coughing in case of abdominal and thoracic surgery patients.
- Respiratory failure due to ventilation perfusion mismatch after the thoracic, abdominal and cardiac surgery (Loscalzo J, 2013).

### Clinical Manifestations

- Increasing respiratory distress
- Dyspnea
- Air hunger
- Central cyanosis
- Agitation
- Anxiousness
- Foam or froth is formed (fluid leaks into the alveoli and mixes with air)
- Sometimes blood tinged with froth (Loscalzo J, 2013).

### Assessment and Diagnostic Findings

- **History collection:** Ask about personal and family history
- **Physical examination:** Observe $O_2$ and $CO_2$ level
- **Auscultation:** Check abnormal heart and lung sound
- **Chest X-ray:** Check for any abnormalities
- **ABG analysis:** Check for any acid-base imbalance.

### Medical Management

- Vasodilators, inotropic medications may be administered
- To treat cardiac problems intra-aortic-balloon pump may be indicated
- A diuretic may be given to control the fluid overload
- Restrict the fluid administer
- To treat hypoxemia oxygen is administered
- To reduce axis anxiousness and control pain morphine is given
- In critical situations, intubation and mechanical ventilation may require

### Nursing Management

- Assist the patient with intubation and mechanical ventilation.
- Assess the patient's respiratory and circulatory status.
- Assess the patient's vital signs, responsiveness or level of consciousness.
- Assess the results of ABGs, Pulse oxymetry chest X-ray and CT-scan reports.
- Assist the patients in skin care, mouth care and exercises of range of motion of extremities.
- Communicate with patient about the needs and health problems.
- Assess the patient's level of understanding and provide health education accordingly (Loscalzo J, 2013).

## Acute Respiratory Distress Syndrome (ARDS)

### Definition

Acute respiratory distress syndrome (ARDS) is a form of respiratory failure characterized by the rapid onset of systemic inflammation in the lungs. ARDS is a serious lung disease. ARDS is a severe lung disease. This happens when the air sac in the lungs are filled with fluid (**Fig. 10.23**). Too much fluid in the lungs will decrease the oxygen concentration or increase the concentration of carbon dioxide in the blood (Chulay Marianne, 2010).

### Causes

The ARDS is caused by lung injury in direct and indirect methods are depicted in **Table 10.15**.

### Pathophysiology

ARDS is a form of fluid deposition in the lungs not related to cardiac failure. It is normally caused by extreme damage to the lungs, referring to the microscopic air sacs of the lungs, which are responsible for exchanging gases such as oxygen and carbon dioxide with capillaries in the lungs. A partial lung failure (atelectasis) and reduced blood oxygen concentrations (hypoxemia) also provide other typical findings in ARDS. Pathological findings such as pneumonia, eosinophilic pneumonia, cryptogenic

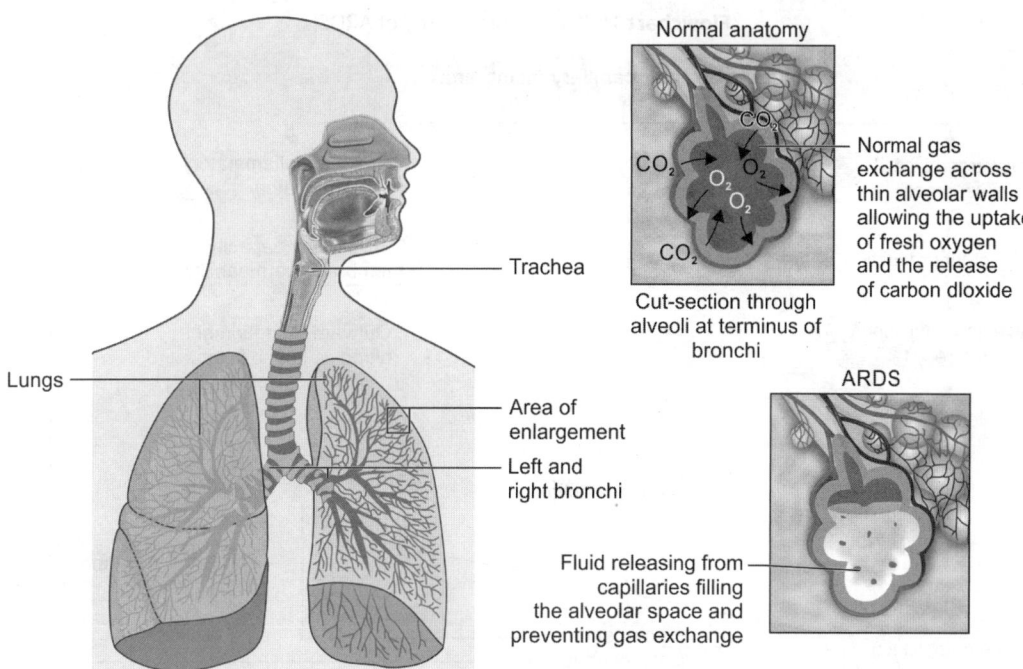

**Fig. 10.23:** Left shows the location of the lungs, trachea, and bronchi within the body. The middle image shows the normal gas exchange of oxygen and carbon dioxide through the air sacs. The image on the right shows the fluid build-up in the air sacs of someone who has ARDS. The fluid build-up prevents gas exchange.

| Table 10.15: ARDS is caused by lung injury in direct and indirect methods. | |
|---|---|
| **Direct lung injury** | **Indirect lung injury** |
| *Common causes:*<br>• Aspiration of gastric contains or other substances<br>• Viral/bacterial pneumonia | *Common causes:*<br>• Sepsis (especially gram-negative infection)<br>• Severe massive trauma |
| *Less common causes:*<br>• Chest trauma<br>• Inhalation of toxic substances<br>• $O_2$ toxicity<br>• Embolism: Fat, air, amniotic fluid, thrombus<br>• Near drowning<br>• Radiation pneumonitis | *Less common causes:*<br>• Acute pancreatitis<br>• Cardiopulmonary bypass<br>• Multiple blood transfusion<br>• Nonpulmonary systemic disease<br>• Anaphylaxis<br>• Disseminated intravascular coagulation<br>• Opioid drug overdose (e.g., heroin) |

organizing pneumonia, fibrinous acute pneumonia, and diffuse alveolar damage (DAD) are consistent with the clinical syndrome. DAD, which is characterized by diffuse inflammation of the lung tissue, is the most common pathology associated with ARDS. Respond to the provocation to the tissues, chemical signals and other inflammatory mediators are typically discharged initially from local epithelial and endothelial cells **(Flowchart 10.7)**.

T-lymphocytes and neutrophils rapidly migrate into the inflamed lung tissue to enhance the phenomenon. Typical histology includes diffuse alveolar injury and formation of hyaline membranes on alveolar walls (Chulay M, Suzanne M, 2020).

### Signs and Symptoms

- Shortness of breath
- Rapid breathing
- Fever
- Low blood pressure
- Tachycardia
- Dry cough and chest pain during inspiration

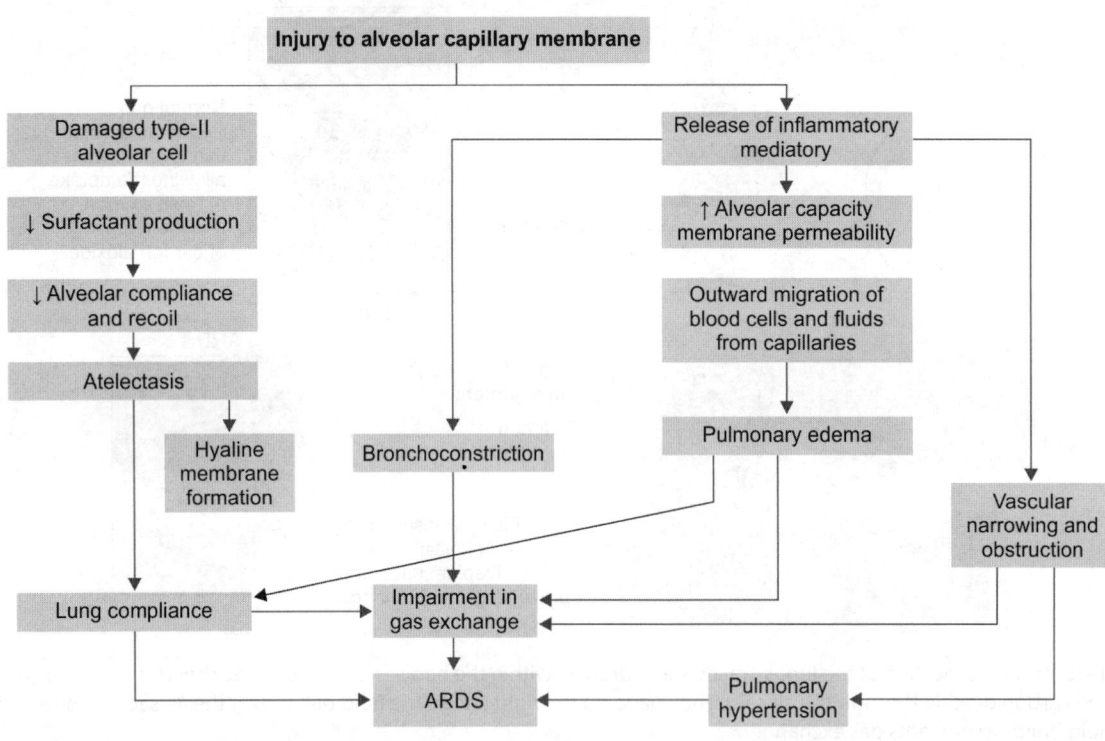

Flowchart 10.7: Pathophysiology of ARDS.

### Diagnostic Evaluation

- History of acute onset of respiratory distress, pulmonary and cardiac disease-associated risk factors
- Physical examination
- **Chest X-ray:** Detects any accumulation of fluids in lungs
- **CT scan of the lungs and thoracic cavity:** To reveals any abnormality of lungs
- Blood test for CBC
- **Pulse oximetry:** Detects the oxygen level in lings
- ABGs analysis
- **Echocardiogram:** Detects the heart function.

### Management

#### Oxygen Administration

- To correct hypoxia by simple mask or nasal cannula
- Initially, a high concentration of $O_2$ required to maximize $O_2$ delivery
- Pulse oximetry required to monitor $O_2$ level continuously
- If the $PaO_2$ cannot maintain at the desired level patient required mechanical ventilation support (Chulay M, Suzanne M, 2020).

#### Mechanical Ventilation

- It is required to maintain the $FiO_2$ level at 60% and $PaO_2$ level at 60 mm Hg or more than that.
- In mechanical ventilation, PEEP mode improves the oxygenations of the patient.
- The goal of mechanical ventilation is to maintain a $PaO_2$ level greater than 60 mm Hg and an $O_2$ level of more than 90% at the lowest possible $FiO_2$ level.
- Positioning of patient
- In acute respiratory distress syndrome, the positioning of the lung infiltration is not uniform. Repositioning into the prone position will oxygenation and relieves atelectasis and improve perfusion. It provides approximately 26% mortality benefits as compared with the supine position in the early stage of treatment (Chulay M, Suzanne M, 2020).

#### Pharmacologic Therapy

Pharmacological management includes as follows:

- Human recombinant interleukin-1 receptor antagonist
- Neutrophil inhibitors
- Pulmonary specific vasodilators
- Surfactant replacement therapy
- Antibiotic therapy
- Antioxidants and corticosteroid therapy

#### Nutrition Therapy

Maintenance of nutrition and fluid volume balance is very much important in the case of ARDS. The patient under this situation requires 35–45 kcal/kg/day to balance the calorie requirement. Enteral feeding is most preferable than parenteral feeding if the patient can take.

### Nursing Management

Patient in critically ill conditions of ARDS requires close monitoring in an ICU setting to avoid life-threatening situations. The primary role of an allotted nurse to provide nursing cares like:
- Oxygen administration
- Nebulization therapy
- Chest physiotherapy
- Assist in endotracheal intubation and tracheostomy procedure
- Mechanical ventilation
- Suctioning
- Bronchoscopy

Nurse has to change the position of the patient frequently to improve ventilation and perfusion and remove secretions. She has to closely monitor the saturation level of the patient. Due to hypoxia and dyspnea patients may be in anxiety. So, provide a calm and suitable environment for the patient. Provide adequate rest to the patient to limit oxygen consumption. Closely monitor the unconscious and breathlessness patient to prevent fall injury. Assess the patient for skin breakdown, muscle atrophy, and deep venous thrombosis. Communicate treatment plan and each procedure to patient and family members (Chulay M, Suzanne M, 2020).

## Chest Trauma

### Definition

"Chest trauma or chest injury is any form of physical injury to the chest including the ribs, heart and lungs. Chest trauma is the leading cause of death, morbidity, hospitalization and disability." It accounts for 25% of all death among traumatic injuries. The CDC (2014) reports that there have been 126–438 deaths from accidental chest injuries. Major chest injury occurs alone or multiple other injuries.

In the United States, chest trauma is accounted every year for over 1,00,000 deaths. Any 33% of these accidents needed treatment to the hospital. Overall, 20–25% of all deaths are caused by the thoracic cavity's blunt trauma (Burns SM, Delgado SA, 2019).

### Causes
- Road traffic accidents
- Fall from height
- Blast injuries
- Gunshot injury
- Stab wound
- Chest compression
- Crush injury

### Types of Chest Trauma

It is classified as two types **Flowchart 10.8**.

### Blunt Trauma

When the body is hit by a blunt object, blunt trauma takes place. It triggers life-threats, such as rupture of the spleen. The harm cannot be externally detected, but the effects can be severe.

### Etiology
- Motor vehicle accident
- Fall from height
- Assault with a blunt object
- Crush injury

### Mechanism of blunt injury
- Declaration – acceleration – injury resulting from the collision between the body part and another object or body part while both are in motion.
- Compression of thoracic structures.
- Shearing (Burns SM, Delgado SA, 2019)

### Pathophysiology

See **Flowchart 10.9**.

**Flowchart 10.8:** Types of chests trauma.

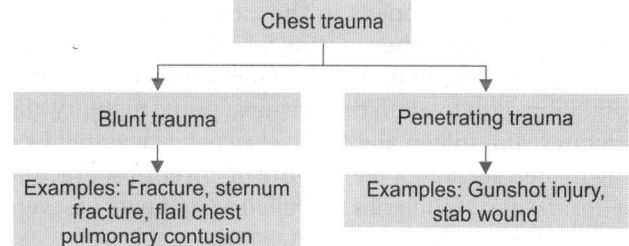

**Flowchart 10.9:** Pathophysiology of chest trauma.

Due to etiology (motor vehicle accident, fall from height)

↓

Blunt chest injuries occur due to mechanism of acceleration, deceleration, shearing and compression

↓

Hypoxia occurs due to disruption of the airway, injuries to lungs parenchyma, rib cage and respiratory muscle

↓

Hypovolemia from massive fluid loss from great vessels, cardiac rupture and hemothorax, cardiac failure from cardiac tamponade, cardiac contusion or increased intrathoracic pressure

↓

Due to these pathogenic states, impairment of ventilator-perfusion leading to acute renal failure and hypovolemic shock and death if not treated properly

### Diagnostic evaluation

Physical examination includes inspection of the airway, breathing and circulation.

### Chest X-ray

- CT Scan
- CBC
- Clotting factors
- Blood grouping and cross match
- Electrolytes
- Oxygen saturation
- ABG analysis
- ECG

### Medical management

- **Airway management:** Provides oxygen support, ET intubation, and ventilator support according to the condition of the patient.
- **Fluid volume management:** Administer IV fluid, blood if essential.
- **Intercostal drainage:** In case of accumulation of blood in the thoracic cavity.

### Sternal and rib fracture

A rib fracture is the most common type of fracture in case of chest trauma. It accounts for sixty percentages of patients who have hospitalized by a blunt trauma of chest. Sternum fracture mostly happens in the case of motor vehicle accidents through the steering wheel. It causes a high mortality rate due to the injury of the subclavian artery or vein. From fifth to ninth ribs are most prone to injury and fractures. The spleen and the liver may be lacerated by a fragmented section of the fracture of lower ribs. Fracture of the first and second ribs are called a "Hallmark of severe trauma" (Burns SM, Delgado SA, 2019).

### Clinical manifestations

**Sternal fracture:**
- Anterior chest pain
- Overlying tenderness
- Ecchymosis, crepitus
- Swelling and possible chest wall deformity

**Rib fracture:**
- Pain at the site of injury
- Shallow breathing
- Localized tenderness
- Crepitus on palpation and auscultation
- Splinting of the chest

### Diagnosis

- History collection
- Physical examination
- Oxygen saturation
- X-ray
- ECG
- ABG analysis
- CT scan
- MRI

### Medical management

- Fractured ribs are usually treated conservatively with effective physiotherapy, fast mobility and adequate pain management.
- Sedation is appropriate for pain relief also allow for deep breathing and coughing.
- The intercostal nerve block is an alternative therapy to reduce pain.
- Chest binder to support the chest wall and provide stability and decreases pain.
- Aggressive pain is managed by epidural analysis, patient-controlled analgesia, or nonopioid analgesia (Lewis SL, Bucher L, Heitkemper MM, Harding MM, Kwong J, Roberts D, 2016).

## Flail Chest

Flail chest is one of the most serious complications of chest trauma. It typically happens if three or four adjacent ribs are separated at two or more places, which results in free-floating rib segments **(Fig. 10.24)**. This leads to paradoxical movement of the chest wall in the flail segment. The paradoxical displacement of the chest wall, related pulmonary contusions and debilitating rib fractures induce the splinting of the chest voluntarily and accidentally (Lewis SL, Bucher L, Heitkemper MM, Harding MM, Kwong J, Roberts D, 2016).

### *Pathophysiology*

See **Flowchart 10.10**.

### *Clinical Manifestations*

- Rapid, shallow respiration
- Tachycardia
- Thoracic movement in asymmetric and uncoordinated pattern
- During inspiration, the affected portion is sucked in and during expiration, it bulged out.
- Pain locally at injury site
- Difficulty breathing

### *Diagnosis*

- Physical examination—ensure the position of injury, abnormal respiratory movement.
- Chest X-ray

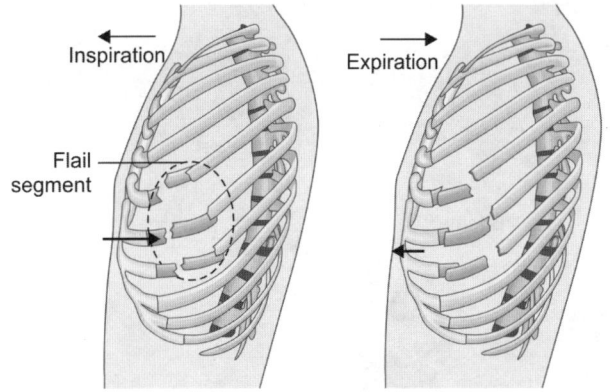

**Fig. 10.24:** Flail chest is when several broken ribs destabilize your chest and make it difficult to breathe.

Multiple rib fractures and disruption of structural components of the chest wall (i.e., bone, cartilage, muscle) leading to a free-floating segment of the chest. The separated segment moves opposite to the rest of the chest wall during the breath cycle (paradoxical movement), creating ineffective ventilation.

**Flowchart 10.10:** Pathophysiology of flail chest.

```
Flail chest injury and breathing in paradoxical manner
                        ↓
Increased dead space, a reduction in alveolar ventilation and
              decreased compliance
                        ↓
Retained airway secretion and causes atelectasis, hypoxemia, etc.
                        ↓
If gas exchange is greatly compromised, respiratory acidosis
occurs as a result of carbon dioxide retention
                        ↓
           Respiratory failure and death
```

- CT scan
- ABG analysis
- ECG
- Pulmonary function test

### Medical Management

- Airway management—oxygen administration, mechanical ventilation.
- Administration of IV fluids.
- Pain management—by analgesic agents, sedatives, and supportive therapy
- Suctioning—to clear secretions from the lungs.
- Pulmonary physiotherapy includes positioning, coughing, and deep breathing.
- Intercostal nerve block
  – Epidural analgesia
  – Intrapleural

– Administration of opioids to relieve or manage thoracic pain (Lewis SL, Bucher L, Heitkemper MM, Harding MM, Kwong J, Roberts D, 2016).

## Pulmonary Contusion

It is one of the severe thoracic injuries related by flail chest pulmonary contusion **(Fig. 10.25)** is defined as "damage to the lung tissues resulting in hemorrhage and localized edema characterized by the development of infiltrates and various degree of respiratory dysfunction and may not evident initially on examination but develops in post-traumatic period." In the case of pulmonary contusion or lung contusion, there is a bruise of the lung, caused by chest trauma as a result of damage to capillaries due to the accumulation of blood and other fluids in the lung tissue. Severe hypoxia develops due to excess fluid accumulation which interferes with gas exchange (Burns SM, Delgado SA, 2019).

### Pathophysiology

See **Flowchart 10.11**.

### Clinical Manifestations

- Cough with an increased amount of secretions
- Bradypnea
- Changes in sensorium
- Tachycardia, tachypnea
- Chest pain
- Hypoxemia
- Blood-tinged secretions
- Respiratory acidosis
- Crackers

### Diagnosis

- Physical examination
- Chest X-ray **(Fig. 10.26)**
- CT Scan **(Fig. 10.27)**
- ABG analysis
- Pulse and oximetry

### Medical Management

- **Airway management:** By adequate oxygenation, mechanical ventilation and controlling pain.
- **IV fluids:** Adequate hydration. It should be closely monitored to avoid hypervolemia.
- **Chest physiotherapy:** For volume expansion of lungs. It includes coughing deep berating.
- **Pain management:** Intercostal nerve block, opioids via patient-controlled analgia.
- **Antimicrobial therapy:** To avoid susceptible infection which damages lung a causes further injury.

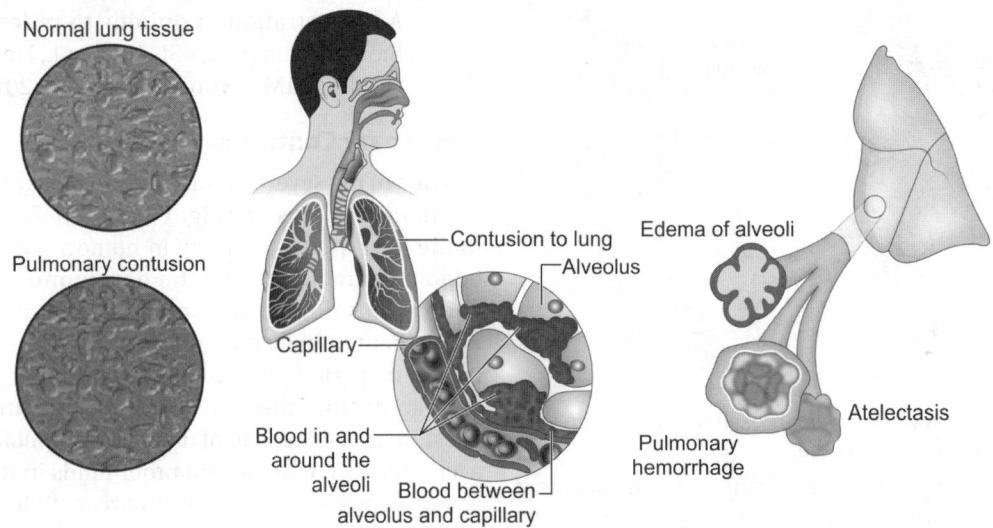

Fig. 10.25: Pulmonary contusion.

**Flowchart 10.11:** Pathophysiology of pulmonary contusion.

```
Due to injury to lung parenchyma and its capillary network
results in leakage of screen protein and plasma
                    ↓
Abnormal accumulation of fluid in the interstitial and
             intra-alveolar space
                    ↓
Their fluid exerts an osmotic pressure that enhances
         loss of fluids from capillaries
                    ↓
Blood and cellular debris enter the lung and accumulate in
bronchioles and alveoli and interfere with gas exchange
                    ↓
As a result, patient has hypoxemia and carbon dioxide retention
                    ↓
     Symptoms of pulmonary contusion develops
```

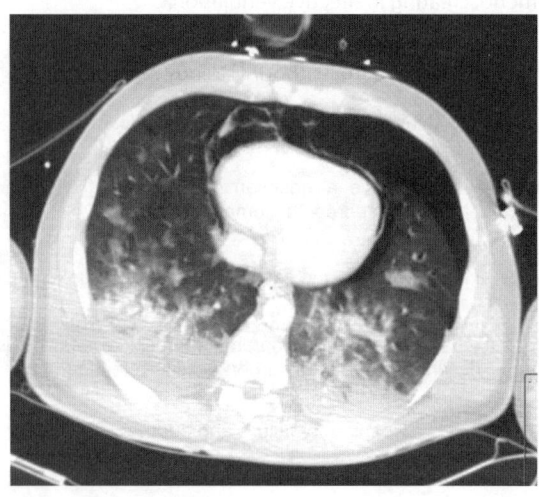

Fig. 10.27: Severe pulmonary contusion with pneumothorax and hemothorax following severe chest trauma.

- **Bronchoscopy:** To remove secretions
- **NG tube insertion:** To relieve gastrointestinal distention
- **Diuretics:** To reduce edema (Burns SM, Delgado SA, 2019)

*Penetrating Trauma*

Penetrating trauma of the chest occurs when a foreign body passes through the thoracic cavity (e.g., gunshot, wound, stabbing).

### Gunshot and stab wounds

It is the most common cause of penetrating trauma. Knives and switch bladder cause most stab wounds. The appearance of the external wound may be deceptive because of pneumothorax, hemothorax, lung contusion, cardiac tamponade along with continuing hemorrhage.

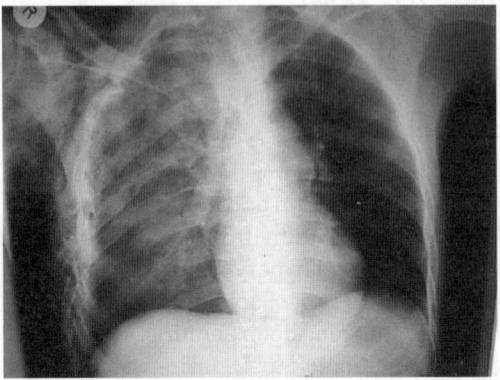

**Fig. 10.26:** Chest X-ray showing right sided (seen on the left of the picture) pulmonary contusion associated with rib fractures and subcutaneous emphysema.

## Diagnostic Evaluation
- Physical examination
- Chest X-ray
- ABG analysis
- ECG
- CT scan

## Medical Management
- Adequate airway ventilation
- Restoration and maintenance of cardiopulmonary functions.
- **Blood transfusion:** To avoid hypovolemic shock
- **IV fluid:** Colloid solutions a crystalloids administration to the patient to treat shock.
- **Chest tube insertion:** For removal of intrathoracic bleeding and to achieve and to achieve continuing re-expansion of lungs.
- **Antimicrobial therapy:** To prevent treat pulmonary infection.

## Emergency Management of Chest Injury

### Initial Management
- Ensure the patency of the airway.
- Provide a semi-fowler position to the patient.
- To provide the patient high flow of oxygen.
- Administer fluid through an intravenous line.
- Assess the injury by removing clothes.
- Cover the wound on chest with non-porous dressing taped on three sides.
- Stabilize the flail rib segment with hand followed by the application of large pieces of tape horizontal across the flail segment.

### Continuous Monitoring
- Monitor vital signs, level of consciousness, oxygen saturation, respiratory status, and urinary output.
- Anticipate intubation for respiratory distress.
- Release dressing of tension pneumothorax develops after a stocking chest wound is covered.

## Nursing Management

### Assessment of respiratory status:
- Dyspnea
- Respiratory distress
- Cyanosis of face, nail beds.
- Tracheal deviation
- Decreased breath sound on the side of injury
- Decreased oxygen saturation
- Frothy secretion

### Cardiovascular status:
- Rapid, therapy pulse
- Decreased blood pressure
- Narrow pulse pressure
- Distended neck vein
- Chest pain
- Dysrhythmias

### In physical examination assess the patient for:
- Brushing
- Abrasion
- Open chest wound
- Asymmetric chest movement

### Nursing care of the patients with chest trauma:
**Breathing pattern**
- Check respiratory status and oxygenation status for significant breathing changes
- Support the hypoxemia patient with oxygen therapy
- Provide the patient with the semi-fowler posture to avoid dyspnea
- Ensure well enough about the attachments of all tubbing and line of patients
- Maintain patients' intake and output status
- To avoid tension pneumothorax, keep the drainage containers under the chest level

**Respiratory status**
- Assess the patient rate, rhythm and respiratory depth.
- Suction if absolutely needed.
- Provide a comfortable position to treat dyspnea.
- To provide the patient with oxygen.
- Provide patients with prescription painkillers to facilitate deep breathing and coughing.
- Assist the intensive spirometry patient.

**Pain management**
- Assessment of pain level by pain scale
- Provide the right position and calm environment to be relaxed in
- Provide the patient the analgesics as recommended by the doctor.

**Assist in self-care activity**
- Assess the extent of patient dependency and encourage in positive reinforcement.
- Encourage for early ambulation and allow the patient to do his/her personal activities.
- Change the position of the patient every two hourly.
- Help the patient in use of incentive spirometry for lung's expansion.

**Avoid the risk of infection**
- Clean hands before and after of every procedure and instruct the caregiver or family members of the patient to wash their hands before contact.

- Instruct the patient to eat diet high in protein and calories.
- Provide antibiotics as per the physician order and if the patient is at high risk, put them in a safe insolation room.
- Allow the patient in coughing and breathe deep breathing exercise (Burns SM, Delgado SA, 2019).

## Hemothorax

Hemothorax is defined as "the accumulation of blood in the pleural cavity." The source of blood may be an injury to the chest wall, great vessels, the lung parenchyma, thoracic cavity, heart, etc., it may develop due to consequence of blunt and penetrating trauma, thoracic procedures, and less commonly by iatrogenic procedures, and maybe spontaneously.

### Etiology

**Traumatic causes:**
- Penetrating injury of lungs, heart, great vessels
- Gunshot injury
- Thoracic procedures (central venous, catheter, thoracotomy, etc.)
- Laceration of internal blood vessels
- Rib fracture

**Non-traumatic or spontaneous causes:**
- Neoplasia
- Blood dyscrasias
- Pulmonary embolism with an infraction
- Bullous emphysema
- Necrotizing infection
- Tuberculosis
- Pulmonary arteriovenous fistula
- Thoracic aortic aneurysm
- Aneurysm of internal mammary artery
- Abdominal pathology (pancreatic pseudocyst, splenic artery aneurysm, or hemoperitoneum)

### Pathophysiology

See **Flowchart 10.12**.

### Clinical Manifestations
- Chest pain
- Difficulty in breathing
- Breathlessness
- Occasionally lightheadedness
- Decreased or absent of breathing sound
- Decreased chest wall movement on the affected side
- Dullness sound on percussion
- Cyanosis
- Tachycardia
- Pale, cool, clammy skin (Chulay M, Suzanne M, 2020).

Due to disruption of tissue in the chest wall, pleural cavity, or intrathoracic structure which results in bleeding to the pleural space and increases the pressure in it. It alters the respiratory and hemodynamic response of the patient. In hemodynamic response, due to heavy blood loss, the symptoms of shock arise like tachycardia, tachypnea, and decrease pulse pressure. In respiratory response, due to the accumulation of a large volume of blood in pleural space which hampers the normal respiration of the patient. This results in abnormal oxygenation and ventilation which causes dyspnea and tachycardia (Chulay M, Suzanne M, 2020).

### Physiologic Resolution of Hemothorax
- Due to severe bleeding, the blood enters into the pleural cavity by the movement of the diaphragm, lunge, and intrathoracic structure which, results in defibrinating of blood and incomplete clotting.
- Due to the lysis of blood, the protein concentration of pleural fluid increases and causes increased osmotic pressure of the pleural cavity. So, later it results in pleural effusion.

### Late Physiologic Sequelae of Unresolved Hemothorax
- In the late stage of hemothorax, it causes two pathological conditions like empyema and fibrothorax.
- Empyema develops due to bacterial growth in retained hemothorax. If it is not treated can lead to septic shock and bacteremia.
- Fibrothorax can develop due to fibrin deposition in both the parietal and visceral surface of the pleural membrane which results in a decrease in lung expansion completely. Later it results in atelectasis and reduces pulmonary function (Chulay M, Suzanne M, 2020).

**Flowchart 10.12:** Pathophysiology of hemothorax.

Due to injury in thoracic cavity blood enters into pleural cavity
↓
It interferes the normal movement of lungs during breathing
↓
Prevent lungs to expand fully which results alteration in ventilation and perfusion
↓
Due to heavy blood loss there is decreased cardiac output and tachycardia
↓
It creates a coat in both visceral and parietal pleura which leads to scarring of pleural cavity called fibro thorax.
↓
It causes pleural effusion and there is increased protein level in pleural fluid

## Diagnostic Evaluation

- Chest X-ray
- Ultrasonography
- CT scan of chest
- Thoracentesis
- MRI to differentiate hemothorax or pleural effusion

## Management

- Antibiotics—to prevent the risk of infection
- Thoracotomy—to drain the fluid by 24–36 F (large bone tubes) which reduces the risk of blood clots obstructing the tube.
- Video-assisted thoracoscopic surgery (VATS) to prevent further bleeding. This procedure is generally performed within 72 hours of the injury. It also helps to remove blood clots.
- Fluid resuscitation by administering iv fluids and blood products.
- Fibrinolytic therapy such as streptokinase or urokinase is given to dissolve the blood clots (Chulay M, Suzanne M, 2020).

## Pneumothorax

### Definition

Pneumothorax is defined as the collapse of the lungs by injury to the parietal and visceral pleura. When an injury occurs to either pleura, the pleural space is exposed to positive atmospheric pressure. Air enters into the pleural space and the lungs or a portion of it becomes collapse. It is otherwise called as "collapsed lungs."

A pneumothorax is the abnormal condition of the lungs that defined as "the presence of air or gas in the pleural cavity which can impair oxygenation and/or ventilation". The clinical signs and symptoms depend on the degree of collapse of the lung (Sharma SK, 2016).

### Causes and Risk Factors

- Smoking
- Genetic factors
- Lungs diseases like COPD, pneumonia, cystic fibrosis, TB
- Mechanical ventilation
- Previous history of pneumothorax
- Chest injury by blunt or entering injury
- Ruptured air blisters
- Cancer of lungs
- Interstitial lung disease like pulmonary fibrosis, sarcoidosis
- Connective tissue diseases of lungs

### Classification of Pneumothorax

See **Flowchart 10.13**.

### Types of Pneumothorax

There are three types of pneumothorax (**Flowchart 10.14**). It includes simple/primary, traumatic and tension pneumothorax.

### Simple or Primary Pneumothorax

It occurs when air enters into the pleural space by the breath of either visceral or parietal pleura. It happens due to the rupture of the bleb, bronchopleural fistula, interstitial lung disease, and in case of severe emphysema (Sharma SK, 2016).

### Traumatic Pneumothorax

Traumatic pneumothorax occurs due to injury of the chest wall and air leakages from the lungs and enters into the pleural space. The causes of the traumatic pneumothorax are blunt trauma like rib fracture, penetrating trauma lime stab wound or gunshot wound, laceration of great vessels, etc., open pneumothorax is one form of it when air enters into the chest wall freely by large injury through a hole. In

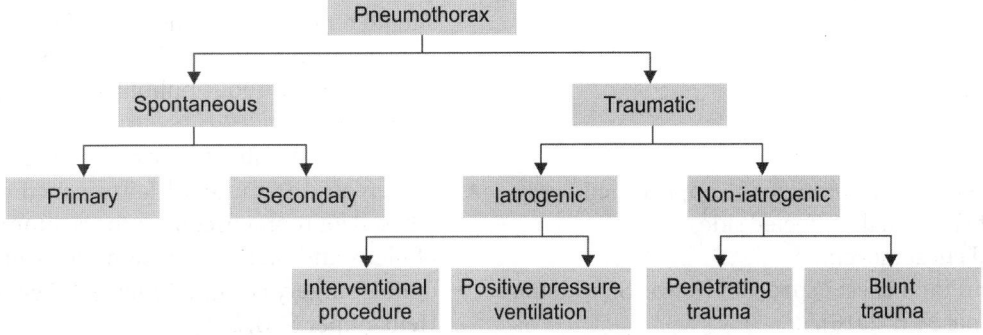

**Flowchart 10.13:** Classification of pneumothorax.

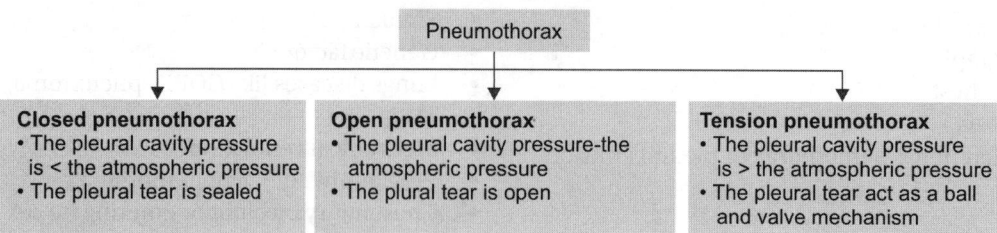

Flowchart 10.14: Types of pneumothorax.

the case of open pneumothorax, a sucking sound produces and the opposite movement of the chest wall occurs during an uninjured site. There is called mediastinal flutter or swing which produces a serious circulatory problem (Sharma SK, 2016).

### Tension Pneumothorax

It occurs when the air is drawn into the pleural space from a laurate lung through a small opening in the chest wall. It is one of the complications of other types of pneumothorax. In this case, air enters into the pleural space and is trapped and can't expel during expiration. So it creates a one-way valve or ball valve mechanism. In the case of breath, it creates tension (positive pressure) in affected pleural space which causes the collapse of the lungs and shifting of the trachea to the unaffected side of the chest. It is called a mediastinal shift. Due to increasing intrathoracic pressure, both respiratory and circulatory functions compromised, and decrease cardiac output occurs which results in decreased. Peripheral circulation and undetectable pulse rate (pulses less electrical activity) (Sharma SK, 2016).

### Clinical Manifestations

- Sudden onset of unilateral pleuritic chest pain
- Respiratory distress
- Tachypnea
- Dyspnea
- Severe hypoxia
- Use of accessory muscle during breathing
- Hypertension
- Tachycardia
- Profuse diaphoresis
- Breathlessness
- Shift of trachea
- The shift of the mediastinum to the opposite side
- Full ness of chest on the affected side
- Diminished chest movement
- Reduction in total chest expansion (Lewis SL, Bucher L, Heitkemper MM, 2016).

### Diagnostic Evaluation

- Physical examination
- Chest X-ray
- Increased radiolucency with the absence of broncho-vesicular marking
- Extend of mediastinal shift
- Presence of pleural fluid
- **CT scan of chest:** It helps to differentiate between large pre-existing emphysematous bullae and pneumothorax. It confirms the size and presence of pneumothorax (Lewis SL, Bucher L, Heitkemper MM, 2016).

### Medical Management

- Medical management depends on the cause and severity of the pneumothorax. The goal of the treatment is to reduce pressure from pleural space by evacuating air and fluid.
- **Primary pneumothorax:** If the lung edge is less than 2 cm from the chest wall and the patient has a normal breathing pattern, it resolves normally without any intervention. But if the patient severe pain and with symptoms, it requires percutaneous needle aspiration. If it will not work then, intercostal tube drainage is to be done.
- **Secondary pneumothorax:** In this case patient requires intercostal tube drainage inserted in the 4th, 5th, and 6th ICS in the midaxillary line and connected to underwater seal drainage. Be sure about not clamping the drainage tube which creat potential danger to the patient. It should remove after 24 hours or after the lung has been fully reinflated and bubbling stopped.
- If there is continuous bubbling for 5–7 days it requires surgery.
- The patient should receive oxygen therapy.
- If intercostal drainage will fail to work the patient is to be advised for thoracoscopy or thoracotomy with stapling of blebs and pleural abrasion. Pleurodesis should be done if surgery is contraindicated (Lewis SL, Bucher L, Heitkemper MM, 2016).

## Tension Pneumothorax

- It is a medical emergency where the pressure of the pleural cavity is reduced by the insertion of a large-bore needle into the pleural space through 2nd ICS.
- Supplementary oxygen therapy is to be provided to the patient.
- Aspiration of fluid needs to be done by tube thoracotomy.
- In the case of recurrent spontaneous pneumothorax surgical pleurodesis is advised to the patient following 2nd pneumothorax (Lewis SL, Bucher L, Heitkemper MM, 2016).

## Nursing Management

- Provide a comfortable position to the patient
- Assess the patient for hypoxia, measure the $SpO_2$ level
- Provide oxygen therapy
- Assess the ABG value of the patient
- Assess the drainage site regularly
- Administer analgesic to reduce pain as prescribed
- Administer antibiotics to prevent infection as prescribed (Lewis SL, Bucher L, Heitkemper MM, 2016)

## Management Modalities of Pneumothorax

See **Flowchart 10.15**.

## Airway Management

Airway management **(Flowchart 10.15)** is the group of maneuvers and medical procedures used to prevent and relived from airway obstruction. It is the vital aspect to provide oxygen and maintain ventilation. These are divided into two categories (Alía I, Esteban A, 2000):

1. **Basic technique:** Noninvasive, no use of advanced medical equipment and advanced training.
2. **Advanced technique:** Requirement of advanced and specialized training and equipment.

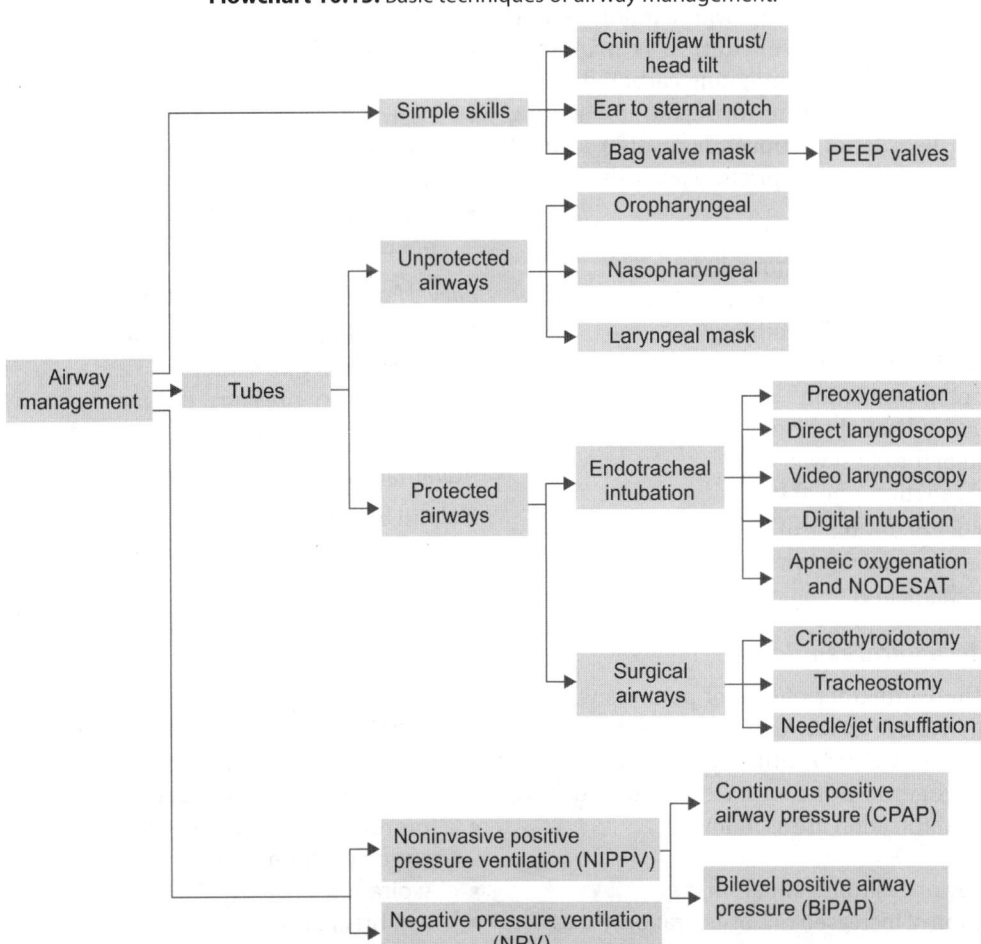

**Flowchart 10.15:** Basic techniques of airway management.

## Causes of Airways Difficulty

- Inadequate ventilation
- Esophageal intubation
- Airway obstruction
- Bronchospasm
- Aspiration
- Premature extubation
- Unintended extubation
- Inadequate $FiO_2$
- Endobronchial intubation
- **Infections:** Bronchitis, pneumonia, croup, epiglottitis, etc
- **Trauma:** Maxillofacial trauma, laryngeal injury, cervical injury, etc
- **Endocrine disorders:** Acromegaly, morbid obesity, DM, etc. (Alía I, Esteban A, 2000)

## Ventilatory Management

### Mechanical Ventilation

Mechanical ventilation is the process by which the patient is assisted for the breathing process who cannot breathe independently. Mechanical ventilation is primarily directed at supplying oxygen, eliminating carbon dioxide, reduced breathing activity, and restoring life-threatening symptoms like a disorder of hypoxemia or poor arterial blood oxygenation, and acute respiratory acidosis.

*Purposes of Mechanical Ventilation*

- Relief of symptoms of respiratory distress
- Rest for the fatigued muscle of respiration
- A decrease in the work of breathing
- Improvement in oxygenation
- Improvement in ventilation
- Restoration of aid base balance
- Stabilization of the chest wall
- Provision of sedation/anesthesia

Current technology of mechanical ventilation are two types:
1. Noninvasive mechanical ventilation
2. Invasive mechanical ventilation

### Noninvasive Mechanical Ventilation

NIV supports the ventilatory efforts of patients without the insertion of invasive airway devices. It has been used effectively in case of COPD, obesity hypoventilation syndrome, cardiogenic pulmonary edema, and lung confusions contraindication are as follows:

- Apnea
- Recent airway or gastrointestinal surgery
- In the condition of increased risk of aspiration, excessive secretion, swallowing impairment, inadequate airway protection, severe hypoxia or acidosis multiorgan failure, hepatic congestion, low cardiac output.

It provides mechanical ventilation without the use of an artificial airway.

There are two modes of NIV:
1. Continuous positive airway pressure
2. Bilevel positive airway pressure

*Continuous Positive Airway Pressure (CPAP)*

It delivers one continuous positive pressure throughout inspiration and expiration. The pressure setting of CPAPs is between 5–15 cm $H_2O$. It helps to open alveoli and prevent atelectasis during expiration. It helps the alveoli for gas exchange and increases the partial pressure of oxygen in facilitating oxygen diffusion into the bloodstream.

Advantages

- Avoids intubation of patient
- Improves arterial oxygenation and functional residual capacity noninvasively
- Without interrupting positive pressure, the patient can speak and cough

Disadvantages

- Feels discomfort due to tight fit
- High-risk of aspiration in case of vomiting of patient
- Increased risk of gastric distension, decreased cardiac output and pneumothorax
- Contraindicated in patients with COPD, tension pneumothorax and low cardiac output

*Bilevel Positive Airway Pressure (BiPAP)*

In the case of BiPAP, there is higher inspiratory pressure and lower expiratory pressure.

Inspiratory pressure reduces the work of breathing further and is more effective than CPAP.

Advantages

Helpful in the patients with the diseases of neuromuscular diseases, cardiopulmonary disorder and sleep apnea.

Disadvantages

Bleeding of nose, skin irritation, dryness of nasal mucosa and skin irritation.

### Complication of Noninvasive Ventilation

- Reduces preload and afterload by decreasing venous return and decreasing left ventricular systolic wall stress.
- Improve stroke volume without increasing myocardial oxygen consumption.
- Aspiration
- Skin breakdown
- Gastric insufflation

- Barotrauma
- Dryness and discomfort
- Anxiety (Alía I, Esteban A, 2000)

### Invasive Mechanical Ventilation

Invasive mechanical ventilation is a specific life-saving intervention procedure which can assist the hospitalized patients with difficulty breathing and respiratory problems. The word "invasive" is used because an instrument which penetrates through the mouth, (e.g., a pipe of the endotracheal), nose or skin (e.g., a tracheostomy tube via a stoma, an operational hole in the windpipe).

### Classification of Ventilators

- **Negative-pressure ventilators:** Exert negative pressure on external chest. It decreases the intrathoracic pressure during inspiration allows air to flow into the lungs, filling its volume.
- **Positive-pressure ventilators:** Inflate the lungs by exerting positive pressure on the airway, forcing the alveoli to expand during inspiration.

### Cycles of mechanical ventilators

- **Pressure-cycled ventilators:** The pressure-cycled ventilator ends inspiration when a preset pressure has been reached.
- **Time-cycled ventilators:** The time-cycled ventilator ends inspiration when a preset time has been reached.
- **Volume-cycled ventilators:** The volume-cycled ventilator ends inspiration when a preset volume has been reached (Alía I, Esteban A, 2000).

### Settings on Mechanical Ventilators

Ventilator settings **(Table 10.16)** are the inputs on a mechanical ventilator that determine how much support is provided for the patient. This is important in determining the volume, rate, and speed of ventilation, as well as the amount of oxygen that is delivered. Ventilator settings are the controls on a mechanical ventilator that can be set or adjusted in order to determine the amount of support that is delivered to the patient. Ventilatory support can be provided in the form of ventilation and oxygenation. Therefore, the ventilator settings will affect both the patient's breathing and the amount of oxygen that is delivered to the lungs.

### Types of ventilator settings

There are several types of ventilator settings that a practitioner must be familiar with, including the following:
- Mode
- Tidal volume
- Frequency (rate)
- $FiO_2$
- Flow rate
- I:E ratio
- Sensitivity
- PEEP
- Alarms

Each parameter can be controlled or adjusted depending on the patient's condition and needs. This is a job duty that should only be performed by qualified physicians and respiratory therapists.

**Table 10.16:** Settings on mechanical ventilators.

| Setting | Description | Standard range |
|---|---|---|
| Oxygen concentration ($FiO_2$) | Amount of oxygen in gas delivered to patient | 21–60% lowest setting allowing for $SaO_2$ over 90%, and $PaO_2$ greater than 60 |
| Total volume ($V_T$) | Volume of gas delivered in one cycle | 6–10 mL/kg of predicted body weight |
| Rate | Minimal number of breaths per minute | 6–12 breaths per minute |
| Inspiratory: Expiratory ratio | Ratio of time of inspiration to time of expiration; may be reversed in conditions where lungs are noncompliant | 1:2 |
| Flow rate | Rate at which tidal volume is delivered to patient | 60–100 liters/minute |
| Sensitivity | The negative aspiratory pressure or flow a patient must generate in order to trigger the ventilator to deliver a breath | –1 to –2 cm $H_2O$ |
| High pressure limit | Ventilator will not exceed this pressure in delivering volume; pop-off mechanism prevents excessive pressure | 10–20 cm $H_2O$ above peak inspiratory pressure |
| Pressure support | Positive pressure used to decrease patient's work of breathing | 5–10 cm $H_2O$ |
| Positive end-expiratory pressure (PEEP) | Positive pressure left in lungs at end of expiration; prevents atelectasis and may enhance oxygenation at higher levels | 3–10 cm $H_2O$ |

## Modes of mechanical ventilators

A ventilator mode is a way of describing how the mechanical ventilator assists a patient with inspiration. The characteristics of a particular mode control how the ventilator functions.

There are several types of ventilator modes, including the following:
- Assist/control (A/C)
- Synchronous intermittent mandatory ventilation (SIMV)
- Pressure support ventilation (PSV)
- Continuous positive airway pressure (CPAP)
- Volume support (VS)
- Control mode ventilation (CMV)
- Airway pressure release ventilation (APRV)
- Mandatory minute ventilation (MMV)
- Inverse ratio ventilation (IRV)
- High-frequency oscillatory ventilation (HFOV)

When selecting a ventilator mode, must first determine if the patient needs full or partial ventilatory support. In general, the assist/control (A/C) mode can be used if the patient needs full ventilatory support. If they only need partial support, synchronous intermittent mandatory ventilation (SIMV) would be recommended. After intubating a patient and connecting to the ventilator, it is time to select the mode of ventilation (**Table 10.17**) to be used. Several principles need to be grasped in order to do this consistently for the patient's benefit.

## Weaning from the ventilator

This is the process of removing the patient from ventilatory support, when patient breath spontaneously and being extubated. Mechanical ventilation weaning can be described as a process of replacing the ventilation support suddenly or gradually. The weaning (**Table 10.18**) from mechanical ventilation typically involves the elimination of all artificial airway and closely connected aspects of treatment to patient (Alía I, Esteban A, 2000).

### Nursing Care of Patient under Mechanical Ventilators

Establish a therapeutic communication with the patient

- It is very much essential to communicate with patient under mechanical ventilator. Provide a communication board or writing tools to patient to express his/her need.
- Ask questions to patient and tell him to answer by nonverbally by shaking head/hand.
- It is also important to communicate with other healthcare team members like doctors, pharmacist, respiratory therapist regarding the present health condition and health need of patient.

**Table 10.18:** Conditions of indication for weaning.

| Parameters | Values |
|---|---|
| Respiratory rate | Less than 25 breaths per min |
| Tidal volume | Greater than 5 mL/kg |
| Vital capacity | Greater than 10 mL/min. |
| Minute ventilation | Less than 10 L/min |
| $PaO_2/FiO_2$ | Greater than 200 |
| Shunt (Qs/Qr) | Less than 20% |
| Negative inspiratory force (NIF) | Less than 25 cm water |
| f/Vt (respiratory frequency to tidal volume) | Less than 105 (in case of adults) Less than 130 (in case of elderly) |

**Table 10.17:** Common modes of mechanical ventilation.

| Mode | Description | Target population | Nursing implications |
|---|---|---|---|
| Controlled mandatory ventilation | Tidal volume delivered at a set rate independent of patient effort, rarely used | Apneic patients or those with little or no respiratory drive | Patients may be heavily sedated or have induced paralysis |
| Assist-control ventilation (AC) | Tidal volume delivered at a set rate in response to patient effort, if patient fails to breathe at predetermined time, ventilator will deliver a breath | Patients able to breathe spontaneously with weak respiratory muscles | Patient is able to hyperventilate if volume controlled or may become hypercapneic if pressure controlled |
| Synchronized intermittent mandatory ventilation (SIMV) | Tidal volume delivered at a low set rate in response to patient effort while allowing spontaneous breaths between | Patients who cannot sustain spontaneous ventilation for extended periods | Provides better synchrony and preserves some respiratory muscle function |
| Continuous positive airway pressure | Applies positive pressure during spontaneous breaths | Effective as a weaning trial or training mode in patients capable of spontaneous ventilation | Patient must be monitored for respiratory distress |

- Allow family members to communicate with patient if possible or the nurse can provide information to family members regarding the health condition of the patient (Alía I, Esteban A, 2000).

Frequently check ventilator modes and setting
- Assess the patient's vital signs, $O_2$ saturation, breathing sound, pain and amunity level and compare with previous record and report any abnormality found to physician.
- Nurse has to always alert to alarm of ventilator.
- Always check the situation equipment for leakage, bag value mask and oxygen cylinder and pipe of supply.
- Always check the mode of the ventilation patients receiving airflow.
- Check the waveforms of the monitor of the mechanical ventilator to observe and identify the abnormal situation (Alía I, Esteban A, 2000).

Suction the patient appropriately
- In case of positive pressure mechanical ventilation patient may have NG tube, ET tube and tracheostomy tube. So suction is needed to clear the airway from deposition of secretions.
- Before situation hyper oxygenate the patient to prevent hypoxia.
- Limit the pressure of the suction and do for shortest duration as possible.
- Assess the connection of the tube before and after the suction
- Maintain the record after the procedure.

Assessment of pain and sedation level
- Assess the pain level of patient through pain scale provide analgesic as prescription order pain and anxiety can be reduced through nonpharmacological methods like presence of family member, therapeutic communicator, music therapy, etc.
- To measure the sedation level two scales are used such as Richmond Agitation sedation scale and Ramsay sedation scale.

Prevention of infection
- The major complication of mechanical ventilation is ventilator-associated pneumonia (VAP).
- Provide oval care 2 times daily through chlorhexidine solution.
- Provide the patient an intermittent compression device to prevent peripheral edema and DVT.
- Provide histamine-2 blocker which prevents the patient from peptic ulcer.
- Check the vital signs every 4 hourly to assess any signs of infection like fever redness, etc.
- Elevate the head of the bed 30 to 45 degrees to prevent lungs infection.
- Provide antibiotics therapy to avoid ICU related/nosocomial infection.
- Maintain aseptic technique during any procedure.
- Regularly do the passive exercises like range of motion exercise and change the position of the patient and change the position of the patient to increase peripheral circulation.
- Provide protein rich and highly fiber diet which helps for healing of body tissue and maintain the immunity of the patient.

Prevent the patient from hemodynamic instability
- Monitor the BP of the patient every 2-4 hourly.
- Administer the TV fluid to stabilize the hemodynamic status of the patient.
- Provide modification like dopamine or norepinephrine to stabilize the heart rate normal if prescribed by physician.
- Pneumothorax and Barotrauma may cause due to high inspiratory pressure with PSV and PEEP. To identify the complications, check the breath sounds and oxygenation status regularly.

Management of the airways
- Check the cuff pressure or leakage of the cuff of ET tube or tracheostomy tube to minimize the complication.
- To clear the secretion, suction the patient and avoid the blockage of the airway.
- Check the position of the tracheostomy tube to avoid accidental extubation.

Provide adequate nutrition to the patient

Ventilator patient should be well nourished. Those patients can't shallow they need the parenteral therapy for nutrition or by nasal tube feeding.

Weaning from ventilator appropriately
- Nurse has to check the criteria for wearing from mechanical ventilation.
- Before extubating check the respiratory and circulatory status of the patient.
- Some factors can affect the wearing such COPD, peripheral vascular disease pain and anxiety, etc. So, check this status of the patient.
- Wearing process is a team work. So, communicate with other healthcare providers such as respiratory therapist, nutritionist, physician, etc., to avoid any complication.

Health education to patient and family members
- Communicate with family members regarding the treatment plan each procedure to reduce their anxiety

- Establish a therapeutic communication with relatives of patient and allow them in care the patient if possible
- Allow the family members to visit the patient at least once in a day to reduce anxiety of both patient and family members
- Educate the family members about the post discharge medication and follow-up to patient
- Teach them for healthy diet and active and passive exercise for improvement of lungs function of the patient
- Advise them for healthy habits and quit of smoking if patient is taking better function of the lung (Alía I, Esteban A, 2000)

## Bronchial Hygiene

Bronchial hygiene means the clearance of airway in various technique, which include chest physiotherapy (which consist of postural drainage, vibration, coughing and suctioning, breathing exercises such as huffing and diaphragmatic breathing) much hyperventilation (used in incubating patients) and giving bronchodilators and mucus thickening medications. Several techniques help the patients clear the mucus from their airways and improve respiration. These techniques are used in patients who have thick and copious sputum production due to respiration diseases like bronchiectasis, cystic fibrosis, occluded endotracheal tubes, and some types of pneumonia. This is the technique to prevent respiratory complications and treat pulmonary infections (Civetta JM, Taylor RW, Kirby RR, 1990).

### *Purposes*

- Improve the clearance of secretions
- Increase lung volume
- Maintaining airways
- Warm humidify aiming at enhancing ventilation and gas exchange

### *Indication of Bronchial Hygiene Therapy*

- In the case of COP
- Pneumonia
- Cystic fibrosis
- Pre and post thoracic surgery to prevent atelectasis and respiratory infection

### *Contraindication*

- Increased intracranial pressure (>20 mm Hg)
- Any spinal injury in acute condition
- Active hemoptysis
- Pulmonary embolism
- Pulmonary edema and congestive heart failure (Civetta JM, Taylor RW, Kirby RR, 1990).

### *Types of Bronchial Hygiene*

#### *Nebulization Therapy*

Nebulization therapy is an effective and efficient way to believer medication directly into the lung by inhalation. Doctors prescribe a variety of different medications for that warrant nebulizer therapy. The nebulizer is the type of drug delivery device used to administer medication in the form of a mist inhaled into the lungs. Patients with conditions such as asthma, pneumonia, cystic fibrosis, and COPD can all benefit from nebulizer therapy.

#### *Deep Breathing Exercise*

Deep breathing exercises of breathing training as the breathing practice to achieve more efficient and controlled ventilation and reduce the work of breathing. It is indicated in patients with COPD and dyspnea. It promotes the maximum alveolar inflation and relaxation of respiratory muscles. It reduces the anxiety and decreases ineffective, uncoordinated patterns of respiration, decrease respiration rate. Thus, specific breathing exercises include diaphragmatic and pursed-lip breathing.

Goal of diaphragmatic breathing

Strengthen the diaphragm during breathing.

Goal of pursed-lip breathing

- Improves oxygen transport
- Helps induce a slow, deep breathing pattern
- Assist the patient to control breathing during the period of stress
- Helps prevent the airway to collapse
- Helps to train the expiratory muscle to prolong exhalation
- Increase airway pressure during expiration.

Indication

- The patient required additional oxygen
- Respiratory diseases like emphysema
- Elderly patients who are prolong hospitalized due to lower respiratory diseases
- Postoperative patient
- To reduce anxiety and stress

Nursing management

- The nurse has to instruct patients regularly
- Breath slowly and rhythmically in a released manner and exhale completely to empty the lunge
- Inhale through the nose because of filtration, humidification and warm air

- Concentration on prolonging the light of exhalation than inhalation
- Avoidance of dust environment
- Adequate diet and healthy nutrition and atmosphere
- Small and frequent diet
- Adequate rest and good sleeping pattern which conserves energy (Civetta JM, Taylor RW, Kirby RR, 1990)

### Chest Physiotherapy

"Chest physiotherapy is a group of therapy which includes postural drainage, training along with effective coughing technique" (Chulay M, Suzanne M, 2020).

### Goal
- Removal of bronchial secretion
- To improve ventilation
- To increase the efficiency of respiratory muscle

### Postural drainage

Postural drainage or segmented bronchial drainage is a procedure that improves the removal of bronchial secretions by a specific position. By use of specific positions **(Fig. 10.28)** that allow the force of gravity to assist in the removal of secretions from the lunge and trachea-bronchial tree. It is used to prevent or relieve bronchial obstruction caused by the accumulation of secretions. By postural drainage, the secretions move from the lungs and smaller bronchial airways to the main bronchi and trachea by the force of gravity, and then secretions removed by coughing. Before the procedure, the nurse has to instruct patients to inhale bronchodilators and mucolytic agents if prescribed, because these are improved to liquefy and drainage of secretions of the bronchial tree. Generally, five positions are used in postural drainage. These are head down, prone, right and left lateral, and sitting upright. (one for drainage of each lunge) (Chulay M, Suzanne M, 2020).

### Nursing management
- The nurse should be known about the diagnosis of patients and the involvement of lobes of lunges of the patient.
- Aware of the cardiac status, structural deformities of the chest wall and spine.
- Involvement of family members during the procedure.
- Auscultation of chest before and after the procedure to assess the effectiveness of therapy.
- Perform procedure four times before meals to prevent nausea, vomiting and aspiration.
- Use bronchodilation, nebulization, mucolytics to decrease the thickness of sputum and prevent edema of the bronchial wall.
- Provide a comfortable position as possible in each position.
- Provide an emesis basin, sputum cup and paper tissue.
- Teach patient how to cough and breath during the procedure.
- If the patient can't cough arrange a suction machine to remove secretions mechanically.
- After the procedure, the nurse has to note the amount color, odor, viscosity and character of expelled sputum.
- Evaluate the patient skin color and pulse during the initial time of the procedure to the assessment of hypoxemia.
- If required provide oxygen during the procedure.
- After the procedure, the patient may need mouth wash before resting for freshness (Chulay M, Suzanne M, 2020).

### Chest Percussion and Vibration

Chest percussion and vibration are the procedure to vibrate the lunge by cupping the hands and lightly striking the chest wall in a rhythmic manner over the lung segment to help the removal of mucus adhering to the tracheobronchial tree.

The wrists are alternately flexed and extended so that the chest is cupped or clapped painlessly. During the procedure, a soft towel placed or cloth placed over the segment to prevent skin irritation and redness. If performed for 5–10 minutes for each position. The patient was advised for diaphragmatic breathing during the procedure for relaxation. Thus, the procedure is avoided if the patient has any type of drainage in the chest, sternum, spine, liver, kidney spleen or breast (in women). It is avoided in the case of an elderly patient because of rib fracture and osteoporosis. Vibration is applied by manual compression and tremor on the chest wall during exhalation. After vibration, the patient is asked to cough by using the abdominal muscle to clear the secretion (Chulay M, Suzanne M, 2020).

### Nursing management
- Provide a comfortable position and environment for the patient.
- Provide medication for pain as prescribed.
- Provide pillow to support below the area of striking.
- Stop the procedure in case of increased pain, shortness of breath, weakness, lightheadedness and hemoptysis.
- This therapy is safe to continue up to normal respiration and breath sound and until chest X-ray finding is normal (Nettina SM, Msn AB, 2013).

### Intercostal drainage

Intercostal drainage or chest drainage is a type of intervention for improving as exchange and management of chest drainage to enhance breathing during the

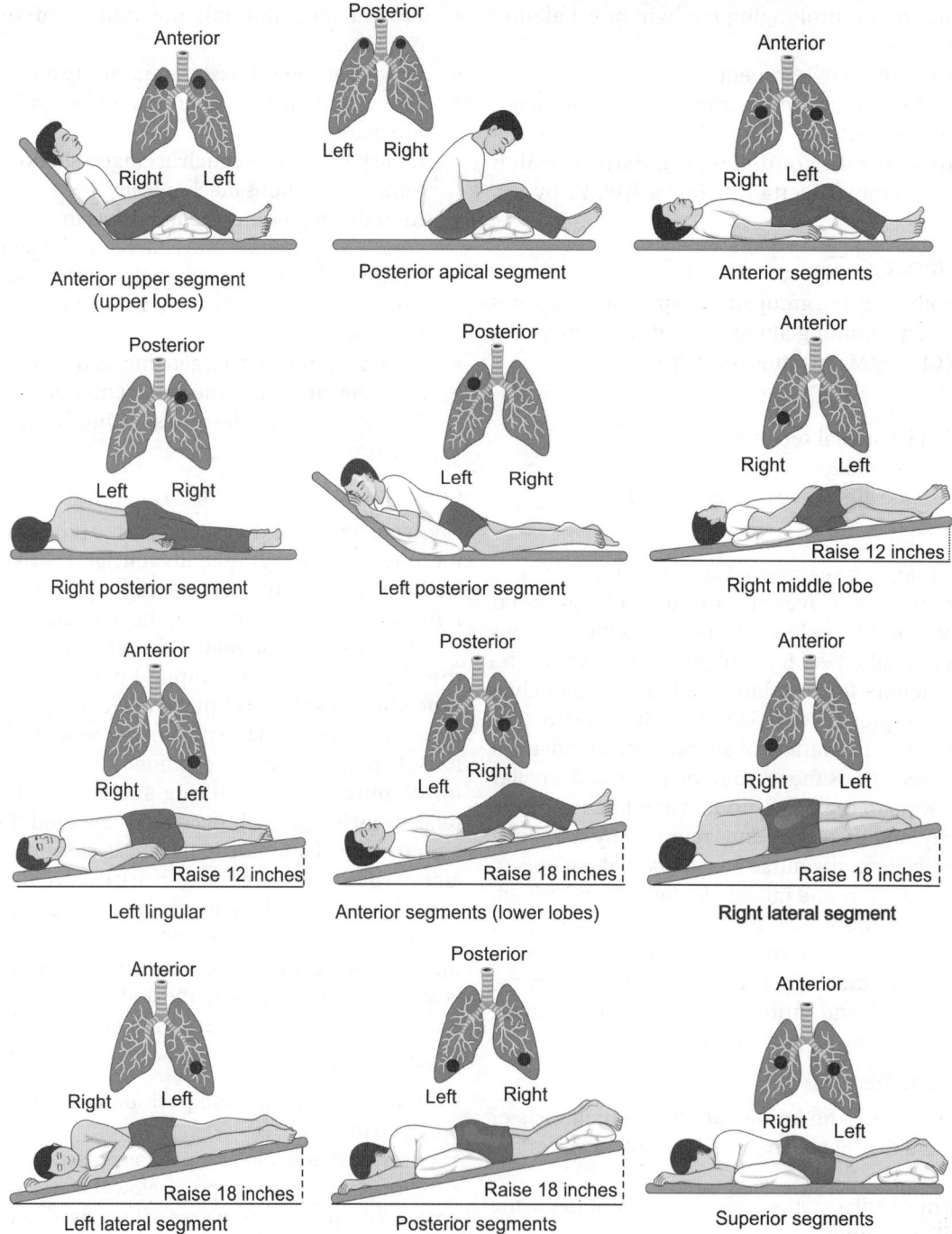

**Fig. 10.28:** Different positions of postural drainage.
*Source:* John Landry BS, 2023.

post-operative period. It is indicated in the case of thoracic surgery to remove fluid, blood, and excess air to re-expand the involved lung. It is also used in the case of spontaneous pneumothorax and trauma resulting in a pneumothorax. Placement of a chest tube in the pleural space restores the negative intrathoracic pressure needed for lung re-expansion after surgery or trauma. (Nettina SM, Msn AB, 2013)

## Thoracic Surgeries

Thoracic surgeries are broadly classified into two categories. These are thoracic incisions and pulmonary resections.

### Thoracic incisions

Thoracic incisions are the surgery to assess the pleural space and thoracic cavities. The following are the surgeries which includes in thoracic incisions.

### Posterolateral thoracotomy

It is still expected that the posterolateral thoracotomy is the most common incision used in a general thoracic incision. It is the historical gold standard of chest incisions that offers outstanding visibility for most general chest procedures. Posterolateral thoracotomies are an optimal option. However, large muscles with all their inherent drawbacks need transaction; thus, muscle saving variants should be considered. This is an operation that not only has outstanding access to the lung, hilum, mediastinum in the middle and posterior, trachea in the endothoracic, and esophagus in the endothoracic region, but it also makes it possible to safely monitor pulmonary blood vessels during pulmonary resection. Posterolateral thoracotomy procedure provides all areas of the thorax with greater accessibility as for every other incision for thoracotomy. The two possible drawbacks of posterolateral thoracotomy are that it is painful and that, by separating the respiratory muscles and decreasing chest wall mobility, it can affect the respiratory mechanics. Definitely, in older patients with compromised cardiopulmonary activity, these drawbacks are magnified. However, using current postoperative treatment methods, such as epidural analgesia, these problems can be reduced.

Posterolateral thoracotomy provides the pleural space and its contents with excellent visibility. This approach deals with patient positioning, which must be performed carefully if one is to prevent shoulder or brachial plexus injuries. The incision of the skin must be correctly positioned and slightly oblique in the center. The muscle of the serratus must not be divided and the pleural space must be entered through the proper intercostal space. This space should be extended slowly to prevent rib fractures. The pleural space and its contents have excellent visibility by posterolateral thoracotomy. This process deals with the patient positioning that must be carried out cautiously because shoulder or brachial plexus injuries are to be avoided. The skin incision must always be located appropriately and slightly oblique in the center. The serratus muscles must not be split and the pleural space through the right intercostal space must be reached. To avoid rib fractures, this space must be expanded slowly (Chulay M, Suzanne M, 2020).

### Axillary thoracotomy

For the following procedures, an axillary thoracotomy may be used:
- Upper thoracic sympathectomy.
- Drainage for emphysematous bulla.
- Apical pleurectomy.
- Access into axilla lesions.

An incision is created with a knife with the lowest axillary skin plug with the patient in a lateral position. The incision is made deeper by diathermy through the fat until the chest wall is reached. The incision reaches the axillary space between the pectoral and latissimus dorsal muscles and does not have to be cut either. In the third intercostal region, the chest is entered. Diathermy is incised into the periosteum over the third rib. There is a cut at the base of the periosteum and pleura. The incision is carried to the degree needed to ensure sufficient exposure. The wound is covered with an intercostal muscle layer by nylon stitch, with the fat layer and skin sutures being absorbed. The pleural space must be drained (Nettina SM, Msn AB, 2013).

### Anterior thoracotomy

The thoracotomy anterolateral offers excellent access to the upper, right and middle lobes. It may spread to the opposite chest (clamshell incision) through the sternum. Our ideal approach for unilateral lung transplantation is anterolateral thoracotomy. Bilateral sequential pulmonary transplants can normally be performed without sternal division by bilateral anterolateral thoracotomy. The benefit of this incision is that the patient remains supine. Cosmetic findings are better than median sternotomy or thoracotomy posterolateral. The posterior pleural space is less exposed than a posterolateral thoracotomy. This incision should be avoided for procedures requiring excellent post-exposure.

With a slight roll under the ipsilateral shoulder, patients are put in the supine position. The arm of the patient is tucked away. Alternatively, you should put the ipsilateral hand under the buttock and the elbow can be padded to prevent any strain on the ulnar nerve. In the fourth or fifth interspace, on the lateral edge of the skin, the incision starts and curves to the anterior axillary line along the sub mammal flap. The second rib will help to locate the fourth interspace by palpating where this meets the sternomanubrial joint. For most resections and lung transplantation, this space provides good visibility. The incision is carried to the pectoral fascia via the subcutaneous tissue. The soft tissue or breast tissues must be increased in heavy patients or women with pendulous breasts, to separate the pectoral muscle up to the level of the fourth interspace. The length of the incision is separated between intercostal muscles. Additionally, the small section of the fourth costal cartilage may be withdrawn or the cost sternal joint disarticulated.

The latter method is used to dissect and tie the mammal vessels to prevent their tearing. The intercostal muscles are subsequently divided to maximize visibility by positioning the retractor and rib spreading. The right angles of the Balfour retractor cause the latissimus and serratus muscles to retract satisfactorily. The incision is closed with 4 peri coastal sutures by approximation of the ribs. Then the pectoral muscle and the subcutaneous tissue and skin are approximated (Nettina SM, Msn AB, 2013).

**Thoracoabdominal incision**

In the large majority of cases, the thoracoabdominal incision is very exposed to thorax, abdominal, and retroperitoneal areas. For distant or proximally stomach operations, the left thoracoabdominal incision offers excellent visibility. It is especially useful for complex reactions, usually very difficult since the stomach, diaphragm, and liver have major adhesions.

The thoracoabdominal incision **(Figs. 10.29A and B)** extends from the 7th intercostal space to the costal arch and then along a paramedian line (2 centimeters from the linea alba) up to the umbilicus. Incision by trunk muscles to eight ribs, the anterior lamina of the rectus sheath paramedian incision (latissimus dorsi, serratus anterior, external oblique muscles). The rectus abdominis is dissected underneath the coastal arc and the muscle laterally is pushed. The arch is cut off by a rib shear. The intercostal region is extended by a thoracic retractor and an external laparotomy retractor is used. The diaphragm is cut close to the beginning until the retroperitoneum is sufficiently exposed. However, this technique can be expanded to make superior visibility and safer operations simpler through a left thoracoabdominal incision.

**Median sternotomy incision**

Median sternotomy is a kind of operation involving a vertical inline incision **(Fig. 10.30)** on the sternum that separates or ruptures the sternum itself. For operations, including cardiac transplant, corrective operations on congenital heart defects, or coronary artery bypass operation, this approach provides access to the heart and lung. Median sternotomy, which is a preliminary stage, is also mistakenly named open-heart surgery. However, the open heart often requires pericardial incisions, which are not required for many median sternotomy procedures (Nettina SM, Msn AB, 2013).

**Transverse thoracosternotomy (Clamshell)**

The standard approach for bilateral lung transplantation (BLT) is transverse thoracosternotomy, but every precaution should be taken to avoid sternal wound breakdown. The longitudinal transverse thoracic incision offers a very strong exposure in double lung transplantation to the mediastinal structures. The placement, along with the use of two longitudinal wires around the sternal division, of modified transverse sternotomy and a figure of 8 with a single monofilament metal wire, contributes to greater stability and equally diffuse oblique strain. (Emadwiandr, 2013)

**Thoracosternotomy (Hemiclamshell)**

A combination of anterolateral thoracotomy and median sternotomy incision **(Figs. 10.31A and B)** is hemiclamshell incision. This incision was typically applied to mediastinal or anterolateral cervicothoracic intersecting vascular injuries and tumor resection in the cervicothoracic region, or anterior mediastinum. One of the benefits of hemiclamshell incision is that hilar and mediastinal vascular systems are optimally exposed. Better observation of vascular systems and potential vascular injuries by hemiclamshells may be more easily treated. In cases where mediastinal, cardiac vascular structures and mass feeding vessels are unable to be accurately assessed by the tumor, it could be safer to monitor vascular structures following tumor removal with circulatory arrest. In the treatment of tumors like this, a multidisciplinary approach is useful. Optimal exposure and manipulation of intrathoracic Giant tumor resections are provided by the hemiclamshell incision. There is no difference in the complication rate compared

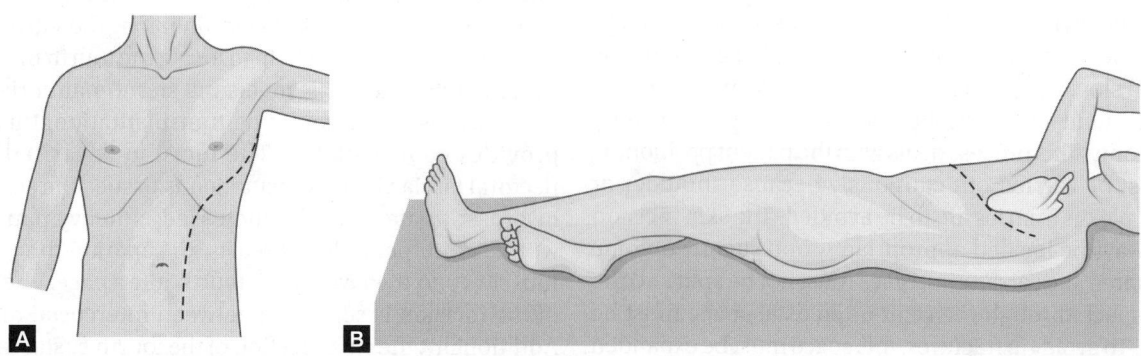

**Figs. 10.29A and B:** (A) Thoracoabdominal incision; (B) Posterior incision extension with patient positioned to expose the left flank.

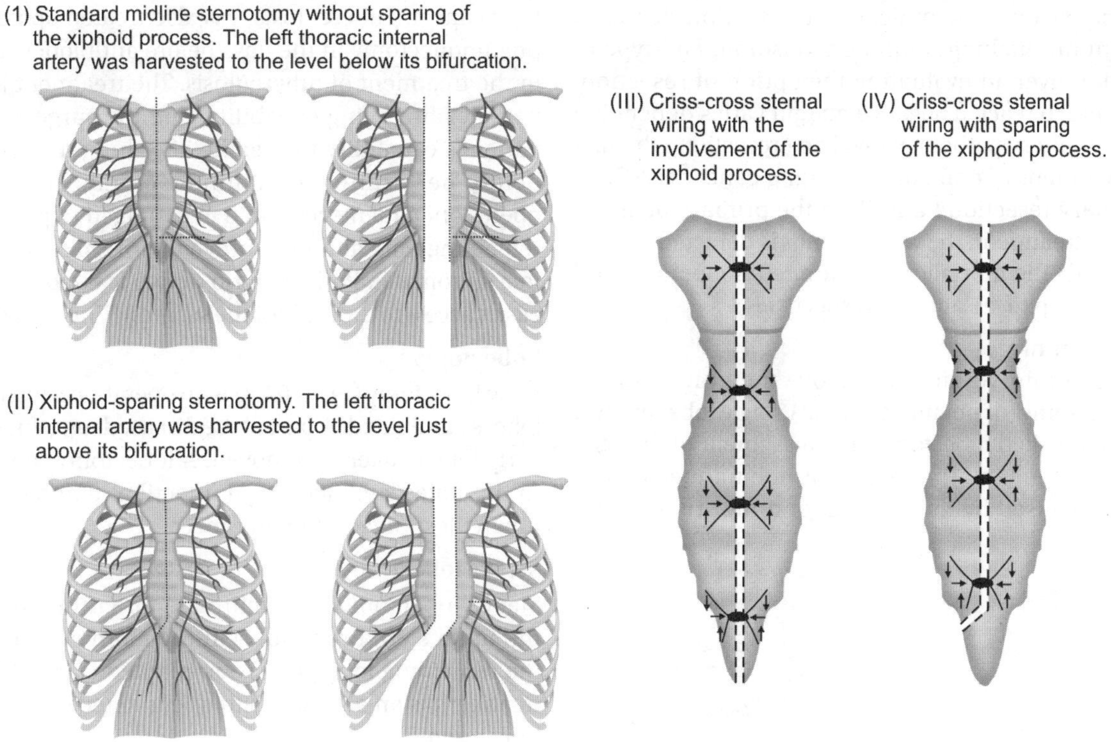

(1) Standard midline sternotomy without sparing of the xiphoid process. The left thoracic internal artery was harvested to the level below its bifurcation.

(III) Criss-cross sternal wiring with the involvement of the xiphoid process.

(IV) Criss-cross sternal wiring with sparing of the xiphoid process.

(II) Xiphoid-sparing sternotomy. The left thoracic internal artery was harvested to the level just above its bifurcation.

**Fig. 10.30:** Illustration of surgical techniques in the xiphoid-sparing and standard midline sternotomy groups.
*Source:* Rashed A, Verzar Z, Alotti N, Gombocz K, 2018.

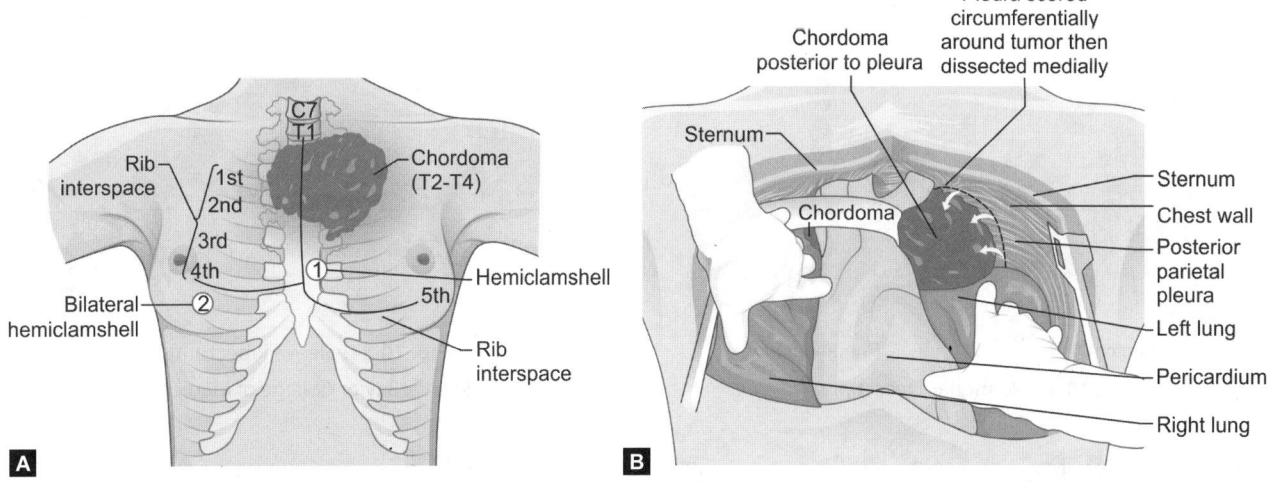

**Figs. 10.31A and B:** Bilateral hemiclamshell thoracotomy. (A) Sequence of bony cuts employed in this case; (B) Overall exposure afforded by the bilateral hemiclamshell thoracotomy.
*Source:* Burke JF, Chan AK, Mayer RR, Garcia JH, Pennicooke B, Mann M, Berven SH, Chou D, Mummaneni PV, 2020.

to conventional incision due to the underlying condition or wound. Patient adherence is essential in postoperative treatment along with all other thoracic incisions to avoid complications (Emadwiandr, 2013).

## Pulmonary resections

Pulmonary resections include the various methods or procedures for the removal of different parts of the lungs. The different lung resections **(Fig. 10.32)** are usually called anatomical or non-anatomical. The resection degree is dependent on the lungs' duration, position, and type of lesion. Moreover, in evaluating the option of resection, the potential to reach a negative margin varies depending on the pulmonary pathology involving resection. The first line of treatment of non-small cell lung cancer (NSCLC) is pulmonary resection I and II. In the primary phase of the NSCLC treatment, the whole tumor is detected, staged and resected. The mortality rate for pneumonectomy and lobectomy is up to 4% and 8%, respectively.

**Pneumonectomy**

The surgical intervention to remove the lung is called pneumonectomy (or pneumectomy). A single lobe removal procedure is called lobectomy, and a segment of the lung a wedge (or segmental) resection. A pneumonectomy is most often caused by the removal of tumor tissue from lung cancer. Tuberculosis was also treated operatively by pneumonectomy in the days before antibiotics were used in the treatment of tuberculosis. The treatment limits the patient's breathing capability, and the surgeon tests the patient's capability to breathe after lung tissue removed before performing a pneumonectomy. Following the operation, patients are often encouraged to practice their remaining lung and to improve their respiratory function in a spirometer. Perhaps a rib or two is cut out to provide easier access to the lung for the surgeon (Emadwiandr, 2013)

**Lobectomy**

Lung lobectomy **(Fig. 10.33)** is an operation in which a lung lobe is eliminated. A part of the diseased lung, for example, early lung cancer, is removed. A lobectomy can also lead to therapies such as fungal infection, emphysema, and tuberculosis in addition to cancer.

**Sleeve lobectomy**

Sleeve lobectomy is a technique for cutting the lobe of the main stem bronchus. On the main stem bronchus, the remaining lobe (s) is re-implanted **(Fig. 10.34)**. This treatment is an alternative to pneumonectomy for central lung tumors.

This is the operation for treating a lung tumor in an airway, lobe, and part of the main bronchus. The bronchial ends are rejoined and the bronchus re-joined to any remaining lobes. This operation is undertaken to conserve

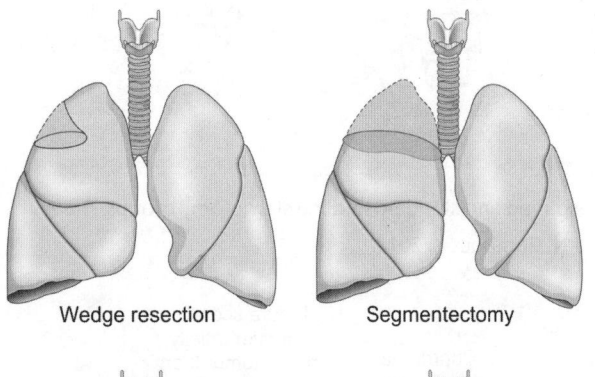
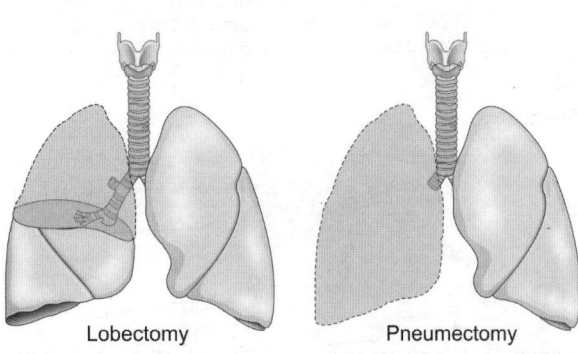

**Fig. 10.32:** Pulmonary resections.

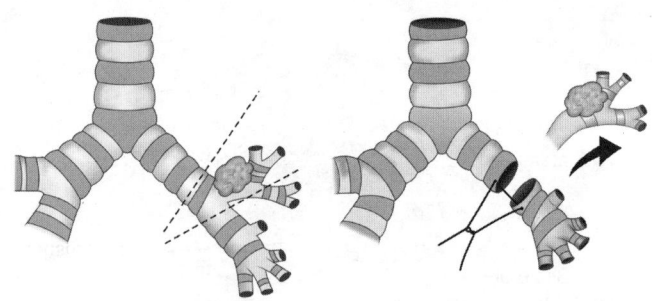

**Fig. 10.34:** Sleeve lobectomy.
*Source:* Baylor College of Medicine.

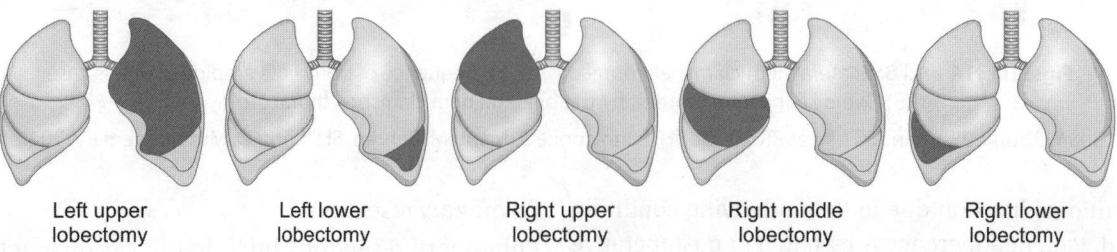

**Fig. 10.33:** Types of lobectomies (gray indicates resected lobe).
*Source:* Baylor College of Medicine.

half of the lung. Sometimes known as resection of the sleeve (Emadwiandr, 2013).

## Segmentectomy

A segmentectomy or segmental resection **(Fig. 10.35)** is an alternative for treating early-stage, non-small cell lung (NSCLC) cancer. It needs the removal of any of the lung lobes to remove a cancerous tumor completely. A segmental lung rection is a technique aimed at eliminating the diseased lung tissue and leaving the stable lung tissue undamaged. Only the diseased portion of a lung lobe is removed during a lung segmentation. In patients with stage 0 non-small cell lung cancer, lung segmentectomy is most frequently performed.

## Wedge resection

Wedge resection is a procedure for the operation of removing a tiny part of tissue **(Fig. 10.36)** in a wedge for the removal of a small tumor or the diagnosis of lung cancer. It is ideal in the treatment of certain forms of lung cancer, in particular NSCLC, which involves the removal of small lesions, known as lung nodules, of cancer cells. But with this surgery, the nodules cannot be firmly rooted in the lung tissue. For patients, wedge resection can also be desired where a substantial reduction in lung function cannot withstand the removal of a significant portion of the lung. Wedge resection can also be done as an alternative to lobectomy, in which the whole lobe is separated from the lungs. This is done where there is a small region of cancer. In combination with chemotherapy and/or radiation, wedge resection is normally performed. It takes around 3 hours

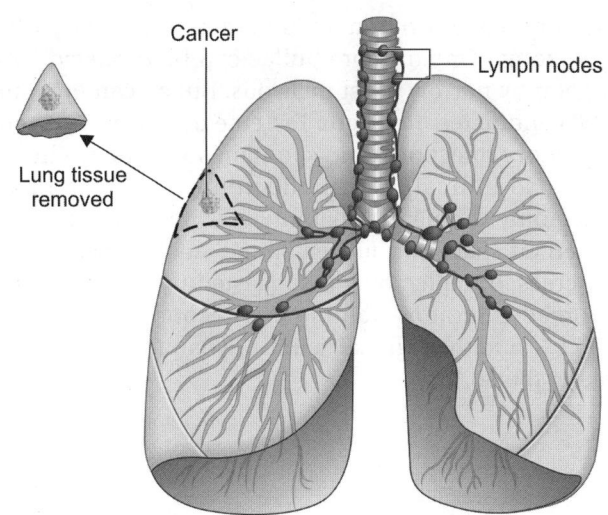

**Fig. 10.36:** Wedge resection of lungs.

to perform the surgery. The surgeons make three small incisions (from 5–15 mm) in the chest and side of a patient with general anesthesia. A thoracoscope and other surgical instruments used during the operation are inserted through the narrow incisions (Emadwiandr, 2013).

## Bullectomy

Bullectomy is an operation that removes dilated air spaces or bullae **(Fig. 10.37)** from the lungs. Chronic obstructive pulmonary disease and emphysema are general causes of dilated airspace. Patients with giant bullae filling half the thoracic volume and compressing comparatively

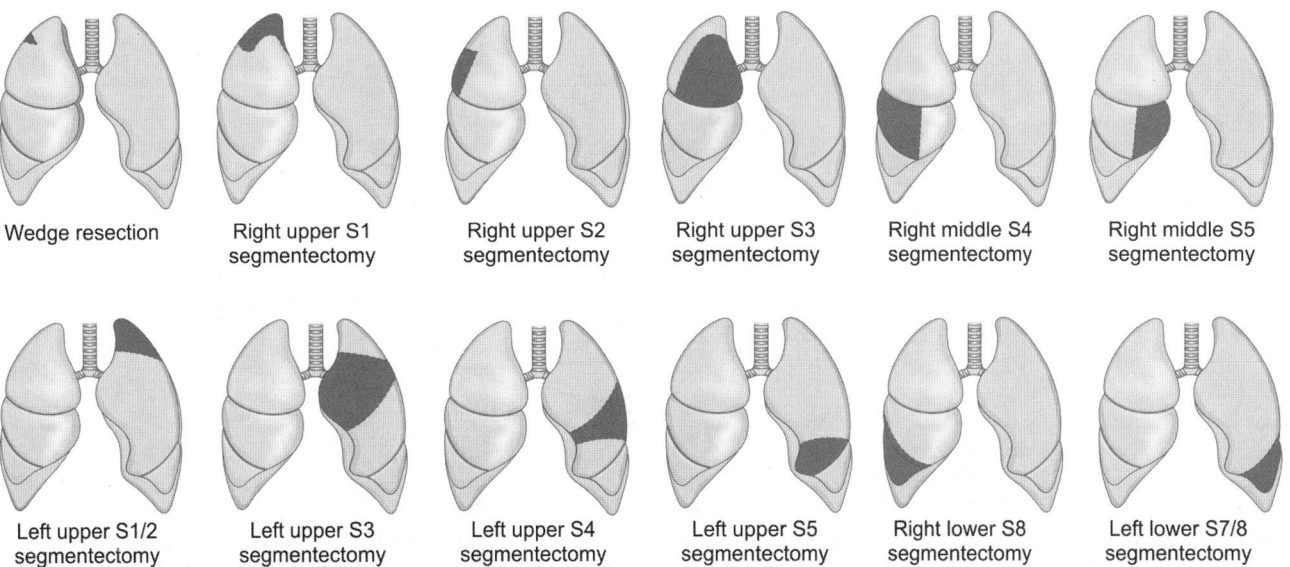

**Fig. 10.35:** Types of segment and wedge resections grey indicates resected area of the lung.

*Source:* Baylor College of Medicine.

normal adjacent parenchyma are recommended for bullectomy. One or more bullae can be removed by a surgeon by narrow chest incisions. Bullae can grow up to 20 centimeters in length. Extreme dyspnea, recurrent respiratory infections, and spontaneous pneumothorax have also indicated for bullectomy. With the post-bullectomy ventilator capability, it is necessary to have dilated air spaces or bullae volume. As the size of bulls is increased, bullectomy is suggested if the proportion of forced expiratory volume in a second exceeds 40% (FEV1%) and the regional volume dynamic ventilation is greater than 0.5.

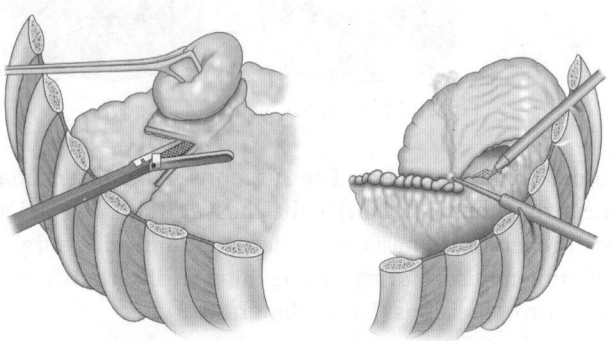

**Fig. 10.37:** Open bulla resection by wedge resection or anatomic resection.
*Source:* Themes UFO, 2017.

### Lung volume reduction surgery

Lung volume reduction surgery (LVRS) is an operation to remove the lung tissue **(Fig. 10.38)** that is diseased and emphysematous. This process decreases the size of the inflated lung and causes the remaining, much more functional, lung to expand (growth). Some patients with extreme emphysema (COPD), disabled dyspnea (shortness of breath, trouble breathing), and extreme air trapped are treated for lung volume restriction operations. The procedure to decrease lung volume has been shown to enhance the breathing capability, lung ability, and overall life quality in selected patients. The outcome depends on when or how much the tissue is involved, the resistance to exercise, and a patient's ability to undergo surgery (Emadwiandr, 2013).

### Video-assisted thoracic surgery (VATS)

VATS, the type of thoracic surgery conducted by the thoracoscope using small incisions and special equipment for trauma to be minimally invasive. It is a minimally invasive thoracic procedure **(Figs. 10.39A to D)**. Thoracoscopy or pleuroscopy are other names for this technique. Three narrow (about 1-inch) incisions, in addition to one long six to eight-inch chest incision used in traditional, "open" thoracic operations, are used during thoracoscopic operations. These small incisions implant surgical instruments and the thoracoscope. The thoracoscope transfers pictures from the operating room to the next screen display (Emadwiandr, 2013).

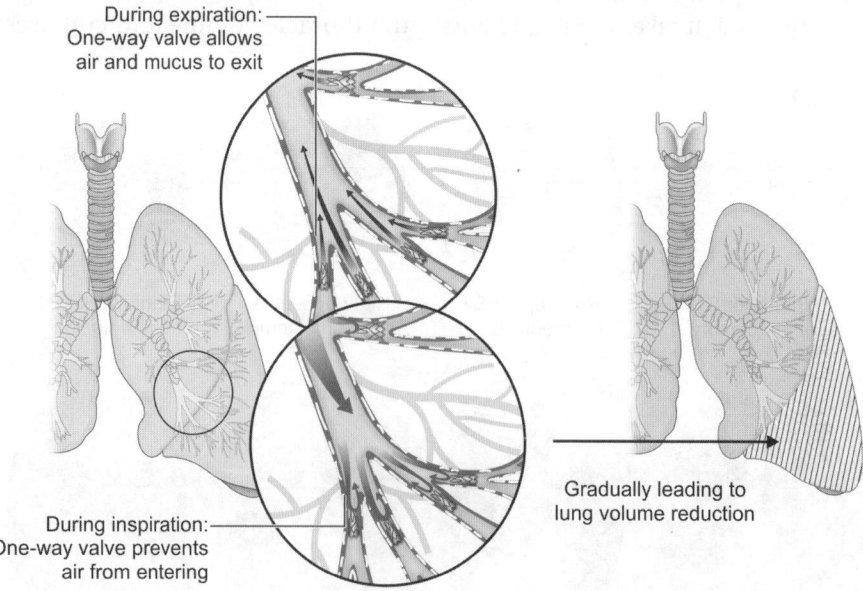

**Fig. 10.38:** Valve therapy for bronchoscopic lung volume reduction involves implantation of 1-way valves to allow airflow and mucus clearance outward to central airways. The 1-way flow leads to selective de-aeration and collapse of treated areas, reducing hyperinflation and air trapping. Unlike lung volume reduction surgery, the procedure is performed unilaterally due to the inherent procedural risk of pneumothorax.

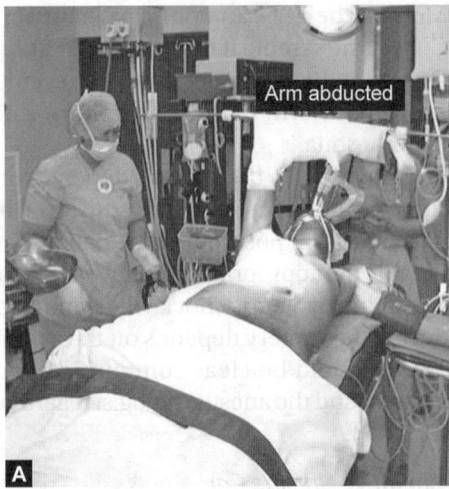
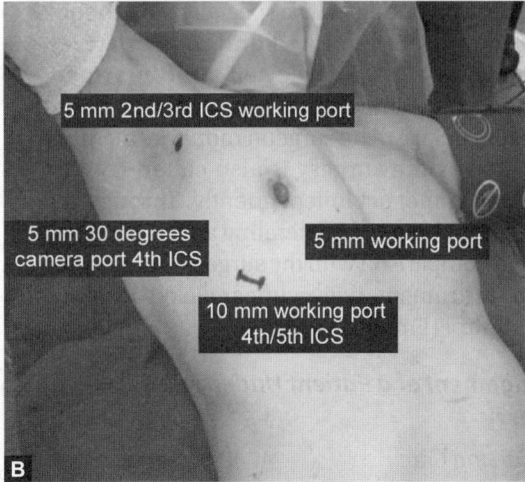
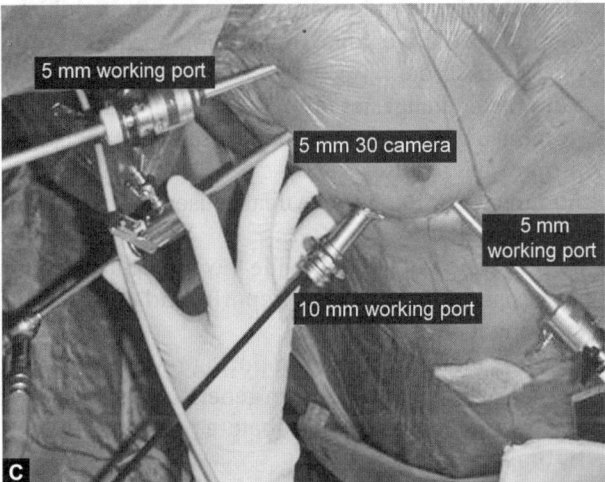
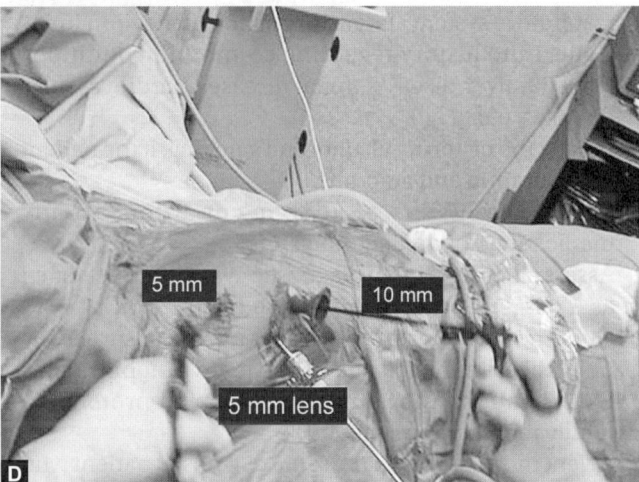

**Figs. 10.39A to D:** (A) Position of pt; (B) Right VATS thymectomy incisions; (C) Camera and port placements; (D) Instrument setup for right VATS.

Patients undergoing the minimally invasive procedure as compared to traditional surgery experiences:
- Decreased postoperative pain
- Limited duration of hospital stays
- Rapid recovery and back to work more easily

Additional potential advantages include lower infection risk and decreased bleeding.

### Robotic thoracic surgery

Robotic surgery **(Fig. 10.40)** has main benefits over the traditional minimally invasive technique by thoracic surgeons, video-assisted thoracic surgery, or VATS. VATS only provides the surgeon with 2D pictures of the operating area and has to use long rigid surgical equipment. Surgeons who use VATS lack the robot's depth vision who offers 3-D views. And the robot uses flexible instruments that simulate and surpass human handling greatly.

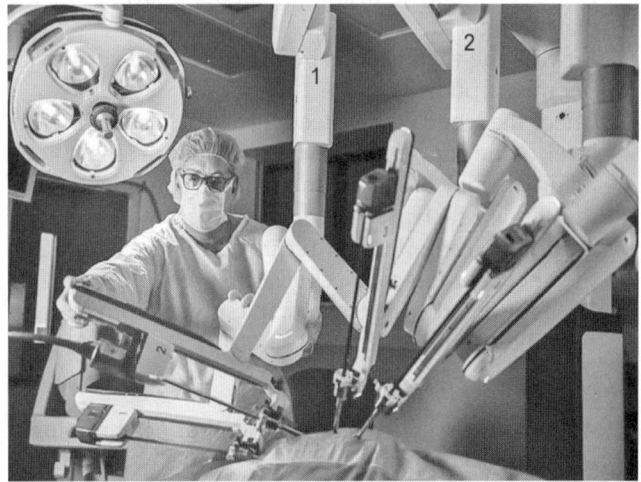

**Fig. 10.40:** Robotic surgery in thoracic patients.

Robot operation is conducted in a specially built robotic surgery suite composed of a hand and foot-operated surgeon console and a 3-D HD viewer, a robot-armed, traveling patient wheelchair, and a three-dimensional magnified imagery display. The surgeon monitors all robot motions. This is why the surgery is also called robotic surgery. The robot cannot act independently. Through the use of a 3-D HD robot vision, the operating area is provided to the surgeon. In comparison with the surgeon's hands, the robot's "wristed" instruments deliver unparalleled dexterity, precision and control (Emadwiandr, 2013).

### Nursing Management of a Patient Undergoing Thoracic Surgery

#### Preoperative Nursing Care

- The nurse to ask about the previous diseases of the respiratory system and history of hospitalization in it.
- Collect the history regarding co-morbid conditions like DM, liver diseases, renal diseases, cardiovascular diseases, etc.
- Collect the history of alcohol and smoking, if the patient has (duration and amount).
- Assess the history of allergic conditions to any medication, foods, and things, etc.
- Assess all the reports of diagnostic evaluation tests such as ABGs, ECG, chest X-ray, PET, etc.
- Nurse has to confirm the patient's ability for surgery by physical examination and postoperative mobilization.
- Explain all the procedures and hospital protocol to family members and patient.
- Orient the patient with the same diagnosed patient who is under treatment to reduce anxiety and going of faith.
- Remove all the dentures, jewellery, hairpins from the patient, and provide hospital clothing to him.
- Instruct the patient overnight not per orally before the day of surgery.
- Provide the medications before the day of surgery as per prescription.
- Check the blood group, bleeding time, clotting time, Hb level, of the patient, and instruct them to arrange blood before the day of surgery to avoid the complications of the surgery such as hypovolemic shock.
- Arrange all medication required for the operation theater according to the checklist.
- Keep the record of consent for the surgery from patients or family members (Booker KJ, 2015).

#### Intraoperative Nursing Care

- Administer oxygen by bagging with the anesthesiologist to promote ventilation.
- Suction the patient in case of any blockage of the ET tube. Assist the surgeon in operation theater.
- Monitor the ECG, and pulse oximetry in all the time.
- Collect the sample if needed during surgery.
- Check the body temperature to prevent hypothermia. Provide a warm blanket and warm saline to reduce hypothermia.
- The position of the patient depends on the types of surgery and the need of the surgeon. The nurse's role has to assist in positioning the patient.
- Provide the appropriate amount of fluid to minimize the risk of hypovolemic shock. The administration of fluid during the surgery depends on the surgical procedure. There should be clear communication between the surgeon and the anesthesiologist regarding this (Booker KJ, 2015).

#### Postoperative Nursing Care

- The nurse has to administer postoperative antibiotics to minimize the chance of infection according to the physician's order.
- Administer analgesics for pain management.
- Administer proton pump inhibitors and H2-blockers as prophylaxis for stress ulcers.
- Administer anti-emetics to treat nausea after the general anesthesia.
- To prevention of DVT, provide low molecular heparin, low dose unfractionated heparin and compression stocking to the patient.
- Provide adequate nutrition during the postoperative period. After recovering from general anesthesia check the patients showing reflex before providing anything by orally.
- Start the food from liquid to semisolid then solid after 6 hours of recovery from general anesthesia.
- Provide chest physiotherapy, postural drainage, incentive spirometry, deep breathing, and coughing exercise to avoid postoperative complications of open thoracic surgery. Encourage and assist the patient in early ambulation.
- Routinely check the incision site for bleeding. Check the discharges from the wound (color, amount) and record it. Check the drainage tubes for any leakage.
- Check the input and output ratio of the patient to check the fluid overload or dehydration.
- Educate the patient regarding pulmonary rehabilitation and follow up visit plans. (Booker KJ, 2015)

### Complications of the Thoracic Surgery

#### Early Complication

- ARDS
- Atelectasis
- Pulmonary edema

- Respiratory failure
- Pneumonia

*Late Complications*
- Bronchovascular fistula
- Bronchopleural fistula
- Wound infection and empyema
- Post-pneumonectomy syndrome
- Post-thoracotomy pain (Davidson JE, 2002)

##  Summary

Respiratory emergencies are the conditions which are associated with the diseases of the thoracic cavity, airways, and pulmonary parenchyma. Asthma and COPD are more common diseases of respiratory system. Bronchoscopic therapies, including laser photodynamic ablation therapy (PDT) and stent placement, can be beneficial to airway blocking. The most frequent form of superior vena cava syndrome (SVCS) is bronchogenic carcinoma and lymphoma. Spiral CT is available today, but ventilation profusion scintigraphy remains the first-line examination for pulmonary embolism (PE). Neoplastic and iatrogenic etiology parenchymal lung disease can occur as a result of infections. In cancer patients, the prevalence of pneumocystis carinii (PCP) is on the increasing, but prophylaxis will prevent it. It have been disappointing to combat acute respiratory distress syndrome (ARDS) by altering inflammatory mediators and the prognosis is poor.

##  Points to Ponder

- Functional residual capacity (FRC) is lowered in supine position and reduced further by anesthesia. Acute lung injury (ALI)/acute respiratory distress syndrome (ARDS) goes with very low lung volume, frequently below 1 L.
- Airway resistance is increased in obstructive lung disease, but also during anesthesia and in ALI/ARDS because of reduced lung volume with decreased airway dimensions.
- Both pulse oximetry and capnography are essential monitors in the intensive care unit (ICU), particularly during intubation, ventilation and transport.
- In case of an unexpected difficult airway, the number of intubation attempts should be limited to two and an alternative approach to maintain oxygenation and ventilation, such as extraglottic airway (EGA) devices, needs to be chosen.
- The intubating laryngeal mask airway (ILMA) is a useful back-up tool for both ventilation and intubation if tracheal tube placement fails.
- Cricothyrotomy is an emergency surgical airway used to save a life when all attempts at securing a patent airway fail and arrest is eminent.
- Hypercapnia can suppress the immune response to bacterial infection.
- Acute respiratory failure placed an increased metabolic demand on the cardiovascular system.
- In heart and/or respiratory failure patients, continuous positive airway pressure (CPAP) application can provide favorable hemodynamic and respiratory effects.
- Positive end-expiratory pressure (PEEP) is usually one of the first ventilator settings chosen when mechanical ventilation (MV) is initiated.
- Prone positioning optimizes lung recruitment and ventilation-perfusion matching, resulting in an improvement of gas exchange in 70–80% of acute respiratory distress syndrome (ARDS) patients. For this effect, patients with profound life-threatening hypoxemia may be treated with prone positioning as a rescue maneuver.
- The current clinical evidences support the use of prone position in the most severe form of ARDS (e.g., $PaO_2/FiO_2$<150 mm Hg, need of high plateau pressure and high positive end-expiratory pressure (PEEP) level, diffuse pulmonary infiltrates), while it should be avoided in less severe patients for its potential adverse effects.
- Risk factors for life-threatening asthma include chronic severe asthma, taking ≥3 asthma medications, previous intensive care unit admissions, previous invasive ventilation and psychosocial factors.
- Oxygen therapy is used for the hypoxia in acute exacerbation of chronic obstructive pulmonary disease (AECOPD). The objective is to reach $PaO_2$ 60 mm Hg (8 kPa; $SpO_2$ 90%). Venturi mask is the best method for administering oxygen.
- Respiratory alkalosis is usually a sign of an underlying pulmonary or central nervous system disease.
- Hypoxemia is a key element in pathogenesis, diagnosis, and prognosis of ventilator-associated pneumonia (VAP).
- Posture change, chest percussion, incentive spirometry and manual hyperinflation are the most common techniques applied in the intensive care unit to improve mucus clearance and prevent pulmonary complications.
- Small bore chest tubes are as effective as large ones and should be used initially.
- Thoracotomy is the procedure of choice for chest surgical exploration when massive hemothorax or persistent bleeding is present.

##  Abbreviations

- LVF : Left Ventricular Failure
- $ETCO_2$ : End-tidal Carbon Dioxide
- NPPV : Noninvasive Positive Pressure Ventilation
- BOOP : Bronchiolitis Obliterans with Organizing Pneumonia
- GOLD : Chronic Obstructive Lung Disease
- PFT : Pulmonary Function Test
- PT : Pulmonary Tuberculosis
- ARF : Acute Respiratory Failure

- ALI : Acute Lung Injury
- DAD : Diffuse Alveolar Damage
- ABG : Arterial Blood Gas
- CPAP : Continuous Positive Airway Pressure
- BiPAP : Bilevel Positive Airway Pressure
- VAP : Ventilator Associated Pneumonia
- DVT : Deep Vein Thrombosis
- BLT : Bilateral Lung Transplantation
- NSCLC : Non-small Cell Lung Cancer
- FEV : Forced Expiratory Volume
- LVRS : Lung Volume Reduction Surgery
- VATS : Video-assisted Thoracic Surgery
- PDT : Photodynamic Ablation Therapy
- SVCS : Superior Vena Cava Syndrome
- PE : Pulmonary Embolism
- ARDS : Acute Respiratory Distress Syndrome

### Short Answer Questions

1. Define lung compliance.
2. List two brain stem centers that regulate respiration.
3. Describe the key features of the oxygen dissociation curve.
4. Define high frequency positive pressure ventilation.
5. List three criteria for weaning of a patient from a ventilator.
6. Define respiratory failure.
7. Define five indications of mechanical ventilation.
8. Define is Adam's apple.
9. Define acute respiratory failure.
10. Define atelectasis.

**Write Short Note on:**

1. Status asthmaticus.
2. Pathophysiology of COPD.
3. Positive pressure ventilation.
4. Pathophysiology of ARDS.
5. Noninvasive ventilation.
6. Potential complications of mechanical ventilators.
7. Modes of mechanical ventilator.
8. Respiratory system assessment.
9. Weaning from ventilator.
10. Pulmonary embolism.

### Long Answer Questions

1. Define COPD. Write the etiology, clinical manifestations and pathophysiology of the disease.
2. Define pneumonia. Write the pathophysiology and diagnostic evaluation of the pneumonia.
3. Write briefly about the medical and nursing management of status asthmaticus.
4. Define ARDS. Write the medical and nursing management of a patient of ARDS.
5. Describe the different types of thoracic surgery with nursing management.
6. Define pulmonary tuberculosis. Write its pathophysiology, clinical manifestations and diagnostic evaluation. Describe briefly regarding DOTS therapy.
7. Define chest physiotherapy. Briefly describe the steps of physiotherapy.
8. Briefly write about the chest trauma, its types and nursing management.
9. Define pulmonary embolism. Write the etiology, clinical manifestations and pathophysiology of the disease. Write the nursing management of pulmonary embolism.
10. Briefly describe the modes of mechanical ventilator. Write the nursing management of patient under mechanical ventilator.

### Bibliography

1. Alía I, Esteban A. Weaning from mechanical ventilation. Critical Care. 2000;4 (2):1-9.
2. Angell ML. Fast Facts for the Critical Care Nurse. 1st edition. Newyork: Springer Publishing Company; 2012:1–272.
3. Booker KJ. Critical Care Nursing: Monitoring and Treatment for Advanced Nursing Practice. Critical Care Nursing Monitering Treateatment Advance Nursing Practices. 2015:1–272.
4. Bristle TJ, Collins S, Hewer I, Hollifield K. Anesthesia and Critical Care Ventilator Modes: Past, Present, and Future. AANA Journal. 2014;82 (5).
5. Brown D, Edwards H, Seaton L, Buckley T. Lewis's Medical-Surgical Nursing: Assessment and Management of Clinical Problems. Elsevier Health Sciences; 2015.
6. Burns SM, Delgado SA. AACN Essentials of Progressive Care Nursing. McGraw Hill Education; 2019.
7. Chulay M, Suzanne M. AACN Essentials of Critical Care Nursing Pocket Handbook (80). Stikes Perintis Padang; 2020.
8. Chulay Marianne BSM. Essential of Critical Care Nursing. 2nd Edition. The McGraw Hill Companies, 2010; 1389:1–208.
9. Civetta JM, Taylor RW, Kirby RR. Introduction to Critical Care. Critical Care Medicine. 1990;18 (11):1308.
10. Davidson JE. Essentials of Critical Care Nursing. J Cardiovascular Nursing. 2002;7(1):78.
11. Emadwiandr. Essential Of Critical Care Nursing A Holistic Approach. Vol. 53, Wolters Kluwer Health. 2013: 1689–1699.
12. Hsu KY, Lin JR, Lin MS, Chen W, Chen YJ, Yan YH. The Modified Medical Research Council Dyspnoea Scale is a Good Indicator of Health-Related Quality of Life in Patients with Chronic Obstructive Pulmonary Disease. Singapore Med J. 2013;54 (6):321-7.
13. Häggström, Mikael (2014). "Medical Gallery of Mikael Häggström 2014". WikiJournal of Medicine 1 (2).

14. Lewis SL, Bucher L, Heitkemper MM, Harding MM, Kwong J, Roberts D. Medical-Surgical Nursing-E-Book: Assessment and Management of Clinical Problems, Single Volume. Elsevier Health Sciences; 2016.
15. Light RW. Pleural effusion. New England Journal of Medicine. 2002;346 (25):1971–7.
16. Loscalzo J. Harrison's Pulmonary and Critical Care Medicine, 2nd Edn. McGraw-Hill Education; 2013.
17. Malarvizhi S, Gugan R, editors. Black's Medical-surgical Nursing. Elsevier Health Sciences; 2019.
18. Marty AT. Oxford Textbook of Critical Care. 2nd Edn, Oxford Publication, Oxford University Press; 2016:1–1903.
19. Nettina SM, Msn AB. Lippincott Manual of Nursing Practice. Lippincott Williams and Wilkins; 2013.
20. Patwa A, Shah A. Anatomy and Physiology of Respiratory System Relevant to Anaesthesia. Indian Journal of Anesthesia. 2015;59 (9):533-41.
21. Perrin KO, MacLeod CE. Understanding the Essentials of Critical Care Nursing. Pearson Prentice Hall; 2009.
22. Pratt P, O'Riordan B. Critical Care Nursing. Nursing Standard (through 2013). 1999;13 (48):59.
23. Qureshi H, Sharafkhaneh A, Hanania NA. Chronic Obstructive Pulmonary Disease Exacerbations: Latest Evidence and Clinical Implications: Their Advance Chronic Diseases, (2014); Vol. (5):212–27.
24. Rashed A, Verzar Z, Alotti N, Gombocz K. Xiphoid-sparing Midline Sternotomy Reduces Wound Infection Risk after Coronary Bypass Surgery. Journal of Thoracic Disease. 2018; 10 (6):3568.
25. Remington LA, Goodwin D. Clinical Anatomy and Physiology of the Visual System E-Book. Elsevier Health Sciences; 2021.
26. Rothstein, JM, SH Roy, and SL Wolf. The Rehabilitation Specialist's Handbook. 2nd Edn. Philadelphia: FA Davis Co., 1998.
27. Sharma SK. Lippincott Manual of Medical-Surgical Nursing Adaptation of Nettina: Lippincott Manual of Nursing. Wolters Kluwer India Pvt Ltd; 2016.
28. Stephens G. Using a Structured Clinical Assessment to Identify the Cause of Chest Pain. Nursing Standard. 2019; 34 (4).
29. Stocks J, Hislop AA. Structure and Function of the Respiratory System. Drug Delivery to the Lung. New York: Marcel Dekker. 2002:47-104.
30. Suzanne C Smeltzer, Brenda G Bare, Janice L Hinkle KHC. Burrner and Suddarth'S Textbook of Medical Surgical Nursing. 12th ed. Vol. 1, Wolters Kluwer Health. Lippincott Williams and Wilkins; 2013:1–2364.
31. Thim T, Krarup NH, Grove EL, Rohde CV, Løfgren B. Initial Assessment and Treatment with the Airway, Breathing, Circulation, Disability, Exposure (ABCDE) Approach. International Journal of General Medicine. 2012;5:117.
32. Vincent JL, Abraham E, Kochanek P, Moore FA, Fink MP. Textbook of Critical Care E-Book. Elsevier Health Sciences; 2016.
33. Waugh A, Grant A. Ross and Wilson Anatomy and Physiology in Health and Illness E-book. Elsevier Health Sciences; 2014.
34. Waugh Anne GA. Anatomy and Physiology. 9th Edn. Vol. 53, Elsevier Publisher. Elsevier; 2013:1689–1699.

# Chapter 11

# Endocrine System Emergencies and Management

*Pratibha Khosla*

## CHAPTER OUTLINE

- Anatomy and Physiology of Endocrine System
- Assessment of Endocrine System
- Hypoglycemia
- Hyperglycemia
- Diabetic Ketoacidosis
- Thyroid Crisis/Storm
- Myxedema
- Adrenal Crisis
- Antidiuretic Hormone Dysfunctions

## Learning Objectives

At the end of the chapter, the students will be able to:

- Describe the basic anatomy and physiology of the endocrine system.
- Perform the assessment of a patient with endocrine disorders with history collection and physical examination.
- Describe the purposes and nurses; responsibilities of different diagnostic procedures involved to study endocrine system disorder.
- Describe the etiology, clinical manifestations, assessment and management of hypoglycemia.
- Describe the etiology, pathophysiologic mechanisms, clinical manifestations, diagnosis, and management of hyperglycemia.
- Describe the classification, etiology, risk factors, pathophysiology, clinical manifestations, diagnosis, and emergency management of diabetic ketoacidosis.
- Describe the etiology, classification, diagnosis and management of thyroid crisis.
- Describe the causes, types, pathophysiology, diagnosis, complications and management of myxedema.
- Describe the types, etiology, pathophysiology, clinical manifestations, diagnosis, and management of adernal crisis.
- Describe the etiology, pathophysiology, clinical features, diagnosis, complications and management of antidiuretic hormone dysfunction.

## ANATOMY AND PHYSIOLOGY OF ENDOCRINE SYSTEM

Nervous system and the interconnected network of glands known as the endocrine system control body systems. **Endocrine glands** (EN-do⁻krin; *endo* = within) secrete their products (hormones) into the interstitial fluid surrounding the secretory cells rather than into ducts (Baker GF, 2006).

The endocrine glands include the pituitary, thyroid, parathyroid, adrenal, and pineal glands. In addition, several organs and tissues are not exclusively classified as endocrine glands but contain cells that secret hormones. These include the hypothalamus, thymus, pancreas, ovaries, testes, kidneys, stomach, liver, small intestine, skin, heart, adipose tissue, and placenta. Taken together, all endocrine glands and hormone-secreting cells constitute the **endocrine system (Fig. 11.1)**.

The chemical substances secreted by the endocrine glands are called hormones. Hormones help to regulate organ function in concert with the nervous system. This dual regulatory system, in which rapid action by the nervous system is balanced by slower hormonal action, permits precise control of organ functions in response to varied changes within and outside the body. The hypothalamus is a brain region which regulates homeostasis by mediating endocrine, autonomic and behavioral functions. It is comprised of several nuclei containing distinct neuronal populations producing neuropeptides

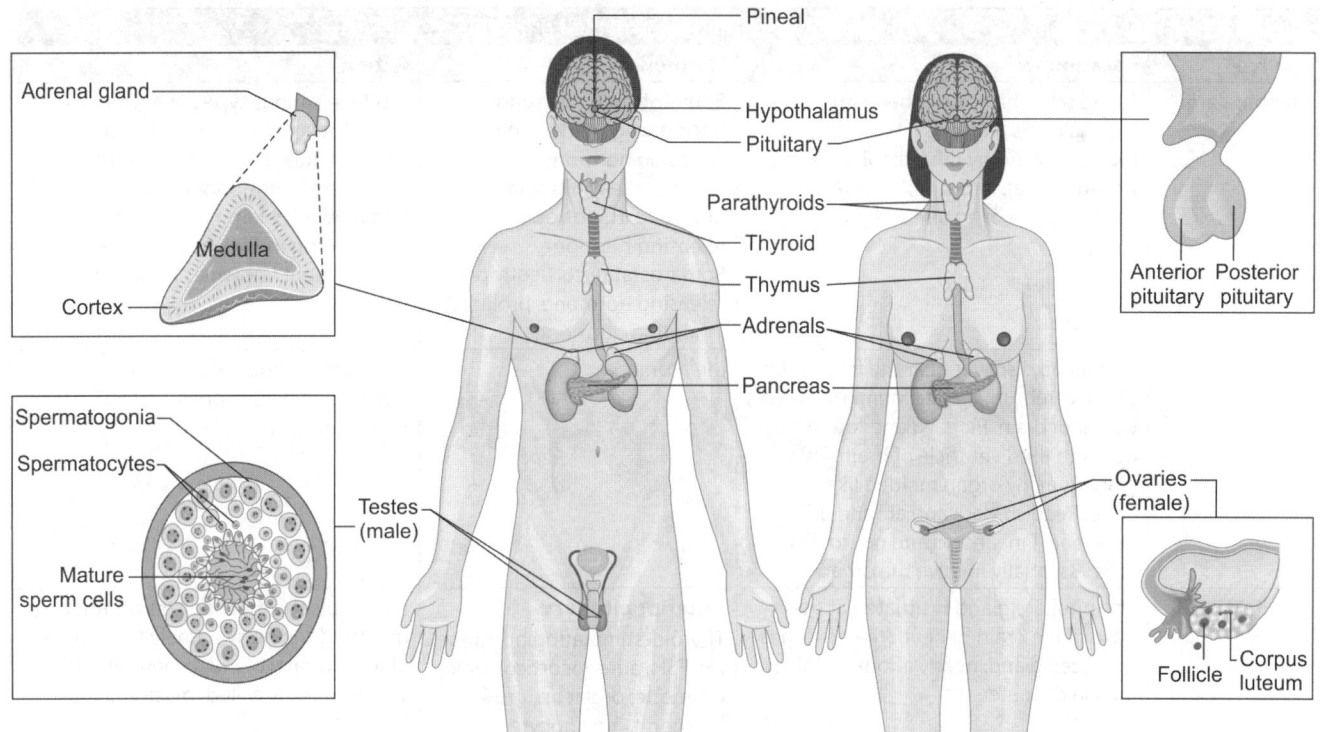

**Fig. 11.1:** Endocrine system.

and neurotransmitters that regulate fundamental body functions including temperature and metabolic rate, thirst and hunger, sexual behavior and reproduction, circadian rhythm, and emotional responses (Stephen Kemp M, 2017). **Table 11.1** lists the major hormones, their target tissue, and some of their properties.

## ASSESSMENT OF ENDOCRINE SYSTEM

Each cell in our body is impacted by our endocrine framework. The endocrine framework acts to keep up harmony at the cell level and is a crucial connection in homeostasis. **Figure 11.2** shows the pituitary gland, the relationship of the brain to pituitary action, and the hormones secreted by the anterior pituitary and the posterior pituitary. At the point when variations from the norm happen, sickness can result. Treatment typically requires dealing with a freak hormone by either diminishing or expanding its creation or emission from its related endocrine organ. A careful understanding of the endocrine framework and how it is important in precisely assessing and treating endocrine issues.

The symptoms of an endocrine disorder vary widely depend on the specific gland involved. Changes in energy level and fatigue are common to many endocrine imbalances, the detail history and any unusual change that affects the daily life is looked for. Some of the major endocrine disturbances and their clinical features has been described in the **Table 11.2** for better understanding.

### Examination of Endocrine System

When conducting a focused endocrine assessment, begin with a thorough history of chief complaints. Elicit information about any experienced signs or symptoms of endocrine disease or disorders. Endocrine disorders and diseases usually manifest according to which endocrine hormone is being overproduced and secreted, or under-produced, at any given age. The key to discovering the nature of the symptoms lies in understanding of the functions of the endocrine hormones.

### Symptoms-centered Endocrine Assessment

The symptoms-centered endocrine assessment indicates a potential endocrine malfunction. Any deviation from the last assessment then consider a specific endocrine assessment. Specific assessment for specific symptoms helps in identifying specific gland malfunction of endocrine system. It helps in saving time.

Detailed past and present history of patients is needed while conducting an endocrine assessment, which may include:

**Table 11.1:** Lists of the major hormones, their target tissue, and some of their properties.

| Source | Location | Hormones | Action |
|---|---|---|---|
| Hypothalamus | Gland hypothalamus is beneath the thalamus and gets linked to pituitary gland by infundibulum (stalk like structure). It resembles to the configuration of an almond | Somatotropin releasing hormone, gonadotropin-releasing hormone, melanocyte-inhibiting hormone, thyrotropin-releasing hormone, Somatostatin, corticotropin-releasing hormone, prolactin-inhibiting hormone | Produce various types of hormones (somatotropin, somatostatin, etc.) which regulates the production of different hormones all over the body. Hypothalamus also helps in maintaining individual's internal environment known as homeostasis |
| Pineal gland | This gland discover near the focal point of the cerebrum, hence found between center of brain. Pineal gland found beneath third ventricle of brain. This gland is a tiny organ molded like a pine cone. Reddish-dark and around 0.33 inch long. Pineal cells and neuroglial cells essentially involve the organ | Melatonin | Regulate circadian rhythm and reproductive hormones |
| Pituitary gland | The pituitary gland is situated at the base of the brain beneath the nose. It is pea sized gland, nearly about 1/3 of an inch in diameter | **Anterior pituitary** Thyroid-stimulating hormone, LH, FSH, adrenocorticotropic hormone, prolactin, growth hormone, melanocyte-stimulating hormone **Posterior pituitary** Vasopressin, oxytocin | It controls the mechanisms of other glands of the body namely thyroid gland, adrenal gland, ovaries and testes. That's why it is called "master gland" |
| Thyroid gland | Situated in front of the trachea and beneath the larynx. This gland looks like butterfly | Triodothyronine ($T_3$), thyroxine ($T_4$), calcitonin | Regulates metabolism. The $T_3$ and $T_4$ are two main thyroid hormones |
| Parathyroid glands | Parathyroids are typically located on the back of the thyroid. They resemble of a grain of rice in size and shape | Parathyroid | Four small gland combines to make parathyroid gland. It regulates the calcium level of blood |
| Thymus | Located in the upper anterior part of chest between lungs directly behind sternum. Has two thymic lobes and is a pinkish-gray organ | Thymosin hormone Thymopoietin Thymulin | It strengthens the immune system. Stimulates growth hormone production. Helps in differentiation of T cells |
| Adrenal gland | Each kidney possesses triangular shaped organs of height 1.5 inches and 3 inches in length | Glucocorticoids Mineralocorticoids | Secrets hormone adrenaline, which triggers the body's fight or flight response |
| Pancreas | Pancreas is situated beneath the stomach, retroperitoneal in position, nearer to L1 and L2. It is 6-inch-long gland and its ducts opens to duodenum of small intestine | Insulin Somatostatin Glucagon | Primary hormones of the pancreas include insulin and glucagon, and both regulate blood glucose |
| Ovaries | Oval shaped organ attached to uterus by ligament, two in number | Estrogen Progesterone | Maturation of primary oocytes into secondary oocytes. Maintenance of pregnancy. Helps in lactation |
| Testes | Primary male reproductive organ, two in number. Situated inside the scrotum | Testosterone | Helps in development of secondary sexual character of men. Regulate libido, muscle strength, and bone density |

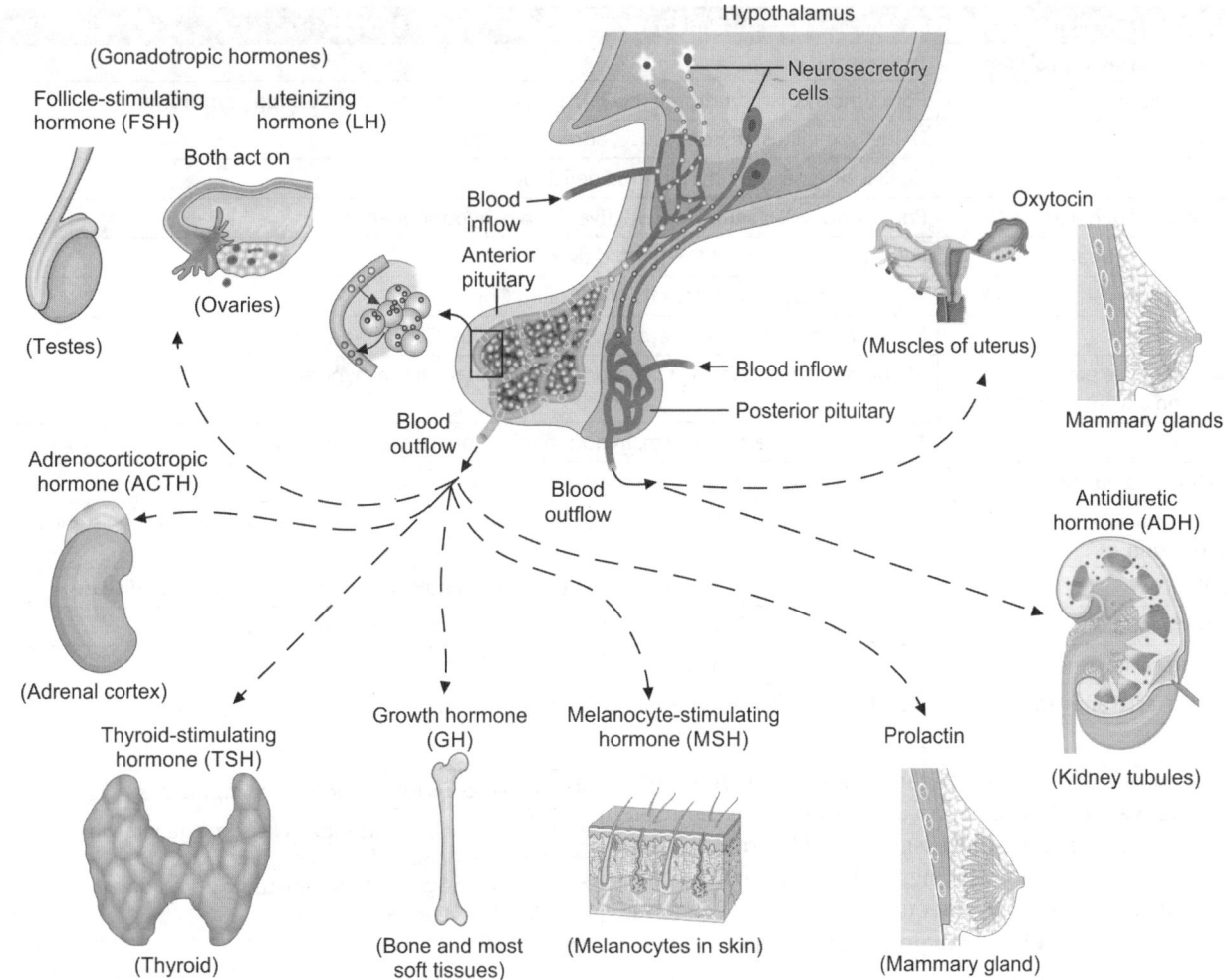

**Fig. 11.2:** The pituitary gland, the relationship of the brain to pituitary action, and the hormones secreted by the anterior pituitary and the posterior pituitary.

*Source:* Baker GF, Tortora GJ, Nostakos NPA. Principles of Anatomy and Physiology. Vol. 76, The American Journal of Nursing. 2006: 477.

## Chief Compliant

It may include nausea and vomiting, fatigue or lethargy, underweight or obese, dizziness, low feeling, tantrum, or anxiety, pain, decreased libido, irregularities in urinary or bowel habits, changes in vision, intolerance to heat or cold, or change in appetite.

## Present Health Status

Allow patients to verbalize themselves. Be an active listener, Ask patients how they are doing? Patients detailed history reveals endocrine cause of symptoms. The patient's vocal pitch may give a clue. A hypogonadal male has a high-pitched voice, while an androgenized female may have a deeper voice than expected. Body fat distribution gives important clues to the presence of adrenal steroid excess, while excessive wasting may imply adrenal steroid insufficiency or hyperthyroidism. Observation of skin color, pattern of wrinkling, distribution of skin pigment, and body hair can yield useful historical clues.

Past health history and current lifestyle plays a vital part in the assessment of endocrine disorders so it is of utmost importance to have a clear picture so that diagnosis and treatment may made so that the desired goals can be achieved.

- **Psychological status:** Impaired mental status is a common presentation in the emergency department, and can be caused by endocrine emergencies. Disorientation, awareness, and consciousness can be maintained by the interaction among the brainstem reticular core, the thalamus, and the cerebral cortex.

**Table 11.2:** Describing the common clinical features of endocrine disturbance.

| Symptom, sign or problem | Differential diagnoses |
|---|---|
| Gain in weight | Polycystic ovarian syndrome (PCOS), underactive thyroid and Cushing's syndrome |
| Loss in weight | Diabetes mellitus, thyrotoxicosis, adrenal insufficiency |
| Dwarfness | Coeliac disease, growth hormone deficiency |
| Late onset of puberty | Primary gonadal failure, underactive thyroid, hypopituitarism |
| Irregular menstruation | Hyperprolactinemia PCOS, thyroid dysfunction |
| Diffuse inflammation in neck | Thyrotoxicosis, Hashimoto's thyroiditis and Goiter |
| Polydipsia | Hyperparathyroidism, diabetes mellitus/insipidus, Conn's syndrome |
| Unwanted male pattern hair growth on a women's face | Idiopathic, PCOS, Cushing's syndrome, congenital adrenal hyperplasia |
| Sweating | Acromegaly, hyperthyroidism, hypogonadism, pheochromocytoma |
| Sweating and flushing of skin | Carcinoid syndrome, hypogonadism (especially menopause) |
| Medicine tolerated hypertension | Pheochromocytoma, Conn's syndrome, acromegaly, Cushing's syndrome, renal artery stenosis |
| Impotence | Diabetes mellitus, primary or secondary hypogonadism, non-endocrine systemic disease |
| Muscle fatigue or myasthenia | Thyrotoxicosis, Cushing's syndrome, hyperparathyroidism, osteomalacia |
| Pathological fracture of bone | Hypogonadism, thyrotoxicosis, Cushing's syndrome |
| Impaired facial appearance | Acromegaly, hypothyroidism, Cushing's syndrome, PCOS |

Impaired consciousness means a significant alteration in the wakefulness and the awareness of self and of the environment. It is necessary to find the root causes and to maintain the vital signs. Diabetic coma is one of critical diagnosis in the emergency room. Diabetic ketoacidosis (DKA) and hyperglycemic hyperosmolar syndrome are the most serious acute hyperglycemic emergency. Checking the blood glucose, calcium and electrolytes imbalances is the first step to evaluate altered mentality.

- **Family history:** Family history is an vital component of the assessment of endocrine patients. Ask the patient about their family history having endocrine disorder. Family tree should be drawn and link should be established. Genetic counseling should arranged for such patients.

*Physical Assessment*

Endocrinology is interesting area of medical field which provides challenging opportunity to assess the patient's physical change. Endocrinology is not the matter of study of only one organ. It compromises various gland. Most of endocrinological gland are not palpable except thyroid and the testicles. Detailed and prompt physical examination helps in clarify the diagnosis. Endocrine diagnosis involves the sequence of history, physical examination, laboratory, and radiologic evaluation.

**How to Proceed for Endocrine Examinations?**

- Take time at the outset to make some general observations.
- The initial handshake may suggest a diagnosis.
- Measure the patient's height, using a stadiometer in children and adolescents and weight.
- Assess the face for unusual hair growth and pigmentation.
- Is the patient slow and lethargic (hypothyroidism), or restless and anxious (hyperthyroidism)?
- Assess the entire skin surface, looking for abnormal pallor (hypopituitarism), vitiligo, plethora (Cushing's or carcinoid syndrome) or pigmentation (Addison's disease).
- Calculate the body mass index.
- If the patient having more weight than height (obese), is the adiposity centrally distributed (Cushing's syndrome and growth hormone deficiency) (Cushing's syndrome and growth hormone deficiency)?
- Psychiatric assessment may be helpful in Cushing Syndrome patients. Two-thirds of patients with Cushing's syndrome have psychological or psychiatric features.
- Is the hair growth normal in quantity and quality? Look for extra hair growth in females with menstrual disturbance, especially on the face, chest and abdomen (polycystic ovary syndrome (PCOS).
- Test the urine for glycosuria (diabetes mellitus) and proteinuria (hypertensive renal damage).
- Assess the hands for excessive sweating, skin crease pigmentation (Addison's disease) soft tissue overgrowth (acromegaly), and wasting of the muscles due to carpal tunnel syndrome (hypothyroidism, acromegaly). Cushing's syndrome patients often have thin skin and fragile bone.

- Check the pulse rate, volume and rhythm. Raised pulse rate and atrial fibrillation may suggest thyrotoxicosis.
- Record the blood pressure. Raised blood pressure is a characteristics of various endocrine conditions, such as pheochromocytoma and Conn's syndrome (primary hyperaldosteronism). Check for postural hypotension with lying and standing blood pressures if you suspect adrenal insufficiency.
- Examine the eyes in all thyroid patients for external inflammation, proptosis, diplopia and visual function. Optic chiasm compression lead to bitemporal hemianopia in case of pituitary tumors patients.
  Longstanding optic pathway compression leads to optic atrophy. Assess the fundus of eyes for it.
- Assess the neck for goiter. Record its circumference, surface, and consistency. Measures with help of calipers if discrete nodule is present. While palpation, consider patient's privacy and their comfort.
- Ascult for a thyroid bruit with stethoscope.
- Look for gynecomastia in men (common in Klinefelter's syndrome 47XXY, and for evidence of milk production in a man or non-breastfeeding woman (galactorrhea). In case of galactorrhea, gently palpate the breast in the direction of the nipple, to check the discharge of milk. Privacy of patients is mandatory and before procedure explain about it.
- Inspect the axillae for acanthosis nigricans or loss of axillary hair.
- Inspect for a Kyphosis, which may be a sign of osteoporotic vertebral collapse.
- Inspect the abdomen. In carcinoid syndrome, liver becomes massively big which can be palpable for nodule. In case of pheochromocytoma, restricted palpation should be done as it may leads to hypertensive paroxysm.
- Inspect the male external genitalia for the quantity of pubic hair and Tanner gradings should use for pubertal staging of all adolescents. Monitor and record testicular consistency and volume (use an Orchidometer).
- Assess the lower extremities for pretibial myxedema (Graves disease), proximal muscle wasting and weakness (Cushing's syndrome and hyperthyroidism).

*Investigation Techniques*

Broad range of diagnostic tests can be used in the diagnostic findings. There are mainly three categories of diagnostic test in common. They are blood sample, urine sample and stimulation and evocative test.

Endocrine disease diagnostic findings have been briefly explained.

### Bedside

- **Urine test:** Diabetes mellitus—traces of glucose in urine
- **Hypertensive renal damage:** Traces of protein in urine
- **Random blood sugar:** High in diabetes mellitus.

### Blood

- **$Ca^{+2}$:** Hypercalcemia in hyperparathyroidism.
- **T4 test:** Raised in hyperthyroidism, decline in hypothyroidism.
- **Thyroid-stimulating hormone:** Insignificant in hyperthyroidism, raised in primary hypothyroidism.
- **Serum cortisol level:** Go down in hypoadrenalism, usually with reduced tetracosactide response, loss of circadian rhythm and corticosteroid in Cushing's syndrome.
- **Human chronic gonadotrophins (HCG):** Raised in primary hypogonadism in both male and female.

### Imaging

- **USG:** FNAC (fine needle aspiration cytology) and imaging of thyroid, parathyroid, ovary and testis, etc.
- **MRI:** Pituitary, pancreas
- **CT:** Pancreas, adrenal
- **Radionuclide:** Thyroid (123 I), parathyroid (99m Tc-sesta-MIBI), adrenal (123 I-mIBG), neuroendocrine tumors (123 I-octreotide)
- **PET CT:** Thyroid and neuroendocrine tumors.

### Invasive

- **FNAC:** Thyroid
- **Inferior petrosal sinus sampling (IPSS):** Adrenocorticotropic hormone testing in case of Nelson's syndrome.

## HYPOGLYCEMIA

Hypoglycemia frequently described as plasma glucose level less than 70 mg/dL; nevertheless, manifestations may or may not be seen prior to plasma glucose levels drop to be lower than "55 mg/dL." (Mathew P, 2022). The symptoms of Whipple's triad have been used to describe hypoglycemia since 1938.

Whipple's triad clinically characterizes insulinomas: episodic hypoglycemia, central nervous system (CNS) dysfunction temporarily related to hypoglycemia (confusion, anxiety, stupor, paralysis, convulsions, coma), and dramatic reversal of significant jumpy system abnormalities by glucose administration. To use "Whipple's triad", a physician has to initially confirm the signs of hypoglycemia, and after that get low blood glucose, and ultimately, show quick reduction of signs after regulation of the blood glucose.

In the course of fasting, serum glucose measures are managed with the help of gluconeogenesis and glycogenolysis in liver. "Gluconeogenesis is the pathway in which glucose is produced from non-carbohydrate sources, these non-carbohydrate sources could be protein, lipids, pyruvate or lactate". Whereas "glycogenolysis is the breakdown of glycogen into glucose product". Substantial amount of glycogenolysis takes place in hepatocytes (liver) and myocytes (muscles).

"Hypoglycemia" is commonly found among individuals with diabetes under pharmacologic management. In individuals having type 1 diabetes are at threefold increased risk to suffer hypoglycemia in contrast to individuals having type 2 diabetes through getting treated.

## Etiology

Among individuals without diabetes, hypoglycemia is rare, and if it is seen, it is due to some crucial reasons of hypoglycemia: Pharmacologic, alcohol, chronic diseases, counter-regulatory hormonal insufficiencies and non-islets celli malignancies.

Incidents of true hypoglycemia in a patient without diabetes is primarily because of the effect of medications like overt intake of insulin. Several possible sources of hypoglycemia are critical sickness, liquor, cortisol insufficiency and nutritional deficiencies.

Alcoholic consumption slows down the process of gluconeogenesis, which has no influence on glycogenolysis. Hence, hypoglycemia happens post long time alcohol intake and post glycogen reserves are diminished.

In serious disease conditions, such as, terminal hepatic illness, sepsis, fasting, or kidney failure, glucose usage is more than glucose consumption, glycogenolysis/gluconeogenesis. The imbalance results in hypoglycemia. Counter-regulatory hormonal insufficiencies may be seen in conditions with adrenal insufficiency. Hypoglycemia related to these insufficiencies are uncommon. "Non-islet cell tumours may also be a cause of hypoglycemia through increased secretion of insulin-like growth factor 2 (IGF-2) (Stephen Kemp M, 2007). IGF-2 increases glucose utilization, which can lead to hypoglycemia".

## Epidemiology

Hypoglycemia is frequently seen with type 1 diabetes, usually among individuals getting rigorous insulin treatment. Serious hypoglycemia is described around "62 to 320" incidents every "100" individuals-annually among type I diabetics.

Individuals with type 1 diabetes need insulin treatment completely; individuals having type 2 diabetes suffer hypoglycemia infrequently in compare to individuals having type 1 diabetes. The reason for this is partly, because of pharmacotherapy which possibly will not cause hypoglycemia such as metformin. Occurrence of hypoglycemia among individuals having type 2 diabetes is outlined around 35 incidents for 100 individuals-year. Gender related differences are not evident.

## Pathophysiology

Basic counterregulatory efficiency block hypoglycemic occurrences. "All of these counterregulatory mechanisms include an interplay of hormones and neural signals to regulate the release of endogenous insulin, to increase hepatic glucose output, and to alter peripheral glucose utilization" (Cryer PE, 2016). Amongst the counter-regulatory measures, synchronization of insulinsecretion takes a vital part. Reduction of insulin formation due to lowered serum glucose exists as bodies first line of defence in response to hypoglycemia.

The internal glucose to be produced, mainly the liver glycogenolysis, lower insulin measure is required. Along with decline in plasma glucose measure, beta cell release of insulin declines, which results in increase liver/kidney gluconeogenesis with liver glycogenolysis. Glycogenolysis keeps serum glucose measure above "8 to 12 hours" till glycogen reserves get diminished. With time, liver gluconeogenesis accord to maintain euglycemia in time of need.

Reduction of insulin manufacturing takes place when glucose measures are at low-normal level. That provides a distinguishing characteristic in comparison with different counterregulatory mechanisms. Further counterregulatorymechanisms generally occur if serum glucose measures reduce more than physiological level. In further counterregulatory measures, pancreatic alpha cells release of glucagon as next line of defence opposed to hypoglycemia. In case elevated glucagon fails in accomplishing euglycemia, adrenomedullary epinephrine will be released. Collectively three counterregulatory mechanism take place in the acute phase of hypoglycemia.

Previous referred counter-regulatory measures may be unsuccessful in resolving hypoglycemia. Additionally counterregulatory mechanisms are used such as growth hormone and cortisol. The secretion of both growth hormone and cortisol occur in cases of long-term hypo-glycemic conditions.

## History and Physical Assessment

Signs and symptoms concerning hypoglycemia may be categorized under neuroglycopenic and neurogenic. Neuroglycopenic manifestations are those which is due to immediate central nervous system (CNS) distress of glucose. There may be behavior change, confusions, fatigue, seizure, coma, and potentially death if not promptly checked. Neurogenic manifestations be like adrenergic (tremor, palpitations, fear) or cholinergic (hunger, diaphoresis, paresthesia). Neurologic manifestations rise due to sympathoadrenal association (either norepinephrine or acetylcholine secretion) because of feedback of perceived hypoglycemia.

Thorough history is crucial while assessing hypoglycemia. Important concerns that are to be looked into during a patient's history taking are:
- Thorough history of medications
- Alcohol and/or drug usage
- Any present or past mental health issues
- "History of diabetes mellitus or multiple endocrine neoplasia syndromes (MEN) in family"
- Uninitiated weight fluctuations
- Change of medications
- Any acute renal trauma or kidney failure
- Symptoms of other hormone deficiencies.

It is additionally critical to take note of the setting of the hypoglycemic scene comparative with diet or activity.

Laboratory estimate that defines hypoglycemia has not yet been established. Hypoglycemia is considered to be existing if an individual reports of manifestations corresponding to hypoglycemia with further lower serum glucose measure (<70 mg/dL). Hypoglycemia arise with medical complications integrated with laboratory results of lower serum glucose alternatively to 100% biochemical detection. Generally neurogenic and neuroglycopenic manifestations of hypoglycemia arise in glucose measures equal to or less than 50 to 55 mg/dL, but this threshold may differ through different patients.

Individuals having diabetes may come with manifestations of hypoglycemia in comparatively grater serum glucose measures. Chronic hyperglycemias modify the "set point" so that neuroglycopenic/neurogenic signs have clear manifestations. This event is termed as "pseudohypoglycemia" as the serum glucose could possibly have been in usual measure in spite of the clinical manifestations.

## Evaluation

As mentioned earlier, documentation of "Whipple's triad" used as effective measure for hypoglycemia, but some basic lab tests must affirm hypoglycemia. Many relevant tests may be considered to involve insulin, proinsulin, and C-peptide measures throughout any incident of probable hypoglycemia. In cases where C-peptide measure reduces due to high levels of insulin, an individual should be given insulin externally. Insulin in its initial state is produced in the system and is adhered with "C peptide". "The body then cleaves C peptide from the pro form of the molecule to create active insulin. Elevated C-peptide levels and insulin levels can be seen with secretagogue agents such as sulfonylureas or insulin secretagogues since both classes of agents stimulate endogenous insulin secretion."

After ruling out any usage of exogenous insulin regimen, origin of endogenous hyperinsulinemia has to be reviewed. Localization can generally be done by abdominal computed tomography (CT) along with MRI.

## Management

Recognizing an individual with hypoglycemia seems difficult because of the possible detrimental consequences like coma and/or death. Serious hypoglycemic should be managed by intravenous (IV) dextrose along with infusion of glucose. In case of responsive individuals capable of taking medication orally (PO), quick digestible glucose containing food (like fruit juice) must be advised. In individuals those are not able to eat orally, 1-mg intramuscular (IM) injection of glucagon can be administered (Joel Thome DB, 2019).

When the individual reaches an awake state, any form of food sources rich in glucose can be given to the individual so as to reach balanced euglycemia. Vigilant blood glucose monitoring must be done so as to prevent low glucose levels in future.

Nonmedical treatment for frequently occurring episodes of hypoglycemia comprises of health awareness and lifestyle modification. Many of them are not aware of the critical consequences of continuous hypoglycemia. Also, health education should be given on significance of regular blood glucose track and how to recognize of the initial signs of hypoglycemia.

In cases lifestyle modifications does not affect in controlling incidents, opt for pharmacological interventions must be changed. Individuals at risk should be counseled "to wear a medical alert bracelet and to carry a glucose source like gel, candy or tablets in case symptoms arise". During outpatient department visit, assessing blood sugar logs and food logs have been found beneficial in recognizing concerns of the individual.

## Differential Diagnosis

In cases where hypoglycemia has been established, then main objective is to correct first hypoglycemia along with recognizing the associated factors. While treating hypoglycemia, background must involve drugs and nutritional compliance, modification of medicines, doubt of presence of serious renal trauma and knowingly or unknowingly administration of medicines more than advised dosage.

## Complications

If not treated promptly hypoglycemia results in severe neurologic complications, even may lead to coma or loss of life.

Almost all patients with hypoglycemia are managed conservatively. Repetitive attacks of hypoglycemia without any evidence or noticeable effect sometimes call for specialist by senior endocrinologist. Discussion with diabetic health education provider will prove helpful to manage and prevent future complications. Hypoglycemia has been frequently found among newborn children, especially among women having uncurbed diabetes.

### Integrated Approach

A multidisciplinary perspective towards treating hypoglycemia is advocated. Appropriate course of action on minimizing hypoglycemia episodes includes partaking and persuasive advice among "primary care physicians, physician assistant, nurse practitioner, endocrinologists, diabetes educators, pharmacists, diabetic nurses, the patient's family and the patient". The key person in managing is none other than the patient themselves. Non-compliance to medications and dietary advises frequently lead to nonfulfillment of the objective. Individuals must stick to a workable exercise with proper diet which will help prevent sudden increase or decrease of hourly blood glucose levels. A multidisciplinary perspective towards hypoglycemia, will result in optimum management which results in healthier quality of living in patients (Amy Hess-Fisch, 2019).

### Nursing Management

The nursing diagnosis of risk for unstable blood glucose level, according to the North American Nursing Diagnosis Association International 9 (NANDA-I), poses several additional dangers and nursing diagnoses for the patient. The nurse's role is to diagnose human responses that are within the scope and level of skill of the nurse. Critical thinking is required to identify and comprehend the risk factors of unstable blood glucose levels, notably low levels for the purposes of this study, as well as the accompanying signs and symptoms upon patient presentation.

Nursing diagnoses are critical because they influence the nursing care plan and determine the patient's prognosis. Clear nursing diagnoses are essential for each patient and should be tailored to the patient's specific presentation. Nurses must also make nursing diagnoses rather than medical diagnoses, which are made by advanced physicians and clinicians.

It is critical to know whether the patient has type I or type II diabetes, any current pharmacologic therapy, a history of unstable blood glucose or hypoglycemia, adherence to a special diet or medications, current or recent illnesses that could affect the glucose, and social history in the case of unstable blood glucose. Alcohol consumption (which may alter gluconeogenesis and glycogenolysis) and drug usage (which may decrease the patient's desire to eat in addition to creating unfavorable physiologic effects) are examples of physical activity and other social history. A precise nursing diagnosis is critical to establishing a stable blood glucose level and preventing undesirable outcomes such as organ damage, coma and death. During an episode of unstable or low blood glucose, it is critical to monitor the patient's glucose level on a regular basis.

Pharmacologic and nonpharmacologic nursing interventions may be used to treat hypoglycemia episodes. Any patient exhibiting signs of unstable blood sugar, especially hypoglycemia, requires immediate and frequent glucose monitoring. For the aware patient, nursing care may involve giving them three or so glucose tablets, glucose gel, or carbs. 4 to 6 ounces of fruit juice or soda (not sugar-free), saltine crackers, or hard candies (only if the patient is awake) are acceptable forms of carbohydrates. Nursing management of hypoglycemia for an unconscious patient comprises securing appropriate intravenous access and, if necessary, administering 50% dextrose or glucagon in accordance with facility procedure or a healthcare provider's order.

Monitoring and maintaining blood glucose levels within normal ranges as well as the remission of hypoglycemic signs and symptoms should be expected nursing outcomes for patients who are experiencing hypoglycemia promptly. The nurse should anticipate that patients who underwent neurological alterations or lost consciousness will return consciousness without any disabilities, such as paresthesia or aphasia. This involves the reversal of behavioral alterations, perplexity, and occasionally stroke-mimicking convulsions. Before leaving the patient unattended, the nurse should be confident that the hypoglycemic episode has passed.

The following long-term outcomes for the patient should be expected: regular glucose monitoring, maintenance of normal glucose levels, maintenance of normal hemoglobin A1c levels, adherence to medications, diet, and medical appointments, evidence of the patient's capacity to recognize the signs and symptoms of hypoglycemia, self-management of hypoglycemia, and comprehension of when and what information to report to the provider.

## HYPERGLYCEMIA

"The term hyperglycemia derived from the Greek hyper (high) + glykys (sweet/sugar) + haima (blood). Hyperglycemia is blood glucose greater than 125 mg/dL while fasting and greater than 180 mg/dL 2 hours postprandial". An individual having altered glucose tolerance, or pre-diabetes, if fasting plasma glucose is "100 mg/dL to 125 mg/dL". An individual is said to be diabetic if the fasting blood glucose is higher than "125 mg/dL" (Mouri Mi, 2019).

In cases where "hyperglycemia" is not tackled, which may result in several critical threat to the life conditions which involves eye damage, renal, neurological, cardiovascular system. Hence, it is becoming very important to treat 'hyperglycemia' promptly and successfully to abet difficulties related to the disease and enhance patient outcomes.

## Etiology

The main contributing factors towards "Hyperglycemia" are reduced insulin release, decreased glucose usage, subsequently elevated glucose manufacture. "Glucose homeostasis is a balance between hepatic glucose production and peripheral glucose uptake and utilization". Insulin plays most vital role in regulating the glucose homeostasis.

Secondary cause of hyperglycemia include the following:
- Wrecking the pancreas from long standing pancreatitis, hemochromatosis, pancreatic cancer and cystic fibrosis.
- Endocrine complications which leads to "peripheral insulin resistance such as Cushing syndrome, acromegaly and pheochromocytoma".
- Usage of medicines such as "glucocorticoids, phenytoin, and estrogens".
- Diabetes during gestation is established among more than 4% of all gestations and is commonly because of reduced insulin reactivity.
- Absolute TPN or hyperalimentation and dextrose infusions.
- Responsiveness observed post-surgery and among basically sick patients.

Prime risks for causing hyperglycemia:
- Obesity greater or equal to 120 percent off required healthy bodyweight.
- History of type II diabetes in family.
- "Native Americans, Hispanics, Asian Americans, Pacific Islanders, or African Americans".
- Existing conditions of hyperlipidemia or hypertension.
- History GDM.
- Existing conditions like PCOD/PCOS.

## Epidemiology

Increasing rate of "hyperglycemia" has been alarming throughout past 20 years because of multiplying rate of obesity, lowered physical activity, and a growing old age group. The prevalence is similar among both genders. "The nations having the higher count of patients with diabetes included China, India, United States, Brazil, and Russia". "Hyperglycemia" has been quite evident among below to middle-earning family.

"The latest data released by the centers for disease control and prevention indicate that there are nearly 30.5 million Americans with diabetes and nearly 84 million Americans with pre-diabetes". The count is predicted to rise in the coming years.

## Pathophysiology

"Hyperglycemia" of an individual having type I diabetes occur as an outcome of "genetic, environmental, and immunologic" elements. Which results in wrecking off pancreatic beta cells and insulin insufficiency. An individual having type II diabetes, insulin resistance and disrupted insulin secretions results in "hyperglycemia".

As per current research, metabolic diseases like type II diabetes mellitus elevates chances of cognitive disorders and Alzheimer's dementia". "Alzheimer's dementia" is a significant result of diabetes type II current research has shown that the diseases are interrelated one to the other at clinically as well molecularly. As peripherally insulin resistance results in type II diabetes, cerebral insulin resistance is connected with neurologic disorder and cognitive deterioration in "Alzheimer's dementia". **Flowchart 11.1** explains the pathogenesis of hyperglycemia.

## History and Physical Assessment

Signs of serious "hyperglycemia" are polyuria, polydipsia, and weight dropping. If an individuals blood glucose rises, nervous system complications may evolve. An individual possibly feel lethargic, central neurological deficiencies, and altered mental status. An individual may advance into coma.

Individuals having diabetic ketoacidosis can come complaining of nausea, vomiting and abdominal discomfort including the above mentioned manifestations. Patients breath may have a fruity smell and have rapid superficial breathing, contemplating compensatory hyperventilation due to acidosis.

Physical assessment may show symptoms of hypovolemia like hypotension, tachycardia and parched mucosa.

### Clinical Assessment

During assessment for a patient for hyperglycemia, prime attention has to be given to individuals cardiorespiratory function, mental state and volume level. In addition serum glucose should be taken promptly. Tests comprise serum electrolytes along with the estimation for the anion gap, blood urea nitrogen and creatinine, and CBC. Urine test

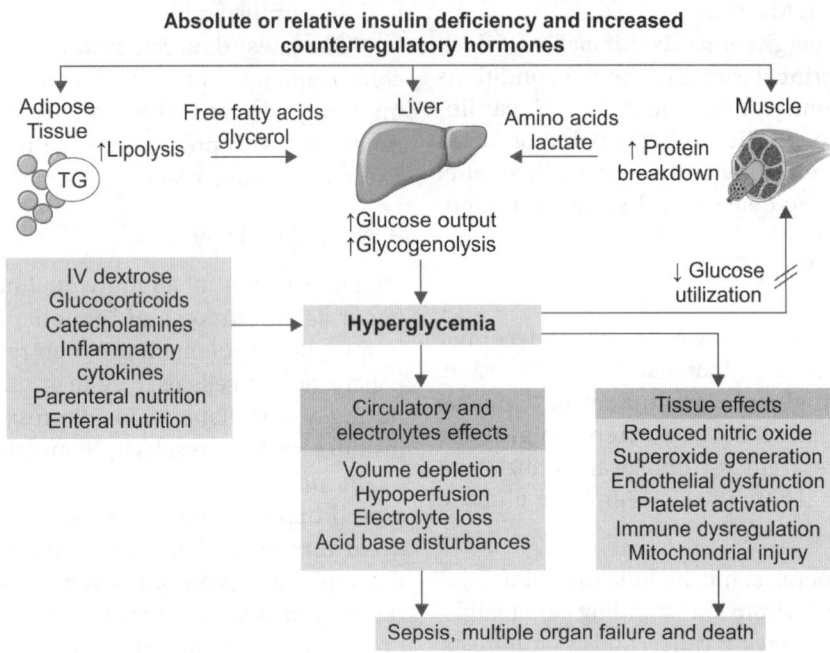

**Flowchart 11.1:** Pathogenesis of hyperglycemia.

with dipstick evaluation for the presence of glucose and ketones bodies in the urine. ABG or VBG are needed in cases where serum bicarbonate is markedly lowered.

*Determining Levels of Blood Glucose*

For ascertaining whether an individual is progressing to type II diabetes an individual requires tests results mentioned:
- Fasting plasma glucose level of 126 mg/dL or higher.
- 2-hour plasma glucose level of 200 mg/dL or higher during a 75 g oral glucose tolerance test (oGTT).
- Random plasma glucose of 200 mg/dL or higher in the presence of symptoms of hyperglycemia.
- Hemoglobin A1c level of 6.5% or higher.

*Treatment/Management*

Important management objective of "hyperglycemia" include terminating manifestations associated with "hyperglycemia" along with lessen abiding difficulty. Glycemic control of individuals having type I diabetes is accomplished with changing insulin routine alongside appropriate nutritional therapy. Individuals having type 2 diabetes are treated by dietary and living style modification along with drugs. Individuals having hyperglycemia required to be monitored for issues like retinopathy, nephropathy, and cardiovascular ailments (Kahn ASA TJA, 2004).

*Objectives of Management*

Management objectives are reducing following complications related with hyperglycemia:
- Renal and optic issues by regulating blood pressure and reducing hyperglycemia.
- Ischemic cardiopathy, stroke and peripheral vasculature disorder by managing hypertension, hyperlipidemia, and termination of smoking.
- Lowering likelihood to "metabolic syndrome and stroke" with controlled weight management and controlling the "hyperglycemia".
- Individuals with "hyperglycemia" while having established status of having type 2 diabetes require referral to an endocrinologist. If there exists no contraindications, the treatment of choice to reduce level of hyperglycemia is metformin. Additionally, many patients need insulin therapy and additional combined medications.

*Preventions for Complications*

The prevention of complications related to "hyperglycemia", following recommended preventative measures:
- Referring for an eye examination annually by an ophthalmologist.
- Monitoring A1c levels within a period of 3–6 month.
- Monitoring urine albumin levels annually.
- Examining feet of the patient at every session.

- Maintaining the blood pressure levels below "130/80 mm Hg".
- Initiating statin therapy in cases an individual is hyperlipidemic.

Several individuals carry the risk of higher glycemic fluctuations of their blood glucose in a 24 hours period along with variations in the similar time on subsequent days, which in turn causes repeated attacks "of hypoglycemia and hyperglycemia". The individuals require meticulous supervision by an endocrinologist followed by strict management regimen aimed in reducing equally the risks or to minimum sustain one while lowering associated risks.

### Differential Diagnoses

Differential diagnoses of "hyperglycemia" comprise:
- Diabetes mellitus type I and II.
- Stress induced "hyperglycemia".
- Medication inducedex. steroids.
- Acromegaly.
- Cushing's syndrome.
- Iatrogenic (parenteral nutrition).

### Treatment of Hyperglycemia in a Hospital Setting

See **Table 11.3**.

### Prognosis

Prognosis of patients having hyperglycemia is dependent on what extent the levels of blood sugar are under control. Persistent hyperglycemia has potential to produce serious lifeand limb-threatening conditions. Modifications in lifestyle, routine physical activity and dietary modifications are vital for an improved prognosis. Patients who manage euglycemia has reported significantly improved prognosis and better quality of life in contrast to those patients who fail to manage hyperglycemia. If the complexities of hyperglycemia once develop, almost always they are pretty-much permanent. Numerous researches reported unmanaged hyperglycemia reduces longevity and detetoriate the quality of life. Hence, combative reduction of hyperglycemia is started, and individuals should carefully be tracked. Researches indicated that focus should be to accomplish an A1C of less than 7%. However, containing blood glucose very firmly may lead to hypoglycemia which is not properly endured by older patients who are currently having a diagnosed cardiomyopathy (Kitabchi AE, Umpierrez GE).

### Complications

Problems resulting from unmanaged and unchecked "hyperglycemia" for an extended duration:

*Microvascular*
- Diabetic retina disorder
- Renal diseases
- Neurological disorders

*Macrovascular*
- Cerebrovascular impairments
- Peripheral vascular impairments
- Postoperative and rehabilitation care.

"Hyperglycemia" a frequent postoperative complication. High blood glucose in postoperative period is related with greater intraoperative complexities so the aimed blood glucose level has to be maintained about 140–180 mg/dL. **Figure 11.3** describes the pharmacological treatment of hyperglycemia according to site of action. Multidisciplinary care approach postoperatively is provided to individual throughout medical staying, thereby creating a follow-up protocol to manage hyperglycemia and reduce intraoperative complexities.

### Nursing Management

Impaired skin integrity if a superficial rash is present, impaired tissue integrity if a wound is present, deficient knowledge, imbalanced nutrition, and ineffective health maintenance are some nursing diagnoses that may be appropriate for patients with a medical diagnosis of diabetes mellitus. If the disease is not properly managed, it can lead to hospitalization, a fluid volume deficit with extreme hyperglycemia such as diabetic ketoacidosis, a risk of falls in the presence of dizziness, peripheral neuropathy, or vision changes, a risk of infection with chronic hyperglycemia, especially in the presence of an open wound, a risk of injury if there is nerve damage such as peripheral neuropathy, and a risk of unstable blood glucose if blood glucose fluctuates.

The most prevalent life-threatening condition that necessitates rapid nursing care is hypoglycemia. Extreme hyperglycemia is uncommon, but it is a possibility. As a result, nurses must notice clinical signs of elevated blood glucose levels in patients and incorporate blood glucose monitoring into their care plan. Nursing management also includes assessing the patient for type 2 diabetes mellitus problems and giving patient education on the plan of care, as well as good dietary intake, activity guidelines, and the recommended medication regimen as needed.

## DIABETIC KETOACIDOSIS

Diabetic ketoacidosis (DKA) is a fatal condition is a complication of diabetes. Increase in metabolic rate of fat is the main reason behind DKA. End product of fat metabolisms by liver is ketones which is acidic in nature. Diabetic acidosis may be mild, moderate, or severe based on rate of fat metabolisms. **Table 11.4** shows the classification of DKA. More ketone in body more worst will be the mental condition.

## Symptoms of Diabetic Acidosis

Diabetic acidosis itself is a symptom of type 1 diabetes than disease.

Typical symptoms of diabetic acidosis include:
- Emesis
- Dehydration
- An abnormal odor of the breath – fruity odor
- Heavy breathing (called kussmaul breathing) or hyperventilation
- Palpitation

**Table 11.3:** Major guidelines for treatment of hyperglycemia in a hospital setting.

| | ICU | Non-ICU |
|---|---|---|
| ADA/AACE | • Initiate insulin therapy for persistent hyperglycemia (glucose >180 mg/dL [>10 mmol/L])<br>• Treatment goal: For most people, target a glucose level between 140–180 mg/dL (7.8–10.0 mmol/L)<br>• More stringent goals (110–140 mg/dL [6.1–7.8 mmol/L]) may be appropriate for selected individuals, if achievable without significant risk for hypoglycemia | • No specific guidelines<br>• If treated with insulin, pre-meal glucose targets should generally be <140 mg/dL (<7.8 mmol/L), with random glucose levels <180 mg/dL (<10.0 mmol/L)<br>• More stringent targets may be appropriate for those with previously tight glycemic control. Less stringent targets may be appropriate in people with severe comorbidities |
| ACP | • Recommends against intensive insulin therapy in those with or without diabetes in surgical/medical ICUs<br>• Treatment goal: Target glucose between 140–200 mg/dL (7.8–11.0 mmol/L), in people with or without diabetes, in surgical/medical ICUs | |
| Critical care society | • Glucose >150 mg/dL (>8.3 mmol/L) should trigger insulin therapy<br>• Treatment goal: Maintain glucose <150 mg/dL (<8.3 mmol/L) for most adults in ICU<br>• Maintain glucose levels <180 mg/dL (10.0 mmol/L) while avoiding hypoglycemia | |
| Endocrine society | | • Pre-meal glucose target <140 mg/dL (<7.8 mmol/L) and random blood glucose <180 mg/dL (<10.0 mmol/L). A lower target range may be appropriate in people able to achieve and maintain glycemic control without hypoglycemia. A glucose of <180–200 mg/dL (<10.0–11.0 mmol/L) is appropriate in those with terminal illness and/or with limited life expectancy or at high risk for hypoglycemia.<br>• Adjust antidiabetic therapy when glucose falls <100 mg/dL (<5.6 mmol/L) to avoid hypoglycemia |
| Society of thoracic surgeons (guidelines specific to adult cardiac surgery) | • Continuous insulin infusion preferred over SC or intermittent intravenous boluses.<br>• Treatment goal: Recommend glucose <180 mg/dL (<10.0 mmol/l) during surgery (≤10 mg/dL [≤6.1 mmol/L] in fasting and pre-meal states) | |
| Joint British Diabetes Society for inpatient care | | Target blood glucose levels in most people of between 108–180 mg/dL (6.0–10 mmol/L) with an acceptable range of between 72–216 mg/dL (4.0–12.0 mmol/L) |

AACE/ADA: American Association of Endocrinologists and American Diabetes Association joint guidelines; ACP: American College of Physicians; ADA: American Diabetes Association; ICU: intensive care unit

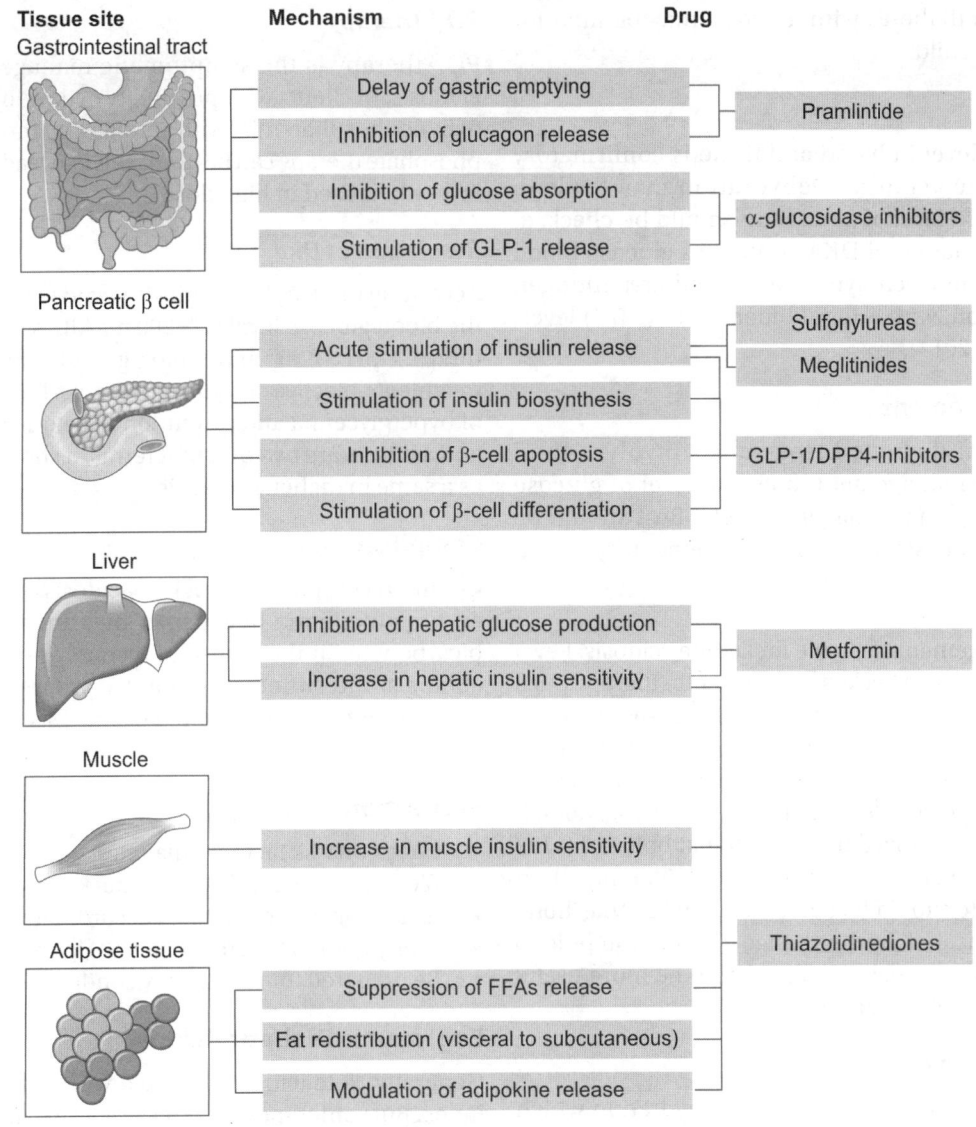

Fig. 11.3: Pharmacological treatment of hyperglycemia according to site of action.

| Table 11.4: Classification of DKA. | | | |
|---|---|---|---|
| **Parameters** | **Mild** | **Moderate** | **Severe** |
| Serum bicarbonate (mmol/L) | 15–18 | 10<15 | <10 |
| Arterial pH | 7.25–7.30 | 7.0–7.24 | <7.0 |
| Anion gap | >10 | >12 | >12 |
| Mental status | Alert | Alert/Drowsy | Stupor/Coma |

- Confusion and disorientation
- Coma

Diabetic acidosis appears due to high blood glucose level since long period of time (hyperglycemia).

## Causes

Lack of insulin in body impaired glucose metabolisms.

Diabetic acidosis have various of etiology:
- Having over 15 mmol/L consistently blood glucose levels
- Forgetting insulin shots
- Development of a fault in insulin pen or insulin pump
- As an outcome of illness or infections
- Higher or continuous levels of stress
- Uncontrolled alcohol intake
- Illicit drug consumption

DKA can possibly happen preceding the identification of type 1 diabetes.

Gestational diabetes with acidosis may be fatal for mother and her child.

## Diagnosis

Raised ketone level in blood and urine is confirmatory test for diabetic acidosis. Dehydration may leads to hypokalemia and level of potassium should be checked. Laboratory evaluation of DKA comprises glucose blood evaluation, serum electrolyte levels, blood urea nitrogen (BUN) evaluation, with arterial blood gases (ABG) levels (Gosmanov AR, 2014).

## Clinical Management

Management of diabetic ketoacidosis involves fluid and electrolyte management, increase level of glucose management, ketone management, etc. Rest should be done accordingly to symptomatic management.

### Insulin Therapy

Insulin is management of choice for ketone acidosis. Level of potassium must be checked before insulin therapy (>3.3 mmol/L). In diabetic acidosis, regular insulin should be 0.1 u/kg body weight insulin should given intravenous (IV) and in continous infusion per hourly. Aim of insulin therapy is to reduce blood glucose level at the rate 50–70 mg/hour. If condition is not improved then additional bolus of 0.1u/kg should administer till it reaches 200–250 mg/dL in DKA, insulin rate should be decreased to 0.05 U/kg/hour, followed, as indicated, by the change in hydration fluid to D5 ½ NS. Insulin through IV route would be more useful than regular dose of insulin.

### Potassium Therapy

Client having ketoacidosis may have dehydration which leads to hypokalemia. Therefore potassium therapy should start immediately and insulin should withhold till potassium level raised to >3.3 mmol/L. Low level of potassium may leads to respiratory distress and arrythmias.

### $HCO_3$ Therapy

$HCO_3$ therapy is used to correct the alter pH level of the body. Raised pH of blood stops fat metabolisms and hence helps insulin to treat ketoacidosis. $HCO_3$ therapy can leads to low potassium level, decreased tissue perfusion and cerebral edema and slow down in the correction of ketosis. Nevertheless, clients having critical ketoacidosis (bicarbonate <10 mEq/L, or $PCO_2$ <12) could possibly encounter decrease pH if failed to manage with $HCO_3$.

### $PO_4^3$ Therapy

$PO_4^3$ therapy is the symptomatic management of ketoacidosis. In clients with possibility of developing problems of hypophosphatemia, with cardiac and muscle weakness, phosphate therapy can be used. This can lead to low calcium level when used in high dose.

### Resolution of Dka

According to ADA, ketoacidosis is said to be resolved upon the blood glucose level is "<200 mg/dL", serum $HCO_3$ " ≥15 mEq/L", "pH >7.30" and "anion gap ≤12 mEq/L". Thus, the treatment objective of ketoacidosis must focus on correction of hyperglycemia and resolution of ketone bodies. Ketosis and acidosis are two different terms, it should not be taken as a same in diabetic acidosis.

## Complications

Common complications of ketoacidosis are hypoglycemia and hypokalemia because of overdose of insulin and bicarbonate. In the course of recovery period of diabetes acidosis, the sufferer frequently progress to a passing hyperchloremic non-anion gap acidosis, which typically got fewer clinical significance.

## Prevention

- Check on risk factor of diabetes.
- Blood glucose level should check at regular interval.
- Insulin dose should taken accordingly.
- Fruity odor of breath should not ignore.
- Be prepared for emergency condition.

## Euglycemic Diabetic Acidosis

Generally, ketoacidosis is linked with high hyperlycemic index. But sometimes in few case it also happen with usual blood glucose. This condition normally called euglycemic diabetic ketoacidosis and it is due to irregular maintenance of insulin intake.

### Nursing Management

The most common nursing diagnosis are nausea and vomiting, pain in the abdomen, extreme thirst, dyspnea and malaise, urination that is too frequent, confusion, high blood sugar levels, breath that smells like fruit, ketone levels in the urine are extremely high.

- Monitor vitals
- Check blood sugars and treat with insulin as ordered
- Start two large-bore IVs
- Administer fluids as recommended
- Check electrolytes as potassium levels will drop with insulin treatment

- Check renal function
- Assess mental status
- Look for signs of infection (a common cause of DKA)
- Educate the patient on the importance of compliance with diabetic medications
- Educate the patient on the importance of follow-up
- Check urine output
- Encourage patient to quit smoking and abstain from alcohol
- Encourage a healthy diet
- Ask the patient to wear an ID bracelet signifying that he or she has had a DKA episode
- Check urine and blood cultures
- Listen to the lungs for rales and crackles.

# THYROID STORM

Thyroid storm, or thyrotoxic crisis, is an acute, debilitating, hypermetabolic condition caused by unrestrained secretion of thyroid hormones (THs) in persons with thyrotoxicosis. Thyroid storm may be the primary display of thyrotoxicosis in unidentified case of children, particularly in newborn. The clinical symptoms comprise "pyrexia, tachycardia, hypertension, and neurological and GI abnormalities". High blood pressure may lead to cardiac arrest that is related with hypotension and shock. Because thyroid storm is practically every time deadly if not treated, early diagnosis and prompt treatment are critical. Thankfully, it is very infrequent among young (healthline.com, 2019).

Identification is fundamentally based on clinical symptoms, and no particular diagnostic procedures are fixed. Many elements could potentially accelerate development of thyrotoxicosis to thyroid storm. Previously, thyroid storm was frequently discovered in the course of a thyroid surgery, often in grown up young ones and mature persons, but advanced presurgical treatment has remarkably reduced the occurrence of this problem. Presently, thyroid storm is seen frequently as a medical problem in lieu of a surgical crisis.

## Diagnosis

The assessment of thyroid storm depends on clinical symptoms, instead of laboratory assessments. If the person's signs and symptoms are in line with thyroid storm, without any hold up start treatment till laboratory support of thyrotoxicosis.

Outcomes of thyroid assessments are almost always in line with hyperthyroidism and are helpful in cases where the sufferer has not been identified previously.

Frequent results include high levels of triiodothyronine ($T_3$), thyroxine ($T_4$), and free $T_4$ values; higher $T_3$ resin absorption; subdued thyroid-stimulating hormone (TSH) values; and an increased 24-hour iodine absorption. TSH values are not subdued in infrequent occasions of increased TSH production. **Flowchart 11.2** shows an algorithm for diagnostic considerations in thyroid storm TS, thyroid storm; ICU, intensive care unit; $T_3$, triiodothyronine; $T_4$, thyroxine; US, ultrasound examination; TRAb, anti-thyroid stimulating hormone receptor antibody.

Cardiac enlargement because of congestive heart failure can be seen in chest radiographic assessment. Radiographic assessment could possibly make clear pulmonary edema as a result of cardiac failure indicated by pulmonary inflammation.

Computed tomography (CT) of the head will be vital to rule out any neurologic infirmities if assessment is unsure following the primary equilibrium of a patient who had come with disorientation.

## Pathophysiology

Thyroid storm is an undermined condition of thyroid hormone–effect, serious hypermetabolism including numerous organs and is considered as the majorly maximal condition of thyrotoxicosis. The signs and symptoms associated to extremely elaborate consequences of THs related to over secretion (unrelated to raised production) or, infrequently, surge consumption of TH.

Intolerance to heat with perspiration can be seen frequently in uncomplicated thyrotoxicosis but evident as high fever in thyroid storm. Unusually increased metabolism demands a rise in oxygen and energy requirement. Cardiovascular detection of temperate abnormally rapid sinus rythm in thyrotoxicosis increase to advanced tachycardia, increased blood pressure, increased-output heart failure, and a tendency to arise cardiopathy. In the same manner, irritation and confusion in thyrotoxicosis advances to extreme deliriousness, rage, convulsions, and can become comatose. Gastro intestinal demonstration of thyroid storm are diarrhea, emesis, hepatitis and enteralgia, in contradiction to just light increase of transaminases and plain improvement of enteral transfer in thyrotoxicosis (healthline.com, 2019).

## Etiology

Thyroid storm is triggered by the features mentioned below in patients having thyrotoxicosis:
- Septicemia
- Any invasive procedure
- Anesthesia induction
- Radioactive iodine (RAI) therapy
- Drugs like anticholinergic and adrenergic drugs, pseudoephedrine; salicylates; nonsteroidal anti-inflammatory drugs (NSAIDs); chemotherapy

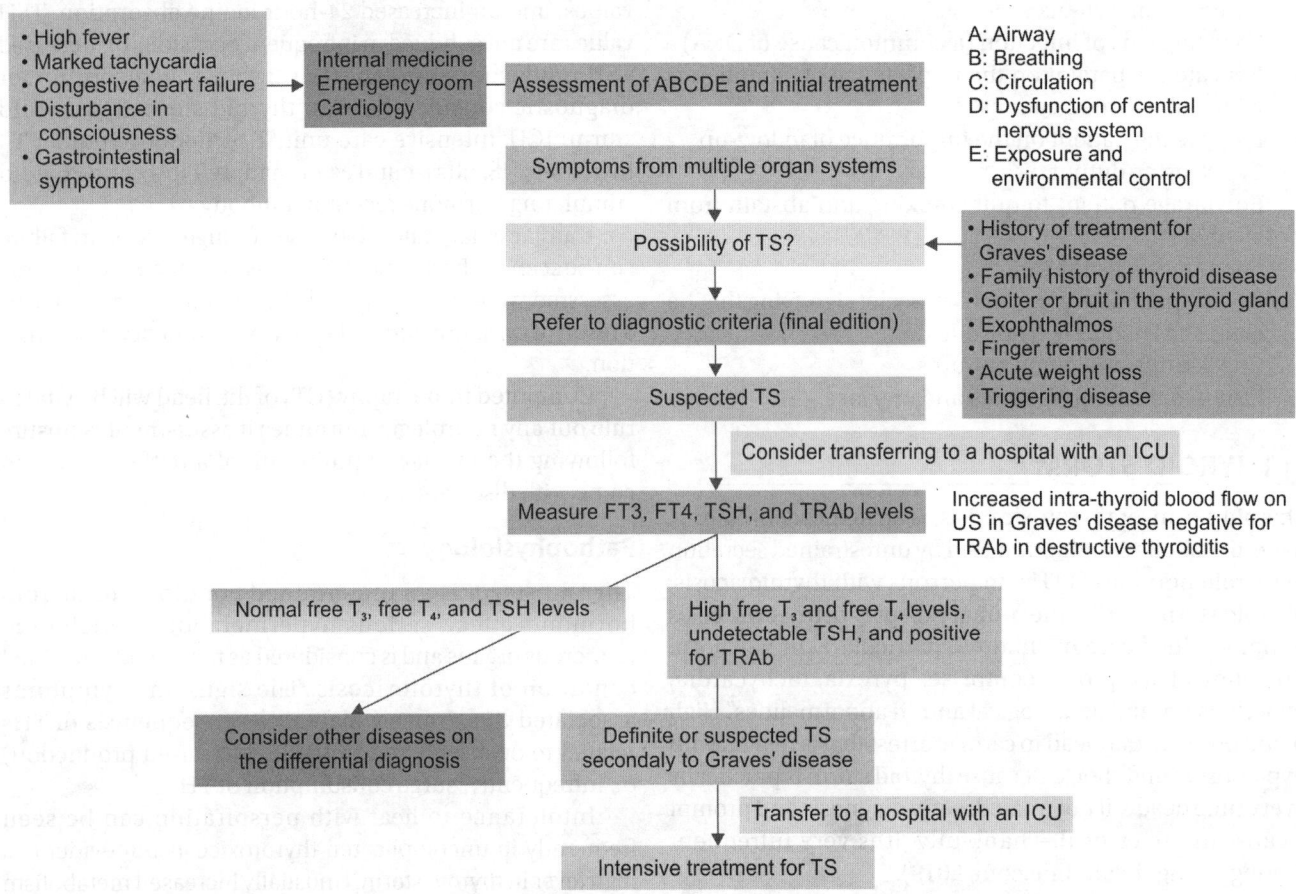

Flowchart 11.2: An algorithm for diagnostic considerations in thyroid storm.

(TS: thyroid storm; ICU: intensive care unit; $T_3$: triiodothyronine; $T_4$: thyroxine; US: ultrasound examination; TRAb: anti-thyroid stimulating hormone receptor antibody).

- Overt thyroid hormone (TH) ingestion
- Termination of or withholding antithyroid medications
- Diabetic ketoacidosis
- Injury to the thyroid gland
- Repeated stimulation of an expanded thyroid by palpation
- Toxemia of pregnancy and labor in teens; molar pregnancy
- Thyroid storm can arise among young with thyrotoxicosis from any cause but is frequently related with Graves disease.
- Transplacental passage of maternal thyroid-stimulating immunoglobulins in neonates
- McCune-Albright syndrome with autonomous thyroid function
- Hyperfunctioning thyroid nodule
- Hyperfunctioning multi nodular goiter
- Thyroid-stimulating hormone (TSH)—secreting tumor.

Thyrotoxicosis found to be "3–5 times" more frequent in women compared to men, mostly among adolescents. Thyroid storm attack a less percent of individuals having thyrotoxicosis. The occurrence is probably more in women; but, there is no evidence based data about gender-distinct occurrences are available.

The occurrences of thyrotoxicosis is frequently through the 30 to 40 years of age. As young age thyrotoxicosis commonly seen in adolescents, thyroid storm is frequently seen among adolescent age group, despite it is seen in all ages.

Thyroid storm is a critical, lethal crisis. If not treated, thyroid storm is universally deadly among elderly (90% mortality rate) frequently known to give rise to comparably serious consequences among young. Loss of life from thyroid storm frequently are result of cardiac arrhythmia, congestive cardiac failure, high fever, multiple system disorder, or various causes, frequently the culminating elements are mostly the reason behind death (Remonti, 2014).

## Management

Treatment plan for thyroid storm is as the following:
- Supportive measures
- Antiadrenergic drugs
- Thionamides
- Iodine preparations
- Glucocorticoids
- Bile acid sequestrants
- Management of the coexisting diseases
- Infrequently plasmapheresis

Persons having medical reasons to avoid thionamides should be treated with "supportive measures, combative beta blockade, iodine preparations, glucocorticoids, and bile acid sequestrants" is given for a period of one week prior to a thyroidectomy. Plasmapheresis could be considered otherwise if regular plans are not beneficial. **Figure 11.4** describes specific and supportive therapy in patients with thyroid storm.

## Nursing Management

The nursing diagnosis may include tiredness, tremor, sweating, hyperactive, palpitations caused by anxiety heat sensitivity, nervous, diarrhea.
- Administer dextrose-containing intravenous fluids as ordered to correct fluid and glucose deficits.
- Carefully assess the patient for heart failure or pulmonary edema.
- Dopamine may be used to support blood pressure.
- Provide supplemental oxygen as ordered to help meet increased metabolic demands.
- Once the patient is hemodynamically stable, provide pulmonary hygiene to reduce pulmonary complications.
- If the patient is in heart failure, typical pharmacologic agents for treatment of heart failure may also be indicated.
- Reduce oxygen demands by decreasing anxiety, reduce fever, decrease pain, and limit visitors if necessary.
- Anticipate aggressive treatment of precipitating factor.
- Institute pressure ulcer strategies.

# MYXEDEMA

The term myxedema is generally used to describe serious condition of hypothyroid disorders. Dermatological modifications which are seen in hypothyroid and rarely hyperthyroid conditions are also called myxedema. **Figure 11.5** skin changes in hyperthyroidism, myxedema is the accumulation of mucopolysaccharides in the layers of skin, leading to inflammation of the inflicted part. Usually in Graves disease, change in skin is seen in hyperthyroidism, it is called pretibial myxedema.

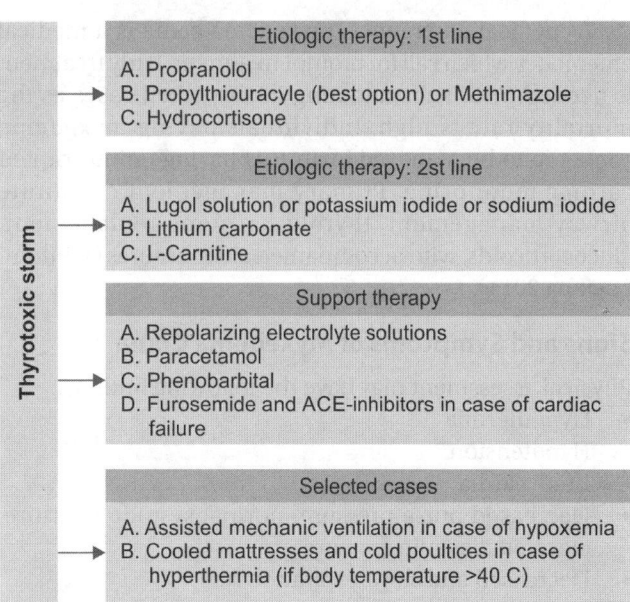

**Fig. 11.4:** Specific and supportive therapy in patients with thyroid storm.

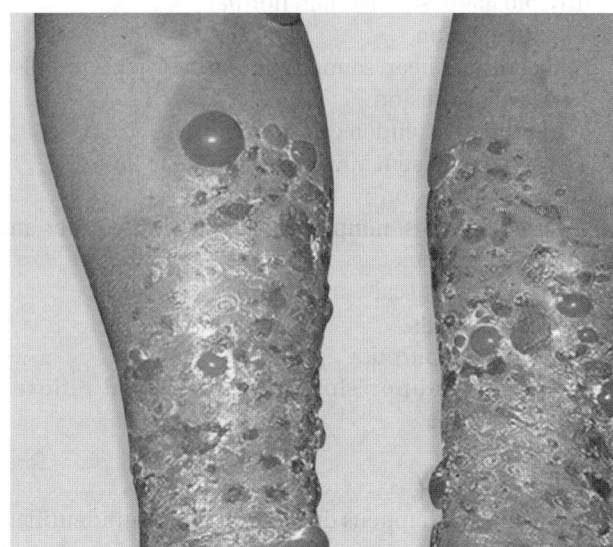

**Fig. 11.5:** Skin changes in hyperthyroidism.

Myxedema coma, sometimes termed as myxedema crisis, is an unusual and a grave medical disorder which represents serious hypothyroid disorder accompanied by physiological deterioration. This disorder is generally seen among individuals having chronic, unidentified hypothyroid disorder and almost always is caused due to infections, cerebrovascular disorders, cardiac arrest, injury, or medications. Individuals having myxedema coma usually are seriously ailing, accompanied by remarkable hypothermia and altered mental condition.

A medical emergency, myxedema coma is a medical emergency which call for prompt treatment. Early treatment is needed prior substantiating in suspected cases as the mortality rate is high. Individuals having myxedema coma are to be managed in an ICU having uninterrupted cardiac monitoring. Primary management constitute airway management, thyroid hormone replacement, glucocorticoids, with accompanied aid measures (Remonti Luciana 2014).

## Signs and Symptoms of Myxedema Coma

Physical assessment may have the following findings:
- Hypothermia
- Hypotension
- Bradycardia
- Decreased pulse pressure, normal systolic pressure, elevated diastolic pressure
- Decreased and slow respiration rate
- Periorbital puffiness
- Macroglossia
- Coarse hair
- Thyroid gland smaller than normal
- Pleural effusion
- Soft or distant heart sounds, diminished apical impulse, pericardial effusion
- Abdominal distention due to ascites
- Decrased or absent bowel sounds due to ileus
- Bladder distension
- Cold extremities, nonpitting edema of the upper and lower extremities
- Cool, pale, dry, scaly, and thickened skin
- Dry, brittle nails
- Ecchymoses, purpura
- Confusion, stupor, slow speech, delayed reflexes, seizures, coma.

## Pathophysiology

Myxedema coma happens due to prolonged, unidentified, and unmanaged hypothyroid disorder which is generally aggravated due to any pre-existing complications. Myxedema coma may occur due to various factors of hypothyroid disorders.

The role of thyroid hormones is vital in cell metabolism, chronic hypothyroid disorders is related to reduce in metabolic rate and lowered oxygen utilization, as a result total body systems are affected adversely. It leads to hypothermic conditions, it serves as a strong factor of mortality. Also results in reduced metabolism of drug resulting in over intake of drugs especially sedatives, hypnotics, and anesthetic agents; which potentially aggravate myxedema coma.

### Cardiovascular

Impaired cardiac contractility, results in decreased stroke volume, lowered cardiac output, bradycardia and occasionally hypotension. Decreased stroke volume in serious patients may be a consequence of pericardial effusions due to the deposition of fluid rich in mucopolysaccharides in the pericardial space. In the absence of any pre existing cardiac disorders congestive cardiac failure is unusual.

Electrocardiographic diagnosis include bradycardia, blockage of varying degrees, low voltage, nonspecific ST-segment changes, flattened or inverted T-waves, prolonged Q-T interval, and ventricular or atrial arrhythmias.

Decreased effect of beta-adrenergic receptors results in long-term effect of "alpha-adrenergic receptors, increased catecholamines, and increased systemic vascular resistance, causing some patients to have diastolic hypertension and a narrowed pulse pressure". "Plasma volume is decreased, and capillary permeability is increased, leading to fluid accumulation in tissue and spaces and pericardial effusions."

### Neurologic

Regardless of the tag myxedema coma, in many cases individuals do not pass into a real coma stage, however shows different levels of state of mind. Brain function is affected by reduced oxygen supply and hence decreased intake, diminished glucose use and decreased cerebral blood supply. Hyponatremia may also lead to altered mental status.

### Pulmonary

Central recession of ventilatory drive with diminished sensitivity to hypoxia and hypercapnia leads to the most significant pulmonary impairment of myxedema coma. hypoventilation. Respiratory muscle weakness, mechanical obstruction by a large tongue, and obesity-hypoventilation syndrome are among various contributing factors to hypoventilation. Fluid accumulation causes pleural effusions and reduced dispensing volume.

### Renal

With decreased glomerular filtration rate due to reduced cardiac output and peripheral vasoconstriction or as a result of rhabdomyolysis renal function may be compromised. As a result of elevated serumi antidiuretic hormone and decreased water elimination in patients with myxedema coma hyponatremia is commonly seen.

### Gastrointestinal

In myxedema coma the gastrointestinal tract has marked infiltration of mucopolysaccharides along with edema.

Additionally, malabsorption, gastric atony, impaired peristalsis, paralytic ileus, and megacolon occurs due to neuropathic modifications. Increased capillary permeability, cardiac arrest, and various other factors results in asites. Secondary to a related blood disorder gastrointestinal bleeding may occur.

### Hematologic

High-risk of bleeding because of coagulopathy linked with an acquired "Von Willebrand Syndrome (Type I)" and decline in factors like "V, VII, VIII, IX, and X" is associated with myxedema coma. Secondary to hemorrhage patients may also have "microcyticanemia, or macrocyticanemia caused by vitamin B12 deficiency, or normocytic normochromic anemia, which may be secondary to decreased oxygen requirement and reduced erythropoietin" (Yang Q., 2011).

## Diagnosis

Laboratory assessments are vital to validate the determination of myxedema coma. Result includes the following:
- Thyroid-stimulating hormone (TSH) is increased in almost all cases, specifying an initial thyroid disorders
- Free thyroxine ($T_4$) and free triiodothyronine ($T_3$) levels are decreased.
- Hyponatremia with reduced serum osmolality
- Because of reduced renal perfusion, serum creatinine levels are generally increased
- Evaluation of adrenal functions must be carried out as well as complete blood count (CBC).
- Leukocytosis may not be found due to hypothermia. A white blood cell count may prove guiding in the existing of infection.
- Chest radiography may picture features of cardiomegaly, pericardial effusion, congestive cardiac failure, or pleural effusion.
- Electrocardiography may show sinus bradycardia, low-amplitude QRS complexes, a prolonged QT interval, flattened or inverted T waves, or arrhythmias.

## Management of Myxedema Coma

Medical care of myxedema coma includes the following:

### Airway Management

- **Thyroid hormone replacement:** Due to the uncommonness of the disease and unavailability of clinical trial hence the absolute approach of treatment and dosage of thyroid hormonal replacement in myxedema coma still remains contentious.
- **Glucocorticoid therapy:** Primary adrenal insufficiency may be seen in patients having primary hypothyroid disorder, whereas hypopituitary disorders and secondary adrenal insufficiency is seen in patients having secondary hypothyroid disorders; corticosteroids are preferred for treatment as there are chances of aggravating acute adrenal insufficiency due to increased metabolic rate of cortisol that results after giving $T_4$ therapy.
- **Supportive measures:** Maintaining the temperature by treating hypothermia; treating concomitant infections; Administer saline and free water restriction for correcting serious hyponatremia; Infuse intravenous dextrose for correcting hypoglycemia; thyroid hormone therapy is commonly used to correct hypotension.

### Nursing Management

Slow metabolic rate, a lack of thyroid hormone, reduced thyroid hormone production, autoimmune illnesses such as Hashimoto's thyroiditis, surgery to remove the thyroid gland, head and neck radiation therapy, thyroid hormone-lowering medications, hypothyroidism at birth, reduced iodine levels.

- Monitor vital signs, including heart rate and rhythm.
- Administer thyroid replacement, levothyroxine sodium (synthroid) is most commonly prescribed.
- Instruct the client about thyroid replacement therapy.
- Instruct the client in low-calorie, low-cholesterol, low-saturated-fate diet.
- Assess the client for constipation; provide roughage and fluids to prevent constipation.
- Provide a warm environment for the client.
- Avoid sedatives and narcotics because of increase sensitivity to these medications.
- Monitor for overdose of thyroid medications, characterized by tachycardia, restlessness, nervousness, and insomnia.
- Instruct the client to report episodes of chest pain immediately.

### Patient Education

Monitoring of thyroid hormone levels by testing regularly and daily intake of thyroid medications has to be explained to the patients who are diagnosed with hypothyroidism.

Counseling should be provided to patients with history of thyroiditis, thyroid irradiation or thyroid surgery about the recurrence of hypothyroidism in future. Health education should be provided on the signs and symptoms of hypothyroidism and the importance of timely medical advise, diagnosis and assessment has to be explained.

## ADRENAL CRISIS

'Adrenal crisis', is a severe 'adrenal insufficiency' is a serious deadly state with a death rate of 0.5/100 annually (Vikas Sharma, 2014). It is regarded as one of the endocrine crisis aggravated by both inner and outer activity in the situation of identified or unidentified decrease in secretion of cortisol the 'adrenal hormone', the key 'glucocorticoid'. Prompt recognition and early treatment can be life saving for a patient and effect living. The diagnosis should be done to draw a line to separate adrenal insufficiency and adrenal crisis as adrenal crisis is life-threatening if not treated. As the disorder is thoroughly explained, it is frequently hard to identify, and starting the management perhaps the hold up causing marked morbidity and mortality.

Anatomic destruction of the gland may be the cause of primary adrenal insufficiency, both acute or chronic. Tuberculosis or fungal infections, other diseases having effect on the adrenal glands may lead to the destruction of the gland, and causes hemorrhage. Although, the commonest factor is idiopathic degradation, most probably which is autoimmune disorder in origin. **Figure 11.6** represents how bodily stress and adrenal insufficiency lead to an adrenal crisis.

Metabolic failure like insufficient hormone production and secretion can also lead to primary adrenal insufficiency, congenital adrenal hyperplasia (CAH), enzyme inhibitors like metyrapone, or cytotoxic agents like mitotane may be the reason of this kind of failure. Primary adrenocortical insufficiency is uncommon which may occur at any age. Affects both the genders equally 1:1.

Hypopituitarism due to hypothalamic-pituitary disease or suppression of the hypothalamic-pituitary axis by exogenous steroids or endogenous steroids like tumors may lead to secondary adrenal insufficiency. Secondary adrenocortical insufficiency is comparatively prevalent. Long-term treatment with steroidal drugs has significantly caused in the increase of cases.

Chronic insufficiency from an acute aggravation may lead to adrenal crisis, generally as a result of sepsis or surgical stress. Adrenal hemorrhage commonly septicemia-induced, water house Friderichsen syndrome (fulminant meningococcemia) and anticoagulation complication may lead to acute adrenal insufficiency. With drawing steriod therapy is the commonest cause which results in acute adrenocortical insufficiency and is significant cause of glucocorticoid deficiency.

"Tertiary causes refer to disruption of the hypothalamus which in turn affects ACTH release".

### Pathophysiology

The pathophysiology leading to adrenal crisis is still obscure. Often it is due to the imbalance in the demand and supply of the hormone cortisol. Increased level of stress from hypothalamic-pituitary axis stimulation which causes rise in ACTH which results in rise of the cortisol. However the contract is also seen in some cases (Remonti Luciana, 2003).

The main function of the adrenal glands is production of glucocorticoids and mineralocorticoids, other hormones are also secreted by adrenal glands are like precursors of sex hormones and catecholamines. The pituitary glands produce ACTH and it plays a vital role in stimulating the release of hormone cortisol from adrenal glands. On the basis of primary insufficiency or secondary insufficiency, which may lead to deficiency of both mineralocorticoid or glucocorticoid or only glucocorticoid. The primary function of aldosterone is potassium secretion and sodium retention. Gluconeogenesis, increased sensitivity to catecholamines, and regulation of the immune system is promoted by hormone cortisol.

In cases where an individual with primary insufficiency gets adrenal crisis, they may also have hyponatremia and hyperkalemia along with being hypoglycemic and hypotensive as a result of both aldosterone and cortisol insufficiency, correspondingly.

Due to reduced sensitivity to catecholamines, hypotension and due to impaired gluconeogenesis, only hypoglycemia is seen among individuals having isolated cortisol deficiency. This is the reason hypotension is all most always refractory to vasopressors. Cortisol function is regulating the cytokines like inflammatory cytokines including tumor necrosis factor.

In cases where there is no release of hormone cortisol in adrenal insufficiency, the TNF-alpha secretion and increased sensitive condition leads to cortisol resistance as a result it increases the mortality of individuals suffering from adrenal crises even after prompt management.

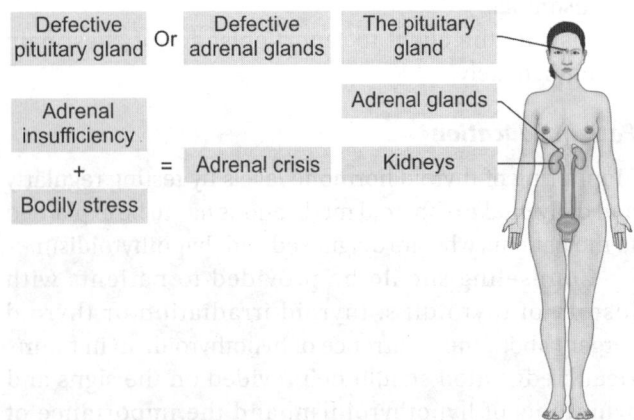

**Fig. 11.6:** Representing how bodily stress and adrenal insufficiency lead to an adrenal crisis.

Among individuals having good health, glucocorticoids increases production of an enzyme which changes norepinephrine to epinephrine. In patients with adrenal insufficiency, the basal and stress-induced epinephrine secretion may be defective and may lead to hypotension or hypoglycemia in crisis condition.

## History and Physical Assessment

An accurate history taking is the primary focus in the evaluation process of patients who are suspicious of adrenal crisis. A detailed of past medical and surgical history is a must.

**Figure 11.7** describes different signs and symptoms of adrenal fatigue syndrome. Any medication prescription has to be reviewed by the evaluating physician. Any use of steroids for a prolonged period has to be reported as an abrupt withdrawal potentially lead to adrenal crisis.

History of autoimmune disease has to be made clear as individuals with autoimmune polyglandular endocrine disorders may have several autoimmune diseases. Among individuals having type I diabetes taking insulin repeated episodes of hypoglycemia should serve as a warning of adrenal insufficiency.

Among young, excessive loss of weight in "61–100%" and various signs like hypoglycemia emergency with seizures. Other symptoms as "anorexia, orthostatic hypotension and tachycardia can be seen in 88–94% of the patients while skin and mucosal hyperpigmentation in 80–94%". GI symptoms like nausea, vomiting and diarrhea which is seen among "75–86%" or episodes of abdominal pain in 31% cases. "The less common presentation are a surgical emergency, amenorrhea, libido reduction, depression in less than 40% of the patients and the least common presentation is salt-craving which is only seen in 9–16% of the patients.

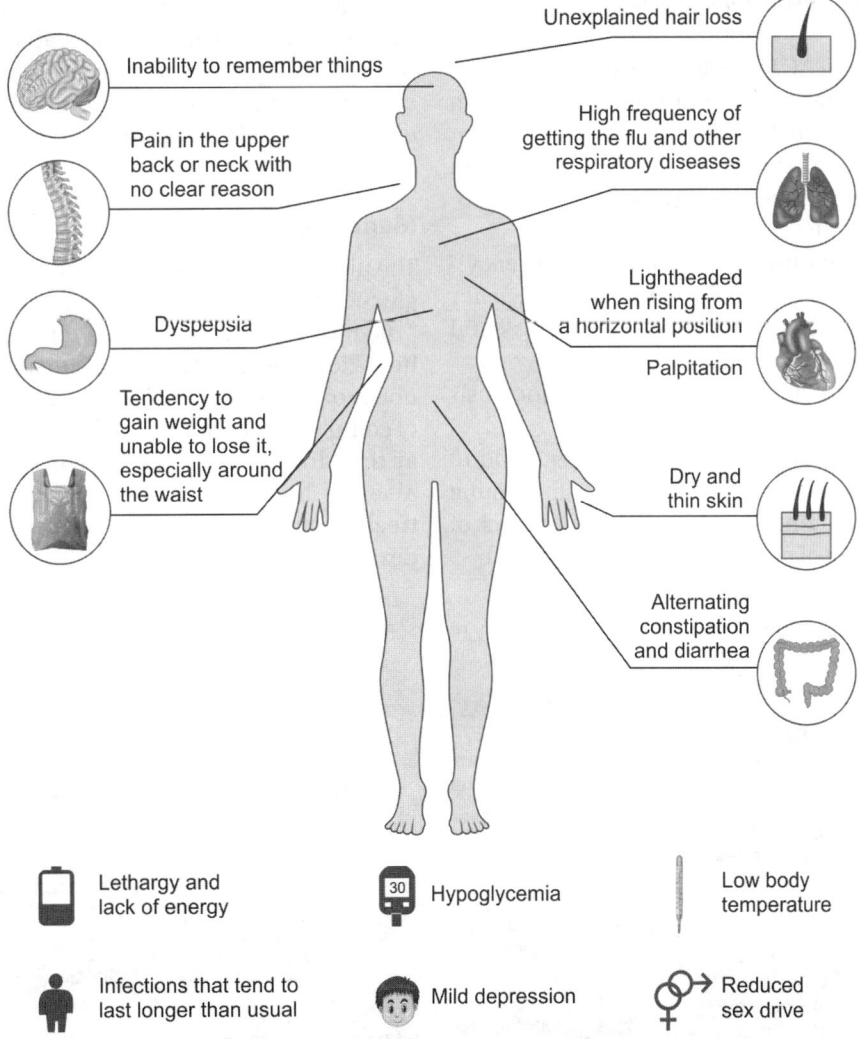

**Fig. 11.7:** Different signs and symptoms of adrenal fatigue syndrome.

Pregnant patients, patients with meningitis and patients with a headache and vision changes represent a small subset of patients that may present with occult adrenal crisis secondary to Sheehan syndrome, Waterhouse-Friedrichsen syndrome, and pituitary apoplexy respectively. Patients with pituitary apoplexy may present with a headache and bitemporal hemianopsia in addition to signs of adrenal crisis." **Flowchart 11.3** diagrammatically representing the Addition's crisis pathway.

## Diagnosis and Management of Adrenal Insufficiency

### Number of Disturbances is Seen in Case of Adrenal Crisis

The basic lab tests shows:
- "Hyponatremia (due to mineralocorticoid deficiency)"
- "Hyperkalemia (due to mineralocorticoid deficiency)"
- "Hypoglycemia (due to decreased gluconeogenesis and glycogenolysis)"
- "Low or low normal ACTH level in secondary adrenal insufficiency and high or high normal ACTH level in primary adrenal insufficiency"
- "Hypercalcemia (due to increased intestinal absorption and decreased renal excretion of calcium)"
- "Prerenal failure with elevated creatinine level"
- "Low aldosterone (due to mineralocorticoid deficiency)"
- "High renin is expected in primary adrenal insufficiency as there is an increase in urinary sodium loss and decreases in the blood volume)"
- "Normocytic normochromic anemia, lymphocytosis and eosinophilia"
- "TSH levels may be increased, usually between 4 and 10 IU/L (due to coexisting hypothyroidism in autoimmune polyglandular endocrine disorders or due to the lack of the inhibitory effect of cortisol on TSH production)"

Confirmatory tests may be scheduled, among individuals where clear assessment of adrenal crisis is difficult but it should not be done before empirical management of a suspected case. An ACTH stimulation test would confirm the diagnosis but should not be done in the acute cases. Laboratory tests like ACTH, serum cortisol, aldosterone, dehydroepiandrosterone sulphate, and renin should be drawn before the administration of hydrocortisone for review at a later time. Sometimes an arbitrary cortisol level preceding the treatment can omit or reinforce the diagnoses of adrenal insufficiency and crisis; despite, it should never stop the treatment with glucocorticoids if the assessment is unclear. "A high cortisol level of >20 mg/dL (550 nmol/L) can exclude the diagnosis, while a low cortisol level of <5 mg/dL in the early morning and in the setting of acute illness support the diagnosis". Investigations for the aggravating causes like infection, infiltrating disorders, metastasis has to be treated. Additionally, patient has to be tested for hyponatremia, autoimmune disorders and thyroid functions. Adrenal imaging evaluations generally are rarely needed if suspicious of bilateral adrenal hemorrhage or carcinoma or in unique situations. **Flowchart 11.4** shows an algorithm for diagnosis and management of adrenal insufficiency.

### Management

The ultimate management of adrenal crisis is treating with glucocorticoids, especially hydrocortisone. The dosage is "100 mg IV/IM" as first bolus then "100 to 300 mg" in 24 hours for a period of 2–3 days either as boluses in every six hours or as uninterrupted administration in expectation of complete restoration. Hydrocortisone from this infusion at this dosage will yield adequate mineralocorticoid also. As hydrocortisone is the treatment of choice, treating with prednisolone or methylprednisolone, and dexamethasone is beneficial. These patients need prompt

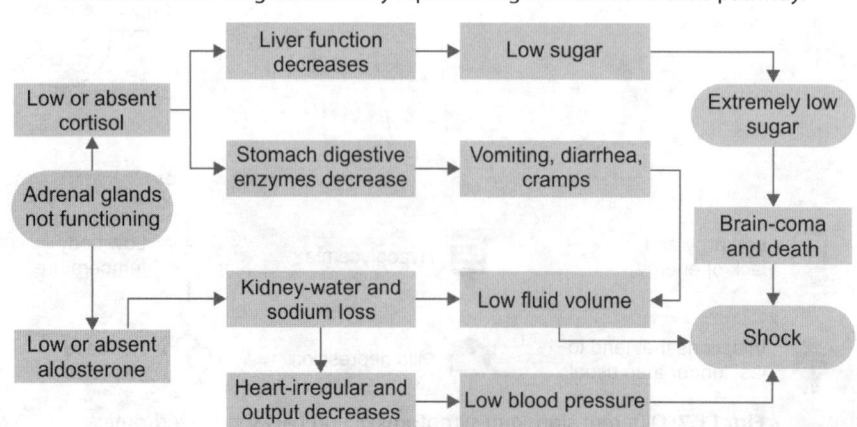

**Flowchart 11.3:** Diagrammatically representing the Addition's crisis pathway.

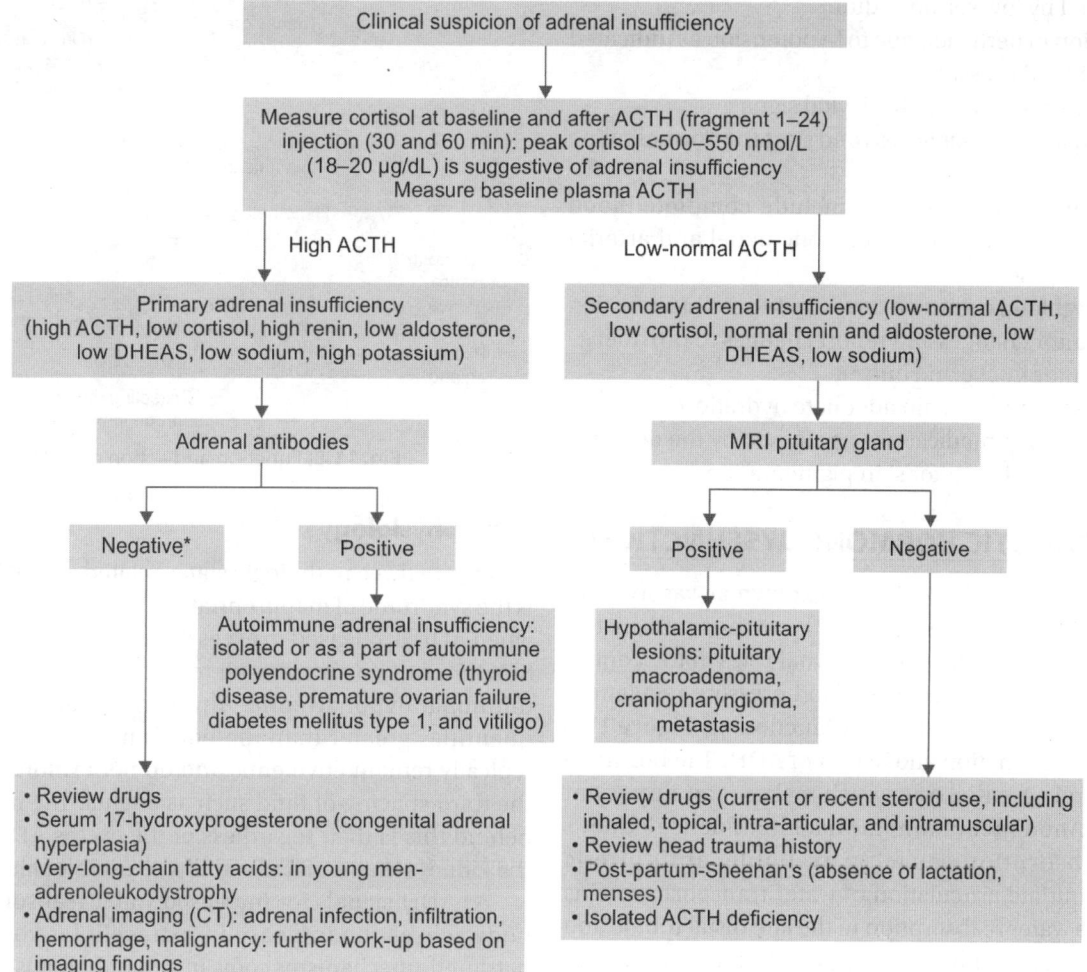

**Flowchart 11.4:** Algorithm for diagnosis and management of adrenal insufficiency (Baker GF, 2006).

fluid and vasopressor administration additionally. Detailed assessment is to be done to find out the leading factors, and empiric antibiotics are prescribed. Focused observation in the intensive care unit (ICU) is needed. In women with pregnancy, hydrocortisone is the choice and should be discharged on hydrocortisone rather than cortisone acetate.

### Guide to Manage Adrenal Crisis in an Emergency

- Administer 100 mg hydrocortisone intravenous in every 6-8 hour if the features of adrenal crisis are evident clinical and laboratory findings.
- Rehydration of the patient with normal saline 0.9% is important (it will also correct the hypovolemia and the prerenal failure) as dehydration and hypovolemia are regular features. Normal saline to be administered during the initial treatment then the need for further IV fluid resuscitation has to be managed as per the hemodynamic level of the patient (generally 4–6 liters are required in the initial 24 hours)
- Treating hypoglycemia with IV dextrose with repeated observation of the blood glucose level is vital.
- Do not manage hyponatremia rapidly (>6-8 mEq in the initial 24 hours) to not get into osmotic demyelination syndrome (consider that cortisol substitution may promote water diuresis along with suppression of antidiuretic hormone)
- Monitoring of the urine output is essential.
- Consult an endocrinologist at the earliest.
- On clinical enhancement taper steroids and the tapering has to be gentle.

### Nursing Management

Nursing diagnosis includes the following:
- The threat of infection due to immunocompromised immunity, as evidenced by fever

- The risk of volume depletion due to salt wasting as indicated by low serum sodium
- Alteration in perfusion due to hypotension as indicated by low blood pressure
  - Assess patient and check vital signs
  - Gain intravenous access and start the normal saline infusion
  - Monitor lab values that include complete blood count, lactate, basic metabolic panel and arterial blood gases
  - Draw blood cultures to investigate possible infection
  - Monitor changes and report changes to provider
  - Monitor intake and output
  - Assess and maintain adequate hydration
  - Administer medications as advised by the doctor
  - Assess and monitor skin pigmentation

## ANTIDIURETIC HORMONE DYSFUNCTION

Antidiuretic hormone (ADH) also known as vasopressin and arginine vasopressin (AVP) synthesized in the hypothalamus. It is known to play vital roles in the control of the body's osmotic balance, blood pressure regulation, sodium homeostasis, and kidney functioning. **Figure 11.8** shows various function and action of ADH. The hormone plays several essential role which makes it an important hormone. Antidiuretic hormone mainly influence kidney's water reabsorption capacity; available, antidiuretic hormone initiate articulation of water transport proteins to enhance water reabsorption in the late distal tubule and collecting duct. Antidiuretic hormone imbalance leads to multiple disease conditions.

ADH is the essential hormone accountable for constitution homeostasis. Hyperosmolar states most firmly trigger its delivery. ADH is put away in neurons inside the hippocampus. These neurons express osmoreceptors that are perfectly receptive to blood osmolarity and react to changes as meager as two mOsm/L. Therefore, slight heights in osmolarity bring about the discharge of ADH. ADH at that point demonstrations principally in the kidneys to build water reabsorption, in this way restoring the osmolarity.

ADH emission additionally happens during conditions of hypovolemia or volume exhaustion. In these states, diminished baroreceptors sense blood vessel blood volume in the left chamber, carotid conduit, and aortic artery. Stimulus about low circulatory strain detected by these receptors is communicated to the vagus nerve, which straightforwardly stimulate the secretion of ADH. ADH at that point advances water reabsorption in the kidneys and will likewise cause vasoconstriction.

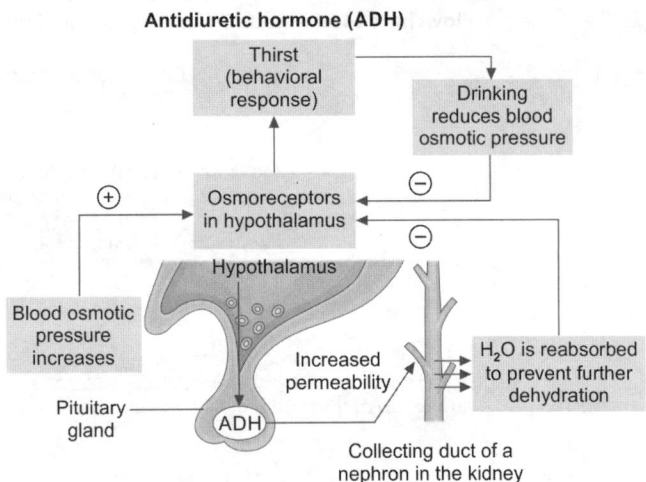

**Fig. 11.8:** Function and action of ADH.

## Pathophysiology

"There are three pathologic states related to ADH. The first is the syndrome of inappropriate ADH (SIADH) and occurs when ADH is released in excessive unregulated quantities. SIADH results in excess water reabsorption and thus creates dilutional hyponatremia. Although water is retained in quantities greater than the body's needs, these patients typically remain euvolemic and do not exhibit features of the third spacing of fluid such as edema. The mechanism behind this is that, regardless of the excess ADH present, the kidneys maintain their ability to excrete salt.

As ADH signals for increased water reabsorption, the body senses the increase in extracellular volume, and natriuretic mechanisms come into play that cause increased salt excretion via the kidneys. The increased salt in the urine will osmotically attract water to be excreted as well, thus keeping the body in a euvolemic state. This increase in salt excretion also contributes to the hyponatremia seen in SIADH.

Settings in which SIADH arises include malignancies (most often by autonomous production of ADH by small cell lung cancer), central nervous system (CNS) disturbances (e.g., stroke, hemorrhage, infection, trauma, etc.), drugs (e.g., selective serotonin reuptake inhibitors, carbamazepine, and others), surgery (most likely secondary to pain), and more.

Patients with SIADH may be asymptomatic or present with a spectrum of severity of complaints based on their level of hyponatremia. Nausea and malaise are typically the earliest presenting symptoms and present when the sodium acutely falls below 125 to 130 mEq/L. Lower levels of sodium are associated with headache, obtundation, seizure, and even coma and respiratory arrest. These symptoms arise due to the increased movement of water into neurons as the extracellular osmolarity falls. The intracellular swelling causes neuronal dysfunction".

"Unlike the excess ADH seen in SIADH, the remaining two pathologic states related to ADH result from either decreased ADH or resistance to its effects. A failure of ADH secretion causes central diabetes insipidus. In this scenario, ADH levels are low; thus, the collecting tubules are impermeable to water, resulting in excess water excretion.

In nephrogenic diabetes insipidus, ADH secretion is normal, but there is a defect in the V receptor or other signalling mediators that makes the kidneys unresponsive to ADH. In either disease, the net effect is increased excretion of water. The depletion of water causes the production of large volumes of dilute water and the concentration of body fluids leading to hypernatremia and hyper osmolarity. This status results in polyuria, polydipsia, and the effects of electrolyte imbalances that ensue".

"Central diabetes insipidus is the more common form and often seen after brain trauma or surgery that damages either the hypothalamus or posterior pituitary. Other cerebral infiltrative processes such as infection, autoimmune disease, or neoplastic disease may also cause central diabetes insipidus. Nephrogenic diabetes insipidus can be either inherited or acquired. The most common inherited form is attributed to mutations in the V receptor and often manifests in childhood. Acquired causes of nephrogenic diabetes insipidus are more often at play in adulthood expression of the disease. Most often, acquired nephrogenic diabetes insipidus is due to drugs, notably lithium and some antibiotics such as tetracyclines".

## Laboratory Testing

The laboratory tests frequently used to diagnose conditions related to ADH abnormalities include serum osmolality, urine osmolality, urine electrolytes, thyroid function tests, cortisol levels, liver function tests, and serum uric acid.

## Treatment

Treatment of the syndrome of inappropriate antidiuretic hormone secretion (SIADH) and the rapidity of correction of hyponatremia depend on the degree of hyponatremia, on whether the patient is symptomatic, and on whether it is acute (< 48 hours) or chronic.

The urine osmolality and creatinine clearance also must be considered when choosing the type of therapy. If no history is available to determine the duration of hyponatremia and if the patient is asymptomatic, it is reasonable to presume the condition is chronic. Diagnosis and treatment of the underlying cause of SIADH is also important.

Correcting hyponatremia too rapidly may result in central pontine myelinolysis (CPM) with permanent neurologic deficits. It is important to remember that even severe hyponatremia can correct rapidly with just fluid restriction if the hyponatremia is associated with absent ADH secretion (e.g., psychogenic polydipsia).

European guidelines for the treatment of syndrome of inappropriate antidiuresis include the following recommendations for management of moderate or profound hyponatremia:
- Restrict fluid intake as first-line treatment
- Second-line treatments include increasing solute intake with 0.25–0.50 g/kg per day of urea or a combination of low-dose loop diuretics and oral sodium chloride
- Use of lithium, demeclocycline, or vasopressin receptor antagonists is not recommended
- Recommendations on the treatment of SIADH from an American Expert panel included the following
  - If chronic, limit rate of correction
  - Fluid restriction should generally be first-line therapy
  - Consider pharmacologic therapies if serum Na+ is not corrected after 24-48 hours of fluid restriction or if patient has a low urinary electrolyte free water excretion
  - Patients being treated with vaptans should not be on a fluid restriction initially
  - Water, 5% dextrose or desmopressin can be used to slow the rate of correction if the water diuresis is profound.

### Emergency Care

Prompt management of hyponatremia without fail has to be contemplated with the threat of giving rise to CMP. An uncommon at the same time consequential condition, CMP may appear one to many days following prompt management of hyponatremia. Prompt treatment of hyponatremia is recommended among individuals having critical manifestations like "seizures, stupor, coma, and respiratory arrest, regardless of the degree of hyponatremia". Emergency management also should be vigorously taken into consideration for patients having "moderate-to-severe hyponatremia" with a recorded period of 48 hours or less.

Aim is to rectify hyponatremia in such a manner that it does not lead to any neurological conditions. The point is to raise serum Na+ levels by 0.5-1 mEq/h, and not more than 10-12 mEq in the initial 24 hours, to bring the Na+ incentive to a greatest degree of 125–130 mEq/L. Organization of 3% hypertonic saline should be limited to these developing conditions, and both neurological side effects and serum Na+ should be observed oftentimes to accomplish the ideal objective and to forestall overcorrection. Adjustment of serum Na+ levels by 6 mEq/L in 24 hours has been named the "rule of sixes." The rule states that, "six a day makes sense for safety; 6 in 6 hours for severe symptoms and stop."

### Nursing Management

Nursing diagnosis includes excess fluid volume related to disease progression, excessive fluid consumption, a weakened regulatory mechanism, dysregulation of the endocrine system and renal impairment.

- Restrict fluid as ordered, generally <500 mL/day in severe cases and 800 to 1000 mL/day in moderate cases.
- Administer potassium supplements as ordered, assess renal function and ensure adequate urine output before administering potassium.
- As adjuncts to water restriction, demeclocycline may be ordered to inhibit the renal response to ADH in patients with lung malignancies.
- Avoid hypotonic enemas to treat constipation because water intoxication can be potentiated.
- Institute pressure ulcer prevention strategies.

## Summary

Nurses are the largest group of healthcare workers, their training and awareness in the management of endocrine emergency patients are vital. Patients in adult and pediatric age group present to the emergency department or intensive critical care unit with varieties of lethal conditions like diabetic ketoacidosis, thyroid crisis, and adrenal crisis which need immediate interventions. The nurse must work with multidisciplinary team to provide a comprehensive care to these critically ill patients. As an emergency nurse require adequate knowledge on prompt identification of illness, diagnostic methods, initial stabilization and management are crucial to save the life of patients.

## Points to Ponder

- Endocrine disorders and diseases usually manifest according to which endocrine hormone is being overproduced and secreted, or under-produced, at any given age.
- Diabetic coma is one of critical diagnosis.
- Diabetic ketoacidosis (DKA) and hyperglycemic hyperosmolar syndrome are the most serious acute hyperglycemic emergency.
- Detailed and prompt physical examination helps in clarify the diagnosis.
- Endocrine diagnosis involves the sequence of history, physical examination, laboratory, and radiologic evaluation.
- There are mainly three categories of diagnostic tests, blood sample, urine sample and stimulation and evocative test.
- Glucose is the principal metabolic propellant of cerebellar function in physiological state. The cerebrum is immensely finite in providing its glucose not like other, organs of the body. Hence, the brain cells need a continuous provision of arterial glucose to maintain normal metabolic role.
- Hypoglycemia is commonly found among individuals with diabetes under pharmacologic management.
- Insulinomas are overactive islets cells malignancies related to elevated insulin production.
- The main contributing factors towards hyperglycemia are reduced insulin release, decreased glucose usage, subsequently elevated glucose manufacture.
- Diabetic acidosis itself is a symptoms of type 1 diabetes than disease.
- Client having ketoacidosis may have dehydration which leads to hypokalemia.
- Ketoacidosis is linked with high hyperlycemic index.
- Thyroid storm may be the primary display of thyrotoxicosis in unidentified case of children, particularly in newborn.
- Dermatological modifications which are seen in hypothyroid and rarely hyperthyroid conditions are also called myxedema.
- Myxedema coma, sometimes termed as myxedema crisis, is an unusual, is a grave medical disorder which picture serious hypothyroid disorder accompanied by physiological deterioration.
- Anatomic destruction of the gland may be the cause of primary adrenal insufficiency, both acute or chronic.
- ADH is the essential hormone accountable for constitution homeostasis.
- Diabetes insipidus is an important cause of hypernatremia

## Abbreviations

- AC : Adrenal Cortex
- FSH : Follicle-stimulating Hormone
- ACTH : Adrenocorticotropic Hormone
- ADH : Antidiuretic Hormone
- DI : Diabetes Insipidus
- DKA : Diabetic Ketoacidosis
- DM : Diabetes Mellitus
- GH : Growth Hormone
- HCG : Human Chorionic Gonadotropin
- LH : Luteinizing Hormone
- HGF : Human Growth Factor
- ICSH : Interstitial Cell-stimulating Hormone
- IDDM : Insulin-dependent Diabetes Mellitus
- IGT : Impaired Glucose Tolerance
- JOD : Juvenile-Onset Diabetes
- MEA : Multiple Endocrine Adenomatosis
- MEN : Multiple Endocrine Neoplasia
- MSH : Melanocyte-stimulating Hormone
- NIDD : Noninsulin-dependent Diabetes Mellitus

- PTH : Parathyroid Hormone
- SIADH : Syndrome of Inappropriate ADH
- STH : Somatotropic Hormone
- $T_3$ : Triiodothyronine
- $T_4$ : Thyroxine
- TFT : Thyroid Function Test
- TSH : Thyroid-stimulating Hormone
- OGTT : Oral Glucose Tolerance Test
- CAH : Congenital Adrenal Hyperplasia

### Short Answer Questions

1. Emergency management of hypoglycemia.
2. Dietary management of hypoglycemia.
3. Precautionary measures in cases of hypoglycemia.
4. Diagnosis of hypoglycemia.
5. Dietary management for DK.
6. Primary adrenal insufficiency.
7. Physical assessment in adrenal crisis.
8. Assessment of myxedema.
9. Prevention of diabetic ketoacidosis.

### Long Answer Questions

1. Describe in details about the etiology and pathophysiology of ADH.
2. Write in details about the treatment and management of ADH.
3. Describe in details about the etiology and pathophysiology of myxedema.
4. Write in details about the management of myxedema.
5. Describe in details about the etiology and pathophysiology of hypoglycemia.
6. Write in details about the management of the hypoglycemia.
7. Describe in details about the etiology and pathophysiology of diabetic ketoacidosis.
8. Write in details about the management of diabetic ketoacidosis.
9. Describe in details about the etiology and pathophysiology of adrenal crisis..

### Bibliography

1. Amy Hess-Fischl MS, RD, LDN, BC-ADM CR by BGM. Hypoglycemia Treatment for Low Blood Glucose Depends on your Symptoms and Causes [Internet]. [cited 2019 Oct 8].
2. Baker GF, Tortora GJ, Nostakos NPA. Principles of Anatomy and Physiology. Vol. 76, The American Journal of Nursing. 2006: 477.
3. Bancos I, Hahner S, Tomlinson J, Arlt W. Diagnosis and Management of Adrenal Insufficiency. Lancet Diabetes Endocrinol [Internet]. 2015;3 (3):216–26.
4. Boone M, Deen PMT. Physiology and Pathophysiology of the Vasopressin-Regulated Renal Water Reabsorption [Internet]. Vol. 456, Pflugers Archiv European Journal of Physiology. Pflugers Arch; 2008 [cited 2020 Sep 1]. p. 1005–24.
5. Cryer PE, Arbeláez AM. Hypoglycemia in Diabetes. In: Textbook of Diabetes [Internet]. Chichester, UK: John Wiley and Sons, Ltd; 2016 [cited 2019 Oct 8]. p. 513–33.
6. Diabetic Ketoacidosis (DKA): Practice Essentials, Background, Pathophysiology [Internet]. [cited 2019 Dec 4].
7. Edmunds MR, Denniston AK, Boelaert K, Franklyn JA, Durrani OM. Patient information in Graves' Disease and Thyroid-Associated Ophthalmopathy: Readability Assessment of Online Resources. Thyroid. 2014;24 (1):67–72.
8. Gosmanov AR, Gosmanova EO, Dillard-Cannon E. Management of Adult Diabetic Ketoacidosis. Vol. 7, Diabetes, Metabolic Syndrome and Obesity: Targets and Therapy. Dove Medical Press Ltd.; 2014:255–64.
9. How are Mild, Moderate, and Severe Diabetic Ketoacidosis (DKA) Defined? [Internet]. [cited 2019 Dec 5].
10. Joel Thome DB. Addressing Hypoglycemic Emergencies [Internet]. [cited 2019 Oct 8].
11. Kahn ASA TJA. Evaluation of a Bedside Blood Ketone Sensor: The Effects of Acidosis, Hyperglycaemia and Acetoacetate on Sensor Performance. Diabet Mdicine. 2004;21 (7):782–5.
12. Kitabchi AE, Umpierrez GE, Fisher JN, Murphy MB SF. Thirty Years of Personal Experience in Hyperglycemic Crises: Diabetic Ketoacidosis and Hyperglycemic Hyperosmolar State. J Clin Endocrinol Metab. 93 (5):1541–52.
13. Mathew P, Thoppil D. Hypoglycemia. In Treasure Island (FL); 2022.
14. Mouri Mi, Badireddy M, Heffner A, Murin S, Sandrock C. Hyperglycemia. StatPearls [Internet]. 2019 [cited 2019 Oct 8].
15. Remonti Luciana Reck, KramerCaroline Kaercher, Leitão Cristiane Bauermann, Pinto Lana Catani F. GJL. Thyroid Ultrasound Features and Risk of Carcinoma: A Systematic Review and Meta-Analysis of Observational Studies. Thyroid Radiol Nucl Med. 2014;25 (5).
16. Shlomo Melmed, Kenneth S. Polonsky, P. Reed Larsen and HMK. Larsen: Williams Textbook of Endocrinology, 10th ed., Copyright © 2003 Elsevier By OkDoKeY. 2003:3196.
17. SL L. Endocrine System. In: Medical-surgical Nursing: Assessment and Management of Clinical Problems. 7th ed. p. 225–51.
18. Stephen Kemp M. Anatomy of the Endocrine System [Internet]. EMedicine Heath. 2017 [cited 2019 Jul 5].
19. Thyroid Storm: Causes, Symptoms, and Diagnosis [Internet]. [cited 2019 Dec 5].
20. Vikas Sharma, Papori Borah, Lakshya J. Basumatary, Marami Das, Munindra Goswami AKK. Myopathies of Endocrine Disorders: A Prospective Clinical and Biochemical Study. Ann Indian Acad Neurol. 2014;17 (3):298–302.
21. Yang Q. Harrison's Endocrinology. Vol. 84. The Yale Journal of Biology and Medicine. 2011.

# Chapter 12

# Obstetrical Emergency and Management

 Debajani Nayak

## CHAPTER OUTLINE

- Types of Obstetrical Emergency
- Antepartum Hemorrhage
  - Placenta previa
  - Abruptio placentae
- Pregnancy-induced Hypertension
  - Gestational hypertension
  - Pre-eclampsia
  - Eclampsia
- Obstructed Labor
- Postpartum Hemorrhage
- Ruptured Uterus
- Puerperal Sepsis
- Obstetrical Shock

### Learning Objectives

At the end of the chapter, the students will be able to:
- Identify the causes and diagnosis of common obstetric emergencies.
- Understand the feto-maternal complication in obstetric emergency cases.
- Explain the protocols for the management of common obstetric emergencies.

## INTRODUCTION

Many of the illnesses associated with pregnancy that can worsen the condition of both mother and fetus. From that some of the emergency situation may arises during pregnancy, labor, and puerperium. Special hospital care is needed for the conditions. Pregnancy-related health issues are those that develop while a woman is pregnant. There are a number of pregnancy-related illnesses and disorders that can endanger both the mother's and the child's health. During active labor and after delivery, obstetrical crises can arise (postpartum) (Leta M, 2022).

### Definition of Obstetrical Emergency

Obstetric emergency is the life-threatening health conditions for pregnancy women and their babies that occur anytime during pregnancy, labor and postpartum. The mother to be, the fetus, or both may be in danger of dying during obstetric emergencies. Severe bleeding may also occur, and timely intervention is important (Crochetière C, 2003).

## TYPES OF OBSTETRICAL EMERGENCY

### Obstetrical Emergency during Pregnancy

- **Ectopic pregnancy:** Implantation of fertilized egg in the fallopian tube rather than the uterine wall is called ectopic, or tubal, pregnancy. The pregnancy may be complicated with rupture of the fallopian tube causing internal hemorrhage (Tamai K, 2007).
- **Placenta previa:** Placenta is implanted over the lower uterine segment either partially or completely resulting premature bleeding and possible postpartum hemorrhage.
- **Abruptio placentae:** Premature separation of placenta from the uterus prematurely, causing bleeding from the vagina leads to risk for both the fetus and mother.
- **Pre-eclampsia/eclampsia:** These are the conditions of pregnancy-induced hypertension (PIH) where, elevation of blood pressure after 20 weeks of pregnancy can lead to Pre-eclampsia. Its severe complication leads to eclampsia which is dangerous for both mother and baby.

- **Premature rupture of membranes (PROM):** The rupture of amniotic sac before labor begins, normally before thirty-seven weeks of pregnancy resulting leakage and infection of the amniotic fluid.

## Obstetrical Emergencies during Labor and Delivery

- **Rupture of uterus:** It is the spontaneous tear of the uterine muscle that may result in the expulsion of the fetus through peritoneal cavity which can occur during late pregnancy or active labor.
- **Placenta accreta:** It is an emergency condition where, the placenta attaches abnormally to the myometrium of uterine wall causing severe blood loss after delivery.
- **Cord prolapsed:** When the umbilical cord descent through the cervix out of the uterus before the presenting part of the baby. So that the prolapsed cord will compromise the blood flow which may occur death of the baby.
- **Shoulder dystocia:** Shoulder dystocia occurs, when the anterior shoulder unable to pass through the birth canal after delivery of head.

## Obstetrical Emergencies during Postpartum

- **Postpartum hemorrhage:** Postpartum hemorrhage is defined as the loss of more than 500 mL of blood in the first 24 hours following delivery.
- **Puerperal sepsis:** It is defined as infection of the genital tract due to pathogens occurring at anytime after rupture of membranes within postpartum period.
- **Obstetric shock:** It is the condition during perinatal period resulting from in ability of circulatory system to deliver oxygen and nutrient for normal.

# ANTEPARTUM HEMORRHAGE

## Definition

Antepartum hemorrhage is the bleeding from the genital tract after the 28th week of pregnancy and includes the first and second stage of labor. It is considered as a medical emergency can lead to death of the mother as well as the baby.

## Classification

The total amount of blood loss and signs of circulatory shock due to blood determine the severity of the antepartum hemorrhaging **(Table 12.1)**. There are 4 degrees of antepartum hemorrhaging (Perth, 2015).

## Causes of Antepartum Hemorrhage

No definite cause is diagnosed in about 50% of all women who present with antepartum hemorrhage, however, placenta previa and placental abruption are the major identifiable causes **(Flowchart 12.1)** (APH, 2011).

## Placenta Previa

Placenta previa and placenta previa accreta are associated with significant 1-11 maternal and fetal morbidity and mortality, as well as substantial demands on healthcare resources. The moment is right to update the guidelines for this condition since placenta previa and associated consequences, such as placenta accreta, will continue to rise in instances due to the rising cesarean section rate and ageing mothers. 7, 8,12–24 vasa previa is also listed in this recommendation for the first time since, despite being uncommon, it is linked to high perinatal morbidity and mortality (No GT, 2011).

**Table 12.1:** Classification of antepartum hemorrhaging.

| Stage | Amount of blood loss |
|---|---|
| Spotting | Stains, streaking, or spotting of blood |
| Minor hemorrhage | Less than 50 mL |
| Major hemorrhage | 50–1000 mL without signs of circulatory shock |
| Massive hemorrhage | Greater than 1000 mL with or without signs of circulatory shock |

**Flowchart 12.1:** Causes of antepartum hemorrhage.

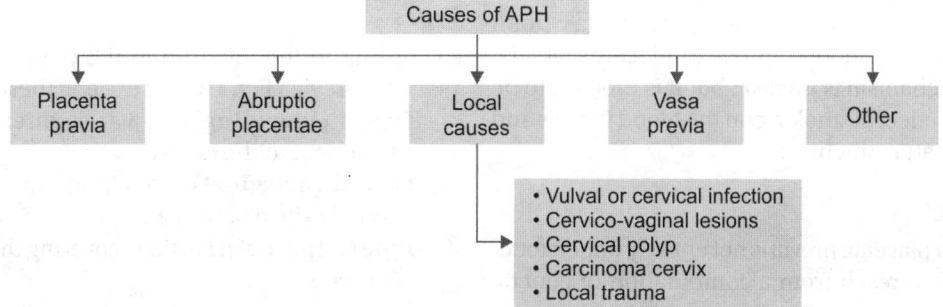

## Definition

Placenta previa refers to when the placenta of a growing fetus is attached abnormally low within the uterus. Intermittent antepartum hemorrhaging occurs in 72% of women living with placenta previa (Love, C, 1996). The severity of a patient's placenta previa depends on the location of placental attachment.

## Etiology

The exact cause of placenta previa is unknown. It is hypothesized to be related to abnormal vascularization of the endometrium caused by scarring or atrophy from previous trauma, surgery, or infection (Dashe JS, 2022). The etiology of placenta previa includes:

- **Abnormal placental implantation:** Placenta previa occurs when the placenta implants abnormally low in the uterus, near or covering the cervix. This abnormal implantation can occur due to various factors, including:
  - *Previous uterine surgeries:* Women with a history of cesarean section, uterine surgeries, or uterine curettage have a higher risk of developing placenta previa. Scar tissue from previous surgeries can disrupt the normal implantation of the placenta.
  - *Uterine abnormalities:* Certain uterine abnormalities, such as a bicornuate uterus or a septate uterus, can increase the risk of placenta previa. These abnormalities can affect the location and attachment of the placenta.
- **Advanced maternal age:** Placenta previa is more common in older mothers, particularly those over the age of 35. The exact reasons for this association are not well understood but may be related to changes in the uterine environment or increased rates of uterine scarring from previous pregnancies or procedures.
- **Multiparity:** Women who have had multiple pregnancies have a higher risk of developing placenta previa. The repeated stretching and thinning of the uterine wall with each pregnancy may contribute to abnormal placental implantation.
- **Previous placenta previa:** Women who have previously had placenta previa in a previous pregnancy are at a higher risk of recurrence in subsequent pregnancies.
- **Smoking:** Smoking during pregnancy has been associated with an increased risk of placenta previa. The exact mechanism is unclear, but it is thought to be related to the effect of smoking on the blood vessels and the placental attachment.

## Pathophysiology

The exact cause of placenta previa is not entirely understood, but it is believed to result from a combination of genetic

**Flowchart 12.2:** Pathophysiology of placenta previa.

| The factors may reduce differential growth of lower segment, resulting in less upward shift in placental position as pregnancy advances. |
| --- |
| ↓ |
| With placenta previa, the placenta attaches lower in the uterus |
| ↓ |
| This results in some portion of the placental tissue covering the cervix |
| ↓ |
| It can result in bleeding during the pregnancy or during or after delivery |

and environmental factors. Here's a brief overview of the pathophysiology of placenta previa (**Flowchart 12.2**):

- **Implantation abnormality:** During a normal pregnancy, the fertilized egg implants itself into the lining of the uterus, away from the cervix. However, in placenta previa, the placenta implants in the lower portion of the uterus, near or over the cervix.
- **Abnormal trophoblastic invasion:** Trophoblasts are specialized cells of the placenta that invade the uterine lining to establish the maternal-fetal blood circulation. In placenta previa, these trophoblasts may not adequately invade or penetrate the uterine lining, leading to improper anchoring of the placenta.
- **Reduced decidua formation:** The decidua is the part of the uterine lining that is modified during pregnancy to support the growing placenta. In placenta previa, the formation of decidua in the lower part of the uterus may be reduced or disrupted, further contributing to improper placental attachment.
- **Placental vessel disruption:** As the cervix begins to dilate and thin out in preparation for childbirth, the placental vessels overlying the cervix can be torn or disrupted, leading to bleeding.
- **Increased pressure:** As the uterus expands with the growing fetus, the placenta may experience increased pressure, which can cause it to detach from the uterine wall and result in bleeding.

## Types

According to the location of the placenta four types of placenta previa (**Fig. 12.1**) are seen. These are:

1. **Type I (low lying):** Lower segment of uterus, no attachment to the cervix
2. **Type II (marginal):** Touching but not covering the internal orifice of the cervix
3. **Type III (partial):** Partially covering the internal orifice of the cervix

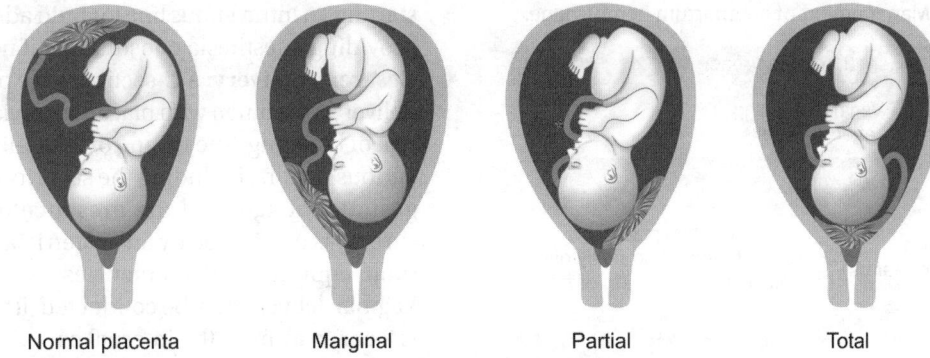

**Fig. 12.1:** Types of placenta previa.

4. **Type IV (complete):** Completely covering the internal orifice of the cervix.

## Clinical Features

### Symptoms
Sudden onset with painless and recurrent vaginal bleeding.

### Signs
- Signs of anemia with visible blood loss.
- Height of the uterus is according to the gestational week.
- Feeling as nontender, relaxed, soft and elastic uterus.
- Presence of fetal heart sound.
- Visible bright red colored blood-stained clothings.
- Occurs around 32 weeks of gestation, but can be as early as late mid-trimester.

### Diagnosis (Warren, 2009)
- **History:** May reveal antepartum hemorrhage.
- **Abdominal examination:** Usually finds the uterus nontender, soft and relaxed.
- **Leopold's maneuvers:** May find the fetus in an oblique or breech position or lying transverse as a result of the abnormal position of the placenta.
- Malpresentation is found in about 35% cases.
- **Vaginal examination:** It is avoided in known cases of placenta previa.

## Complications of Placenta Previa

### Maternal Complications

#### Antenatal period
- Antepartum hemorrhage
- Abnormal presentation
- Preterm labor

#### Intranatal period
- Premature membrane rupture
- Prolapse of umbilical cord
- Less dilation of cervix
- Intranatal hemorrhage
- Moreuse of instrumental delivery
- Retained bits of placenta

#### Postnatal period
- Postpartum hemorrhage
- Postpartum sepsis
- Subinvolution
- Embolism

### Fetal Complications in Placenta Previa
- Low birth weight
- Intrauterine fetal death
- Congenital malformation
- Birth injuries to the newborn

### Management
The APH management depends on the types and severity of bleeding, week of gestation, and fetal condition. If it finds placenta previa early in the second trimester, it can get better on its own. The position of the placenta can change as the uterus expands to accommodate the growing baby. There is often less of a chance that the placenta will move higher in the uterus (**Flowcharts 12.3 and 12.4**).

#### Medical Management
If the placenta is near or covering just part of the cervix and not bleeding:
- Reducing strenuous activities like running, lifting and exercising.
- Bed rest at home.
- No sexual intercourse, tampons or douching.
- More frequent prenatal appointments.
- Repeat the USG for placental location
- The treatment is carried up to 37 weeks of pregnancy.
- CS usually is scheduled to minimize the risk of hemorrhage.

**Flowchart 12.3:** Management of antepartum hemorrhage.

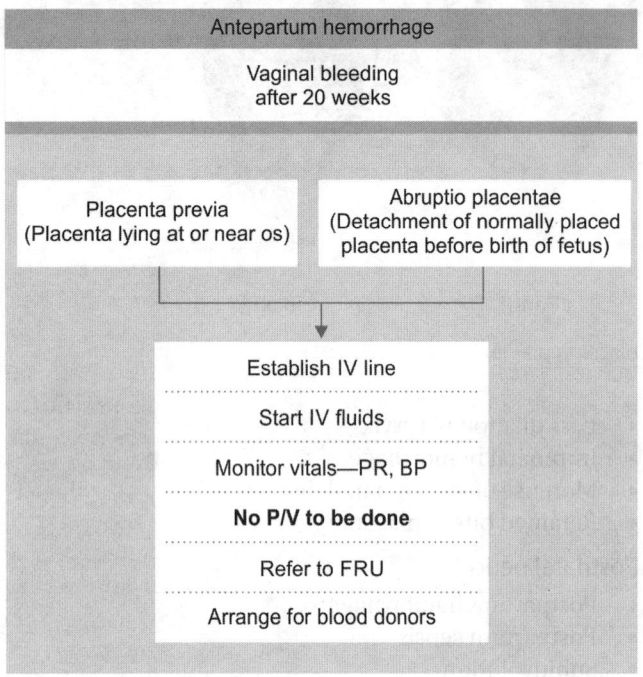

*Source:* SBA Quality Protocol Poster, NHM, Ministry of Health and Family Welfare, GOI.

- **Diagnosis and assessment:** Placenta previa is usually diagnosed through ultrasound examination. The degree of placental coverage and the proximity to the cervix are determined to assess the severity of the condition.
- **Strict bed rest:** Women with placenta previa are usually advised to be on strict bed rest to minimize the risk of bleeding. They may be hospitalized if the condition is severe or if bleeding occurs.
- **Monitoring:** Close monitoring of the mother and the fetus is crucial. Vital signs, including blood pressure and heart rate, are regularly checked. Fetal monitoring is performed to assess the well-being of the baby.
- **Blood transfusion preparation:** Due to the risk of significant bleeding during delivery, blood products, such as packed red blood cells and fresh frozen plasma, are often prepared in case transfusion is required.
- **Medications:** Medications may be administered to delay delivery and allow for fetal lung maturation. These may include corticosteroids (such as betamethasone) to promote fetal lung development if preterm delivery is anticipated.
- **Preoperative preparation:** In cases of significant bleeding or if the placenta previa persists close to term, a planned cesarean delivery (C-section) is usually scheduled. Preoperative preparations include fasting, starting an intravenous line for fluid administration, and providing anesthesia consultation if needed.
- **Cesarean delivery:** A C-section is the preferred mode of delivery for women with placenta previa to minimize the risk of bleeding. The timing of the delivery depends on various factors, including the severity of the condition, gestational age, and the presence of bleeding. The surgery is performed by an obstetrician in an operating room equipped for emergencies.
- Vaginal delivery may be conducted, if the placenta edge is 2 cm away from the internal os
- Contraindications of vaginal examination
  - Patient in exsanguinated state
  - Diagnosed cases of major degree of placenta previa
  Associated complicating factors such as malpresentation, elderly primigravidae, pregnancy with history of previous cesarean section, contracted pelvis, etc.
- **Postoperative care:** Following a C-section, the mother is closely monitored for bleeding and other complications. Pain management is provided, and antibiotics may be administered to prevent infection. The newborn is assessed by a pediatrician for any immediate medical needs.
- **Postpartum recovery:** After delivery, the mother's recovery is monitored, and steps are taken to ensure her well-being. Close observation continues for any signs of bleeding or infection.
- **Discharge planning:** Once the mother's condition stabilizes, she and the newborn are discharged with appropriate instructions for postpartum care. Follow-up appointments are scheduled to monitor their health.

*Nursing Management*

The nursing management of placenta previa involves providing comprehensive care and support to women with this condition. Here are some key aspects of nursing management:

- **Assessment and monitoring:** Nurses play a vital role in assessing and monitoring the mother and the fetus. This includes monitoring vital signs, assessing for signs of bleeding, and documenting the frequency and severity of contractions. Fetal heart rate monitoring is important to evaluate the well-being of the baby.
- **Education and counseling:** Nurses provide education and counseling to the woman and her family about placenta previa, its risks, and the importance of adhering to activity restrictions. They explain the signs and symptoms of bleeding or complications that should prompt immediate medical attention. Nurses also provide emotional support and address any concerns or anxieties the woman may have.

**Flowchart 12.4:** Scheme of management of placenta previa in a hospital.

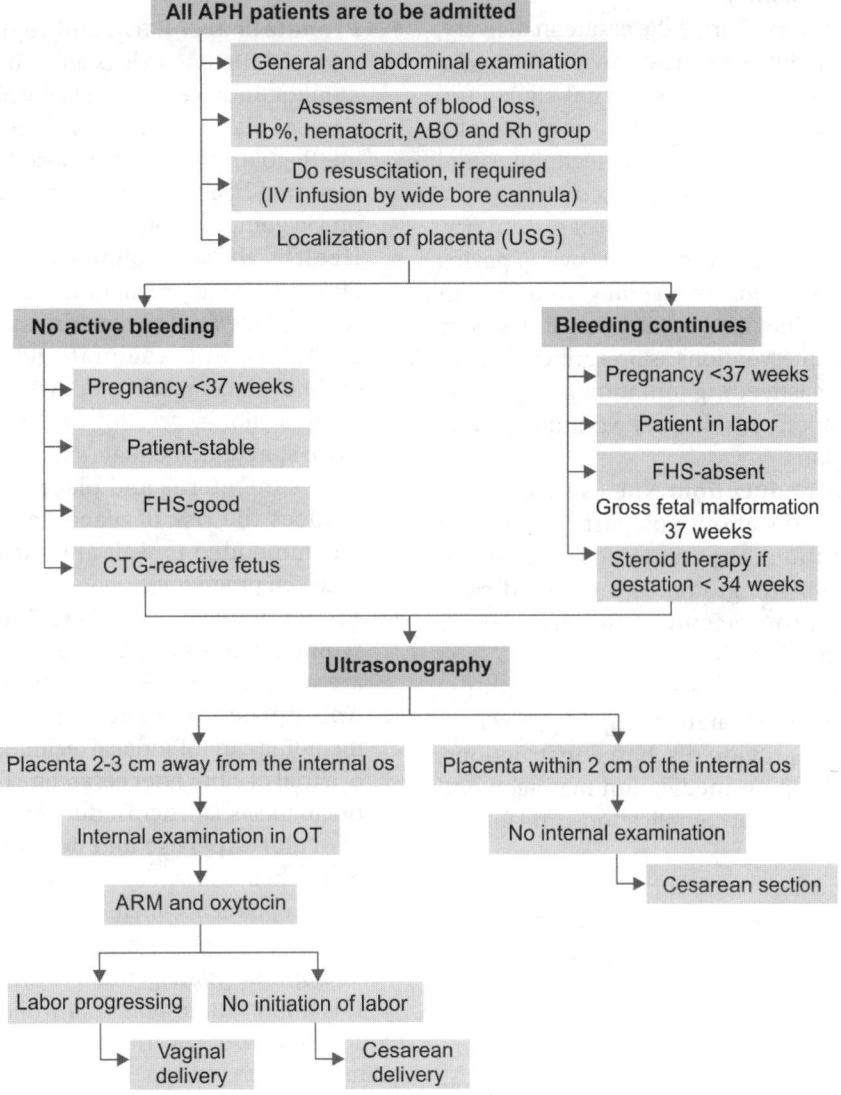

- **Bed rest and activity restriction:** Nurses assist in implementing and reinforcing the prescribed bed rest and activity restriction measures. They educate the woman about the importance of limiting physical exertion, avoiding heavy lifting, and refraining from sexual intercourse.
- **Bleeding assessment and management:** Nurses closely monitor for any signs of bleeding, such as vaginal bleeding or spotting. They assess the amount and characteristics of the bleeding and promptly report any significant changes to the healthcare provider. Nurses may assist in obtaining blood samples for laboratory tests, such as complete blood count (CBC), coagulation studies, and blood typing and cross-matching, in preparation for potential transfusions.
- **Emotional support:** Placenta previa can be emotionally distressing for women and their families. Nurses provide emotional support, reassurance, and encouragement throughout the pregnancy. They create a caring and empathetic environment, actively listen to the woman's concerns, and provide appropriate counseling and referrals if needed.
- **Preoperative preparation:** In cases where a planned cesarean delivery is necessary, nurses play a crucial role in preparing the woman for surgery. This includes ensuring fasting guidelines are followed, establishing an

intravenous line for fluid administration, and providing preoperative skin preparation.
- **Intraoperative support:** During the cesarean delivery, nurses assist the healthcare team by providing essential supplies, monitoring the woman's vital signs, and offering emotional support. They ensure a safe and sterile environment, maintain aseptic technique, and document the procedure and events accurately.
- **Postoperative care:** After the cesarean delivery, nurses closely monitor the woman's recovery, paying particular attention to signs of bleeding, infection, or other complications. They assess pain levels and provide pain management interventions as prescribed. Nurses also assist with breastfeeding initiation and provide postpartum education on self-care, wound care, and contraception options.
- **Patient and family education:** Nurses educate the woman and her family about postpartum care and signs of complications that may require medical attention. They provide guidance on wound care, pain management, contraception options, and the importance of follow-up visits.
- **Discharge planning:** Nurses collaborate with the healthcare team to ensure a safe discharge for the woman and her baby. They provide discharge instructions, including information on medication management, activity restrictions, signs of complications, and follow-up appointments.

Throughout the nursing management process, effective communication and collaboration with the healthcare team are essential to ensure coordinated and holistic care for women with placenta previa.

## Prevention

Placenta previa is a condition that cannot be completely prevented, as it is primarily determined by the placental implantation site. However, there are certain factors that can potentially reduce the risk of placenta previa or minimize its severity. Here are some considerations for prevention:

- **Preconception care:** It is important for women to receive preconception care, which includes a comprehensive evaluation of their overall health and medical history. This allows healthcare providers to identify and address any potential risk factors for placenta previa, such as previous cesarean deliveries, uterine surgeries, or multiple pregnancies.
- **Avoidance of risk factors:** Some risk factors for placenta previa include advanced maternal age, smoking, and illicit drug use. By avoiding these risk factors, women can potentially reduce their chances of developing placenta previa.
- **Prenatal care:** Early and regular prenatal care is essential. Prenatal visits allow healthcare providers to monitor the development of the placenta and detect any signs of placenta previa or other complications early on. Regular prenatal care also helps optimize overall maternal health, reducing the likelihood of placenta previa complications.
- **Healthy lifestyle choices:** Maintaining a healthy lifestyle during pregnancy, including a balanced diet, regular exercise (as recommended by the healthcare provider), and adequate rest, can contribute to optimal placental development and reduce the risk of complications.
- **Birth spacing:** Adequate spacing between pregnancies allows the uterus and placenta to fully recover and reduces the risk of placenta previa. It is generally recommended to wait at least 18 months to 2 years between pregnancies.
- **Proper management of previous cesarean sections:** Women who have had previous cesarean deliveries are at a higher risk of developing placenta previa. Appropriate management of cesarean sections, including careful surgical techniques and consideration of a trial of labor after cesarean (TOLAC) in subsequent pregnancies, can help reduce the risk of placenta previa.
- **Provider expertise and decision-making:** Choosing a healthcare provider experienced in managing high-risk pregnancies, including placenta previa, can help ensure appropriate monitoring, timely interventions, and optimal management of the condition.

It is important to note that while these measures may reduce the risk or severity of placenta previa, they cannot guarantee its prevention. The placenta's location is primarily determined by biological factors, and in some cases, placenta previa may still occur despite taking preventive measures. Regular prenatal care and close monitoring by healthcare professionals remain crucial in identifying and managing placenta previa to optimize outcomes for both the mother and the baby.

## Abruptio Placentae (Accidental Hemorrhage)

One of the main reasons of vaginal bleeding in the second half of pregnancy is placental abruption, which is traditionally defined as the premature separation of the placenta before birth. Placental abruption causes complications in 0.4–1% of pregnancies. One of the main factors contributing to maternal morbidity and perinatal mortality is placental abruption. Obstetric hemorrhage, the requirement for blood transfusions, an emergency hysterectomy, disseminated intravascular coagulopathy, and renal failure are among the dangers for mothers. Even though maternal deaths are uncommon, they occur seven times more frequently than average (Tikkanen M, 2010).

## Definition

Abruptio placentae, also known as placental abruption, is a serious medical condition during pregnancy where the placenta separates prematurely from the inner wall of the uterus before the baby is born. This separation can be partial or complete and can lead to various complications for both the mother and the baby **(Fig. 12.2)**.

## Causes

The exact cause of abruptio placentae (placental abruption) is often unknown. However, several factors and risk factors have been associated with an increased likelihood of experiencing this condition. The causes of abruptio placentae can include:

- **Trauma or injury:** Trauma or injury to the abdomen during pregnancy, such as from falls, motor vehicle accidents, or physical assaults, can increase the risk of placental abruption. The forceful impact can cause the placenta to separate from the uterine wall (Tikkanen, M, 2006).
- **Hypertension or pre-eclampsia:** High blood pressure, particularly chronic hypertension or pregnancy-induced hypertension (pre-eclampsia), has been associated with an increased risk of placental abruption. Hypertension can lead to vascular changes and damage to the placental tissues, potentially triggering placental abruption (Tikkanen, M, 2010).
- **Maternal risk factors:** Certain maternal factors may contribute to the development of placental abruption, including advanced maternal age (over 35), a history of previous placental abruption, chronic hypertension, diabetes, or clotting disorders (Ananth, 1999).
- **Substance abuse:** Substance abuse, especially cocaine use, has been identified as a significant risk factor for placental abruption. Cocaine can cause vasoconstriction and disrupt blood flow to the placenta, leading to placental abruption (Kelsey, 2014).
- **Uterine factors:** Uterine abnormalities, such as fibroids (noncancerous growths in the uterus), uterine rupture (a tear in the uterus), or a previous cesarean section, can increase the likelihood of placental abruption.
- **Multiple pregnancies:** Carrying twins, triplets, or a higher-order multiple pregnancy increases the risk of abruptio placentae compared to singleton pregnancies.

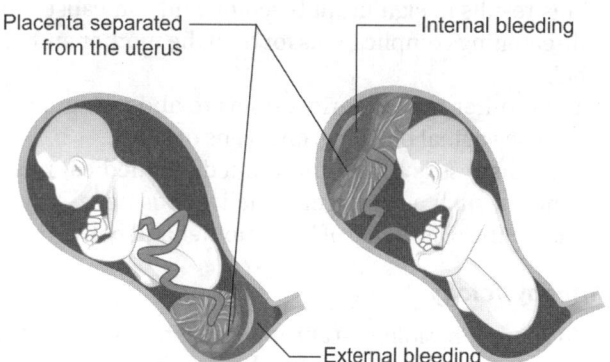

**Fig. 12.2:** Abruptio placentae.

- **Fetal factors:** Certain fetal conditions, such as genetic abnormalities or fetal growth restriction, may contribute to placental abruption.

## Classification

Abruptio placentae can be classified into different types based on the severity and extent of placental separation. The common classification system used is based on the degree of separation and is divided into three categories (Binod GC, 2020).

### Grade 1—Mild

- In Grade 1 abruptio placentae, there is a small amount of placental separation, and the symptoms may be relatively mild.
- The bleeding may be minimal or occult (hidden), and the mother and baby may not exhibit severe distress.
- However, close monitoring is still necessary to ensure the condition does not worsen.

### Grade 2—Moderate

- Grade 2 abruptio placentae refers to a moderate degree of placental separation.
- In this case, the bleeding is typically more pronounced, and the symptoms may be more severe.
- The mother may experience abdominal pain, uterine tenderness, and potentially more noticeable vaginal bleeding.
- Fetal distress may also be present, and closer monitoring and medical intervention are required.

### Grade 3—Severe

- Grade 3 abruptio placentae is the most severe form of placental separation. It involves complete separation of the placenta from the uterine wall.

- This results in significant bleeding and can cause life-threatening complications for both the mother and the baby.
- The mother may experience severe abdominal pain, intense vaginal bleeding, and signs of shock.
- Fetal distress is likely, and immediate medical intervention, such as emergency delivery, is necessary to ensure the well-being of both mother and baby.

### Pathophysiology

- The pathophysiology of abruptio placentae involves the premature separation of the placenta from the uterine wall before delivery.
- This separation disrupts the normal blood flow between the mother and the fetus, leading to various clinical manifestations and potential complications.
- The exact cause of abruptio placentae is not always clear, but several factors can contribute to its development. Here is an overview of the pathophysiology of abruptio placentae:
  - *Placental detachment:* The placenta normally attaches to the uterine wall and receives oxygen and nutrients from the maternal blood supply. In abruptio placentae, the placenta separates partially or completely from the uterine wall, disrupting the normal blood flow.
  - *Disruption of blood supply:* Placental detachment leads to the disruption of blood vessels that supply the placenta. This can result in bleeding within the uterine cavity, between the placenta and the uterine wall, or concealed behind the placenta. The severity of bleeding can vary, ranging from mild to severe, and may be overt or covert.
  - *Compromised fetal oxygenation and nutrient supply:* With placental separation and bleeding, the exchange of oxygen and nutrients between the mother and the fetus is compromised. This can lead to fetal hypoxia (insufficient oxygen supply) and reduced nutrient delivery, affecting the baby's well-being.
  - *Maternal and fetal complications:* The severity of abruptio placentae determines the potential complications for both the mother and the fetus. Maternal complications include hemorrhagic shock, disseminated intravascular coagulation (DIC), and renal failure. Fetal complications can range from fetal distress, growth restriction, preterm birth, to stillbirth.
  - *Contributing factors:* Various factors can increase the risk of abruptio placentae, including advanced maternal age, high blood pressure (hypertension), Pre-eclampsia, previous history of abruptio placentae, trauma to the abdomen (such as from motor vehicle accidents or domestic violence), smoking, drug use (particularly cocaine), multiple pregnancies (such as twins or triplets), and certain genetic or vascular disorders.

It is important to note that the exact mechanisms underlying placental separation in abruptio placentae are not fully understood and may vary between cases. The condition can present with varying degrees of severity, ranging from mild cases with minimal symptoms to severe cases with life-threatening complications. Prompt recognition, accurate diagnosis, and appropriate management are essential in mitigating the risks associated with abruptio placentae and optimizing outcomes for both the mother and the baby.

### Signs and Symptoms

The signs and symptoms of abruptio placentae can vary depending on the severity of the condition. Common signs and symptoms include:

- **Vaginal bleeding:** Dark red or purple vaginal bleeding may occur, although in some cases, bleeding may not be apparent or may be concealed behind the placenta.
- **Abdominal pain:** Women with abruptio placentae often experience severe, continuous abdominal pain. The pain may be localized or spread across the abdomen, and it may not subside or may worsen over time.
- **Uterine tenderness:** The uterus may feel tender or painful when touched or palpated by a healthcare provider.
- **Back pain:** Some women may experience persistent, intense back pain that may radiate from the lower back to the abdomen.
- **Uterine contractions:** Women with abruptio placentae may experience frequent, painful uterine contractions, often described as a constant tightening or cramping sensation.
- **Fetal distress:** The baby may show signs of distress, such as decreased fetal movement, an abnormal heart rate (either too fast or too slow), or a non-reassuring pattern on fetal monitoring.
- **Signs of shock:** In severe cases of abruptio placentae, signs of shock may be present, including rapid heartbeat, low blood pressure, pale and cool skin, lightheadedness, and confusion.

### Complications of Abruptio Placentae

#### Maternal Complications

- Maternal mortality
- Hypovolemic shock

- Postpartum hemorrhage
- Blood coagulation disorders
- Oliguria and anuria
- Renal failure
- Multiple organ failure
- Puerperal sepsis

*Fetal Complications*

- Prematurity
- Congenital anomalies
- Intrauterine growth restriction (IUGR)
- Hypoxia to the fetus
- Disseminated intravascular coagulation (DIC)

## Management

### Medical Management

The medical management of abruptio placentae, also known as placental abruption, involves prompt assessment, stabilization, and appropriate interventions to ensure the well-being of the mother and the baby. The specific management approach depends on the severity of the condition and the gestational age of the pregnancy. Here are the key aspects of medical management for abruptio placentae **(Flowchart 12.5)**:

- **Assessment and monitoring:** The healthcare team will assess the severity of the abruptio placentae through physical examination, evaluation of vital signs, and monitoring of fetal well-being. Continuous fetal heart rate monitoring may be initiated to assess the baby's condition.
- **Intravenous fluid resuscitation:** If the mother is experiencing signs of shock, intravenous fluids are administered to stabilize her blood pressure and improve perfusion to vital organs.
- **Blood transfusion:** In cases of significant blood loss, blood transfusion may be necessary to replace the lost blood and maintain adequate oxygen-carrying capacity.
- **Emergency delivery:** In severe cases of abruptio placentae or if the mother or baby's life is at immediate risk, an emergency delivery may be performed. The mode of delivery depends on various factors, including gestational age, maternal stability, and fetal well-being. A cesarean delivery (C-section) is often the preferred method to expedite delivery and minimize the risk of further bleeding.

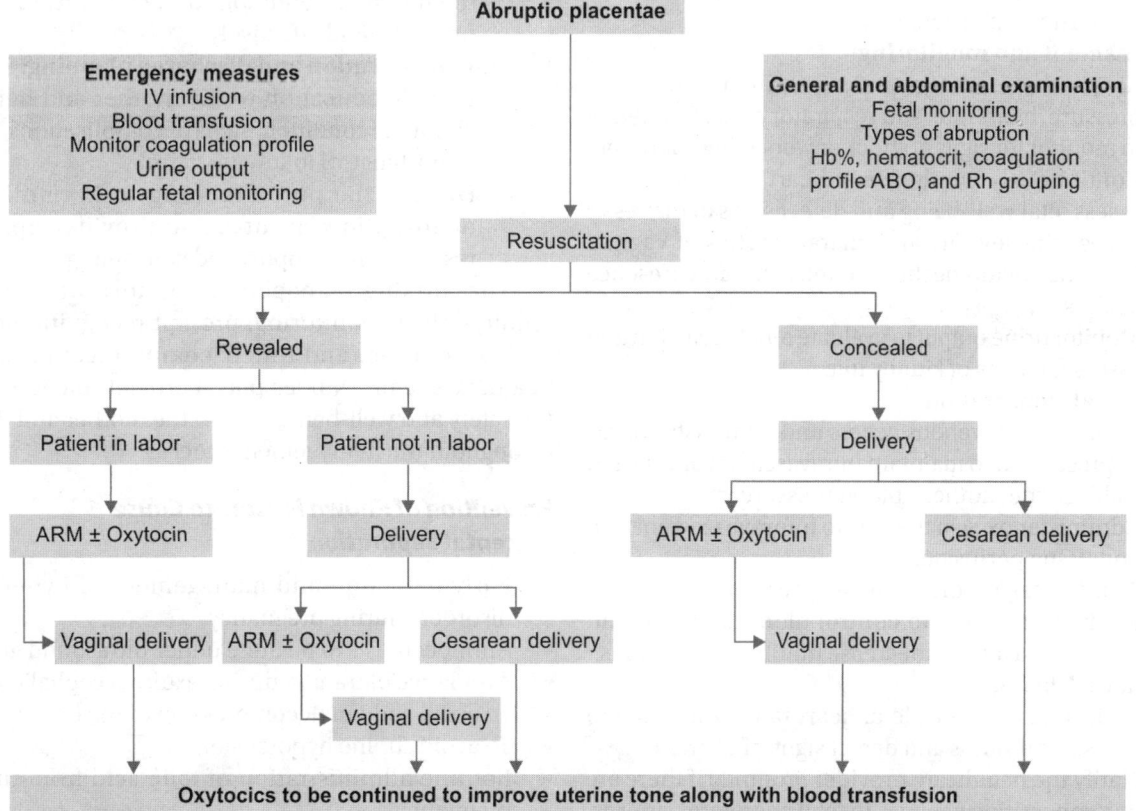

**Flowchart 12.5:** Scheme of management of abruptio placentae.

- **Coagulation management:** Coagulation factors may be assessed through laboratory tests, such as coagulation profile and platelet count. If there are abnormalities, the healthcare team may administer blood products, such as fresh frozen plasma or platelets, to correct coagulation deficits and prevent excessive bleeding.
- **Maternal stabilization:** Hemodynamic stability of the mother is crucial. Medications may be administered to manage blood pressure, control bleeding, and prevent complications associated with abruptio placentae.
- **Fetal well-being:** Continuous monitoring of the baby's heart rate is essential. If there are signs of fetal distress or compromised well-being, expedited delivery may be necessary.
- **Postpartum care:** Following delivery, the mother's recovery is closely monitored. Vital signs, bleeding, and coagulation parameters are assessed. Pain management, fluid balance, and close observation for any signs of infection or complications are provided.

*Nursing Management*

The nursing management of abruptio placentae, focuses on providing immediate and comprehensive care to the mother and the baby. The nursing interventions aim to stabilize the mother's condition, monitor fetal well-being, and prevent complications. Here are the key nursing considerations for managing abruptio placentae:

- **Assessment and monitoring:**
  - Assess the mother's vital signs, including blood pressure, heart rate, and respiratory rate, frequently to monitor for signs of shock or worsening condition.
  - Continuously monitor fetal heart rate patterns to assess fetal well-being and detect signs of distress.
  - Assess the severity and characteristics of vaginal bleeding, including the amount, color, and presence of clots.
  - Monitor urine output to evaluate renal perfusion and assess for signs of kidney injury.
- **Maternal stabilization:**
  - Establish intravenous access and administer fluids as prescribed to maintain intravascular volume and stabilize the mother's blood pressure.
  - Administer oxygen therapy to improve oxygenation and tissue perfusion.
  - Administer medications as prescribed, such as antihypertensives to control blood pressure and uterine relaxants to decrease uterine contractions.
- **Fetal well-being:**
  - Perform continuous fetal heart rate monitoring to assess fetal status and detect signs of distress.
  - Notify the healthcare provider promptly if there are any concerning changes in fetal heart rate patterns.
  - Assist with non-stress tests or other fetal monitoring tests as indicated.
- **Emotional support and communication:**
  - Provide emotional support to the mother and her family, as abruptio placentae can be a distressing and potentially life-threatening condition.
  - Communicate clearly and compassionately about the condition, treatment plan, and potential outcomes.
  - Involve the family in decision-making processes and ensure they have access to necessary information and resources.
- **Collaboration and teamwork:**
  - Collaborate with the healthcare team, including obstetricians, anesthesiologists, and other specialists, to ensure a coordinated approach to care.
  - Facilitate effective communication among team members to share information, monitor the progress of the condition, and promptly address any changes or concerns.
- **Documentation and reporting:**
  - Document the assessments, interventions, and the mother's response to treatment accurately and in a timely manner.
  - Communicate important findings and changes in the mother's condition to the healthcare provider promptly and effectively.
- **Patient education and discharge planning:**
  - Provide education to the mother and her family about the condition, signs of complications, and the importance of follow-up care.
  - Discuss the potential long-term implications of abruptio placentae and provide appropriate resources for support and counseling.

The nursing management of abruptio placentae requires close monitoring, prompt recognition of signs of deterioration, and timely communication with the healthcare team. Nurses play a crucial role in ensuring the safety and well-being of both the mother and the baby throughout the management process.

### Prevention of Known Factors to Cause Placental Separation

- Early detection and management of hypertensive disorders during pregnancy
- Amniocentesis to be done under ultrasound guidance
- Avoidance of trauma during external cephalic version
- To avoid sudden decompression of the uterus
- To avoid supine hypotension
- Routine administration of folic acid from the early pregnancy

## Conclusion

Antepartum hemorrhage is a major cause of maternal morbidity and mortality all over the world. The timely managing of placenta previa and abruptio placentae can be contingent upon the severity of the problem and also on the duration of pregnancy. It is important to note that the management of abruptio placentae may differ based on the individual circumstances, the severity of the condition, and the healthcare provider's judgment. The goal is to stabilize the mother, optimize fetal well-being, and provide timely interventions to minimize potential complications. The healthcare team, including obstetricians, nurses, and other specialists, collaborate closely to ensure appropriate management and ongoing care.

### Scheme of Management of Abruptio Placentae

See **Flowchart 12.5**.

# PREGNANCY-INDUCED HYPERTENSION (PIH)

Hypertension in pregnancy is a common cause of maternal and perinatal morbidity and mortality. There is a wide variation in the incidence of hypertension in pregnancy due to differences in the definition and the diagnostic methods. Pre-eclampsia and eclampsia seem to create more concern than others; however, any form of hypertension in pregnancy increases the risk of adverse pregnancy outcomes (Gbala MO, 2021).

## Definition

- PIH is defined as the presence of new-onset hypertension (blood pressure ≥140/90 mm Hg) during pregnancy without the presence of proteinuria.
- Pregnancy-induced hypertension (PIH), also known as gestational hypertension, is a condition characterized by the development of high blood pressure during pregnancy. It typically arises after 20 weeks of gestation and usually resolves after delivery. PIH is one of the most common complications of pregnancy, affecting a significant number of women worldwide.
- Gestational hypertension is characterized by elevation of blood pressure after mid-pregnancy for the first time and without presence of proteinuria. Later this may leads to pre-eclampsia. Increased blood pressures without proteinuria or other signs of pre-eclampsia are found in the gestational hypertensive patients. Up to 1/3 of those who are thought to have gestational hypertension are later found to have pre-eclampsia.

## Incidence

- It is one of the most common complications of pregnancy, affecting approximately 5–10% of pregnancies worldwide (ACOG, 2019).
- Hypertension, complicating 5 to 7% of all pregnancies, is a leading cause of maternal and fetal morbidity, particularly when the elevated blood pressure (BP) is due to pre-eclampsia, either alone (pure) or "superimposed" on chronic vascular disease (Program NH, 2000).
- PIH can range from mild to severe, with severe cases posing a higher risk of complications.

## Risk Factors

Several risk factors have been associated with the development of PIH, these are (Roberts, 2003):
- Primi mothers
- Advanced maternal age (over 35 years)
- Pre-existing hypertension
- Obesity
- Multiple pregnancies (e.g., twins or triplets)
- Certain medical conditions such as diabetes and kidney disease.

## Clinical Types

Pregnancy-induced hypertension (PIH), can be categorized into different clinical types based on its progression and associated features. The clinical types of PIH include the following:
- **Gestational hypertension:** This is the mildest form of PIH. It is diagnosed when a woman develops high blood pressure (systolic blood pressure of 140 mm Hg or higher and/or diastolic blood pressure of 90 mm Hg or higher) after 20 weeks of gestation, without the presence of proteinuria (excess protein in the urine). Blood pressure returns to normal within 12 weeks postpartum, and there is typically no evidence of end-organ damage.
- **Pre-eclampsia:** Pre-eclampsia is a more severe form of PIH. It is diagnosed when a woman develops high blood pressure after 20 weeks of gestation along with proteinuria (urinary protein excretion of 0.3 g or higher in a 24-hour urine collection or a protein/creatinine ratio of 0.3 or higher). Pre-eclampsia can also manifest with other signs and symptoms, including headache, visual disturbances, upper abdominal pain, and laboratory abnormalities (such as liver or kidney dysfunction). It can lead to complications for both the mother and the baby.
- **Eclampsia:** Eclampsia is the most severe form of pre-eclampsia and is characterized by the occurrence of seizures or convulsions in a woman with pre-eclampsia.

These seizures are unrelated to pre-existing neurological conditions and can present during pregnancy, childbirth, or the postpartum period. Eclampsia requires immediate medical attention due to the potential risks to the mother and the baby.

## Gestational Hypertension

Gestational hypertension is a type of pregnancy-induced hypertension (PIH) characterized by the development of high blood pressure (systolic blood pressure of 140 mm Hg or higher and/or diastolic blood pressure of 90 mm Hg or higher) after 20 weeks of gestation in a previously normotensive woman. It is diagnosed when elevated blood pressure is present without the concurrent presence of proteinuria (excess protein in the urine) or other signs of organ damage.

- **Onset and resolution:** Gestational hypertension typically arises after 20 weeks of gestation and resolves within 12 weeks after delivery.
- **Absence of proteinuria:** Unlike Pre-eclampsia, gestational hypertension is characterized by the absence of significant proteinuria (urinary protein excretion of 0.3 g or higher in a 24-hour urine collection or a protein/creatinine ratio of 0.3 or higher).
- **Blood pressure management:** The management of gestational hypertension aims to control blood pressure to prevent complications. Lifestyle modifications, such as regular physical activity, a balanced diet, and adequate rest, may be recommended. In some cases, antihypertensive medications may be prescribed to keep blood pressure within a safe range.
- **Monitoring and follow-up:** Regular monitoring of blood pressure and fetal well-being is essential for women with gestational hypertension. Prenatal visits may be more frequent to closely monitor the condition and evaluate potential complications.
- **Potential progression:** Gestational hypertension can progress to pre-eclampsia, a more severe form of PIH. Therefore, close monitoring is crucial to detect any signs of worsening hypertension or the development of proteinuria or other pre-eclampsia-related symptoms.

## Pre-eclampsia

### Definition

One of the hypertensive disorders of pregnancy, pre-eclampsia is typically described as new-onset hypertension with proteinuria after 20 weeks of pregnancy. However, it is today recognized as a complex, progressive, multisystem condition with a highly varied course and a number of grave consequences. As a result of the pre-eclampsia pathophysiology becoming better understood, the American College of obstetricians and gynecologists task force on hypertension in pregnancy has improved pre-eclampsia diagnostic criteria. New goals for screening, diagnosis, prevention, and treatment have also developed (Anderson CM, 2017). Pre-eclampsia is the hypertension of 140/90 mm Hg or more found after 20 weeks of pregnancy with substantial proteinuria in aearlier normotensive and nonproteinuric woman.

### Incidence

The incidence of pre-eclampsia in hospital setting varies from 5 to 15%. The incidence is about 10% in case of primigravida whereas 5% in multigravida.

### Risk Factors for Pre-eclampsia

- Primigravida
- Maternal age (<20 or >35)
- Multiple gestation
- New paternity
- Family history: Hypertension, pre-eclampsia
- Abnormalities of placenta
- Obesity
- Pre-existing vascular disease
- Chronic hypertension
- Chronic renal disease

### Etiology for Pre-eclampsia

- **Placental dysfunction:** Abnormal placentation and inadequate remodeling of uterine spiral arteries are key factors in pre-eclampsia development. This leads to impaired placental perfusion and compromised nutrient and oxygen exchange (Roberts, 1999).
- **Genetic factors:** Genetic predisposition plays a role in pre-eclampsia susceptibility, with familial clustering and heritability observed (Saleh, 2020).
- **Immune maladaptation:** Dysregulation of the maternal immune response and abnormal placentation contribute to the pathogenesis of pre-eclampsia (Redman, 2005).
- **Endothelial dysfunction:** Pre-eclampsia is associated with endothelial dysfunction, characterized by impaired vascular relaxation, increased vasoconstriction, and systemic inflammation (Roberts, 2012).
- **Abnormal trophoblast invasion:** Deficient invasion of trophoblast cells into maternal spiral arteries results in inadequate remodeling, leading to reduced uteroplacental blood flow and pre-eclampsia.
- **Maternal factors:** Various maternal factors increase the risk of pre-eclampsia, including primiparity, advanced

maternal age, obesity, pre-existing hypertension, diabetes, and certain autoimmune disorders (Duley, 2009).

## Pathophysiology

It involves multiple mechanisms that contribute to vascular dysfunction, inflammation, oxidative stress, and endothelial damage. Here is an overview of the pathophysiology of pre-eclampsia.

- **Placental factors:** Abnormal placental development and inadequate invasion of trophoblast cells into the maternal spiral arteries lead to impaired remodeling of the uterine vasculature (Redman, 2005).
- **Placental ischemia/hypoxia:** In pre-eclampsia, the compromised uteroplacental blood flow results in placental ischemia and subsequent release of factors, such as soluble fms-like tyrosine kinase 1 (sFlt-1) and soluble endoglin (sEng), into the maternal circulation. These factors contribute to endothelial dysfunction, reduced nitric oxide (NO) bioavailability, and increased vasoconstriction (Maynard, 2003).
- **Endothelial dysfunction:** Pre-eclampsia is characterized by widespread endothelial dysfunction, with impaired vasodilation, increased vascular permeability, and altered coagulation.
  Dysregulated release of vasoactive substances, such as endothelin-1, thromboxane A2, and angiotensin II, contributes to vasoconstriction and increased blood pressure (Roberts, 2012).
- **Inflammation and oxidative stress:** Pre-eclampsia involves an exaggerated inflammatory response and increased oxidative stress.
  Activated leukocytes, cytokines, and pro-inflammatory factors contribute to systemic inflammation, endothelial activation, and tissue damage.
  Oxidative stress, resulting from an imbalance between reactive oxygen species (ROS) production and antioxidant defenses, further promotes endothelial dysfunction and organ injury (Sankaralingam, 2016).
- **Systemic manifestations:** Pre-eclampsia can affect multiple organ systems, including the liver, kidneys, brain, and hematological system, leading to complications such as liver dysfunction, renal impairment, neurological symptoms, and coagulopathy (Roberts, 2001).

## Diagnostic Criteria of Pre-eclampsia

### Hypertension

The hallmark feature of pre-eclampsia is the development of high blood pressure. The diagnostic criteria for pre-eclampsia include a systolic blood pressure of 140 mm Hg or higher and/or a diastolic blood pressure of 90 mm Hg or higher on two occasions, at least four hours apart, in a previously normotensive woman during pregnancy (ACOG, 2019).

### Proteinuria

Proteinuria, the presence of excess protein in the urine, is a common finding in pre-eclampsia. It is typically assessed by a 24-hour urine collection, with a protein excretion of 0.3 g or higher considered significant (Brown, 2019).

- Thrombocytopenia (platelets < 100 000/mm$^3$)
- Impaired LFT (2 × normal)
- Renal insufficiency (Cr = 1.1 mg/dL)
- Pulmonary edema
- New onset cerebral disturbance or visual impairment

## Clinical Features

Pre-eclampsia is principally a syndrome of signs and when symptoms appear, it is usually late.

### Symptoms

- Slight swelling over the ankles which persists on rising from the bed in the morning or tightness of the ring on the finger is the early manifestation of pre-eclampsia edema. Gradually, the swelling may extend to the face, abdominal wall, vulva feet, and even the whole body (ACOG, 2019).
- **Headaches:** Persistent or severe headaches can occur in pre-eclampsia and should be evaluated.
- **Visual disturbances:** Visual changes such as blurred vision, flashing lights, or floaters may be indicative of pre-eclampsia.
- **Abdominal pain:** Epigastric pain (upper abdominal pain, just below the ribs) can be a sign of liver involvement in pre-eclampsia.
- **Nausea and vomiting:** Some women with pre-eclampsia may experience persistent nausea and vomiting (Magee, 2014).

### Signs

- Abnormal weight gain
- Rise in blood pressure
- Visible edema over the ankles
- Pulmonary edema
- Abdominal examination may reveal evidence of chronic placental insufficiency, such as scanty liquor or growth retardation of the fetus
- Thus, the manifestations of pre-eclampsia usually appear in the following order, rapid gain in weight visible edema and/or hypertension, and proteinuria.

## Complications of Pre-eclampsia

### Maternal Complications during the Prenatal Period
- Eclampsia
- Accidental hemorrhage
- Oliguria/anuria
- Dullness in vision
- Preterm labor
- HELLP syndrome
- Cerebral hemorrhage
- Acute respiratory distress syndrome (ARDS)

### During Labor
- Eclampsia
- Postpartum hemorrhage

### Puerperium
- Eclampsia within 48 hours of delivery
- Shock
- Puerperal sepsis

### Fetal Complications
- Intrauterine death
- Intrauterine growth restriction
- Asphyxia
- Prematurity

## Medical Management

### Antenatal Management (Before 37 Weeks)
The management of pre-eclampsia before 37 weeks of gestation aims to:
- Prevent complications
- Stabilize the mother's condition
- Optimize fetal well-being

The specific approach to management may vary based on the severity of pre-eclampsia and the gestational age of the fetus. Here are the key components of pre-eclampsia management before 37 weeks.

### Antenatal care and monitoring
- Regular antenatal visits are crucial to monitor blood pressure, assess symptoms, and evaluate fetal well-being.
- Blood pressure should be monitored frequently, and laboratory tests, including complete blood count, liver function tests, and renal function tests, may be performed to assess the severity of pre-eclampsia and detect complications.
- Fetal well-being should be evaluated through regular fetal movement assessments, non-stress tests, and/or ultrasound evaluations (Magee, 2014).

### Blood pressure management
- Blood pressure control is an essential aspect of pre-eclampsia management.
- Mild to moderate hypertension may be managed through lifestyle modifications, such as rest, reduced sodium intake, and increased fluid intake.
- In severe cases or when blood pressure remains uncontrolled, antihypertensive medications may be prescribed (ACOG, 2019).

### Magnesium sulfate therapy
- Magnesium sulfate is commonly administered to women with pre-eclampsia before 32–34 weeks of gestation to prevent eclamptic seizures.
- It is typically given intravenously and continued for a specified duration, usually until 24 hours postpartum (Duley, 2010).

### Fetal surveillance
- Close monitoring of the fetal condition is essential in pre-eclampsia management.
- Serial ultrasound examinations, non-stress tests, and/or umbilical artery Doppler studies may be performed to assess fetal growth, amniotic fluid levels, and umbilical artery blood flow.
- The timing of delivery may be determined based on the severity of pre-eclampsia, gestational age, and fetal well-being (Brown, 2018).

### Corticosteroids for fetal lung maturation
- If preterm delivery is anticipated due to severe pre-eclampsia, corticosteroids (e.g., betamethasone) may be administered to promote fetal lung maturation and reduce the risk of respiratory distress syndrome.
- The timing and dosing of corticosteroids are based on gestational age and individual patient factors (ACOG, Bulletin 207, 2019).

### Hospitalization and expert care
- Women with severe pre-eclampsia, evidence of end-organ damage, or severe hypertension may require hospitalization for closer monitoring and specialized care.
- Consultation with obstetric specialists, such as maternal-fetal medicine specialists or obstetric critical care specialists, can provide expert management in complex cases (ACOG, 2019).

### Intranatal Management
Intrapartum management of pre-eclampsia involves careful monitoring and interventions to ensure the safety and well-being of both the mother and the baby during the labor and

delivery process. The specific intrapartum management approach may vary based on the severity of pre-eclampsia, gestational age, and the clinical condition of the mother and the baby. Here are key aspects of intrapartum management of pre-eclampsia, along with references for further reading:

- **Continuous maternal and fetal monitoring:**
  - Close monitoring of the mother's blood pressure, heart rate, and oxygen saturation is essential throughout labor.
  - Continuous electronic fetal monitoring is typically performed to assess the baby's heart rate and detect any signs of fetal distress (Magee, 2014).
- **Blood pressure management:**
  - Blood pressure control is crucial during labor to prevent severe hypertension and minimize the risk of complications.
  - Antihypertensive medications may be administered if blood pressure remains elevated or if there are signs of end-organ damage (ACOG- 202, 2019).
- **Magnesium sulfate for seizure prophylaxis:**
  - Magnesium sulfate is typically continued intravenously during labor and delivery to prevent eclamptic seizures in women with pre-eclampsia.
  - The dosage and administration may vary based on the hospital protocol and individual patient factors (Duley, 2010).
- **Labor induction and augmentation:**
  - In cases of severe pre-eclampsia or when there are signs of maternal or fetal compromise, labor induction may be recommended to expedite delivery.
  - Oxytocin augmentation may be used to enhance labor progress when necessary (ACOG- 107, 2019).
- **Mode of delivery:**
  - The mode of delivery (vaginal or cesarean) is determined based on various factors, including the severity of pre-eclampsia, gestational age, fetal well-being, and the clinical condition of the mother.
  - **Vaginal delivery** is generally preferred when maternal and fetal conditions allow.
  - **Cesarean delivery** may be indicated in cases of fetal distress, severe maternal hypertension, placental abruption, or other obstetric indications (Brown, 2018).

## Anesthesia Considerations

- Anesthesia options, such as epidural or spinal anesthesia, may be used for pain relief during labor. However, the decision should be individualized based on the patient's condition and preferences.
- Anesthesia providers should be aware of the patient's diagnosis of pre-eclampsia and collaborate with the obstetric team to ensure safe administration (SOAP, 2016).

### Antihypertensive Therapy

The use of antihypertensive drugs in the management of pre-eclampsia should be determined by healthcare professionals based on the severity of hypertension, gestational age, presence of end-organ damage, and individual patient factors. Antihypertensive treatment aims to lower blood pressure to safe levels while considering the potential impact on placental perfusion. Here are some commonly used antihypertensive drugs for pre-eclampsia **(Table 12.2)**:

Labetalol

- Labetalol is considered a first-line antihypertensive medication for the management of pre-eclampsia.
- It is a non-selective beta-blocker with additional alpha-blocking properties.
- Labetalol is generally well tolerated and can be administered orally or intravenously (Brown, 2018).

Nifedipine

- Nifedipine, a calcium channel blocker, is commonly used for the management of hypertension in pre-eclampsia.
- It acts primarily as a vasodilator, reducing peripheral vascular resistance and lowering blood pressure.
- Immediate-release nifedipine is often preferred over the extended-release formulation due to concerns about rapid blood pressure lowering.

Methyldopa

- Methyldopa is considered safe and effective for the management of hypertension in pre-eclampsia.
- It acts centrally to lower blood pressure and is generally well tolerated during pregnancy.
- Methyldopa is commonly used when other antihypertensive medications are not preferred or contraindicated (ACOG-202, 2019).

Hydralazine

- Hydralazine is an arterial vasodilator that can be used for the management of severe hypertension in pre-eclampsia.
- It is typically administered intravenously and can rapidly lower blood pressure.
- Hydralazine may be used when other antihypertensive agents are contraindicated or ineffective (ACOG-202, 2019).

**Table 12.2:** Antihypertensives in pre-eclampsia with severe symptoms (Odigboegwu O, 2018).

| Drugs | Indication | Dose | Comment |
|---|---|---|---|
| **First line** | | | |
| Methyldopa | PE with severe symptoms hypertension in pregnancy | 0.5–3 g/day PO in 2 divided doses | Established long-term safety. Breast milk compatible mild hypertensive effect and slow onset of action, hence may not be used alone |
| Labetalol | PE with severe symptoms, usually IV formulation | Start with 20 mg IV bolus may require double dose 10 min later | Rapid onset of action studies confirm safety in pregnancy may cause maternal hepatotoxicity |
| Hydralazine | PE with severe symptoms, usually IV formulation. Long-acting nifedipine | 5 mg IV slowly over 1 to 2 min 30–90 mg once daily. May be increased at 7- to 14-day intervals, to maximum dose of 120 mg a day | Usually breast milk compatible. More adverse effect than labetalol hypotensive effect is less predictable |
| Nifedipine | PE with severe symptoms, immediate release oral formulation | Start with 10 mg PO. May repeat the dose 30 min later | Use particularly when IV access is not available. May cause rapid drops in BP. Concern of serious side effects when used simultaneous with magnesium sulfate. |
| **Second line** | | | |
| Nicardipine | Resistant acute-onset severe hypertension when first line has failed | Give as IV infusion of 3 to 9 mg/hour | Delay onset of action (5–15 min). Titrate slowly to avoid overdose |
| Sodium Nitroprusside | Acute life-threatening hypertension associated with PE | Start with 0.24 µg/kg/min. May titrate to maximum dose of 5 µg/kg/min | Rarely used in dire emergency. Give for shortest amount of time to avoid toxicity (cyanide and thiocyanate) |

(IV: intravenous; PE: Pre-eclampsia; PO: per oral)

### Postpartum Management

The postpartum management of pre-eclampsia focuses on monitoring and supportive care to ensure the well-being of the mother and the prompt resolution of the hypertensive disorder. The key aspects of postpartum management of pre-eclampsia:

- **Blood pressure monitoring:**
  - Blood pressure should continue to be monitored regularly in the immediate postpartum period to ensure that it returns to normal levels.
  - The frequency of blood pressure monitoring may vary based on the severity of pre-eclampsia and the clinical judgment of the healthcare provider.
- **Observation for signs of complications:**
  - Close observation for signs and symptoms of complications associated with pre-eclampsia, such as postpartum eclampsia, stroke, pulmonary edema, or renal dysfunction, is essential.
  - Symptoms such as severe headache, visual disturbances, shortness of breath, chest pain, or worsening edema should be promptly reported to healthcare providers.
- **Management of residual symptoms:**
  - Postpartum women with residual symptoms of pre-eclampsia, such as persistent hypertension, proteinuria, or edema, may require ongoing medical management.
  - Antihypertensive medications may be continued or adjusted as necessary to control blood pressure.
  - Reference: American College of Obstetricians and Gynecologists. (2019). Hypertension in pregnancy. Practice Bulletin No. 202.
- **Assessment of renal and liver function:**
  - Evaluation of renal function through laboratory tests, such as serum creatinine and urine protein analysis, may be performed to assess renal recovery.
  - Liver function tests may be ordered to monitor for improvement in liver function following resolution of pre-eclampsia-related liver involvement.
- **Psychological support and education:**
  - Women who have experienced pre-eclampsia may benefit from psychological support and counseling to address any emotional or psychological concerns.
  - Education on the signs and symptoms of pre-eclampsia and the importance of long-term follow-up should be provided.
- **Contraception counseling:**
  - Contraception counseling and guidance on family planning options should be provided to postpartum women with a history of pre-eclampsia.

- Guidance on the choice of contraception methods that are safe and appropriate for the individual's health status should be discussed.

### Nursing Management

Nursing management plays a crucial role in the care of women with pre-eclampsia, ensuring their safety, monitoring for complications, and providing support throughout the pregnancy and postpartum period. Some important aspects of nursing management of pre-eclampsia:

- **Assessment and monitoring:**
  - Regular assessment of vital signs, including blood pressure, pulse, respiratory rate, and temperature, is essential to monitor the mother's condition.
  - Monitoring urine output, proteinuria levels, and laboratory values such as liver function tests and renal function tests are important in evaluating the severity of pre-eclampsia and assessing organ involvement.
  - Monitoring fetal well-being through regular fetal heart rate monitoring, nonstress tests, or ultrasound examinations is crucial.
- **Blood pressure management:**
  - Nurses play a vital role in monitoring and managing blood pressure levels in women with pre-eclampsia.
  - Regular blood pressure measurements should be taken using appropriate techniques and equipment.
  - Nurses may administer antihypertensive medications as prescribed by the healthcare provider, monitor the response to treatment, and report any significant changes or adverse effects.
- **Symptom management and comfort measures:**
  - Providing comfort measures to alleviate symptoms associated with pre-eclampsia, such as headaches or edema, is important.
  - Assisting with position changes, providing a quiet and calm environment, and promoting rest and relaxation can help reduce discomfort and stress.
- **Fluid and nutrition management:**
  - Nurses collaborate with the healthcare team to ensure adequate fluid and nutritional intake for women with pre-eclampsia.
  - Monitoring fluid balance, including intake and output, is important to prevent fluid overload or dehydration.
  - Educating women about a healthy diet, including foods low in sodium, is essential to manage blood pressure and promote overall well-being.
- **Medication administration:** Nurses are responsible for administering prescribed medications, such as antihypertensive drugs or magnesium sulfate for seizure prophylaxis, while ensuring accurate dosing, proper administration routes, and monitoring for potential side effects or adverse reactions.
- **Patient education and support:**
  - Providing comprehensive education to women and their families about pre-eclampsia, its signs and symptoms, the importance of regular prenatal care, and the need for adherence to prescribed medications is crucial.
  - Offering emotional support, addressing concerns or fears, and promoting open communication contribute to the overall well-being of women with pre-eclampsia.
- **Collaboration and communication:**
  - Nurses play a vital role in interdisciplinary collaboration, working closely with obstetricians, midwives, and other healthcare professionals to ensure coordinated and comprehensive care for women with pre-eclampsia.
  - Clear and timely communication regarding the woman's condition, any changes or concerns, and the plan of care is essential for effective management.

Nurses are at the forefront of providing care and support to women with pre-eclampsia. Their vigilant monitoring, skillful assessment, effective communication, and compassionate care significantly contribute to positive outcomes for both the mother and the baby.

### Prevention

Prevention of pre-eclampsia focuses on identifying and managing risk factors, promoting healthy lifestyle choices, and providing appropriate prenatal care. While pre-eclampsia cannot always be prevented, certain strategies may help reduce the risk or mitigate its severity.

#### Regular Prenatal Care

- Early and regular prenatal care is essential to monitor the mother's health and identify any risk factors or signs of pre-eclampsia.
- Regular prenatal visits allow healthcare providers to assess blood pressure, monitor urine for proteinuria, and perform necessary laboratory tests to detect and manage pre-eclampsia early.

#### Healthy Lifestyle Choices

- Encourage women to adopt a healthy lifestyle before and during pregnancy.
- Advise them to maintain a balanced diet rich in fruits, vegetables, whole grains, and lean proteins.

- Promote regular physical activity, such as walking or prenatal exercises, unless contraindicated.
- Encourage women to avoid excessive weight gain during pregnancy.

*Calcium Supplementation*
- Calcium supplementation during pregnancy has been associated with a potential reduction in the risk of pre-eclampsia, especially in populations with low dietary calcium intake.
- Healthcare providers may recommend calcium supplementation based on individual risk factors and regional guidelines.

*Aspirin Prophylaxis*
- Low-dose aspirin (75–150 mg/day) may be recommended for women at high risk of pre-eclampsia.
- This includes women with a history of pre-eclampsia, multiple gestations, chronic hypertension, renal disease, autoimmune disorders, or other risk factors.
- Aspirin prophylaxis is typically started between 12 and 28 weeks of gestation, after excluding contraindications.

*Management of Chronic Conditions*
- Effective management of pre-existing conditions, such as chronic hypertension or diabetes, is crucial in preventing or minimizing the impact of pre-eclampsia.
- Women with chronic conditions should receive appropriate medical management and regular monitoring during pregnancy.

*Smoking Cessation and Alcohol Avoidance*

Encourage women to quit smoking and avoid alcohol during pregnancy, as these substances have been associated with an increased risk of pre-eclampsia.

It is important to note that while these preventive measures may help reduce the risk or severity of pre-eclampsia, they may not completely eliminate the possibility of developing the condition. Each woman's individual risk factors and medical history should be taken into account when determining the appropriate preventive strategies.

The management decisions in pre-eclampsia should be individualized based on the patient's specific circumstances, gestational age, the severity of pre-eclampsia, and the expertise of the healthcare team. It is important for women with PIH to receive regular prenatal care and closely follow their healthcare provider's recommendations. With proper management and monitoring, most women with PIH can have successful pregnancies and healthy outcomes for both themselves and their babies.

## Eclampsia

Eclampsia is a serious and life-threatening complication that can occur during pregnancy. It is characterized by the onset of seizures or convulsions in a woman who has pre-eclampsia, a condition marked by high blood pressure and organ damage. Eclampsia typically occurs after the 20th week of pregnancy and can be a medical emergency requiring immediate intervention (ACOG, 2013).

### Definition

Eclampsia is a severe and potentially life-threatening condition that occurs during pregnancy or in the immediate postpartum period, characterized by the onset of seizures or convulsions in a woman with pre-eclampsia. Pre-eclampsia is a disorder marked by high blood pressure and organ damage, typically affecting the liver, kidneys, and blood clotting system. Eclampsia is considered the most severe complication of pre-eclampsia (ACOG, 2013), (Magee, 2014).

### Incidence

- Eclampsia is more prevalent in developing countries and regions with limited access to healthcare resources.
- According to the World Health Organization (WHO, 2014), eclampsia affects approximately 1 in 1,000 pregnancies worldwide.
- Eclampsia is a leading cause of maternal and perinatal morbidity and mortality, particularly in low- and middle-income countries.

### Etiology

The exact causes of eclampsia are not fully understood, it is believed to share similar underlying factors with pre-eclampsia. Some key causes of eclampsia along with references for further reading:

*Placental Dysfunction and Poor Placental Perfusion*

Impaired development and dysfunction of the placenta, leading to reduced blood flow and oxygen supply to the fetus, are considered significant factors in the pathogenesis of eclampsia (Redman, 2005).

*Abnormalities in the Immune System*

Dysregulation of the maternal immune response to the placenta, involving inflammation and vascular dysfunction, is thought to contribute to the development of eclampsia (Sargent, 2006).

## Endothelial Dysfunction

Eclampsia is associated with widespread endothelial dysfunction, affecting various organs and systems, leading to vasoconstriction, increased blood pressure, and organ damage (Redman, 2003).

## Genetic Factors

Genetic factors are thought to play a role in the development of eclampsia, as evidenced by familial clustering and genetic variations associated with the condition (Roberts, 2001).

## Other Risk Factors

In addition to the shared risk factors with pre-eclampsia, such as maternal age, obesity, and pre-existing medical conditions, other factors like first pregnancy, multiple pregnancies, and a history of pre-eclampsia/eclampsia increase the risk of developing eclampsia (Ananth, 2013).

## Clinical Features of Eclampsia

Eclampsia is a serious condition characterized by the onset of seizures or convulsions in a woman with pre-eclampsia during pregnancy or in the postpartum period. These seizures are typically generalized tonic-clonic seizures, involving loss of consciousness, convulsions, and muscle rigidity. Here are some key clinical features of eclampsia:

- **Seizures:** The hallmark feature of eclampsia is the occurrence of seizures. These seizures can manifest as convulsions characterized by rhythmic muscle contractions and relaxations. They can be generalized, affecting the entire body, and may last from a few seconds to several minutes (Magee, 2018).
- **Preceding symptoms of pre-eclampsia:** Eclampsia typically follows the development of pre-eclampsia. Pre-eclampsia is characterized by high blood pressure (hypertension) and the presence of protein in the urine (proteinuria). Women with eclampsia often have exhibited symptoms of pre-eclampsia prior to the onset of seizures, including (Brown 2018).
  - *Hypertension:* Elevated blood pressure readings, often above 140/90 mm Hg.
  - *Proteinuria:* The presence of excess protein in the urine, usually measured by a urine dipstick or a 24-hour urine collection.
  - *Edema:* Swelling, particularly in the hands, feet, and face, caused by fluid retention.
  - *Headache:* Persistent or severe headaches.
  - *Visual disturbances:* Vision changes, such as blurred vision, double vision, or flashing lights.
  - *Abdominal pain:* Discomfort or pain in the upper abdomen, typically on the right side.
- **Altered consciousness and neurological symptoms:** During eclamptic seizures, the affected individual loses consciousness and may exhibit various neurological symptoms, including (Roberts, 2001).
  - *Altered mental status:* Confusion, disorientation, or loss of consciousness.
  - *Muscle rigidity:* Stiffness and rigidity of muscles during seizures.
  - *Loss of bladder or bowel control:* Involuntary release of urine (urinary incontinence) or feces (fecal incontinence) during seizures.
  - *Postictal state:* After a seizure, there may be a period of confusion, drowsiness, and fatigue.
- **Systemic complications:** Eclampsia can lead to complications affecting various organ systems, including (Sibai, 2005):
  - *Cardiovascular system:* High blood pressure can strain the heart, leading to cardiac issues such as myocardial infarction or heart failure.
  - *Central nervous system:* Seizures can cause brain damage, stroke, or cerebral hemorrhage.
  - *Renal system:* Impaired kidney function and damage can occur due to reduced blood flow and increased strain on the kidneys.
  - *Hepatic system:* Liver dysfunction or hepatic rupture may arise as a result of compromised blood flow.
  - *Coagulation system:* Eclampsia can lead to abnormalities in blood clotting, potentially causing disseminated intravascular coagulation (DIC).

## Diagnosis

The diagnosis of eclampsia, a condition characterized by the occurrence of seizures in a woman with pre-eclampsia, is primarily based on clinical evaluation and the presence of characteristic symptoms. Here are some key points regarding the diagnosis of eclampsia:

## Clinical Presentation

Eclampsia is typically diagnosed in women with pre-eclampsia who develop seizures during pregnancy or in the postpartum period (Sibai, 2005).

- **Premonitory stage:**
  - The patient becomes unconscious.
  - The muscles of the face, tongue, and limbs becomes twitch. The stage remains for approximately 30 seconds.
- **Tonic stage:** The entire body undergone tonic spasm, the extremities are stretched and finger straightened. There is ends with respiration and the tongue projects among the teeth. Cyanosis may appear. Eye balls become static. This stage continues for about 30 seconds.

- **Clonic stage:** The voluntary muscles experience alternative contraction and relaxation. The twitch starts in the face followed by the extremities and entire body with convulsion. Chances of tongue bite, stertorous breathing are found; cyanosis becomes dissolves. This stage persists for 1 to 4 minutes.
- **Stage of coma:** Next the fit, the patient undergoes coma stage which remains for a short-term period. On instance, the patient may confused resulting the fit and forget about the events.

### History and Physical Examination

- History of pre-eclampsia symptoms (e.g., hypertension, proteinuria, edema), previous pregnancy history, and risk factors, is important for the diagnosis.
- Physical examination may reveal signs of pre-eclampsia, such as high blood pressure, edema, or evidence of end-organ damage (Ananth, 2013).

### Laboratory Investigations

- Laboratory tests are used to assess the severity of pre-eclampsia and to evaluate potential complications in eclampsia. These may include blood tests to assess liver and kidney function, complete blood count, and measurement of coagulation parameters.
- Urine tests, such as dipstick analysis or 24-hour urine collection, help detect proteinuria (ACOG Practice Bulletin No. 202).

### Imaging Studies

In some cases, imaging studies may be performed to assess organ damage or complications. These may include ultrasound examination of the kidneys, liver, or fetal well-being (ACOG 2013).

### Maternal Complications of Eclampsia

- **Injuries:** Tongue bite, injuries due to fall from bed, bed sore.
- **Pulmonary complications:**
  - Edema due to leaky blood capillaries
  - Pneumonia due to aspiration, hypostatic or infective
  - Adult respiratory distress syndrome
  - Embolism
- **Cardiac:** Acute left ventricular failure
- **Renal failure**
- **Hepatic:** Necrosis, subcapsular hematoma
- **Cerebral:** Edema (vasogenic) hemorrhage
- **Neurological deficits**
- **Disturbed vision:** Due to retinal detachment or occipital lobe ischemia

- **Hematological**
  - Thrombocytopenia
  - Disseminated intravascular
  - Coagulopathy
- **Postpartum**
  - Shock
  - Sepsis
  - Psychosis

### Medical Management

The primary goals of medical management of eclampsia are to control seizures, lower blood pressure, prevent complications, and deliver the baby **(Flowchart 12.6)**.

Here are the key components of medical management for eclampsia:

- **Stabilization:** The first step is to ensure the safety and stability of the mother and the baby. This involves maintaining a clear airway, providing oxygen if needed, and monitoring vital signs.
- **Seizure control:** Controlling seizures is crucial to prevent further complications. Intravenous administration of anticonvulsant medications is typically used to stop seizures. The most commonly used medication is magnesium sulfate, which is given as an initial loading

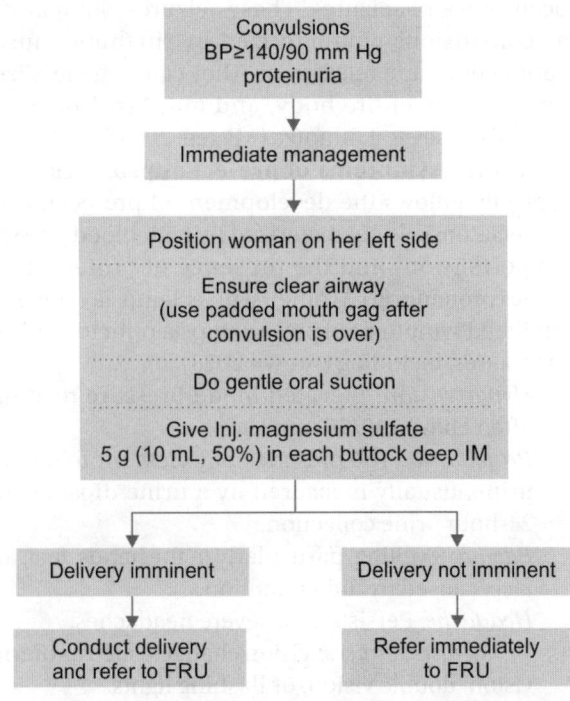

**Flowchart 12.6:** Management of eclampsia.

*Source:* SBA Quality Protocol Poster, NHM, Ministry of Health and Family Welfare, GOI.

dose followed by a maintenance infusion. Magnesium sulfate also helps prevent recurrent seizures.
- **Blood pressure control:** High blood pressure is a characteristic feature of eclampsia. Antihypertensive medications may be used to bring blood pressure under control, but careful monitoring is essential to avoid excessively lowering blood pressure, which could reduce placental perfusion.
- **Monitoring and evaluation:** Close monitoring of the mother and the baby is necessary to detect any signs of worsening condition or complications. This includes frequent blood pressure measurements, urine output monitoring, laboratory tests (such as blood tests and urine analysis), fetal heart rate monitoring, and ultrasound examinations.
- **Delivery:** Delivery of the baby is typically the definitive treatment for eclampsia. Depending on the gestational age, the urgency of the situation, and the maternal and fetal condition, the healthcare team will determine the most appropriate method of delivery. In some cases, an emergency cesarean section may be performed, while in others, induction of labor may be attempted.
- **Postpartum care:** After delivery, close monitoring and care continue to ensure the mother's recovery. Blood pressure control is important during the postpartum period, and magnesium sulfate may be continued for a period of time to prevent recurrent seizures. The healthcare team will also assess for any signs of complications, such as postpartum hemorrhage or organ dysfunction.

**The guidelines for management of eclampsia according to FOGSI are as follows (FOGSI, 2019):**
- **Need for help:** Avoid tongue bite, insert airway/mouth gag
- **Avoid injury:** Padded bed rails, restraints
- **Maintain $O_2$ saturation:** Pulse oximetry
- **Minimize aspiration:** Lateral decubitus position, oral suction
- Initiate magnesium sulfate.
- Control blood pressure.
- Delivery (LSCS is preferred for obstetric/fetal indications only).

1. The optimal drug for the treatment of eclampsia is $MgSO_4$. Initially loading dose of 4 g in slow IV at 4 mL/5 min by 20 mL syringe is given.
2. Maintenance dose of 5 g deep IM injection is given in every 4 hours in alternate buttocks.
3. Monitor the respiration rate, patellar reflexes and urine output.
4. Initiation of labor is done immediately after stabilization of the patient followed by vaginal delivery. Cesarean section is indicated in case of obstetric complications. Continue the antihypertensive drugs like labetalol, nifedipine, and hydralazine during labor.

It is important to note that the management of eclampsia requires specialized medical expertise and should be performed in a healthcare facility equipped to handle obstetric emergencies. Prompt and appropriate medical care significantly improves the outcome for both the mother and the baby.

*Nursing Management*

Nursing management plays a vital role in the care of a woman with eclampsia. Nurses are responsible for monitoring the patient, providing immediate interventions, and ensuring her safety and well-being. The key nursing interventions for the management of eclampsia:

Assessment and monitoring

- Perform a thorough initial assessment, including vital signs, oxygen saturation, and neurologic status.
- Continuously monitor vital signs, including blood pressure, heart rate, respiratory rate, and temperature.
- Assess and document the frequency, duration, and characteristics of seizures.
- Monitor fetal heart rate and uterine activity if the pregnancy is viable.
- Assess and document urine output, as oliguria (reduced urine output) may occur.
- Conduct regular neurological assessments to evaluate for changes in level of consciousness, motor function, and reflexes.

Seizure precautions

- Ensure a safe environment for the patient by padding the bed rails and removing any objects that could cause injury during seizures.
- Place the patient in a side-lying position to prevent aspiration and maintain a patent airway.
- Administer oxygen as prescribed to ensure adequate oxygenation during and after seizures.

Medication administration

- Assist with the administration of medications prescribed by the healthcare provider, such as anticonvulsants (e.g., magnesium sulfate) and antihypertensive agents.
- Monitor the patient's response to medications, including the effectiveness of seizure control and blood pressure reduction.

Fluid and electrolyte balance
- Monitor intake and output closely to assess fluid status.
- Monitor laboratory results, including electrolyte levels (such as serum magnesium, calcium, and sodium levels), renal function, and coagulation studies.
- Assist with intravenous fluid therapy as prescribed.

Emotional support and comfort
- Provide emotional support and reassurance to the patient and her family, as eclampsia can be a frightening and stressful experience.
- Maintain a calm and quiet environment to minimize triggers for seizures.
- Offer pain relief measures if the patient experiences headache or other discomfort.

Health education and discharge planning
- Educate the patient and her family about eclampsia, its signs and symptoms, and the importance of adhering to prescribed medications and follow-up appointments.
- Provide information about self-care measures and signs of potential complications to watch for after discharge.
- Collaborate with other healthcare professionals to develop a safe and appropriate discharge plan.

Eclampsia is a serious condition for both mother and the fetus. The condition requires prompt diagnosis and treatment for pregnant women. So, a preventive approach and proper emergency management of eclampsia is the key to reduce maternal mortality and morbidity. The collaborative work by the healthcare team is essential to manage proficiently for the best outcome. The health care giver should follow the clinical guidelines, updated and oriented their knowledge with the emergency management of eclampsia so that will get a better perinatal outcome to a great extent.

# OBSTRUCTED LABOR

Obstructed labor, also known as cephalopelvic disproportion (CPD), occurs when the size or position of the fetus prevents it from passing through the birth canal. This condition can lead to prolonged labor, fetal distress, and maternal complications. Prompt recognition and management are essential to ensure the well-being of both the mother and the baby. Here is an overview of obstructed labor with references to support the information provided.

## Definition

Obstructed labor occurs when the presenting part of the fetus cannot progress through the birth canal, despite strong uterine contractions (WHO, 2018).

Obstructed labor, refers to a condition in which the normal progression of labor is hindered or obstructed, leading to difficulties in the delivery of the fetus through the birth canal. It is characterized by the inability of the baby's head or body to pass through the pelvis or birth canal, resulting in prolonged labor or an inability to deliver the baby vaginally.

## Incidence

In the developing countries, the prevalence is about 1–2% in the referral hospitals.

## Etiology

Obstructed labor can have various causes, including fetal, maternal, and uterine factors. Here are some common causes:

### Fetal Factors
- **Malpresentation:** When the fetus is not in the normal head-down (vertex) position, it can lead to obstructed labor. Examples include breech presentation (buttocks or feet first), transverse lie (sideways position), or face presentation.
- **Fetal macrosomia:** A condition where the fetus is significantly larger than average, making it difficult to pass through the birth canal.
- **Fetal abnormalities:** Certain congenital anomalies or genetic conditions can interfere with the progress of labor.

### Maternal Factors
- **Pelvic abnormalities:** An abnormally shaped or contracted pelvis may impede the passage of the fetus. This can be due to conditions like pelvic dystocia, android pelvis, platypelloid pelvis, or tumors/growths blocking the birth canal.
- **Previous pelvic surgeries or fractures:** Scarring or deformities resulting from previous surgeries or fractures can restrict the space available for the baby to descend through the birth canal.
- **Pelvic inflammatory disease (PID):** Inflammation and scarring of the pelvis due to infections can cause narrowing or obstruction.

### Uterine Factors
- **Uterine inertia:** Weak or inadequate uterine contractions that do not effectively push the baby through the birth canal.
- **Uterine abnormalities:** Certain conditions, such as fibroids (benign tumors in the uterus) or uterine septum

(a malformation of the uterus), can obstruct labor by affecting the normal uterine function.

## Clinical Features

Obstructed labor is typically associated with specific clinical features that indicate difficulties in the progress of labor. The clinical presentation may vary depending on the underlying cause and severity of the obstruction. Some common clinical features of obstructed labor are (WHO, 2018) (Cunningham, 2018):

- **Prolonged labor:** Obstructed labor often leads to an abnormally prolonged duration of labor beyond the expected time frame.
- **Ineffective uterine contractions:** Insufficient or ineffective uterine contractions may occur, resulting in slow or halted progress of labor.
- **Failure to progress:** Despite strong uterine contractions, there is a failure of the presenting part of the fetus to descend through the birth canal.
- **Maternal exhaustion:** Prolonged and obstructed labor can cause severe exhaustion in the mother due to the prolonged physical exertion and pain.
- **Fetal distress:** The obstruction can lead to signs of fetal distress, such as abnormal fetal heart rate patterns or meconium-stained amniotic fluid.
- **Abnormal pelvic examination:** A physical examination of the pelvis may reveal signs of obstruction, such as inadequate cervical dilation, fetal malposition, or an inability to feel the presenting part of the fetus.
- **Maternal discomfort/pain:** The mother may experience severe and prolonged pain, which may not be relieved by analgesics or other comfort measures.

## Diagnosis

### History

- Prolonged labor
- Increase frequency and intensity of uterine contractions
- Rupture of the membranes

### General Examination

- Maternal distress, exhaustion
- Rise in body temperature and pulse
- Dryness of tongue, cracked lips

### Abdominal Examination

- Hard and tender uterus
- Regular and robust uterine contractions without reduction
- Presence of retraction ring

### Fetus

- Difficult to find the fetal parts
- FHS are absent or slow
- Fetal distress may be there
- Caput formation on the vertex presentation
- Cord prolapses
- Shoulder dystocia

### Vaginal Examination

- Edematous vulva
- Dry and hot vagina
- Fully or partially dilated cervix
- Ruptured membranes
- Nonengagement of the presenting part

## Complications

### Maternal

- Rupture of uterus
- Necrotic vesicovaginal fistula
- Intrauterine infections
- Peritonitis
- Puerperal sepsis
- Postpartum hemorrhage
- Injury to the birth canal

### Fetal

- Birth asphyxia
- Intracranial hemorrhage
- Birth injuries
- Neonatal infections

## Management

### Medical Management

The medical management of obstructed labor aims to safely resolve the obstruction and facilitate the delivery of the baby. The specific approach depends on the underlying cause, severity of the obstruction, and available resources. Here are some common medical management strategies (WHO, 2018) (Cunningham, 2018) (Gizzo, 2014):

### Non-surgical Interventions

- **Positional changes:** Adjusting the mother's position, such as changing from lying down to an upright or lateral position, may help optimize the pelvic dimensions and facilitate fetal descent.
- **Augmentation of labor:** Administering oxytocin or other medications to strengthen uterine contractions and promote progress in labor.
- **Amniotomy:** Artificial rupture of membranes to facilitate the descent of the baby's head and stimulate labor progression.

*Assisted Vaginal Delivery Techniques*
- **Vacuum extraction:** A vacuum device is used to apply suction to the baby's head, assisting in its descent through the birth canal during contractions.
- **Forceps delivery:** Obstetric forceps are used to gently grasp the baby's head and guide it through the birth canal.

*Cesarean Section*

Emergency cesarean section is performed when vaginal delivery is not possible or if there are indications of fetal distress, cephalopelvic disproportion, or other complications.

### Nursing Management

Nursing management plays a crucial role in supporting the healthcare team and providing comprehensive care for women experiencing obstructed labor. Here are some key aspects of nursing management in cases of obstructed labor:

*Assessment and Monitoring*
- Regular assessment of vital signs, including blood pressure, pulse, and temperature.
- Continuous monitoring of maternal and fetal well-being, including fetal heart rate monitoring and assessing for signs of fetal distress.
- Monitoring uterine contractions, including frequency, duration, and strength.
- Assessment of maternal pain levels and providing appropriate pain management interventions.

*Emotional Support and Communication*
- Providing emotional support to the woman and her family, as obstructed labor can be distressing and overwhelming.
- Communicating effectively with the woman, explaining the situation, procedures, and interventions to alleviate anxiety and promote informed decision-making.

*Collaboration with the Healthcare Team*
- Collaborating closely with the obstetrician, midwife, and other members of the healthcare team to ensure coordinated care and effective management of the obstructed labor.
- Facilitating clear communication and information exchange among team members.

*Positioning and Comfort Measures*
- Assisting the woman in finding comfortable positions during labor that may aid in promoting optimal fetal descent.
- Providing comfort measures such as relaxation techniques, breathing exercises, massage, and heat/cold therapy to alleviate pain and promote relaxation.

*Documentation and Record-keeping*
- Ensuring accurate and timely documentation of labor progress, vital signs, interventions, and outcomes.
- Recording information related to the woman's physical and emotional well-being and any complications that arise during the labor process.

*Preparation for Interventions*
- Assisting with the preparation for and during procedures such as vacuum extraction, forceps delivery, or cesarean section.
- Ensuring that all necessary equipment, medications, and supplies are readily available.

*Postpartum Care and Monitoring*
- Providing postpartum care to the woman and monitoring for any signs of complications, such as postpartum hemorrhage, infection, or trauma.
- Supporting breastfeeding initiation and providing guidance on newborn care and maternal recovery.

Nursing management in cases of obstructed labor involves a collaborative and multidisciplinary approach to ensure the safety and well-being of the woman and her baby. It is essential for nurses to have a thorough understanding of obstetric emergencies, effective communication skills, and the ability to provide compassionate care.

### Prevention
- Antenatal detection of the factors causing prolonged labor
- Intranatal monitoring of progress of labor, use of partograph
- Timely intervention of a prolonged labor

Obstructed labor is one of the important cause of both maternal and fetal mortality as well as morbidity. Various clinical strategies should be implemented to early diagnosis and management of prolonged labor. The choice of intervention depends on factors such as the stage of labor, maternal and fetal conditions, available resources, and healthcare provider expertise.

## POSTPARTUM HEMORRHAGE

Postpartum hemorrhage is one of the leading causes of maternal morbidity and mortality worldwide. It is life-threatening and is one of the obstetric emergencies.

## Incidence

Approximately 3 to 5% of obstetric cases are seen with postpartum hemorrhage. Worldwide, one-fourth and 12% of in the United States maternal deaths can occur due to postpartum hemorrhage annually.

## Definition

Postpartum hemorrhage (PPH) is defined as excessive bleeding following childbirth, typically within 24 hours of delivery which may adversely affects the general condition of the women (WHO, 2012).

## Types

- **Primary postpartum hemorrhage:** Primary PPH refers to excessive bleeding that occurs within the first 24 hours after childbirth.
- **Secondary postpartum hemorrhage:** Secondary PPH refers to excessive bleeding that occurs between 24 hours and 6 weeks after childbirth.

## Causes

### Primary Postpartum Hemorrhage

- **Uterine atony:** Uterine atony is the most common cause of primary PPH. It occurs when the uterus fails to contract effectively after delivery, leading to ongoing bleeding.
- **Traumatic PPH:** Traumatic PPH results from tears or lacerations in the birth canal, cervix, or uterus. These injuries can occur during labor, delivery, or instrumental delivery (e.g., forceps or vacuum extraction).
- **Retained placental tissue:** Primary PPH can also be caused by the incomplete expulsion of the placenta or placental fragments. Retained placental tissue prevents the uterus from contracting fully, resulting in continued bleeding.
- **Coagulation disorders:** Coagulation disorders, such as disseminated intravascular coagulation (DIC), hemophilia, von Willebrand disease, or thrombocytopenia, can contribute to primary PPH. Impaired clotting mechanisms lead to excessive bleeding following childbirth.

### Secondary Postpartum Hemorrhage

#### Subinvolution of the Placental Site

In some cases, the placental site fails to heal properly, resulting in ongoing bleeding. This can occur due to retained placental tissue or infection.

#### Retained Products of Conception

Secondary PPH can also be caused by the incomplete removal of placental fragments or other products of conception during the initial management of primary PPH.

#### Infection

Infections of the uterus, such as endometritis, can lead to secondary PPH. The inflammation and tissue damage associated with infection can cause persistent bleeding.

#### Coagulation Disorders

Similar to primary PPH, coagulation disorders can contribute to secondary PPH if clotting mechanisms are impaired.

## Pathophysiology

### Uterine Atony

- Uterine atony, the most common cause of PPH, refers to the inability of the uterus to contract effectively after delivery.
- It can occur due to factors such as overdistension of the uterus (e.g., multiple gestations or polyhydramnios), prolonged labor, use of certain medications (e.g., magnesium sulfate), or uterine infections.
- Inadequate uterine contractions lead to the inability to compress blood vessels, resulting in continued bleeding.

### Trauma

- Traumatic causes of PPH include lacerations or tears in the birth canal, cervix, or uterus.
- These tears can occur during labor or delivery, particularly in cases of instrumental delivery (e.g., forceps or vacuum extraction) or precipitous deliveries.
- Trauma-related bleeding may be arterial or venous in nature, depending on the site and extent of the injury.

### Retained Placental Tissue

- In some cases, PPH can occur due to the incomplete expulsion of the placenta or placental fragments.
- Retained placental tissue prevents the uterus from contracting fully, leading to ongoing bleeding.
- It can be caused by placenta accreta, increta, or percreta (abnormal placental implantation), placental adhesions, or improper management of the third stage of labor.

### Coagulation Disorders

- Disorders of coagulation can contribute to PPH. Conditions such as disseminated intravascular coagula-

tion (DIC), hemophilia, von Willebrand disease, or thrombocytopenia (low platelet count) impair the body's ability to form stable blood clots.
- Without effective clot formation, excessive bleeding can occur following childbirth.

## Clinical Features

The clinical features of PPH can vary depending on the severity of the bleeding and the underlying cause. Here are the common clinical features of PPH:
- **Excessive or prolonged bleeding:** The hallmark sign of PPH is the presence of excessive or prolonged bleeding after delivery. Blood loss of 500 mL or more within the first 24 hours is considered significant. In severe cases, blood loss can exceed 1,000 mL or be rapid and life-threatening.
- **Signs of hypovolemia:** Due to the significant blood loss, women with PPH may exhibit signs and symptoms of hypovolemia, including:
  - Rapid heart rate (tachycardia)
  - Low blood pressure (hypotension)
  - Pale skin and mucous membranes
  - Cool and clammy skin
  - Weakness and dizziness
  - Reduced urine output
- **Abnormal uterine firmness:** Uterine atony, which is the most common cause of PPH, can result in a soft and boggy uterus that fails to contract properly. The uterus may feel enlarged and lack the expected firmness after childbirth.
- **Large blood clots:** Passage of large blood clots, either spontaneously or during massage of the uterus, is a common sign of PPH. These clots indicate the presence of excessive bleeding and the need for immediate medical attention.
- **Back pain or lower abdominal discomfort:** Traumatic causes of PPH, such as tears or lacerations, may result in localized pain in the back or lower abdominal region.
- **Signs of shock:** In severe cases of PPH, women may exhibit signs of shock, which include:
  - Altered mental status or confusion
  - Rapid and shallow breathing
  - Bluish skin or lips (cyanosis)
  - Reduced consciousness or loss of consciousness
  - Weak or absent peripheral pulses.

## Diagnosis

The diagnosis of postpartum hemorrhage (PPH) involves a combination of clinical assessment, measurement of blood loss, and laboratory investigations. Prompt recognition and diagnosis are crucial to initiate appropriate management. The key aspects of diagnosing PPH are:
- **Clinical assessment:** The healthcare provider will conduct a thorough clinical evaluation to assess the signs and symptoms of PPH. This may include:
  - Evaluation of vital signs, including heart rate, blood pressure, and respiratory rate.
  - Examination of the uterus to assess firmness, size, and position.
  - Assessment of the amount and character of bleeding, including the presence of large blood clots.
  - Evaluation of the patient's overall clinical condition, including signs of hypovolemia and shock.
- **Measurement of blood loss:** Accurate measurement of blood loss is crucial in diagnosing PPH. While visual estimation can be helpful, it is often inaccurate. Quantitative measurement of blood loss can be achieved by:
  - Using calibrated drapes or collection devices to collect and measure blood.
  - Weighing soaked items (e.g., pads, towels) and subtracting the dry weight.
  - Using blood collection bags or graduated containers for direct measurement.
- **Laboratory investigations:** Laboratory tests can provide additional information to aid in the diagnosis and management of PPH. Common investigations include:
  - *Hemoglobin and hematocrit levels:* These tests assess the degree of anemia due to blood loss.
  - *Coagulation profile:* Assessing coagulation factors and platelet count can help identify coagulation disorders that may contribute to PPH.
  - *Blood typing and cross-matching:* In cases where blood transfusion may be necessary, determining the patient's blood type and ensuring compatibility with potential blood products is important.
- **Imaging studies:** In certain situations, imaging studies may be utilized to evaluate the underlying cause of PPH. For example, ultrasound may be used to assess for retained placental tissue or identify abnormalities in the uterus or blood vessels.

## Prevention

Postpartum hemorrhage cannot always be prevented. But the incidence can be reduced by assessing the risk factors during antenatal and intranatal period.

### Antenatal

- Improve the health status of the woman
- Monitor hemoglobin level to be normal (>10 g/dL)

- Screening of high-risk patients
- Refer and deliver the high-risk mothers in a well-equipped hospital
- Routine blood grouping to be done for all antenatal mothers
- Localization of placental should be done through USG for all antenatal women.

### Intranatal
- Routine active management of the third stage labor.
- The infusion to be continued for minimum one hour after the delivery incase of induced or augmented labor by oxytocin.
- Oxytocin 5 IU slow IV is to be given to reduce blood loss for delivery by cesarean section.
- Routine observation for at least two hours after delivery
- Examination of the placenta and membranes.

## Management
### Primary Postpartum Hemorrhage
The management of primary postpartum hemorrhage (PPH) involves a systematic approach aimed at stabilizing the patient, controlling bleeding, and addressing the underlying cause. Here are the general principles and interventions commonly employed in the management of primary PPH (**Flowchart 12.7**).

### Initial Stabilization
- Ensure patient safety and activate the emergency response team.
- Establish intravenous access and initiate fluid resuscitation with crystalloids or blood products as needed.
- Monitor vital signs, oxygen saturation, and urine output.
- Provide supplemental oxygen if necessary.

### Uterine Massage and Bimanual Compression
- Perform uterine massage to stimulate uterine contractions and aid in the control of bleeding.
- If uterine atony is present, apply bimanual compression by placing one hand inside the vagina and the other on the lower abdomen to compress the uterus.

### Medications
- Administer uterotonic medications to enhance uterine contractility and control bleeding. The preferred first-line agent is oxytocin, followed by other options such as intravenous or intramuscular ergometrine, carboprost tromethamine, or misoprostol.
- In cases of refractory or severe bleeding, additional medications such as tranexamic acid or recombinant factor VIIa may be considered, depending on the clinical situation.

### Surgical and Procedural Interventions
If conservative measures fail or are contraindicated, surgical interventions may be necessary, including:
- Manual removal of retained placental tissue or blood clots.
- Uterine tamponade using balloon devices, such as the Bakri balloon or the Foley catheter balloon.
- Uterine artery embolization (UAE), which involves blocking the blood vessels supplying the uterus to control bleeding.
- Surgical procedures like uterine artery ligation or hysterectomy, as a last resort in life-threatening cases.

### Consultation and Multidisciplinary Care
- Involve a multidisciplinary team, including obstetricians, anesthesiologists, hematologists, and interventional radiologists, as needed, to manage complex cases.
- Consultation with a senior obstetrician or maternal-fetal medicine specialist is advisable in severe or refractory cases.

### Secondary Postpartum Hemorrhage
The management of secondary postpartum hemorrhage (PPH) involves identifying and addressing the underlying cause of the bleeding. It typically occurs between 24 hours and 6 weeks after childbirth. The specific management strategies depend on the cause of secondary PPH. Here are the general approaches and interventions used in the management of secondary PPH (ACOG Bulletin No. 194, 2019) (RCOG Guideline No. 52, 2019).

### Evaluation and Diagnosis
- Conduct a thorough clinical evaluation to determine the cause of secondary PPH. This may involve a physical examination, imaging studies (e.g., ultrasound), and laboratory investigations.
- Identify the underlying cause, such as retained placental tissue, infection, subinvolution of the placental site, or coagulation disorders.

### Medical Interventions
- **Antibiotic therapy:** If an infection is identified as the cause of secondary PPH, administer appropriate antibiotic therapy to treat the infection.
- **Uterine stimulants:** In cases of subinvolution of the placental site, uterine stimulants like oxytocin may be used to promote uterine involution and control bleeding.
- **Coagulation support:** In secondary PPH associated with coagulation disorders, appropriate management includes correcting the underlying coagulation defect with blood products (e.g., fresh frozen plasma, platelet

**Flowchart 12.7:** Management of postpartum hemorrhage.

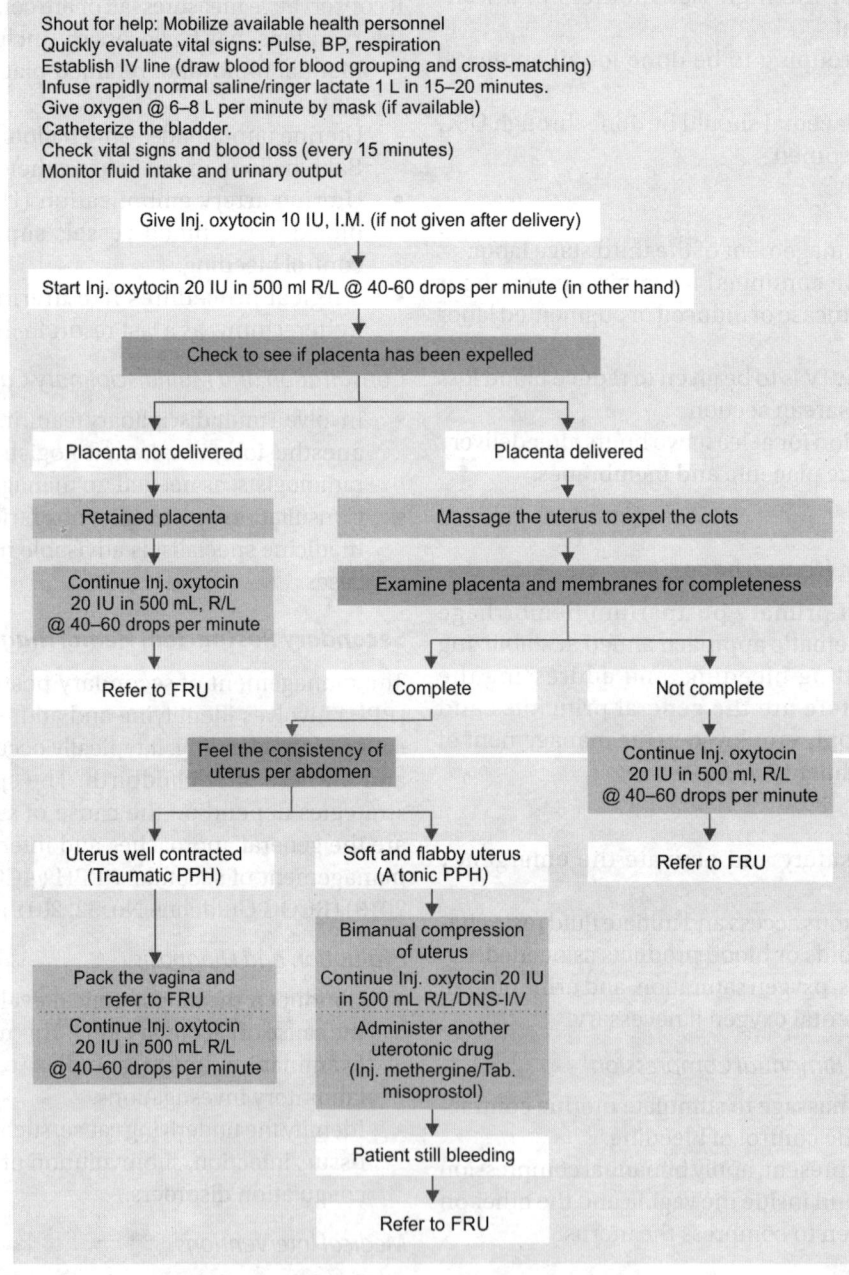

*Source:* SBA Quality Protocol Poster, NHM, Ministry of Health and Family Welfare, GOI.

transfusion) or specific coagulation factor replacement therapy.

*Surgical Interventions*

- **Manual removal of retained placental tissue or blood clots:** If retained placental tissue is identified as the cause of secondary PPH, it may need to be manually removed under appropriate anesthesia.

- **Hysteroscopy:** In cases of persistent or recurrent bleeding due to retained products of conception or uterine adhesions, hysteroscopy may be performed to visualize and treat the uterine cavity.

- **Uterine artery embolization (UAE):** In certain cases, UAE may be used to selectively block the blood vessels supplying the uterus to control bleeding.

*Consultation and Multidisciplinary Care*
- Involve a multidisciplinary team, including obstetricians, interventional radiologists, hematologists, and infectious disease specialists, as needed, to manage complex cases.
- Consult with senior obstetricians or maternal-fetal medicine specialists for guidance in challenging situations.

### Nursing Management

Nursing management plays a crucial role in the assessment, monitoring, and supportive care of women experiencing postpartum hemorrhage (PPH). Nurses are involved in early recognition of PPH, providing immediate interventions, coordinating care, and ensuring the overall well-being of the mother. Here are key aspects of nursing management in PPH:

*Early Recognition and Assessment*
- Nurses should be vigilant in recognizing signs and symptoms of PPH, such as excessive bleeding, changes in vital signs, and signs of hypovolemia.
- Conduct a thorough assessment of the woman's condition, including monitoring vital signs, assessing uterine firmness, quantifying blood loss, and evaluating the woman's overall well-being.

*Emergency Response and Communication*
- Activate the emergency response system and inform the healthcare team about the suspected or confirmed PPH.
- Communicate effectively with the healthcare team, including obstetricians, anesthesiologists, and other necessary specialists, to ensure a coordinated and prompt response.

*Supportive Care and Patient Monitoring*
- Ensure the woman's safety and comfort during the management of PPH.
- Administer supplemental oxygen as needed.
- Maintain intravenous access and assist with fluid resuscitation.
- Continuously monitor vital signs, including blood pressure, heart rate, respiratory rate, oxygen saturation, and urine output.
- Assess the woman's level of consciousness and mental status.
- Observe for signs of complications, such as disseminated intravascular coagulation (DIC) or infection.

*Medication Administration*
- Assist in the administration of uterotonic medications, such as oxytocin, ergometrine, carboprost tromethamine, or misoprostol, as prescribed by the healthcare provider.
- Ensure proper medication administration techniques, including correct dosage, route, and rate of administration.
- Monitor the woman for any adverse effects or allergic reactions to medications.

*Emotional Support and Communication*
- Provide emotional support and reassurance to the woman and her family during this stressful situation.
- Offer clear and concise explanations of procedures, treatments, and interventions to alleviate anxiety and facilitate informed decision-making.

*Documentation and Reporting*
- Document all assessments, interventions, and responses to treatment accurately and promptly.
- Report the progress and changes in the woman's condition to the healthcare team, ensuring continuity of care.

In conclusion, postpartum hemorrhage (PPH) is a serious and potentially life-threatening condition characterized by excessive bleeding following childbirth. It can occur due to various causes such as uterine atony, retained placenta, uterine rupture, trauma, or coagulation disorders. Routine active management of the third stage of labor should be used to reduce its incidence. Prompt recognition and management of PPH are essential to prevent complications and ensure the well-being of the mother.

## RUPTURED UTERUS

A ruptured uterus is considered a critical event due to the potential complications that can arise. It can lead to internal bleeding, hemorrhage, maternal shock, damage to surrounding organs, and compromised oxygen supply to the fetus. In some cases, it may result in fetal distress, stillbirth, or neonatal complications.

### Definition

A ruptured uterus refers to a tear or disruption in the wall of the uterus, which can occur during labor, delivery, or the immediate postpartum period. It involves a complete or partial tear in the uterine wall, which can result in life-threatening complications for both the mother and the fetus.

### Etiology

- **Previous uterine surgery:** Previous uterine surgeries, particularly cesarean sections (C-sections), are

significant risk factors for uterine rupture. The scar tissue from the previous surgical incision may weaken the uterine wall, making it more susceptible to rupture during subsequent pregnancies and labor.
- **Prolonged or obstructed labor:** Prolonged labor or difficulties in the progress of labor can increase the risk of uterine rupture. The excessive pressure and stretching of the uterine wall during prolonged contractions can lead to rupture.
- **Uterine trauma or injury:** Trauma or injury to the uterus, such as a uterine rupture during a previous delivery, uterine instrumentation, or external trauma to the abdomen, can weaken the uterine wall and predispose it to rupture in subsequent pregnancies.
- **Uterine anomalies:** Structural abnormalities or congenital malformations of the uterus can increase the risk of uterine rupture. These anomalies may affect the strength and integrity of the uterine wall.
- **Induction or augmentation of labor:** The use of medications or procedures to induce or augment labor, such as the administration of prostaglandins or the use of oxytocin (Pitocin), can increase the risk of uterine rupture, especially in women with a previous uterine scar.
- **Uterine overdistension:** Conditions that cause excessive stretching or distension of the uterus can increase the risk of rupture. This can occur with multiple gestations (such as twins or triplets), polyhydramnios (excessive amniotic fluid), or large fetal size.

## Pathophysiology

The pathophysiology of a ruptured uterus involves a disruption or tear in the uterine wall, which can have serious consequences for both the mother and the fetus. The specific pathophysiological processes that occur during a ruptured uterus are as follows:
- **Uterine wall integrity:** The uterus is composed of three layers: the inner endometrium, the middle myometrium (thick muscular layer), and the outer serosa. The integrity and strength of the uterine wall are crucial for maintaining the structural integrity of the uterus during pregnancy and labor.
- **Uterine rupture:** A ruptured uterus occurs when there is a partial or complete tear in the uterine wall. The tear can involve the myometrium, the serosa, or both. The rupture may occur in a scarred area from a previous uterine surgery (such as a cesarean section) or in an unscarred uterus **(Fig 12.3)**.
- **Causes of rupture:** Several factors can contribute to the rupture of the uterine wall. These include previous uterine surgeries (particularly prior cesarean sections), prolonged or obstructed labor, trauma to the uterus, uterine anomalies, and the use of medications or procedures to induce or augment labor.
- **Hemorrhage:** Rupture of the uterine wall can result in significant bleeding. The blood loss can occur within the uterus (intracavitary hemorrhage) or into the peritoneal cavity (intraperitoneal hemorrhage). The extent and severity of hemorrhage depend on the size and location of the rupture.
- **Maternal consequences:** A ruptured uterus can lead to maternal complications, including hypovolemic shock due to blood loss, hemodynamic instability, and disseminated intravascular coagulation (DIC). The rupture can also cause damage to surrounding structures, such as nearby blood vessels or the bladder.
- **Fetal consequences:** The fetus is at risk of compromised oxygen and nutrient supply due to uterine rupture. The disruption of the uterine blood supply can lead to fetal distress, asphyxia, or even fetal demise.
- **Secondary complications:** A ruptured uterus can result in additional complications, such as infection (due to exposure of the peritoneal cavity), injury to other organs (e.g., bladder or intestines), or the formation of adhesions within the pelvis.

## Clinical Features

- **Sudden, severe abdominal pain:** Women with a ruptured uterus often experience intense and localized abdominal pain that may be constant or intermittent. The pain is usually described as sharp, tearing, or stabbing.
- **Abnormal bleeding:** Vaginal bleeding may or may not be present in cases of uterine rupture. If bleeding occurs,

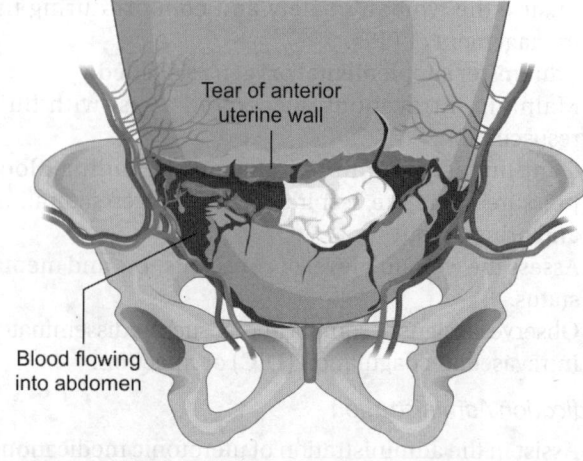

**Fig. 12.3:** Transverse uterine rupture.

it can range from light spotting to heavy and persistent bleeding.
- **Hemodynamic instability:** A ruptured uterus can cause significant blood loss, leading to hypovolemic shock. Signs of hemodynamic instability may include hypotension (low blood pressure), tachycardia (rapid heart rate), and pallor.
- **Fetal distress:** The fetus may show signs of distress due to compromised oxygen and nutrient supply. This can manifest as abnormal fetal heart rate patterns, decreased fetal movement, or meconium-stained amniotic fluid.
- **Uterine tenderness:** Palpation of the uterus may reveal uterine tenderness or localized pain upon examination.
- **Signs of peritonitis:** In cases of extensive rupture, the spillage of uterine contents into the abdominal cavity can lead to peritonitis, an inflammation of the peritoneum. Signs of peritonitis may include abdominal rigidity, guarding, rebound tenderness, or generalized abdominal pain.

## Diagnosis
- **Clinical assessment:**
  - Evaluate the patient's presenting symptoms and medical history, including previous uterine surgeries, obstetric history, and any known risk factors for a ruptured uterus.
  - Perform a thorough physical examination, assessing for signs of shock, abdominal tenderness, abnormal bleeding, and fetal distress.
- **Vital signs monitoring:**
  - Monitor vital signs, including blood pressure, heart rate, respiratory rate, and oxygen saturation, frequently and consistently.
  - Note any signs of hemodynamic instability, such as hypotension, tachycardia, or pallor.
- **Imaging studies:**
  - *Ultrasound:* Transabdominal or transvaginal ultrasound can be used to assess the presence of a uterine rupture, evaluate the fetus, and identify any signs of internal bleeding or fluid accumulation.
  - *Magnetic resonance imaging (MRI):* In certain cases, an MRI may be performed to provide more detailed imaging and assess the extent of the uterine rupture.
- **Intraoperative findings:** In cases where the diagnosis of a ruptured uterus is uncertain or when immediate surgical intervention is necessary, exploration of the abdomen and uterine inspection during an emergency laparotomy can confirm the diagnosis.

It is important to note that the diagnosis of a ruptured uterus can be challenging as the clinical presentation can be variable, and the signs and symptoms may overlap with other obstetric emergencies. The presence of risk factors, clinical suspicion, and the degree of clinical instability should guide the diagnostic approach.

## Management

### Medical Management of Ruptured Uterus
Medical management alone is not sufficient for the management of a ruptured uterus. A ruptured uterus is a critical obstetric emergency that requires immediate surgical intervention. However, medical interventions are an important component of the overall management strategy to stabilize the patient and support them before, during, and after surgical repair. The medical management of a ruptured uterus includes:

*Stabilization and Resuscitation*
- Ensure a patent airway and provide supplemental oxygen, if needed.
- Establish intravenous access for fluid resuscitation and administer crystalloids or blood products to restore circulating volume.
- Monitor vital signs closely, including blood pressure, heart rate, respiratory rate, oxygen saturation, and urine output.
- Correct any electrolyte abnormalities, such as hypovolemia-induced electrolyte imbalances.

*Blood Transfusion*
- Assess the need for blood transfusion based on the severity of hemorrhage and the patient's hemodynamic status.
- Cross-match blood or use emergency O-negative blood if the need is urgent.
- Transfuse blood products, such as packed red blood cells and fresh frozen plasma, to correct anemia and restore coagulation factors as needed.

*Pharmacological Interventions*
- Administer medications to control uterine contractions and minimize bleeding before and during surgical repair.
- Uterotonic agents, such as oxytocin or prostaglandins, may be used to promote uterine contraction and decrease bleeding.

*Antibiotic Therapy*
- Initiate broad-spectrum antibiotic therapy to reduce the risk of infection, considering the potential contamination of the peritoneal cavity.
- Select antibiotics based on local guidelines and the patient's specific risk factors.

*Pain Management*
- Provide appropriate pain management to alleviate the patient's discomfort.
- Administer analgesics as needed, considering the patient's pain severity, individual response, and any contraindications.

*Supportive Care*
- Monitor the patient closely for signs of complications, such as infection or organ dysfunction, and provide appropriate supportive care as necessary.
- Provide emotional support and counseling to the patient and her family during this traumatic event.

## Surgical Management of Ruptured Uterus

The surgical management of a ruptured uterus is the mainstay of treatment for this obstetric emergency. It involves immediate surgical intervention to repair the uterine tear, control bleeding, and address associated complications. The specific surgical approach may vary depending on the extent and severity of the rupture, the stability of the patient, and the gestational age of the fetus. Here are the key components of surgical management:

*Emergency Laparotomy*
- An emergency laparotomy is the primary surgical procedure performed for a ruptured uterus.
- The patient is taken to the operating room urgently for surgical intervention.
- A midline or transverse incision is made in the abdomen to access the uterus and evaluate the extent of the rupture.

*Uterine Repair*
- The uterine tear is identified and repaired. The repair technique may involve suturing the uterine wall, reinforcing the uterine incision if present, or removing devitalized tissue.
- The repair should be performed with appropriate sutures and surgical techniques to ensure proper hemostasis and integrity of the uterine wall.
- In cases of extensive rupture or irreparable damage, a decision for hysterectomy (removal of the uterus) may be made based on clinical judgment, patient's condition, desire for future fertility, and other factors.

*Hemostasis*
- Control of bleeding is crucial in the surgical management of a ruptured uterus.
- Hemostasis is achieved by ligating bleeding vessels, using sutures or surgical clips, and ensuring proper closure of any torn blood vessels.
- In cases of severe hemorrhage, additional measures such as blood transfusion, use of hemostatic agents, or even embolization of uterine arteries may be necessary.

*Associated Complications*
- Other associated complications, such as bladder injuries, lacerations, or adhesions, are addressed during the surgery.
- Bladder injuries can be repaired, and additional procedures may be performed to address any other injuries or conditions discovered during the surgical exploration.

*Postoperative Care*
- Following surgery, the patient is closely monitored in the postoperative period.
- Vital signs, blood loss, urine output, and laboratory values are monitored to assess the response to treatment and identify any ongoing complications.
- Pain management, wound care, infection prevention, and thromboprophylaxis are important components of postoperative care.

## Nursing Management of Ruptured Uterus

The nursing management of a patient with a ruptured uterus is crucial for providing comprehensive care and supporting the patient's recovery. Nurses play a vital role in the immediate assessment, monitoring, and ongoing care of the patient. Here are key aspects of nursing management for a patient with a ruptured uterus:

*Assessment and Monitoring*
- Conduct a thorough initial assessment, including vital signs, level of consciousness, pain assessment, and assessment of uterine bleeding.
- Monitor vital signs closely, including blood pressure, heart rate, respiratory rate, oxygen saturation, and urine output.
- Assess the patient's pain level and provide appropriate pain management interventions.
- Continuously monitor the patient's uterine bleeding, keeping track of the amount and characteristics of vaginal bleeding.

*Hemodynamic Support*
- Assist in the administration of intravenous fluids and blood products as prescribed to restore circulating blood volume and maintain hemodynamic stability.
- Monitor for signs of fluid overload or inadequate resuscitation and communicate any concerns to the healthcare team.

*Surgical Care and Wound Management*
- Collaborate with the surgical team to prepare the patient for surgery, ensuring proper identification, and obtaining informed consent.
- Assist in positioning the patient for surgery, maintaining aseptic technique, and providing necessary surgical instruments and supplies.
- After surgery, monitor the patient's wound for signs of infection or dehiscence, and provide wound care as prescribed.

*Postoperative Care*
- Monitor vital signs, including blood pressure, heart rate, respiratory rate, oxygen saturation, and urine output closely in the postoperative period.
- Administer prescribed medications, such as analgesics, antibiotics, and uterotonics, and monitor for their effects and side effects.
- Assist the patient with activities of daily living, such as hygiene, mobilization, and nutrition, as tolerated.
- Educate the patient and family about signs of complications, self-care measures, and the importance of follow-up care.

*Psychosocial Support*
- Provide emotional support and reassurance to the patient and family members, as they may experience anxiety, fear, or distress.
- Encourage open communication and address any concerns or questions they may have.
- Collaborate with the healthcare team to provide appropriate counseling or referrals to support services if needed.

*Ongoing Monitoring and Education*
- Continuously monitor the patient's condition, including vital signs, pain level, bleeding, and urine output.
- Educate the patient and family about signs and symptoms of potential complications, such as infection, excessive bleeding, or wound problems.
- Provide information about contraception, family planning, and the implications for future pregnancies.

In conclusion, a ruptured uterus is a rare but critical obstetric emergency that requires prompt recognition, immediate intervention, and multidisciplinary management. It involves a tear or disruption in the uterine wall, which can lead to significant maternal and fetal morbidity and mortality if not promptly diagnosed and managed. The successful management of a ruptured uterus relies on prompt recognition, immediate access to emergency obstetric care, close collaboration among healthcare professionals, and a well-coordinated approach. Timely diagnosis and appropriate interventions are essential to improve outcomes and ensure the well-being of the mother and the baby.

## PUERPERAL SEPSIS

A considerable portion of postpartum maternal morbidity and mortality is still attributed to puerperal sepsis. It is a potentially life-threatening condition that requires immediate medical attention. A pelvic abscess, pelvic thrombophlebitis, or septic shock can all happen to patients who have a puerperal genital tract infection.

### Incidence

About 6 to 7% of women experience febrile morbidity after a vaginal birth, which is defined as a temperature of at least 100.4°F (38°C) for more than two days in a row (excluding the first postpartum day) during the first 10 postpartum days. The frequency of febrile morbidity after primary cesarean delivery is around twice as high as after vaginal delivery.

### Definition

According to WHO, puerperal sepsis was characterized as the infection of genital tract within 42 days of the postpartum period.

### Etiology

Puerperal sepsis is usually caused by bacteria that enter the uterus through the birth canal during delivery or through medical interventions such as cesarean sections or uterine procedures.
- **Group A streptococcus (GAS):** This bacterium is one of the most common causes of severe puerperal sepsis and can rapidly lead to septic shock.
- **Escherichia coli (E coli):** This bacterium is normally present in the digestive tract but can cause infection if it enters the genital tract during childbirth.
- **Other bacteria:** Various other bacteria, including *Staphylococcus aureus, Klebsiella, Enterococcus*, and anaerobic bacteria, can also cause puerperal sepsis.

### Pathophysiology

Puerperal sepsis, also known as postpartum sepsis or childbed fever, is primarily caused by bacterial infections that occur in the genital tract of women after childbirth or miscarriage. The pathophysiology of puerperal sepsis involves the following processes:
- **Bacterial entry:** Bacteria can enter the genital tract during childbirth through various routes. This can occur

due to prolonged or difficult labor, invasive procedures (such as cesarean section or episiotomy), manual removal of the placenta, or the presence of pre-existing infections.
- **Infection and inflammatory response:** Once bacteria enter the genital tract, they can colonize and multiply in the uterine lining (endometrium) or other areas of the reproductive system. This colonization triggers an immune response and the release of inflammatory mediators.
- **Spreading infection:** The infection can spread from the initial site of colonization to surrounding tissues, leading to a wider infection of the genital tract. The bacteria can invade the uterine wall, fallopian tubes, ovaries, or nearby structures.
- **Systemic inflammatory response:** The presence of a widespread infection triggers a systemic inflammatory response throughout the body. The immune system releases pro-inflammatory cytokines and activates immune cells, leading to systemic manifestations of sepsis.
- **Endotoxin and exotoxin effects:** Bacterial toxins, such as endotoxins and exotoxins, are released by the infecting bacteria. Endotoxins are produced by Gram-negative bacteria and can cause a strong inflammatory response. Exotoxins are produced by various bacteria and can cause tissue damage and organ dysfunction.
- **Vasodilation and increased vascular permeability:** The release of inflammatory mediators leads to vasodilation and increased vascular permeability. This results in leakage of fluid and proteins from blood vessels into the surrounding tissues, leading to edema and impaired tissue perfusion.
- **Organ dysfunction:** In severe cases, the systemic inflammatory response can progress to septic shock, characterized by widespread tissue hypoperfusion and organ dysfunction. Multiple organs, including the lungs, liver, kidneys, and cardiovascular system, can be affected.
- **Coagulation abnormalities:** Puerperal sepsis can also disrupt the normal coagulation process. The release of pro-inflammatory cytokines and bacterial toxins can lead to a prothrombotic state, causing abnormal clotting and disseminated intravascular coagulation (DIC) in some cases.

Overall, the pathophysiology of puerperal sepsis involves the initial entry of bacteria into the genital tract, followed by infection, systemic inflammatory response, vascular changes, and potential organ dysfunction. Early recognition and prompt treatment are crucial to prevent complications and improve outcomes for women affected by puerperal sepsis.

## Risk Factors of Puerperal Sepsis

### Antepartum Factors
- Under nutrition
- Anemia in pregnancy
- Preterm labor
- Premature rupture of the membranes
- Chronic illness

### Intrapartum Factors
- Frequent vaginal examinations
- Prolonged rupture of membranes
- Operative delivery
- APH and PPH
- Retained bits of placenta or membranes
- Placenta previa
- Cesarean delivery

## Clinical Symptoms
- Fever (temperature of 38°C or more)
- Increase pulse rate
- Chills and general malaise
- Lower abdominal pain
- Tender uterus
- Subinvolution of the uterus
- Offensive and copious vaginal discharge
- Pale skin, which can be a sign of large volume blood loss
- Fatigue and weakness
- Nausea and vomiting
- Headache
- Confusion or altered mental status (in severe cases)
- Shock

## Diagnosis
- A thorough *history and physical examination* should be part of the evaluation of a febrile postpartum patient.
  - Assess the high-risk factors for puerperal sepsis during antenatal, intranatal and postnatal periods.
  - It is important to rule out **extrapelvic causes** of fever like breast engorgement, mastitis, aspiration pneumonia, atelectasis, pyelonephritis, thrombophlebitis, or wound infection.
- A **pelvic examination** may allow the probing of painful, thrombosed, and edematous ovarian, parauterine, or iliac veins even if it is typically ineffective in the diagnosis of pelvic thrombophlebitis.
  - Examinations of abdomen and pelvic for signs of involution of genital organs.
  - Examine the infection site for degree and severity.
- A **computed tomography scan or ultrasonogram** of the abdomen and pelvis may be beneficial. However,

this diagnosis is typically made by excluding other possibilities and by the quick regression of fever after the start of heparin anticoagulant medication (Kim MA, 2009).

- **Other investigations of puerperal pyrexia**
  - Culture of vaginal and endocervical swabs.
  - Urine analysis for culture and sensitivity by clean catch method.
  - Blood sample collection for culture.

## Management

### Medical Management

Puerperal sepsis requires immediate medical treatment to prevent complications. The following steps are typically taken:

- **Antibiotic therapy:** Broad-spectrum antibiotics are administered intravenously to target the infection and cover a wide range of potential bacteria.
- **Intravenous fluids:** Fluids and electrolytes are given to maintain hydration and stabilize blood pressure.
- **Source control:** If there are abscesses or retained placental tissue, surgical intervention may be necessary to remove or drain the infected material.
- **Supportive care:** Supportive measures such as pain relief, fever management, and monitoring of vital signs are provided to ensure the patient's comfort and stability.
- **Blood cultures:** Blood samples may be collected to identify the specific bacteria causing the infection and guide antibiotic selection.
- **Intensive care:** In severe cases, patients may require admission to the intensive care unit (ICU) for close monitoring and organ support.
- **General measures:**
  - The women should be isolated
  - Maintenance of fluid and nutritional status
  - Correction of anemia
  - Administration of indwelling catheter
  - Monitor and record pulse, respiration, temperature, lochia, fluid intake, and output
  - Management of bacteremia or septic shock
- **Surgical treatment of:**
  - Perineal wound
  - Retained uterine products
  - Pelvic abscess
  - Hysterectomy is indicated in cases with rupture or perforation

### Nursing Management

The nursing management of puerperal sepsis focuses on prompt recognition of the condition, early intervention, and supportive care to promote the recovery of the patient. Here are some key aspects of nursing management for puerperal sepsis:

### Assessment and Monitoring

- Monitor vital signs closely, including temperature, heart rate, blood pressure, and respiratory rate.
- Assess the patient's level of consciousness, mental status, and urine output.
- Monitor laboratory values, including complete blood count, blood cultures, and inflammatory markers.
- Assess the incision site (if applicable) for signs of infection or poor wound healing.
- Monitor the patient's response to antibiotic therapy and any adverse reactions.

### Infection Control

- Implement strict infection control measures, including proper hand hygiene before and after patient contact.
- Follow standard precautions and wear appropriate personal protective equipment (gloves, gown, mask) when providing care.
- Ensure a clean and sterile environment for procedures and wound care.
- Educate the patient and family members about infection prevention strategies.

### Medication Administration

- Administer antibiotics as prescribed, ensuring timely administration and appropriate dosing.
- Monitor for any adverse reactions or allergies to medications.
- Provide education to the patient regarding the importance of completing the full course of antibiotics.

### Fluid and Electrolyte Management

- Monitor fluid balance and administer intravenous fluids as prescribed to maintain hydration and hemodynamic stability.
- Monitor electrolyte levels and provide appropriate supplementation as needed.
- Assess for signs of fluid overload or dehydration and adjust fluid therapy accordingly.

### Wound Care and Drainage

- Perform careful and aseptic wound care for any surgical incisions or perineal lacerations.
- Monitor wound healing and assess for signs of infection or dehiscence.
- Ensure proper functioning of any wound drains or catheters and maintain their integrity.

*Pain Management*
- Assess and manage the patient's pain effectively using appropriate pain assessment tools.
- Administer analgesics as prescribed and reassess their effectiveness.
- Implement nonpharmacological pain management strategies, such as relaxation techniques or positioning.

*Emotional Support and Education*
- Provide emotional support to the patient and family members during a stressful and challenging time.
- Offer clear and concise explanations of the patient's condition, treatment plan, and progress.
- Educate the patient and family about signs and symptoms of infection, the importance of adherence to medication regimen, and strategies for preventing future infections.

*Collaboration and Communication*
- Collaborate with the healthcare team to ensure coordinated care and timely interventions.
- Communicate any changes in the patient's condition or response to treatment promptly.
- Involve the patient and family in the care planning process and encourage their active participation.

It is crucial for nurses to closely monitor patients with puerperal sepsis, promptly identify any deterioration, and provide comprehensive care to prevent complications and promote recovery. Regular assessment, effective communication, and patient education are essential components of nursing management in these cases.

In conclusion, puerperal sepsis is a serious and potentially life-threatening condition characterized by bacterial infection in the genital tract after childbirth or miscarriage. Timely recognition and appropriate management are essential in the management of puerperal sepsis. Early identification, prompt intervention, and comprehensive care are crucial in managing puerperal sepsis to prevent complications and ensure the well-being and recovery of women affected by this condition.

## OBSTETRICAL SHOCK

Obstetrical shock (OS), the most major contributor to high maternal mortality (MM) throughout human history, is a life-threatening circulatory collapse condition connected to pregnancy, childbirth, and puerperium (obstetric causes). Indirect causes of non-obstetric reasons in pregnancy, labor, and puerperium are referred to as shock in obstetrics (SIO) (polytrauma, aesthetic incidents, cardiovascular or cerebrovascular incidents, other septic syndromes). The objectives of OS treatment are to promptly identify the site or cause of bleeding, damage, or inflammation, stop the spread of shock, avoid major blood transfusions, protect the uterus (and adnexa), and, if feasible, preserve fertility (Cerovac A, 2022).

### Definition

Obstetric shock refers to a life-threatening condition characterized by severe circulatory insufficiency and organ dysfunction during pregnancy or shortly after childbirth.

### Etiology

- **Hemorrhage:** Excessive bleeding is the most common cause of obstetric shock. It can result from complications such as placental abruption (premature separation of the placenta), placenta previa (implantation of the placenta over the cervix), uterine rupture, or postpartum hemorrhage.
- **Sepsis:** Infection can lead to septic shock during pregnancy or postpartum. It may occur due to infections of the genital tract, urinary tract, or surgical site (such as cesarean section). In severe cases, the infection can spread throughout the body, causing systemic inflammation and organ dysfunction.
- **Pre-eclampsia and eclampsia:** These are pregnancy-related conditions characterized by high blood pressure, proteinuria (presence of excess protein in the urine), and, in the case of eclampsia, seizures. Severe forms of pre-eclampsia and eclampsia can lead to shock due to impaired organ perfusion.
- **Amniotic fluid embolism:** This rare but potentially fatal condition occurs when amniotic fluid or fetal material enters the maternal circulation, triggering an allergic or inflammatory response. It can lead to cardiovascular collapse and shock.
- **Cardiac events:** Conditions such as myocardial infarction (heart attack) or cardiomyopathy (weakening of the heart muscle) can cause shock during pregnancy or shortly after delivery.
- **Anaphylaxis:** Severe allergic reactions to medications or substances during pregnancy can lead to anaphylactic shock, which can have obstetric implications.
- **Trauma:** Accidents, falls, or physical trauma during pregnancy or childbirth can cause shock if there is significant blood loss or internal injury.
- **Thromboembolism:** Blood clotting disorders or the formation of blood clots in the deep veins (deep vein thrombosis) or lungs (pulmonary embolism) can lead to shock.

## Pathophysiology

The pathophysiology of obstetric shock involves a complex interplay of various factors and underlying causes. The common thread in obstetric shock is inadequate tissue perfusion and oxygen delivery due to a compromised circulatory system. Here is a general overview of the pathophysiological processes involved in obstetric shock:

- **Decreased blood volume:** Obstetric shock often occurs due to significant blood loss. This can result from conditions such as hemorrhage, placental abruption, uterine rupture, or postpartum hemorrhage. The decrease in blood volume reduces the circulating fluid available for organ perfusion.
- **Inadequate tissue perfusion:** With decreased blood volume, there is a reduction in oxygen and nutrient delivery to the organs and tissues. This leads to impaired cellular metabolism and function, contributing to organ dysfunction.
- **Activation of compensatory mechanisms:** In response to decreased tissue perfusion, the body activates compensatory mechanisms to maintain blood pressure and perfusion to vital organs. These mechanisms include an increase in heart rate (tachycardia), constriction of blood vessels (vasoconstriction), and redistribution of blood flow to critical organs.
- **Cellular oxygen deprivation:** In obstetric shock, insufficient oxygen delivery to cells leads to a state of tissue hypoxia. Cells switch to anaerobic metabolism, resulting in the production of lactic acid as a byproduct. Accumulation of lactic acid contributes to metabolic acidosis, further impairing cellular function.
- **Systemic inflammatory response:** Certain causes of obstetric shock, such as sepsis or amniotic fluid embolism, can trigger a systemic inflammatory response. This response involves the release of inflammatory mediators, activation of clotting factors, and endothelial dysfunction. It can lead to microvascular thrombosis, impaired blood flow, and organ damage.
- **Organ dysfunction:** Prolonged inadequate tissue perfusion can result in multiorgan dysfunction. Organs commonly affected in obstetric shock include the heart, kidneys, liver, lungs, and brain. Depending on the underlying cause and severity of shock, complications such as acute respiratory distress syndrome (ARDS), acute kidney injury, coagulopathy, or disseminated intravascular coagulation (DIC) may occur.

## Types of Obstetric Shock (Miller DA, 2017)

- **Hemorrhagic shock:** This type of obstetric shock occurs due to excessive bleeding during pregnancy, labor, or postpartum. It can result from conditions such as placental abruption, placenta previa, uterine rupture, or postpartum hemorrhage.
- **Septic shock:** Obstetric septic shock is caused by severe infection, usually resulting from infections of the genital tract, urinary tract, or surgical site. Common sources of infection include chorioamnionitis (infection of the placental membranes), endometritis (infection of the uterine lining), or urinary tract infections.
- **Hypovolemic shock:** This type of shock occurs when there is a significant loss of blood or fluids, leading to decreased blood volume. It can be caused by hemorrhage, fluid loss from severe vomiting or diarrhea, or inadequate fluid replacement during labor or postpartum.
- **Cardiogenic shock:** In rare cases, obstetric shock can result from cardiac events such as myocardial infarction (heart attack), cardiomyopathy (weakening of the heart muscle), or arrhythmias (abnormal heart rhythms).
- **Anaphylactic shock:** Although rare, obstetric shock can occur due to a severe allergic reaction known as anaphylaxis. This can be triggered by medications, anesthesia, or substances used during pregnancy or childbirth.

## Clinical Features of Shock

The clinical features of obstetric shock can vary depending on the underlying cause and the stage of pregnancy or postpartum period. Some common clinical features of obstetric shock include:

- **Hypotension:** Low blood pressure is a hallmark sign of shock. The blood pressure may be significantly reduced, and the person may appear pale or have cool and clammy skin.
- **Tachycardia:** The heart rate is typically increased as the body tries to compensate for the decreased blood volume and maintain organ perfusion. The pulse may feel rapid and weak.
- **Altered mental status:** As shock progresses, the person may experience confusion, restlessness, or even loss of consciousness. This is due to inadequate oxygen and nutrient supply to the brain.
- **Weakness and fatigue:** The person may feel extremely weak and fatigued due to decreased perfusion of vital organs, including muscles.
- **Decreased urine output:** In severe shock, the kidneys receive reduced blood flow, leading to decreased urine production. The person may have oliguria (low urine output) or anuria (absence of urine production).

- **Respiratory distress:** As shock progresses, the person may experience rapid and shallow breathing, shortness of breath, or even respiratory failure. This can occur due to inadequate oxygen delivery to the lungs.
- **Signs of bleeding:** If the underlying cause of shock is hemorrhage, there may be visible signs of bleeding, such as vaginal bleeding, or signs of internal bleeding, such as abdominal pain or distension.
- **Other signs:** Depending on the cause of shock, additional symptoms may be present. For example, in septic shock, there may be signs of infection such as fever, elevated heart rate, and localized tenderness.

## Diagnosis

The diagnosis of obstetric shock involves a combination of clinical assessment, vital signs monitoring, laboratory investigations, and imaging studies. Prompt recognition and early diagnosis are crucial for timely intervention and appropriate management. Here are some key components of diagnosing obstetric shock:

### Clinical Assessment

- Evaluate the patient's presenting symptoms and medical history, including obstetric history and any known risk factors for obstetric complications.
- Perform a thorough physical examination, assessing for signs of shock, such as hypotension, tachycardia, altered mental status, and decreased urine output.
- Assess for signs of underlying causes of shock, such as vaginal bleeding, signs of infection, or signs of cardiac events.

### Vital Signs Monitoring

- Monitor vital signs, including blood pressure, heart rate, respiratory rate, and oxygen saturation, frequently and consistently.
- Note any abnormal trends or significant deviations from baseline values.

### Laboratory Investigations

- Order blood tests, including complete blood count (CBC), coagulation profile, blood chemistry (electrolytes, renal function tests, liver function tests), and blood typing and cross-matching for potential transfusion.
- Measure arterial blood gases to assess oxygenation, acid-base balance, and metabolic status.
- Additional tests may be ordered based on suspected or confirmed underlying causes, such as cultures for infection, troponin levels for suspected cardiac events, or D-dimer levels for suspected thromboembolism.

### Imaging Studies

- Depending on the suspected cause and clinical presentation, imaging studies may be ordered. For example, ultrasound can be used to assess the presence of placental abnormalities, evaluate for uterine rupture, or identify potential sources of bleeding.
- In cases of suspected pulmonary embolism, a computed tomography (CT) scan of the chest may be performed.
- Echocardiography can be helpful in assessing cardiac function and identifying structural abnormalities.

### Fetal Monitoring

- If applicable, continuous electronic fetal monitoring is important to assess the well-being and response to maternal resuscitation.
- Monitoring the fetal heart rate can help determine the need for urgent delivery if the fetal condition is compromised.

## Management

### Medical Management

The medical management of obstetric shock involves a comprehensive approach that aims to stabilize the patient, address the underlying cause, restore blood volume, and optimize organ perfusion. The specific management will depend on the cause of shock and the individual patient's condition. Here are some general principles and interventions commonly used in the medical management of obstetric shock:

### ABCDE Approach

- The initial management follows the ABCDE approach (airway, breathing, circulation, disability, and exposure).
- Ensuring a patent airway, providing oxygen supplementation, and initiating respiratory support if needed are the first steps.
- Monitoring vital signs, including blood pressure, heart rate, and oxygen saturation, is essential.

### Intravenous Fluid Resuscitation

- Administering intravenous fluids is crucial to restore circulating blood volume. Crystalloids (such as normal saline or lactated Ringer's solution) are typically used as the initial fluid of choice.
- The volume and rate of fluid administration will depend on the severity of shock and ongoing losses.
- Blood products (packed red blood cells, fresh frozen plasma) may be required if hemorrhage is a cause of shock.

### Transfusion
- If severe hemorrhage is present, blood transfusion may be necessary to replace lost red blood cells and maintain oxygen-carrying capacity.
- Cross-matched blood or emergency O-negative blood can be used if necessary.

### Medications
- Depending on the cause and specific circumstances, medications may be administered.
- Examples include uterotonic agents (such as oxytocin or misoprostol) to promote uterine contraction and control bleeding, antibiotics in cases of suspected or confirmed infection, and medications to manage hypertensive emergencies or cardiac conditions.

### Surgical Interventions
- In cases of uncontrolled bleeding or certain obstetric emergencies, surgical interventions may be required.
- These can include procedures like uterine artery embolization, uterine compression sutures, or emergency cesarean section.

### Supportive Care
- Close monitoring of vital signs, oxygen saturation, urine output, and laboratory values is essential.
- Additional interventions may include supplemental oxygen, monitoring of central venous pressure or pulmonary artery catheterization, and correction of electrolyte imbalances.

### Consultation and Multidisciplinary Approach
- Obstetric shock management often requires a multidisciplinary approach involving obstetricians, anesthesiologists, critical care specialists, and blood bank personnel.
- Prompt consultation and collaboration among the healthcare team are crucial for optimal management.

## Nursing Management

Nursing management plays a vital role in the care of a patient with obstetric shock. Nurses have a crucial responsibility in the early recognition of shock, prompt initiation of interventions, and ongoing monitoring of the patient's condition. Here are key aspects of nursing management in obstetric shock:

### Assessment and Monitoring
- Perform a thorough assessment of the patient, including vital signs (blood pressure, heart rate, respiratory rate), oxygen saturation, temperature, and level of consciousness.
- Monitor fetal well-being if applicable, including fetal heart rate monitoring.
- Assess and document the presence of any signs of bleeding, such as vaginal bleeding or signs of internal bleeding.
- Monitor urine output and laboratory values, including hemoglobin, hematocrit, coagulation profile, and blood gases.
- Continuously assess the patient's response to interventions and reassess the severity of shock.

### Prompt Intervention and Resuscitation
- Initiate immediate resuscitation measures following the ABCDE approach (airway, breathing, circulation, disability, and exposure).
- Ensure a patent airway and administer oxygen as necessary.
- Establish intravenous access for fluid administration and blood products if needed.
- Assist in administering intravenous fluids, ensuring appropriate infusion rates based on the severity of shock and ongoing losses.
- Assist in transfusion administration if indicated, ensuring compatibility and monitoring for transfusion reactions.
- Collaborate with the healthcare team in the administration of medications, such as uterotonic agents, antibiotics, or other medications specific to the cause of shock.

### Supportive Care
- Position the patient appropriately, ensuring comfort and adequate perfusion.
- Monitor and support respiratory function, providing supplemental oxygen as needed.
- Provide emotional support and reassurance to the patient and her family.
- Educate the patient and her family about the condition, treatment options, and signs of complications.

### Ongoing Monitoring and Evaluation
- Continuously monitor vital signs, including blood pressure, heart rate, respiratory rate, and oxygen saturation.
- Monitor urine output closely to assess renal perfusion.
- Assess for signs of improved perfusion, such as improved mental status, stable vital signs, and increased urine output.
- Monitor for signs of complications, such as infection, coagulopathy, or organ dysfunction.

*Collaboration and Communication*

- Collaborate closely with the healthcare team, including obstetricians, anesthesiologists, and other specialists, to ensure coordinated care.
- Communicate relevant information to the team, including changes in the patient's condition, response to interventions, and any concerns or complications.
- Provide clear and concise documentation of assessments, interventions, and the patient's response to treatment.

In conclusion, obstetric shock is a life-threatening condition that can occur during pregnancy or shortly after childbirth. It is characterized by severe circulatory insufficiency and organ dysfunction. Prompt recognition, immediate resuscitation, and appropriate medical management are crucial to improve outcomes for the mother and the baby.

## Summary

Emergency care is given to a woman who is facing a pregnancy or birthing issue in order to treat her (and ultimately save her life). Using a vacuum extractor or forceps to assist a vaginal birth, manually removing a placenta, removing the products of conception after a miscarriage or abortion, and for comprehensive emergency obstetric care (CEmOC), performing a cesarean section surgery to deliver a baby or administering a blood transfusion are all examples of EmOC components.

## Points to Ponder

- Painless antepartum vaginal bleeding is the sign of placenta previa.
- Ultrasound is the confirmatory investigation to assess placenta previa before doing digital or speculum examination.
- Transvaginal sonography is the best diagnostic method to detect APH.
- Management based on the degree of placenta previa, gestational week, and fetal presentations.
- Early detection and treatment of antepartum hemorrhage will improve perinatal outcome.
- If placenta previa is diagnosed in early gestation, repeat sonography is advised.
- Call for help, if the patient has signs of high blood pressure.
- The symptoms of pregnancy-induced hypertension can include a blurred vision, swelling, or making less urine output.
- The goal of treatment is to prevent the condition from getting of poorer and developing complications.
- A cesarean section should be preferred in emergency obstetric conditions.

## Abbreviations

- EmOC : Emergency Obstetric Care
- CEmOC : Comprehensive Emergency Obstetric Care
- PIH : Pregnancy-induced Hypertension
- APH : Antepartum Hemorrhage
- PPH : Postpartum Hemorrhage
- PROM : Premature Rupture of Membrane
- TAS : Transabdominal Ultrasound
- TVS : Transvaginal Ultrasound
- TPS : Transperineal Ultrasound
- MRI : Magnetic Resonance Imaging
- NICU : Neonatal Intensive Care Unit
- IV : Intravenous
- IM : Intramuscular
- USG : Ultrasonography
- CTG : Cardiotocography
- CS : Cesarean Section
- IUGR : Intrauterine Growth Retardation
- DIC : Disseminated Intravascular Coagulation
- HELLP : Hemolysis, Elevated Liver Enzymes, and Low Platelet Count
- ARDS : Acute Respiratory Distress Syndrome
- MgSO$_4$ : Magnesium Sulfate
- BP : Blood Pressure
- LSCS : Lower Segment Cesarean Section
- CPD : Cephalopelvic Disproportion
- WHO : World Health Organization
- RCOG : Royal College of Obstetricians and Gynecologists
- CT : Computed Tomography
- ECG : Electrocardiogram

## Short Answer Questions

1. Describe the etiopathology of pre-eclampsia.
2. Differentiate placenta previa from abruptio placentae.
3. Write a note on obstetric shock.
4. What is puerperal sepsis?
5. Write the signs and symptoms of eclampsia.
6. What are the types of placenta previa?
7. What is abruption placentae?

## Long Answer Questions

1. What are the causes of per vaginal bleeding in third trimester of pregnancy? Discuss the management of a case of abruptio placentae.
2. Discuss various conservative techniques available for the treatment of postpartum hemorrhage.
3. What is antepartum hemorrhage? Explain placenta previa and its types. Explain abruption placentae, its types and management.

4. Define pre-eclampsia. Write down its etiology, clinical manifestations and management in detail.
5. What is eclampsia? Write down its etiology, clinical manifestations, diagnostic evaluations and management in detail.
6. Define postpartum hemorrhage (PPH) and list down the types of PPH. Explain the causes of PPH and discuss the management of PPH.
7. Define obstructed labor. Describe the diagnosis of obstructed labor. Explain the management of obstructed labor.

## Bibliography

1. American College of Obstetricians and Gynecologists. Hypertension in pregnancy: Report of the American College of Obstetricians and Gynecologists' Task Force on Hypertension in Pregnancy. Obstetrics and Gynecology; 2013;122(5):1122-1131.
2. American College of Obstetricians and Gynecologists. ACOG Practice Bulletin No. 194: Postpartum Hemorrhage. Obstetrics and Gynecology; 2019;133(5): e327-e343
3. American College of Obstetricians and Gynecologists. Antenatal corticosteroid therapy for fetal maturation. Practice Bulletin No. 207; 2019.
4. American College of Obstetricians and Gynecologists. Hypertension in Pregnancy. Practice Bulletin No. 202; 2019.
5. American College of Obstetricians and Gynecologists. Induction of Labor. Practice Bulletin No. 107; 2019.
6. Ananth CV, Keyes KM. Prevention of Pre-eclampsia: A Strategic Approach. Best Practice and Research Clinical Obstetrics and Gynaecology; 2013;27(3):363-376.
7. Ananth CV, Wilcox AJ, Savitz DA. Effect of maternal age and parity on the risk of uteroplacental bleeding disorders in pregnancy. Obstetrics and Gynecology; 1999;94(5):721-727.
8. Anderson CM, Schmella MJ. CE: Preeclampsia: Current Approaches to Nursing Management. AJN The American Journal of Nursing. 2017;117(11):30-8.
9. Antepartum Hemorrhage; Royal College of Obstetricians and Gynecologists; 2011.
10. Brown MA, Magee LA, Kenny LC, Karumanchi SA, McCarthy FP, Saito S, Hall DR. The Hypertensive Disorders of Pregnancy: ISSHP Classification, Diagnosis and Management Recommendations for International Practice. Pregnancy Hypertension; 13:291-310.
11. Cerovac A, Habek D, Cerovac E, Habek JČ. Obstetric Shock and Shock in Obstetrics–steady Obstetrical Syndrome. MedicinskiGlasnik. 2022;19(2).
12. Crochetière C. Obstetric Emergencies. Anesthesiology Clinics of North America; 2003;21(1):111-25.
13. Cunningham FG, Leveno KJ, Spong CY, Dashe JS, Casey B M, Bloom SL (Eds.). Williams Obstetrics (25th ed.). McGraw-Hill Education; 2018.
14. Dashe JS, McIntire DD, Ramus RM, Santos-Ramos R, Twickler DM, "Persistence of Placenta Previa According to Gestational Age at Ultrasound Detection". Obstetrics and Gynecology; 2002; 99 (5 Pt 1):692–7.
15. Duley L. The Global Impact of Pre-eclampsia and Eclampsia. Seminars in Perinatology; 33(3); 130-137.
16. Duley L, Gülmezoglu AM, Henderson-Smart DJ, Chou D. Magnesium Sulfate and Other Anticonvulsants for Women with Pre-eclampsia. Cochrane Database of Systematic Reviews; 2010 (11):CD000025.
17. FOGSI-GESTOSIS-ICOG, Hypertensive Disorders in Pregnancy (HDP) Good Clinical Practice Recommendations; 2019.
18. Gbala MO, Adegoke AI. Hypertension in Pregnancy. Contemporary Obstetrics and Gynecology for Developing Countries; 2021:289-98.
19. Gizzo S, Di Gangi S, Saccardi C, Patrelli TS, D'Antona D. Diagnosis, Prevention and Management of Prolonged and Obstructed Labor. Womens Health (Lond Engl); 2014;10(4):385-398.
20. Kelsey JA, Forouzan I. Placental Abruption in Cocaine-Exposed Gravidas. Journal of Maternal-Fetal and Neonatal Medicine; 2014; 27(17):1810-1813.
21. Kim MA, Hayashi RH, Gambone JC. Obstetric Hemorrhage and Puerperal Sepsis. Hacker and Moore's Essentials of Obstetrics and Gynecology; 2009:128-38.
22. Leta M, Assefa N, Tefera M. Obstetric Emergencies and Adverse Maternal-perinatal Outcomes in Ethiopia; A systematic Review and Meta-analysis. Frontiers in Global Women's Health; 2022;3:942668.
23. Love C, Wallace E. Pregnancies Complicated by Placenta Praevia: What is Appropriate Management?. BJOG: An International Journal of Obstetrics and Gynaecology; 1996;103(9):864-867.
24. Magee LA, Pels A, Helewa M, Rey E, von Dadelszen P. Canadian Hypertensive Disorders of Pregnancy Working Group. Diagnosis, Evaluation, and Management of the Hypertensive Disorders of Pregnancy: Executive Summary. Journal of Obstetrics and Gynecology Canada; 2014;36(5):416-438.
25. Maynard SE, Min JY, Merchan J, Lim KH, Li, J, Mondal S, Karumanchi, SA. Excess Placental Soluble fms-like tyrosine kinase 1 (sFlt1) may contribute to endothelial dysfunction, hypertension, and proteinuria in preeclampsia. Journal of Clinical Investigation; 2003;111(5):649-658.
26. Miller DA, Chollet JA, Goodwin TM. Rupture of the Uterus. In Gabbe's Obstetrics: Normal and Problem Pregnancies, 8th ed., Elsevier; 2017:731-742.
27. No GT. Placenta Praevia, Placenta Praevia Accreta and Vasa Praevia: Diagnosis and Management. London: RCOG. 2011: 1-26.
28. Odigboegwu O, Pan LJ, Chatterjee P. Use of Antihypertensive Drugs During Preeclampsia. Frontiers in Cardiovascular Medicine. 2018;5:50.

29. Perth, Antepartum Hemorrhage. Western Australia: Department of Health Western Australia; 2015:3-6.
30. Program NH. Report of the National High Blood Pressure Education Program Working Group on High Blood Pressure in Pregnancy. American Journal of Obstetrics and Gynecology; 2000;183(1):s1-22.
31. Redman CW, Sargent IL. Latest Advances in Understanding Preeclampsia. Science; 2003;300(5621):1591-1594.
32. Redman CW, Sargent IL. Latest Advances in Understanding Preeclampsia. Science; 2015;308(5728);1592-1594.
33. Redman CW, Sargent IL. Placental Stress and Pre-eclampsia: A Revised View. Placenta; 2005;26(2-3):97-105.
34. Roberts JM, Cooper DW. Pathogenesis and genetics of Pre-eclampsia. The Lancet; 2001;357(9249):53-56.
35. Roberts JM, Escudero C. The Placenta in Preeclampsia. Pregnancy Hypertension; 2012;2(2):72-83.
36. Roberts JM, Hubel CA. The Two-stage Model of Preeclampsia: Variations on the Theme. Placenta, 20(Suppl A):S32-S37.
37. Roberts JM, Bell MJ. If we know so much about Preeclampsia, why haven't we cured the disease? Journal of Reproductive Immunology, 2003;59(1):1-9.
38. Royal College of Obstetricians and Gynecologists. Management of postpartum hemorrhage (Green-top Guideline No. 52), 2019.
39. Sankaralingam S, Arenas IA, Lalu MM, Davidge ST, Consortium CPR. Preeclampsia: Current Understanding of the Molecular Basis of Vascular Dysfunction. Expert Reviews in Molecular Medicine, 18, e9.
40. Sargent IL, Borzychowski AM, Redman CW. Immuno-regulation in Normal Pregnancy and Pre-eclampsia: An Overview. Reproductive Biomedicine Online; 2006; 13(5):680-686.
41. Sibai BM. Eclampsia. Obstetrics and Gynecology; 2005; 105(2):402-410.
42. Society for Obstetric Anesthesia and Perinatology. Management of Obstetric Patients with known or Suspected COVID-19: Society for Obstetric Anesthesia and Perinatology (SOAP) Interim Considerations. Anesthesia and Analgesia; 2016;131(2):323-326.
43. Tamai K, Koyama T, Togashi K. MR Features of Ectopic Pregnancy. European Radiology; 2007;17(12):3236-46.
44. Tikkanen M, Nuutila M, Hiilesmaa V. Incidence of Placental Abruption in Relation to Cigarette Smoking and Hypertensive Disorders During Pregnancy: A Systematic Review and Meta-Analysis. Obstetrical and Gynecological Survey; 2010;65(12):804-810.
45. Tikkanen M, Nuutila M, Hiilesmaa V, Paavonen J. The Impact of Fetal-Maternal Trauma on Pregnancy Outcome. Acta Obstetricia et Gynecologica Scandinavica; 2006;85(6):680-684.
46. Tikkanen M. Placental Abruption: Epidemiology, Risk Factors and Consequences. Acta Obstetricia et gynecologica Scandinavica. 2011;90(2):140-9.
47. Warren Richard, Arulkumaran Sabaratnam. Best Practice in Labor and Delivery (1st ed., 3rd Printing. ed.). Cambridge: Cambridge University Press; 2009:142–146.
48. World Health Organization (2012), Postpartum Hemorrhage: Prevention and Treatment, https://www.who.int/reproductivehealth/publications/maternal_perinatal_health/9789241548502/en/
49. World Health Organization (WHO). (2018). WHO Recommendations: Intrapartum Care for a Positive Childbirth Experience. Retrieved from https://apps.who.int/iris/bitstream/handle/10665/260178/9789241550215-eng.pdf
50. World Health Organization. WHO Recommendations for Prevention and Treatment of Pre-eclampsia and Eclampsia: Implications and Actions. World Health Organization; 2014.

### Internet Source

- https://kwmidwifery.ca/prenatal-care/placenta-previa/
- https://thesciencenotes.com/abruptio-placentae-types-classification-signs-prevention-and-treatment/
- https://www.who.int/reproductivehealth/publications/maternal_perinatal_health/9789241548502/en/
- https://nhm.gov.in/images/pdf/guidelines/nrhmguidelines/sba_guildelines_final_unfpa.pdf

# Chapter 13

# Neonatal and Pediatric Emergencies and Management

*Dinabandhu Barad*

## CHAPTER OUTLINE

- **Neonatal emergencies:** Asphyxia neonatorum, pathological jaundice in neonates, neonatal seizures, metabolic disorders, intracranial hemorrhage, neonatal sepsis, RDS/HMD (respiratory distress syndrome/hyaline membrane disease).
- **Congenital disorders:** Cyanotic heart disease, tracheoesophageal fistula, congenital hypertrophic pyloric stenosis, imperforate anus.
- **Pediatric emergencies:** Dehydration, acute bronchopneumonia, acute respiratory distress syndrome, poisoning, foreign bodies, seizures, traumas, status asthmatics.
- **Common congenital disorders:** Cleft lip and palate, hypospadias, epispadias, gastroschisis.

## Learning Objectives

At the end of the chapter, the students will be able to:
- Identify the neonatal and pediatric emergencies.
- Describe etiology, clinical features, diagnosis and management of asphyxia neonatorum.
- Explain the causes, clinical features, pathophysiology, diagnosis and management of pathological jaundice in neonate.
- Compare various common neonatal surgical conditions and their management.
- Recall the types and management of metabolic disorders.
- Describe intracranial hemorrhage in terms of types, clinical features, diagnosis and management.
- Describe management of neonatal sepsis.
- Explain various respiratory emergencies like respiratory distress syndrome, acute bronchopneumonia, status asthmaticus and their management.
- Compare various common congenital disorders in terms of clinical features and management.
- Explain different types and management of fluid and electrolyte disturbances.
- Identify various toxic agents and their antidotes.
- Discuss management of foreign body aspiration.
- Explain medical and nursing management of seizure.
- Discuss various types of trauma and their management.

## INTRODUCTION

Neonatal and pediatric emergencies encompass a specialized and critical branch of health care dedicated to addressing urgent medical situations that affect infants and children. These emergencies require immediate assessment, intervention, and treatment to prevent severe complications and ensure the well-being of the young patients. The neonatal phase primarily focuses on newborns, typically from birth up to the first 28 days of life. During this period, infants are particularly vulnerable due to their immature physiological systems and susceptibility to various medical conditions. Neonatal emergencies often demand specialized care and equipment tailored to the unique needs of these fragile patients. In contrast, pediatric emergencies extend beyond the neonatal period and encompass children of various ages, typically up to 18 years old. These emergencies can range from acute illnesses and injuries to chronic conditions that suddenly worsen. Providing timely and appropriate care is essential for pediatric patients, as their bodies continue to grow and develop, influencing how they respond to medical interventions. Neonatal and pediatric emergencies encompass a wide spectrum of conditions, including respiratory distress, infectious diseases, cardiac issues, traumatic injuries, neurological disorders, and toxic exposures, among others. Recognizing and effectively managing these emergencies require healthcare providers to have specialized knowledge, training, and experience in pediatric medicine. Due to the unique physiology and psychological considerations associated with caring for infants and children, healthcare providers involved in neonatal and pediatric emergency care must possess not only clinical expertise but also the ability to communicate effectively with both the young patients and their parents or caregivers. Additionally, a multidisciplinary approach involving pediatric specialists, nurses, respiratory therapists, and other healthcare professionals is often necessary to provide comprehensive and coordinated care.

## NEONATAL AND PEDIATRIC EMERGENCIES

Neonatal and pediatric emergencies are the injury or illness that potentially life-threatening. Management of these innate fragile group are quite complex as compare to the adult. In recent years, the mortality and morbidity due to emergency conditions markedly dropped due to advancement in the knowledge and technology. Following are the common neonatal and pediatric emergencies listed below.

- **Neurological emergencies**
  - Seizure
  - Shaken baby syndrome
- **Respiratory emergencies**
  - Brief resolved unexplained event (BRUE)
  - Airway obstruction
- **Gastrointestinal emergencies**
  - Necrotizing enterocolitis
  - Intussusception
- **Cardiac emergencies**
  - Tet spell
  - Cyanotic heart lesions
- **Endocrine emergencies:** Thyrotoxicosis
- **Infective emergencies:** Sepsis
- **Environmental emergencies**
  - Burn
  - Drowning
  - Poisoning
  - Anaphylaxis

### Neurological Emergencies

#### Seizure

Neonatal seizure is most of the time less identified and complex to treat. More than 50% of the neonate with hypoxic ischemic encephalopathy develop neonatal seizure and for rest of the 40–50% have unspecific etiological factors. During seizure activity neonate may present abnormal mouth and eye movement, excessive drilling, apnea, pedalling movement of leg, shaking extremities and lip smacking, fixed staring. EEG can be used to record the electrical activity and neuroimaging with CT and MRI will provide crucial information regarding hemorrhage, tumor, brain injury or other anatomical deviations. CSF and Blood examination may help in identifying bacteremia, meningitis or electrolyte imbalance. Management often includes administration of benzodiazepine (diazepam, lorazepam, midazolam), phenobarbital and phenytoin. Close monitoring of respiratory status and vitals are crucial to prevent further complication (A Parthasarathy et.al., IAP Textbook of Pediatrics, 7th Ed 2019).

#### Shaken Baby Syndrome (SBS)

It is a form of abusive brain injury caused by violent shaking of the baby by parents or caregiver. Also called as shaken impact syndrome or abusive head trauma. Forceful shaking causes injury to the skull, brain parenchyma, nerve branches, ribs clavicle, etc., resulting intracranial hemorrhage and retinal hemorrhage. The clinical features of the child with SBS may be irritability, bluish discoloration of skin, poor feeding, seizure, irregular respiration, emesis, dilated pupil, coma, altered alertness, poor feeding, trouble sucking, sluggish and brady cardia, etc., diagnosis often made by thorough physical examination to identify the signs of SBS like retinal hemorrhage, lacerations, bone fractures, chest or abdominal injury, brushing of skin, swelling, etc. For further in-depth investigation history, fundoscopy, X-ray, CT, MRI, ultrasonography, routine urine and blood examination may be required to establish a strong evidence. Immediate management like CPR, surgical intervention for ICH, restoration of respiratory and circulatory status may be required to save the life of the child (A Parthasarathy et. al., IAP Textbook of Pediatrics, 7th Ed., 2019).

### Respiratory Emergencies

#### Brief Resolved Unexplained Events (BRUE)

BRUE may be defined as the combination of clinical features such as apnea, altered skin and muscle tone, gagging, or choking. Previously, it was called as apparent life-threatening event (ALTE). Infants between the age of 1–3 months usually develop BRUE. Approximately half (50%) of the infant develop BRUE without any identifiable reason but the remaining 50% of the infants may have gastrointestinal (50%), neurological (30%), respiratory (20%), cardiovascular (5%), metabolic and endocrine (2–5%) issues. As there is no definitive guideline and the root cause of BRUE is variable, diagnosis often require detailed history taking, thorough clinical examination and extensive lab investigation like routine blood examination, blood culture, nasopharyngeal swab culture, routine and microscopic examination of urine, serum electrolyte, CSF study, X-ray, CT, MRI, ECG, EEG, ultrasonography, esophageal PH monitoring, etc., are required. Management includes immediate restoration of patency of air way, prevention of aspiration, CPR and treatment of underlying causes.

### Airway Obstruction

Airway obstruction is common among the children below 5 years of age due to ingestion of foreign body. Obstruction may also occur in upper or the lower respiratory tract. The cause of upper respiratory tract obstruction may be due to deviated nasal septum, choanal atresia, nasal pyriform aperture stenosis, glossoptosis, macroglossia, Laryngomalacia, vocal cord paralysis, laryngeal atresia, subglottic stenosis, subglottic hemangioma, etc. Similarly, lower airway obstruction may be due to tracheal stenosis, tracheomalacia, congenital lobar emphysema, bronchogenic cyst, diaphragmatic hernia, etc. The child with obstructive airway may present apnea, coughing, wheezing, excessive drooling, stridor and cyanosis. History taking from the parents, physical examination, laryngoscopy, bronchoscopy, endoscopy, chest X-ray, CT and MRI may reveal the underlying reason of obstruction. Immediate management to restore the respiration is crucial (A Parthasarathy et.al., 2019).

## Gastrointestinal Emergencies

### Necrotizing Enterocolitis (NEC)

NEC is the most common GI emergency among the premature infants characterized by damage of the intestinal tract. This is more prevalent among the formula feed babies. Immature gut, hypoxia, inflammatory mediators, microorganisms are the contributing factor in the development of NEC. The extent of damage of the intestine is variable from mucosal damage to the damage of full intestinal wall or perforation. GI manifestation may be the abdominal distention, vomiting, poor feeding, frequent loose stool, blood in stool, blue or black color skin over abdomen, ascites. Systemic clinical presentation are the apnea, decreased heart rate, shock. Platelet count should be advised to identify thrombocytopenia as it will help to predict the necrosis of diagnosed NEC neonates. CBC, serum electrolyte level also should be monitored. Abdominal X-ray is the reliable and specific to detect the NEC. Management often include cessation of oral feeding, and combination of multiple antibiotic therapy (Ramesh Agarwal, Ashok Deorari et. al.).

### Intussusception

It is a condition in which a part of intestine slides into the adjacent intestinal lumen making a telescopic appearance. It is of two types as follows:
1. **Idiopathic intussusception:** Commonly occurs among infants and toddlers at ileocecal junction.
2. **Enteroenteral intussusception:** It is commonly found among older children between ilium and jejunum.

Only one-third of the affected infants show vomiting, abdominal pain and hematochezia as the classical triad of intussusception and other features include lethargy, diarrhea and fever. Diagnosis of this condition require ultrasonography, abdominal X-ray, barium swallow and barium enema. If immediate management will not be taken then blood supply will be ceased resulting necrosis and perforation of the affected part of intestine.

## Cardiac Emergencies

### Tet Spell

The infant with Tetralogy of Fallot Tet spell if expose to certain triggering factors but this can happen even if the triggers are absent. This lethal hypoxic spell has a classical presentation, i.e., shortness of breath, cyanosis, uncontrollable crying or panic, and syncope. Knee chest positing during Tet spell to elevate systemic vascular resistance, hence decrease right to left shunt of blood inside the heart and allow more blood to enter lung. Sedative may be administered to reduce the oxygen demand and to supress the respiratory center there by help in managing shortness of breath (Parul Dutta and Piyush Gupta, 2021).

### Cyanotic Heart Lesions

These are a group of defects resulting right to left shunt of the blood resulting poor oxygenation and cyanosis. Tetralogy of Fallot, transposition of great artery, truncus arteriosus, total anomalous pulmonary venous connection, single ventricle, etc., are the example of cyanotic heart lesions (Piyush Gupta, 2021).

## Endocrine Emergencies

### Thyrotoxicosis

It is a life-threatening condition characterized by clinical syndrome due to high level of free thyroid hormone of any source. Where the mortality rate of thyrotoxicosis without treatment is between 80–100% with treatment the percentage drops to 10–50%. Heat intolerance, sweating, tachycardia, fever, diarrhea are the features of thyrotoxicosis. Antithyroid medications or thyroidectomy are the choice of treatment (A Parthasarathy et.al, 2019).

## Infective Emergencies

### Sepsis

According to the IAP sepsis can be defined as "systemic bacterial infections of the newborn are termed as neonatal sepsis and include overwhelming infection without localization (septicemia), or pneumonia, meningitis, urinary tract infection". Sepsis that occurs within 72 hours of birth is called early onset sepsis otherwise called as late onset sepsis. CBC, ESR, CRP, blood culture, chest X-ray, blood sugar investigation are required for diagnosis of sepsis. Supportive and antimicrobial treatment are the key treatment in this case (Ramesh Agarwal, Ashok Deorari et. al., AIIMS Protocols in Neonatology, 2nd Edition).

## Environmental Emergencies

### Burn

It is a type of injury to the skin or muscle by heat, electricity, chemical, radiation or friction, socioeconomic status, child abuse medical conditions like seizure are the contributing factors of burn injury.

Types of burn injury can be as follows:
- Chemical burn
- Thermal burn
- Electrical burn
- Scald burn

Based on the depth of the injury burn can be classified as follows:
- Superficial burn/first degree burn (damage confined to the epidermis only)
- Superficial partial thickness burn/2nd degree burn (involve epidermis and superficial dermis)
- Deep partial thickness burn/2nd degree burn (involve epidermis and dermis in depth along with blood vessels)
- Full thickness burn/3rd degree burn (involvement of all skin layers)
- Fourth degree burn: involving full thickness of skin and underlying muscles, tendons and subcutaneous fat.

### Management

Assessment of surface are of rectal injury Lund Browder diagram for pediatric population is used. Fluid electrolyte balance, wound care, infection control, pain management and nutrition are the areas of treatment.

### Drowning

Drowning is defined by the World Health Organization as "a process resulting in primary respiratory impairment from submersion/immersion in a liquid medium". Children between the age of 1–4 years have the highest mortality rate. It is of four types as follows:
1. Dry drowning
2. Wet drowning
3. Secondary or near drowning
4. Immersion syndrome

Prompt management at the emergency room with CPR, intubation, thermoregulation, fluid electrolyte balance and neuro protective strategies can help in the survival of the life.

### Anaphylaxis

According to WHO, "anaphylaxis is a severe, life-threatening systemic hypersensitivity reaction characterized by being rapid in onset with potentially life-threatening airway, breathing, or circulatory problems and is usually, although not always, associated with skin and mucosal changes".

—**WHO**

"Anaphylaxis is a serious systemic hypersensitivity reaction that is usually rapid in onset and may cause death. Severe anaphylaxis is characterized by potentially life-threatening compromise in breathing and/or the circulation, and may occur without typical skin features or circulatory shock being present." —**Revised definition by WAO**

Among pediatric population food are the most common triggering factors of anaphylactic reaction. Whereas other triggering factors also can cause with or without IgE mediated anaphylaxis. Milk, egg, fish, sea foods, bee stings, snake bite, vaccines, antibiotics, NSAIDS anesthetic agents are the common causative factors of anaphylaxis among children. The common clinical presentation of the child may be redness of the skin, swelling, nausea, vomiting, abdominal cramping, diarrhea, hypotension, arrhythmia, seizure, loss of consciousness, difficulty in breathing, etc. Epinephrine is the first drug of choice along with specific antidotes. Administration of corticosteroids, antihistamines are required. CPR may be required for some of the children.

## Asphyxia Neonatorum and Hypoxic Ischemic Encephalopathy

**Asphyxia neonatorum or perinatal asphyxia** is a hypoxic insult to the fetus resulting from deprived gas exchange. According to WHO about 25 lakhs new born died in 2018 globally because of several causes, where perinatal asphyxia is one of the leading causes resulting death of the baby during first 28 days of life. Perinatal asphyxia leads to multiorgan failure including brain, heart, kidney, liver, lungs and intestine, etc. CNS dysfunction related to perinatal asphyxia is called as **hypoxic ischemic encephalopathy (HIE)**.

## Definition

"A failure to initiate and sustain breathing at birth"—**WHO**
"Gasping or ineffective breathing or lack of breathing at one minute of life." —**NNF India**

As per American Academy of Pediatrics (AAP) and American College of Obstetrician and Gynecologists (ACOG) all of the following features must be present for designation of perinatal asphyxia.
- Umbilical artery blood PH <7.0
- 5-minute APGAR score <3
- Neonatal neurological manifestation (e.g., seizures, hypotonia or coma in the immediate neonatal period)
- Evidence of multiorgan dysfunction (e.g., kidney, lungs, liver, heart, intestine).

As per the National Neonatal Perinatal Database (NNPD) network the definition for classifying moderate and severe perinatal asphyxia as follows based on APGAR score (Table 13.1):
- **Moderate:** Slow or gasping breathing or an APGAR score of 4–6 at 1 minute.
- **Severe:** No breathing or an APGAR score of 0–3 at 1 minute.

## Risk Factors

Perinatal asphyxia can happen anytime during antepartum, intrapartum, and postpartum period due to following factors:
- **Maternal hypoxia**
  - Hypo/hypertension
  - Maternal infection
  - Gestational diabetic mellitus
  - Respiratory diseases

**Table 13.1:** APGAR score.

| | Parameters | 0 | 1 | 2 |
|---|---|---|---|---|
| A | Activity (muscle tone) | Absent | Arms and legs flexed | Active movement |
| P | Pulse | Absent | <100 bpm | >100 bpm |
| G | Grimace (reflex response) | No response to stimulation | Grimace on stimulation | Cry on stimulation |
| A | Appearance (skin color) | Blue, pale | Body pink extremities blue | Whole body pink |
| R | Respiration | Absent | Slow and irregular | Vigorous cry |

*Source:* Adapted from the American College of Obstetricians and Gynecologists (ACOG).

- Cardiac diseases
- Cocaine use
- **Placental factors (impaired exchange of $O_2$ and $CO_2$ across placenta)**
  - Placenta previa
  - Abruptio placentae
- **Reduced blood flow from placenta to fetus**
  - Umbilical cord abnormality
  - Cord prolapse
  - Umbilical cord entanglement
  - Cord compression
  - Umbilical artery or vein abnormality
- **Fetal factors (increase demand by fetus)**
  - Anemia
  - Infection
  - Cardiomyopathy.

*Interpretation*

| Score | Status |
|---|---|
| 0–3 | : Severe perinatal asphyxia |
| 4–7 | : Mild and moderate perinatal asphyxia |
| 8–10 | : Normal |

## Classifications

There are several classification systems available for HIE but the most reliable and practiced systems are the Levene classification system. Based on this HIE can be classified into mild, moderate and severe based on 4 parameters (consciousness, tone, seizure and sucking/respiration). To measure the severity of the HIE Thompson scoring system also is used in clinical practice. There are 9 parameters in Thomson scoring (tone, level of consciousness, fits, posture, moro reflex, grasp reflex, sucking reflex, respiration and fontanel) and has a minimum score 0 representing normal and maximum 22 which indicates severe HIE. Score between 1–10 indicates mild, 11–14 represents moderate and 15–22 indicates severe HIE.

## Pathophysiology

In perinatal asphyxia placental blood flow is compromised resulting multiorgan failure. Neonatal brain is the common victim of perinatal asphyxia as it requires adequate oxygen and blood supply continuously. When blood flow to the fetus is compromised a protective mechanism called **diving seal reflex** redistribute the blood to the vital organs like brain, adrenal gland, etc., by reducing the blood flow to the less vital organs like skin, muscle, intestine, etc.

The diving seal reflex act as a protective mechanism for the vital organs but there are studies claiming that all neonates don't exhibit similar kind of adaptive mechanism consistently. Phelan and colleagues carried out a study on 14 patients of hypoxic ischemic encephalopathy and found that all the neonates develop cerebral palsy without multi-organ failure. So, it was postulated that the mechanism associated in the development of cerebral palsy among these 14 cases did not allow sufficient time for the adaptive mechanism to redistribute the blood to the vital organs. Several studies are also claiming that intermittent asphyxia for less than 60 mins unlikely to develop brain injury. Hence severe, prolonged and total asphyxia results brain damage more quickly as compare to intermittent asphyxia for short period of time (Piyush Gupta, 2021).

The pathophysiological event in cases of perinatal asphyxia occurs in two phases:
1. Primary energy failure
2. Secondary energy failure

*Primary Energy Failure*

When adaptive mechanism failed and cerebral blood flow become insufficient to meet the demand, a complex series of biochemical event begins. In asphyxiate newborn hypoxia forces anaerobic metabolism resulting increase lactic acid, decrease in PH, reduced ATP. Decreased energy production leads to impairment of ATP dependant ion channels which in turn causes accumulation of sodium, calcium and chloride and water inside the cell and potassium, glutamate, aspartate outside the cell. The consequence of imbalance of ions and influx of water leads swelling, lysis and necrotic death of cells.

*Secondary Energy Failure*

It occurs 6–48 hours after the initial insult. Although the specific mechanism of secondary energy failure is illusive it is strongly associated with oxidative stress, inflammation and excitotoxicity. During hypoxic ischemic encephalopathy the irons bound with the proteins are released and become free to react with peroxidase to make free radicals. As the neonatal brain has insufficient antioxidants and lack of ability to clear the oxygen free radicals it become vulnerable to neuronal tissue damage. Excitotoxicity occurs when excessive production and accumulation of neurotransmitters like glutamate occurs extracellularly and over stimulate the excitatory receptors. As a result of overexcitation sodium and calcium influx occurs worsening the tissue damage. Although inflammation is found to be associated with HIE the mechanism is still unclear (Piyush Gupta, 2021 and A Parthasarathy et. al., 2019).

**Clinical features of perinatal asphyxia**
- Respiratory distress or apnea
- Bluish discoloration of skin
- Brady cardia
- Poor muscle tone

- Poor reflex response
- Acidosis PH<7
- APGAR score <3
- Meconium stained amniotic fluid
- Neurological features like seizure, coma, etc.
- Symptoms of multiorgan failure

**Features of perinatal asphyxia associated with HIE depends on severity as follows:**

*Mild HIE*
- Poor feeding
- Irritability
- Excessive cry
- Increased muscle tone
- Dilated pupil
- Increased deep tendon reflex

*Moderate HIE*
- Hypotonia
- Lethargic
- Increased deep tendon reflex
- Constricted pupil
- Seizure
- Bradycardia

*Severe HIE*
- **Birth–12 hours:** Depressed level of consciousness, periodic breathing or respiratory failure, hypotonia, seizure, normal pupillary response.
- **12–24 hours:** Variable change in the consciousness, seizure, apnea spells, jitteriness, weakness in the proximal extremities.
- **24–72 hours:** Stupor or coma, respiratory failure, change in the pupillary response, intraventricular hemorrhage and periventricular hemorrhage (preterm).
- **>72 hours:** Stupor or coma, poor reflex response, hypotonia occurs more common than hypertonia, weakness in proximal extremities.

## Diagnosis

There are no specific investigations available for confirmatory diagnosis of perinatal asphyxia but some investigations can help to identify the severity of neural damage and multiorgan failure. The common investigations are as follows:
- Blood sugar
- Arterial blood gas analysis
- $SPO_2$
- Serum electrolyte level
- Blood urea and nitrogen
- Serum creatinine
- Liver function test
- CT scan
- MRI
- EEG

## Management

The management of perinatal asphyxia is primarily supportive. But initial resuscitation and stabilization can prevent its incidence. The supportive management includes maintenance of fluid electrolyte balance, thermoregulation, blood glucose, monitoring and controlling seizure, etc. Although most of the neonate don't require any intervention to breathe approximately 1% require extensive resuscitation. The guidelines for neonatal resuscitation is given by the American Heart Association (AHA) the concepts in these guidelines may be applied to newborns during the neonatal period (birth to 28 days). As initial resuscitation can prevent adequate care should be taken for immediate and effective management which depends on—(1) anticipating the need of resuscitation and (2) adequate preparation of personnel and delivery room.

### Anticipating the Need of Resuscitation

Although perinatal asphyxia is unpredictable there are certain antepartum and intrapartum history which can provide us crucial information to anticipate it. It is also found that approximately 50% of the asphyxiate neonate have no risk factors hence one should always be ready for resuscitation while attending delivery. Following are some of the risk factors to anticipate perinatal asphyxia in the neonate (NVSSK Basic Newborn Care and Resuscitation Program Training Manual, 2020).
- Gestational hypertension
- Meconium-stained amniotic fluid (MSAF)
- Eclampsia
- Prolapsed umbilical cord
- Prolonged labor
- Abnormal presentation of the fetus
- Assisted delivery
- Rh incompatibility
- PROM (prolonged rupture of membrane)
- Multiple gestation
- Presence of congenital anomaly
- Maternal sedation, anesthesia or analgesia.

### Adequate Preparation of Personnel and Delivery Room

Before the delivery a helper should be identified to assist in the resuscitation process. The helper can be a nursing officer, hospital staff or family member of the mother based on the availability at the setting. The helper should be educated about his/her role during resuscitation (NVSSK Basic Newborn Care and Resuscitation Program Training Manual, 2020).

The temperature of the delivery room should be ≥25°C and draught free. The delivery surface and resuscitation surface should be warm clean and dry. While preparing the equipment it is important to ensure following points:
- Cleanliness of the equipment
- Working condition of the equipment
- Appropriate size
- Mucus extractor with a bulb should not be used and it should have a big trap (20 mL)
- The volume of the bag should be between 250–500 mL not more than that
- While doing suction negative pressure should be below 100 mm Hg
- Radiant warmer should be turned on before 30 mins to keep the environment warm
- All the equipment should be tested priorly.

### Equipment for Resuscitation

**Suction equipment**
- Mucus aspirator
- Suction device
- Suction catheter (10F/12F)
- Feeding tube 6F

**Positive pressure ventilation equipment's**
- Face mask
- Bag and mask equipment (240–500 mL)
- Oxygen source with flow meter
- Laryngeal mask airway (LMA)

**Intubation equipment**
- Laryngoscope with straight blade (00: extremely preterm, 0: preterm, 1: term)
- Endotracheal tubes of internal diameter

**Medication**
- Epinephrine
- Normal saline

**Miscellaneous**
- Radiant warmer
- Linen
- Shoulder roll
- Clock with second-hand
- Stethoscope
- Syringes
- Gauze
- Umbilical catheters 3.5, 5F
- Three-way stopcocks
- Gloves
- Nasogastric tubes
- Two clean, warm towels/clothes
- Adhesive tape

### Initial Steps of Resuscitation
(NVSSK Basic Newborn Care and Resuscitation Program Training Manual, 2020 and Piyush Gupta, 2021).

- **Provide warmth:** The neonate should be received in a prewarmed towel and placed under the preheated radiant warmer. For stabilization and maintenance of temperature of the healthy neonate some the techniques are prewarming the linen, drying the skin, swaddling, skin to skin contact, covering the baby, etc. The very low birth weight baby is more susceptible to hypothermia therefore additional care should be taken such as continuous monitoring, prewarming the radiant warmer, prewarming delivery room to 26°C, covering the baby with plastic wrap, etc.
- **Positioning:** The child should be placed in supine position with neck slightly extended. Hyperextension or flexion position are inappropriate as these may interfere with air entry. To maintain the position shoulder roll (½ to 1 inch thick) can be used.
- **Clear air way:** Clearing the airway depends on the type of amniotic fluid (clear or meconium-stained). If the amniotic fluid is clear, then mouth should be suctioned first then nose. The negative pressure for suctioning should not exceed 100 mm Hg. Vigorous suctioning should be avoided as this may cause brady cardia. In case of meconium-stained amniotic fluid, mouth should suction first followed by nose and suctioning from trachea may require endotracheal intubation. But direct suction to trachea should be avoided.
- **Dry, stimulation and reposition:** After clearing the airway the neonate should be dried using prewarmed towel. All the wet linen and clothes should be removed to prevent heat loss.
- **Tactile stimulation:** Usually suctioning and drying stimulates breathing. If the neonate still not responding the tactile stimulation can be given by flicking or slapping the soles of the feet or by rubbing back, trunk or extremities. The maximum limit of tactile stimulation is twice and the baby with primary apnea usually respond to this stimulation. If the baby doesn't respond to tactile stimulation, then it indicates that the baby is in secondary apnea, and it warrant immediate positive pressure ventilation.
- **Oxygen supplementation:** If the child is not maintaining saturation or heart rate is not increasing in room air then higher concentration of oxygen should be administered using mask.
- **Evaluation:** After supplemental oxygen it is important to evaluate heart rate, respiration, oxygen saturation, skin color.

## Positive pressure ventilation (PPV)

NVSSK Basic Newborn Care and Resuscitation Program Training Manual, 2020.

- Positive pressure ventilation is required when the child is apneic or gasping or heart rate below 100 bpm or persistent cyanosis (in spite of oxygen administration) even after initial stabilization.
  - Positive pressure ventilation can be provided by self-inflating bag, laryngeal mask airway or with a T-piece resuscitator.
  - The absolute contraindication of bag and mask ventilation is diaphragmatic hernia, and the relative contraindication is meconium aspiration syndrome. In these cases, intubation is preferred for positive pressure ventilation.
  - Self-inflating bag has two inlets at the posterior part: A smaller one for attachment of oxygen source and a bigger one for air entry. It possesses a safety valve at the anterior part called pop off valve which opens when excess pressure generates inside the bag during ventilation. The pop off valve opens when pressure exceeds 30–40 cm $H_2O$ to prevent barotrauma of the lung.
  - A mask should be attached to the anterior part of the bag and should be of appropriate shape and size. The size of the mask for preterm are 0 or 00 and for term neonate size 1. The correct mask should cover the tip of the chin, nose and mouth. Too big mask may extend up to eye resulting possible damage and air leakage. Too small mask may not cover the nose and mouth appropriately and additionally it may depress the nose blocking the air flow.
  - Before initiating bag and mask ventilation clear the air way and position the baby on the back with neck slightly extended (sniffing position). Shoulder roll can be used to keep the neck in stable position for patent air way.
  - The person who will provide PPV should position himself/herself at the side or at the head of the baby for better visualization of chest and for holding the mask comfortably. Mask should be placed on the face covering the tip of the chin, nose and mouth. Mask should be held using thumb, index and middle finger around the edge making a shape of letter 'C'. Ring and little finger should be placed under the chin to bring it forward for slight extension of the neck.
  - To initiate ventilation, squeeze the bag just enough to generate gentle chest rise as during normal breathing. The rate of ventilation should be between 40–60 per minute. To maintain the rate, say "Breathe-- two--three", "Breathe--two--three". Squeeze the bag while saying **'Breathe'** and release when saying **'two'**, **'three'**.
- Chest should rise during ventilation. If absent then ensure application of adequate pressure while squeezing the bag, check for any air leakage, fitting of the mask, positioning of the neck and clear the secretions. Then start ventilating again with corrective measures for next 30 seconds and check for any sign's improvement. The most important sign of improvement is the spontaneous breathing if exists then gradually reduce the rate and volume of ventilation. The signs of successive ventilation are as follows:
  - Spontaneous breathing (regular and rate between 30–60 breaths/min)
  - Bilateral chest movement
  - Absence of grunting or chest indrawing
  - Crying

If the baby shows signs of successive ventilation, then stop ventilating. If the baby has no signs of improvement even after 30 seconds of ventilation, then add oxygen and assess heart rate and call for help. If the heart rate is normal (> 100 bpm) then continue ventilation with oxygen for another 30 seconds and reassess breathing. If the baby is still not breathing well then advance support like chest compression, intubation and medication may be required. If the heart rate is below 100 bpm, then also advance support is required.

## Intubation

Endotracheal (ET) intubation is indicated in following conditions:

- When bag mask ventilation is ineffective or prolonged more than 2 mins
- Before initiating chest compression
- When endotracheal administration of medication is required
- If bag mask ventilation is contraindicated
- ELBW baby <1000 g.

As a nurse gather all the equipment prior to the procedure and check the working condition. While choosing appropriate size of the ET tube based on birth weight as discussed below take two additional ET tubes one above and one below the anticipated size. ET tube intubation should be performed only by the skillful neonatologist or anesthesiologist. As a nurse positioning the baby on a flat surface, assisting during the procedure and selecting appropriate size of the laryngoscope blade and ET tubes are important. Intubation should be performed quickly as possible within 20 seconds. Confirm the placement of the ET tube in the air way and start ventilating by attaching the

bag. The following are the indicators of appropriate tube placement:
- During ventilation chest should rise bilaterally and symmetrically.
- Increase in the heart rate.
- Detection of end tidal $CO_2$.
- Presence of mist air during exhalation.

| Birth weight (g) | ET tube size (internal diameter in mm) |
|---|---|
| <1000 | 2.5 |
| 1000–2000 | 3.0 |
| 2000–3000 | 3.5 |
| >3000 | 4.0 |

### Chest compression

NVSSK Basic Newborn Care and Resuscitation Program Training Manual, 2020 and Piyush Gupta, 2021.

Chest compression is indicated when heart rate is below 60 bpm even after positive pressure ventilation for 30 seconds. But chest compression is a common practice if heart rate is between 60–80 bpm and is not increasing. Chest compression should be continued along with ventilation and 100% oxygen. Compression should be delivered over the lower third of the sternum (roughly around 1 cm below the inter nipple line) at a depth of approximately one-third of the anteroposterior diameter of the chest. Therefore, two rescuers are required, one for chest compression and other for PPV. The two acceptable techniques for chest compression are:
1. Two thumb technique (two thumbs are placed adjacent to each other with fingers encircling around the chest)
2. Two finger technique

The ratio of chest compression and PPV is 3:1 where 90 chest compression and 30 PPV should be performed within one minute. One rescuer provides 3 compressions and the second rescuer provide one PPV by following one and two and three and breathe as shown in **Figure 13.1**. If the heart rate is >100 then stop chest compression and gradually discontinue ventilation if the baby is breathing spontaneously. If the heart rate is between 60–100 bpm then stop chest compression and continue PPV at a rate of 40–60 breaths/min. If the heart rate is still below 60 bpm then medications should be administered.

### Medication

Epinephrine is administered when heart rate remains <60 bpm despite of PPV and chest compression. It is a sympathomimetic drug which increases heart rate, cardiac output. It can be administered via intravenous route or into the endotracheal tube at a dose of 0.1–0.3 mg/kg.

### Post Resuscitation Management

- After resuscitation the baby should be transferred to the NICU for observation and care. Care should be taken on following aspects after resuscitation:
    - Maintenance of body temperature
    - Monitoring vital signs
    - Maintenance of blood glucose level
    - Assessment of skin color, breathing
    - Identification of any complications
- IV fluid can be administered with 10% dextrose at 60 mL/kg/day.
- Blood glucose level should be maintained within 75–100 mg/dL for uninterrupted supply of glucose to the brain. If hypoglycemia is detected then a bolus of 2 mL/kg of 10% dextrose should be administered followed by continuous infusion at a rate of 6 mg/kg/minute.
- Anticonvulsants can be used if the baby has seizure activity.
- Therapeutic hypothermia (33.5°C–34.5°C) can be provided to the baby with moderate to severe HIE and gestational age ≥36 weeks as a neuroprotective management. The treatment should be started within 6 hours of life for maximum protection of the CNS. The treatment is provided in two phases a total period of 84 hours (Piyush Gupta, 2021).
    - *Phase 1:* Active cooling—for 72 hours from the initiation of cooling
    - *Phase 2:* Rewarming—12 hours of gradual rewarming after completion of 72 hours of cooling. Temperature is gradually increased by 0.5°C every 2 hours until the core body temperature reaches 37°C +/- 0.2. It is important to monitor temperature frequently following rewarming to prevent rebound hyperthermia.

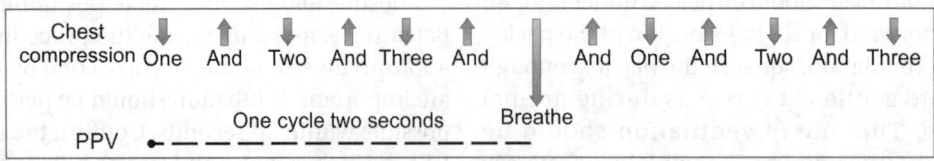

**Fig. 13.1:** Methods to maintain chest compression to ventilation ratio.

## Nursing Management

### Nursing Diagnosis - 1

Ineffective breathing pattern related to immature respiratory organs as evidenced by gasping, APGAR score.

Interventions

- Position the newborn in supine position with neck slightly extended
- Clear the air way if required use suction
- Administer supplemental oxygen as prescribed
- Keep the resuscitative equipment and emergency drugs near the bed side
- Monitor heart rate, respiration, oxygen saturation and skin color
- Assess ABG level to monitor oxygen and ventilation status
- Monitor rate and depth of breathing pattern every 4 hourly
- Auscultate breath sound to identify any adventitious breath sound
- Monitor chest indrawing or retraction and nasal flaring to identify increase in respiratory effort
- Use pulse oximeter to detect $SPO_2$ and pulse rate
- Monitor the level of consciousness

### Nursing Diagnosis - 2

Risk of hypothermia related to impaired thermoregulation as evidenced by fluctuation in the body temperature.

Interventions

- During delivery receive the newborn in a prewarmed towel
- Dry the neonate and remove all wet linen and clothes to prevent heat loss
- Encourage skin to skin contact
- Place the baby under radiant warmer if indicated
- Monitor vitals specially temperature regularly
- If not contraindicated encourage breastfeeding
- Postpone weighing the baby until uninterrupted skin to skin contact is done
- At the time of weighing the baby place a warm towel on the scale
- Avoid bathing which may cause hypothermia

### Nursing Diagnosis - 3

Risk for infection related to inadequate immunity/environmental exposure as evidenced by invasive procedures, broken skin and low WBC count.

Interventions

- Assess vitals every 4 hourly or as required
- Assess the factors which might lead to neonatal sepsis like rupture of membrane, prolonged labor, number of clean and unclean vaginal examinations, spontaneous preterm labor, etc.
- Encourage breastfeeding which can deliver passive immunity to the newborn
- Avoid unnecessary handling of the newborn
- Strictly follow infection control practice while providing care and doing invasive procedures
- Protect the newborn from iatrogenic and cross-infection
- Monitor lab results specially WBC count, CRP, ESR, blood culture, CSF culture, etc.
- Assess and monitor nutritional status and weight of the newborn
- Administer antibiotics as prescribed
- Assess immunization history and administer as per requirement.

## Pathological Jaundice in Neonate

Neonatal jaundice is the yellowish discoloration of the skin and sclera of the new born during first few weeks of life. This is the most common medical emergency if there is an underling pathological cause behind it. The incidence of jaundice among the term and preterm neonates is about 60% and 80% respectively. Although jaundice sometime can be harmless (physiological jaundice) but it can warrant immediate medical attention if it is a pathological one (Ramesh Agarwal, Ashok Deorari et. al. AIIMS Protocols in Neonatology, 2nd Edition).

### Definition

The yellowish discoloration of the skin and sclera as a result of excessive accumulation of bilirubin (hyperbilirubinemia) during first few weeks of life is called neonatal jaundice.

### Types

Neonatal jaundice can be categorized based on underlying causes as physiological and pathological jaundice. The differences between both the types are explained in the **Table 13.2**.

### Etiology

- **Increased production**
- **Hemolytic causes**
    - Immune mediated hemolysis (Coombs positive)
        - Rh in compatibility
        - ABO incompatibility
    - Nonimmune mediated hemolysis (Coombs negative)
        - RBC membrane defect (hereditary spherocytosis, elliptocytosis)

**Table 13.2:** Differences between pathological and physiological jaundice.

| Parameters | Pathological | Physiological |
|---|---|---|
| Onset | Occurs within 24 hours | Occurs after 24 hours |
| Cause | Pathological condition | Normal heme breakdown |
| Resolves | Automatically | Requires medical treatment |
| TSB | >15 mg/dL | <15 mg/dL |
| Direct bilirubin | >2 mg/dL | <2 mg/dL |
| Rate of bilirubin rise | >5 mg/dL/24 h or >0.5 mg/dL/h | <5 mg/dL/24 hours |
| Persists | Beyond 2 weeks | Don't persists beyond 2 weeks |
| Palm and sole | Yellowish discoloration | No discoloration |

- RBC enzyme defect (pyruvate kinase deficiency, G6PD deficiency)
- Hemoglobinopathies (sickle cell disease, thalassemia)
- **Nonhemolytic causes**
  - Trauma
    - Cephalohematoma
    - Intraventricular hemorrhage
  - Others
    - Hypothyroidism
    - Gestational diabetic mellitus
    - Cystic fibrosis
- **Bilirubin clearance**
  - Obstructive jaundice
  - Biliary atresia
  - Choledocholithiasis
- **Genetic abnormality**
  - Gilbert syndrome
  - Crigler Najjar syndrome
  - Rotor syndrome
  - Dubin Johnson syndrome

*Bilirubin Metabolism*

Bilirubin is produced as a metabolite of heme **(Flowchart 13.1)**. It is crucial to excrete this toxic substance out of the body through renal and GI system/the metabolism of bilirubin can be well understood through following steps.

- **Production:** About 75% of bilirubin is produced from the breakdown of heme in the reticuloendothelial system and remaining 25% of the bilirubin are derived from the heme containing proteins like cytochrome, catalase, peroxidase, myoglobin, etc., production of heme takes place in two steps where hemeoxygenase and biliverdin reductase enzymes are essential **(Flowchart 13.1)**. About 34 mg of bilirubin is produced when 1 g of heme breaks down. A healthy newborn produces approximately double amount of bilirubin as compared to the healthy adult.
  - Healthy newborn : 3–4 mg/kg/day
  - Healthy adult : 6–10 mg/kg/day
- **Transportation:** Bilirubin once released from the site of production (reticuloendothelial system) and reaches the plasma they combine with albumin to make bilirubin albumin complex. Bilirubin makes a complex with high density lipoprotein (HDL) in case of hypoalbuminemia very rarely. The advantages of albumin binding are as follows:
  - Reduces the chance of leaving blood vessels
  - Minimize its filtration through glomerulus
  - Prevent its deposition in tissue
- **Uptake and conjugation:** Bilirubin albumin complex dissociates into individual components leaving unconjugated bilirubin which is taken up by the hepatocytes. Conjugation is crucial to convert aqueous insoluble (unconjugated) to soluble (conjugated) bilirubin. In hepatocytes bilirubin is conjugated with two molecules of glucuronic acid by the enzyme glucoronyl transferase.
- **Excretion and enterohepatic circulation:** The conjugated bilirubin then excreted to the bile canaliculi and transported through bile to the small intestine. The intestinal bacteria then degrade the conjugated bilirubin to urobilinogen. Approximately half of the urobilinogen reabsorbed to the portal circulation and remaining half convert to stercobilin.

Assessment and Diagnosis

Jaundice in the new-born can be when the serum bilirubin level crosses 5 mg/dL. Visible jaundice progresses in cephalocaudal direction where the face and sclera becomes

**Flowchart 13.1:** Bilirubin metabolism.

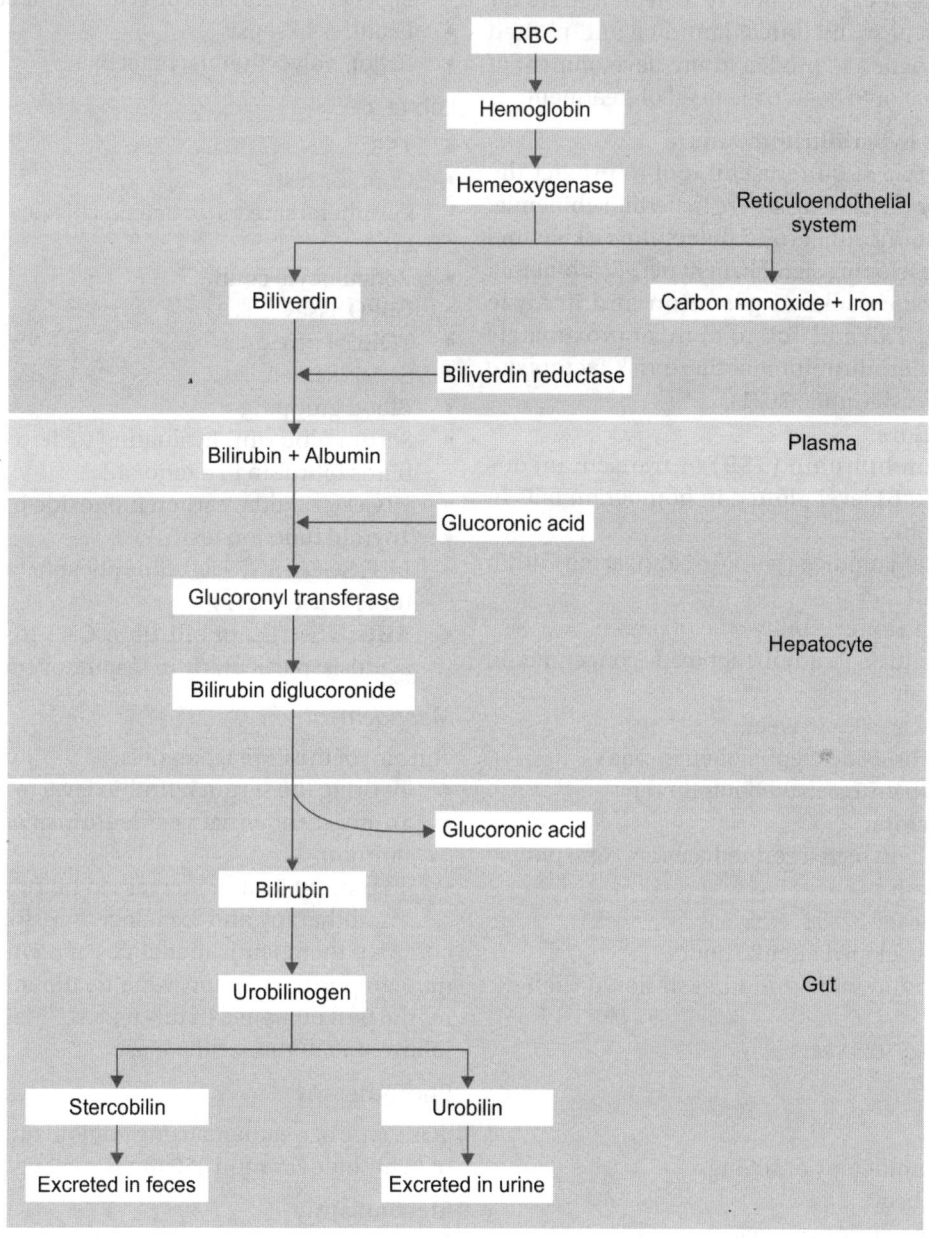

yellowish first and the end based on increased intensity of serum bilirubin. The skins of face and sclera are thin as compare to the palm and sole this might be a possible explanation to the cephalocaudal progression of yellowish discoloration of skin.

**Clinical assessment of neonatal jaundice (Kramer's rule)**
The clinical evaluation of the jaundice should always be done under natural light. The pulp of the finger or thumb is pressed against the baby's skin preferably a bony part till it blanches to detect yellowishness of the skin. The whole body of the baby is divided in to 5 zones which provides rough estimation serum bilirubin level. The five zones body areas and the serum bilirubin levels are as follows:

1. Zone 1 : Face (4–8 mg/dL)
2. Zone 2 : Chest and upper abdomen (5–12 mg/dL)
3. Zone 3 : Lower abdomen, thigh (8–16 mg/dL)
4. Zone 4 : Arms, lower legs (11–18 mg/dL)
5. Zone 5 : Palm and sole (>18 mg/dL)

As per the American Academy of pediatrics, total serum bilirubin should be measured hourly instead of days for the new-born infant with clinical jaundice and plotted on Bhutani's nomogram to predict future development of Hyperbilirubinemia or to decide the need of treatment.

**Predicting severe hyperbilirubinemia**

Although nomogram is quite useful tool to predict the newborn at risk for developing severe hyperbilirubinemia. It is also a paramount concern to detect the risk factors associated with developing significant hyperbilirubinemia among infants <35 weeks of gestation and analyze combiningly with TSB and TcB to more approximately predict severe hyperbilirubinemia these risk factors are categorized as (Piyush Gupta, 2021).

- **Major risk factors:**
  - Total serum bilirubin (TSB) or transcutaneous bilirubin (TcB) level plotted in nomogram falls in high risk zone.
  - Pathological jaundice (jaundice appearing within 24h of birth)
  - ABO or Rh incompatibility
  - Increased end tidal carbon monoxide concentration in exhaled air
  - Gestational age 35–36 weeks
  - Significant bruising (cephalohematoma)
  - If previous baby received phototherapy
- **Minor risk factors:**
  - TSB and TcB in high intermediate risk zone plotted in nomogram
  - Gestational age 37–38
  - Jaundice developed after 24 hours
  - A macrosomia baby due to gestational diabetic mellitus
  - Maternal age ≥25 years
  - Male child.

History taking
- History of phototherapy of sibling
- Onset of jaundice
- Maternal illness during pregnancy
- Type of delivery
- Any injury to the baby during delivery
- Any delay in the passage of urine and meconium
- Delay in cord clamping
- Urine and stool color

Physical examination
- Weight (to detect excessive loss weight)
- Injury to head and other body parts
- Identify prematurity
- Signs of hepatosplenomegaly
- Neurological manifestations
- Signs and symptoms of TORCH infection
- Features of sepsis
- Pallor, polycythemia, petechiae.

Lab test
- TSB
- Coombs test
- Peripheral smears (to detect schistocytes, spherocytosis, etc.)
- Reticulocyte count
- G6PD assay
- TORCH titre
- Sepsis screen
- Blood grouping
- Serum albumin: Evaluating toxicity level as albumin binds bilirubin in a ratio of 1:1
- ETCO (end tidal carbon monoxide in breath)
- Thyroid function test
- **LFT:** SGOT, SGPT, alkaline phosphatase and Y-Glutanyl transferase (GGT)
- **ABG:** The risk of bilirubin CNS toxicity increase in acidosis, particularly in respiratory acidosis.

*Management*

The aim of the management is:
- To bring the serum bilirubin level to the safe range
- To prevent brain damage due to increase in unconjugated bilirubin
- To prevent further increase in bilirubin level

Phototherapy and exchange transfusion are the most common therapeutic modalities of neonatal jaundice. It is quite important to choose the treatment options carefully for the best outcome. In this regard, "Maisels chart" can be followed to minimize the bias.

*Phototherapy*

It is a type of treatment using nonionizing visible spectrum of light (blue) around 450 nm wave length.

**Mechanism**

In 1958 Cremer et al., observed that there is and significant effect of light in reducing serum bilirubin. Since then, different light sources were developed and even now are working effectively.

Phototherapy works by converting water insoluble toxic, unconjugated bilirubin to water soluble isomers which can be excreted through urine and feces without conjugation with glucuronic acid.

Phototherapy causes following three reactions:
1. **Configurational isomerization:** It is a reversible reaction in which the normal bilirubin 4Z,15Z converts

into an isomer 4Z,15E which is water soluble compound therefore can be excreted through bile without hepatic conjugation **(Flowchart 13.2)**.
2. **Structural isomerization:** It is an irreversible reaction. The reaction converts native 4Z, 15Z bilirubin mainly to Z-lumirubin which is excreted through bile and urine **(Flowchart 13.2)**.
3. **Photo-oxidation:** The absorption of the photon from phototherapy light produces unstable, excited bilirubin which then react with oxygen to produce colorless products like biliverdin dipyroles and monopyroles **(Flowchart 13.2)**. These photo-oxidation product are mainly excreted through urine. This is a very slow process as compare to photo-isomerization.

### Devices
- Fluorescent tubes (CFL)
- Light emitting diodes (LED)
- Halogen lamps
- Fibro-optic system

### Types of phototherapy unit
- Single surface
- Double surface
- Triple surface

### Potential side effects
- Dehydration
- Loose stool
- Skin rashes
- Hyperthermia

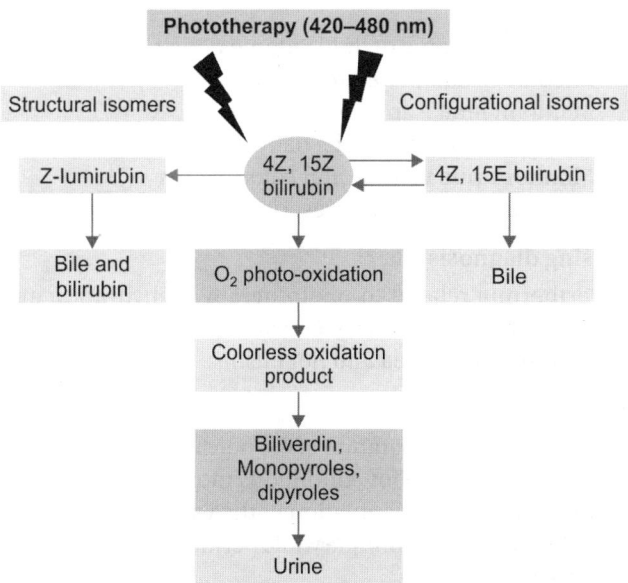

**Flowchart 13.2:** Mechanism of phototherapy.

### Procedure (Piyush Gupta, 2021)
- Wash hands
- Place the baby naked in the phototherapy unit
- Use appropriate eye patches to protect the eye from intense light. Cover the genitalia of the male infants.
- Remove the eye patches every 4–6 hours for eye care.
- Ensure the distance between the baby and light source not more than 30.5 cm when LED light is used. But in case of neo blue light distance can be as close as 15 cm.
- During phototherapy baby's skin should be exposed as much as possible for maximum effectiveness. Therefore, position of the baby should be changed every 2–3 hours.
- As dehydration is a potential complication, daily fluid requirement should be monitored.
- At regular interval (4 hourly/more often as needed) temperature and vital signs should be monitored as baby may develop hypo/hyperthermia.
- Duration and frequency of breastfeeding depends on the severity of the jaundice to reduce the timeout of the phototherapy.

### Role of nurse in phototherapy (Rimpal Sharma, 3rd Edition)
- Explain the parents about the need and action of phototherapy
- Protect the eyes of the infant from intense bright light by placing appropriate eye patches
- Observe any discharge from the eye and give eye care every 4–6 hours
- Monitor the vitals at regular interval
- Monitor total serum bilirubin level every 12–24 hours
- Monitor signs of dehydration
- Maintain input output chart for follow up
- Change the position of the baby every 2–3 hours
- Weight the baby daily to monitor nutritional well-being
- Maintain ambient temperature 25–28°C
- Ensure optimal breastfeeding
- Monitor rebound TSB rise after stopping phototherapy
- Promote family centered care

### Exchange transfusion
Exchange transfusion is quite effective method in reducing serum bilirubin level. In this patients' blood is removed and replaced with the donors bloods or its products.

### Aims
- To decrease TSB
- To prevent kernicterus in case of unconjugated hyperbilirubinemia
- To reduce circulating antibodies
- To minimize hemolysis due to autoimmune disorder

## Indication of exchange transfusion
- Rise in the TSB >1 mg/dL/hour despite of phototherapy
- TSB 20 mg/dL in hemolytic jaundice
- TSB >25–30 mg/dL in nonhemolytic jaundice
- At birth cord blood hemoglobin <11g/dL
- At birth cord blood bilirubin >4.5 mg/dL
- Clinical suspicion of bilirubin encephalopathy

## Types of exchange transfusion

### Single volume exchange transfusion (SVET)
Single volume exchange transfusion (SVET) means removal of the blood equivalent to the circulating blood volume of the patient. The blood volume of the patient therefore is important to calculate before exchange transfusion to decide the amount of blood to be removed during exchange transfusion.

*Calculation*
- In term infants the approximate circulating blood volume = 80 mL/kg
- In preterm infants the approximate circulating blood volume = 100 mL/kg.

*Example*
If a term infant is 3 kh weight then the total circulating blood volume is approximately

$$3 \text{ kg} \times 80 \text{ mL} = 240 \text{ mL}$$

Therefore, in single volume exchange for the above infant 240 mL of blood should be removed and the same amount should be replaced with the donors' blood.

Similarly, if a preterm infant is 2 kg weight then the amount of blood to be removed is approximately = 2 kg × 100 mL = 200 mL

### Double volume exchange transfusion
DVET refers to removal of double amount of the circulating blood volume of the patient.

*Calculation*
In term infant the approximate circulating volume is = 80 mL/kg

So, the double volume = 2 × 80 mL = 160 mL/kg
Similarly for preterm infant the approximate circulating blood volume = 100 mL
So, the double amount = 2 × 100 mL = 200 mL

*Example*
- If a term infant is 3 kg weight then the amount of blood in DVET to be removed = 3 kg × 160 mL = 480 mL
- If a preterm infant is 2 kg weight, then the amount of blood in DVET to be removed = 2 kg × 200 mL = 400 mL

## Nursing management

### Nursing diagnosis - 1
Neonatal hyperbilirubinemia related to underlying cause like (hemolytic, nonhemolytic, decrease bilirubin clearance or genetic causes, delay in meconium passage, inadequate nutrition, traumatic birth injury, etc.) as evidenced by abnormal liver function test results, yellow sclera and mucus membrane.

*Interventions*
- Assess and document the degree of jaundice in skin and sclera
- Promote adequate hydration and nutrition
- Maintain intake and output chart and monitor nutritional status
- Investigate the causes of the hyperbilirubinemia
- Monitor the lab results specifically bilirubin level and liver function tests
- During phototherapy protect the eyes of the infant from intense bright light by placing appropriate eye patches and change the position of the baby every 2–3 hours.
- Perform exchange transfusion and administer IVIg as prescribed
- Encourage breastfeeding unless contraindicated
- Teach the parents regarding phototherapy at home, possible issues and safety

### Nursing diagnosis - 2
Deficient fluid volume related to inadequate breastfeeding, phototherapy or malnutrition as evidenced by dry skin, sunken fontanels, no tears when crying, lack of bowel activity, oliguria.

*Interventions*
- Assess the degree of fluid volume deficit
- Encourage adequate breastfeeding
- Maintain intake and output chart
- Monitor the weight of the baby daily
- Monitor urine volume and color
- Administer IV fluid as prescribed

### Nursing diagnosis - 3
Hyperthermia related to phototherapy, dehydration and infection as evidenced by elevated body temperature, tachycardia, tachypnea and hot flushes.

*Interventions*
- Assess body temperature of the newborn every 4 hourly or use skin probe for continuous monitoring
- Maintain proper ventilation in the ward
- Follow aseptic technique while performing any invasive procedure

- Provide cold compress to the child
- Provide antipyretics and antibiotics as prescribed
- Encourage breastfeeding to increase immunity of the newborn
- Monitor lab results like WBC count, CRP level, ESR, blood and CSF culture, etc.

## Neonatal Seizure

Seizure is defined as paroxysmal involuntary disturbance of brain function that may manifest as an impairment or loss of consciousness, abnormal motor activity, behavioral abnormality, sensory disturbances or autonomic dysfunction. Seizure happens during the course of acute clinical illness is called as provoked seizure. Provoked seizure affects approximately 3–5% of all children. Epilepsy is defined as two or more unprovoked seizures occurring more than 24 hours apart. Febrile seizure is very common affecting 2–4% of all children below 5 years. It refers to occurrence of seizure between the age of 6–60 months associated with fever but without evidence of intracranial infection of defined cause.

## Classification

As per International League Against Epilepsy (ILAE) seizure is classified as generalized, focal, unknown unset and unclassified.

### Generalized Seizure

- **Motor:**
  - Tonic-clonic
  - Clonic
  - Myoclonic
  - Myoclonic-tonic-clonic
  - Myoclonic-atonic
  - Atonic
  - Epileptic spasm
- **Nonmotor:**
  - Typical
  - Atypical
  - Myoclonic
  - Eyelid myoclonia

### Focal Seizure

- **Motor:**
  - Aware
  - Impaired awareness
  - Unknown awareness
  - Automatism
  - Atonic
  - Clonic
  - Epileptic spasm
  - Hyperkinetic
  - Myoclonic
  - Tonic
  - Focal to bilateral tonic-clonic
- **Nonmotor:**
  - Aware
  - Impaired awareness
  - Unknown awareness
  - Autonomic
  - Behavioral arrest
  - Cognitive
  - Emotional
  - Sensory
  - Focal to bilateral tonic-clonic

### Unknown Onset Seizure

- **Motor:**
  - Tonic-clonic
  - Epileptic spasm
- **Nonmotor:** Behavioral arrest

### Unclassified Seizure

### Common etiological factors

- **Neonatal period:**
  - Birth asphyxia
  - Trauma to CNS
  - Hypoglycemia
  - Infections (meningitis, septicemia)
  - Inborn errors of metabolism
  - Maternal withdrawal of medications
- **Beyond neonatal period:**
  - Febrile convulsion
  - Infections (meningitis, encephalitis, etc.)
  - Electrolyte imbalance
  - Neoplasm
  - Brain abscess
  - Trauma
  - Cerebral malformation
  - Toxic/metabolic injury

### Phases of Seizure Activity are Prodromal, Aural, Ictal, and Postictal

- **Prodromal phase:** This phase begins before few hours to days before onset of actual seizure. During this phase, the child may have mood or behavior changes.
- **Aural phase:** This is also known as pre-ictal phase. It lasts from few seconds to an hour. This phase begins just before the ictal with symptoms like visual changes, abnormal sounds, altered taste, involuntary movement, tingling sensation, etc.

- **Ictal stage:** This is the visible phase of seizure. It lasts from few seconds to few minutes. During this phase, the child may experience altered consciousness, involuntary muscle movement, etc.
- **Postictal stage:** This is the period after ictal phase and the duration of this phase is variable from seconds to days. This is the recovery phase where the child may be in conscious or unconscious state.

### Clinical Features

The clinical features of seizure vary depending on the types and underlying causes but the common symptoms are as follows:
- Staring or rapid eye blinking
- Jerking movements of extremities
- Muscle stiffness
- Altered consciousness
- Abnormal breathing or apnea
- Loss of bowel or bladder control
- Falling suddenly
- Not responding to noise or words for brief periods
- Confusion
- Nodding head rhythmically
- Loss of memory
- **Generalized seizure:** This is the type of seizure where the abnormal electrical activity involves both hemisphere of the brain.
- **Tonic seizure:** The term tonic means continuous stiffness of the extremities.
- **Clonic:** It means rhythmic alternative contraction and relaxation of muscles.
- **Tonic-clonic:** It refers to the seizure commence with continuous stiffening of the muscles followed by rhythmic alternative contraction and relaxation of muscles.
- **Myoclonic:** It refers to sudden shock like contraction involving extremities and head.
- **Atonic:** It refers to sudden loss of muscle tone. It is also called as akinetic seizure/drop attack/drop seizure.
- **Absence seizure:** It is characterized by brief and sudden loss of consciousness. It is also called as petit mal seizure.
- **Focal seizure:** This is the type of seizure where the abnormal electrical activity involves only one hemisphere of the brain.

### Investigations

- Electroencephalography
- Neuroimaging (CECT, MRI)
- Blood electrolyte level
- Blood glucose level
- Blood culture
- Lumbar puncture to identify CNS infections

### Management

Firstline antiepileptic drugs:
- Phenobarbitone: 3–5 mg/kg/day
- Phenytoin: 3–8 mg/kg/day
- Carbamazepine: 10–30 mg/kg/day
- Sodium valproate: 10–60 mg/kg/day

The most common antileptics used based on specific types of seizure are mentioned below:
- **Seizure type:** Choice of antiepileptic
- **Generalized tonic clonic:** Phenytoin, sodium valproate
- **Focal seizure:** Carbamazepine
- **Absence seizure:** Sodium valproate, ethosuximide, lamotrigine
- **Myoclonic seizure:** Sodium valproate, benzodiazepine
- **Infantile spasm:** ACTH, sodium valproate, benzodiazepine
- **Mixed:** Sodium valproate.

Child with febrile seizure should be treated similar to any other acute seizure. Child with first febrile seizure should be hospitalized if any of the following features are present:
- Lethargy beyond postictal phase
- Clinically unstable
- Age less than 18 months
- Complex features
- Uncertain home situation
- Unclear follow-up
- Child suspected of meningitis.

Simple febrile seizure last <15 mins and onset is within 24 hours without any focal features. Lumbar puncture is strongly recommended to rule out meningitis. Although antipyretics are not effective should be administered to make the child comfortable. Tepid sponging should be done to reduce body temperature. Benzodiazepines are the drug of choice in this case which can be administered rectally or orally. Diazepam is usually advised at a dose of 0.3–0.5 mg/kg and repeated every 8–12 hours for 3 days if temperature ≥ 38°C. Intermittent clobazam (1 mg/kg/day for 3 days) can be given orally to prevent recurrence of febrile seizure.

### Nursing Management

*Nursing Diagnosis - 1*

Risk for injury related to altered psychomotor performance, sensory integration dysfunction as evidenced by:

Interventions

- Elevate the side rails of the bed if prodromal signs are experienced to prevent fall.

- Place the child on a soft flat surface of the floor if the child is out of the bed.
- Avoid restraining the child which may cause injury.
- Remove the sharp instruments and clear the surroundings.
- Avoid taking temperature orally during seizure episode as this may lead to breakage of the thermometer, if necessary, then tympanic temperature can be taken.
- Administer antiepileptic drugs as prescribed after confirming the dose, frequency, route, etc.
- Monitor the side effects of the medication.
- Review the underlying pathological conditions and lab investigations for future nursing management and need of the specific medication management.

### Nursing Diagnosis - 2

Ineffective airway clearance related to retained secretions as evidenced by altered respiratory rhythm, adventitious breath sounds, cyanosis, hypoxemia, nasal flaring, subcostal retraction, tachypnea, uses accessory muscle to breathe.

### Interventions

- Assess the patency of the air way specially in case of trauma or neurological injury.
- Auscultate for detection of abnormal breath sound and recording of vitals, $SPO_2$ are also important.
- Suctioning should be done as required to clear the airway.
- Place the child in lying position with head slightly turn to one side to prevent aspiration.
- Loose the clothes if any from neck, chest and abdominal area.
- After the seizure activity identify the need of suction, oxygen administration and positive pressure ventilation.

### Nursing Diagnosis - 3

Deficient knowledge related to inadequate access to resources as evidenced by inaccurate follow-through of instruction and inaccurate statements regarding seizure management.

### Interventions

- Assess the current knowledge of the parents.
- Assess the level of understanding.
- Identify the barriers in the learning process.
- Encourage the parents and family members to ask questions.
- Educate the parents and family members regarding the disease, triggering factors, treatment plan, home care and prognosis, etc.
- Encourage the family members to spend time with the child to minimize the stress of the child related to hospitalization.
- Teach the family regarding the diet plan after consulting with dietitian.
- Provide positive reinforcement to adhere to the treatment regimen.
- Educate using multiple media like diagram, animations, posters to facilitate the understanding.
- Focus on single topic at once rather than multiple topics.

## Metabolic Disorders

Metabolism is the aggregate of the chemical reactions that are continuously occurring in the living organisms to keep them alive. The principal function of the metabolism are the production of energy, elimination of the nitrogen wastes, making building blocks for carbohydrate, protein and fat. Numerous chemical reactions are occurring at the subcellular level at the same time that are controlled by specific proteins or enzymes. Any defect in these proteins or enzymes may lead to defect in the metabolic process and in turn leads to the disorders.

The metabolic disorders or the inborn errors of metabolism are the group of rare genetic disorders most of which are autosomal recessive, some are X-linked recessive and few are autosomal dominant. Although these are very rare kind of genetic defects till now more than 500 in born errors of metabolism diseases are identified.

The common groups of in born errors of metabolism with example are listed below:

- **Amino acid metabolism defect**
  - Defective metabolism (phenylketonuria, maple syrup urine disease (MSUD), alkaptonuria, tyrosinemia, albinism)
  - Defective transport (cystinosis, cystinuria, Hartnup disease, lysinuric protein intolerance)
- **Carbohydrate metabolism defect**
  - Galactosemia
  - Glucose 6 phosphate dehydrogenase (G6PD) deficiency
  - Pyruvate dehydrogenase deficiency
  - Carbohydrate intolerance disorders (lactose intolerance, hereditary fructose intolerance)
  - Fructosuria
  - Pentosuria
  - Mucopolysaccharidosis and oligosaccharidosis
  - Glycogen storage disorders.
    - Type I (Von Gierke's disease)
    - Type II (Pompe's disease)
    - Type III (Cori's disease)
    - Type IV (Anderson's disease)
    - Type V (Mc Ardle's disease)
    - Type VI (Her's disease)
    - Type VII (Tauri's disease)

- **Lipid metabolism defect**
  - *Fatty acid oxidation defects:* Zellweger's syndrome, Carnitine deficiency, Refsum's disease
  - *Lipid storage defects:* Tay-Sachs disease, Gaucher's disease, Niemann pick disease, Farber's disease, Fabry's disease, Krabbe's disease
  - *Lipoprotein metabolism defects:* Hyperlipoproteinemias, Hypolipoproteinemias (Tangier's disease, A- beta Lipoproteinemia)
- **Mineral metabolism defect:** Wilson disease, Menkes Kinky hair disease, hemochromatosis
- **Purine and pyrimidine metabolism defect:** Lesch-Nyhan disease.
- **Mitochondrial diseases:** Leigh disease, myoclonic epilepsy ragged red fibers (MERRF), Leber hereditary optic neuropathy.

### Phenylketonuria

It is an autosomal recessive disorder caused by defective metabolism of the amino acid phenylalanine. Normally phenylalanine converts to tyrosine by the enzyme called phenylalanine hydroxylase **(Flowchart 13.3)**. This enzyme is encoded by the gene PAH located in the q arm of chromosome 12 (Chr. 12q23.2). Therefore, mutation in this locus causes the deficiency of the enzyme which leads to failure of conversion and finally there is accumulation of phenylalanine in the blood, CSF and other tissues. The severity of the hyperphenylalaninemia depends on the degree of enzyme deficiency which may differ from very high plasma concentrations >20 mg/dL (Classic PKU) to mild elevation 2–6 mg/dL. The excess amount of phenylalanine is metabolized and converted to phenylketones (phenyl pyruvate and phenyl acetate) that are excreted through urine thus justifies the name phenylketonuria (Nelson Textbook of Pediatric, 21st Edition).

### Types of PKU

Based on the defect of the enzymes PKU can be classified as follows:
- **Type I (classical):** Complete deficiency of the enzyme phenylalanine hydroxylase (PAH)

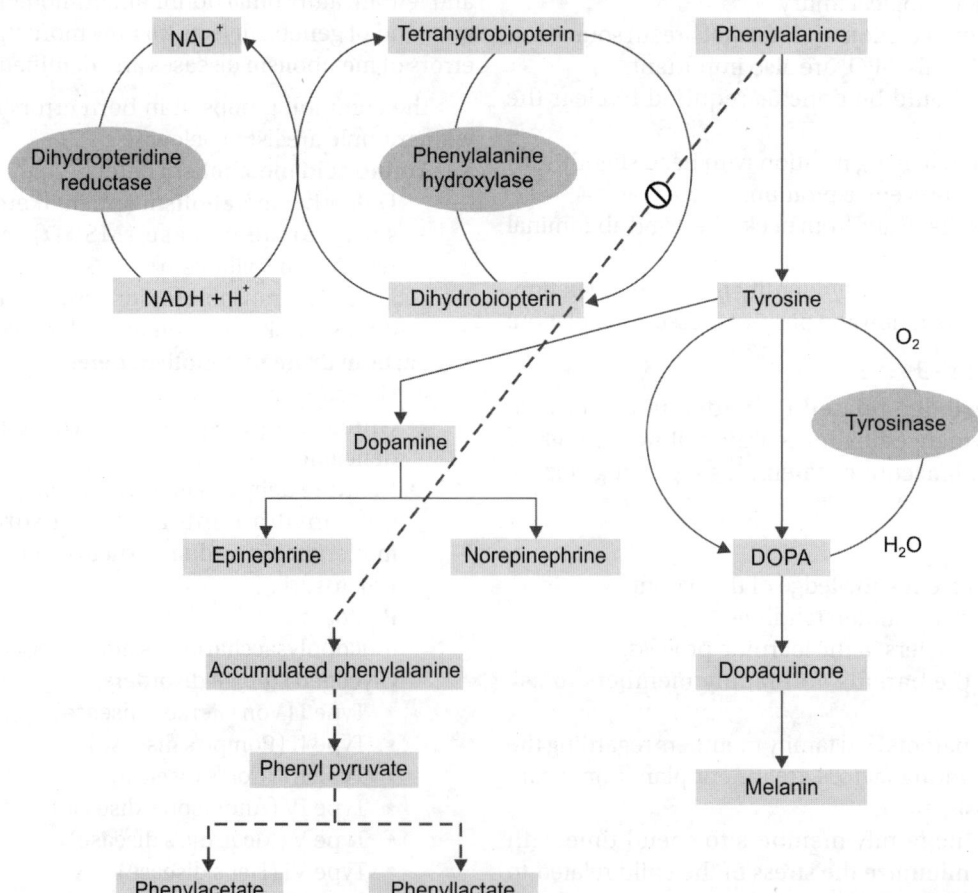

**Flowchart 13.3:** Phenylalanine metabolism pathway.

- **Type II (variant):** Partial deficiency of enzyme PAH
- **Type III (transient):** Delayed maturation of PAH
- **Type IV:** Deficiency of dihydrobiopterin reductase
- **Type V:** Deficiency of dihydrobiopterin synthetase lead to defective biosynthesis of dihydrobiopterin.

*Etiology*

Approximately 97% of the cases are affected with the phenylalanine hydroxylase deficient PKU in which the enzyme PAH is partially or completely deficient and, in few cases, there is immature phenylalanine hydroxylase which has altered function. The deficiency of PAH is due to the mutation in the gene PAH which provides instructions to make the enzyme phenylalanine hydroxylase. PAH gene is located in the q arm of the chromosome 12 at the locus 12q23.2 between 102,836,889bp-102,958,410 bp. There are more than 500 mutations identified till now in the PAH gene which leads to PKU. Most of the mutations are the point mutation which replaces single codon on the DNA sequence thereby change the corresponding amino acid. The most common point mutation is the replacement of the amino acid arginine with tryptophan at the position 408 (written as Arg408Trp or R408W). (Nelson Textbook of Pediatric, 21st Edition).

*Classic phenylketonuria*

When severe hyperphenylalaninemia (>20 mg/dL in plasma) remain untreated it shows sign symptoms of classic PKU except rare cases.

**Clinical features:**

The infants affected with classic PKU do not show sign symptoms at birth but gradually begin to develop neurological manifestations due to accumulation of excess phenylalanine in the brain which causes destruction of myelin sheath. The neurological features can be intellectual disability, seizure, behavioral problems, delayed development, etc. Excess phenylalanine also interferes with the neurotransmitters like dopamine and serotonin causing depression. Deficiency of PAH also impedes the melanin production **(Flowchart 13.3)** that leads to light color of the eye, skin and hair. Excretion of the phenylacetic acid (phenyl ketone) in urine and sweat causes musty or mousy odor of the body (Nelson Textbook of Pediatric, 21st Edition).

*Mild hyperphenylalaninemia*

When the plasma concentration of phenylalanine is between 2–20 mg/dL is called mild hyperphenylalaninemia or non-PKU hyperphenylalaninemia. The infants suffering from mild hyperphenylalaninemia have partial deficiency of the phenylalanine hydroxylase enzyme or tetrahydrobiopterin (BH4).

**Clinical features**

Clinically these infants don't reveal any sign symptoms but progressive brain damage may occur with age.

**Diagnosis**

Physical examination for classical PKU: the affected infants have lighter eye, skin and hair color as compare to the normal infants. They may have Musty or mousy body odor. Microcephaly, growth retardation, wide gap between the teeth also can be seen.

*Lab Investigations*

According to the recommendation of American academy of pediatric PKU screening should be repeated by two weeks of age if it is performed before the newborn was 24 hours of age. However, a second test is not required if the initial PKU test is done with:

Blood test

**Plasma phenylalanine level**

Nelson Textbook of Pediatric, 21st Edition.

The normal level in plasma is 0.5–1 mg/dL but when cut off value is 2 mg/dL most of the infants remain unidentified. Plasma level between 2–20 mg/dL is called mild form of hyperphenylalaninemia and more than 20 mg/dL is diagnosed as classic PKU.

Once the diagnosis of hyperphenylalaninemia is established deficiency of the Tetrahydrobiopterin (BH4) should be excluded.

*PKU screening*

As there is gradual development of the sign symptoms in the affected infant early diagnosis can only be done through mass screening. PKU screening can be performed by the following methods:
- Guthrie bacterial inhibition assay
- McCamon Robins flurometric test
- Tandem mass spectrometry

PKU screening test is accurate when performed between 24 hours to 7 days of age of the infant. If the screening test is performed within 24 hours then repeat test by two weeks is required for diagnosis.

**$BH_4$ loading test**

This test is done to identify the tetrahydrobiopterin ($BH_4$) deficiency. To carry out the test sapropterin dihydrochloride (tetrahydrobiopterin) is administration orally at a dose of 20 mg/kg to the affected infant with elevated phenylalanine level. If the hyper phenylalanine level in the blood comes to the normal range within 4–8 hours of administration then the result is called positive. If the infant is under diet therapy then it should be discontinued at least before 2 days or phenylalanine should be administered at a dose of

100 mg/kg 3 hours prior to the test to elevate level before administration of $BH_4$ (Nelson Textbook of Pediatric, 21st Edition).

**Urine test**
- **Ferric chloride test:** The test is performed by taking 5 mL of urine in the test tube and then 3–4 drops of ferric chloride is added to it. If phenylketones will be in the urine then addition of ferric chloride react with them and change the urine color from yellow to green/blue giving a positive result otherwise the test is called negative.
- **Dinitrophenylhydrazine (DNPH) test:** For this test 2 mL of urine sample is taken in the test tube and equal amount of DNPH reagent is mixed with it. If there will be phenylketones in the urine then DNPH reagent reacts with them and makes yellow precipitation indicating positive result (Nelson Textbook of Pediatric, 21st Edition).

**DNA analysis**
It is useful to detect specific mutation in the affected gene for which following methods are used:
- Sanger sequencing
- Next generation sequencing (NGS)
- Multiplex ligation dependent probe amplification (MLPA)
- Whole exome sequencing
- PCR based technique

Imaging study
In research studies cranial CT scan on patients with 6-pyruvoyl tetrahydropterin synthase (PTPS) deficiency revealed calcification in the lentiform nuclei and in patients with dihydropteridine reductase (DHPR) deficiency there was severe cortical and subcortical atrophy.

MRI studies on patients with $BH_4$ deficiency showed white matter changes and on patients with PTPS deficiency showed delayed myelination and abnormal high intensity signals in cerebral white matter. So imaging study can be used to understand and monitor the neurophysiological changes of the affected patients but this may not be appropriate for a newborn.

Treatment
Diet therapy
The aim of the treatment is to lower and maintain the plasma phenylalanine level between 2–6 mg/dL at least till 12 years of age. The infant with persistent plasma phenylalanine level >6 mg/dL are treated with phenylalanine restricted diet. But infant having plasma phenylalanine level between 2–6 mg/dL are not required any diet restriction. The treatment of PKU mostly based on the diet therapy where diet containing phenylalanine are restricted and tyrosine containing diets are provided as supplement. The foods that contains high amount of phenylalanine are fish, meat, eggs, nuts, legumes, wheat, milk, beans, etc., therefore should be avoided. As the body do not produce phenylalanine the infant should not be over treated when the infant is under diet restriction otherwise it may leads to phenylalanine deficiency. There is a controversy regarding the duration of the diet restriction as discontinuation of the therapy leads to IQ deterioration and cognitive impairment. Current recommendation says diet restriction should be continued lifelong. (Nelson Textbook of Pediatric, 21st Edition) and (Piyush Gupta, Textbook of Pediatrics, 5th Ed. 2021).

Pharmacological therapy
In case of mild form of hyperphenylalanine oral administration of **sapropterin dihydrochloride** (tetrahydrobiopterin) is effective in reducing plasma phenylalanine level. It is also effective in case of $BH_4$ deficient PKU (Piyush Gupta, Textbook of Pediatrics, 5th Ed. 2021).

**Phenylalanine ammonia lyase** (PAL) is currently under clinical trial which is used as an alternative to the PAH enzyme therefore can be used in case of classic form of phenylketonuria.

### Maple Syrup Urine Disease (MSUD)

It is an autosomal recessive aminoacidopathy occurs due to deficiency of the enzymes required to metabolize branched chain amino acids valine, leucine, and isoleucine. The enzyme needed for catalyses of these three amino acids is called BCKD ((branched chain ketoacid dehydrogenase) complex. This complex is composed of 4 subunits E1 alpha, E1 Beta, E2 and E3 which work together for the catalyses **(Table 13.3)**. This complex is regulated by the regulators like BCKDK and PPM1K (protein phosphatase 1K mitochondrial). The complex also need following coenzymes for its optimal functioning [Maple Syrup Urine Disease—NORD (National Organization for Rare Disorders)]:
- CoA (Coenzyme A)
- Alpha lipoic acid also called lipoic acid/thioctic acid/lipoate
- Cocarboxylase also called thiamine pyrophosphate (TPP)
- Flavin adenine dinucleotide (FAD)
- Nicotinamide adenine dinucleotide (NAD).

Pathophysiology
BCKD complex along with the regulators and cofactors are responsible for the catalyses of the valine, leucine, and

**Table 13.3:** BCKD complex.

| Sub unit | Name | Gene | Locus |
|---|---|---|---|
| $E_{1\alpha}$ | Branched chain ketoacid dehydrogenase E1 subunit alpha | BCKDHA | Ch19q13.2 |
| $E_{1\beta}$ | Branched chain ketoacid dehydrogenase E1 subunit beta | BCKDHB | Ch6q14.1 |
| $E_2$ | Dihydrolipoyl transacetylase | DBT | Ch1p21.2 |
| $E_3$ | Dihydrolipoamide dehydrogenase | DLD | Ch7q31.1 |

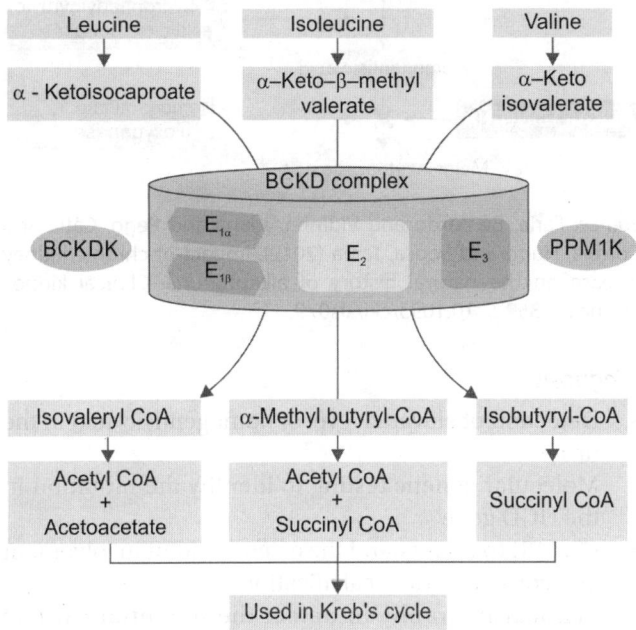

**Flowchart 13.4:** Biochemical pathway of MSUD.

*Source*: Blackburn PR, Gass JM, Vairo FPE, Farnham KM, Atwal HK, Macklin S, et al. Maple syrup urine disease: mechanisms and management. Appl Clin Genet. 2017;10:57–66.

isoleucine. This complex composed of four subunits which are encoded by the gene BCKDHA, BCKDHB, DBT and DLD. Any mutation in these genes lead to deficiency of the BCKD complex as a result metabolism of the branched chain amino acids is stopped and there is accumulation of the leucine, isoleucine and valine in the body **(Flowchart 13.4)**. When excreted specially in urine, the odor is quite similar to maple syrup therefore the name 'maple syrup urine disease' [Maple Syrup Urine Disease - NORD (National Organization for Rare Disorders)]

### Types of MSUD

MSUD is classified in five types based on the clinical presentation and response to thiamine treatment. They are as follows [Maple Syrup Urine Disease—NORD (National Organization for Rare Disorders)]:

### Classic MSUD

This is the most severe form of the MSUD where BCKD complex activity <2% of normal is present. The affected infant in this type shows symptoms within 7 days of age. As there is excess amount of branched chain amino acids aggregated in the brain the child initially present the neurological signs like seizure, dystonia, hypo/hypertonia, etc. The infant may have feeding intolerance, hypoglycemia, lethargy and coma.

### Intermittent MSUD

In this type of MSUD, the residual enzymatic activity of BCKD complex may vary between 5–20% of the normal. The affected infant usually remain asymptomatic unless exposed to stress or any catabolic activity like surgery, fasting or infection, etc. The infant may show the symptoms like lethargy, poor feeding, vomiting, maple syrup odor (ear wax, urine and sweat) ataxia and coma.

### Intermediate (Mild) MSUD

This is a milder type of MSUD where the BCKD activity is higher than the classic and intermittent form. The dehydrogenase activity may range between 3–30% of the normal. The clinical features usually insidious and confined to the CNS like mental retardation with or without seizure. The affected infants have odor of maple syrup.

### Thiamine Responsive MSUD

The residual dehydrogenase activity in this form of MSUD is between 2–40% of the normal. These infant respond to the thiamine treatment and show clinical improvement therefore the name thiamine responsive MSUD. It is found that some infants respond to thiamine at 10 mg/24 hour where as others may need as much as 200 mg/24 hour.

### $E_3$ Subunit Deficient MSUD

This is a rare form of MSUD due to deficiency of the $E_3$ subunit (dihydrolipoamide dehydrogenase) of BCKD complex. In addition to the sign symptoms of the intermediate form of MSUD these infants develop lactic acidosis.

### Diagnosis

- The infant may be suspected of MSUD if there is typical maple syrup odor of the sweat, urine and the ear wax.

- **Amino acid analysis:** There is elevation in the levels of amino acids (leucine, isoleucine, and valine) in urine and plasma.
- Detection of BCKD enzyme activity in the lymphocytes and fibroblasts.
- Molecular testing for detection of mutation in the genes BCKDHA, BCKDHB, DBT and DLD.
- Prenatal diagnosis by detecting BCKD activity in amniocytes and chorionic villus cells.

*Management*
- **Dietary restriction:** As there is no specific treatment available dietary restriction of branched chain amino acid is the main stay of management. These infants remains under dietary restriction throughout their life.
- **Dialysis:** The goal of the hemodialysis or peritoneal dialysis is to remove the excess amount of branched chain amino acids from the body as renal clearance of these compounds are very poor.
- **Hydration:** Fluid management is also important which reduces the plasma concentration of the leucine, isoleucine and valine but this alone is not effective.
- **Thiamine therapy:** Some children respond to thiamine therapy and show improvement in their clinical status. The dose of thiamine therapy may vary between 2 mg/24 hours to 200 mg/24 hours.
- Treatment of cerebral edema can be done with hypertonic saline or diuretics like Mannitol and Lasix.

### Alkaptonuria (Black Urine Disease)

It is an autosomal recessive genetic disorder characterized by accumulation of homogentisic acid due to deficiency of the enzyme homogentisic acid 1, 2 dioxygenases. This enzyme is encoded by the gene called HGD which is located at chr3q13.33. Therefore, mutation of this gene leads to deficiency of the enzyme homogentisic acid 1, 2 dioxygenases. The accumulated homogentisic acid is rapidly excreted through urine and when comes in contact with the air during micturition it is oxidized and turns the urine into black color hence the name black urine disease. The biochemical pathway of phenylalanine and Alkaptonuria is described in the **Flowchart 13.5** [Alkaptonuria—NORD (National Organization for Rare Disorders)].

*Clinical Features*
Early in the infancy the child may be suspected if there will be black color staining of the diaper. There may be blue, black or gray color of the sclera, ear cartilages due to widespread accumulation of the homogentisic acid in the cartilages. Later in the life there may be joint involvement showing features similar to osteoarthritis (Piyush Gupta, Textbook of Pediatrics, 5th Ed., 2021).

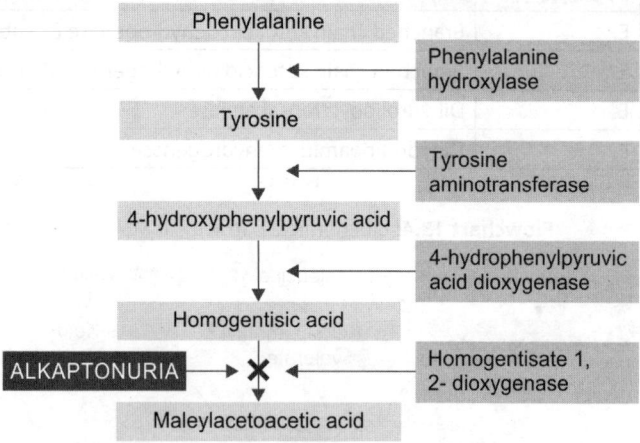

**Flowchart 13.5:** Biochemical pathway of phenylalanine in alkaptonuria.

*Source*: Faria, Bernardo and Vidinha, Joana and Pêgo, Cátia and Correia, Hugo and Sousa, Tânia (2012). Impact of chronic kidney disease on the natural history of alkaptonuria. Clinical kidney journal. 5. 352-5. 10.1093/ckj/sfs079.

*Diagnosis*
- Detection of elevated level of homogentisic acid in the urine
- Molecular genetic testing to identify the mutation in the HGD gene
- CT, MRI to understand the extend of joint involvement and coronary artery calcification
- Echocardiography to detect the potential cardiac complications.

*Management*
- NSAID to reduce pain and inflammation
- Narcotics are administered in worst case scenario
- Dietary restriction (protein) may not help in reducing plasma homogentisic acid level
- High dose of vitamin C is effective in reducing the level of homogentisic acid
- A drug called 'Nitisinone' is under clinical trial but some studies proved that it is significantly effective in lowering the plasma homogentisic acid level (Piyush Gupta, Textbook of Pediatrics, 5th Ed., 2021).

### Galactosemia

Galactosemia is an autosomal recessive metabolic disorder characterized by accumulation of Galactose in the blood due to inadequate metabolism. The mutation in the genes leads to deficiency of three different enzymes essential for conversion of Galactose to glucose in a pathway called Leloir pathway **(Flowchart 13.6)**.

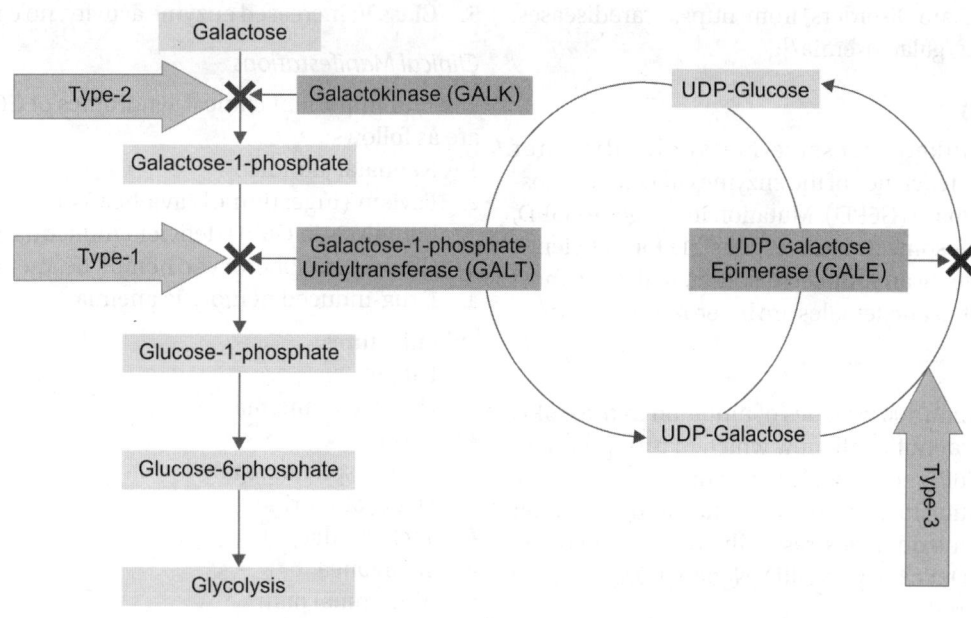

**Flowchart 13.6:** Biochemical pathway of galactosemia.

*Source*: UKEssays. Galactosemia Disorder: Causes, Forms and Treatments November 2018.

## Types

The principal types of galactosemia are as follows:
- **Type 1: Classic galactosemia:** This is the most common form of galactosemia occurs due to deficiency of the enzyme Galactose-1-phosphate uridyltransferase (GALT) which is required to convert the Galactose-1- phosphate to glucose-1-phosphate. The gene which codes for this enzyme is located in the chromosome 9, therefore mutation in the locus 9p13 leads to deficiency of GALT enzyme. Primary clinical features of galactosemia include hepatic failure, cataract, failure to thrive, etc.
- **Type 2: Galactokinase deficiency:** In this type, there is a mutation in the GALK1 gene located at ch17q24 resulting deficiency of the enzyme Galactokinase essential for conversion of galactose to galactose-1-phosphate. Cataract is the exclusive clinical feature which is treatable or preventable.
- **Type 3: Galactose epimerase deficiency:** It is caused by mutation in the GALE gene present at ch1p36 which leads to deficiency of the enzyme called UDP galactose epimerase. This enzyme is important to convert UDP Galactose to UDP glucose which is an important step if galactose metabolism.

## Clinical Manifestations

Galactosemia—NORD (National Organization for Rare Disorders) from: https://rarediseases.org/rare-diseases/galactosemia/

- Feeding intolerance
- Vomiting
- Jaundice
- Irritability
- Lethargy
- Poor growth
- Hepatomegaly and liver dysfunction
- Sometime cataract may appear as early as few days of life
- Sepsis due to *E. coli*
- Seizure
- Brain edema
- Ascites in some cases
- Hemorrhage due to coagulopathy
- Learning disability and neurological manifestations later in the life
- Premature ovarian insufficiency (POI) in most of the females with classic or severe form of galactosemia.

## Management

The affected infant primarily under goes dietary restriction, basically the dairy products and other foods having high lactose content. Some of the children also have speech problem therefore long-term speech therapy is advised for them. Antibiotics may be administered to control the infection. Genetic counseling to the family members also to be done to assess and predict the nature of the disease transmission along generations, to calculate the risk for future generation, etc. [Galactosemia - NORD (National Organization for Rare Disorders) from: https://rarediseases.org/rare-diseases/galactosemia/].

### G6PD Deficiency

This is an X-linked recessive metabolic disorder characterized by deficiency of the enzyme Glucose-6-phosphate dehydrogenase (G6PD). Mutation in the gene G6PD, located in chromosome Xq28 is responsible for deficiency of the enzyme. Being an X-linked disorder, males are most commonly affected and females are heterozygous carriers.

*Cause*

There are more than 400 varieties of mutation in the G6PD gene have been identified till now which in turn produces less functional G6PD enzymes. Hence mutation in the gene leads to interruption in the chain of reaction and RBC suffer destruction from oxidative stress [Glucose-6-Phosphate Dehydrogenase Deficiency - NORD (National Organization for Rare Disorders)].

*Pathophysiology*

Free radicals and reactive oxygen species (ROS) are the by-product of normal metabolic process of human cells including RBC. They are highly unstable and reactive. Hence should be neutralized to prevent damage of the cells. But there are certain factors like infections, drugs, etc., can accelerate the production of free radicals and ROS with significant damage of RBC called oxidative stress. Fortunately, RBC has 2GSH (reduced glutathione) which is capable of neutralizing free radicals and ROS. The production of reduced glutathione from oxidized glutathione (GSSG) require NADPH and conversion of NADPH from $NADP^+$ depends on G6PD enzyme **(Flowchart 13.7)**. Hence in case of G6PD enzyme deficiency whole biochemical process is disrupted and accumulation of free radicals and ROS increases oxidative stress and hemolysis of RBC.

*Classification*

The World Health Organization classifies G6PD genetic variants into five classes, as follows (Glucose-6-phosphate dehydrogenase deficiency. WHO Working Group. Bull World Health Organ. 1989).

1. **Class I:** Severe deficiency (<10% activity) with chronic (nonspherocytic) hemolytic anemia
2. **Class II:** Severe deficiency (<10% activity), with intermittent hemolysis
3. **Class III:** Moderate deficiency (10–60% activity), hemolysis with stressors only
4. **Class IV:** Nondeficient variant, no clinical sequelae
5. **Class V:** Increased enzyme activity, no clinical sequelae

*Clinical Manifestations*

The four important clinical syndromes of G6PD deficiency are as follows:
1. Neonatal jaundice
2. Favism (ingestion of fava beans cause intravascular hemolysis in G6PD deficient individual)
3. Chronic no spherocytic hemolytic anemia
4. Drug-induced hemolytic anemia

Other features:
- Fatigue
- Hemolytic anemia
- Fever
- Hepatosplenomegaly
- Dark color urine
- Tachycardia
- Tachypnea
- Abdominal pain

*Diagnosis*

- **Screening/qualitative tests:** In qualitative tests, a predetermined threshold is estimated for specific diagnostic tests (30–40% of normal activity) then patients' sample is tested for the G6PD level. Hence positive result indicates there is deficiency of the G6PD and the level is below the threshold. Similarly, negative result indicates there is no deficiency and the enzyme activity is above the threshold. Following are the example of qualitative test:
  - Ultraviolet spot test
  - Methemoglobin reduction test
  - Brilliant cresyl blue decolorization test
- **Definitive/quantitative test:** Quantitative tests help to quantify the activity of the G6PD in the blood. For example, if the test result shows <10% of normal activity of G6PD then it indicates severe deficiency and >100% of normal represents high activity. For instance, spectrophotometric analysis.
- **Molecular diagnostic testing and DNA analysis**

*Management*

The aim of the management is to:
- Prevent the development of hemolysis
- Treatment of anemia
- Management of neonatal jaundice

As a preventive strategy, avoiding factors that might lead to oxidative stress like drugs, fava beans, infections, etc., is crucial. Blood transfusion during hemolysis can correct the anemia along with fluid therapy to prevent kidney

**Flowchart 13.7:** Pentose phosphate pathway in RBC.

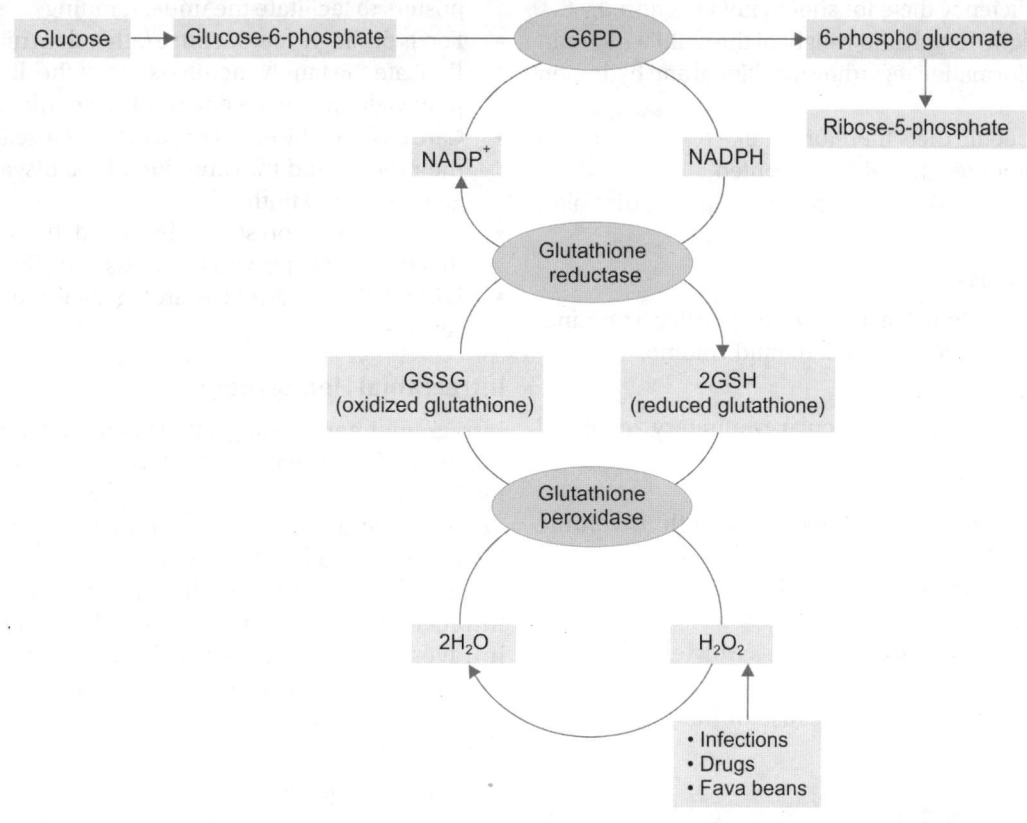

*Source*: Tiwari M. Glucose-6-phosphatase dehydrogenase (G6PD) and neurodegenerative disorders: Mapping diagnostic and therapeutic opportunities. Genes Dls. 2017 Dec 1;4(4):196–203.

failure. Splenectomy may be required for the children with splenomegaly or to reduce the need of transfusion. For the management of neonatal jaundice phototherapy and exchange transfusion are recommended.

Nursing management of metabolic disorders

Nancy T Hat field, Broadribb's Introductory Pediatric Nursing.

**Urine analysis:** Monitoring and interpreting the urine analysis for PH, specific gravity, ketones, glucose, etc., are important to identify metabolic acidosis/alkalosis and kidney function.

- **Color:** The color of the urine also provides clues of many metabolic disorders as follows:

| Urine color | Disorder |
| --- | --- |
| Dark brown/black | Alkaptonuria/hemoglobinuria/myoglobinuria |
| Blue | Hartnup disease |
| Blue/brown | Alkaptonuria |

- **Odor:** Odor of the urine also should be considered as is associated with several metabolic diseases.

| Urine odor | Disorders |
| --- | --- |
| Maple syrup/burnt sugar | MSUD |
| Sulfur | Cystinuria |
| Boiled cabbage | Tyrosinemia type I |
| Cat's urine | Multiple carboxylase deficiency |
| Mousy | PKU |

Nursing diagnosis - 1

Imbalanced nutrition less than body requirements related to abnormal metabolism as evidenced by lethargy, altered urine color and odor, hypoglycemia, muscle hypotonia, etc.

**Interventions**
- Monitor vital signs upon admission to the hospital for baseline information for future diagnosis and treatment.
- Assess skin color, texture, intactness, condition and peripheral perfusion may provide crucial signs of shock or protein deficiency related to metabolic disorders.

- Assess for dry and brittle hair which may indicate protein or zinc deficiency there for should not be ignored.
- Assess height/length and weight of the child which can provide information regarding nutritional and hydration status.
- Restrict specific diets therefore intake of precursors to toxic metabolites should be prevented.
- Consult with dietitian for preparing special diet plan for the child.

Nursing diagnosis - 2

Risk for electrolyte imbalance related to diarrhea, vomiting, excessive fluid volume, insufficient fluid volume.

**Interventions**
- Assess vital signs, cardiovascular, respiratory, renal and mental status routinely
- Monitor and record intake and output
- Measure child's weight daily to detect fluid volume excess at early stage
- If the child is dehydrated provide ORS or IV fluid as prescribed
- Monitor lab reports like serum electrolyte, ABG, urine analysis, etc.
- Investigate to find out the cause of fluid electrolyte imbalance
- Monitor the signs of shock
- Administer blood products to correct fluid loss as prescribed
- Encourage to drink plenty of fluid if dehydrated
- Educate the child and family members regarding preventive measures of fluid electrolyte imbalance
- Demonstrate methods of input and output measurement and instruct to monitor at home
- Provide antidotes or electrolyte supplements based on prescription

Nursing diagnosis - 3

Deficient knowledge related to inadequate access to resources as evidenced by inaccurate follow-through of instruction and inaccurate statements about metabolic disorders.

**Interventions**
- Assess the current knowledge of the parents
- Assess the level of understanding
- Identify the barriers in the learning process
- Encourage the parents and family members to ask questions
- Provide positive reinforcement to adhere to the treatment regimen
- Demonstrate the skills in the management of foreign body aspiration
- Educate using multiple media like diagram, animations, posters to facilitate the understanding
- Focus on single topic at once rather than multiple topics
- Educate the family members about the diet containing phenylalanine, need and duration of the restriction
- Care givers of the infant need to be counselled regarding the process and transmission of the disease from one generation to another
- Emotional support should be provided to the parents so that they can cope with the stress and adverse situation
- Educate the caregivers regarding safety measures during seizure

## Intracranial Hemorrhage

Intracranial hemorrhage (ICH) can be defined as accumulation of blood within the brain tissue or the surrounding meningeal spaces. Hemorrhage within meninges can be classified as extradural hemorrhage, subarachnoid hemorrhage and subdural hemorrhage whereas hemorrhage within brain parenchyma can be categorized as intracerebral hemorrhage, cerebellar hemorrhage and intraventricular hemorrhage **(Fig. 13.2)** (Intracranial Hemorrhage - Stat Pearls - NCBI Bookshelf).

### Classification

*Extradural Hemorrhage*

Extradural hemorrhage is the accumulation of blood between the inner layer of the skull bone and the dura matter. In majority of the cases hemorrhage occurs due to rupture of the meningeal artery as compare to the veins. The primary cause of extradural hemorrhage is the skull injury but there are rare cases when spontaneous hemorrhage occurs among pediatric population. Although adults are the

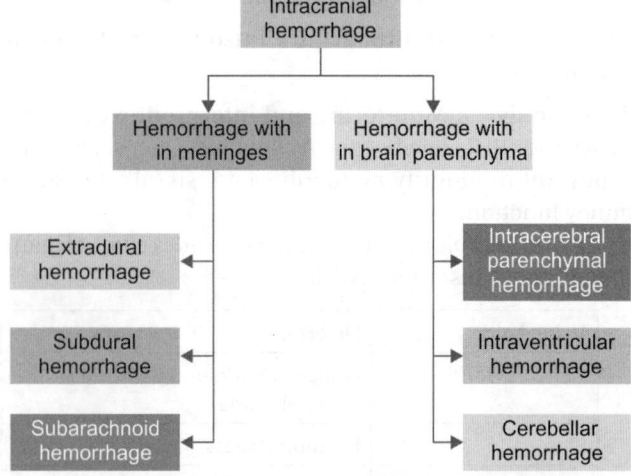

**Fig.13.2:** Classification of intracranial hemorrhage.

major victims of stroke, infants can suffer as well. There are certain cases reported in scientific papers that stroke during perinatal period may also cause epidural hemorrhage. The young children suffering from epidural hemorrhage may have altered consciousness, emesis, dilated pupils, excessive drooling and seizure (Intracranial Hemorrhage - Stat Pearls - NCBI Bookshelf).

## Subdural Hemorrhage

Bleeding into the space between dura and arachnoid matter is called as subdural hemorrhage. The incidence of subdural hemorrhage is between 5–10% as compare to the ICH as a whole. Rupture of the veins, sinus, tentorium cerebri and falx cerebri are primarily associated with the subdural hemorrhage. Child with subdural hemorrhage may exhibit seizure, altered consciousness, abnormal motor activity, macrencephaly, frontal bossing, protruding fontanelle. Diagnosis can be made using cranial USG, CT or MRI but lumbar puncture is usually avoided to prevent the risk of herniation of brain tissue. Although USG is radiation free, can be performed at the bedside to detect the subdural hemorrhage, but not always reliable. Further evaluation by CT and MRI therefore required to confirm the diagnosis. MRI is always preferred over CT as radiation is not required for evaluation depending upon feasibility. But it is tough to distinguish between subdural and intracerebellar hemorrhage from CT and MRI when bleeding is in the posterior cranial fossa. Where subdural hemorrhage in posterior fossa is frequently found in term babies, Intracerebellar hemorrhage is more prevalent among preterm infants. Surgical intervention like craniotomy or subdural tap (by inserting a needle through lateral margin of anterior fontanelle) indicated in this case to drain the accumulated blood to improve the clinical status. (Intracranial Hemorrhage - Stat Pearls - NCBI Bookshelf)

## Subarachnoid Hemorrhage

Bleeding into the subarachnoid space is rare and initially don't reveal any sign symptoms. As the hemorrhage increases the infant develop seizure and then neurological deterioration. In this case, lumbar puncture is significantly important to identify the increasing number of red blood cells in CSF. Accumulation of blood in sulci and longitudinal fissure can easily be identified through CT and MRI. Usually, ultrasonography is not advised for diagnosis (Intracranial Hemorrhage - Stat Pearls - NCBI Bookshelf).

## Intracerebral Parenchymal Hemorrhage

Intracerebral parenchymal hemorrhage is the bleeding into the brain substance commonly among the preterm infants. Germinal matrix hemorrhage and periventricular hemorrhagic infarction are the primary causes of the parenchymal hemorrhage. Sporadic parenchymal hemorrhage is rarely found as most of the parenchymal hemorrhage are associated with germinal matrix hemorrhage and intraventricular hemorrhage. The infants with a history of parenchymal hemorrhage show developmental delay, altered motor activity, cognitive and behavioral problem in later life. Cranial imaging using ultrasonography or CT are useful in detecting and grading the hemorrhage. As definitive treatment is not available supportive care is the main stay of management. Immediate surgical intervention is required in case of midline shift of the brain beyond 5 mm.

## Intraventricular Hemorrhage (IVH)

Hemorrhage into the brain ventricular system is more common among preterm than term infants. According to Sanders, "bleeding in the ventricular system without discernible parenchymal component or arising within 15 mm from the ventricular wall is called intraventricular hemorrhage". During prenatal period the mitotic activity of glial cells and neural cells take place in the germinal matrix before migrating to different parts of the brain. Germinal matrix is enriched with a network of premature microvasculature which are very delicate and fragile hence slight increase in pressure may cause rupture and hemorrhage. Towards the term when the cell proliferation completes the germinal matrix progressively regress. In case of preterm infants, the regression of germinal matrix is not completed and become the primary source of hemorrhage due to rupture of premature blood vessels. Therefore, the primary source of hemorrhage is the germinal matrix in the preterm babies whereas in case of term infants the source of hemorrhage is inconsistent. In term infants the root of hemorrhage may be the remnant non-regressed germinal matrix, choroid plexus, periventricular venous infarcts, tumor and arteriovenous malformation, etc.

### Cause

Although the cause of IVH is still illusive it is believed that disruption in the cerebral autoregulation, abnormal blood flow or pressure of the cerebral blood vessels are the factors leading to hemorrhage. Cerebral autoregulation ability is more among term infants as compare to the preterm because of the structural and functional maturity of the regulatory system. In case of impaired autoregulation brain cannot control the pressure and flow of the blood through the blood vessels. So, abrupt increase or decrease in blood flow or pressure can easily rupture the immature micro blood vessels of the germinal matrix. Following are some factors associated with IVH:

- Rapid fluid administration
- Increased blood volume and pressure
- Seizure
- Respiratory distress syndrome
- Pneumothorax
- Alteration in blood PH, $PaCO_2$ or $PaO_2$
- Vascular malformation
- Thrombocytopenia
- Instrumental delivery
- Chorioamnionitis

### Classification of IVH

Based on the physical extent of hemorrhage and ventriculomegaly in cranial imaging IVH is classified into four grades. Dilation of the ventricle is called ventriculomegaly which can range from mild to severe. (mild: 0.5–1 cm dilation, moderate: 1.0–1.5 cm dilation, or severe: >1.5 cm dilation).
- **Grade I:** Germinal matrix hemorrhage
- **Grade II:** Hemorrhage fills less than 50% of the lateral ventricle
- **Grade III:** Hemorrhage fills and enlarges the lateral ventricle
- **Grade IV:** Intraparenchymal hemorrhage.

*Source*: Akman İ, Galip N. Pretermde Germinal Matriks İntraventriküler Kanama. J Istanbul Fac Med 2011 Nov 10.

### Clinical Manifestation

The infant with Grade-I or Grade-II intraventricular hemorrhage do not present any clinical feature. But the infant having Grade-III or Grade-IV intraventricular hemorrhage start to exhibit symptoms like cyanosis, pallor, poor feeding, anemia, abnormal neuromotor response, convulsion, shock, abnormal cry, metabolic acidosis, etc. after 2–3 days of birth. Although IVH is rare at birth or after first month of life, some infants present clinical signs of IVH between 2nd to 4th week after birth.

### Diagnosis

Since clinical features are silent in many cases of IVH routine screening through ultrasonography is important for diagnosis. Infants <32 weeks of gestation or <1500 g are highly prone to the IVH, hence routine ultrasonography through anterior and posterior fontanelle is recommended for early detection and evaluation. Similarly, if an infant is suspected for IVH during physical examination or assessment of clinical symptoms then CT scan or MRI is indicated for confirmatory diagnosis. Although cranial ultrasonography is safe and radiation free it is not sensitive to detect edema, intracerebral hemorrhage and infarcts. In such cases CT and MRI are the most preferred and reliable diagnostic methods. Nowaday's research has been shifted to find a biomarker to detect IVH as early as possible. Researchers have found that certain biomarkers like **S100B, erythropoietin (EPO), activin A** level increases in the cord blood among the infants with IVH. In future if theses biomarkers will be found to be very sensitive and reliable then the possibility of early detection and prevention of IVH will be wider.

### Management

There is no definitive treatment available for IVH therefore preventive and symptomatic management are the key to treat the condition. As a prophylaxis measure indomethacin 0.1 mg/kg/day for 3 consecutive days is administered to the VLBW babies to minimize the occurrence of IVH. Infant showing seizure activity is treated with anticonvulsants. Blood transfusion is required for the infants with low hematocrit and thrombocytopenia. Infants with premature lung are treated with surfactant. Drainage of CSF from the ventricle is crucial for the infants with posthemorrhagic hydrocephalus (PPH) along with regular follow up by cranial ultrasonography. CSF drainage can be done by several methods like ventriculoperitoneal shunt, lumbar tap, ventriculosubgaleal shunt, etc., to lower the elevated intracranial pressure and its associated complications.

### Nursing Management

Nursing diagnosis - 1

Risk for ineffective cerebral tissue perfusion related to cerebral vasospasm secondary to intracranial hemorrhage as evidenced by poor feeding, abnormal neurological response, speech problem and difficulty swallowing, etc.

**Interventions**
- Assess the level of consciousness and neurological status
- Assess protective reflexes like swallowing, gagging and coughing
- Positioning the head in midline and elevating to 30° will reduce the intracranial pressure
- Monitor ICP and inform the healthcare provider immediately if >15 mm Hg
- Monitor oxygen saturation continuously and assess ABG as prescribed to detect hypoxia in advance
- Assess ICP and mean arterial pressure (MAP) to calculate cerebral perfusion pressure
- Impaired cerebral autoregulation on blood flow and pressure can anytime increase or decrease and may lead to hemorrhage from the delicate blood vessels of germinal matrix. Continuous monitoring of blood pressure and other vitals are essential to trace the pattern of fluctuation and to prevent IVH

- Most of the preterm suffering from pneumothorax develop IVH therefore close monitoring of clinical signs like tachycardia, alteration in breath sound, reduced $PaO_2$, elevated $PaCO_2$ is essential
- Vigorous tracheal suctioning induces germinal matrix hemorrhage hence, should be avoided if not required
- Whenever possible invasive interventions to be avoided as these may induce cry that leads to increase intracranial pressure.
- It is also important to monitor the blood PH as metabolic acidosis and $PaCO_2$ are associated with IVH.

### Nursing diagnosis - 2
Impaired physical mobility related to cognitive dysfunction secondary to intracranial hemorrhage as evidenced by decreased muscle control, restricted movement.

**Interventions**
- Assess the functional levels of mobility
- Assess the patient's ability to carry out the activities of daily living
- Evaluate the ability to perform range of motion of joints
- Take measure to prevent skin breakdown and development of pressure ulcer
- Keep the skin clean, dry to maintain skin integrity
- Take precautionary measures to avoid fall injury or injury during seizure activity
- Use comfort devices and anti-embolic stockings as applicable
- Perform passive ROM exercise to maintain muscle strength
- Demonstrate the use of mobility devices like crutches, cane walkers, etc.
- Encourage the child to do activities herself/himself if safe to perform.

### Nursing diagnosis - 3
Impaired verbal communication related to cognitive dysfunction as evidenced by aphasia, dysarthria, dysphonia, slurred speech, difficulty using body expressions, difficulty maintaining communication and absence of eye contact, etc.

**Interventions**
- Assess the communicative ability of the child
- Assess the ability of the child to follow and perform simple tasks like closing and opening eyes, mouth, etc.
- Use alternative methods of communication like hand gestures, pictures and symbols, etc.
- Provide positive reinforcement to the child during communication
- Allow sufficient time to the child to answer.

## Neonatal Sepsis
Neonatal sepsis is one of the commonest causes of death among newborn worldwide. Most of the deaths have been reported from the low and middle-income countries because of poor hygiene and inadequate infection control practice. Neonates are highly vulnerable to sepsis due to immature immune defense mechanism. According to WHO about 1 million death occurs because of neonatal sepsis out of which approximately 42% are during the first week of life. In India, the major contributing factor of neonatal mortality is the sepsis which accounts approximately 30–50% of neonatal death. The higher incidence of infection may be due to increase rate of maternal infection, unhygienic practice during delivery, increases prevalence of LBW babies, poor adherence to exclusive breastfeeding practice, etc.

### Definition
Neonatal sepsis is characterized by sign and symptoms of infection with or without accompanying bacteremia during first 28 days of life. It includes several systemic infections such as septicemia, pneumonia, meningitis, urinary tract infection, arthritis and osteomyelitis. Superficial infections like conjunctivitis and oral thrush are excluded from neonatal sepsis. (Ramesh Agarwal, Ashok Deorari et. al., AIIMS Protocols in Neonatology, 2nd Edition).

### Classification
Based on the age of onset neonatal sepsis are categorized into two broad groups:
1. **Early onset sepsis:** In this type, the onset of sign and symptoms of sepsis appear within 72 hours of birth. The pathogens might be acquired from maternal genital tract or the place of delivery.
2. **Late onset sepsis:** In this, the sign and symptoms of sepsis appear after 72 hours of birth. The source of pathogens in late onset sepsis may be from the community or hospital (nosocomial).

### Risk Factors
The risk factors of neonatal sepsis are of two categories:
1. **Perinatal risk factors:**
    - Rupture of membranes >24 hours
    - Spontaneous preterm labor
    - Chorioamnionitis (intra-amniotic infection)
    - Prolonged labor
    - Unclean per vaginal examinations
    - Perinatal asphyxia
2. **Extreme risk factors:**
    - Rupture of membranes >72 hours
    - Chorioamnionitis (intra-amniotic infection)
    - Foul smelling liquor

## Etiology

In western countries, the primary cause of sepsis is the Group B *Streptococcus* where as in India the leading cause of neonatal sepsis are the gram-positive (*Staphylococcus aureus, Staphylococcus albus* and *Enterobacter*) and gram-negative pathogens (*Klebsiella pneumoniae, E. coli*, acinetobacter baumannii, pseudomonas, citrobacter). *Candida albicans* and *Candida tropicalis* rarely cause sepsis although few cases have been isolated.

## Clinical Manifestations

Clinical manifestation of neonatal sepsis can be described under two heading as follows:

### Nonspecific Clinical Manifestations

Early features of sepsis are highly variable and nonspecific. The affected neonate may present one or more from the following features:
- Hypo/hyperthermia
- Hypo/hyperglycemia
- Increase or decrease heart rate
- Lethargy
- Poor cry
- Irritability
- Refusal to suck
- Respiratory distress
- Apnea
- Gasping
- Metabolic acidosis
- Inadequate weight gain
- **System specific clinical manifestations:** Respiratory: apnea, brady/tachypnea, retraction, grunting
- **Cardiac:** Brady/tachypnea, shock, hypotension, poor perfusion
- **Renal:** Oliguria due to acute renal failure
- **Gastrointestinal:** Vomiting, abdominal distension, feeding intolerance, diarrhea, hepatosplenomegaly, paralytic ileus, necrotizing enterocolitis
- **Hematological:** Pallor, DIC and bleeding
- **Skin:** Cellulitis, petechiae, purpura, impetigo, sclerema, umbilical redness and discharge, multiple pustules, abscess
- **CNS:** Hyperirritability, bulging fontanel, seizure, hypo/hypertonia.

## Diagnosis

- **Blood culture:** It is the gold standard method to identify the pathogen directly in the blood hence help in deciding specific antimicrobial agent for administration. In all suspected cases of neonatal sepsis blood culture should be done before initiating any antimicrobial agent.
- **Lumbar puncture:** In case of early onset sepsis LP is indicated if the blood culture shows positive result or if clinical presentation strongly associated with septicemia all case of late onset sepsis lumbar puncture should be done before starting antibiotics. Abnormal findings suggestive of sepsis include the following:
  - Elevated level of polymorphs >30 WBC/cumm
  - CSF proteins >150 mg%
  - CSF/blood glucose ratio <50%
  - Positive gram stain
  - Positive CSF culture
- **Sepsis screen:** Sepsis screen is a combination of multiple tests carried out primarily to exclude the infection rather than confirming the diagnosis of sepsis. If repeat screen at 12–24 hours after the 1st screen shows negative result then infection can be excluded confidently. The components of sepsis screen are as follows:
  - Total WBC count <5000/mm$^3$
  - Absolute neutrophil count <1800/mm$^3$
  - Immature (band cells + myelocytes + metamyelocytes) to total neutrophils ratio >0.2
  - Increased micro–erythrocyte sedimentation rate (> 15 mm/h)
  - Elevated C-reactive protein > 1 mg/dL

  (If two or more components shows positive result with maternal risk factors then antibiotic can be initiated after blood culture.)
- **Complete blood count:** Although leucopenia (<5000/mm$^3$) and leucocytosis (>25000/mm$^3$) both are associated with neonatal sepsis leucopenia is much more common. Additional neutropenia (<1800/mm$^3$) and thrombocytopenia (<100000/mm$^3$) also should be taken into consideration for the diagnosis.
- **Urine culture:** Urine culture can be done to exclude urinary tract infection.
- **Imaging study:** Chest X-ray is indicated for the neonate with respiratory distress and apnea and abdominal X-ray if necrotizing enterocolitis is suspected. All the meningitis suspected neonates should undergo Ultrasound and CT scan of head.

## Management

- **Supportive management:**
  - *Thermoregulation:* To avoid hypo/hyperthermia the ambient environment where the newborn will receive the care should be thermoneutral.
  - *Maintenance of oxygen saturation:* SPO$_2$ should be maintained between 91–95% for which oxygen therapy or ventilatory support may be required. During oxygen therapy continuous SPO$_2$ monitoring is mandatory using fingertip pulse oximeter for both

preterm and term neonates. It is also important to avoid hyperoxygenation for a prolonged period as this may lead to retinopathy of prematurity, bronchopulmonary dysplasia, periventricular leukomalacia, necrotizing enterocolitis and cerebral palsy.
  – *Maintenance of hemodynamic stability:* Administration of intravenous fluid, volume expanders are required if the infant is hemodynamically unstable. Administration of packed RBC may also be necessary to treat anemia. Monitoring blood pressure, blood glucose level, capillary refill time and measurement of urine output are required to assess hemodynamic stability of the neonate.
- **Antimicrobial treatment:** Antibiotics should be initiated after the diagnostic tests are complete. But it is not always crucial to wait for the laboratory tests for starting antibiotics. Antibiotics can be started if any one of the following is present.

  **For early onset sepsis**
  – Presence of >3 risk factors for early onset sepsis
  – Presence of foul-smelling liquor
  – Positive sepsis screen plus one or two risk factors
  – Clinically suspected neonate for sepsis

  **For late onset sepsis**
  – Positive sepsis screen
  – Clinically suspected neonate for sepsis

The duration of antibiotic therapy varies based on the underling condition. The duration of antibiotic therapy is 28 days for osteomyelitis/arthritis, 21 days for meningitis, 14 days if blood culture positive, 5–7 days if culture negative sepsis. (Ramesh Agarwal, Ashok Deorari et. al., AIIMS Protocols in Neonatology, 2nd Edition).

*Nursing Management*
- **Assessment:** Monitoring vital signs continuously is helpful to identify minor changes in the infant's health status or behavior. It also crucial to observe for any signs of distress like reduced muscle tone, lethargy, pallor skin color abnormal or diminished response to stimuli, etc., monitoring the trends of the baseline data and input output should be strictly done.
- **Hand hygiene and aseptic technique:** The best method to prevent further infection of the sepsis child is the hand hygiene and performing procedures under strict aseptic techniques are important. Hence the caregivers should adhere to the infection control practice as per the institutional policy.
- **Maintain neutral thermal environment:** Fluctuation in the body temperature is very common in the infants diagnosed with sepsis. This happens as much needed energy diverts away from growth and the body's ability to fight the infection. Hence to maintain neutral thermal environment the infant may need to be placed in a warmer or incubator, and temperature must be regularly monitored.
- **Maintain fluids and electrolytes:** A special diet plan for maintenance of nutritional requirement, fluid balance and electrolyte balance may be required for the neonate with sepsis. Some of the infants may be kept under NPO as they have an increase chance of aspiration, paralytic ileus and necrotizing enterocolitis. Total parenteral nutrition should be provided to the infant under NPO to meet the nutritional requirement.
- **Provide adequate oxygenation and ventilation:** Continuous monitoring oxygen saturation is required for the infant with sepsis as hypoxemia is very common among them. The affected infant may need supplemental oxygen, continuous positive airway pressure (CPAP) or mechanical ventilation based on the severity of the condition and level of oxygen saturation.
- **Monitoring and treatment of seizures:** Seizure is one of the common complications of the neonatal sepsis. Therefore, monitoring the infant's behavior is crucial to identify the types of seizure. Administer the antiepileptic medications as prescribed by the consultant and preventing aspiration during seizure episode are the primary nursing management.
- **Monitoring of lab results:** Nurses should monitor the lab investigations like CBC, blood culture, electrolytes, ABG analysis, blood glucose, CSF analysis and urine analysis are helpful to identify the specific organism, severity of the disease, selection of the antimicrobial agent, treatment of the hypoglycemia and maintenance of fluid electrolyte balance.
- **Parental support:** Parents of the affected child should be counselled as this is a unique situation for them and they might be undergoing emotional crisis. As a nurse educate the parents and other family members regarding disease like risk factors, treatment options available, prognosis, importance of practicing hand hygiene, etc.

*Nursing diagnosis - 1*

Hyperthermia related to inflammatory process secondary to infection as evidenced by skin warm to touch, infant does not maintain suck, tachycardia, tachypnea, lethargy, elevated WBC count.

**Interventions**
- Assess body temperature of the newborn every 4 hourly or use skin probe for continuous monitoring
- Maintain proper ventilation in the ward

- Follow aseptic technique while performing any invasive procedure
- If possible, avoid unnecessary invasive procedures
- Provide cold compress to the child
- Provide antipyretics and antibiotics as prescribed
- Encourage breastfeeding to increase immunity of the newborn
- Monitor lab results like WBC count, CRP level, ESR, blood and CSF culture, etc.

Nursing diagnosis - 2

Deficient fluid volume related to excessive fluid loss as evidenced by dry skin and mucus membrane, decrease skin turgor, sunken fontanels, no tears when crying, lack of bowel activity, oliguria.

**Interventions**
- Monitor vitals and oxygen saturation for baseline data
- Assess the degree of fluid volume deficit
- Encourage adequate breastfeeding
- Maintain intake and output chart
- Monitor the weight of the baby daily
- Monitor urine volume and color
- Administer IV fluid as prescribed
- Review the lab results like urine specific gravity, serum electrolytes, blood glucose level, etc.
- Monitor the signs of shock

Nursing diagnosis - 3

Ineffective peripheral tissue perfusion related to reduced oxygen supply as evidenced by capillary refill time >3 seconds, decreased peripheral pulses, altered skin characteristics.

**Interventions**
- Assess the signs of reduced peripheral tissue perfusion like skin color, capillary refill time, peripheral pulses, oxygen saturation, etc.
- Review laboratory data like arterial blood gas, blood coagulation studies, PCV, kidney function test, serum electrolytes, etc.
- Monitor respiratory status including rate, depth, pattern, any abnormal breath sounds
- Observe any changes in skin color
- Administer oxygen as prescribed
- Provide calm and quiet environment
- Administer IV fluid and blood products as prescribed.

## Respiratory Distress Syndrome (RDS)

It is one of the common causes for NICU admission of the neonate. The prevalence of RDS is higher among preterm neonates as compare to the term babies. This was previously called as hyaline membrane disease.

### Definition

According to National Neonatal Perinatal Database of India (NNPD) presence of any two of the following characteristics in a neonate can be diagnosed as respiratory distress syndrome:
- Respiratory rate > 60/minute
- Subcostal/intercostal recessions
- Expiratory grunt/groaning

### Causes
- Transient tachypnea of newborn
- Pneumonia
- Sepsis
- Meconium aspiration syndrome
- Perinatal asphyxia
- Persistent pulmonary hypertension
- Diaphragmatic hernia
- Tracheoesophageal fistula
- Laryngo tracheomalacia
- Arrythmia
- Congenital heart disease
- Cardiomyopathy
- Birth trauma
- Anemia
- Polycythemia

### Clinical Features

The onset of clinical features can be within few minutes to hour after birth. Following are the clinical presentation of the neonate suffering from respiratory distress syndrome:
- Tachypnea (RR >60/minute)
- Nasal flaring
- Grunting
- Chest retraction
- Cyanosis
- Lethargy
- Irregular breathing
- Apnea

### Assessment of the Severity of RDS and Diagnosis

The clinical judgment of severity of RDS can be done by one of the two widely used scoring system called Silverman Anderson scoring system and Downe's scoring system. The parameters of Silverman Anderson score are upper chest, lower chest, xiphoid retractions and grunting. Each parameter has a score ranging from 0–2 where minimum score is 0 and maximum score 10. Severity of respiratory distress is classified as severe (score >7), moderate (score 5–7) and mild (score <5).

The parameters of Downe's score are respiratory rate, cyanosis, air entry, grunt and retraction. Each parameter has a score range from 0–2, minimum score 0 and maximum 10. Severity of RDS classified as impending respiratory failure (score >7), respiratory distress (score 4–7), No respiratory distress (score <4).

## Diagnosis

Diagnosis of the neonate may require multiple investigations like:
- Gastric aspirate shake test
- Transillumination test
- Chest radiography
- Ultrasonography
- Arterial blood gas analysis
- Sepsis screen if sepsis is suspected
- CSF examination to rule out meningitis
- ECG to exclude congenital heart disease.

*Source*: Ramesh Agarwal, Ashok Deorari et. al., AIIMS Protocols in Neonatology, 2nd Edition.

## Treatment

### Antenatal Corticosteroids

Administration of corticosteroid during 24–34 weeks of gestation can prevent RDS by enhancing lung maturity. A complete dose of either betamethasone or dexamethasone can be administered during this period. In Indian setting based on the cost, availability and effectiveness betamethasone is used and is thought to be safer than dexamethasone. Betamethasone 12 mg IM at 24-hour interval two doses.

Dexamethasone 6 mg IM at 12-hour interval four doses.

### Oxygen Therapy

The target of oxygen therapy is to maintain the $SPO_2$ level between 88–95 %. During oxygen therapy, it is also important to monitor $SPO_2$ continuously by fingertip pulse oximeter to prevent hypo/hyperoxia.

### Surfactant Therapy

This therapy is quite effective in reducing mortality rate, complications and duration of ventilatory support. Surfactant is directly administered to the lungs by endotracheal tube at a dose of 100–200 mg/kg. Although a single dose is enough, it can be repeated after 6–12 hours if respiratory distress persists.

### Mechanical Ventilation

The mechanical ventilation can be considered if:
- The neonate has moderate to severe respiratory distress
- Persistent intractable apnea
- $SPO_2$ remaining below the normal range with CPAP.

### Antibiotics

It can be started after obtaining the blood culture or sepsis screen.

### Supportive Therapy

The neonate should be treated under radiant warmer to prevent hypothermia and if not required handling should be avoided. In case of a hemodynamically stable neonate expressed breast, milk can be provided at a volume of 10–20 mL/kg 4 hourly. IV fluid can be administered with 10% dextrose at a dose of 60–80 mL/kg/day. It also important to monitor the urine output weight and serum electrolyte. Monitoring vitals, ABG, $SPO_2$ level, blood glucose and capillary refill time are also important.

## Nursing Management

### Nursing Diagnosis - 1

Ineffective breathing pattern related to pulmonary immaturity and decreased surfactant production as evidenced by nasal flaring, cyanosis, hypercapnia, hypoxia, chest retraction, grunting, tachypnea.

Interventions
- Assess respiratory status for presence of any adventitious breath sound, rate, chest retraction, etc.
- Assess oxygen saturation continuously
- Administer oxygen as prescribed and maintain $SPO_2$ between 91–95%. Avoid hyperoxygenation for prolonged period as this may lead to retinopathy of prematurity, bronchopulmonary dysplasia, periventricular leukomalacia, necrotizing enterocolitis and cerebral palsy.
- Assess signs of hypoxia regularly
- Suction the air way as required to clear the secretions
- Administer antibiotics, bronchodilators, steroids as prescribed
- Review the ABG results and other lab results
- Ensure the ventilator and emergency respiratory support equipments are available at bedside.

### Nursing Diagnosis - 2

Ineffective thermoregulation related to immature thermoregulatory center and less body adipose tissue as evidenced by increased/decreased body temperature from normal range, flushed skin, skin warm/cool to touch, slow capillary refill time, tachycardia.

Interventions
- Assess body temperature of the newborn every 4 hourly or use skin probe for continuous monitoring
- Maintain proper ventilation in the ward
- Place the baby under radiant warmer if hypothermic
- Dry and cover the baby with warm clothes if hypothermic

- Follow aseptic technique while performing any invasive procedure
- If possible, avoid unnecessary invasive procedures
- Provide cold compress to the child
- Provide antipyretics and antibiotics as prescribed
- Encourage breastfeeding to increase immunity of the newborn
- Monitor lab results like WBC count, CRP level, ESR, blood and CSF culture, etc.

*Nursing Diagnosis - 3*

Ineffective airway clearance related to retained secretions as evidenced by altered respiratory rhythm, adventitious breath sounds, cyanosis, hypoxemia, nasal flaring, subcostal retraction, tachypnea, uses accessory muscle to breathe.

Interventions

- Assess the patency of the air way specially in case of trauma or neurological injury.
- Auscultate for detection of abnormal breath sound and recording of vitals, $SPO_2$ are also important.
- Provide prone position which is found to be beneficial in improving lung oxygenation and function hence should be provided if possible.
- Suctioning should be done as required to clear the airway.
- Chest physiotherapies are also quite helpful to remove excess secretions but should be performed if indicated.
- Maintenance of fluid balance along with recording input and output is also required.

## Congenital Disorders

### Cyanotic Heart Disease

**Congenital heart disease (CHD)** comprises a range of structural or functional heart abnormalities present at birth, affecting approximately 1 in 100 newborns. These defects can involve heart chambers, valves, arteries, or veins and can vary in severity from minor issues to life-threatening conditions. While the precise causes often remain elusive, genetic and environmental factors, or a combination of both, may contribute to CHD. Timely diagnosis, advanced medical technology, and surgical interventions have significantly improved the prognosis. Many individuals with CHD can lead fulfilling lives with appropriate care, including medications, catheter-based procedures, and, in some cases, open-heart surgery, underscoring the importance of early detection and comprehensive management.

**Cyanotic heart disease** is a subset of congenital heart disease characterized by a bluish or cyanotic tint to the skin, lips, and nails due to insufficient oxygen levels in the blood. This condition typically results from structural heart defects that allow deoxygenated blood to mix with oxygenated blood, reducing the overall oxygen content in the bloodstream.

### *Classification of Congenital Heart Disease*

*Cyanotic Heart Disease*

- Tetralogy of fallot (TOF)
- Tricuspid atresia (TA)
- Transposition of great arteries (TGA)
- Total anomalous pulmonary venous connection (TAPVC)

*Acyanotic Heart Disease*

- Ventricular septal defect (VSD)
- Atrial septal defect (ASD)
- Patent ductus arteriosus (PDA)
- Aortic stenosis
- Pulmonary stenosis
- Coarctation of aorta

### *Tetralogy of Fallot*

Tetralogy of Fallot is a congenital heart defect that was first described by the French physician Étienne-Louis Arthur Fallot in 1888. It is a complex condition characterized by the presence of four distinct heart abnormalities, which collectively result in inadequate oxygenation of the blood. These four abnormalities are:

1. **Ventricular septal defect (VSD):** This is a hole in the septum, or wall, that separates the two lower chambers of the heart, known as the ventricles.
2. **Pulmonary stenosis:** In TOF, the pulmonary valve or the pulmonary artery is narrowed, restricting the flow of blood from the right ventricle to the lungs.
3. **Right ventricular hypertrophy:** Due to the increased workload caused by the narrowed pulmonary valve or artery, the right ventricle becomes thickened and enlarged.
4. **Overriding aorta:** The aorta, the main artery that carries oxygen-rich blood from the heart to the rest of the body, is positioned directly over the VSD, allowing it to receive blood from both the right and left ventricles.

*Etiology*

While the exact cause of TOF remains a subject of ongoing research, it is generally believed to result from a combination of genetic and environmental factors.

- **Genetic factors:** There is evidence to suggest that TOF can be hereditary, with a genetic predisposition playing a role in its development.
- **Environmental factors:** Exposure to certain environmental factors during pregnancy can increase the risk

of TOF in the developing fetus. Maternal infections, exposure to toxins, or certain medications taken during pregnancy may all be contributing factors.
- **Chromosomal abnormalities:** In some cases, TOF may be associated with chromosomal abnormalities, such as down syndrome. These chromosomal anomalies can contribute to the development of congenital heart defects.
- **Maternal health:** The overall health of the mother during pregnancy can also influence the risk of TOF. Poorly controlled maternal diabetes or the use of specific medications during pregnancy may increase the likelihood of the condition.

*Clinical Features*
- **Cyanosis:** Cyanosis, or a bluish or purple discoloration of the skin, lips, and nail beds, is a hallmark sign of TOF. It results from reduced oxygen levels in the blood.
- **Difficulty breathing:** Infants with TOF may exhibit rapid breathing and experience episodes of breathlessness, particularly during feeding or crying.
- **Tet spells:** These are sudden, severe episodes of cyanosis and difficulty breathing that can be triggered by crying, feeding, or other activities. Tet spells are considered medical emergencies and require immediate attention.
- **Failure to thrive:** Infants with TOF may have difficulty gaining weight and growing at a normal rate due to the increased energy expenditure required to compensate for the heart's inefficiency.
- **Clubbing of fingers and toes:** Over time, the fingers and toes of individuals with TOF may become enlarged and rounded at the tips. This condition, known as clubbing, is a result of chronic low oxygen levels.
- **Irritability:** Infants with TOF may appear irritable and fussy, particularly during episodes of cyanosis and discomfort.
- **Fatigue:** Older children and adults with TOF may experience fatigue, particularly during physical activity, as their hearts struggle to provide adequate oxygen to meet the body's demands.

*Diagnosis*

Diagnosing TOF typically involves a combination of prenatal testing, physical examinations, and various imaging studies.
- **Prenatal screening:** In some cases, TOF may be detected during routine prenatal ultrasounds, although a definitive diagnosis is usually made after birth.
- **Physical examination:** A thorough physical examination of the newborn is essential. The presence of cyanosis, a heart murmur, or other abnormal findings can raise suspicion of TOF.
- **Echocardiogram:** Echocardiography is a noninvasive imaging test and primary tool for diagnosing TOF and assessing the severity of the defects.
- **Electrocardiogram (ECG or EKG):** An ECG records the electrical activity of the heart and can help identify any irregularities in the heart's rhythm.
- **Chest X-ray:** Boot shaped heart is the radiological finding in a child with TOF.

*Medical Management*

Before surgical intervention, medical management may be initiated to stabilize the child and prepare them for the upcoming surgery. Several medications can be employed in the management of TOF, each serving a specific purpose:
- **Prostaglandin E1 (PGE1):** This medication helps maintain the ductus arteriosus open, a fetal blood vessel connecting the pulmonary artery to the aorta. Keeping it open temporarily improves blood flow to the lungs, alleviating cyanosis.
- **Diuretics:** Diuretics may be prescribed to reduce fluid buildup in the body, which can occur due to heart-related issues and help manage symptoms such as edema.
- **Beta-blockers and anti-arrhythmic medications:** In cases where arrhythmias are present, medications such as beta-blockers or other anti-arrhythmics may be used to manage heart rhythm abnormalities and ensure cardiovascular stability.

*Surgical Management*

The cornerstone of TOF management is surgical repair. This procedure, often performed when the child is between 3 to 6 months old, aims to correct the anatomical abnormalities associated with TOF. The primary objectives of TOF repair surgery are:
- **Closing the ventricular septal defect (VSD):** During the surgery, the VSD, a hole in the septum between the heart's ventricles, is meticulously closed. This is a crucial step in preventing the mixing of oxygen-poor and oxygen-rich blood.
- **Pulmonary valve repair or replacement:** The narrowed pulmonary valve is addressed during the surgery. Depending on the specific case, the valve may be enlarged or replaced with an artificial valve to improve blood flow to the lungs.
- **Additional repairs:** If there are other associated heart defects, such as right ventricular outflow tract obstruction or aortic override, they are repaired simultaneously during the surgical procedure.

In cases where the child is too small or not stable enough for a full repair, palliative procedures may be considered.

These include the Blalock-Taussig shunt, which creates a connection between the subclavian artery and the pulmonary artery to increase blood flow to the lungs, or alternatives like the Waterston or Potts shunt.

Management of tet spell

- Early recognition is crucial. Be alert to signs such as sudden worsening of cyanosis, increased irritability, restlessness, or lethargy, and altered consciousness.
- Quickly position the child in a knee-chest or squatting position. This helps increase systemic vascular resistance (SVR) and reduce the right-to-left shunting of blood.
- Provide the child with 100% oxygen via a mask or nasal cannula. The increased oxygen concentration helps increase oxygen saturation levels in the blood.
- **Administer morphine sulfate:** A vasodilator that can help reduce the spasm of the infundibulum (muscular outlet of the right ventricle). It also has a sedative effect, which can calm the child. The usual dose of morphine sulfate for a Tet spell is 0.1–0.2 mg/kg IV.
- Beta-blockers like propranolol can help reduce the severity and frequency of Tet spells by decreasing the heart rate and reducing the force of ventricular contractions. The usual dose of propranolol is 0.01–0.03 mg/kg IV.
- **Prepare for emergent surgical intervention:** If the Tet spell is not responding to medical management emergency interventions may include balloon atrial septostomy (Rashkind procedure) to improve blood flow or even immediate surgical correction of the cardiac defect.

### Tricuspid Atresia

Tricuspid atresia is characterized by the absence or severe underdevelopment of the tricuspid valve, which is normally situated between the right atrium (the upper right chamber of the heart) and the right ventricle (the lower right chamber of the heart). This valve plays a crucial role in regulating the flow of blood from the right atrium to the right ventricle. Due to the absence or extreme underdevelopment of the tricuspid valve, there is no direct passage for blood to flow from the right atrium into the right ventricle. This leads to several important pathophysiological consequences:

- **Reduced blood flow to the right ventricle:** The right ventricle may remain hypoplastic (underdeveloped) because it doesn't receive the usual volume of blood from the right atrium.
- **Obstructed flow from the right atrium:** The absence of the tricuspid valve obstructs the normal flow of blood from the right atrium.
- **Atrial and ventricular septal defects:** To compensate for the lack of direct communication between the right atrium and right ventricle, individuals with tricuspid atresia often have associated heart defects, such as atrial septal defects (ASDs) and ventricular septal defects (VSDs). These defects provide pathways for blood to flow from the right atrium to the left side of the heart and then to the lungs for oxygenation. While these defects help supply oxygenated blood to the body, they also lead to a mixing of oxygenated and deoxygenated blood, resulting in cyanosis (blueness of the skin).

*Clinical Features*

- Cyanosis
- Tachypnea
- Difficulty feeding
- Failure to thrive
- Clubbing of fingers and toes
- Heart murmur
- Increased risk of infection
- **Congestion:** In severe cases, individuals with tricuspid atresia can develop symptoms of heart failure, such as fluid retention, swollen legs or abdomen, and difficulty breathing.

*Diagnosis*

- **Echocardiogram (Echo):** This is a primary diagnostic tool for assessing heart defects. An echocardiogram uses sound waves to create images of the heart's structure and function. It can reveal the absence or abnormality of the tricuspid valve, as well as the anatomy of the other heart structures.
- **Electrocardiogram (ECG or EKG):** An ECG records the electrical activity of the heart and can help identify abnormalities in heart rhythm and conduction.
- **Chest X-ray:** A chest X-ray may be performed to assess the size and shape of the heart and to look for signs of congestion in the lungs.
- **Cardiac catheterization:** In some cases, a cardiac catheterization procedure may be necessary to obtain more detailed information about the heart's anatomy and function. This involves inserting a thin tube (catheter) into the heart's chambers and blood vessels.

*Medical Management*

- **Prostaglandin E1:** Prostaglandin E1 (PGE1) infusion is often initiated to maintain patency of the ductus arteriosus, a fetal blood vessel that helps bypass the defective tricuspid valve and allows blood to flow from the right atrium to the left atrium. This helps in mixing oxygenated and deoxygenated blood and improving oxygen levels in the body.
- **Diuretics:** Diuretics may be prescribed to manage fluid buildup in the body, particularly in cases of congestive

heart failure. Diuretics help reduce excess fluid and reduce the workload on the heart.
- **Anticoagulation:** Some patients with tricuspid atresia may be at risk of developing blood clots, particularly those with Fontan circulation (a surgical procedure used in some cases of congenital heart disease). Anticoagulant medications, such as warfarin, may be prescribed to prevent clot formation.

*Surgical Management*

The mainstay of treatment for tricuspid atresia is surgical repair. The specific surgical approach can vary depending on the individual case and associated defects. Common surgical procedures include the Glenn shunt, the Fontan procedure, and various palliative surgeries to improve circulation. These surgeries are performed to redirect blood flow, bypass the defective tricuspid valve, and optimize oxygenation.

- **Glenn shunt:** A surgical connection is created between the superior vena cava (SVC) and the pulmonary artery. The superior vena cava is one of the main veins that return deoxygenated blood from the upper part of the body to the heart. By connecting the SVC directly to the pulmonary artery, deoxygenated blood from the upper body can bypass the right ventricle and flow directly to the lungs. This improves the oxygenation of blood without the need for the right ventricle to pump it.
- **Fontan shunt:** The Fontan procedure redirects blood flow from the upper and lower body directly to the pulmonary arteries, bypassing the right ventricle. There are variations of the Fontan procedure, including the lateral tunnel Fontan and the extracardiac Fontan. In both methods, a connection is created between the superior vena cava (SVC) and the pulmonary arteries, allowing oxygen-poor (deoxygenated) blood returning from the body to flow directly into the lungs.
  - *Lateral Tunnel Fontan:* In this approach, a tunnel is created inside the right atrium to connect the SVC and the pulmonary arteries. This tunnel allows for a controlled flow of blood to the lungs.
  - *Extracardiac Fontan:* In this method, a conduit (tube) is used to connect the SVC and inferior vena cava (IVC) directly to the pulmonary arteries outside of the heart. This approach can be used when the anatomy of the heart makes the lateral tunnel technique challenging.

## Transposition of Great Arteries

Transposition of the great arteries (TGA) is a complex congenital heart defect where the two main arteries leaving the heart, the aorta, and the pulmonary artery, are switched or "transposed." In TGA, the aorta arises from the right ventricle, and the pulmonary artery arises from the left ventricle. This results in oxygen-poor blood circulating through the body and oxygen-rich blood recirculating to the lungs.

*Clinical Features*
- Cyanosis
- Dyspnea
- Poor feeding
- Tachypnea
- Signs of congestive cardiac failure
- Clubbing of finger and toes
- Murmur

*Diagnosis*
- **Chest X-ray:** A chest X-ray can provide information about the size and shape of the heart and the position of the great arteries. However, it may not definitively diagnose TGA but can help rule out other conditions.
- **Echocardiogram (Echo):** An echocardiogram is uses to visualize the abnormal position of the aorta and pulmonary artery and assess the associated defects, such as ventricular septal defects (VSD) or atrial septal defects (ASD).
- **Additional imaging:** In some cases, additional imaging studies such as magnetic resonance imaging (MRI) or computed tomography angiography (CTA) may be used to provide more detailed information about the heart's anatomy.
- **Cardiac catheterization:** It allows for direct measurement of pressures and oxygen levels in the heart's chambers and great arteries. It is often used to confirm the diagnosis and may be performed prior to surgical correction.

*Medical Management*
- **Prostaglandin E1 (PGE1) administration:** To maintain the patency of the ductus arteriosus (a fetal blood vessel that normally closes shortly after birth), prostaglandin E1 may be administered intravenously. This helps ensure adequate oxygenated blood is circulated to the body.
- **Oxygen therapy:** Oxygen may be administered to improve oxygen saturation levels in the baby's blood. This helps alleviate cyanosis (bluish skin discoloration due to low oxygen levels).

*Surgical Management*
- **Balloon atrial septostomy (Rashkind procedure):** In some cases, a balloon atrial septostomy may be performed as an emergency procedure. This involves

threading a catheter through the baby's atrial septum (the wall between the atria) and then inflating a balloon to create or enlarge a hole (atrial septal defect) to allow for better mixing of oxygenated and deoxygenated blood.

- **Surgical correction:** The definitive treatment for TGA is surgical correction, which is typically performed in the first few days to weeks of life. The most common surgical procedure is the arterial switch operation (Jatene procedure). During this surgery, the aorta and pulmonary artery are repositioned to their correct locations, and the coronary arteries are re-implanted to ensure adequate blood supply to the heart muscle. This procedure effectively "switches" the great arteries back to their proper positions.

### Total Anomalous Pulmonary Venous Connection (TAPVC)

TAPVC stands for "total anomalous pulmonary venous connection," which is a congenital heart defect (a heart condition present at birth) that affects the way oxygen-rich blood from the lungs returns to the heart. In a normal heart, the pulmonary veins carry oxygenated blood from the lungs and connect to the left atrium of the heart. In TAPVC, the pulmonary veins connect abnormally to the right atrium or another location within the heart, causing oxygen-rich blood to mix with oxygen-poor blood. This mixing of oxygenated and deoxygenated blood can lead to inadequate oxygen supply to the body, resulting in symptoms such as cyanosis and dyspnea.

### Clinical Features

- Tachypnea
- Poor feeding
- Cyanosis
- Failure to thrive
- Congestive heart failure
- Pulmonary edema
- Pulmonary hypertension
- Recurrent chest infection

### Diagnosis

- **Clinical evaluation:** A detailed medical history, including any symptoms or signs that might suggest a heart problem. Common symptoms in infants may include cyanosis (bluish skin and lips), rapid breathing, difficulty feeding, and poor growth.
- **Physical examination:** A physical examination can reveal clinical signs such as abnormal heart sounds or murmurs, and signs of heart failure in some cases.
- **Chest X-ray:** A chest X-ray may show enlargement of the heart and abnormal blood flow patterns, which can be suggestive of TAPVC.
- **Echocardiogram (Echo):** An echocardiogram is a key diagnostic tool for TAPVC. It uses ultrasound waves to create images of the heart and its blood flow. An echocardiogram can often reveal the abnormal connections of the pulmonary veins and assess the extent of the defect.
- **Doppler ultrasound:** Doppler ultrasound is a specific type of echocardiogram that can help assess blood flow through the heart and pulmonary veins.
- **Cardiac catheterization:** In some cases, a cardiac catheterization may be performed. This involves threading a thin tube (catheter) through a blood vessel to the heart to obtain more detailed information about the anatomy and blood flow within the heart.
- **MRI or CT scan:** These imaging studies can provide more detailed information about the heart's structure and blood flow. They are often used in conjunction with other tests to confirm the diagnosis and assess the anatomy.
- **Oxygen saturation measurement:** Blood oxygen saturation levels are typically lower than normal in individuals with TAPVC, which can be detected using a pulse oximeter.

### Medical Management

- **Stabilization and support:** When TAPVC is diagnosed in a neonate or infant, immediate stabilization and supportive care are crucial. This may include oxygen supplementation, intravenous fluids, and medications to support cardiac function.
- **Prostaglandin E1 (PGE1) infusion:** In some cases, PGE1 infusion may be initiated to maintain or reopen the ductus arteriosus, a fetal blood vessel that allows some oxygenated blood to bypass the heart and reach the systemic circulation. This can help improve oxygenation until surgical correction can be performed.
- **Nutritional support:** Infants with TAPVC may experience feeding difficulties due to their cardiac condition. Nutritional support, often with high-calorie formula or breast milk, may be necessary to ensure adequate growth and nutrition.
- **Antibiotics:** Prophylactic antibiotics are usually administered before surgery to reduce the risk of infection.
- **Continuous monitoring:** Close monitoring of vital signs, oxygen saturation levels, and cardiac function is essential. This can be done in a neonatal intensive care unit (NICU) or a pediatric cardiac intensive care unit (CICU).

## Surgical Management

- **Timing of surgery:** The timing of TAPVC surgery depends on various factors, including the patient's age, size, and clinical condition. In most cases, surgery is performed as soon as possible after diagnosis, especially if the patient is a neonate or infant.
- **Surgical approach:** There are different surgical techniques to repair TAPVC, and the choice of approach depends on the specific anatomy of the anomaly. The most common approaches include:
  - *Supracardiac:* In this approach, the pulmonary veins are redirected to the back of the left atrium via an incision in the superior vena cava (SVC) or the right atrium.
  - *Cardiac:* This approach involves opening the left atrium directly to connect the pulmonary veins to it.
  - *Infracardiac:* The pulmonary veins are connected to the posterior or diaphragmatic part of the left atrium through an incision in the inferior vena cava (IVC).

## Nursing Management

### Nursing diagnosis - 1

Ineffective airway clearance related to airway obstruction or fistula as evidenced by altered respiratory rhythm, adventitious breath sounds, cyanosis, hypoxemia, nasal flaring, subcostal retraction, tachypnea, uses accessory muscle to breathe.

**Interventions**

- Assess the patency of the air way specially in case of cleft lip and palate, tracheoesophageal fistula.
- Auscultate for detection of abnormal breath sound and recording of vitals, $SPO_2$ are also important.
- Assess skin color and capillary refill time.
- Assess respiratory status as pneumonia and respiratory distress are common among these children.
- Assess abdominal distension which occurs due to entry of air in to stomach in TEF.
- Suctioning should be done as required to clear the airway.
- Keep the baby nil per oral as there is high chance of aspiration.
- Administer supplemental oxygen as prescribed.
- Elevate the head end of the bed to 30–45 degree to prevent the tongue from falling back and air way obstruction.
- Prepare the child and infant for surgical intervention.

### Nursing diagnosis - 2

Acute pain related to surgical incision as evidenced by expressive behavior, facial expression of pain, positioning to ease pain, reports intensity using standardized pain scale, altered physiological parameter, guarding behavior, etc.

**Interventions**

- Assess the characteristics of pain like onset, location, intensity, duration.
- If the child cannot verbalize assess the level of pain using pain assessment tool (premature infant pain profile, neonatal facial coding system, wong-baker faces pain rating scale, neonatal/infant pain scale, FLACC scale, behavioral pain scale, nonverbal pain scale, visual analogue scale, adolescent pediatric pain tool) as appropriate for the child.
- Provide comfortable position and calm and quite environment.
- Provide wound care to alleviate pain.
- Monitor vitals at regular interval as physiological parameter fluctuates during pain.
- Initiate nonpharmacological measures of pain management like distraction techniques, relaxation methods, etc.
- Administer analgesics as advised to the child.
- Evaluate the effectiveness and side effect of the analgesics.

### Nursing diagnosis - 3

Risk for infection related to impaired tissue integrity, difficulty managing wound care, difficulty managing long term invasive device.

**Interventions**

- Assess vitals every 4 hourly or as required specially temperature.
- Assess the sign and symptoms of infection and any purulent discharge from the incision.
- Provide wound care as needed.
- Apply sterile dressing to reduce infection and promote wound healing.
- Change the position the child every 2 hourly to prevent pressure ulcer if required place comfort devices below the bony prominences.
- Encourage breastfeeding unless contraindicated.
- Avoid unnecessary handling of the newborn.
- Strictly follow infection control practice while providing care and doing invasive procedures.
- Follow the 5 moments of hand hygiene.
- Protect the newborn from iatrogenic and cross-infection.
- Monitor lab results specially WBC count, CRP, ESR, blood culture, CSF culture, urine analysis and culture, etc.
- Assess and monitor nutritional status and weight of the newborn.
- Administer antibiotics as prescribed.

- Assess immunization history and administer as per requirement.
- Provide adequate rest and sleep, limit visitors.

**Esophageal atresia (EA) with or without tracheoesophageal fistula (TEF)**

It is a congenital anomaly characterized by abnormal communication between esophagus and trachea. There are five different types of TEF (**Fig 13.3**) as follows:
1. A: EA without fistula
2. B: EA with proximal TEF
3. C: EA with distal TEF
4. D: EA with proximal and distal TEF
5. E: TEF without esophageal atresia also called H-type fistula.

Clinical features
- Excessive drooling
- Frothy salivation
- Cyanosis and choking during first feed
- Abdominal distension
- Coughing
- Respiratory distress
- Regurgitation

Diagnosis

Inserting an orogastric tube may get arrested at a distance of 10–12 centimetres from the mouth if EA or TEF might be present. For further investigation chest X-ray can be done to confirm the diagnosis.

Management

The baby should be placed in supine position with head end elevated to 45 degree to prevent aspiration of aspiration of refluxed gastric content. It is also important to suction the esophageal pouch regularly. IV fluids and antibiotics are also necessary to administer (Piyush Gupta, 2021).

Decision about the surgery of a new born with esophageal atresia includes following:

- Immediate gastrotomy is required in EA newborns to relieve abdominal distension. There are several operative procedures available for repairing of the EA, e.g., Kimura, Scharli, Fokers and Livaditis.
- Possible time duration to wait for approximation of the blind ends of the esophagus.
- Whether to perform an esophageal substitution procedure, with or without the formation of a cervical esophagostomy.
- Whether to use a gastric tube (reversed and proximally based or antegrade and distally based).

**Congenital Hypertrophic Pyloric Stenosis**

It is characterized by the narrowing or obstruction of the pylorus due to hypertrophy, or thickening, of the pyloric muscle.

*Etiology*

The exact cause of hypertrophic pyloric stenosis is not fully understood, but it is believed to have a multifactorial etiology with genetic, hormonal and developmental factors playing a role. Here are some key factors that contribute to the development of HPS:

- **Genetic factors:** There is evidence to suggest that there may be a genetic predisposition to hypertrophic pyloric stenosis. It often runs in families, and infants born to parents who have had HPS are at a higher risk of developing the condition themselves.
- **Hormonal factors:** An imbalance in certain hormones, such as gastrin, may play a role in stimulating the excessive growth of the pyloric muscles.
- **Developmental factors:** HPS typically becomes evident in the first few weeks of life, suggesting that it may be related to a developmental issue during fetal development or shortly after birth. It is possible that factors affecting the development of the pyloric muscles or the nerves controlling them could contribute to the condition.

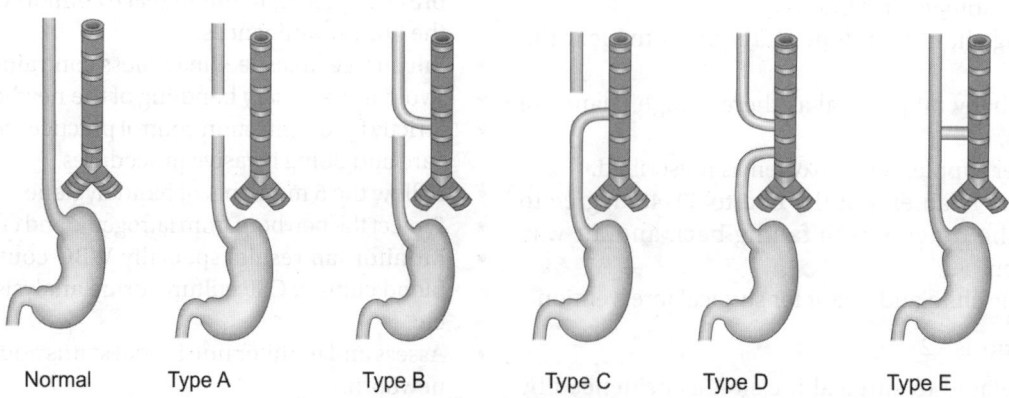

**Fig. 13.3:** Types of esophageal atresia and tracheoesophageal fistula.

## Clinical Features

- **Projectile vomiting:** Infants with HPS often experience forceful and persistent vomiting, typically after feeding.
- **Persistent hunger:** Despite frequent vomiting, affected infants remain hungry and may want to feed more often.
- **Weight loss or poor weight gain:** Due to the vomiting and decreased ability to digest and absorb nutrients, affected infants may fail to thrive and lose weight.
- **Dehydration:** Excessive vomiting can lead to dehydration, which may result in dry mouth, sunken fontanelles (soft spots on the head), and reduced urine output.
- **Palpable "olive-like" mass:** In some cases, a healthcare provider can feel a small, firm lump in the infant's upper abdomen, which corresponds to the enlarged pylorus.
- **Dehydration:** Repeated vomiting can lead to dehydration, which can manifest as dry mouth, dry skin, sunken fontanelles (soft spots on the infant's head), decreased urine output, and increased irritability.
- **Visible peristalsis:** In some cases, visible peristaltic waves (wave-like movements of the stomach muscles) may be observed across the infant's abdomen, especially after feeding.
- **Electrolyte imbalances:** Repeated vomiting can lead to imbalances in electrolytes, such as low levels of potassium (hypokalemia), which can result in muscle weakness and other symptoms.

## Diagnosis

### Medical History and Physical Examination

Detailed medical history, including information about the infant's feeding patterns, vomiting, and weight loss. During the physical examination, the healthcare provider may palpate the infant's abdomen to feel for an olive-shaped mass in the upper abdomen.

- **Abdominal radiograph:** The typical signs associated with congenital hypertrophic pyloric stenosis are as follows:
  - Double/triple track sign
  - Shoulder sign
  - Diamond sign
  - Mushroom sign
  - Caterpillar sign
  - Beak sign
  - Teat sign
- **Upper gastrointestinal (UGI) series:** In some cases, a barium swallow or upper gastrointestinal series may be ordered. This involves having the infant swallow a contrast solution (barium), which can be visualized on X-rays. The test can show the narrowing and elongation of the pyloric canal.

## Management

Infants with HPS often present with dehydration and electrolyte imbalances due to excessive vomiting. Infants with HPS may have low levels of potassium (hypokalemia) and other electrolyte disturbances due to vomiting. These imbalances need to be corrected before surgery.

### Pyloromyotomy

Under general anesthesia the surgeon makes a small incision in the infant's abdomen, typically in the upper right quadrant then the surgeon performs a myotomy, which involves making a longitudinal incision in the thickened muscle of the pylorus. This incision relieves the obstruction and allows the stomach contents to pass into the small intestine. After the myotomy is completed, the surgeon carefully closes the incision with dissolvable sutures or surgical staples.

### Nursing diagnosis - 1

Acute pain related to surgical incision as evidenced by expressive behavior, facial expression of pain, positioning to ease pain, reports intensity using standardized pain scale, altered physiological parameter, guarding behavior, etc.

**Interventions**

- Assess the characteristics of pain like onset, location, intensity, duration
- If the child cannot verbalize assess the level of pain using pain assessment tool (premature infant pain profile, neonatal facial coding system, wong-baker faces pain rating scale, neonatal/infant pain scale, FLACC scale, behavioral pain scale, nonverbal pain scale, visual analogue scale, adolescent pediatric pain tool) as appropriate for the child
- Provide comfortable position and calm and quite environment
- Provide wound care to alleviate pain
- Monitor vitals at regular interval as physiological parameter fluctuates during pain
- Initiate nonpharmacological measures of pain management like distraction techniques, relaxation methods, etc.
- Administer analgesics as advised to the child
- Evaluate the effectiveness and side effect of the analgesics.

### Nursing diagnosis - 2

Deficient fluid volume related to excessive fluid loss as evidenced by dry skin and mucus membrane, decrease skin turgor, sunken fontanels, no tears when crying, lack of bowel activity, oliguria.

### Interventions
- Assess the degree of fluid volume deficit
- Encourage adequate breastfeeding
- Maintain intake and output chart
- Monitor the weight of the baby daily
- Monitor urine volume and color
- Administer IV fluid as prescribed
- Review the lab results like urine specific gravity, serum electrolytes, blood glucose level, etc.

## Anorectal Malformation (ARM)

It is a congenital defect characterized by abnormal development of anus, rectum and urogenital tract. The incidence of ARM is about 1 in 5000 and male babies are more affected than the females. The cause of ARM is unknown.

### Classification

The types of anorectal malformation and postoperative outcomes were evaluated using the Krickenbeck classification. As per the classification system ARM is classified into two major groups:
1. Major clinical groups
2. Rare/regional variants

Both the groups have many other subgroups as described below:

#### Major clinical group
- Perineal fistula
- Rectourethral fistula
- Bulbar
- Prostatic
- Rectovesical fistula
- Vestibular fistula
- No fistula
- Anal stenosis

#### Rare/regional variants
- Pouch colon
- Rectal atresia/stenosis
- Rectovaginal fistula
- Cloaca
- H-type fistula
- Others

### Clinical Manifestations
- Absence of anal opening
- Presence of anal opening in the abnormal location
- Unable to pass meconium
- Passing of meconium through urine
- Abdominal distension
- Vomiting.

### Diagnosis
- Physical examination
- Invertogram
- Cross table radiograph
- Ultrasonography
- CT scan
- MRI

### Management

Medical management of anorectal malformation is not effective. The initial management includes the symptomatic treatment and protective colostomy. Surgical management of ARM vary in male and female (Gangopadhyay AN, Pandey V 2015).

#### Krickenbeck classification of surgical procedures
- Perineal operation
- Anterior sagittal approach
- Sacroperineal approach
- Posterior sagittal anorectoplasty (PSARP)
- Abdominal sacroperineal pull through
- Abdominoperineal pull through
- Laparoscopic-assisted pull through

#### Male newborn
- Posterior sagittal anoplasty or limited PSARP is required for the newborn with rectoperineal fistula. In this case, colostomy is not required.
- The newborn with fistula between rectum and urinary tract requires colostomy to divert the fecal matter.
- PSARP is need for the infant with rectobulbar or rectoprostatic fistula.
- Abdominal approach is needed for patients with rectobladder neck fistula and pouch colon.

#### Female newborn
- The decision about the surgery depends on various factors like length of clinical presentation, number of openings at the vestibule, etc.
- The infant with one opening, sepsis, and abdominal distention requires a colostomy to divert the fecal matter.
- The newborn with rectovestibular anomaly require diversion colostomy and PSARP.
- PSARP is needed to repair the persistent cloaca.

#### Preoperative care

Parul Dutta Pediatric Nursing, 5th Edition and Nancy T Hatfield.

Parent should be counseled and explained regarding the surgical procedure and its requirement.
- Consent from the parent should be taken as per the hospital guideline.

- Previous health history and other relevant information should be collected and documented.
- Assessment of general health status like length, weight, appearance, level of consciousness, etc. should be appropriately mentioned in the document.
- Recording and monitoring of BP, oxygen saturation, temperature, ABG are mandatory.
- All the investigation reports should be collected and attached with the patient file.
- Prior to the surgery baby should be nil per oral (6 hours before if formula feed, 4 hours before if breastfeed and 2 hours before if taken fluid).
- Surgical site should be prepared if required.
- As a nurse ensure that everything is ready as per pre-operative checklist.

**Postoperative care**

Nancy T Hat field, Broadribb's Introductory Pediatric Nursing.
- Immediately after surgery monitoring vitals (BP, $SPO_2$, temperature, respiratory rate) are important for nurses.
- If any postoperative complications arise then surgeon should immediately be informed.
- Maintain respiratory stability and monitor $SPO_2$ regularly.
- If the child is intubated then monitor and record arterial blood gas along with chest radiograph to ensure proper positioning of the tube.
- As the newborn remains nil per oral, hence adequate fluid electrolyte balance should be maintained.
- Input and output chart should be strictly maintained.
- Antibiotic and analgesics should be administered as prescribed.
- Total parental nutrition (TPN) can be provided for the baby with nil per mouth.
- Parents should be explained and educated regarding the treatment.

## Pediatric Emergencies

### Fluid Electrolyte Disturbance

A major portion of the human body is composed of fluid and electrolyte. Therefore, appropriate proportion of both is crucial to maintain homeostasis and optimal physical and mental performance. Dysregulation of fluid and electrolyte is a common issue among all age group during illness. At birth about 75% of body weight is composed of water which reduces to 65% by one year of age. The reduction of body weight is due to the loss of water from the extracellular space. There are two major compartments of the body water called Intracellular water (ICW) and extracellular water (ECW) spaces. The ratio of ICW to ECW is about 2:1 after one year of age and remain constant. Further the extracellular water space has two compartments called interstitial and intravascular space which are at a ratio of 3:1 (Nelson Textbook of Pediatric, 21st Edition).

There are several factors like water intake and output, hydrostatic pressure, oncotic pressure, osmolality, etc., that control the movement and distribution of water in different compartments. Osmolarity refers to the number of solute particles per litter solution whereas osmolality means number of solute particles per kg solvent. The role of the kidney in regulation of water and osmolality is to control the excretion or reabsorption of solute and water under the influence of anti-diuretic hormone and natriuretic peptides. The water gain in the body can be from both endogenous (ingested water, liquid foods and water in solid food) and exogenous (water from oxidation of carbohydrate, protein and fat) sources. Similarly, the water loss from the body occurs in two different ways named as sensible and insensible water loss. Sensible water loss occurs through urination, feces, vomitus, blood loss, etc., and insensible water loss occurs through sweat and respiration. Insensible water loss tends to be higher among preterm neonates as compare to the sensible water loss. As skin of the preterm babies are very thin about 70% of the insensible water loss occurs through it and remaining 30% are from the respiratory tract.

Electrolyte level in the body fluid of different compartment are tightly regulated within a very narrow range. These are important for nerve conduction, functioning of body organs, muscle contraction, maintenance of blood pressure, rebuilding of damaged tissue, etc. Osmolality of the ICF, interstitial fluid and intravascular fluid are in equilibrium state except for transient change. The movement of water or electrolyte across the compartment occurs depending on the difference in the concentration. Usually water moves from low osmolality to high osmolality compartment through permeable membrane. There are five mechanism associated with the derangement of electrolyte level as follows:
1. Underlying disease process
2. End organ injury
3. Fluid and electrolyte interventions
4. Use of medications with potential of electrolyte derangements
5. Application of critical care technology

### Fluid Disturbances

The equilibrium between the intake and output of water depends on various factors like dietary intake, physical activity, age, environmental conditions, etc. Although the total body water is tightly regulated, fluid derangements like dehydration and overhydration are commonly encountered. Dehydration occurs due to lack of fluid intake or too much excretion whereas overhydration occurs as a result of excessive fluid intake.

## Dehydration

Dehydration is a common form of fluid imbalance as a result of excessive water loss. The major cause of dehydration among children are the diarrhea, vomiting, burn, excessive blood loss, congenital adrenal hyperplasia, thyrotoxicosis, cystic fibrosis, diabetic ketoacidosis, diabetic insipidus and diabetic mellitus, etc. Dehydration due to acute diarrheal disease is a significant cause of childhood morbidity and mortality.

### Types of dehydration based on osmolarity

Based on the osmolarity dehydration can be categorized as isotonic, hypotonic and hypertonic.

- **Isonatremic/isotonic:** It occurs when equivalent amount of water and sodium are lost from the extracellular fluid without changing osmolarity (serum sodium: 130–150 mEq/L).
- **Hyponatremic/hypotonic:** It occurs when sodium loss is higher in proportion to the water resulting reduced osmolarity (serum sodium: <130 mEq/L) of the extracellular fluid.
- **Hypernatremic/hypertonic:** It occurs when water loss is higher in proportion to the sodium resulting increased osmolarity (serum sodium: >150 mEq/L) of extracellular fluid.

### Types of dehydration based on severity (as per IMNCI)

- **Severe dehydration:** When two of the following signs are present called severe dehydration.
  - Lethargic or unconsciousness
  - Sunken eyes
  - Not able to drink
  - Skin pinch goes back slowly
- **Some dehydration:** When two of the following signs are present called some dehydration.
  - Restless, irritable
  - Sunken eyes
  - Drinks eagerly, thirsty
  - Skin pinch goes back slowly
- **No dehydration:** Not enough signs to classify as some or severe dehydration.

### Severity of dehydration based on weight loss:

- **Mild dehydration:** When fluid loss is <5% of total body weight.
- **Moderate dehydration:** When fluid loss is 5–10% of total body weight.
- **Severe dehydration:** When fluid loss is >10% of total body weight.

### Clinical features

**Mild dehydration**
- Thirst
- Dry skin
- Oliguria
- Yellowish discoloration of urine
- Muscle cramping
- Dry lips, tongue and mouth
- Crying without tears
- Weakness
- Irritable
- Sleepy

**Moderate dehydration**
- Hypotension
- Yellowish urine
- Faint
- Severe muscle contraction seizure
- Sunken eyes
- Headache
- Dry and loose skin with lack of elasticity
- Tachypnea
- Tachycardia

**Severe dehydration**
- Altered level of consciousness
- Tachycardia
- Hypotension
- Lethargy, irritability
- Cold extremities
- Unable to urinate
- Shock

### Diagnosis

History and clinical examination are the important aspect of diagnosis but lab investigations are also required to specifically classify the dehydration. Investigations are also needed to decide the type and amount of fluid required for the management of dehydration.

- Blood urea
- Serum creatinine
- Serum sodium
- Urine analysis

### Management

Fluid electrolyte management depends on various factors like age, weight, total fluid loss, degree of dehydration and underlying condition, etc.

Based on the gestational age and birthweight the fluid therapy for neonate may be as follows:

**Term baby (>1500 g)**
- **Day 1:** The water loss of a term baby of more than 1500 g through urine is around 50 mL/kg/day and insensible water loss is approximately 10 mL/kg/day. Hence to keep a balance with the output the neonate should receive fluid (10% dextrose) between 60–70 mL/kg/day.
- **Day 2–7:** During this period, the baby excretes more urine and in addition to that passage of stool also contributes to the loss of water. Hence additional 15–20 mL/kg/day of fluid are required to maintain the balance but the maximum fluid input should be within 150 mL/kg/day.
- **After 7 days:** After 7 days the requirement of fluid is higher therefore should be administered at 150–160 mL/kg/day.

**Preterm baby (1000–1500 g)**
- **Day-1:** Although the urine output is same for both preterm and term babies it has been found that the preterm newborn tend to lose more water as compare to the term in the form of insensible water through skin (as preterm neonates have thin skin). Therefore, in addition to the fluid replacement covering the body (cap, sucks. plastic coverings) is also required as it can prevent the loss of water. Hence fluid requirement of preterm neonates is about 80 mL/kg/day in the form of 10% dextrose.
- **Day 2–7:** The fluid requirement of the preterm baby during this period is similar to that of a term baby as the skin becomes mature and there is a reduction in the amount of insensible water loss. But sodium and potassium supplement should be started.
- **After 7 days:** The preterm baby receives fluid similar to the term baby during this period but sodium supplementation should be added and continued up to 32–34 weeks of gestational age.

### Management of dehydration based on severity from 2 months to 5 years

As per the IMNCI guideline the management of dehydration depends on the severity.

- **No dehydration:**
  - According to the guideline child with no dehydration should be treated at home but care should be taken to prevent dehydration.
  - Hence children less than 2 years should receive oral rehydration therapy (ORT) of 50–100 mL after each loose stool and children above 2 years should receive ORT of 100–200 mL after each loose stool.
  - Exclusive breastfeeding should be continued along with ORT.
  - Zinc supplement should be provided as ½ tablet (one tablet = 20 mg) for 14 days for child less than six month of age and 1 tablet for 14 days for child older than six months.

- **Some dehydration:**
  - Child with signs of some dehydration should be given ORS at the clinical setting over 4 hours based on age and weight **(Table 13.4)**.
    If age is not known then use following formula to calculate approximate amount of ORS requirement:
    Approximate ORS requirement = Weight in kg × 75
  - After four hours of ORS therapy child should be assessed again for degree of dehydration. And further treatment should be adopted based on type of dehydration.
  - Breastfeeding should be continued.
  - Extra fluid should be provided.
  - Zinc supplement should be provided as ½ tablet (one tablet = 20 mg) for 14 days for child less than six month of age and 1 tablet for 14 days for child older than six months.

- **Severe dehydration:**
  - Immediate administration of IV fluid is required for child with severe dehydration to restore the intravascular volume quickly. For an infant below 1 year of age administer 30 mL/kg of Ringer lactate solution or normal saline over 1 hour followed by 70 mL/kg over 5 hours. Similarly, for child between 1–5 years of age administer 30 mL/kg of Ringer lactate solution or normal saline over 30 minutes followed by 70 mL/kg over 2 hours 30 minutes.
  - Reassess the child to identify the rehydration status every 1–2 hours.
  - After restoration of the intravascular volume total fluid deficit should be corrected by ORT.
  - If diarrhea persists even after restoration of rehydration then fluid replacement is required to

| Table 13.4: ORS requirement as per age and weight (as per WHO). | | | | |
|---|---|---|---|---|
| Age | Up to 4 months | 4 months to 1 year | 1–2 years | 2–5 years |
| Weight in kg | <6 | 6–<10 | 10–<12 | 12–19 |
| ORS in mL | 200–400 | 400–700 | 700–900 | 900–1400 |

compensate the ongoing loss of water through stool. The fluid replacement for large amount of watery stool should be as followings

- After rapid restoration of intravascular volume, correction of fluid deficit and replacement of ongoing loss next step is the maintenance of fluid and electrolyte balance. To calculate the amount of fluid to be administered for maintenance Holliday – Segar method can be followed:
  - 100 mL per kg/day or 4 mL/kg/hour for first 10 kg
  - Then 50 mL for each kg for next 10 kg
  - Then 20 mL/kg for each subsequent kg.

  *Example:*
  - A child of 7 kg weight should receive 7 × 100 mL = 700 mL/day.
  - Similarly, a child of 25 kg should receive (10 × 100 mL) + (10 × 50 mL) + (5 × 20 mL) = 1600 mL/day.

### Water Intoxication

It is a very rare condition which occurs when intake of water is much higher than excretion. Excessive water intake dilutes the blood and as a result this hyponatremia develops. Due to osmosis the water crosses the blood brain barrier and accumulates inside the brain causing edema and neurological symptoms.

In infants, water intoxication can happen while feeding the baby with excessive diluted formula, juice, etc. But in case of older children this may be due to unhealthy mental condition, child abuse, excessive drinking during exercises to replenish the water loss, etc.

### Clinical features

- Irritability
- Excessive urination
- Vomiting
- Muscle cramps
- Edema
- Hypothermia
- Drowsiness
- Poor coordination
- Lethargy

### Diagnosis

Diagnosis can be made by taking detailed history of the patient specifically about amount of fluid intake. In addition to that serum electrolyte should be assessed as excessive water intake causes hyponatremia.

### Management

- The amount of fluid intake should be restricted
- Intake and output chart should be strictly followed
- To treat hyponatremia hypertonic saline should be started
- In severe cases like child with neurological symptoms diuretics should be used to excrete excess water.

### Electrolyte Disturbances

The most common electrolyte derangements in children are the hypo/hypernatremia and hypo/hyperkalemia.

### Hyponatremia

Sodium is one of the electrolytes which is required in a large amount from external sources. It helps in nerve conduction, regulation of muscle contraction and maintenance of fluid balance in the body, etc. The normal range of serum sodium is about 135–145 mEq/L. Hyponatremia is defined as serum sodium level below 135 mEq/L. Based on the level of sodium in the blood serum hyponatremia can be classified as follows: (Hyponatremia: Practice Essentials, Pathophysiology, Epidemiology from: https://emedicine.medscape.com/article/242166-overview).

- **Mild hyponatremia:** Serum sodium 130–134 mEq/L.
- **Moderate hyponatremia:** Serum sodium 125–129 mEq/L.
- **Severe hyponatremia:** Serum sodium <125 mEq/L.

### Etiology

- Hyperglycemia
- Vomiting
- Diarrhea
- Burn
- Cirrhosis of liver
- Water intoxication
- Administration of diuretics
- Polycystic kidney disease
- Nephrotic syndrome
- Obstructive uropathy
- Hypothyroidism
- Syndrome of inappropriate antidiuretic hormone (SIADH)
- Deficiency of glucocorticoid.

### Clinical features

Hyponatremia results decrease in the ECF osmolality therefore water moves through the blood brain barrier and accumulate inside the brain causing edema. Cerebral edema causes neurological manifestation which is one of the dangerous features of the hyponatremia. The child with hyponatremia may have following clinical presentations (Nelson Textbook of Pediatric, 21st Edition):

- Apnea due to brain stem herniation
- Anorexia
- Nausea and vomiting
- Lethargy

- Confusion
- Irritability
- Seizure
- Coma
- Reduced reflexes
- Hypothermia
- Weakness
- Muscle cramps

## Diagnosis

Diagnosis of hyponatremia can be done by detecting plasma/serum sodium level. A detailed history may help to identify the underline cause of hyponatremia. The common laboratory investigations are the plasma osmolality, urine osmolality and urine sodium.

## Management

The management of hyponatremia depends on variety of factors like cause of hyponatremia, severity of the symptoms, duration of hyponatremia, etc.

- Child with severe neurological symptoms like seizure, altered level of conscious ness should be immediately treated with 3–5 mL/kg of 3% normal saline (hypertonic saline) as initial therapy. After initial therapy serum sodium should be assessed to decide further treatment. If the child still has seizure, then initial treatment should be repeated and if the neurological symptom of the child is reduced then treatment should be started to correct the sodium level at a rate of 6–8 mEq/L over 24 hours.
- Child with mild to no symptoms don't require rapid correction/initial hypertonic saline infusion. Such children need supervision and monitoring of new neurological symptom. The goal of the initial treatment for these children is to resolve the underlying cause of hyponatremia. The target of hyponatremia correction among these children is about 6–8 mEq/L over 24 hours.
- Central pontine myelinolysis (CPM) is very common among chronic hyponatraemic patients as compare to acute patients. CPM develops when attempt is made for rapid serum sodium correction at a rate > 12 mEq/L/24 hours or >18 mEq/L/48 hours.
- Child with SIADH should be under fluid restriction. Furosemide is effective in these patients as it causes excretion of water. Vasopressin antagonists also can be administered to counteract the action of ADH.

## *Hypernatremia*

Hypernatremia is defined as elevated serum sodium level greater than 145 mEq/L. The three basic mechanism that leads to hypernatremia are the following:
1. Sodium intoxication
2. Water deficit
3. Water and sodium deficit but the deficit of water is higher than sodium.

**Types based on serum concentration:**
- Mild (148–150 mEq/L)
- Moderate (151–154 mEq/L)
- Severe (≥155 mEq/L).

**Etiology**
- **Sodium intoxication:**
  - Excessive addition of sodium in to formula
  - Excessive administration of hypertonic saline
  - Hyperaldosteronism (causes retention of sodium)
  - Intake of excess sodium bicarbonate (baking soda)
- **Water deficit:**
  - Diabetic insipidus
  - Wolfram syndrome
  - Excessive insensible water loss
  - Inadequate water intake (lack of breastfeeding, child abuse or neglect)
- **Water and sodium deficit:**
  - Diarrhea
  - Vomiting
  - Burns
  - Excessive sweating
  - Diabetic mellitus
  - Chronic kidney disease
  - Treatment with osmotic diuretics

## Clinical features

**Acute hypernatremia**

In acute hypernatremia, there is a transient increase in the sodium concentration in the ECF causes efflux of water from the intracellular compartment resulting cellular dehydration. When this phenomenon occurs in the CNS brain size shrinks and cerebral vasculatures start to rupture causing hemorrhage and neurological symptoms. Following are some of the clinical features of acute hypernatremia (Piyush Gupta, 2021):
- Irritability
- Fever
- High pitched cry
- Lethargy
- Altered level of consciousness
- Coma
- Seizure
- Oliguria
- Weakness
- Tachypnea
- Cerebral hemorrhage
- Hypovolemia
- Features of dehydration
- Delayed capillary refill time

## Chronic hypernatremia (>48 hours)

The children with chronic hypernatremia are usually asymptomatic because of the CNS adaptive ability. During adaptive phase water moves from CSF to the brain to compensate the fluid loss. In addition to that the intracellular solutes start to increase either by uptake from outside or by intracellular synthesis. Elevation of osmolytes inside the cell draws water and prevent cellular dehydration.

**Diagnosis**
- Serum sodium
- Urinary sodium
- Serum osmolarity
- Urea and creatinine
- Brain imaging (CT/MRI) to rule out intracranial space occupying lesion and other pathological conditions
- Serum aldosterone
- Serum cortisol
- ADH (to detect or exclude diabetic insipidus)

## Management

**Correction of hypernatremia**

Correction of hypernatremia should be done with hypotonic saline (0.45% of normal saline) to replenish the water deficit. In case of chronic hypernatremia, the cerebral adaptation mechanism corrects the intracellular dehydration and restores the cerebral volume. Therefore, rapid infusion of hypotonic saline should be avoided as it may cause accumulation of water in the brain causing cerebral edema. The recommended rate of correction of serum sodium is below 0.5 mEq/L per hour or 10–12 mEq/L/day. Due to safety concern the rate of correction is also same in case of acute hypernatremia. Once the child passes urine potassium should be administered at a dose of 20 mEq/L to facilitate influx of water into the cell. If serum sodium is above 180 mEq/L then peritoneal dialysis should be initiated.

**Fluid resuscitation**

Any child with marked hypovolemia should be treated immediately with isotonic solution (0.9% normal saline) to replenish the fluid deficit. The amount of fluid to be replaced can be calculated using following formula:

Replacement volume (in L) = TBW deficit × 1 ÷ [1 − (Na concentration in replacement fluid in mEq/L ÷ 154 mEq/L)]

The total body water (TBW) in children is about 60% of the total body weight.
Hence TBW = 0.6 × Weight.

**Other modalities**
- Peritoneal dialysis should be done if the child is having renal failure, obstructive uropathy, serum sodium >180 mEq/L.
- Surgery should be performed in case of polycystic kidney disease, renal dysplasia and reflux nephropathy.

### Hypokalemia

Potassium is the second most cation which is abundant in the body. About 98% of the potassium are present in the ICF and remaining 2% are in the ECF. The concentration of the potassium in the serum is between 3.5–5.5 mEq/L. Hypokalemia is defined as serum potassium level <3.5 mEq/L. Based on the serum concentration the severity of hypokalemia can be as follows:
- **Mild hypokalemia:** Serum potassium 3.0–3.5 mEq/L.
- **Moderate hypokalemia:** Serum potassium 2.5–3.0 mEq/L.
- **Severe hypokalemia:** Serum potassium <2.5 mEq/L.

### Etiology

- **Reduced intake:**
  - Anorexia nervosa
  - Starvation
  - Pica
  - Dysphagia
  - Alcoholism
- **Excessive loss:**
  - Diarrhea
  - Vomiting
  - Excessive sweating
  - Nasogastric aspiration
  - Severe burn
  - Laxative abuse
  - Diuretics use
  - Bartter syndrome
  - Cushing syndrome
  - Diabetic ketoacidosis
  - Dialysis
- **Transcellular shift from ECF to ICF:**
  - Insulin therapy
  - Alkalosis
  - Hyperthyroidism
  - Barium poisoning
  - Periodic paralysis
  - Refeeding syndrome
- **Drugs:**
  - Theophylline
  - Hydroxychloroquine
  - Verapamil
  - Ampicillin
  - Cisplatin
  - Amphotericin B
  - Aminoglycosides

## Clinical features

- Muscle weakness starts from limb then trunk and respiratory muscles
- Paralytic ileus
- Ventricular fibrillation
- Tachycardia
- Muscle cramps
- Reduced GI motility: Constipation
- Polyuria
- Polydipsia

## Diagnosis

- Serum potassium level
- Urine potassium level
- ECG changes: Flattened 'T' wave, depressed ST segment, appearance of 'U' wave
- Abdominal ultrasound or CT scan if adrenal tumor or hyperplasia is suspected

## Management

The aim of the treatment is to correct the potassium deficiency and its underlying cause. The child with mild hypokalemia may recover spontaneously but in some cases oral potassium is administered at a dose of 2-4 mEq/kg/day with maximum dose of 120-240 mEq/day. The child with severe hypokalemia or with symptoms should be administered with intravenous potassium supplement at a dose of 0.5-1.0 mEq/kg over 1 hour. The child receiving IV potassium should be monitored continuously for ECG changes.

### Hyperkalemia

Hyperkalemia is defined as a serum potassium level greater than 5.5 mEq/L. It can be classified into three types based on the serum concentration as follows:
- **Mild hyperkalemia:** Serum potassium 5.5-6.5 mEq/L
- **Moderate hyperkalemia:** Serum potassium 6.5-7.5 mEq/L
- **Severe hyperkalemia:** Serum potassium >7.5 mEq/L.

## Etiology

- **Excessive intake:**
  - Iatrogenic increase of potassium
  - Blood transfusion
  - Excessive dietary intake
- **Transcellular shift from ICF to ECF:**
  - Metabolic acidosis
  - Tissue injury: Rhabdomyolysis, tumor lysis syndrome, burn, surgery, tissue necrosis
  - Hemolysis
  - Exercise
  - Deficiency of insulin
  - Digitalis poisoning
- **Reduced excretion:**
  - Renal failure
  - Adrenal failure: Hypoaldosteronism, congenital adrenal hyperplasia, Addison disease
  - Sickle cell disease
  - Obstructive uropathy
  - *Drugs:* ACE inhibitors, potassium sparing diuretics, heparin, NSAIDs, angiotensin II blockers.

## Clinical features

- Tachycardia
- Ventricular fibrillation
- Nausea
- Vomiting
- Paresthesia
- Changes in the ECG
- Muscle weakness
- Ascending paralysis

## Diagnosis

- Serum potassium
- Urine analysis
- Serum urea and creatinine
- **ECG changes:** Peak 'T' wave, prolonged PR interval, Widen QRS complex, ST segment depression

## Management

The aims of the management of hyperkalemia are to prevent arrythmia by stabilizing the heart and removal of excessive potassium.

To stabilize the heart 10% calcium gluconate at a dose of 0.5-1.0 mL/kg over 1-3 minutes should be administered IV under cardiac monitoring. Calcium stabilizes the heart and there by prevent arrythmia, its action is very rapid. Sodium bicarbonate also helps to prevent arrhythmia by shifting the potassium from ECF to ICF. Insulin also helps to move the potassium intracellularly there by lowers the concentration in ECF. Insulin administration can cause hypoglycemia hence should be given along with glucose. Nebulized beta-adrenergic drugs like salbutamol or terbutaline also helps in reducing serum potassium concentration.

For excretion of potassium from the body diuretics should be administered if patient is not anuric. Dialysis may be required in patients with severe renal failure or severe hyperphosphatemia resistant to drug therapy. Sodium polystyrene sulfonate is an exchange resin administered rectally or orally. The sodium part of the resin is exchanged with potassium and then potassium polystyrene sulfonate is excreted from the body. Some patient may require dietary modification as a long-term management.

## Nursing Management

### Nursing diagnosis - 1

Deficient fluid volume related to excessive fluid loss as evidenced by dry skin and mucus membrane, decrease skin turgor, sunken fontanels, no tears when crying, lack of bowel activity, oliguria.

**Interventions**
- Monitor vitals and oxygen saturation for baseline data
- Assess the degree of fluid volume deficit
- Encourage adequate breastfeeding
- Maintain intake and output chart
- Monitor the weight of the baby daily
- Monitor urine volume and color
- Administer IV fluid as prescribed
- Review the lab results like urine specific gravity, serum electrolytes, blood glucose level, etc.
- Monitor the signs of shock.

### Nursing diagnosis - 2

Risk for electrolyte imbalance related to diarrhea, vomiting, excessive fluid volume, insufficient fluid volume.

**Interventions**
- Assess vital signs, cardiovascular, respiratory, renal and mental status routinely
- Monitor and record intake and output
- Measure child's weight daily to detect fluid volume excess at early stage
- If the child is dehydrated provide ORS or IV fluid as prescribed
- Provide supplemental oxygen as prescribed
- Monitor lab reports like serum electrolyte, ABG, urine analysis, etc.
- Investigate to find out the cause of fluid electrolyte imbalance
- Monitor the signs of shock
- Administer blood products to correct fluid loss as prescribed
- Encourage to drink plenty of fluid if dehydrated
- Educate the child and family members regarding preventive measures of fluid electrolyte imbalance
- Demonstrate methods of input and output measurement and instruct to monitor at home
- Provide antidotes or electrolyte supplements based on prescription.

## Acute Bronchopneumonia

It is one of the oldest diseases and number one cause of mortality in developing countries. Each year 150 million of childhood pneumonia cases are reported globally, out of which developing countries contribute approximately 95% and India alone is contributing one fourth of the total global cases.

### Pneumonia

It is defined as an inflammation of lung parenchyma due to infection. Noninfective inflammation of lung parenchyma is called as pneumonitis.

### Definition

It is defined as acute (less than 3 weeks) exudative and suppurative peribronchiolar inflammation resulting multi focal patchy consolidations in one or more lobules of the lung. This is also called as lobular pneumonia and commonly caused by bacteria.

### Etiology

A Parthasarathy et. al., IAP Textbook of Pediatrics, 7th Ed., 2019.

Acute bronchopneumonia primarily caused by bacteria and rarely caused by viruses.

Based on age following pathogens causes bronchopneumonia among newborn and children:

- **0–3 months:** Gram negative enterobacteriaceae, enterococci, *Chlamydia trachomatis*, Group B streptococci, *Hemophilus influenzae*, Listeria monocytogens.
- **1–5 years:** *Streptococcus pneumoniae, Hemophilus influenzae, Staphylococcus, Mycoplasma pneumoniae.*
- **>5 years:** *Streptococcus pneumoniae, Staphylococcus, Staphylococcus pyogenes, Mycoplasma pneumoniae.*

### Grading of Pneumonia

As per WHO pneumonia is classified in to three different types based on clinical presentations as described in the:

*Pneumonia*
- Cough
- Fast breath
- Fever <38.5°C
- No feeding difficulty
- No dehydration

*Severe Pneumonia*
- Fever >39°C
- Fast breath
- Retraction
- Grunting
- Bronchial breath sound with or without crackle
- Poor feeding
- Dehydration
- $SPO_2 \geq 92$ at room air
- Chest X-ray with or without opacity

## Very Severe Pneumonia
- Poor feeding
- Altered sensorium
- Intermittent apneic spell
- Cyanosis
- Excessive sweating
- Narrow pulse pressure
- Decreased PH
- $SPO_2$ < 92 at room air

## Clinical Features

The classical triad of affected child are the fever, tachypnea/dyspnea and cough (fever and cough are the rare presentation of the neonate but are common among infant and children). But the clinical presentation varies based on the age of the child as described in the:

### Neonate
- Tachypnea (>60 breaths/min)
- Grunting
- Retraction
- Hypoxemia
- Hyperirritability
- Lethargy
- Feeding intolerance
- Intermittent apnea
- Cyanosis
- Cough and fever are the rare manifestation

### Infants
- Fever
- Cough
- Tachypnea (>50 breaths/min)
- Grunting (rare in older infant)
- Excess irritability
- Poor feeding
- Hypoxemia
- Lethargy
- Vomiting
- Wheezing

### Older Children and Adolescents
- Fever
- Cough
- Tachypnea (1–5 years: >40 breaths/min, 6–12 years: >30 breaths/min, 12 years or older: >20 breaths/min)
- Dyspnea
- Chest pain
- Lethargy
- Headache
- Vomiting
- Diarrhea
- Dehydration
- Abdominal pain
- Otalgia

## Diagnosis
- Diagnosis of pneumonia is primarily based on the clinical presentation and very rarely require laboratory investigations.
- Sputum and blood culture can be done to identify the specific pathogen.
- Bronchoscopy and lung aspiration are highly reliable invasive procedure but are not routinely performed as these are too invasive.
- Chest X-ray may reveal multifocal patches in the lobules.
- Additionally, CBC, ESR and CRP can be done but are not specifically indicate pneumonia.
- Monitoring $SPO_2$ is mandatory during hospitalization of all affected children.

## Nursing Management

### Nursing Diagnosis - 1

Ineffective breathing pattern related to decreased lung function as evidenced by altered tidal volume, decreased inspiratory and/or expiratory pressure, decreased vital capacity, hypercapnia, hypoxemia, hypoxia, orthopnea, uses accessory muscles to breathe.

### Interventions
- Assess respiratory status for presence of any adventitious breath sound, rate, chest retraction, etc.
- Assess oxygen saturation continuously
- Assess function of accessory muscle of respiration
- Provide high fowlers position to the child to promote optimal lung expansion and oxygenation
- Administer humidified supplemental oxygen as prescribed
- Assess signs of hypoxia regularly
- Suction the air way as required to clear the secretions
- Administer antibiotics, bronchodilators, steroids as prescribed
- Review the ABG results and other lab results
- Ensure the ventilator and emergency respiratory support equipment are available at bedside.
- Monitor ventilator alarms and settings
- Educate the child about appropriate technique of coughing (after taking deep breath hold for 2 seconds then cough 2/3 times)
- Demonstrate breathing exercise using incentive spirometer
- Advise intermittent rest during ambulation and activities.

## Nursing Diagnosis - 2

Ineffective thermoregulation related to inflammatory body response secondary to infection as evidenced by increased body temperature from normal range, flushed skin, skin warm to touch, slow capillary refill time, tachycardia.

### Interventions
- Assess body temperature of the newborn every 4 hourly or use skin probe for continuous monitoring
- Maintain proper ventilation in the ward
- Follow aseptic technique while performing any invasive procedure
- If possible, avoid unnecessary invasive procedures
- Provide cold compress to the child
- Remove excessive clothing
- Provide antipyretics and antibiotics as prescribed
- Monitor lab results like WBC count, CRP level, ESR, blood and CSF culture, etc.

## Nursing Diagnosis - 3

Ineffective airway clearance related to retained secretions as evidenced by altered respiratory rhythm, adventitious breath sounds, cyanosis, hypoxemia, nasal flaring, subcostal retraction, tachypnea, uses accessory muscle to breathe.

### Interventions
- Assess the patency of the air way specially in case of trauma or neurological injury.
- Auscultate for detection of abnormal breath sound and recording of vitals, $SPO_2$ are also important.
- Provide prone position which is found to be beneficial in improving lung oxygenation and function hence should be provided if possible.
- Suctioning should be done as required to clear the airway.
- Chest physiotherapy are also quite helpful to remove excess secretions but should be performed if indicated.
- Maintenance of fluid balance along with recording input and output is also required
- Encourage the child for adequate fluid intake as hydration can liquify the tenacious secretions in the respiratory tract and can help in easy clearance
- Educate family members about the need of hydration, appropriate technique of taking medications, need of breathing exercise and diet requirement, etc.
- Advise patient and family members to avoid overcrowding places and polluted environments
- Educate the parents for timely immunization specially haemophilus influenzae b and pneumococcal vaccine

## Nursing Diagnosis - 4

Imbalanced nutrition less than body requirement related to inadequate interest in food, inadequate knowledge of nutrient requirement as evidenced by food intake less than recommended daily allowance, lethargy.

### Interventions
- Calculate BMI and assess the nutritional status of the child
- Investigate the cause of imbalanced nutrition
- Monitor weight of the child daily and plot on the graph
- Provide oral care to improve appetite
- Assist the child while eating if required
- Provide small all frequent meals which can be well tolerated and digested
- Provide nutritional supplements as appropriate
- Educate the family members and the child if applicable about the type of nutrition and recommended daily allowance as appropriate
- Consult nutritionist for individualized diet plan
- Administer enteral feeding and if indicated total parenteral nutrition in critical cases.

## Acute Respiratory Distress Syndrome

Pediatric acute respiratory distress syndrome (PARDS) is a significant cause of morbidity and mortality in children. Children with PARDS often require intensive care admission and mechanical ventilation. Acute respiratory distress syndrome (ARDS) is a clinical syndrome caused by injury of the alveolar endothelium which increase permeability of the alveolar capillary barrier unrelated to cardiogenic pulmonary edema.

### Causes

There are several pulmonary and nonpulmonary causes resulting disruption of the alveolar endothelium as follows:
- Sepsis
- Pneumonia
- Bronchiolitis
- Aspiration of vomitus
- Chest trauma
- Burn
- Inhalation of harmful fumes
- Transfusion related acute lung injury (TRAIL)
- Pancreatitis
- Drug reaction
- Lung cancer

### Clinical Features

Although in many cases clinical feature develops within hours but it may gradually take 1-5 days. The affected neonate may show following features:
- Tachypnea
- Cough

- Hypoxemia
- Pulmonary edema
- Crackle sound on auscultation
- Fever
- Abdominal pain in case of pancreatitis
- Fatigue

### *Pathophysiology*

In a healthy individual, the alveolar epithelium consists of two types of cells called type-I and type-II pneumocytes. Type-I cells are the thin and squamous making approximately 95% of the internal surface. These cells help in gas exchange and regulation of ion and fluid balance. The type-II pneumocytes are the larger and cuboidal cells found in between the type-I cells. These cells have sodium dependant channels for excretion of excess amount of alveolar fluid. They also secret pulmonary surfactants and help in the repairing of alveolar epithelium after injury. The alveolar epithelium is in close approximation with the pulmonary capillary endothelial network making a thin gas blood barrier allowing for gas exchange. Disruption in the integrity of alveolar epithelium and capillary endothelium due to direct or indirect lung injury increases permeability and edema. There pathophysiological mechanism of pulmonary edema are multi-faceted but the major mechanism are as follows (Matthay MA, Zemans RL, 2019):

- Decreased excretion of alveolar fluid due to injury of type-II pneumocytes
- Increase permeability of alveolar epithelium and capillary endothelium
- Disruption of epithelial and endothelial barrier due to necrosis or apoptosis.

### *Diagnosis*

- **History and physical exam:** A detailed inquiry about the fever, cough, chest pain, hemoptysis, known aspiration, abdominal pain along with inspection of trauma, surgery, recent medications are crucial.
- **Laboratory investigations:** CBC, blood chemistry, liver function test, coagulation profile, ABG analysis.
- **Imaging:** Chest radiograph, CT scan, chest ultrasound (currently under investigation).
- **Other:** ECG, sputum or endotracheal aspirates for culture.

### *Management*

#### *Ventilation*

Ventilation is the main stay of treatment for ARDS in critical care unit. The Pediatric Acute Lung Injury Consensus Conference (**PALICC**) recommends tidal volume 3–6 mL/kg for patients with poor compliance and 5–8 mL/kg for patients with preserved compliance. Additionally, SPO$_2$ should be maintained between 92–97% for mild and 88–92% for patient with PEEP 10 cm H$_2$O by administering oxygen.

#### *Surfactant therapy*

Although there are several clinical trials showing improvement in the oxygenation with surfactant therapy but is not always consistent. Therefore, PALICC does not recommend routine administration of exogenous surfactant.

#### *Fluid Balance*

As fluid over load and pulmonary edema are the frequent complains in ARDS maintenance of fluid balance is crucial. There are several studies supporting that maintaining fluid balance for longer than 7 days improves lung functions.

#### *Nutrition*

PALICC recommends optimal nutritional balance to meet metabolic need, adequate growth and early recovery.

#### *Corticosteroids*

Inflammation has a major role in the development of ARDS hence corticosteroid is administered in 20–60% of patients.

### **Nursing Management**

#### Nursing Diagnosis - 1

Ineffective breathing pattern related to decreased lung function as evidenced by altered tidal volume, decreased inspiratory and/or expiratory pressure, decreased vital capacity, hypercapnia, hypoxemia, hypoxia, orthopnea, uses accessory muscles to breathe.

#### Interventions

- Assess respiratory status for presence of any adventitious breath sound, rate, chest retraction, etc.
- Assess oxygen saturation continuously
- Assess function of accessory muscle of respiration
- Provide high fowlers position to the child
- Administer supplemental oxygen as prescribed
- Assess signs of hypoxia regularly
- Suction the air way as required to clear the secretions
- Administer antibiotics, bronchodilators, steroids as prescribed
- Review the ABG results and other lab results
- Ensure the ventilator and emergency respiratory support equipments are available at bedside
- Monitor ventilator alarms and settings
- Encourage coughing and deep breathing
- Demonstrate breathing exercise using incentive spirometer
- Advise intermittent rest during ambulation and activities.

*Nursing Diagnosis - 2*

Ineffective thermoregulation related to inflammatory body response secondary to infection as evidenced by increased body temperature from normal range, flushed skin, skin warm to touch, slow capillary refill time, tachycardia.

Interventions

- Assess body temperature of the newborn every 4 hourly or use skin probe for continuous monitoring
- Maintain proper ventilation in the ward
- Follow aseptic technique while performing any invasive procedure
- If possible, avoid unnecessary invasive procedures
- Provide cold compress to the child
- Remove excessive clothing
- Provide antipyretics and antibiotics as prescribed
- Monitor lab results like WBC count, CRP level, ESR, blood and CSF culture, etc.

*Nursing Diagnosis - 3*

Ineffective airway clearance related to retained secretions as evidenced by altered respiratory rhythm, adventitious breath sounds, cyanosis, hypoxemia, nasal flaring, subcostal retraction, tachypnea, uses accessory muscle to breathe.

Interventions

- Assess the patency of the air way specially in case of trauma or neurological injury.
- Auscultate for detection of abnormal breath sound and recording of vitals, $SPO_2$ are also important.
- Provide prone position which is found to be beneficial in improving lung oxygenation and function hence should be provided if possible.
- Suctioning should be done as required to clear the airway.
- Chest physiotherapy are also quite helpful to remove excess secretions but should be performed if indicated.
- Maintenance of fluid balance along with recording input and output is also required.
- Educate the child if possible about appropriate technique of coughing (after taking deep breath hold for 2 seconds then cough 2/3 times).

## Poisoning

Poisoning is when cells are injured or destroyed by the inhalation, ingestion, injection or absorption of a toxic substance. Poisoning among pediatric population is commonly accidental in nature. Children are highly vulnerable as they put items in their mouth because of curiosity and explorative nature. Boys are more affected as compare to the girls all over the globe may be due to the difference in the socialization.

### Common Poisoning Agents

A poison can enter the body through inhalation, ingestion, direct contact with the skin, or injection. Following are the most common poisoning agents identified in the south-east Asia region:

- Pesticides, insecticides, rodenticides, herbicides
- Kerosene
- Prescribed medications/drugs (paracetamol, vitamins, iron tablets, antihistamines, NSAIDS, narcotics, antidepressants, etc.)
- Household chemicals (bleach, detergent, vinegar)
- Paraffin
- Cosmetic products
- Poisonous plants and seeds
- Bite and stings of animals or insects (snake, scorpion, bees, spiders)
- Metals (lead found in battery; mercury found in thermometer)

*Acute vs Chronic Exposure*

Acute exposure means one time contact with the poisoning agent for seconds, minutes or hours or multiple exposures for a day or less.

Chronic exposure means contact with the poisoning agent for a prolonged period from several days, months or years.

### Clinical Features and Associated Poisoning Agent

- Difficulty in breathing (narcotics, organophosphates, barbiturates, benzodiazepines)
- Diarrhea (antibiotics, arsenic, iron, boric acid)
- Constipation (lead, narcotics, botulism)
- Tachypnea (amphetamines, aspirin, ethylene glycol, cyanide)
- Bradypnea (alcohol, narcotics, barbiturates)
- Skin rashes (boric acid, cyanides, mercury, anticholinergics)
- Fever (Anticholinergics, cocaine)
- Mydriasis (atropine, alcohol, cocaine, carbon monoxide)
- Myosis (organophosphate, phenol, morphine, nicotine, barbiturates)
- Seizure (organochlorines, chlorinated hydrocarbons, cocaine, isoniazid, phenothiazine, carbon monoxide, theophylline)
- Cyanosis (nitrate, organophosphates, aniline dyes, dapsone)
- Cardiac arrythmias (tricyclic antidepressants, amphetamine, aluminum phosphide, digitalis, theophylline, arsenic, cyanide, chloroquine)
- Excessive salivation (organophosphates, salicylates, corrosives)

- Dysphasia (due to ingestion of corrosive substance)
- Diaphoresis (organophosphates, nitrates, aspirin, cocaine)
- Dry or hot skin (anticholinergics, botulism)
- Coma (sedatives, narcotics, lead poisoning, organophosphate).

### *Management*

The initial assessment of a suspected patient with unknown toxin exposure should be aimed to treat the patient rather than treating poison. The highest priority should be given to the airway assessment, breathing and circulation. Assessment of $SPO_2$ by pulse oximeter, vitals, ABG, blood glucose, serum electrolyte and other potential life-threatening abnormality are also important. As antidotes are not available for all the toxins the primary treatment should be non-specific and symptomatic. The principles of management of poisoning are as follows:

#### *Principles of Management*

#### Emergency stabilization measures

Clearing the airway, maintaining patency and ventilation are the emergency procedure for stabilizing oxygen saturation. To prevent aspiration specially if the patient is unconscious then transportation should be done by head down semi prone position. Emergency stabilization of seizure, arrythmia, metabolic abnormality, agitation, hypoglycemia, hyperkalemia is important concern. Assessment of vitals and level of consciousness at regular interval is also required.

#### Removal of toxin

- **Eye decontamination:** Exposure to hydrocarbon, detergents, alcohol, acids or alkali may cause serious damage to the tissue therefore immediate local decontamination is required by irrigating the eye with normal saline or water at least for 30 mins. The solution used for irrigation should be PH neutral, acid or alkali should not be used for irrigation. Irrigation should be done till the PH of conjunctival sac reaches 7.4.
- **Skin decontamination:** Immediately remove the clothes and irrigate the whole body with soap and water or only water or normal saline at least for 15 minutes. Physically remove the contaminant. If skin is exposed to sodium and phosphorus then should not be irrigated with water. Skin decontamination also can be done by specific agents like mineral oil for sodium, neosporin for super glue and calcium gluconate for hydrofluoric acid.
- **GI decontamination:** This can be done by gastric emptying, adsorbent administration and catharsis. Gastric emptying should be performed within 1 hours of exposure for optimal effectiveness. Emesis and gastric lavage are the preferred methods of gastric emptying. Vomiting can be triggered by administering large amount of warm water or by administration of emetic drug like syrup ipecac. For induction of emesis ipecac should be administered at a dose of 10 mL in children >6 months, 15 mL for children >1 year. Vomiting should not be induced in case of corrosive agent poisoning, kerosine poisoning, unconscious patient. Gastric lavage is preferred if vomiting is contraindicated or for quick removal of poison. Usually 4/5 washes are performed using tap water for gastric lavage. The volume of each aliquot should be at least 10-15 mL/kg until clear. Ingestion of activated charcoal in for conscious and active patient is indicated for gastric decontamination.
- **Adsorbent:** It is the agent which can effectively bind the toxin in the gut. Activated charcoal is the widely used adsorbent. If the patient is conscious then can be ingested orally but for unconscious patients can be administered via orogastric or nasogastric route within 1-2 hours of exposure to toxic material. Activated charcoal should be administered at least 10 times the dose of toxin. Generally, the dose is 1-2 g/kg for both adult and children.
- **Catharsis:** These are the laxatives and purgatives indicated when the toxic material is not corrosive. Sorbitol, mannitol, magnesium sulfate and sodium sulfate are the commonly used cathartics. These agents increase gastric motility there by minimize the absorption via gastric mucosa.

#### Specific antidote administration

Antidotes are the agents administered to counteract the toxin (**Table 13.5**). These can be classified as mechanical, chemical and physiological antidotes based on mechanism of action. Mechanical antidotes prevent absorption by adsorbing, coating or dissolving the toxin. Chemical antidotes counteract the toxins by altering the chemical nature of the toxin by complex formation and metabolic conversion. Physiological antidotes work by producing opposite effect that of the toxin. Some of the important toxins and their antidotes are discussed below.

#### Enhancing excretion of toxin

- **Forced diuresis:** It is induced by administering a fluid overload and a diuretic simultaneously. The patient with anuria or significant oliguria should not undergo forced diuresis. The aim of the forced diuresis is to increase urine flow rates to 3-5 mL/kg/hr in order to facilitate the renal clearance of the toxin. The drug of choice are furosemide (5 mg/kg every 6 to 8 hours) and mannitol (1 to 2 g/kg IV every 6 hours). Bromide,

Table 13.5: Important toxins and their antidotes.

| Toxin | Antidote |
|---|---|
| Acetaminophen | N-acetylcysteine |
| Amino acid analogues | Amino acids |
| Anticholinergic | Neostigmine |
| Arsenic, mercury, heavy metals | Dimercaprol |
| Benzodiazepines | Flumazenil |
| Beta blocker | Glucagon |
| Botulinum | Botulinus antitoxin, guanidine |
| Bromide | Chloride |
| Carbon monoxide | Oxygen |
| Chloroquine | Diazepam |
| Copper | Penicillamine |
| Coumarin anticoagulants | Vitamin K |
| Cyanide | Sodium nitrite |
| Digoxin | Antidigoxin Fab |
| Ethylene glycol | Ethanol fomepizole |
| Fluoroacetate | Acetate, monoacetin |
| Formaldehyde | Ammonia (by mouth) |
| Heparin | Protamine |
| Hydrofluoric acid | Calcium gluconate |
| Insulin | Glucose |
| Iron, aluminum | Deferoxamine |
| Irritant gases | Budesonide |
| Isoniazid | Pyridoxine (vitamin B6) |
| Lead | Calcium sodium edetate |
| Methanol | Ethanol |
| Morphine and opioids | Naloxone |
| Neuromuscular blocking agents | Neostigmine, edrophonium |
| Organophosphates | Atropine, Pralidoxime |
| Paracetamol | Methionine |
| Phenol | Polyethylene glycol |
| Phosphorous white | Copper solution |
| Selenocystthionine | Cystine |
| Strontium, radium | Calcium salts |
| Thallium | Potassium salts |
| Tricyclic antidepressants | $NaHCO_3$, physostigmine |
| Warfarin | Clotting factors |

lithium, amphetamine, phenobarbital and salicylate intoxication are most likely to respond to forced diuresis. The basic problem associated with forced diuretics is the chance fluid overload and dyselectrolytemia. Hence close monitoring of fluid and electrolyte level, water intoxication, cerebral edema, pulmonary edema is crucial. In addition to that intoxication of few toxins like tricyclic antidepressants and many sedative-hypnotics may induce pulmonary edema. Hence, forced diuretics is contra indicated in this case (Piyush Gupta, 2021).

- **Dialysis and hemoperfusion:**
  - Barbiturates, carbamazepine, salicylates, theophylline, dapsone, lithium, methanol, charcoal hydrate and ethylene glycol are the drugs which can be effectively excreted by dialysis and hemoperfusion.
  - Hemoperfusion with charcoal or exchange resins is more effective than hemodialysis but for removal of drugs like menthol, lithium and ethylene glycol hemodialysis is the preferred method. Peritoneal dialysis is rarely used method as it is less effective. The advantage of peritoneal dialysis is that it doesn't require special facility.

## Supportive therapy

- Some of the children develop encephalopathy due to intoxication of certain toxins therefore maintenance of patent airway is vital along with administration of oxygen if required.
- Maintenance and close monitoring of fluid electrolyte level.
- The child with seizure event should be treated with benzodiazepine and phenobarbitone. If seizure is still not under control then increased ICP may be suspected.
- Fever and pain can be managed by antipyretics and analgesics.
- Antibiotics should be administered in case of infection.

## Prevention of re-exposure

- Toxic materials, chemicals, cleaners, potentially harmful cosmetics and medications should be stored in a secure place where child cannot reach.
- Poisonous substances and food materials should not be kept in same cabinet.
- Medications and poisonous substances should be kept in their original packet and label should not be removed as that might have some important information.
- Kerosine, caustic soda, etc., should not be stored in a beverage bottle.
- Left over or expired medications should be appropriately discarded.

- Parent should not leave the child alone and unsupervised.
- Parents must aware about the potential poisoning substance.
- Tobacco and cigarettes should be kept out of reach and should not be consumed in front of the child.
- Remote controls should be kept out of reach as the small batteries in them have the toxic materials.

*Nursing Management*

Nursing diagnosis - 1

Risk for aspiration related to decreased level of consciousness, depressed gag reflex.

**Interventions**

- Remove unabsorbed poisoning substance from the child if any along with the contaminated clothes.
- Whole-body including nail bed, groin area, etc., should be cleaned to remove any leftover toxins.
- If the child is unconscious then nothing should be given orally
- Evaluate the condition of the child such as level of consciousness, clinical presentations, etc.
- Patency of the air way should be assessed and maintained.
- Provide semi prone position to the child to prevent aspiration.

Nursing diagnosis - 2

Risk for poisoning related to access to dangerous product, access to pharmaceutical preparations, inadequate precautions against poisoning, inadequate knowledge of poisoning prevention.

**Interventions**

- Assess the child's risk for poisoning at home and at hospital.
- Perform environmental safety surrounding the child to prevent accidental poisoning.
- Educate the family members regarding signs of poisoning and prevention.
- Advise the parents about home safety check.
- Advise the parents to keep chemicals and toxic materials away from the child's reach.
- Ensure that the toys do not have batteries which can be removed easily or toxic paints.

Nursing diagnosis - 3

Risk for injury related to exposure to toxic chemicals.

**Interventions**

- Monitor temperature, BP, pulse and $SPO_2$ as toxin intoxication may lead to fluctuation in the vital signs.
- Encourage increased fluid intake to facilitate removal of toxin through urine.
- Administer appropriate antidotes as prescribed.
- Assess the need of supplemental oxygen, IV fluid and medications.
- Administer phenobarbitone and benzodiazepine to the child with seizure as prescribed.
- Maintain input and output chart to monitor the fluid balance.
- Monitor the electrolyte and glucose level of the child as dyselectrolytemia is a major problem of the forced diuretic therapy.
- Educate the parents about the need of child supervision and prevention of poisoning.

**Foreign Body Aspiration (FBA)**

Foreign body aspiration is a potentially life-threatening condition occurring primarily in children between the age of 6 months to 60 months. If not treated appropriately then may cause lung injury, pulmonary infections bronchiectasis and lung abscess. It is one of the leading causes of childhood mortality and morbidity. The signs and symptoms of FBA are often confused with asthma so careful assessment and evaluation are quite important. Commonly aspirated foreign bodies by the children are both organic and inorganic matters as listed below:

*Organic*

- Peanuts
- Popcorn
- Seeds
- Vegetables
- Bones
- Chewing gum
- Hard candy
- Whole grape
- Groundnut
- Chickpeas
- Custard apple seed
- Betel nut
- Tamarind seed
- Coconut

*Inorganic*

- Toy parts
- Crayons
- Pen parts
- Pins
- Nails
- Screws
- Bullet and casings

- Tacks
- Buttons
- Pebbles
- Nuts
- Coins
- Metal ball

### Clinical Features

The symptoms of foreign body aspiration into the air way appears in three stages as follows:
1. **Initial event:** This occurs immediately when foreign body is aspirated. The symptoms include coughing, choking, gagging, and airway obstruction.
2. **Asymptomatic interval:** After the initial event foreign body lodged in the airway, reflexes diminished, and the immediate symptoms alleviate. Child comes to the hospital during this stage and therefore accounts for delayed diagnosis (as the symptoms subsides).
3. **Complications:** At this stage air way obstruction, erosion, or infection develops in the air way or lungs therefore complications like fever, cough, hemoptysis, pneumonia, atelectasis always directs the attention again towards the presence of a foreign body.

### Diagnosis

Diagnosis often is done by imaging study or direct visualization of the object. Chest X-ray, CT scan a, fluoroscopy.

### Management

Management of foreign body aspiration varies depending on the type and location of the lodge. There are various techniques used to remove nasal foreign bodies.
- Direct visualization and extraction are the common methods of foreign body removal. Curettes, alligator forceps, or probes are the common instruments used for extraction of the object from the nasal cavity. The object can be pulled directly out using alligators as in the case of paper or sponge material.
- Forced exhalation is another method that may utilize either the parent or a bag-valve-mask (BVM). The "parent's kiss" utilizes the parent to seal their mouth over the child's mouth with a firm seal, occluding the unaffected are and blowing into the child's mouth in the hope of expelling the object. A BVM can be used in the same fashion with a tight seal.
- Suction can be used to remove or bring an object lower into the nasal passages. In addition, one may use hooks, balloon catheters, and positive pressure to remove the foreign body.
- Bronchoscope can be used to remove the object. Three types of forceps are used for the removal of the foreign material from the airway.
  - *Optical forceps:* It has a telescope to visualize the object for removal.
  - *Nonoptical forceps:* It is used to remove beads, nails, screws, tacks and other objects that are in a distant tiny space.
  - *Biopsy forceps:* If a foreign body remains for a prolonged period then new tissue forms in order to enclose it. So, biopsy forceps are used in this case to remove new tissue masses.

### Nursing Management

#### Complete obstruction of the airway
- Assess the airway patency by directly visualizing through laryngoscope. Inspect the mouth for any foreign body if present remove using Magill's forceps.
- Place the child in prone position and apply 5 blows with the open hand to the interscapular area.
- Turn child face up. Apply 5 chest thrusts using the same technique as for chest compression during CPR.
- Inspect oral cavity to visualize if foreign body has appeared, and remove if possible.
- Continue with alternating back blows and chest thrusts maneuverer if obstruction still persists.

#### Partial obstruction of airway
- In case of partial obstruction above maneuverer should not be performed.
- In this case, upright position of the child is most comfortable.
- If surgical intervention is required then as a nurse all the necessary arrangement should be done along with preparation of operation theater.

### Nursing Diagnosis - 1

Ineffective airway clearance related to foreign body in airway as evidenced by altered respiratory rhythm, adventitious breath sounds, cyanosis, hypoxemia, nasal flaring, subcostal retraction, tachypnea, uses accessory muscle to breathe.

#### Interventions
- Assess the child's level of consciousness and cognitive status
- Assess the patency of the air way directly visualizing through laryngoscope. Inspect the mouth for any foreign body if present remove using Magill's forceps
- Inspect oral cavity to visualize if foreign body has appeared, and remove if possible

- Auscultate for detection of abnormal breath sound and recording of vitals, $SPO_2$ are also important.
- Suctioning should be done as required to clear the airway.
- Administer supplemental oxygen as prescribed
- Monitor respiratory status continuously.

### Nursing Diagnosis - 2

Ineffective breathing pattern related to airway obstruction as evidenced by altered tidal volume, decreased inspiratory and/or expiratory pressure, decreased vital capacity, hypercapnia, hypoxemia, hypoxia, orthopnea, uses accessory muscles to breathe.

### Interventions

- Assess respiratory status for presence of any adventitious breath sound, rate, chest retraction, etc.
- Assess oxygen saturation continuously
- Assess function of accessory muscle of respiration
- Ensure necessary arrangement along with preparation of operation theater if surgical intervention is required.
- Provide high fowlers position to the child to promote optimal lung expansion and oxygenation
- Administer humidified supplemental oxygen as prescribed
- Assess signs of hypoxia regularly
- Suction the air way as required to clear the secretions
- Review the ABG results and other lab results
- Ensure the ventilator and emergency respiratory support equipment are available at bedside
- Monitor ventilator alarms and settings

### Nursing Diagnosis - 3

Deficient knowledge related to inadequate access to resources as evidenced by inaccurate follow-through of instruction and inaccurate statements about foreign body aspiration management.

### Interventions

- Assess the current knowledge of the parents
- Assess the level of understanding
- Identify the barriers in the learning process
- Encourage the parents and family members to ask questions
- Provide positive reinforcement to adhere to the treatment regimen
- Demonstrate the skills in the management of foreign body aspiration
- Educate using multiple media like diagram, animations, posters to facilitate the understanding
- Focus on single topic at once rather than multiple topics.

## Trauma

Trauma is one of the leading causes of mortality and morbidity among pediatric population. Approximately 75% of the children die because of head injury. The causal factors of trauma are not specific because these vary depending on the age. Nonaccidental trauma is common among the infants whereas in case of toddlers fall is the primary cause of trauma. The predominate cause of trauma among older children are related to sports or road traffic accident. About 50% of the children die at the site of trauma due to severe head injury or hemorrhage and around 30% of children die within few hours due to head injury, hemorrhage or air way emergency and the remaining 20% late death are due to organ dysfunction or sepsis. The only good thing in trauma is that more than 30% of deaths are preventable by prompt and aggressive management.

Following are some of the common causes of pediatric trauma injury:
- Road traffic accident (RTA)
- Drowning
- Burn
- Drowning
- Fall
- Animal or insect bite
- Foreign body insertion
- Suffocation
- Child abuse

### Assessment of Severity of Trauma

Pediatric traumatic injury is life-threatening therefore early assessment is vital to minimize the delay of treatment. There are several tools available to quantify the severity of trauma, which provide crucial information for further treatment. The widely used tools for pediatric population are the pediatric Glasgow coma scale and pediatric trauma score (PTS). The maximum and minimum score of Glasgow coma scale is 15 and 3 respectively. Higher the score higher is the response and level of consciousness. The PTS score ranges from -6 to +12, higher the score lesser is the mortality risk. Score <8 indicates significant mortality risk.

### Management

#### Primary Survey

The importance of the primary survey is for rapid identification of life-threatening traumatic injury. This includes ABCDEs: Airway, breathing, circulation, neurological deficit and exposure.
- **Airway:** The risk of airway obstruction is higher among children as compare to the adult because of smaller nasal and oral cavities, larger tongue, larger mass of

tonsillar tissue and slender trachea and larynx. The patients with airway obstruction have abnormal breath sound like stridor or diminished sound. Head injury is the major cause of the airway obstruction as compare to other causes. If airway obstruction is suspected then air way should be opened by jaw thrust maneuver or oropharyngeal air way should be introduced after suctioning the airway to prevent obstruction by mandibular tissue. If obstruction still persists then endotracheal intubation should be performed.

- **Breathing:** Assessment of respiratory rate, movement of chest breath sound are the basics for evaluation of breathing status. Child should be assessed for cyanosis, $SPO_2$ by pulse oximeter and any breathing abnormality like slow irregular breaths, Cheyne-Strokes respiration and apnea. If ventilatory support is required then positive pressure ventilation by bang and mask should be immediately started with 100% oxygen. Use of $CO_2$ detector during endotracheal intubation provides appropriate information regarding placement of the tube.
- **Circulation:** Hypovolemic shock is the commonest feature of trauma which occurs due to excessive hemorrhage. The child with shock may present increased heart rate, weak pulse, delay in capillary refill time, hypothermia, pale skin and altered level of consciousness. To restore the fluid volume rapid infusion of isotonic saline (RL or normal saline) is required and most of the patient become stable without need of further intensive management. If shock persists even after IV fluid resuscitation then blood transfusion is indicated and in extreme cases surgery may be necessary to stop hemorrhage.
- **Neurological deficit:** Immediate neurological evaluation includes assessment of pupillary size and response along with level of consciousness by AVPU (alert, response to verbal stimuli, response to painful stimuli or unresponsive). Use of Glasgow coma scale provides crucial information regarding neurological status and requirement of intubation (score <8 should be intubated) oxygen therapy, adequate ventilation and maintenance of intracranial pressure within normal range are crucial to prevent deterioration of cerebral injury. Hyperventilation, mannitol and hypertonic saline are the treatment of choice for increased ICP. Several studies found that administration of hypertonic saline (3% NS at a dose of 3-5 mg/kg) is more effective than mannitol.
- **Exposure:** Clothing should be removed to inspect any injury and hypothermia should be managed by IV fluids and covering the body with warm blankets.

*Secondary Survey*

Secondary survey is performed after primary survey and stabilization of the patient. It includes focused head to toe examination of the child within 3 mins. It is also important to collect the history using the pneumonic **'SAMPLE'**.

**S**: Signs and symptoms
**A**: Allergies
**M**: Medications
**P**: Past medical history
**L**: Last oral intake
**E**: Event leading to the injury

- **Head trauma:** Head trauma is one of the commonest traumatic injuries leading to death. Scalp injury, skull fracture, concussion, contusion, intracranial hemorrhage are the features of head trauma. Head trauma patients require immediate management of airway, hemorrhage, seizure and increased ICP. If child is not stabilized with initial treatment, then surgical intervention may be required like decompressive surgery and craniotomy, etc. In case of increased ICP due to cerebral edema mannitol and hypertonic saline can be administered. Anticonvulsant should be used to minimize seizure activities. Muscle relaxant (vecuronium) is administered before endotracheal intubation.
- **Cervical spine trauma:** If cervical spine trauma is suspected then radiographic imaging should be done only after stabilizing the patients' condition. CT scan and MRI are helpful in detecting bony injuries or fractures. Spinal cord injury without radiologic abnormality (SCIWORA) is very rare and is identified well in MRI. Methylprednisolone is found to help in improving the motor function in children with spinal cord injury.
- **Thoracic trauma:** Most of the thoracic trauma are due to the blunt trauma from motor vehicle accident. Rib fracture, pulmonary contusion, pneumothorax and hemothorax are the common thoracic trauma among pediatric population. Isolated rib fracture and diaphragm injury are rare among children. Thoracotomy is indicated for children with cardiac tamponade, esophageal injury, diaphragmatic injury, hemothorax and pneumothorax.
- **Abdominal trauma:** Abdominal trauma is mostly blunt, and spleen is the commonest injured organ. CT scan is the reliable imaging study for detection of abdominal organ injury. Following traumatic injury abdominal distention is very common due to accumulation of free air or blood. Spleen injury is the common type of abdominal trauma. Usually, fluid management and

observation are the main stay of treatment but in case of splenomegaly surgical intervention (splenectomy) may be required. Liver injury is treated with fluid therapy and observation without need of surgery. Pancreatic injury occurs as a result of blunt trauma which can be diagnosed by ERCP (endoscopic retrograde cholangiopancreatography)

- **Pelvic trauma:** It is a high energy trauma occurring rarely among children as compared to the adult. The physical signs that are related to pelvic fracture are as follows:
  - *Destot sign:* A large superficial hematoma above the inguinal ligament
  - *Roux sign:* Reduced distance from pubic spine to greater trochanter of femur
  - *Earle sign:* On rectal inspection, a bony prominence or substantial hematoma and tenderness, suggesting a severe pelvic fracture
  
  If it is found that the pelvic ring is unstable then immediate external fixation should be used. CT scan and MRI are the gold standard techniques to identify the location and extent of injury. Surgical intervention is required for correction of fracture.

- **Extremities trauma:** Musculoskeletal structure of children varies significantly as compared to the adult which makes the diagnosis and treatment challenging. Most of the time during assessment extremities injury are missed due to shift of attention towards management of life-threatening problems. The child with extremities trauma may have swelling, tenderness at the site of injury, skin abrasion, etc. During assessment of focus should be given towards neurovascular evaluation. Hence distal pulse, skin color, temperature, capillary refill time and sensory-motor function should be assessed. Doppler ultrasonography should be performed if distal pulses cannot be detected by palpation. Radiographic imaging should be taken to detect the fracture characteristics. Once fracture is conformed immediate immobilization of the hand by using splint will prevent further damage. And the fractured extremity should be elevated above the heart to facilitate fluid drainage. Surgery for fixation of the fractured bone may be required.

## Nursing Management

### Nursing Diagnosis - 1

Risk for bleeding related to trauma.

**Interventions**

- Monitor vital signs specially blood pressure and heart rate
- Administer IV fluid and blood products as prescribed
- Avoid drugs containing salicylate or NSAIDs
- Monitor signs of internal bleeding like black stool, hematuria, etc.
- Review lab reports specially coagulation studies, PCV and Hb level
- Frequently monitor neurological status of the child

### Nursing Diagnosis - 2

Risk for shock related to bleeding, deficient fluid volume, trauma, sepsis.

**Interventions**

- Monitor vitals specially blood pressure and heart rate
- Assess level of consciousness
- Administer IV fluid and blood products as prescribed
- Prepare the patient for surgery if needed
- Administer oxygen if required
- Monitor input and output and maintain chart
- Monitor peripheral pulses, CVP, ECG for prompt identification of shock
- Administer electrolyte to correct electrolyte imbalance.

### Nursing Diagnosis - 3

Acute pain related to physical injury as evidenced by expressive behavior, facial expression of pain, positioning to ease pain, reports intensity using standardized pain scale, altered physiological parameter, guarding behavior, etc.

Interventions

- Assess the characteristics of pain like onset, location, intensity, duration
- If the child cannot verbalize assess the level of pain using pain assessment tool (premature infant pain profile, neonatal facial coding system, Wong-Baker faces pain rating scale, neonatal/infant pain scale, FLACC scale, behavioral pain scale, nonverbal pain scale, visual analogue scale, adolescent pediatric pain tool) as appropriate for the child.
- Provide comfortable position and calm and quite environment
- Provide wound care to alleviate pain
- Monitor vitals at regular interval as physiological parameter fluctuates during pain
- Initiate nonpharmacological measures of pain management like distraction techniques, relaxation methods, etc.
- Administer analgesics as advised to the child
- Evaluate the effectiveness and side effect of the analgesics.

## Status Asthmaticus

Status asthmaticus is defined as a life-threatening form of asthma characterized by hypoxia, hypercarbia and progressive respiratory failure which is unresponsive to standard treatment regimen.

### Types and Etiology

*Type 1: Slow Onset*

- It is more common form of status asthmaticus.
- This can be preventable with strict adherence to the treatment modalities.
- These group of children have history of severe asthma.
- The triggering factors are intrinsic (stress, inadequate inhalation of the prescribed inhaler, under management, etc.)
- Examination shows substantial mucus plugs, edema and infiltration of eosinophil.

*Type 2: Sudden Onset*

- These group of children have no history of hospitalization due to respiratory failure but some may have history of mild form of asthma.
- Abrupt exposer to huge external factors (allergens, sulfites, food, etc.) causes sudden onset.
- Examination shows lack of mucus plugs, empty air ways and infiltration of neutrophils rather than eosinophils.

### Clinical Features

- Signs of respiratory distress (nasal flaring, grunting, retraction, wheezing, etc.)
- Tachypnea
- Hypoxia
- Bradypnea (in case of worsening respiratory failure)
- Tachycardia
- Hypertension
- Pulsus paradox (decrease pulse pressure during inspiration due to decreased stroke volume)
- Irritability
- Disorientation.

### Pathophysiology

The pathophysiology of status asthmaticus is very complex and poorly understood. The physiologic mechanism of this acute asthma is divided in to two phases as follows:

*Early Bronchospasm*

The immune response in acute asthma begins when allergens are inhaled, antigen presenting cells in the epithelium lining of the airways of the lungs and nose express these allergens on their cell surface. The allergens are then presented to other cells involved in the immune response, particularly T-lymphocytes (T-helper cells). Activation of T-helper cells stimulate B-lymphocyte by cell-to-cell interaction that occur between CD40 ligand on the surface of T-helper cell and CD40 protein on B-cell surface. T-cell also releases cytokines, i.e., interleukin (IL), interferon, TNF-beta, etc., which promote further activation of B-cell for antigen specific IgE production. IgE mediated mast cell activation is the central to the pathogenesis of acute asthma. Mast cells are thought to function in homeostasis, including wound healing and in innate and adaptive immunity. In acute asthma IgE-antibodies bind to a specific allergen via its Fab portion and its Fc region bind to the specific high affinity receptor on mast cell called FcεR1. Activation of receptor FcεR1 causes mast cell degranulation. Rapid release of mast cell mediators like histamine, prostaglandin D2, and leukotriene C4 by degranulation induce vasodilation, contraction of the respiratory smooth muscle and mucus secretion. (A Parthasarathy et al., 2019).

*Late Inflammatory Phase*

A late inflammatory phase causing airway swelling and edema due to eosinophils released eosinophilic cationic proteins (ECP) and major basic protein (MBP) (NCBI Bookshelf, from: https://www.ncbi.nlm.nih.gov/books/NBK526070/).

### Diagnosis

Clinical assessment is the corner stone in the diagnosis of severe acute asthma. Assessment of patient with respiratory exacerbation should include general, primary, secondary and tertiary assessment. If life-threatening condition is found at any point of time during assessment, then pediatric advanced life support (PALS) guideline should be strictly followed given by American Heart Association (AHA) to save the life of the patient.

*Becker Asthma Severity Assessment Score*

This scoring system helps in the quick assessment of the severity of asthma, higher the score more the severity The parameters of Becker asthma severity score are respiratory rate/minute, wheezing, I/E ratio and accessory muscle use. Each parameter has score ranging from 0–3, minimum score is 0 and maximum 12. A score >4 considered as moderate form of status asthmaticus and score >7 require ICU admission.

### Laboratory Investigations

CBC, serum electrolytes, serum theophylline, arterial blood gas analysis.

## Imaging

Chest radiograph can be done but is not routinely recommended.

## Management

Management of the patient depend on the severity of the condition which should be done immediately when a child comes to the hospital with acute respiratory exacerbation. clinical assessment and assessment of severity by Becker scoring system, pulse oximetry, chest X-ray, ABG helps in deciding the treatment regimen and need of PICU admission (if Becker asthma score >7). Supportive care, medication and ventilation are the treatment options for status asthmaticus.

### Supportive Care

- Suitable environmental condition
- Maintenance of fluid volume
- Maintenance of electrolyte balance specially potassium
- Oxygen therapy
- Cardiopulmonary monitoring.

### Medications

- **β2 agonists:** Salbutamol (0.15-0.5 mg/kg/hour for continuous nebulization) and Terbutaline (0.5 mg/kg/hour for continuous nebulization) are the drug of choice because of specific action on the β2 adrenergic receptors. β2 agonists causes relaxation of the smooth muscles of the airway by binding the adrenergic receptors. These can be administered via oral, IV, SC or can be inhaled. Nebulization is the most preferred way of delivering the drug.
- **Anticholinergics:** Ipratropium bromide is the widely used anticholinergic agent for acute asthma. It blocks the muscarinic cholinergic receptors there by inhibit bronchial smooth muscle contraction, salivary and mucus gland secretions. Several studies reported that administration of ipratropium bromide alone has no significant effect therefore should be given in conjunction with β2 agonists for quick respiratory improvement and to reduce hospital stay. It should be administered in two or three doses of 250-500 µg via nebulization or 2-3 puffs of 17 µg/puff administered via metered dose inhalers.
- **Corticosteroids:** Corticosteroids are the first line drugs in acute asthma. They work by reducing inflammation, swelling and secretions of airway. In case of moderate to severe asthma exacerbations. Oral prednisone or prednisolone (1-2 mg/kg/day) is taken for a 3-5 day course and dexamethasone (0.3-0.6 mg/kg) is given in either a one or two-dose regimen. Children receiving high-dose b-adrenergic agonist therapy may develop impaired gastric absorption and vomiting, so in these children IV administration may be preferable.
- **Magnesium:** Intravenous magnesium sulphate infusion is found to cause bronchial smooth muscle relaxation there by causes bronchodilation in case of asthma. It can be administered at 50 mg/kg/dose over 30 min or infusion at a rate of 10–20 mg/kg/hours, can repeat once or twice after 4-6 hours.
- **Methylxanthines:** Use of methylxanthines is infrequent in acute exacerbations of asthma because they are less effective than the β2 agonists and associated with severe side effects. Several recent studies, however, suggest that methylxanthines may offer some benefit in children with status asthmaticus. Methylxanthine therapy may be helpful in those critically ill children who are not responsive to steroids, inhaled and IV β2 agonist, and $O_2$. Aminophylline is administered by continuous IV infusion following a loading dose of 5–7 mg/kg infused over 20 min. In general, a loading dose of 1 mg/kg will raise the serum theophylline level by 2 mcg/mL.

### Nursing Management

- **Assessment of general condition:** Assessment of vital signs, respiratory pattern, skin color, breath sound neurological status are vital during preliminary assessment when child comes to the emergency department. Oxygen saturation should be continuously monitored using fingertip pulse oximeter, as the child with acute asthma typically have low $SPO_2$ level.
- **Airway management:** The infant with status asthmaticus usually have bronchospasm and edema in the airway due to inflammation. Hence administration of supplemental oxygen is required to meet the oxygen demand and to maintain oxygen saturation.
- **Monitoring:**
  - After administration of rescue medications monitor its effects.
  - Monitor the symptoms of asthma exacerbation
  - Monitor oxygen saturation, neurological status, response to treatment, etc.
- **Positioning:** Older children may be more comfortable sitting upright or leaning slightly forward supported by a pillow.
- **Supplemental oxygen administration:** Humidified oxygen should be administered to the child with asthma if required then CPAP or mechanical ventilation also should be used to improve the oxygen saturation.
- **Medication administration:** The child with acute asthma exacerbation usually receive corticosteroids, β2 agonists, anticholinergics, methylxanthines and

magnesium. Nurses should check the physician's prescription before administering the medication for name, dose, frequency, etc. Review home medications if any.

- **Family support:** Provide emotional support to the parents and family members. Educate them about the risk factors, allergens, early signs of asthma attack, pathophysiology, treatment regimen, homecare, diet plan, etc. Teach the family members about hygienic measures and its importance.
- **Diet:** Nurses should collect the detailed history to identify the food allergens which might have triggered the asthma so that the specific diet can be avoided. Small and frequent liquid diet should be given for easy digestion. To meet the nutritional requirement dietician should be consulted to prepare a balanced diet. Input and output chart, growth chart, measurement of height and weight should be done to monitor the nutritional status and growth and development.

### Nursing Diagnosis - 1

Ineffective airway clearance related to retained secretions as evidenced by altered respiratory rhythm, adventitious breath sounds, cyanosis, hypoxemia, nasal flaring, subcostal retraction, tachypnea, uses accessory muscle to breathe.

### Interventions

- Assess the patency of the air way specially in case of trauma or neurological injury.
- Auscultate for detection of abnormal breath sound and recording of vitals, $SPO_2$ are also important.
- Provide prone position which is found to be beneficial in improving lung oxygenation and function hence should be provided if possible.
- Suctioning should be done as required to clear the airway.
- Chest physiotherapy are also quite helpful to remove excess secretions but should be performed if indicated.
- Maintenance of fluid balance along with recording input and output is also required.
- Encourage the child for adequate fluid intake as hydration can liquify the tenacious secretions in the respiratory tract and can help in easy clearance.
- Educate family members about the need of hydration, appropriate technique of taking medications, need of breathing exercise and diet requirement, etc.
- Advise patient and family members to avoid overcrowding places and polluted environments.
- Educate the parents for timely immunization specially haemophilus influenzae b and pneumococcal vaccine.

### Nursing Diagnosis - 2

Ineffective breathing pattern related to decreased lung function as evidenced by altered tidal volume, decreased inspiratory and/or expiratory pressure, decreased vital capacity, hypercapnia, hypoxemia, hypoxia, orthopnea, uses accessory muscles to breathe.

### Interventions

- Assess respiratory status for presence of any adventitious breath sound, rate, chest retraction, etc.
- Assess oxygen saturation continuously
- Assess function of accessory muscle of respiration
- Provide high fowlers position to the child to promote optimal lung expansion and oxygenation
- Administer humidified supplemental oxygen as prescribed
- Assess signs of hypoxia regularly
- Suction the air way as required to clear the secretions
- Administer antibiotics, bronchodilators, steroids as prescribed
- Review the ABG results and other lab results
- Ensure the ventilator and emergency respiratory support equipment are available at bedside
- Monitor ventilator alarms and settings
- Educate the child about appropriate technique of coughing (after taking deep breath hold for 2 seconds then cough 2/3 times)
- Demonstrate breathing exercise using incentive spirometer
- Advise intermittent rest during ambulation and activities.

### Nursing Diagnosis - 3

Decreased activity tolerance related to imbalance between oxygen supply and demand as evidenced by easy fatigue, weakness, exertional dyspnea.

### Interventions

- Assess the child's oxygen saturation, vitals and respiratory function regularly
- Assess the ability of the child to perform his/her daily activities
- Assess the nutritional status of the child which might be a cause of decreased activity tolerance
- Provide supplemental oxygen as prescribed
- Provide adequate rest to conserve energy
- Encourage rest between the activities to avoid exertional dyspnea
- Demonstrate breathing exercise to the child to improve lung function
- Administer medications like bronchodilators and steroids as prescribed.

## Common Congenital Disorders

### Cleft Lip and Palate

The formation of lip and palate complete by 5–12 weeks and 12–14 weeks of gestation respectively. Cleft lip and palate are the congenital anomaly of face due to failure of the fusion of 1st branchial arch during intrauterine development. These are the most common birth defects which may occur as both or as isolated. The incidence is approximately 1 in 500–550 births. The cause of cleft lip and palate is unknown but environmental factors and genetic factors together play a major role during embryological development of face. Hence ultrasonography during 2nd trimester can detect the anomaly.

### Classification

A cleft lip and palate may be either unilateral or bilateral and is either complete or incomplete. The most commonly accepted classification systems are the Veau classification and LAHSHAL classification system **(Fig. 13.4)**.

#### Veau classification

| Class | Description |
|---|---|
| I | Defect involving soft palate only |
| II | Defect involving both soft and hard palate but not extending beyond incisive foramen |
| III | Complete unilateral defect beyond incisive foramen involving soft palate, hard palate and lip |
| IV | Complete bilateral defect beyond incisive foramen involving soft palate, hard palate and lip |

*Source:* Al Balushi A, Sahib M, Balushi T. Palatal Fistula 2017.

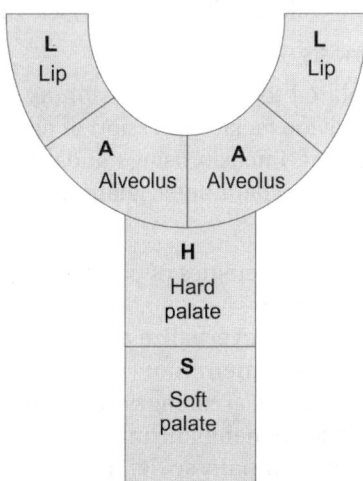

**Fig. 13.4:** LAHSHAL classification (1987).
*Source:* Akram A, McKnight MM, Bellardie H, Beale V, Evans RD. Craniofacial malformations and the orthodontist. Br Dent J 2015 2183 2015 Feb 16;218(3):129–41.

### LAHSHAL classification (1987)

Kriens, 1989 proposed LAHSHAL, an abbreviated documentation system. Lip (L), alveolus (A), hard palate (H), and soft palate (S) were used to form LAHSHAL. Later, it was modified to LAHSHAL on the recommendation of Royal College of Surgeons UK in 2005.

### Surgical Management

The aim of the surgical management of the child with cleft lip and palate are:
- Structural closure of the anomaly
- To create a normal structure for production of speech
- To reduce the dento-alveolar deformities.

Usually, the surgical correction of the child with isolated cleft lip known as cheiloplasty which is done at the age 10 weeks, weight 10 pounds and hemoglobin level 10 g%. Similarly, palatoplasty is the surgical correction of the cleft palate at the age of 9 to 12 months. Surgical techniques for cleft palate are evolving as the knowledge and technology are developing. Following are the common surgical techniques (Agrawal K. Cleft palate repair and variations. Indian J Plast Surg 2009):

- von Langenbeck's bipedicle flap technique
- Veau-Wardill-Kilner Pushback technique
- Bardach's two-flap technique
- Furlow double opposing Z-plasty
- Two-stage palatal repair
- Hole in one repair
- Raw area free palatoplasty
- Alveolar extension palatoplasty (AEP)
- Primary pharyngeal flap
- Intravelar veloplasty
- Vomer flap
- Buccal myomucosal flap

### Hypospadias

This is a congenital anomaly in which the urethral meatus opens abnormally on the ventral surface of the penis anywhere from perineum to the glans penis. The incidence of hypospadias is about 1 in 1000 newborn boys. It is believed that due to influence of endocrine, environmental and genetic factors during 8–20th weeks of embryological development there is certain abnormal changes occur in the urethral structure.

### Classification

According to Duckett classification (1996), there are anterior (50%), middle (30%) and posterior (20%) hypospadias.
- **Anterior form:** Glandular, coronal and distal penile.
- **Middle form:** "Midshaft" and proximal penile.
- **Posterior form:** Penoscrotal, scrotal and perineal.

*Clinical Manifestations*
- Abnormal opening of the urethral meatus on the ventral aspect
- Downward bending of the penis if chordee is present
- At the tip of the penis appearance of penis is resembles like a hood
- Urine spray during micturition is abnormal

*Surgical Management*
- The appropriate age for the surgical correction is between 6 months to 1 year. Before surgery circumcision should be avoided as the foreskin is used in repair
- Glandular hypospadias requires a glandular meatotomy
- Coronal hypospadias requires a meatal advancement and glanduloplasty (MAGPI operation)
- Proximal hypospadias without a chordee can be treated by a skin flap advancement
- If chordee present it should be excised and flap urethroplasty performed

## Epispadias

It is a congenital defect in which the urethral meatus abnormally opens on the dorsal aspect of the penis. The cause of epispadias is unknown but a combination of endocrine, environmental and genetic factors is strongly associated with this anomaly.

*Classification*

**In male:**
- Anterior type without incontinence of urine
  - Glanular epispadias
  - Penile epispadias
- Posterior type with incontinence of urine
  - Penopubic
  - Subsymphyseal

**In female:**
- Bifid clitoris without incontinence of urine
- Subsymphyseal with incontinence of urine

*Surgical Management*

The structural reconstruction of epispadias can be done in single stage or multistaged surgery depending on the location of the opening and associated anomalies. Glanuloplasty is required for the epispadias in which the opening lies at the glans penis. Urethroplasty can be done to create and elongate the urethra along with chordee correction. Similarly, cystoplasty can be done for bladder neck reconstruction and to improve the capacity of the bladder. Modified Cantwell-Ransley technique and Mitchell technique are the common surgical approach in case of male epispadias.

## Esophageal atresia (EA) with or without tracheoesophageal fistula (TEF)

Refer page 480.

## Anorectal malformation

Refer page 482.

*Nursing Management*

Nursing diagnosis - 1

Ineffective airway clearance related to airway obstruction or fistula as evidenced by altered respiratory rhythm, adventitious breath sounds, cyanosis, hypoxemia, nasal flaring, subcostal retraction, tachypnea, uses accessory muscle to breathe.

**Interventions**
- Assess the patency of the air way specially in case of cleft lip and palate, tracheoesophageal fistula
- Auscultate for detection of abnormal breath sound and recording of vitals, $SPO_2$ are also important
- Assess skin color and capillary refill time
- Assess respiratory status as pneumonia and respiratory distress are common among these children.
- Assess abdominal distension which occurs due to entry of air into stomach in TEF
- Suctioning should be done as required to clear the airway
- Keep the baby nil per oral as there is high chance of aspiration
- Administer supplemental oxygen as prescribed
- Elevate the head end of the bed to 30–45° to prevent the tongue from falling back and air way obstruction
- Prepare the child and infant for surgical intervention

Nursing diagnosis - 2

Acute pain related to surgical incision as evidenced by expressive behavior, facial expression of pain, positioning to ease pain, reports intensity using standardized pain scale, altered physiological parameter, guarding behavior, etc.

**Interventions**
- Assess the characteristics of pain like onset, location, intensity, duration
- If the child cannot verbalize assess the level of pain using pain assessment tool (premature infant pain profile, neonatal facial coding system, Wong-Baker faces pain rating scale, neonatal/infant pain scale, FLACC scale, behavioral pain scale, nonverbal pain scale, visual analogue scale, adolescent pediatric pain tool) as appropriate for the child
- Provide comfortable position and calm and quite environment

- Provide wound care to alleviate pain
- Monitor vitals at regular interval as physiological parameter fluctuates during pain
- Initiate nonpharmacological measures of pain management like distraction techniques, relaxation methods, etc.
- Administer analgesics as advised to the child
- Evaluate the effectiveness and side effect of the analgesics

Nursing diagnosis - 3

Deficient fluid volume related to excessive fluid loss as evidenced by dry skin and mucus membrane, decrease skin turgor, sunken fontanels, no tears when crying, lack of bowel activity, oliguria.

**Interventions**
- Assess the degree of fluid volume deficit
- Encourage adequate breastfeeding
- Maintain intake and output chart
- Monitor the weight of the baby daily
- Monitor urine volume and color
- Administer IV fluid as prescribed
- Review the lab results like urine specific gravity, serum electrolytes, blood glucose level, etc.

Nursing diagnosis - 4

Risk for infection related to impaired tissue integrity, difficulty managing wound care, difficulty managing long-term invasive device.

**Interventions**
- Assess vitals every 4 hourly or as required specially temperature
- Assess the signs and symptoms of infection and any purulent discharge from the incision
- Provide wound care as needed
- Apply sterile dressing to reduce infection and promote wound healing
- Change the position the child every 2 hourly to prevent pressure ulcer if required place comfort devices below the bony prominences
- Encourage breastfeeding unless contraindicated
- Avoid unnecessary handling of the newborn
- Strictly follow infection control practice while providing care and doing invasive procedures
- Follow the 5 moments of hand hygiene
- Protect the newborn from iatrogenic and cross-infection
- Monitor lab results specially WBC count, CRP, ESR, blood culture, CSF culture, urine analysis and culture, etc.
- Assess and monitor nutritional status and weight of the newborn
- Administer antibiotics as prescribed
- Assess immunization history and administer as per requirement
- Provide adequate rest and sleep, limit visitors.

### *Gastroschisis*

It is a congenital anomaly in which the abdominal content protrudes through the defective ventral abdominal wall usually on the right side. The opening in majority of the cases are less than 5 CM and usually small and large intestine protrude. The cause or any genetic mutation of this condition is not well understood. The diagnosis of the gastroschisis can be made during prenatal period using ultrasonography. Postnatal diagnosis can be done by physical examination but imaging study may be used to identify the associated anomaly. Management often includes the surgery which may be primary or staged based on the characteristics of gastroschisis.

#### *Primary Surgery*

In cases of mild gastroschisis immediate surgery is performed called primary surgery. Abdominal content is reduced and the opening is closed.

#### *Staged Surgery*

Staged surgery is preferred when primary surgery cannot be performed. Immediately after delivery the protruded abdominal content is wrapped by a sterile moist gauze or a bowel bag. Then the baby is transported to the NICU and sedated with fentanyl and midazolam. Intubation may be required before placing the spring-loaded silo in place. It is also important to choose the appropriate size of the silo (a soft, flexible silicon bag) according to the size of the abdominal wall defect. The silo is available in different sizes (ring size) usually from 3 to 15 cm diameter. Typically, the size of the ring chosen should be 2–3 cm greater than the diameter of the defective abdominal opening. However larger size also may be chosen based on the characteristics of the defective opening.

#### *Procedure*

Ensure the baby is sedated and intubated. Then the wrapped sterile moist gauze or bowel bag should be removed. Examine the exposed gastroschisis like distention of the distal colon with meconium which is good indicator of absence of that the proximal GI atresia. Evacuate the GI and bladder content immediately before placing the silo. Then the skin is prepared with betadine and antiseptic solutions by holding the abdominal content perpendicular to the abdomen. Then the protruded content is gradually placed inside the silo carefully from distal to the proximal colon without making any torsion. Then the ring of the silo is gradually slipped through the opening and placed under the fascia. While the baby is in supine position the silo is then positioned at 90 degrees to the abdominal wall by suspending from the bed. While suspending it is important not to put extra or less pressure to suspend the silo which may cause complications. Then the top of the silo is tighten using umbilical tape which will reduce the abdominal content. Tying the silo is done twice daily below the previous knot to assist in spontaneous reduction of the abdominal content. The surgery to close the defect is done when the content inside the silo is within 2cm from the abdomen. During the final surgery both fascia and the skin are approximated and sutured to close after complete reduction and irrigation of the protruded abdominal content. (Vishwanath Bhat, Matthew Moront, Vineet Bhandari, Gastroschisis: A State of the Art Review).

## Summary

Nurses are the largest group of healthcare workers, their training and awareness in the management of neonatal and pediatric emergency patients are vital. Patients in neonatal and pediatric age group present to the emergency department or intensive critical care unit with varieties/various of lethal conditions like trauma, foreign body aspiration, poisoning, seizure, intracranial hemorrhage and asphyxia, etc., which need immediate interventions. The nurse must work with multidisciplinary team to provide a comprehensive care to these critically ill patients. As an emergency pediatric or neonatal nurse adequate knowledge on prompt identification of illness, diagnostic methods, initial stabilization and management is crucial to save the life of little people.

## Points to Ponder

- **Idiopathic intussusception:** Commonly occurs among infants and toddlers at ileocecal junction.
- **Enteroenteral intussusception:** It is commonly found among older children between ilium and jejunum.
- **Tet spell:** This hypoxic spell has a classical presentation, i.e., shortness of breath, cyanosis, uncontrollable crying or panic, and syncope. Knee chest positing during Tet spell to elevate systemic vascular resistance.
- When blood flow to the fetus is compromised a protective mechanism called diving seal reflex redistribute the blood to the vital organs like brain, adrenal gland, etc., by reducing the blood flow to the less vital organs like skin, muscle, intestine, etc.
- The yellowish discoloration of the skin and sclera as a result of excessive accumulation of bilirubin (Hyperbilirubinemia) during first few weeks of life is called neonatal jaundice.
- Tracheoesophageal fistula is a congenital anomaly characterized by abnormal communication between esophagus and trachea.
- Gastroschisis is a congenital anomaly in which the abdominal content protrudes through the defective ventral abdominal wall usually on the right side.
- PKU is an autosomal recessive disorder caused by defective metabolism of the amino acid phenylalanine.
- MSUD is an autosomal recessive aminoacidopathy occurs due to deficiency of the enzymes required to metabolize branched chain amino acids valine, leucine, and isoleucine.
- Alkaptonuria is an autosomal recessive genetic disorder characterized by accumulation of homogentisic acid due to deficiency of the enzyme homogentisic acid 1, 2 dioxygenase.
- Galactosemia is an autosomal recessive metabolic disorder characterized by accumulation of Galactose in the blood due to inadequate metabolism.
- G6PD deficiency is an X-linked recessive metabolic disorder characterized by deficiency of the enzyme Glucose-6-phosphate dehydrogenase (G6PD).
- Accumulation of blood within the brain tissue or the surrounding meningeal spaces called as intracranial hemorrhage.
- Acute respiratory distress syndrome (ARDS) is a clinical syndrome caused by injury of the alveolar endothelium which increase permeability of the alveolar capillary barrier unrelated to cardiogenic pulmonary edema.
- Pneumonia is an inflammation of lung parenchyma due to infection. Noninfective inflammation of lung parenchyma is called as pneumonitis.
- Status asthmaticus is a life-threatening form of asthma characterized by hypoxia, hypercarbia and progressive respiratory failure which is unresponsive to standard treatment regimen.
- At birth about 75% of body weight is composed of water which reduces to 65% by one year of age.
- The ratio of ICW to ECW is about 2:1 after one year of age and remain constant.
- Foreign body aspiration is a potentially life-threatening condition occurring primarily in children between the age of 6 months to 60 months.
- Seizure is a paroxysmal involuntary disturbance of brain function that may manifest as an impairment or loss of consciousness, abnormal motor activity, behavioral abnormality, sensory disturbances or autonomic dysfunction.
- Trauma is one of the leading causes of mortality and morbidity among pediatric population. Approximately 75% of the children die because of head injury.

## Abbreviations

- ABG : Arterial Blood Gas
- ACOG : American College of Obstetrician and Gynecologists
- ARM : Anorectal Malformation
- BCKD : Branched Chain Ketoacid Dehydrogenase
- BRUE : Brief Resolved Unexplained Event
- BVM : Bag-Valve-Mask
- CBC : Complete Blood count
- CECT : High-dose Contrast-Enhanced Computed Tomography
- CPAP : Continuous Positive Airway Pressure
- CPM : Central Pontine Myelinolysis
- CRP : C-Reactive Protein
- CSF : Cerebrospinal Fluid
- DHPR : Dihydropteridine Reductase
- DIC : Disseminated Intravascular Coagulation
- DNPH : Dinitrophenylhydrazine Test
- DVET : Double Volume Exchange Transfusion
- EA : Esophageal Atresia
- ECF : Extracellular Fluid
- ECP : Eosinophilic Cationic Proteins
- ECW : Extracellular Water
- EPO : Erythropoietin
- ESR : Erythrocyte Sedimentation Rate
- ETCO : End Tidal Carbon Monoxide in Breath
- FAD : Flavin Adenine Dinucleotide
- FBA : Foreign Body Aspiration
- G6PD : Glucose-6-Phosphate Dehydrogenase
- GGT : γ-Glutamyl Transferase
- GSSG : Glutathione
- HIE : Hypoxic Ischemic Encephalopathy
- IAP : Indian Academy of Pediatrics
- ICF : Intracellular Fluid
- ICH : Intracranial Hemorrhage
- ICW : Intracellular Water
- IVH : Intraventricular Hemorrhage
- LFT : Liver Function Test
- LMA : Laryngeal Mask Airway
- MBP : Major Basic Protein
- MERRF : Myoclonic Epilepsy Ragged Red Fibers
- MLPA : Multiplex Ligation Dependent Probe Amplification
- MSAF : Meconium-Stained Amniotic Fluid
- MSUD : Maple Syrup Urine Disease
- NAD : Nicotinamide Adenine Dinucleotide
- NEC : Necrotizing Enterocolitis
- NGS : Next Generation Sequencing
- NNF : National Neonatology Forum
- NNPD : National Neonatal Perinatal Database
- NSAIDs : Nonsteroidal Anti-inflammatory Drugs
- ORT : Oral Rehydration Therapy
- PAH : Phenylalanine Hydroxylase
- PAL : Phenylalanine Ammonia Lyase
- PARDS : Pediatric Acute Respiratory Distress Syndrome
- PHH : Post Hemorrhagic Hydrocephalus
- PKU : Phenylketonuria
- POI : Premature Ovarian Insufficiency
- PPM1K : Protein Phosphatase 1k Mitochondrial
- PPV : Positive Pressure Ventilation
- PROM : Prolonged Rupture of Membrane
- PSARP : Posterior Sagittal Anorectoplasty
- PTS : Pediatric Trauma Score
- RDS : Respiratory Distress Syndrome
- ROS : Reactive Oxygen Species
- RTA : Road Traffic Accident
- SBS : Shaken Baby Syndrome
- SCIWORA : Spinal Cord Injury without Radiologic Abnormality
- SGOT : Glutamic-Oxalacetic Transaminase
- SGPT : Glutamic-Pyruvic Transaminase
- SIADH : Syndrome of Inappropriate Antidiuretic Hormone Secretion
- SVET : Single Volume Exchange Transfusion
- TcB : Transcutaneous Bilirubin
- TEF : Tracheoesophageal Fistula
- TORCH : Toxoplasmosis, Rubella Cytomegalovirus, Herpes Simplex, and HIV
- TPN : Total Parental Nutrition
- TPP : Thiamine Pyrophosphate
- TRAIL : Transfusion Related Acute Lung Injury
- TSB : Total Serum Bilirubin

## Short Answer Questions

1. List out the common toxic agents and their antidotes.
2. Explain the management of foreign body aspiration.
3. Describe the types of fluid disturbances.
4. Explain the management of PKU.
5. List out the types of metabolic disorders.

## Long Answer Questions

1. List out the common pediatric emergencies and explain the management.
2. Define asphyxia neonatorum. Describe the management.
3. Define neonatal sepsis. Describe the screening and management of neonatal sepsis.
4. Describe the nursing management of respiratory distress syndrome.
5. Define status asthmaticus. Enumerate the medical and nursing management.

6. Describe the surgical and nursing management of anorectal malformation.
7. Explain the types, clinical features, diagnosis and management of cleft palate.
8. Define hypernatremia. Write down the clinical features and management of a child with hypernatremia.
9. Describe the types, clinical features, diagnosis and management of childhood seizure.

### Multiple Choice Questions

1. **Dietary treatment of a child with PKU includes:**
   a. Protein free diet
   b. Protein enriched diet
   c. Phenylalanine free diet
   d. Low phenylalanine diet

2. **Dark color urine is associated with which of the following disease:**
   a. Alkaptonuria
   b. Cystinuria
   c. G6PD Deficiency
   d. Tyrosinemia

3. **Which of the following is a common cause of respiratory distress syndrome in preterm babies?**
   a. Lack of nutrient
   b. G6PD deficiency
   c. Poor surfactant
   d. Vitamin B12 deficiency

4. **Which of the following is an antidote of acetaminophen?**
   a. Protamine sulphate
   b. Neostigmine
   c. N-acetylcysteine
   d. Flumazenil

5. **The condition in which a part of intestine slides into the adjacent intestinal lumen making a telescopic appearance.**
   a. Volvulus
   b. Hirschsprung disease
   c. Necrotizing enterocolitis
   d. Intussusception

### Answer Key

| 1. | (d) | 2. | (a) | 3. | (c) | 4. | (c) | 5. | (d) |

### Bibliography

1. Acute Severe Asthma. AHC Media: Continuing Medical. 2013. Available from: https://www.reliasmedia.com/articles/64747-acute-severe-asthma
2. Agarwal R, Deorari AK, Paul V, Sankar MJ, Sachdeva A. AIIMS Protocol in Neonatology. 2nd ed. In: Agrawal R, editor. Noble Publisher; 2019:759.
3. Agrawal K. Cleft Palate Repair and Variations. Indian J Plast Surg;42(Suppl):S102. Available from:/pmc/articles/PMC2825076/
4. Akman İ, Galip N. Pretermde Germinal Matriks İntraventriküler Ka. J Istanbul Fac Med. 2011;74(2):43–6. Available from: https://dergipark.org.tr/en/pub/iuitfd/issue/9263/115872
5. Akram A, McKnight MM, Bellardie H, Beale V, Evans RD. Craniofacial Malformations and the Orthodontist. Br Dent J 2015 2183;218(3):129–41. Available from: https://www.nature.com/articles/sj.bdj.2015.48
6. Al Balushi A, Sahib M, Balushi T. Palatal Fistula Post-Cleft Palate Repair: A Tertiary Center Experience in Oman. Mod Plast Surg. 2017;7:21–30.
7. Alkaptonuria -NORD (National Organization for Rare Disorders). Available from: https://rarediseases.org/rare-diseases/alkaptonuria/
8. Balachandran A, Saxena A, Aggarwal A, Sinha A, Dubey A, Paul AK. IAP Textbook of Pediatrics. 7th ed. Parthasarathy A. New Delhi: Jaypee Brothers Medical Publisher (P) Ltd; 2019.
9. Balık E, Özok G, Ulman I, Demircan M, Sakallı Ü. Pediatric trauma score: Is it Reliable in Predicting Mortality? Pediatr Surg Int. 1993;8:54–5.
10. Blackburn PR, Gass JM, Vairo FPE, Farnham KM, Atwal HK, Macklin S, et al. Maple Syrup Urine Disease: Mechanisms and Management. Appl Clin Genet. 2017;10:57–66.
11. Chanez P, Bourdin A. Pathophysiology of Asthma. Clin Asthma. 2008;23–34.
12. Chawla D, Agarwal R, Deorari AK, Paul VK. Fluid and Electrolyte Management in Term and Preterm Neonates. Indian J Pediatr. 2008;75(3):255–9.
13. Dabas A, Saha A, Jain A, Gupta A, Bajpai A, Kumar A, et al. Textbook of Pediatrics. 5th ed. Gupta P, editor. New Delhi: CBS Publishers and Distributors. 2021.
14. Dutta P. Pediatric Nursing. 5th ed. New Delhi: Jaypee Brothers Medical Publisher(P) Ltd; 2022:538.
15. Galactosemia—NORD (National Organization for Rare Disorders). Available from: https://rarediseases.org/rare-diseases/galactosemia/
16. Glucose-6-phosphate Dehydrogenase Deficiency. WHO Working Group. Bull World Health Organ. 1989;67(6):601–11.
17. Glucose-6-Phosphate Dehydrogenase Deficiency—NORD (National Organization for Rare Disorders). Available from: https://rarediseases.org/rare-diseases/glucose-6-phosphate-dehydrogenase-deficiency/
18. Hyperkalemia: Practice Essentials, Background. Available from: https://emedicine.medscape.com/article/240903-overview.
19. Hypernatremia: Practice Essentials, Pathophysiology, Etiology. Available from: https://emedicine.medscape.com/article/241094-overview.
20. Hypokalemia: Practice Essentials, Pathophysiology, Etiology. Available from: https://emedicine.medscape.com/article/242008-overview.

21. Hyponatremia: Practice Essentials, Pathophysiology, Epidemiology. Available from: https://emedicine.medscape.com/article/242166-overview.
22. Hypospadias: Practice Essentials, Pathophysiology, Etiology. Available from: https://emedicine.medscape.com/article/1015227-overview#a5
23. Intracranial Hemorrhage -StatPearls -NCBI Bookshelf. Available from: https://www.ncbi.nlm.nih.gov/books/NBK470242/
24. Kliegman RM, Stanton B, Geme J St., Schor NF, Behrman RE. Nelson Textbook of Pediatrics. 21st ed. Kliegman RM, editor. Elsevier; 2019: 4264.
25. Lakshmanaswamy A. Clinical Paediatrics. 5th ed. Haryana: Wolters Kluwer (India) Pvt. Ltd; 2021.
26. Manual T. Navjaat Shishu Suraksha Karyakram Basic Newborn Care and Resuscitation Program Training Manual. 2020. Available from: http://www.nihfw.org/pdf/NCHRC-Publications/NavjaatShishuTrgMan.pdf
27. Maple Syrup Urine Disease -NORD (National Organization for Rare Disorders). Available from: https://rarediseases.org/rare-diseases/maple-syrup-urine-disease/
28. Matthay MA, Zemans RL, Zimmerman GA, Arabi YM, Beitler JR, Mercat A, et al. Acute Respiratory Distress Syndrome. Nat Rev Dis Prim. 2019;5(1):18.
29. Neurology: Antiepileptic Medications Available from: https://www.rch.org.au/neurology/patient_information/antiepileptic_medications/
30. Newborn T. Standard Treatment Guidelines 2022 Respiratory Distress in the Term Newborn. 2023.
31. Paneitz DC, Ahmad S. Pediatric Trauma Update. Mo Med. 2018;115(5):438–42.
32. Pediatric Pneumonia Clinical Presentation: History, Physical Examination, Patients with Recurrent Pneumonias. Available from: https://emedicine.medscape.com/article/967822-clinical
33. Rovin JD, Rodgers BM. Pediatric Foreign Body Aspiration. Pediatr Rev. 2000;21(3):86–90.
34. Saharan S, Lodha R, Kabra SK. Management of Status Asthmaticus in Children. Indian J Pediatr. 2010;77(12):1417–23. Available from: https://doi.org/10.1007/s12098-010-0189-8
35. Santhanam S, Anand P, Mohanty PK, Kumar R, Gupta P. Neonatal Sepsis Standard Treatment Guidelines 2022 Upendra Kinjawadekar Under the Auspices of the IAP Action Plan 2022. 2023.
36. Sharma R. Essentials of Pediatric Nursing. 3rd ed. New Delhi: Jaypee Brothers Medical Publisher (P) Ltd; 2021:513.
37. Singhi S, Jain V, Gupta G. Pediatric Emergencies at a Tertiary Care Hospital in India. J Trop Pediatr. 2003;49(4):207–11.
38. Status Asthmaticus—StatPearls -NCBI Bookshelf. Available from: https://www.ncbi.nlm.nih.gov/books/NBK526070/
39. Tiwari M. Glucose 6 Phosphatase Dehydrogenase (G6PD) and Neurodegenerative Disorders: Mapping Diagnostic and Therapeutic Opportunities. Genes Dis. 2017;4(4):196–203.
40. Topjian AA, Raymond TT, Atkins D, Chan M, Duff JP, Joyner BL, et. al. Part 4: Pediatric Basic and Advanced Life Support: 2020 American Heart Association Guidelines for Cardiopulmonary Resuscitation and Emergency Cardiovascular Care. Circulation. 2020;142(16 2):S469–523.
41. Turner NM. Recent Developments in Neonatal and Pediatric Emergencies. Eur J Anaesthesiol; 2011;28(7):471–7.
42. Vasudevan D, SS, Vaidyanathan K. Electrolyte and Water Balance; 2017:410–20.

# Chapter 14

# Other Emergency Conditions and Management

*Madhusmita Nayak*

## CHAPTER OUTLINE

- Assessment and Mechanism of Injuries
  - Thoracic injury
  - Abdominal injury
  - Pelvic fracture
  - Complications of trauma
- Shock
  - Hypovolemic shock
  - Cardiogenic shock
  - Anaphylactic shock
  - Neurogenic shock
  - Septic shock
- Systemic Inflammatory Response Syndrome
- Multiple Organ Dysfunction Syndrome
- Disseminated Intravascular Coagulations
- Drug Overdose and Poisoning
- Acquired Immunodeficiency Syndrome (AIDS)
- Eye Injuries
- Nose Injuries
- Throat Injuries

## Learning Objectives

At the end of the chapter, the students will be able to:
- Assess and understand the mechanism of various trauma or injury.
- Identify the signs of thoracic injury and can manage them.
- Manage abdominal injury.
- Evaluate the signs of pelvic fracture and can able to take precautionary measures while managing it.
- Have idea about the complications of trauma if not treated early.
- Understand various types of shock and ways to manage it.
- Gain knowledge on systemic inflammatory response syndrome and multiple organ dysfunction syndrome.
- Assess a case of disseminated intravascular coagulation and various ways to manage it with nurses role.
- Get an idea about the various drugs overdose signs with poisoning and its emergency treatment.
- Care for patients with HIV and AIDS.
- Diagnose and manage the eye, nose and neck injuries.

## ASSESSMENT AND MECHANISM OF INJURY

### Trauma Assessment

Trauma can be defined as any type of injury to the body organs caused by external forces. The cause can be many like road traffic accidents (RTA), fires explosions, burns, fall injury, any act of violence and crime against vulnerable people (women, children and elderly). Among all the major cause always being the RTAs. Statistics shows that around 5 million of deaths and disability occurs around the world secondary to RTAs **(Fig. 14.1)**. In India alone, the estimated figure is 1 million deaths and around 20 million hospitalization per year. Many times it is seen that the deaths can be prevented through in-time action and keen assessment. Hence all the health professional team members should have knowledge and adequate expertise in doing the trauma assessment as per the guideline to save the lives.

### Objectives

- Decide on appropriate method of trauma assessment.
- Assess the pre-preparation needed for trauma assessment.

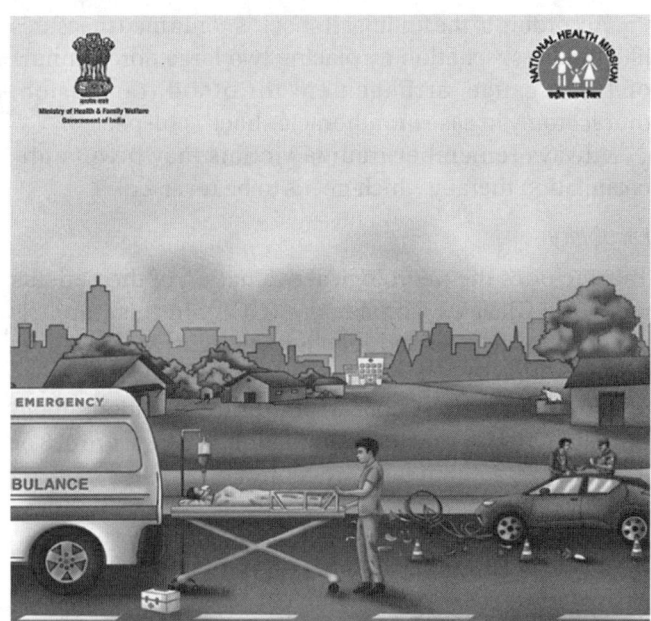

**Fig. 14.1:** Road traffic accident.
*Source:* Training Manual on Management of Common Emergencies, Burns and Trauma for Staff Nurse. NHM Odisha.

- Co-relate the assessment findings with the presence of risk factors and to decide on diagnostics for establishing clinical significance.
- Strengthen the strategies among the inter-professional team members including coordination in care delivery, communication at various level, quick decision-making and prompt action for improving the outcomes.

## Techniques of Assessment

The technique or methods of assessment is an important part of trauma assessment. Every individual both health care and even bystanders who witness an accident victim must know the initial and basic assessment steps which will help to reduce the mortality to a greater extent. **Flowchart 14.1** shows techniques of assessment.

## Pre-hospital Assessment

It is the job of the first responder or the emergency medical service (EMS) team at the place of accident before arrival of the patient to the hospital. The team should contain a physician and nurse and it is ideal to have roles assigned before the arrival of the patient. Usually, the physician is the team leader. The job of team leader is to assign the various roles to the team members and he/she is in-charge of the direction and decision-making upon patient arrival including thorough assessment. Other roles may include history collection, documentation, airway management,

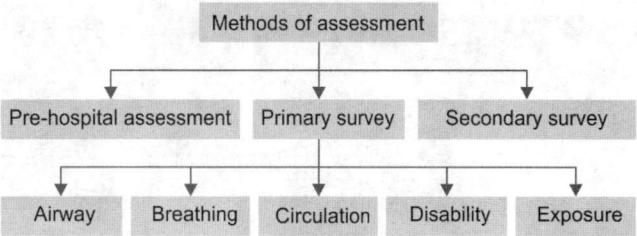

**Flowchart 14.1:** Techniques of assessment.

IV access, attach monitoring devices, and medication administration. The relevant data includes age, gender, mechanism of injury, vital signs, injury sites with intensity, interventions given, etc., as much as possible. Then enquire should be done to identify the possible injury may result in life-threatening conditions. The role of the EMS team is important as they have all revenant information and also, they have prepared equipment for emergency procedure before shifting the patient to the main hospital. It is important to stabilize the patient before transport.

### Primary Survey

Before transportation, the EMS team will inform the tertiary care hospital to prepare the room for patient treatment. Upon arrival of the patient the room should be ready and quiet. The EMS team will brief about the patient's history of injury with emergency management given and also any sign of life-threatening injury. After that the primary survey conducted. It goes in sequence of airway, breathing, circulation, disability, exposure (ABCDE) suggested by advanced trauma life support (ATLS) **(Fig. 14.2)**, developed by the American College of Surgeons.

#### Airway

- Ensuring the patency of airway is the initial step of trauma management and prevents trauma related deaths to maximum extent.
- If the patient is conscious then the patency is ascertained by asking patients questions like name and other this and checking how the patient is responding. This follows the visual inspection of the patient like signs of respiratory distress, presence of stridor, inspecting face, oral cavity, and neck.
- Oral cavity is inspected to see any obstruction like secretion, foreign objects which may interfere with natural air flow and intubation.
- For unconscious patient, tracheostomy is the ideal one. Or else cricothyrotomy can be performed alternatively.
- It is to remember that cervical spine immobilization is a must during and post intubation proper fixation of the tube is highly essential to avoid accidental removal.

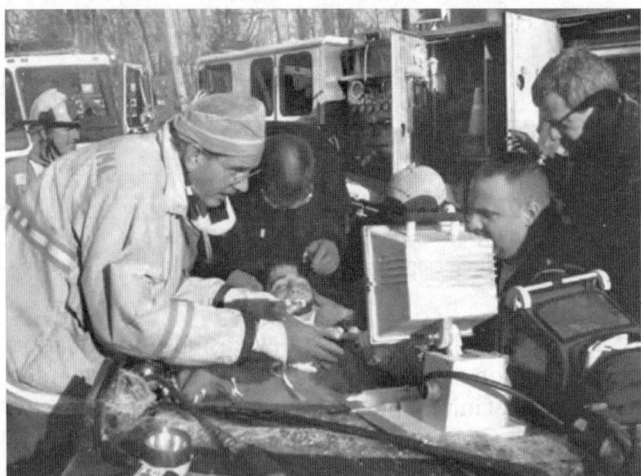

**Fig. 14.2:** ATLS teamwork.

*Source:* National Institute of Health.Gov. Subcommittee AT, International ATLS Working Group. Advanced trauma life support (ATLS®): the ninth edition. The journal of trauma and acute care surgery. 2013 May;74(5):1363-6.

*Breathing*

- My second priority after airway is the breathing assessment. It includes inspection of the patient's chest for pattern of chest rise, any sign of injury, paradoxical chest movement indicating flail chest, penetrating injury, or tracheal deviation.
- Palpate the chest for signs of crepitus and signs of tension pneumothorax. Auscultation for abnormal lung sound. Oxygen saturation to be monitored.
- Diagnostic studies like ultrasonography or chest X-ray can be done along with the physical examination to more confirm the diagnosis.

*Circulation*

The aim is to arrest bleeding and to maintain adequate tissue oxygenation. Start with inspection about any sign of hypovolemic shock like tachycardia and hypotension. This can be confirmed by palpating carotid or femoral pulse.

The 5 locations to look for major hemorrhage include the thorax, peritoneal cavity, retroperitoneal cavity, pelvic or long bone fractures, and external injury.

External bleedings controlled by direct pressure and arterial bleeding from an extremity can be managed by tying tourniquet.

Investigations include focused assessment using sonography in trauma (FAST) examination for evaluation of intra-abdominal bleeding and extended FAST exam (includes pulmonary evaluation) for the evaluation of cardiac tamponade and pneumothorax and cardiac monitoring.

According to the findings if shock is confirmed measures like fluid resuscitation by placing two large bore cannula of 16–18 gauge, arrangement for blood transfusion, thoracotomy in case intrathoracic shock is suspected.

Always remember trauma victims may be on anti-coagulation therapy which needs to be reversed.

*Disability*

This includes the neurological evaluation of the patients using the Glasgow Coma Score (GCS). In this pupils is checked for its size and reactivity to light. Motor ability and sensation in all four extremities are checked for signs of spinal cord injury. Cervical spine immobilization should be maintained during the examination. A GCS score of 8 or less requires definitive airway control.

*Exposure*

It is the final step of the primary survey. It includes minute assessment of the bodily injury which may be skipped during the pre-hospital assessment. This is done by exposing the whole body of the client by removing all cloths. The skin and other areas are examined. But to remember that the patient should be kept warm to prevent hypothermia as it may lead to multiple organ failure.

**Secondary Survey**

It is indicated when the patient is stable and may not need immediate surgical intervention. It is important to perform because there are 4 common conditions which mostly missed during the initial assessment such as "blunt abdominal trauma with internal organ injury, penetrating abdominal trauma, penetrating thoracic trauma, and extremity trauma such as fractures and compartment syndrome".

It includes further detailed history from the patient, a thorough head-to-toe exam, and diagnostic testing.

*History in Detail*

- The history includes patient's past medical and surgical history, medications, and allergies, details of the traumatic event along with mechanism of injury.
- For blunt trauma, important questions may include speed, whether used seatbelt, object damage, and/or height of a fall. For penetrating trauma, it is helpful to know what penetrated the patient, the length of the knife or penetrating objects, and potentially the number of gunshots heard.
- Under medication history, it is important to know if the patient is on anticoagulants or antiplatelet medications or any medications which may affect the physiologic response to hemorrhage.

*Physical Assessment*
- **Head:** For signs of lacerations, abrasions, any foreign body invasion, damage to bones.
- **Ear:** Ear should be inspected for hemotympanum, tympanic membrane rupture, blood within the ear canal, and any other external trauma.
- **Eyes:** Eyes are evaluated for papilledema, globe rupture, unequal pupils, abrasion, and foreign body.
- **Nose:** Bleeding or septal hematoma.
- **Mouth:** Dental injury, bleeding, and posterior oropharynx obstruction, swelling, or edema.
- **Neck:** Palpate for bony injury, crepitus, midline trachea, lacerations, hematomas, and abrasions. Cervical immobilization should be kept in mind while doing such examination.
- **Chest:** Both inspection and palpation of chest is done to detect any sign of deformity, ecchymosis, penetrating wounds, difficult breath, crepitus, and flail chest. Auscultation for abnormal lung sound. Work of breathing can be evaluated through respiratory rate, use of accessory muscles, or inspiratory retractions.
- **Abdomen:** Distension, tenderness, any penetrating injury, abrasions, seatbelt sign, and/or bruising.
- **Flank and back:** Presence of bruising in bilateral flanks or surrounding the patient's umbilicus may represent a retroperitoneal hemorrhage.
- **Rectum and urinary system:** A digital rectal examination done for presence of blood or perineal injury.
- **Genitalia:** Any bleeding, ecchymosis, or lacerations.
- **Musculoskeletal exam:** Extremities evaluated for pain, decreased temperature, or tension that may indicate compartment syndrome. Also look for presence of bruising, laceration, abrasion, open fractures, bony abnormalities, and active bleeding. Pallor in extremity indicates possible blood loss, cyanosis and decreased oxygen perfusion.
- **Neurological examination:** Includes testing the cranial nerves, its strength, sensation, coordination, and reflexes.

*Diagnostic Evaluation*
- **X-rays:** X-rays may be performed for detecting injury to the lungs and pelvis.
- **CT scan:** To evaluate an injury to head, cervical spine, chest or abdomen, and pelvis.

## Mechanism of Injury

First of all with various types of trauma like penetrating/blunt or deceleration, leads to hemorrhage due to tissue injury. This leads to three types of response in the body like activation of coagulation pathway, neuroendocrine stress response and hypoperfused tissue. This ultimately leads to activation of endothelial cells. Wth this inflammatory cells pulled to the injury site lading to immunosuppression and catabolism syndrome (PICS) and systemic inflammatory response syndrome (SIRS). Hence the final outcome is cell injury followed by organ dysfunction. The detailed mechanism in shown in **Flowchart 14.2**.

## Thoracic Injury

Thoracic injury or chest trauma is accounting for around 25% of all deaths occurring from traumatic injury. It usually involves injuries to the bony thorax, intrathoracic organs and thoracic medulla. The most cause of mortality is due to not taking timely measures and delay in reaching the hospital facility. However, many deaths can be prevented with immediate detection and management of the cases. This also prevents incidence of disability secondary to trauma. Anatomically thoracic cavity consists of ribs, spine, sternum with supporting muscles and ligaments. Trauma to the chest wall causes sudden decompression of thorax with pulmonary contusion and in worst cases lung injury. These trauma can be of two types namely blunt and penetrating trauma. The mortality rate of penetrating traumas are higher in comparison to the blunt one. The cause for penetrating traumas **(Fig. 14.3)** are stubbing and gunshot which complicates with direct lungs and other thoracic organ injury. Hence this call for an emergency management.

### Definition

Thoracic injury is defined as a form of injury to the chest wall including ribs, heart, lungs, great vessels, trachea and esophagus.

### Types

The thoracic injury is broadly classified to two main categories named chest injuries and pulmonary injuries. Chet injuries could be blunt and penetrating according to the type of area involved. Whereas the pulmonary injuries involves pneumothorax, hemothorax and cardiac tamponade. The detailed is being explained in **Flowchart 14.3**.

### Causes of Thoracic Injury

The two types of thoracic injury can be cause by various causes. The factors for blunt injury could be all types of road accidents, falls, injuries got during sports, etc., and so also the causes for penetrating injury could be injury or attack by knife, gunshot, arrow also sometime occupational injuries like working with heavy machines in factories. A clear picture has been given in **Figure 14.4**.

**Flowchart 14.2:** Mechanism of injury.

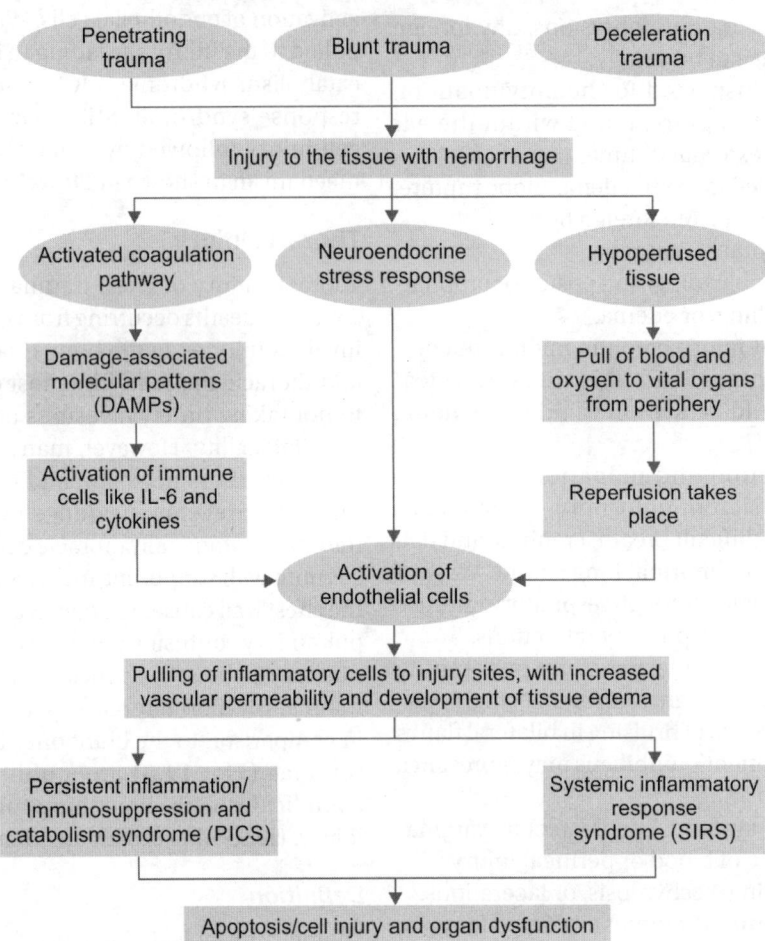

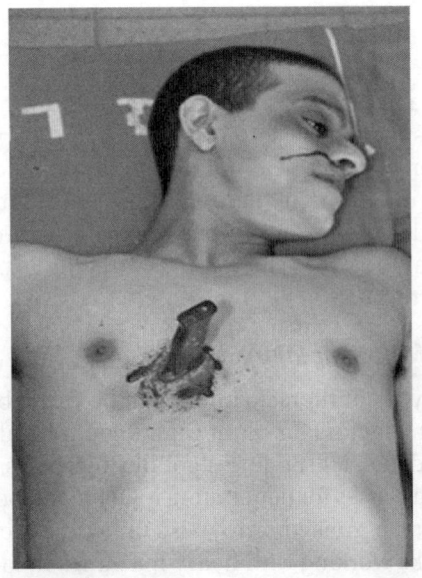

**Fig. 14.3:** Penetrating chest injury.

**Flowchart 14.3:** Classification of injuries.

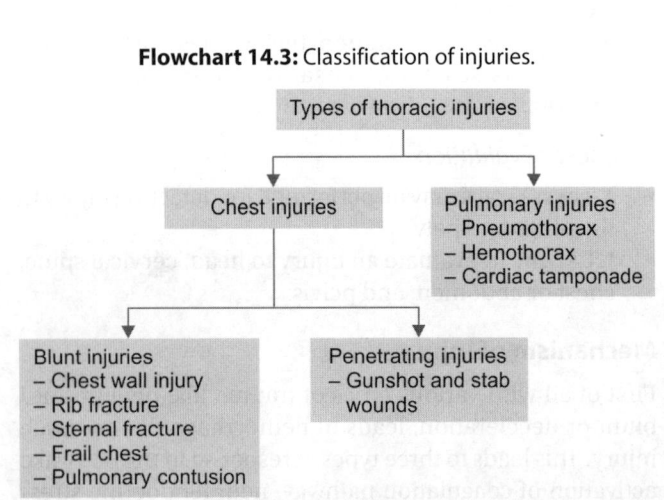

# Chapter 14: Other Emergency Conditions and Management

## Chest Injuries

It includes both blunt and penetrating trauma.

### Defining Blunt Trauma

It occurs when the chest wall gets hit by a blunt object, such as a steering wheel. Externally the injury may look minor, but its impact can be severe and life-threatening leading to internal injuries like splenic rupture.

### Mechanism Involved in Blunt Injury

It is important for every nurse to understand the mechanism how the injury has happened and it is going to do change in body post injury. Basically, three type of action can happen in any chest injuries. Those are acceleration/deceleration, shearing and lastly compression of thoracic organs. The difference between mechanism and pathophysiology here is, in mechanism usually shown how the physical force commence in body with progressing injury and in pathophysiology along with the action of physical force, how the other physiologic response takes place in body is involved. Detailed mechanism is shown in **Flowchart 14.4**.

### Pathophysiology of Blunt Injury

The progression of injury starts with occurrence of injury by various means like accidents and trauma or fall. Then with the three types of mechanism like acceleration/deceleration, shearing and compression of thoracic organs, the trauma to deeper organs and muscles takes place in the order of lungs parenchyma, respiratory muscles, ribs leading to airway obstruction and hypoxia. The further bleeding leads to hypovolemia. If this continues thus inadequate ventilation and perfusion leads to hypovolemic shock, renal failure and death **(Flowchart 14.5)**.

### Chest Wall Injury

#### Etiopathogenesis

The normal physiology of inspiration or air entry to the lungs takes place with the outward expansion of the chest wall muscles and downward compression of the diaphragm.

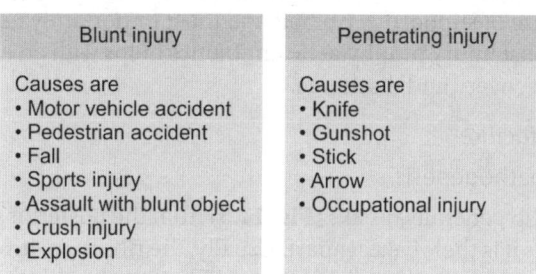

**Fig. 14.4:** Mechanism of thoracic injury.

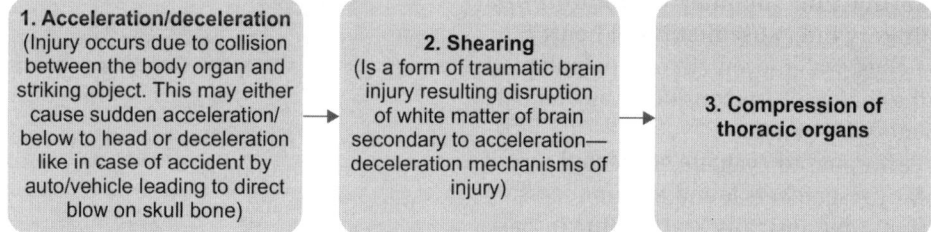

**Flowchart 14.4:** Mechanism of blunt injury.

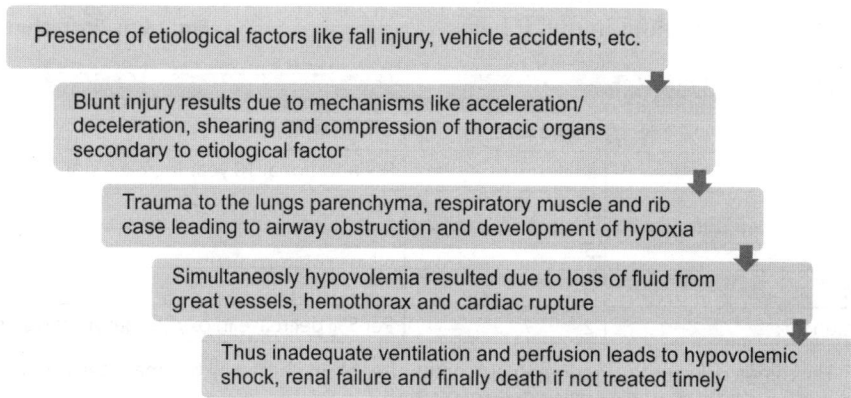

**Flowchart 14.5:** Pathophysiology of blunt injury.

This mechanism creates negative pressure and entry of air to the lungs. But with chest wall trauma with blunt injuries specially interferes with the normal respiration. As per a study the youngsters of age between 20–29 years are the victim for the same. However, some of the casualty have respiratory reserve and can withstand chest wall injury with adequate support. Even then also this type of cases must be treated with urgency to reduce the percentage of morbidity and mortality. The first 72 hours of the post injury is very crucial and decides the recovery of the injury.

### Clinical presentation

- Erythema
- Ecchymosis
- Dyspnea
- Pain during breathing
- Hypoventilation
- Crepitus
- Paradoxical chest wall movement

### Chest injury score

The chest injury score is a standardized scoring system adapted from Battle C, Lovett S, Hutchings H, Evans PA, 2014. This scoring helps to standardize the patients according to the injury risk so that further planning can be done for their immediate response and management **(Table 14.1)**.

### Diagnostic studies

- **Physical examination:** Includes evaluation of a patient's respiratory rate, auscultation of heart rate, observation of chest wall movement and palpation of tenderness in the chest wall. It is considered as adequate for stable patients with trauma.
- **Chest X-ray:** Performed to evaluate suspected risk of rib fracture. Many researchers found this unnecessary if patient is hemodynamically stable. But in case of severity, it help to identify pleural or pulmonary pathology secondary to rib fractures.
- **CT scan:** Computed tomographic scanning is also recommended in case of severe blunt injury. It helps to differentiate chest wall injury from parenchymal or mediastinal injuries. Nowadays 3D CT scans are available and are found helpful regarding decisions on surgical fixation of blunt chest wall trauma.
- **Ultrasonography (USG):** Helps with the identification of rib fractures and pneumothorax secondary to blunt chest wall injury. Also it is found beneficial for situations where X-ray and CT scan is not available.

### Management

- The main aim of management is adequate pain control measures, early mobilization and respiratory care with prevention of progression to complications.
- In case of severity optimal treatment strategies are considered including plan for surgery, ventilatory support, prompt and effective choice of analgesia, use of supportive rib belt and most importantly use of post injury prophylactic antibiotics helps with an early recovery and discharge.

## Rib Fracture

### Etiopathogenesis

- Rib generally breaks **(Fig. 14.5)** from the posterior side as it is the weakest apart. Usually, the ribs from 4th–9th are more prone for fracture than others.

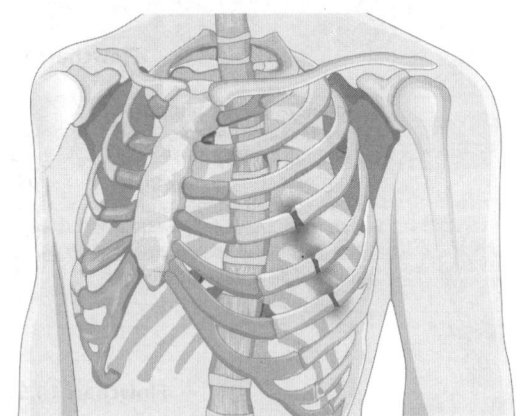

**Fig. 14.5:** Rib fracture.

| Table 14.1: Chest injury risk score. | | |
|---|---|---|
| **Risk factor** | **Risk score** | **Additional notes** |
| Age | 1 | Per additional 10 year increase starting at 10 years of age |
| Number of rib fracture | 3 | Per additional rib fracture |
| Chronic lung disease | 5 | |
| Pre-injury coagulant use | 4 | |
| Level of oxygen saturation | 2 | Per 5% decrease in oxygen saturation starting at 94% |

*Source:* Battle C, Lovett S, Hutchings H, Evans PA. Predicting outcomes after blunt chest wall trauma: development and external validation of a new prognostic model. Critical Care. 2014 Feb;18(1):1-82.

- Adults are at high risk for fracture than children. Elderly with multiple fracture in rib can be complicated with pneumonia and high mortality rate in comparison to the young ones.
- Danger lies with this is not only the breakage to the rib rather penetrating injury to the pleura, lung, liver and spleen.
- Injury to the 9th-11th rib is associated with intra-abdominal injury. And injury of 1st-3rd rib is associated with intrathoracic injury.
- Hepatic injury can be ascertained among patients with right sided rib fracture where as injury to the spleen can be suspected among patient with left sided rib trauma.
- Hence this is the need of the hour to detect early these fractures and treat promptly to prevent long-term complications.

## Clinical picture
- Pain with barrel compression test
- Tenderness
- Bony crepitus
- Ecchymosis
- Spasm of muscles over the rib

**Note:** Barrel compression test is performed by placing the patient in side-line position, then examiner will use both of her hands on the lateral side of the rib cage that is facing upward to compress the ribcage towards the table. Positive if pain or guarding is elicited. Positive test indicated possible rib fracture. It can also be done when the patient is sitting or standing in both anteriorly or posteriorly.

## Diagnostic measures
These types of fractures are commonly diagnosed by using chest X-ray. In case of suspected pulmonary involvement like contusion CT scan is the investigation of choice.

## Complications
Multiple rib fractures can lead to following pulmonary morbidities like:
- Decreased activity of phrenic nerve
- Diaphragmatic dysfunction
- Increased activity of spinal arc activity with intercostal tone
- Reduced functional residual capacity
- Ventricular tachycardia and hypoxemia

## Management
- The goal of treatment is adequate pain relief and maintaining optimum pulmonary function.
- For pain management oral drugs are usually prescribe for young and healthy patients. It is importantly advised to wait for at least 30–45 min before starting any breathing exercise or using incentive spirometry.
- Intercostal nerve blocks with a long-acting anesthetic such as bupivacaine with epinephrine may relieve symptoms up to 12 hours with excellent results.
- For pulmonary health daily activities and deep breathing should be stressed to ensure ventilation and prevent atelectasis.
- Supporting measures like binders, belts, and other restrictive devices are discouraged as they may interfere with adequate ventilation leading to subsequent atelectasis and pneumonia.
- This is to note that more the number of ribs affected greater is the rate of mortality and morbidity. Hence fracture of >3 ribs, even in the absence of other traumatic injuries should immediately be hospitalized to receive aggressive pulmonary therapy and appropriately effective analgesia.
- Also elderly patients with >6 fractured ribs should be admitted to ICU to reduce the incidence of mortality. Oversedation for the purpose of pain relief should be avoided in these cases to prevent respiratory depression and failure.
- Other source of management includes patient-controlled analgesia, parenteral opiates, and thoracic epidural analgesia.

### Sternal Fracture

#### Etiopathogenesis
- Sudden rapid deceleration and forward thrust of the body against the fixed belt during a collision or accident results in sternal fracture.
- It is common among women and older people than younger ones because it is through that young people can transmit effectively the kinetic energy to mediastinum. But possible soft tissue injuries happens in every case in the absence of severity also.
- Complications like myocardial contusion, spinal injury seen in around 6–10% of total cases. Out of which mediastinal injury is considered life-threatening.

#### Clinical presentation
The signs of sternal fracture are chest pain, tenderness, Ecchymosis, crepitus and swelling in chest wall, and that of rib fracture are pain at the injury site, shallow breathing, splinting of chest, etc. (**Table 14.2**).

#### Diagnostic studies
- History and physical assessment
- CT scan
- Chest X-ray (may not be conclusive)
- Ultrasonography
- A 12 lead ECG

| Table 14.2: Clinical presentation of sternal fracture. | |
| --- | --- |
| **Sternal fracture** | **Rib fracture** |
| ◆ Anterior chest pain<br>◆ Overlying tenderness<br>◆ Ecchymosis, crepitus<br>◆ Swelling and possible chest wall deformity | ◆ Pain at the site of injury<br>◆ Shallow breathing<br>◆ Localized tenderness and crepitus on palpation and auscultation<br>◆ Splinting of the chest |

### Management
- Control of pain through proper administration of analgesics. Around 95% of cases can be discharged after this.
- Only a few with severity like overlapping bone fragments showing exaggerated pain, respiratory depression needs immediate surgery.

### Flail Chest
- Flail chest occurs when three or more adjacent ribs are fractured at two points, allowing a freely moving segment of the chest wall to move in paradoxical motion.
- The paradoxical chest movement is the identifying sign of this condition.
- The complications include pulmonary contusion causing respiratory inadequacy, muscular splinting, atelectasis, hypoxemia, and decreased cardiac output.

### Pathophysiology
With a flail chest injury paradoxical breathing occurs due to rib breakage. This leads to low alveolar ventilation and lastly respiratory acidosis. The detailed is given in **Flowchart 14.6**.

### Clinical presentation
- Rapid and shallow breathing
- Tachycardia
- Asymmetrical and un-coordinated chest wall movement
- Dyspnea and chest pain

### Diagnosis
- Collection of history with physical assessment (includes thoracic assessment for paradoxical motion, pain and tenderness)
- Auscultation of lung sound sir any abnormality like crepitus
- Chest X-ray
- CT scan more confirmatory in detecting the presence and extent of underlying injury and contusion to the lung parenchyma
- Atrial blood gas analysis
- ECG and test for cardiac enzyme for suspected tension pneumothorax

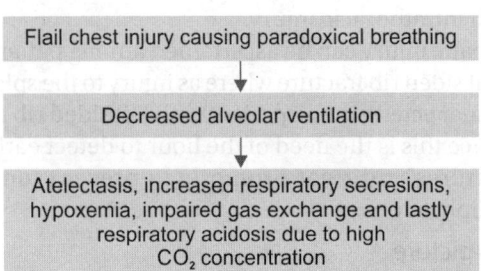

**Flowchart 14.6:** Pathophysiology of flail chest.

- Echocardiogram for significant dysrhythmias, high-grade blocks, or hemodynamic instability unexplained by other causes such as hemorrhage.

### Management
- Emergency care includes immediate administration of oxygen with cardiac and pulse oximetry monitoring.
- The cornerstones of treatment include aggressive pulmonary physiotherapy, effective analgesia, selective use of endotracheal intubation and mechanical ventilation, and close observation in case of respiratory compromise.
- The indication for intubation and ventilator is respiratory decompensation. In case of conscious patient CPAP can be considered.
- Researches show that early operative correction with internal fixation of the flail segment results in a speedier recovery with decreased complication rate, and better cosmetic and functional results, and is cost-effective. Indications for surgery are patients unable to be weaned from the ventilator secondary to flail chest, persistent pain, severe chest wall instability, and a progressive decline in pulmonary functions.
- Future long-term complications may include disability with dyspnea, chronic thoracic pain, and exercise intolerance.

### Pulmonary Contusion
- It was first described by Morgagni in the year 1761. According to Morgagni, "pulmonary contusion is a direct bruise of the lung parenchyma followed by alveolar edema and hemorrhage but without an accompanying pulmonary laceration" **(Fig. 14.6)**.

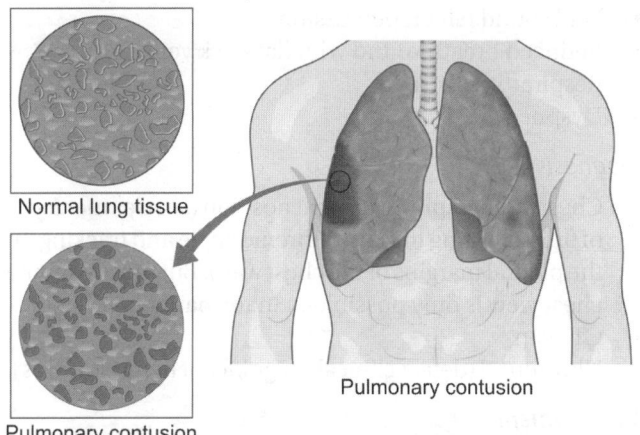

Fig. 14.6: Pulmonary contusion.

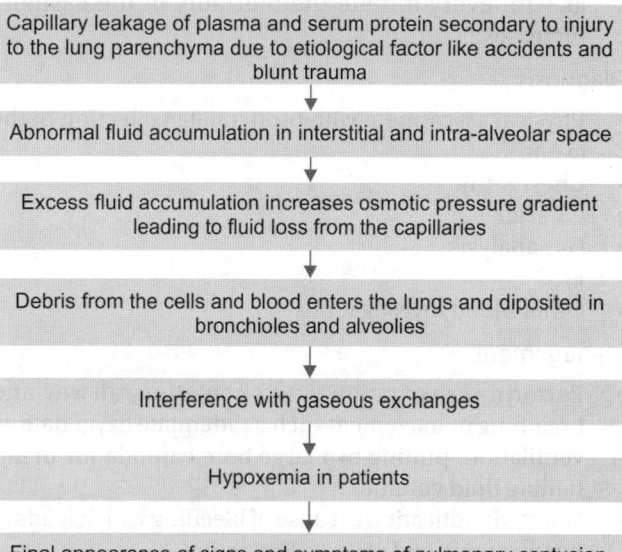

Flowchart 14.7: Pathophysiology of pulmonary contusion.

- Incidence is 30–75%, and commonly seen among children with vehicle accidents.
- It is usually a complication to the flail chest.

Pathophysiology

The pulmonary contusion is the severe injury to the lungs parenchyma due to blunt chest trauma. The disordered physiological process is as below. First due to the causative factors like blunt traumas, direct damage to lung parenchyma occurs. This then leads to leakage of plasma protein and serum protein from the capillary. The result is abnormal fluid accumulation in interstitial and intra-alveolar space. Because of the excess fluid accumulation, the osmotic pressure increased. This leads to loss of capillary fluid. Further debris from the cells and blood enters the lungs and deposited in bronchioles and alveoli. This interferes with the gaseous exchange leading to hypoxia and development of the clinical pictures of pulmonary contusion (Flowchart 14.7).

Clinical presentation

- Respiratory symptoms like dyspnea, tachypnea, hemoptysis and cyanosis
- Cardiovascular symptoms like tachycardia, hypotension and chest wall bruising
- On auscultation absence of breath sounds with rales may be heard
- On palpation fractured ribs may reveal

Diagnosis

- Detailed history with physical assessment
- Chest X-ray
- CT scan
- ABG analysis may show sign of hypoxemia

Treatment

- The first line of treatment is supportive therapy aiming at adequate lung ventilation though intubation and mechanical ventilation. Another reason for this treatment is it prevents overexpansion of one lung and gradual collapse of the other.
- The physician may also consider BPAP or CPAP to avoid invasive procedures.
- Patients with extensive pulmonary contusions and ARDS, extracorporeal membrane oxygenation can be considered for them.
- Certain procedures like fluid restriction, vigorous tracheobronchial toileting, suctioning, and pain management measures helps to combat the symptoms of contusion.
- Note: Use of colloid for these patients is not recommended due to the risk of colloid sequestration within alveoli secondary to capillary leakage.
- The organism sensitive antibiotics are administered to prevent the development of pneumonia.

## Penetrating Injuries

**Definition:** It happens when a foreign body penetrates the body tissues such as stab by a sharp object, gunshot injury, etc.

### Gunshot and Stabbing Wounds

- Most commonly results in penetrating injury.
- Considered life-threatening as it ends up with pneumothorax, hemothorax, contusion of lungs, cardiac tamponade and profuse bleeding leading to shock even the size of the wound is small.

- Hence this requires immediate medical attention as with every minute the mortality of the casualty increases.

### Diagnosis
- Physical assessment with proper data collection of the event
- Chest X-ray
- CT scan
- Gas analysis
- ECG
- Other blood investigations

### Management
- Perform resuscitation with circulation, airway and breathing management such as adequate oxygenation, ventilation, putting two large bore cannula for maintaining fluid volume.
- Quick identification of cause of bleeding which leads to hypovolemia and source elimination.
- Strict intake output monitoring with placing urinary catheter.
- To prevent aspiration, attach the nasogastric tube to a low force suction machine.
- Adequate lungs expansion is commonly affected with penetrating injury, hence consider the insertion of a chest tube for maintaining adequate lungs ventilation.

## Pulmonary Injuries

### Pneumothorax
- **Definition:** Pneumothorax is a complication of thorax injury which means the accumulation of air in the pleural space.
- **Incidence:** It is 10–15% among chest trauma patients.
- **Types of pneumothorax with management:** Pneumothorax is of three types. Those are closed pneumothorax (**Fig. 14.7**), open pneumothorax (**Fig. 14.8**) and tension pneumothorax (**Fig. 14.9**). The details of types of pneumothorax is explained in **Table 14.3**.

## Hemothorax

### Definition
It is defined as accumulation of blood in the pleural space secondary to either blunt or penetrating chest injury. This alters the homeostasis by developing hypovolemic shock (**Fig. 14.10**).

Chylothorax is the accumulation of lymphatic fluid in the pleural space due to leakage in the thoracic duct.

### Signs and Symptoms
- Signs of shock like tachycardia and hypotension, cold and clammy skin
- Dull sound felt on percussion
- Reduced breath sound with flat neck vein
- Respiratory distress
- Dyspnea

### Diagnosis
- Chest radiography in upright position (seen as meniscus of fluid blunting the costophrenic angle and tracking up the pleural margins of the chest wall). But mostly supine chest view is only possible in many patients.
- CT scan
- Ultrasound (detect clinically significant hemothoraces).

### Management
Management of hemothorax is laid out according to the condition of the patient. That is whether the patient is stable or unstable. In case the patient is stable, a series of blood test are advised to see if the amount of blood accumulation. In case when the blood accumulation is >300 mL, then drainage is attached. Then we have to see how much is the drainage coming. If it is >1500 mL in 24 hours or >250 mL/hour, then the patient is categorized as unstable and plan for thoracotomy/VATS is recommended. Similarly if the accumulation blood is <300 mL, which means the patient is less serious hence follow adequate pain control followed by chest X-ray every 4–6 hourly first and then in 24 hours. then if the patient is stable (drain <1500 mL/24 hours or <250 mL/hours), closed tube thoracostomy/thoracotomy/VATS is advised. On the other hand, if the patient is unstable, an urgent thoracotomy is recommended. The detailed pathophysiology is given in **Flowchart 14.8**.

## Cardiac Tamponade

### Definition
It refers to the compression of the heart secondary to the abnormal accumulation of either blood or fluid in the pericardial space (**Fig. 14.11**).

### Etiology
- Iatrogenic-post to any cardiac surgery or procedures
- Trauma
- Malignancy
- Myocardial infraction

### Pathophysiology
In case of cardiac tamponade, there is accumulation of free fluid in cardiac chamber, which interferes with the diastolic filling of ventricles. If the stroke volume decreases, there is decreased cardiac output and appearance of signs of hypovolemic shock. On the contrary, if the venous pressure increased, it can lead to change in various systems leading to

**Table 14.3:** Types of pneumothorax with its management.

| Types | Closed pneumothorax | Open pneumothorax | Tension pneumothorax |
|---|---|---|---|
| Definition | • No external wounds found<br>• Seen among young male with age between 20-40 years with low BMI and smokers (**Fig. 14.7**) | Occurs when air enters and accumulates in pleural space secondary to any open wound to chest wall (**Fig. 14.8**) | • Means progressive accumulation of air under pressure in pleural cavity, leading to shifting of the mediastinum to the opposite side and compressing the contralateral lung and great vessels<br>• Air enters on inspiration cannot exit with expiration (**Fig. 14.9**) |
| Causes | • Fall injury<br>• Vehicle accident<br>• Fractured rib penetrating pleura<br>• During giving CPR | • Penetrating wounds<br>• Accidental pull out of chest tube | Here the injury acts like a one-way valve, which prevents the free bilateral air communication with the atmosphere leading to progressive increase of intrapleural pressure → compresses vena cava leading to decreased cardiac output, hypoxia, acidosis, and shock |
| Pleural cavity pressure | Is less than the atmospheric pressure | Is equal to the atmospheric pressure | Is more than the atmospheric pressure |
| Diagnosis | • If the patient is conscious history and nature of would will help in diagnosis<br>• In case the patient is unconscious, if displacement of heart occurs with diaphragmatic dullness on palpation and percussion. And on auscultation absence of transmitted breath sounds over the pneumothorax can be confirmatory<br>• Chest X-ray | | |
| Management | • **First-aid treatment:** Immediately cover the wound in such a way that it prevents atmospheric air to enter the thoracic cavity during inspiration but at the same it should allow the pleural air to excrete during expiration<br>• **Emergency treatment:** The pressure can be released by a puncture into the tension compartment by inserting the needle between two ribs, with the point away from the heart. But when the patient is unconscious and the diagnosis of tension pneumothorax is uncertain, intubation and positive pressure ventilation may reduce the incidence of respiratory failure<br>• **Definitive treatment:** By tube thoracostomy and ensure to measure the pleural cavity pressure to atmospheric pressure to differentiate between pneumothorax and tension pneumothorax | | |
| Images | 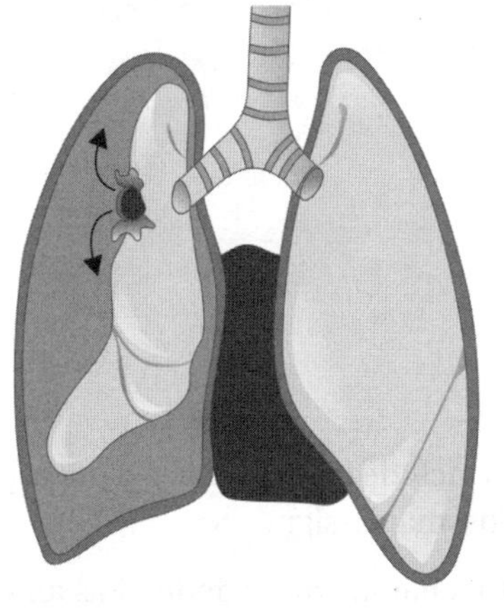 Fig. 14.7: Closed pneumothorax. | 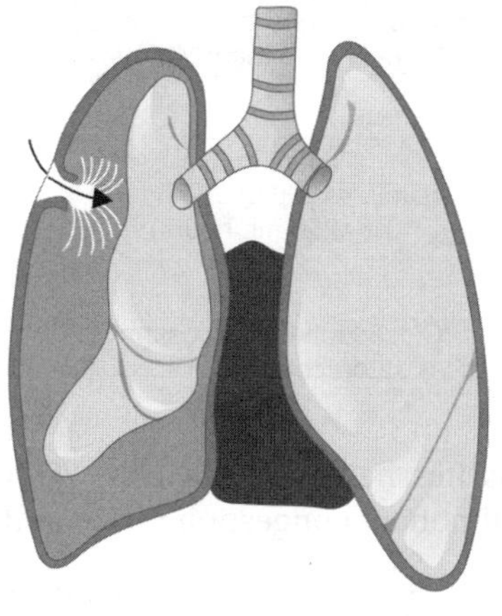 Fig. 14.8: Open pneumothorax. | 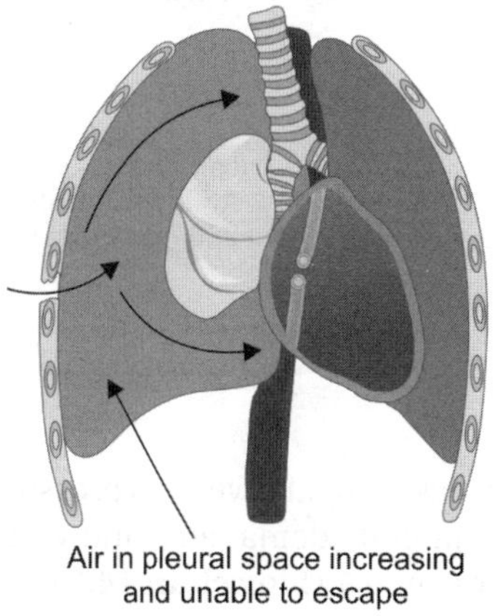 Air in pleural space increasing and unable to escape<br>Fig. 14.9: Tension pneumothorax. |

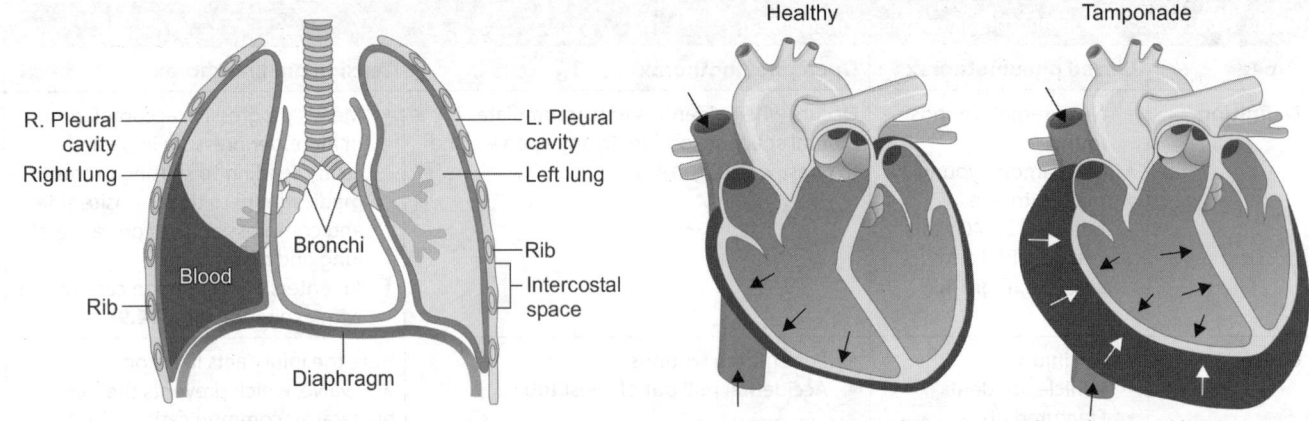

Fig. 14.10: Hemothorax.

Fig. 14.11: Cardiac tamponade with normal heart.

**Flowchart 14.8:** Management of hemothorax.

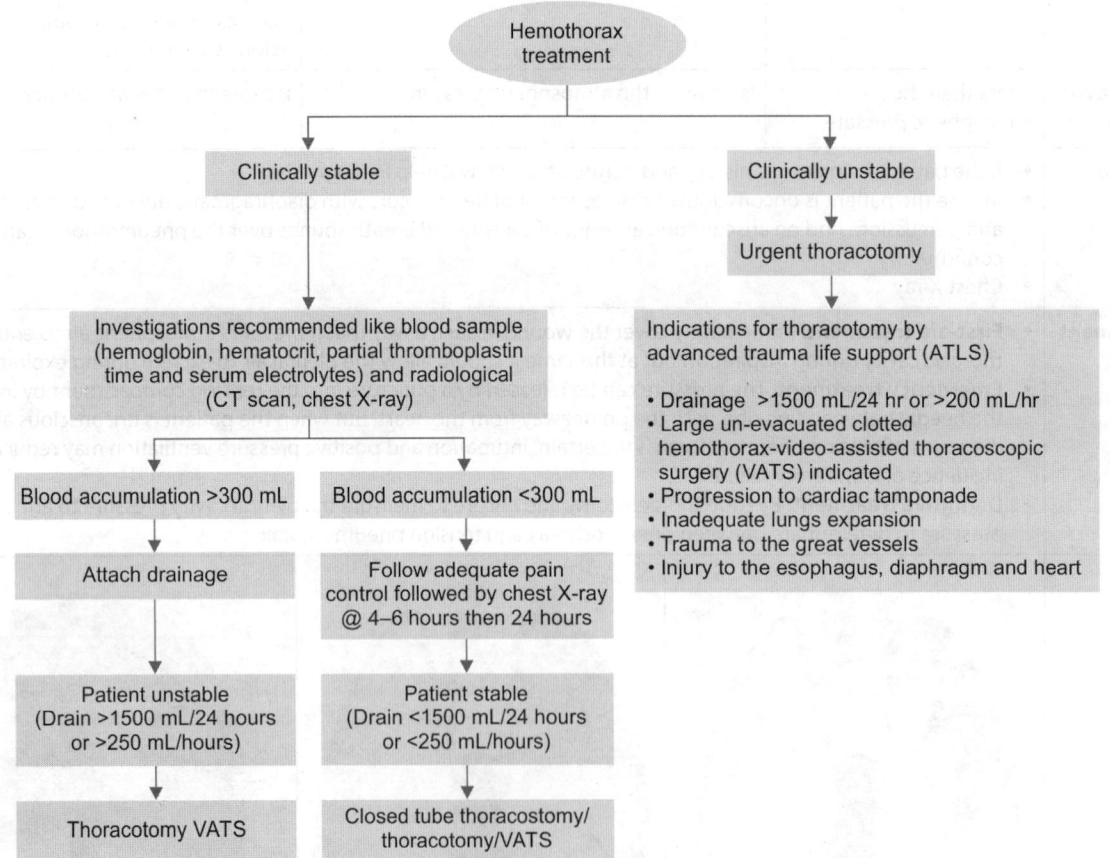

increased jugular venous pressure, ascites, hepatomegaly, peripheral edema, etc., and with pulmonary congestion, rales appear **(Flowchart 14.9)**.

### Clinical Presentation
- Beck's Triad includes distended neck vein/raised JVP, hypotension and muffled heart sound
- Others include tachycardia, dyspnea, pulsus paradoxus and Kussmaul's sign.

**Note:** Pulsus paradoxus is defined as an excessive drop in systolic blood pressure (SBP) during the inspiratory phase of the normal respiratory cycle. Kussmaul's sign is the paradoxical increase in JVP that occurs during inspiration.

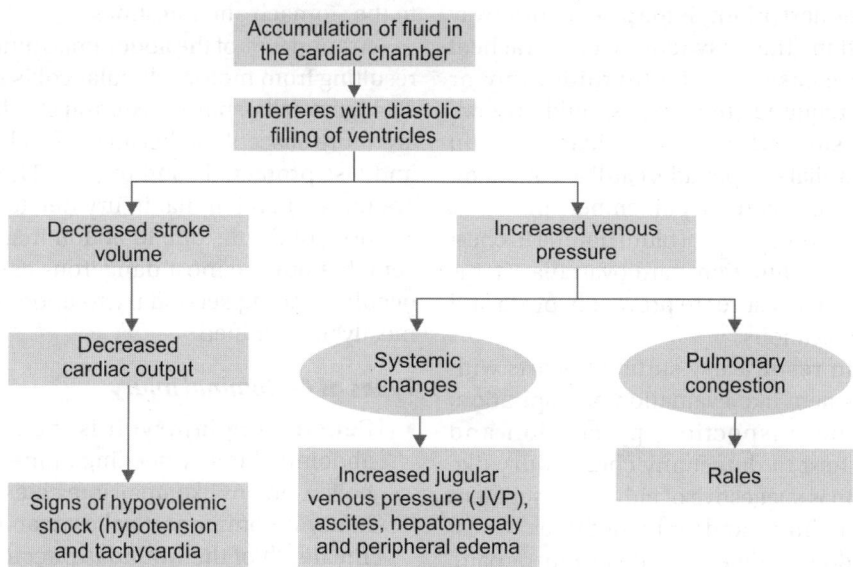

**Flowchart 14.9:** Pathophysiology of cardiac tamponade.

## Diagnostic Measures

- **Ultrasonography (USG):** Finding of abnormal pericardial fluid accumulation with diastolic collapse of the right ventricle or atrium is a highly suggestive feature of cardiac tamponade. A dilated inferior vena cava among hypotensive patients is considered as indirect sign.
- **Electrocardiography (ECG):** *Electrical alternans* are confirmatory signs of cardiac tamponade. This is defined as an ECG change in which the morphology and amplitude of the waves of 'P, QRS, and ST-T' alternate on a single lead in every other beat. Another finding is called "*swinging of heart phenomenon*" or mechanical oscillation of the heart in the pericardial fluid (it means that the heart swings back and forth but again returns to the same position before the next systole).
- **Radiography:** Not helpful in case of mild tamponade but in chronic pericardial effusion case the heart appears like a "water bottle".

## Management

- This calls for an emergency management.
- When the patient admitted to the emergency room, immediately follow the CAB approach. Fluid volume is maintained through the 2–3 large bore cannula (14–16 gauge) for administering crystalloid solution for volume expansion.
- Patency of airway and adequate oxygenation is maintained through face mask.
- Tube thoracotomy is recommended if tamponade is associated with either pneumothorax or hemothorax.
- Pericardiocentesis is done through the aspiration of 5–10 mL of blood for immediate clinical improvement.
- If pericardiocentesis failed or the clinical status deteriorates, then emergency thoracotomy should be done.

**Note:** The recent research evidence shows some controversial finding about the procedure pericardiocentesis. According to the finding this procedure may result in some complications like development of pericardial tamponade, lacerations in coronary artery/lung, and cardiac dysrhythmias. Hence, it is suggested to perform pericardiocentesis procedure under ultrasonographic guidance.

## Nursing Management of Patient with Thoracic Injury

Nurses play an important role in the prompt identification and early nursing assessment with an aim to initiate emergency nursing care for the patients with thoracic injury. This rapid and prompt action is highly essential for early recovery, further deterioration of the condition and development of future complication. Unlike other trauma cases in emergency department, triage care has to be followed, i.e., most life-threatening injuries are to be managed first followed by system wise examination to find out the source, so that best possible outcome can be expected from those patients.

The initial nursing assessment includes evaluation of the breathing pattern, respiratory rate, pattern of chest expansion, oxygen saturation, arterial blood gas (ABG) analysis, chest X-ray. The first aid approach includes establishing CAB that is to maintain the euvolemia through control of hemorrhage and volume replacement by the placement of two large bore cannula to administering crystalloid solution. The next priority is the patency of airway and effective ventilation. This may require endotracheal intubation. In severe cases, a cricothyroidotomy or tracheotomy may be required. The nurse should observe for neck vein distension, which can indicate tension pneumothorax, pericardial tamponade, cardiac contusion or myocardial infarction, or coronary air embolism.

The next nursing priority in case of blunt trauma to chest is maintaining respiratory function, cardiovascular status and adequate pain relief measures to prevent hypoxia and other associated complications.

- **Steps to maintain respiratory status:** It starts with respiratory assessment like evaluation of respiration, oxygen saturation, inspection, percussion and auscultation of chest to detect any chest injury like unequal expansion is suggestive of either flail segment or tension pneumothorax and/or hemothorax. Chest palpation can be done to detect any deformity or pain. The nurse should immediately start oxygen therapy via humidified oxygen via high flow nasal cannula (HFNC) to support respiration, improve hypoxia and reduce the work of breathing. Noninvasive ventilation is considered for patients with respiratory distress.
- **Pain management:** Adequate pain evaluation and management is vital for all patients with chest trauma to enhance lungs expansion and pulmonary toilet. Hence the nurse is responsible for timely and frequent pain evaluation through recommended pain scale to decide on type of analgesics to be effective. Among analgesics inj. Morphine, epidural analgesia and oral drugs (like opioids, paracetamol and nonsteroidal anti-inflammatory drugs) are recommended.
- **Role of breathing exercise:** For increasing adequate air entry to lungs the nurse should encourage physiotherapy, use of incentive spirometry, ambulation under observation and prone position are recommended measures.

| Points to remember |
|---|
| **Pneumonic** |
| **3D's** of Beck's triad in cardiac tamponade |
| • **Distended** neck vein |
| • **Decreased** blood pressure |
| • **Distant/muffled** heart sound |

## Abdominal Injury

### Definition

It is defined as injury to the abdomen causing severe hemorrhage subcutaneously, abdominal wall laceration, intra-abdominal bleeding, hepatic rupture, rupture of the diaphragm, perirenal hemorrhage, and puncture wounds to the stomach and intestines.

Around 90% of the abdominal injuries are blunt trauma resulting from motor vehicular collisions, auto-pedestrian accidents, falls, sports, bike, and child abuse, etc., children are more susceptible because of lack of subcutaneous fat and less protected solid organs. The complication rates are more in abdominal injury due to delay identification. Majority of deaths due to abdominal injuries can be preventable but the most dangerous can be the presence of occult bleeding secondary to abdominal trauma, which mostly unidentified.

### Types of Abdominal Injury

- **Penetrating injury:** It is the most serious type of abdominal injury needing immediate surgery. Mostly hollow organs like small intestines are affected. Hepatic injury is commonest solid organ damage in this case. The depth of the wound is directly proportional to the force/velocity of the external stimuli. The examples are gunshot wounds and stab wounds.
- **Blunt injury:** These are closed injuries commonly results from motor vehicular crashes, falls, blows, or explosions causing extra-abdominal injuries to the chest, head and extremities. It is considered more dangerous as here the identification of injury becomes delayed as external signs may not be present. This may lead to hypovolemic state secondary to massive blood loss into the peritoneal cavity.

### Clinical Presentation

Detailed clinical presentation for both blunt injury and penetrating injury is given in **Table 14.4**.

### Diagnosis

*History*

- Collecting relevant history and relating that with the physical signs are equally important, especially for unconscious patients. The ideal time for history collection is after stabilizing patient post-resuscitation.
- Patient can be asked to tighten the abdomen, if he/she can do so then the injury may not be that much severe.
- History should include the information regarding any solid or liquid intake orally. Because in those cases bladder injury cannot be ignored.
- Having history of hematemesis suggest either patient has swallowed nasopharyngeal bleeding or has sustained a severe stomach injury.
- History of bleeding per rectum suggests trauma to the lower GI tract and pain on the shoulder suggests diaphragmatic irritation.

| Table 14.4: Clinical presentation of abdominal injury. | |
|---|---|
| **Blunt injury** | **Penetrating injury** |
| • Pain in abdomen<br>• Abdominal distension<br>• Discoloration at injury site in abdomen/flank<br>• Signs of shock (tachycardia and hypotension) | • Visible truncal injury along with chest and abdomen<br>• Abdominal pain<br>• Hemorrhage<br>• Penetrating/impaled foreign object<br>• Evisceration<br>• Signs of shock (tachycardia and hypotension) |

## General Physical Examination

- Completely undress the patient. But be careful to identify the early sign of hypothermia. Start with a thorough secondary survey, including examination of all skin folds, the back, and axillae for occult penetrating injuries.
- Never ever attempt to remove the impaled foreign object as this may impair hemostasis causing further bleeding. Hence the removal is only attempted under controlled surgical setting.
- Any form of penetrating injury below nipple line demands the evaluation for intra-abdominal injury. In patients with blunt injuries secondary to motor vehicle collisions, look for ecchymosis or erythema in the area of clavicles or across the abdomen. The classic "seat belt sign" or linear bruising across the lower abdomen is a definite marker for intra-abdominal injury.
- Palpation of abdomen for tenderness, distention, rigidity and guarding.
- Evaluate the pelvis for anteroposterior or lateral instability with gentle pressure, remember repeated examination and application of high force are contraindicated.
- Genital examination is done to see the presence of blood at the urethral meatus, especially in males. If blood at the urethral meatus or a high riding prostate is present, placement of a urinary catheter is contraindicated, and a retrograde urethrogram is required to evaluate for potential urethral injury.
- Digital rectal examinations are performed for every patient with abdominal trauma. Look for gross blood, assess sphincter tone, and note any other evidence of trauma.

## Lab Studies

Baseline examination of hemoglobin, hematocrit, platelet count, blood type are done to evaluate the need for transfusion with packed red cells when required. A raised lactate level and decreased base level indicates shock. Urine examination for gross hematuria, reveals significant injury to the urogenital tract.

## Radiography

As nowadays due to the easy accessibility of CT scanning, X-ray are rarely indicated in such cases. But X-ray of chest, pelvis, and cervical spine can be performed for patients with major abdominal trauma where the facility for CT scan is either unavailable or the patient is unable to go under CT scan machine.

## Ultrasonography

It is the first choice for any type of blunt trauma cases. It has various advantages over others like in case of emergency. It can rapidly and accurately identify intraperitoneal free fluid and also, considered safe in special populations like children and pregnant mothers.

**All about FAST:** Focused assessment with sonography for trauma (FAST) examination is a bedside test that has demonstrated good accuracy with relatively minimal operator experience. it can replace CT scan when needed. It suggests four scan areas: The right upper quadrant, the subxiphoid area, the left upper quadrant, and the pelvis. Unstable patients with a positive FAST examination should undergo urgent exploratory laparotomy.

## CT Scanning

It is a noninvasive and accurate tool for the diagnosis of intra-abdominal injury. However, it is expensive, requires patient transfer and is unsuitable for unstable patients. In case of stable patients, it is the excellent diagnostic tools. It can detect most of the retroperitoneal injuries, but some gastrointestinal injuries may be excluded.

## Diagnostic Peritoneal Lavage (DPL)

Its use has been replaced nowadays due to FAST. It usually detects presence of blood in peritoneal cavity. Drainage of lavage fluid from a chest tube or urinary catheter may indicate a lacerated diaphragm or bladder. It is an invasive procedure which may affect the findings on physical examination, and it should be performed by a surgeon only. Hence due to many disadvantages and availability of more effective method like FAST, CT scanning it is obsoleted.

## Laparoscopy

Suitable for both stable patients with penetrating and blunt abdominal trauma. It can quickly evaluate whether peritoneal penetration has occurred or not. The advantages are—it is less invasive than traditional laparotomy and shortens the hospital stays and decrease patient costs, although it requires surgical consultation.

## Emergency (Exploratory) Laparotomy

It is indicated for hemodynamically unstable patients sustaining blunt or penetrating abdominal trauma with a positive screening test for GAST OR DPL, requires laparotomy to control bleeding and to evaluate further the presence of intra-abdominal injuries. Also patients with obvious diaphragmatic injury confirmed on chest X-ray require emergency laparotomy.

The three main indications for this are peritonitis, unexplained hypovolemia, and the presence of other injuries which may be associated with intra-abdominal injuries.

A quick comparison of all the above diagnostic methods are given in **Table 14.5**, for easy understanding.

## Management

This is an emergency condition demanding immediate hospitalization. The primary focus is the stabilization of the patient through the maintenance of ABCDE (airway, breathing, circulation, disability and exposure) approach.

- **Airway:** Ensure patency of airway and remove any secretion or foreign object. Provide high flow oxygen and intubate if needed. Remember to immobilize the cervical spine till the injury is ruled out.
- **Breathing:** Inspection of thorax for asymmetrical rise, presence of any wound or flail segments. Palpation of chest can be done to evaluate rib fracture or pneumothorax. Auscultation of breath sound for any abnormality. This can be confirmed with pulse oximeter and capnography result.
- **Circulation:** Apply immediate pressure to arrest active bleeding. Adequacy of the blood supply to the vital organs can be assessed through measurement of blood pressure, pulse rate, capillary refill. Fluid resuscitation can be done by putting 2 large bore IV cannula of 16 gauge or more. If not possible due to excessive hypovolemia, a central venous catheter can be placed instead.
- **Disability:** After stabilizing patient assessment for disability is important. It includes a brief but focused neurological examination including Glasgow coma scale (GCS), pupil size along with reactivity, any sign of poor muscle tone/weakness, etc. Remember to perform the neurological examination before administration of analgesics, sedatives, etc.
- **Exposure:** This is to examine minutely by completely undressing the patient for any sign of other physical injury. This includes examination of all skin folds, back, axilla shoulder, etc.

## Management of Blunt Abdominal Trauma

The management of blunt type of abdominal trauma is based on whether the patient is stable or unstable. In-case the patient's SBP is less than 90 mm Hg, the patient is unstable and follows the treatment sequence like fluid resuscitation. After resuscitation, see if the patients responds to the treatment, if yes, then the management for the stable patient is followed. But if the patient do not responds to the fluid infusion, blood transfusion is recommended to replace the lost fluid to treat hypovolemia followed by focussed assessment sonography for trauma (FAST). If the patient is still not stable, an exploratory laparotomy is advised. On the contrary, if the stable with SBP more than and equal to 90 mm Hg, FAST and CT scan id advised to explore cause of bleeding of blunt bleeding like hollow organ perforation, abdominal wall hernia, injury to other solid organs, etc., systemic clinical examination is planned for those patients. But if the clinical condition

| Table 14.5: A quick comparison of diagnostic measures available. | | | |
|---|---|---|---|
| **Method** | **Time** | **Cost** | **Advantage/limitation** |
| General physical examination | Fast | No cost | Useful for baseline examinations. Limitations in depth identification of other associated injuries, coma, drug intoxication, poor sensitivity and specificity |
| Diagnostic peritoneal lavage (DPL) | Fast | Low cost | Gives quick result in unstable patient but invasive and requires expertise. Are nowadays replaced by other methods |
| Focused assessment with sonography for trauma (FAST) | Fast | Low cost | Ideal for detection of intra-abdominal free fluid and pericardial tamponade. Advantageous over DPL. Requires expert hand. Fairly sensitive but not highly specific. |
| CT scanning | Slow | High cost | Most specific for particular sites of injury and can evaluate retroperitoneum, very good sensitivity but may miss bowel injury, risk of reaction to contrast dye |

deteriorates, exploratory laparotomy is planned for stable patients as well **(Flowchart 14.10)**.

## Management of Penetrating Abdominal Trauma

The patients with penetrating abdominal trauma first divided to two groups for management according to some symptoms. If the patient is hemodynamically unstable with the presence of peritonitis, then the patient is directed for exploratory surgery. And on the other hand, if the patient has no sign of peritonitis, but still hemodynamic instability present, CT scan is the investigation of choice to find out if it is a hollow viscus injury or not. A hollow viscus injury refers to blunt force injury specifically to the gastrointestinal system extending from the gastroesophageal junction, stomach, small and large intestine including the rectum. Hence, it is the priority to control the bleeding through exploratory surgery for hollow viscus injury and if there is no sign of such injury, then presence of other injuries like left thoraco-abdominal injury to be evaluated. If the answer is yes, then laparoscopy is done and if no such is present, then the patient is kept for observation **(Flowchart 14.11)**.

## Pelvic Fractures

Pelvic fracture, especially the ring of the pelvis is more prone for fracture secondary to any physical trauma. This is

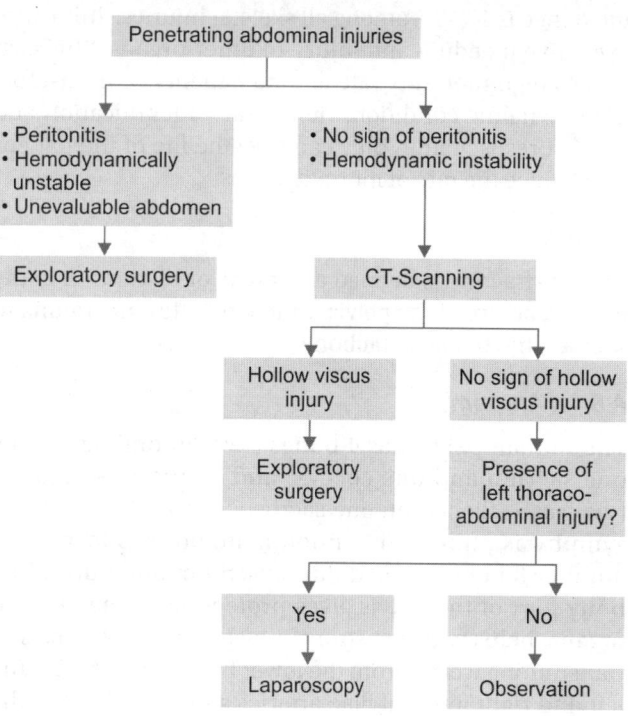

**Flowchart 14.11:** Management of penetrating abdominal trauma.

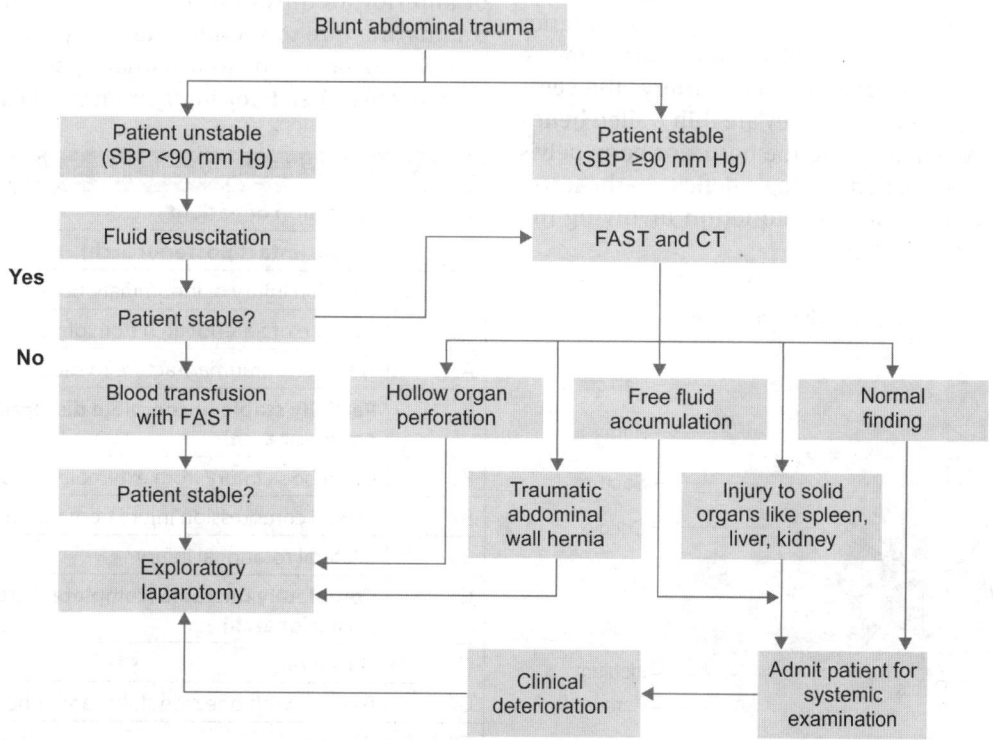

**Flowchart 14.10:** Management of blunt abdominal trauma.

considered as an emergency because it presents immense challenge for the patient and the physician as well. The incidence is 1.5–3% among all skeletal injuries. This cause excessive bleeding and injury to other organs. This also causes high mortality rate among patients with unstable hemodynamic condition. Hence early identification and prompt resuscitation only can save the life of the patient and reduce the rate of mortality.

### Definition

A pelvic fracture is defined as a break or disruption in the bony structure of the pelvis, which includes the trauma to sacrum, hip bones or tailbone.

### A Brief Anatomy

The human pelvis has 4 bones (two innominate bone, one sacrum and one coccyx) and 4 numbers of joints (two sacro-iliac joint, one sacrococcygeal joint and one symphysis pubis). The innominate bone is formed of another 3 bones named ilium, ischium and pubis. The bony part of the pelvis gives protection to the visceral organs, helps with the strong attachment for muscles in transmitting weight from the lower body **(Fig. 14.12)**. The left and right internal iliac arteries supplies blood to the pelvic organs. Posterior arch is the part of the pelvis situated in posterior part which bears the weight bearing force. The superior gluteal artery is the largest branch supplying blood to the pelvis, is commonly gets damaged in case of posterior pelvic arch fracture. Fracture of pelvic ramus cause damage to the obturator and internal pudendal artery. The veins are less likely to get damage as they are thin walled hence don't constrict much. Injury to the posterior bony pelvis and sacrum may result in neurologic deficits in the lower extremities and autonomic dysfunction involving the bowel, bladder, and genitalia.

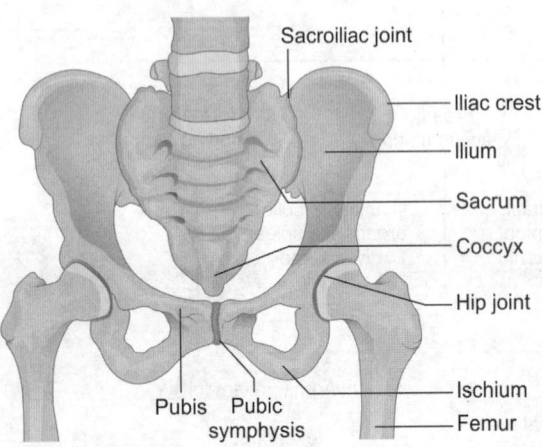

**Fig. 14.12:** Anatomy of pelvis.

### Mechanism of Injury

- **Low energy injury:** Resulted from sudden muscle contraction causing avulsion injury, low energy fall injury or straddle type of injury. It is commonly seen among athletes.
- **High energy injuries:** Resulted from high force from motor accidents, pedestrian injuries, fall from height and crush injuries.

### Classification of Pelvic Fracture

Usually two types of classification:

#### Classification by Tile

The tile classification of pelvic fractures is the precursor of the more contemporary Young and Burgess classification of pelvic ring fractures.

It takes into account stability, force direction, and pathoanatomy. The integrity of the posterior arch determines the grade, with the posterior arch referring to all of the pelvis posterior to the acetabulum. Stability is defined as the 'ability of the pelvis to withstand physiologic force without deformation'.

In tiles classification patients are divided to three categories according to the extent of injury **(Table 14.6)**. First type are quite stable patients including three subgroups like avulsion injuries of two innominate bone (A1), fracture of anterior arch from direct blow (A2) and transverse trauma/fracture to sacrum and coccyx (A3). The second type were patients who were partially stable which included subtypes like open book injury from external rotation (B1),

**Table 14.6:** Pelvic fracture classification by tiles.

| Type | Condition of patient |
|------|----------------------|
| A    | **Stable (intact posterior arch)** |
| A1   | Avulsion injury of innominate bone |
| A2   | Fracture of anterior arch from direct blow |
| A3   | Transverse trauma/fracture to sacrum and coccyx |
| B    | **Partially stable (incomplete disruption of posterior arch)** |
| B1   | Open book injury from external rotation |
| B2   | Lateral compression injury from internal rotation |
| B3   | Bilateral rotational injury |
| C    | **Completely unstable (complete disruption of posterior arch)** |
| C1   | Unilateral |
| C2   | Bilateral with one side stable and other side unstable |
| C3   | Bilateral |

lateral compression injury from internal rotation (B2) and bilateral rotational injury (B3). The last type is completely unstable patient including subtypes like unilateral (C1), bilateral with one side stable and other side unstable (C2) and bilateral (C3). The detailed is illustrated in **Figure 14.13**.

## Classification by Young-Burgess

The Young–Burgess classification **(Fig. 14.14)** is a system of categorizing pelvic fractures based on the vector of applied force at the time of injury and degree of resulting disruption, allowing judgment on the stability of the pelvic ring and prediction of associated blood loss.

The Young and Burgess classification is a modification of the earlier tile classification. It is the widely recommended and mostly used classification system for pelvic ring fractures. It takes into account force type, severity, and direction, as well as injury instability. Three basic mechanistic descriptions are used, each with degrees of severity.

It has three categories as anterior posterior compression, lateral compression and vertical shear **(Table 14.7)**.

## Clinical Presentation

- Unbearable pain with tenderness in pelvic region
- Pain increased when iliac crest pressed together
- Swelling at the site of injury combined with visual or palpable injury
- Discomfort in the lower abdominal region
- Feeling of urgency to urinate.

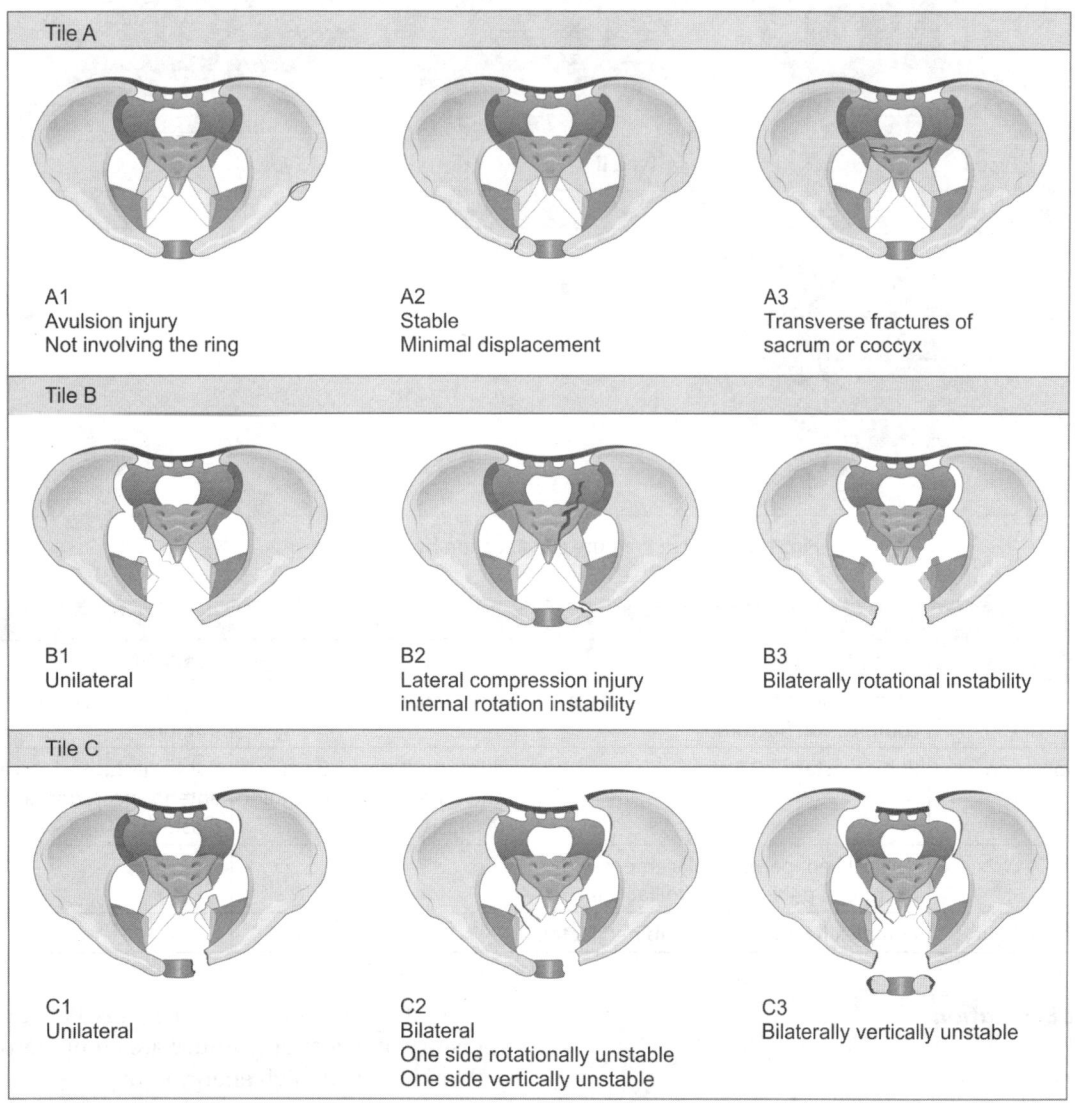

**Fig. 14.13:** Pelvic fracture classification by tiles.

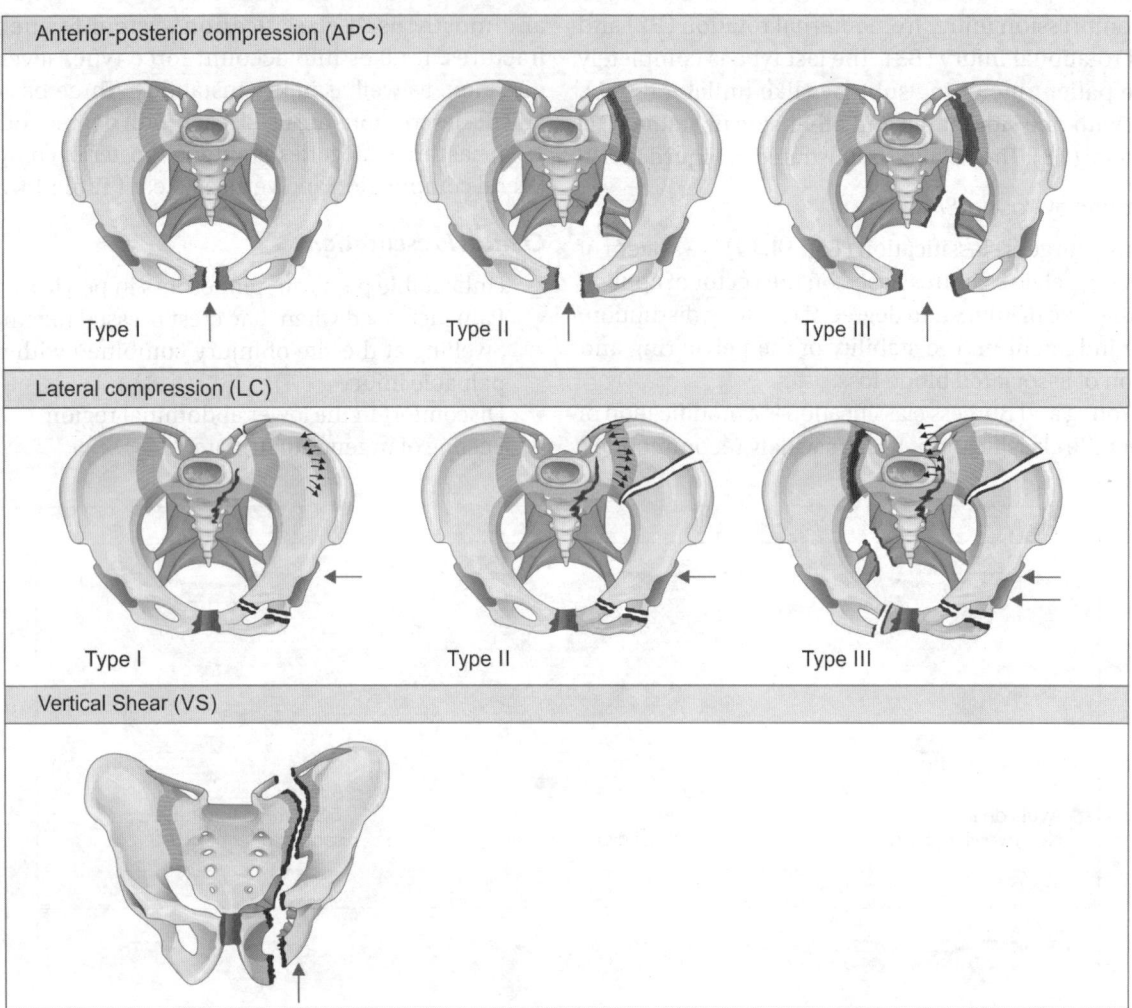

**Fig. 14.14:** Pelvic fracture classification by Young-Burgess.

| Table 14.7: Pelvic fracture classification by Young-Burgess. | | | |
|---|---|---|---|
| **Category of fracture** | **Grade I** | **Grade II** | **Grade III** |
| Anterior-posterior compression (APC) | Pelvic ramus and ipsilateral sacral ala compression fracture | Iliac crescent fracture | Ipsilateral and contralateral APC fracture |
| Lateral compression | Pubic diastasis <2.5 cm | Pubic diastasis >2.5 cm and anterior sacroiliac joint diastasis | Pubic diastasis >5 cm and anterior-posterior sacroiliac joint diastasis |
| Vertical shear | Vertical hemipelvis displacement with fracture of pubis and sacroiliac joint | | |
| Combined force injury | Complex fracture with combined factors | | |

## Diagnostic Evaluation

### History

- To be collected regarding the occurrence and mechanism of injury to get an idea about the severity and extent of involvement of organs. Patient came with history of low energy injury are comparatively stable than those with high energy injury.
- Data regarding direction of force also says about the type of injury. For example, injury with AP force suggest open

book injury of pelvis. Lateral forces damage posterior ligament of pelvis so also the vertical shear causing major pelvic instability.
- The information regarding age should also be considered importantly because elderly patients with osteoporosis are more prone for severe injury eve with a less force.
- The injury to other adjacent organs also common in case of pelvic injury cases, hence while collecting history it is also important to ask the presence of pain, discomfort in any other part of the body.
- In case of female patient history regarding pregnancy should also be asked and of needed pregnancy test can be performed.

## Physical Examination

### Inspection

Observation of iliac crest rotation indicates serious pelvic injury. Careful observation of all the skin folds and skin for open fractures. Presence of ecchymosis/hematoma in perineal area, periumbilical area (Cullen's sign) or flanks (Grey Turner's sign) suggestive of retro-peritoneal bleeding.

### Palpation

- The palpation for detecting pelvic trauma should start at the pubis symphysis anteriorly then proceeds to both pubic rami, the iliac spines and crests laterally, and finally to the sacrum and sacroiliac joints posteriorly. The confirmatory finding is the tenderness in any of this part.
- Remember to do the palpation of pelvis gently with minimal pressure or else this may worsen the hemorrhage.
- In male the bleeding or blood clots in penis is examined by milking it, followed by digital rectal examination to assess for "sensation, sphincter tone, position and consistency of the prostate, presence of a presacral hematoma, bony contour of the sacrum and coccyx, mucosal penetration of bony spicules, and presence of frank or occult blood".
- In female vaginal examination to be done to detect open fracture but be careful while doing so as it may create new open fractures iatrogenically.

### X-ray of Pelvis

Routine X-ray for all cases of pelvis trauma is not necessary especially for conscious and asymptomatic cases with blunt trauma. But according to the guideline issued by advanced trauma life support (ATLS), a X-ray is necessary for patients went through high force injury with severe symptoms and are not conscious.

### CT Scan

It is considered as the investigation of choice. It is able to detect damage to the posterior arch and rotational deformities of pelvis and clear visualization of acetabulum which is not possible in plain radiology.

### Diagnostic Peritoneal Lavage (DPL)

Useful for detecting intra-abdominal hemorrhage. The location for this procedure is infraumbilical region. In case previous abdominal scar present, supraumbilical region is the ideal one.

### Focused Assessment with Sonography in Trauma (FAST)

It is indicated to detect abnormal presence of intraperitoneal fluid in the trauma patient.

## Management

**Primary treatment with resuscitation:** According to the ATLS protocol life saving measures must be initiated immediately in case of pelvic fracture. This includes ensuring patent airway, adequate ventilation and meeting the oxygen demand, immobilization of spine and control of bleeding and to treat hypovolemia if any.

**Controlling bleeding:** Uncontrolled bleeding can be the main cause of death among those patients, which accounts for around 20% of deaths. Methods to control hemorrhage are use of binders, fracture fixation (both internal/external), packing/pelvic tamponade and angiographic embolization.

- **Fluid infusion:** Initial use of crystalloid solutions to stabilize vital signs in the trauma patient is a recommendation by ATLS.
- **Binders:** These are the conventional treatment methods. But to a large extent this may replace the need of fracture fixation. It works by compressing the bleeding arteries and stabilizing and supporting the fracture.
- **Angiography:** Abbreviated injury scale (AIS) is a scoring given any type of physical injury on a 6 point rating scale, where 1 being the mild injury and the 6 being the severe one. According to scientific studies AIS score of >3 with blood transfusion rate of >0.5 units/hour is the actual candidate for angiographic embolization. But this procedure is not safe always and this comes with certain complications like peri-pelvic soft-tissue necrosis and subsequent infection leading to multi-organ failure and death, despite of managements like abscess drainage, necrotic tissue debridement and administration of antibiotics.
- **Packing:** This is another method of controlling bleeding. But it is an invasive procedure and requires surgical facility and expert hands. The packs are placed in preperitoneal and retroperitoneal spaces and usually

removed after 48 hours. It is always combined with external fixation.
- **Internal fixation:** It is ideally considered is patients with multiple injuries in combination with unstable pelvic fracture.
- **Blood transfusion:** Immediate and vigorous transfusion with packed cell RBC is highly advisable. In case of fracture with active bleeding and affected hematocrit status. Many of the research suggest administration of fresh frozen plasma (FFP) and platelets to initiate clot formation and subsequently preventing disseminated intravascular coagulation (DIC).

**Rehabilitation:** The potential candidate for this are patients who can be managed without surgery and may require complete bed rest for a long time. Once the fracture is healed, the rehabilitation can be started to restore the maximum functioning. This includes physiotherapies by experts.

### Nursing Management of Patient with Pelvic Fracture

The role of nurse is very important as they are the key person and are the first line of contact with the patient and their relative. The primary responsibility of them is evaluate the patient, to identify the early signs and symptoms of potential complications.

### Role in Assessment of Trauma Patient

This involves the airway, breathing, circulation, disability, and exposure (ABCDE) approach. The airway and breathing should be assessed for patency and adequacy respectively and according to the finding's oxygen can be administered. Similarly circulation can be assessed through measuring vitals like BP, heart rate, urine output, capillary refill time. This helps to early identify signs of hypovolemic shock secondary to hemorrhage. Followed by assessment and management or disability and any other body part damage in exposure.

The neurological status can be checked by assessing Glasgow coma scale (GCS) and peripheral neurovascular examination.

The nurse should also involve in the management of hypovolemia through adequate and timely fluid infusion and blood transfusion at the same she should be alert to detect volume over load.

- **Pain management** is also an import aspect of nursing management, and this is the right of the patient to be pain and discomfort free. Hence the nurse should first assess the level of pain by pain scale and accordingly management can be given. It is to be remembered poorly managed pain can cause further neurological and respiratory dysfunction.
- **Immobilization of patient** is also an important nursing care. This prevents further complication and aids with the support and early recovery.
- **Inadequate nutrition:** The nurse should also give attention to poor nutrition secondary to difficulties in eating and drinking. This affects the general health of the patient leading to delay recovery.
- **Prevention of venous thromboembolisms** an import action of nurse. This can be achieved by frequent position change, leg exercise, early ambulation and checking Homan sign. The use of thromboprophylaxis is of great help.
- **Risk of pressure ulcer** also adds to the morbidity rate. Hence nurse should give care to pressure areas by frequent assessment, two hourly position change, back care, giving high protein diet for early recovery and use of pressure ulcer prevention mattress.
- **Impaired bowel movement:** Prolonged lying-in bed may develop impaired bowel movement/constipation. This can be managed by increasing the fluid intake, fiber food, ambulation, stool softener if needed, etc.
- **Urine infection:** Another problem with prolonged bed ridden patient is the urinary tract infection secondary to prolonged catheterization. Hence the catheter associated UTI (CAUTI) protocol should be followed like frequent assessment of the catheter insertion site for any sign of infection, asking the patient about any burning sensation, sign of urine retention and changing the catheter in appropriate time can help with the management.

### Complications of Trauma

Remember Pneumonic **"TRAUMATIC"**

T = Poor **T**issue perfusion
R = **R**espiratory difficulties
A = **A**nxiety
U = **U**nstable clotting cascade
M = **M**alnutrition
A = **A**ltered body image
T = **T**hromboembolism
I = **I**nfection
C = **C**oping problems

## SHOCK

### Definition

Shock is an emergency condition secondary to circulatory insufficiency which creates an imbalance between oxygen supply and oxygen demand to the tissue. The end result is tissue hypoperfusion and decreased venous oxygen content leading to metabolic acidosis.

If left untreated, it leads to multiple organ dysfunction syndrome and end stage organ damage with death.

## Classification of Shock

- Hypovolemic shock
- Cardiogenic shock
- Anaphylactic shock ⎫
- Neurogenic shock    ⎬ Circulatory shock
- Septic shock        ⎭

### Hypovolemic Shock

If we split the word 'hypovolemia' it describes hypo meaning low, Vol meaning volume and lastly aemic meaning blood. Hence, it is defined as loss of intravascular blood volume up to 15% or more, leading to inadequate tissue perfusion. Delay in the identification of condition or initiation of treatment leads to ischemia (lack of tissue oxygenation) in the vital organs leading to multiorgan failure and death.

### Pathophysiology

The shock is a very serious illness, if not treated early can lead to deadly complications. First, it starts with hypovolemia due to excessive body fluid or blood loss secondary to injury or trauma. Because of low blood volume, the venous return to the heart decreased leading to decreased preload and cardiac output. This sudden fall of bodies fluid volume lads to hypotension, reduced tissue perfusion, hypoxia and death **(Flowchart 14.12)**.

The fundamental defect in shock is reduced perfusion of vital tissues. Once perfusion declines and oxygen delivery to cells is inadequate for aerobic metabolism, cells shift to anaerobic metabolism with increased production of carbon dioxide and elevated blood lactate levels. Cellular function declines, and if shock persists, irreversible cell damage and death occur.

Due to hypoperfusion during shock, both inflammatory and clotting cascades triggered and also vascular endothelial cells activates white blood cells, which bind to the endothelium and release directly damaging substances (e.g., reactive oxygen species, proteolytic enzymes) and inflammatory mediators (e.g., cytokines, leukotrienes, tumor necrosis factor). Some of these mediators bind to cell surface receptors and activate nuclear factor kappa B (NFκB), which leads to production of additional cytokines and nitric oxide (NO), a potent vasodilator.

Blood pressure is not always low in the early stages of shock (although hypotension eventually occurs if shock is not reversed). Similarly, not all patients with "low" blood pressure have shock. The degree and consequences of hypotension vary with the adequacy of physiologic compensation and the patient's underlying diseases. Thus, a modest degree of hypotension that is well tolerated by a young, relatively healthy person might result in severe cerebral, cardiac, or renal dysfunction in an older person with significant arteriosclerosis.

### Clinical Presentation

- Weak and thready pulse
- Tachycardia and hypotension
- Cold and clammy limbs with delay capillary refilling
- All these symptoms are secondary to excessive fluid loss from the body.

### Treatment

#### Aim

- Assessment and treatment of underlying cause
- Evaluation of electrolyte and acid-base imbalance
- Evaluation and management of volume deficit.

**The management includes:**

**Fluid resuscitation:** Immediate fluid resuscitation is recommended to restore circulating volume and to improve cardiac output. According to National Institute for Health and Care Excellence (NICE), 2017 guideline IV administration of crystalloid solution containing sodium 130–154 mmol/L with one pint (500 mL) bolus over 15 min or less in the absence of active bleeding both internally and externally. In case of active bleeding along with rapid fluid administration blood transfusion is recommended to prevent further complications like tissue hypoxia and multi-organ failure.

### Clinical Consideration

- Evaluation of electrolyte status and acid/base balance is the priority in hypovolemic shock.

**Flowchart 14.12:** Pathophysiology of hypovolemic shock.

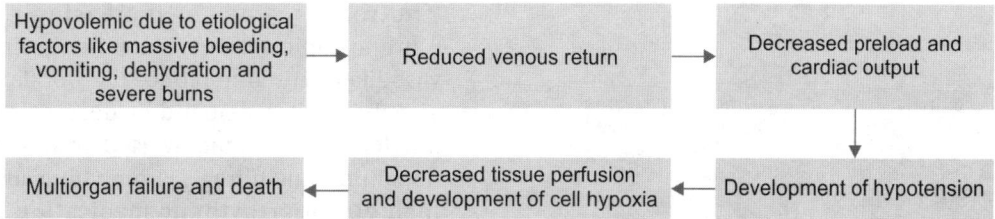

- Hemorrhagic shock should be treated with balanced transfusion of packed red blood cells, plasma and platelets.
- The volume and type of fluid administration should be decided after the complete systematic assessment. For this type of shock crystalloid solution is preferred over colloid.

*Training of Nursing Personnel: Regarding*

- Understanding the normal physiology of fluid and electrolyte balance
- Evaluating the patients' fluid and electrolyte needs (the 5 Rs: Resuscitation, routine maintenance, replacement, redistribution, and reassessment)
- Assessment of risks, benefits, and harms of IV fluids administration
- Administering required amount of fluids and checking the patient response to same
- Documentation of various parameters to track the patient's response and to decide on other measures required.

## Cardiogenic Shock

*Definition*

Cardiogenic shock is defined as inadequate supply of blood and oxygen to vital organs especially heart and other body tissues due to the inability of the heart to pump or contract.

*Risk Factors*

The risk factors are coronary cause including myocardial infraction and noncoronary cause which includes cardiomyopathies, damage to valves, cardiac tamponade and dysrhythmias **(Flowchart 14.13)**.

*Pathophysiology*

The primary etiological factor of cardiogenic shock causes reduced cardiac output, hypotension, systemic vasoconstriction, and cardiac ischemia, which further results in reduction in myocardial contractility. The hallmark is peripheral vasoconstriction and vital end-organ damage, which stems from ineffective stroke volume and insufficient circulatory compensation. Compensatory peripheral vasoconstriction may initially improve coronary and peripheral perfusion; however, it contributes to increased cardiac afterload that overburdens damaged myocardium. This results in diminished oxygenated blood flow to peripheral tissue and, ultimately, the heart. Development of ischemia occurs leading to cardiogenic shock and death **(Flowchart 14.14)**.

*Clinical Presentation*

- Anginal pain
- Dysrhythmias
- Hemodynamic instability

*Management*

Initiation of first line management:

- **Maintaining adequate tissue oxygenation:** Through nasal canula with a rate of 2–6 lt/min. monitoring with ABG analysis and pulse oximeter.
- **Managing chest pain:** For pain control morphine sulfate is administered. Morphine acts by vasodilation and simultaneously decreasing the workload on heart. It also works as antianxiety for patients. Monitoring for level of cardiac enzyme and ECG are recommended.
- **Frequent hemodynamic monitoring:** Evaluation of hemodynamic status is needed for checking the patient's response to treatment. This can be achieved through the placement of an arterial line for the continuous monitoring of blood pressure and also giving easy access for repeated sample collection for gas analysis. A multi-lumen pulmonary artery catheter can be inserted to allow the measurement of pulmonary artery pressures, myocardial filling pressures, cardiac output (CO) with pulmonary and systemic resistance.
- **Role of pharmacotherapy:** The main aim of the treatment is to restore the normal cardiac output. This can be achieved through two opposite kinds of action like simultaneous improvement of cardiac contractility with decreasing the workload on heart. The group of drugs required are sympathomimetic agents for causing cardiac contractility through vasoconstriction. The outcomes are increasing myocardial contractility (inotropic action) or increasing the heart rate (chronotropic action). The other group of drugs are vasodilators used to reduce the workload of the heart and the oxygen demand by decreasing preload and afterload. The commonly used drugs are dobutamine, dopamine, and nitroglycerine. Other supportive drugs include antiarrhythmic medication prescribed to

**Flowchart 14.13:** Risk factors of cardiogenic shock.

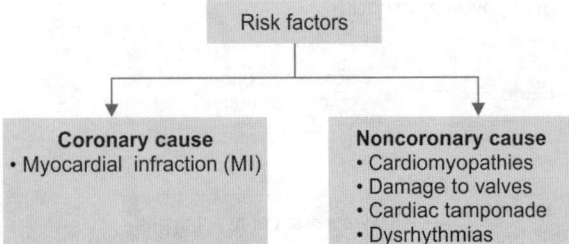

**Flowchart 14.14:** Pathophysiology of cardiogenic shock.

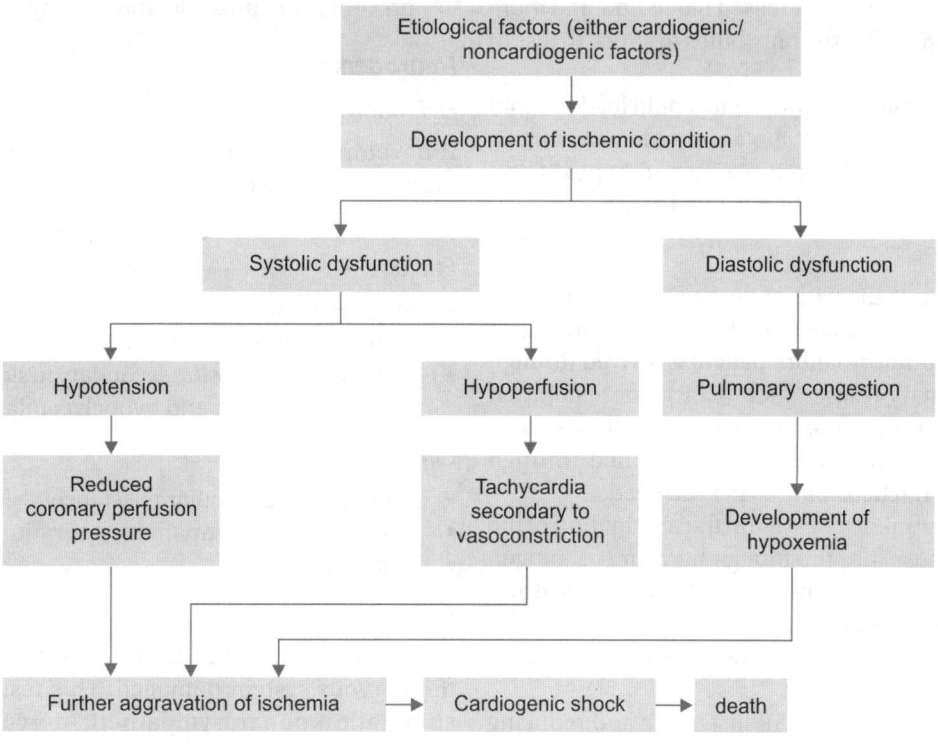

improve hypoxemia, electrolyte and acid-base balances and cardiac dysrhythmias.
- **Fluid therapy:** In addition to the above treatment the appropriate fluid therapy is essential to treat cardiogenic shock. Steps must be taken to monitor the fluid strictly to avoid fluid overload which can increase load on heart leading to cardiac failure.
- **Consideration for mechanical assistive devices:** The decision for use of such device is done when the cardiac output does not improve after the initial first line management. These devices are used temporarily to improve the heart's ability to pump.
  – Intra-aortic balloon counter pulsation is polyurethane balloon catheter is inserted percutaneously through the common femoral artery and advanced into the descending thoracic aorta. It works by inflating the balloon with the beginning of diastole and deflating it just before systole. The objective is to achieve improved stroke volume and coronary artery perfusion with decreased preload, cardiac workload, and myocardial oxygen demand.
  – Ventricular assisted devices both left and right and total artificial hearts. These devices support the heart by ventricular pumping.

### Anaphylactic Shock

#### Definition

It develops secondary to an antigen antibody reaction when someone's body is exposed to certain antigen or allergen or foreign substance and in defense the body produced the antibody.

#### Pathophysiology

Anaphylaxis is caused by exposure to either foreign bodies or any allergen. The body produces antibody in response to this antigen leading to hypersensitivity reaction. This further causes massive release of biochemical mediators from mast cell and basophils. The multiple activation pathways allow for immunologic (e.g., IgE mediated) and/or nonimmunologic activation (e.g., drug directly interacting with receptors). Some antigens may mediate effects via several mechanisms simultaneously (e.g., vespid venom, NSAIDs, opiates). In non-IgE mediated anaphylaxis, symptoms can occur on first exposure to an antigen as prior exposure and sensitization is not required. This then leads to massive vasodilation and abnormal blood distribution. There after reduced venous return causes decreased cardiac output and hypotension.

On the other hand, with massive vasodilation, capillary permeability increases with increased blood flow and more frequent urination. This also contributes to shock to loss of body fluid.

Again raised capillary permeability could lead to rapid fluid shifting, development of whole body edema involving larynx. This cause breathing difficulty and hypoxia and finally loss of consciousness **(Flowchart 14.15)**.

*Management*

- To save the life of the patient immediate resuscitation is recommended through the CAB approach. In case of cardiac or respiratory failure patient is revived through cardiopulmonary resuscitation (CPR). For restoration of circulation intravenous fluid administration is done. The patency of air way can be maintained through intubation or tracheostomy as per the need.
- The actual treatment focusses on the elimination of the underlying cause, i.e., the foreign body or the antigen next to first aid or emergency measures and use of drugs to restore the vascular tone.
- Drug epinephrine is administered in IV route to initiate vasoconstriction.
- For neutralizing the action of histamine and reducing the capillary permeability IV diphenhydramine (Benadryl) is administered.
- Nebulized of drug Albuterol (Proventil) is given to prevent bronchospasm induced by histamine.

### Neurogenic Shock

*Definition*

It develops due to the failure of action of sympathetic nervous system causing vasodilation secondary to spinal cord injury.

*Etiology*

- Spinal cord injury (above T5)
- Complications to spinal anesthesia
- Vasomotor depression secondary to side effect of certain drugs, severe pain and hypoglycemia

*Clinical Presentation*

- Low systemic vascular resistance
- Abnormal parasympathetic activation
- Bradycardia

*Pathophysiology*

In neurogenic shock due to direct trauma to the spinal cord, the nervous system damaged. This results in abnormal stimulation of parasympathetic nervous system. This causes peripheral vasodilation and low vascular tone. With this the systemic vascular resistance reduced. The

**Flowchart 14.15:** Pathophysiology of anaphylactic shock.

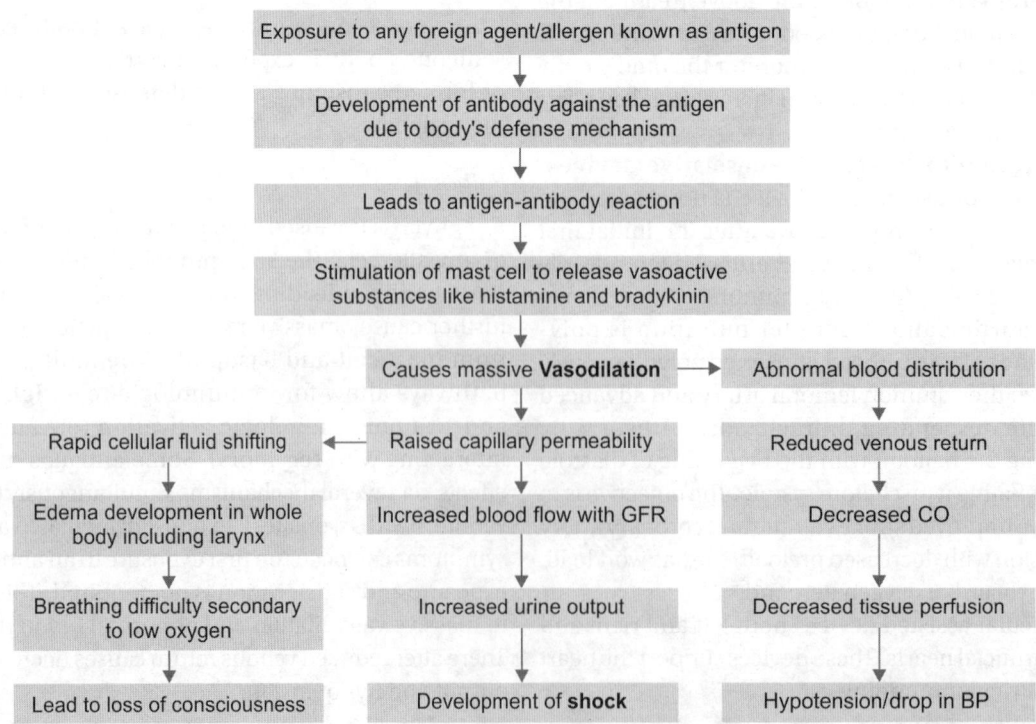

result is inadequate tissue perfusion and impaired cellular metabolism. The last outcome is shock (**Flowchart 14.16**).

*Management*

- Resuscitation of shock done by circulation, breathing and airway (CAB) approach.
- Strict immobilization of spine to avoid further damage.
- Adequate fluid administration and drugs like dopamine and dobutamine are given to improve hypotension.
- Drug atropine is suggested for bradycardia.
- For neurological symptoms steroids can be administered through intravenous route.
- Further management can be planned after a through clinical examination by expert neurologist.

## Septic Shock

Sepsis and septic shock are life-threatening conditions causing morbidity and mortality to millions of patients globally and also leads to multiple organ dysfunction and death in as many as one among four patients even more. Hence early management and appropriate treatment are the need of the hour to improve outcomes and reduce the further adverse outcome.

*Definition*

Earlier, i.e., before 2016, the "sepsis was defined, as the presence of two or more positive systemic inflammatory response syndrome (SIRS) criteria (**Flowchart 14.17**) with a confirmed or suspected infection as the underlying cause. And the presence of organ dysfunction is considered as severe sepsis".

Similarly, "septic shock was defined by the presence of acute circulatory failure and arterial hypotension along with features of sepsis".

**The new definition of sepsis and septic shock given by Third International Consensus, 2016**

"Sepsis as a life-threatening organ dysfunction resulting from dysregulated host responses to infection and defined septic shock as a subset of sepsis in which underlying circulatory, cellular, and metabolic abnormalities are profound enough to substantially increase the risk of mortality".

"Septic shock is also defined as persisting hypotension that requires vasopressors to achieve a mean arterial pressure ≥ 65 mm Hg despite adequate fluid resuscitation and a lactic acid level >2 mmol/L. These new definitions focused on organ dysfunction rather than inflammation".

These above definitions considered quick sequential organ failure assessment (qSOFA) score as shown in **Flowchart 14.18**.

**Flowchart 14.16:** Pathophysiology of neurogenic shock.

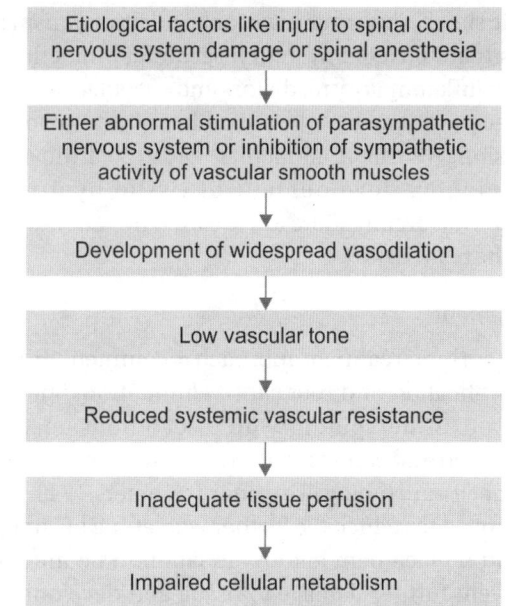

**Flowchart 14.17:** SIRS criteria.

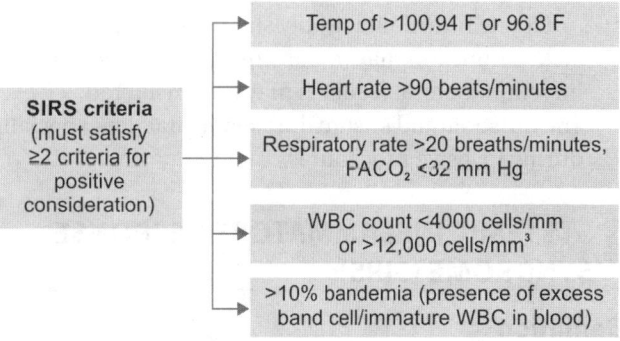

**Flowchart 14.18:** qSOFA score.

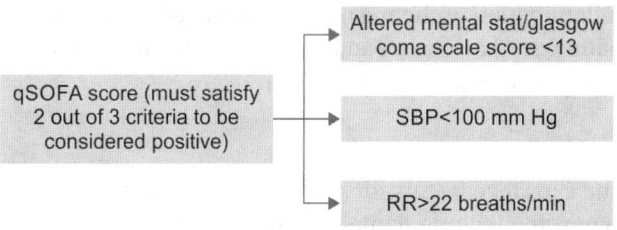

*Risk Factors*

- Immunosuppression
- Advanced age of >65 years
- Malnourishment
- Chronic illness
- Invasive procedures

## Pathophysiology

In septic shock, abnormal invasion of microorganism to the blood stream post to any injury, secondary infection. This activates inflammatory mediators and coagulation cascade. This leads to hypovolemia, vasodilation and myocardial depression. All this triad factors leads to cardiovascular insufficiency, development of tissue hypoxia and multiple vital organ failure and death if not attended early **(Flowchart 14.19)**.

## Management

- The current treatment approach recommends the early identification and root cause elimination. Specimens (blood/urine/sputum/would secretions, etc.) to be collected and send for culture and sensitivity test.
- Unnecessary tubing like urinary catheters, IV lines to be removed to reduce the further worsening of condition.
- Fluid replacement and oxygenation to be initiated to prevent further damage to tissue and development of tissue hypoxia and organ dysfunction.
- Antibiotics like third-generation cephalosporin are recommended.
- Adequate nutritional supply should not be forgotten as lack of nutrition may impair the patient's resistance to infection. Enteral feedings may be considered.
- The nurse should ensure the aseptic practices specially during invasive procedures.

## SYSTEMIC INFLAMMATORY RESPONSE SYNDROME (SIRS)

### Definition

SIRS is defined as an exaggerated defence response of the body to a noxious stressor (infection, trauma, surgery, acute inflammation, ischemia or reperfusion, or malignancy, to name a few) to localize and then eliminate the endogenous or exogenous source of the insult.

### Etiology

The causative factors for systemic inflammatory response syndrome include damage associated molecular pattern (DAMP) and pathogen associated molecular pattern (PAMP). The DAMP includes symptoms like, burns, trauma, acute pancreatitis, substance abuse, adverse drug reaction, ischemia, hematologic malignancies, etc., whereas PAMP includes all type of microbial infection related factors like bacterial, viral and fungal infections and toxic shock syndrome, etc. **(Flowchart 14.20)**.

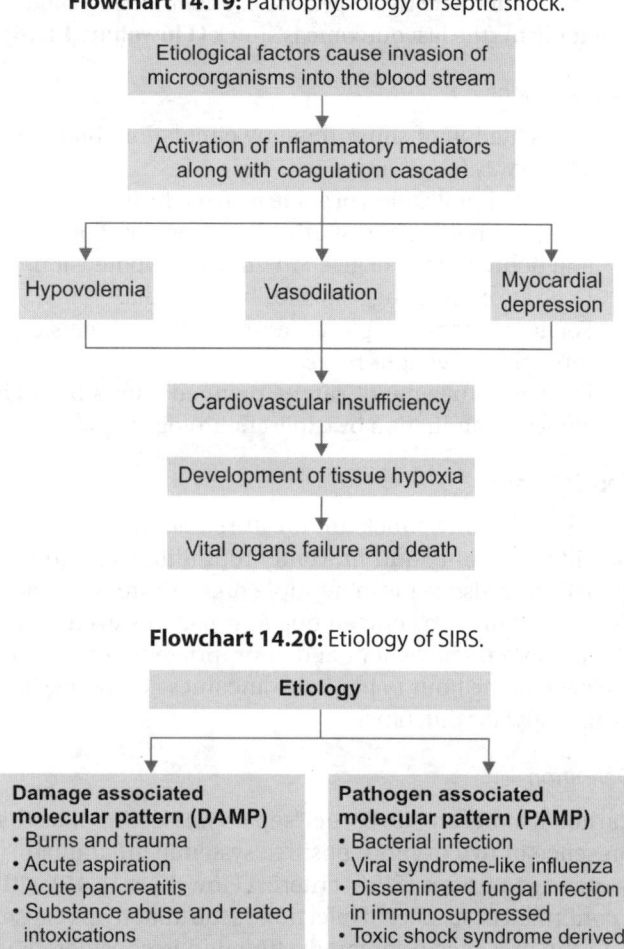

**Flowchart 14.19:** Pathophysiology of septic shock.

**Flowchart 14.20:** Etiology of SIRS.

### Stages of SIRS

Bone R, 1997 has suggested a five-stage approach called "sepsis cascade" which laid down the progression of sepsis process from SIRS to multiple organ dysfunction syndrome (MODS). This is important to take timely action to prevent the serious complications **(Flowchart 14.21)**. Those stages are:

### *Stage 1*

As soon as the pathogen invades the body, the body responds by starting local reaction at the injury site with the aim to prevent the further spread. This is achieved with the release of immune-mediators like cytokines and interleukins. This in turn stimulate reticuloendothelial

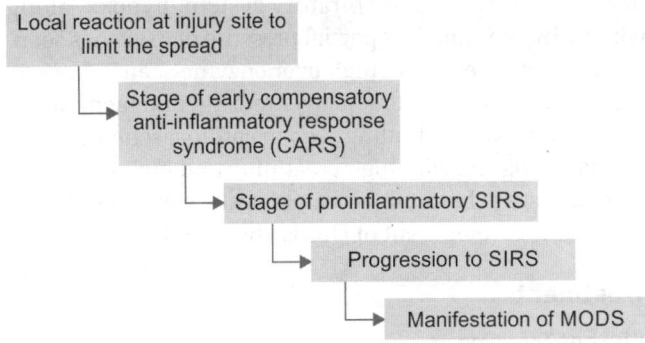

Flowchart 14.21: Stages of SIRS.

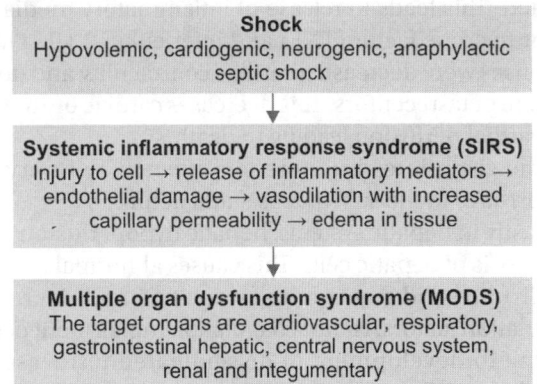

Flowchart 14.22: Relationship between shock, SIRS and MODS.

system to enhance tissue repair. The events for tissue repair goes like local vasodilatation (caused by nitric oxide and prostacyclin) → disruption of endothelial tissue lining allowing leukocyte transfer to the tissue → swelling and heat production due to the leakage of protein rich fluids and cells to extracellular space → local somatosensory nerve stimulation causing pain and loss of function.

*Stage 2*

It is the first compensatory stage called as CARS. In this stage, immunological balance and homeostasis is maintained through the activation of macrophages, growth factors and platelets.

*Stage 3*

It is the stage called proinflammatory SIRS, which includes progressive endothelial dysfunction, coagulopathy, and activation of coagulation cascade eventually leading to end-organ microthrombosis, increased capillary permeability and finally loss of circulatory integrity.

*Stage 4*

In this stage, CARS is taking over SIRS. In this stage, severe immunosuppression takes places leading increased incidence of opportunistic infection.

*Stage 5*

All the manifestation of multiple organ failure seen.

### Relationship between Shock, SIRS and MODS

Hence from the above discussions and explanations, it is clear that shock os an life-threatening emergency which is caused due to various reasons like low body fluid volume, cardiogenic origin, anaphylaxis and septic origin. Due to shock the body tries to compensate by activating systemic inflammatory response syndrome. This causes injury to cell, release of inflammatory mediators, endothelial damage, vasodilation, increased capillary permeability and edema. If after SIRS, the shock is not reversible the last stage is multiple organ dysfunction syndrome (**Flowchart 14.22**).

## MULTIPLE ORGAN DYSFUNCTION SYNDROME

### Definition

Multiple organ dysfunction syndrome (MODS) is defined as the development of potentially reversible physiologic disarrangement involving two or more organ systems not involved in the disorders, resulted in ICU admission, and a potentially life-threatening physiologic insult.

In other words, MODs develops with the combination of direct and reperfusion injury causing the progressive dysfunction of >2 organs secondary to any life-threatening illness or injury.

The most common cause of this is shock, specifically septic shock and patients surviving severe traumatic injury.

### Pathophysiology/Sequences of Events

The multiple organ failure post to shock and systemic inflammatory response syndrome affects various systems of body. In pulmonary system, first increased permeability of lungs parenchyma. Due to this excessive fluid accumulation in alveoli leading to alveolar edema. Development of metabolic acidosis. This leads to low blood PH. This is respiratory acidosis. The respiratory rate increases to compensate the acidosis. The fast respiration leads to hyperventilation and carbon dioxide washout. And lastly progressive hypoxia with lungs injury and acute respiratory distress syndrome.

In renal system, renal perfusion severely affected. This leads to renal insufficiency, tubular necrosis and renal damage. Lastly symptoms of oliguria with raised serum creatinine level appears.

In cardiovascular system, coronary perfusion is severely affected. This leads to release of inflammatory mediators, tumor necrotic factor (TNF) and interleukin-1 (IL-1). The responses were decreasing cardiac contractility and down-regulate beta-receptors. This decreases cardiac output and myocardial perfusion leading to death.

The gastrointestine system is affected by injury and hemorrhage to the sub-mucosal and ileum.

Lastly in hepatic systems, hepatic hypoperfusion leads to necrosis of hepatic cells. This causes abnormal increase of bilirubin and transaminase enzyme and decreased coagulation factors. Hence coagulation impairment occurs leading to development of disseminated intravascular coagulation **(Flowchart 14.23)**.

## Clinical Presentation

The multiple organ dysfunction syndrome, in almost all the system show some of the signs. Those are altered consciousness, state of confusion and development of psychosis in CNS. In respiratory system, hypoxia along with tachypnea and low partial pressure of oxygen is seen. High bilirubin level and high liver enzyme seen in hepatic system. Sign of shock that is hypotension and tachycardia with abnormal ECG finding seen in cardiovascular system. Similarly oliguria with high creatinine and high BUN seen in renal system. Lastly, in hematological system, low platelet count and development of DIC is observed **(Fig. 14.15)**.

## Treatment

### Aims of Treatment

- Prompt identification of the early signs of organ failure
- To find out the cause of the organ failure and systemic inflammation
- Ensure provision for supportive care to maximize the tissue perfusion

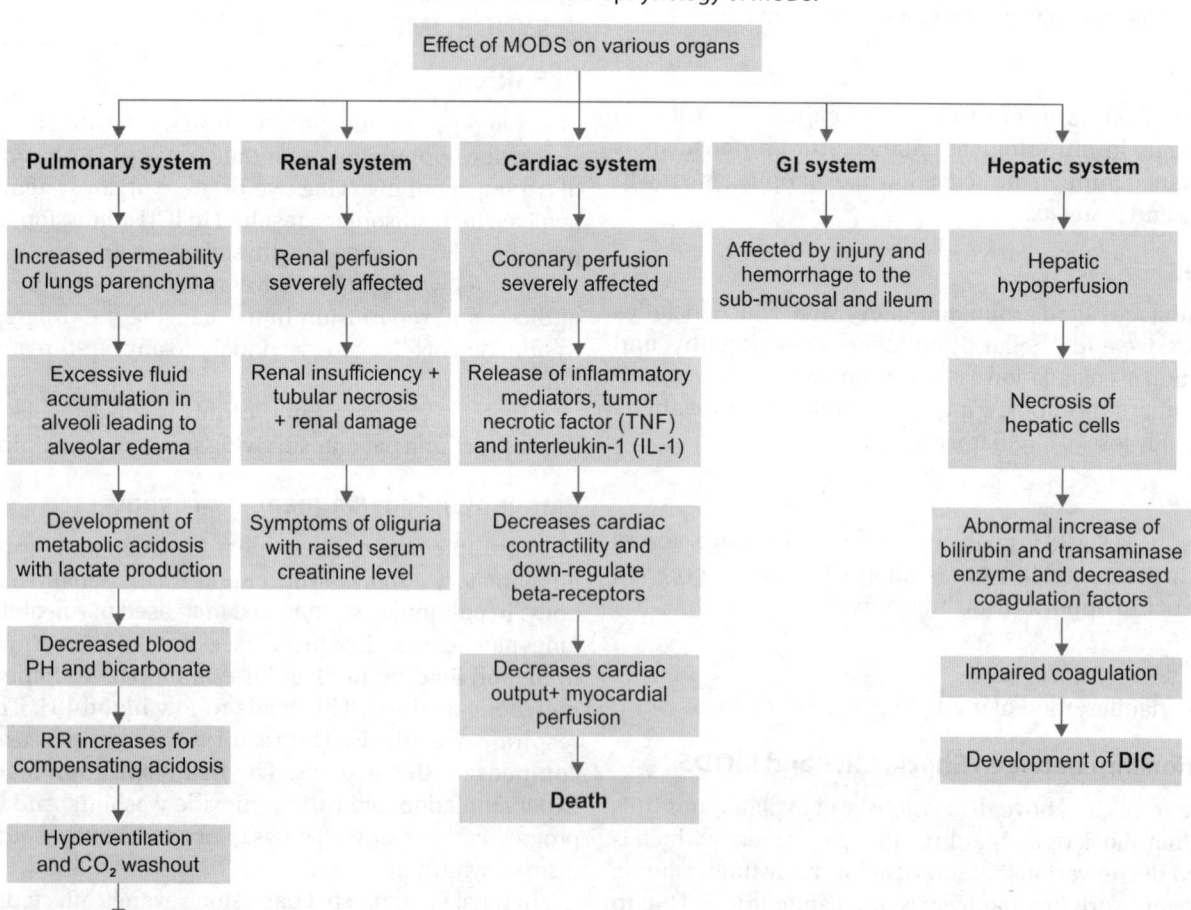

**Flowchart 14.23:** Pathophysiology of MODS.

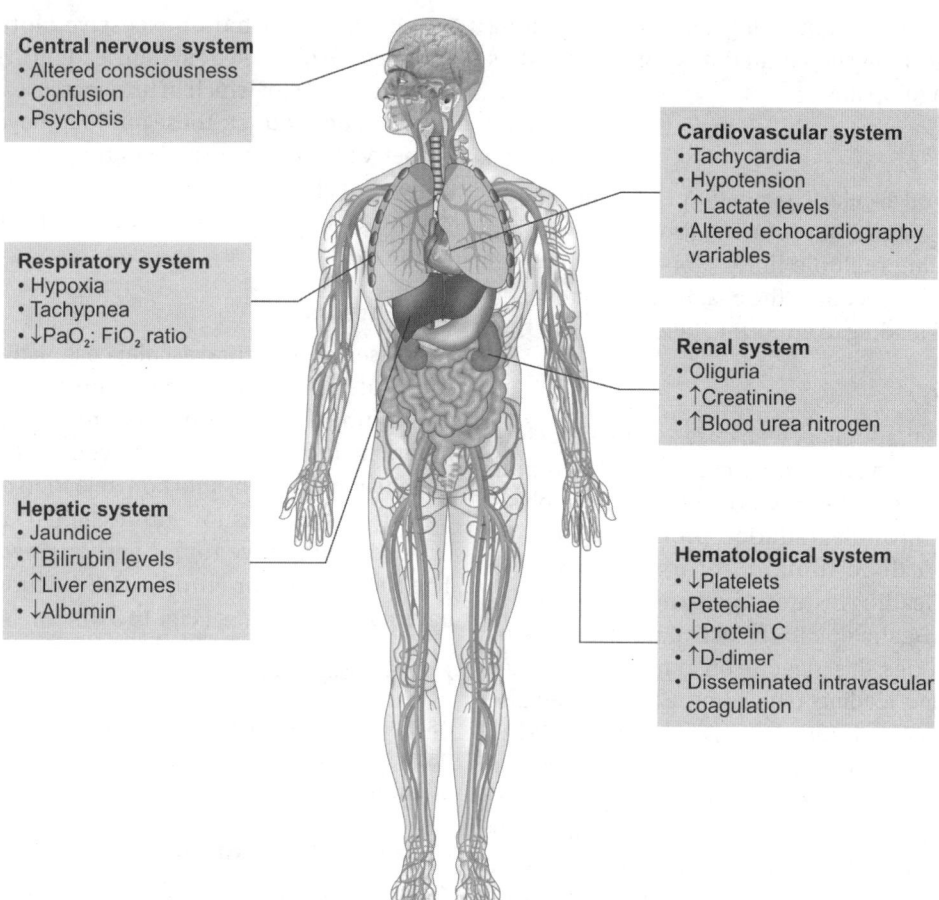

**Fig. 14.15:** Clinical manifestations of MODS.

### Actual Treatment

- Maintaining the state of euvolemia through adequate fluid administration. At the same time, it is to be kept in mind that, the focus is to retain the tissue perfusion without causing tissue edema.
- Inotropes and vasopressors are given for cardiovascular support.
- Airway patency, adequate ventilation and tissue oxygenation are maintained through mechanical ventilation and oxygen therapy.
- Antibiotic therapy for systemic inflammation.
- Antiendotoxin therapy is an recent treatment approach for sepsis management, which includes hyperimmune plasma, polymyxin B and nonsteroidal anti-inflammatory medications (NSAID). They (antibodies) work by binding to endotoxins and thereby preventing the inflammation.
- Also identification and treatment of coagulopathies.
- Simultaneous monitoring of vitals, serum glucose and cortisol level. Insulin may be supplied (0.1–1 IU/kg/h) to maintain normoglycemia. Low-dose corticosteroid therapy may be beneficial for patients with critical illness related to corticosteroid insufficiency.
- Antioxidant therapies like dimethyl-sulfoxide (IV) and vitamin E (IM) are recommended.
- Glutamine may be given to protect GI track by providing nutrition to enterocytes for maintaining GI barrier.
- Proton pump inhibitors are prescribed to reduce the risk of ulcer.

## DISSEMINATED INTRAVASCULAR COAGULATION (DIC)

The term disseminated means 'widespread', intravascular means 'within the bold vessel' and lastly coagulation means 'blood clot formation'. Hence, it is a thrombo-hemorrhagic disorder. It is also called as consumption coagulopathy because due to increase clot formation there is excess consumption of clotting factors and platelets. Hence, the level of platelet and clotting factors were decreased in blood leading to abnormal bleeding. Thus, as the clotting factors were abnormally consumed it is rightly called as consumption coagulopathy.

## Definition

Disseminated intravascular coagulation is a syndrome in which either the extrinsic or intrinsic or both pathways are activated producing multiple fibrin clots in small blood vessels This ultimately reduces the coagulation factors and platelets in blood leading to abnormal bleeding.

## Pathophysiology

In DIC first there is tissue injury with release of tissue factors. This activates the coagulation cascade. Then thrombin converts fibrinogen to fibrin. This further causes fibrinolysis. Then release of fibrin degradation product (FDP) and D-dimer. Further deposition of fibrin and platelet in microcirculation leading to thrombosis and tissue damage due to ischemia. Again, due to the active release of tissue factors post to injuries, this triggers consumption of clotting factors and platelets leading to bleeding. Bleeding can also occur due to homeostatic instability **(Flowchart 14.24)**.

DIC is not basically a disease rather an abnormal response to the normal clotting cascade stimulation by any disorder or disease. This may be acute, sub-acute or chronic. First of all following any tissue injury tissue factor is released at the site of injury to enhance the normal coagulation mechanism. Next to this thrombin, an intravascular coagulant triggers the conversion of fibrinogen to fibrin favoring platelet aggregation. With this there is widespread deposition of the platelet and fibrins in microcirculation resulting clot formation. This process may lead to multiorgan failure and clotting inhibitory factors like antithrombin III and protein C are depressed.

On the other hand, excessive clotting/thrombosis activates the fibrinolytic system leading to breaking down of newly formed clot which in turn increases the level of fibrin degradation product. These products have anticoagulation property inhibiting normal clotting mechanism. The result is bleeding. DIC most commonly seen among the patients with long-term illness like cancer, leukemia and other autoimmune diseases.

## Risk Factors

The disseminated intravascular coagulation could be acute, sub-acute and chronic. The factors for acute DIC includes carcinomas like acute leukemia, metastatic tumors, others includes—abruptio placentae, HELLP syndrome, transfusion reaction, abortion, rejection of transplants, etc.

The risk factors for sub-acute DIC includes, myelo/lymphoproliferative tumor and retained dead fetus, etc. The risk factors for chronic DIC includes, cancers, liver pathologies and SLEs **(Fig. 14.16)**.

## Clinical Presentation

As DIC is having two phase, thrombotic phase and hemorrhagic phase. The symptoms are listed accordingly as shown in **Table 14.8**.

## Diagnostic Evaluation

The laboratory findings to detect DIC are, there is elevated levels of prothrombin time, partial thromboplastin time, thrombin time, D-dimer and fibrin degradation product, where as platelet count and fibrinogen is markedly decreased in DIC **(Table 14.9)**.

There is a scoring system available to detect the severity of DIC, which is given by International Society on Thrombosis and Hemostasis **(Table 14.10)**.

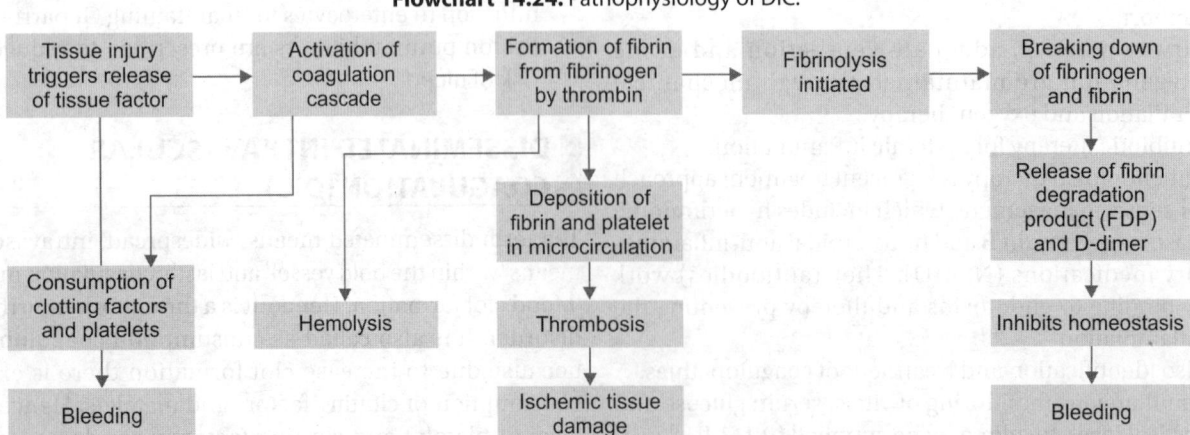

**Flowchart 14.24:** Pathophysiology of DIC.

| Acute DIC | Sub-acute DIC | Chronic DIC |
|---|---|---|
| • Cancer<br>• Acute leukemia<br>• Metastatic tumors<br>• Transfusion reaction<br>• Abruptio placentae<br>• HELLP syndrome<br>• Abortion (septic)<br>• Anaphylactic shock<br>• Advanced degree burn<br>• Transplant rejection | • Myelo/lympho-proliferative tumor<br>• Retained dead fetus | • Cancer<br>• Liver pathology<br>• Systemic lupus erythematus (SLE) |

**Fig. 14.16:** Risk factors of DIC.

**Table 14.8:** Clinical presentation of DIC.

| Symptoms of thrombotic phase | Symptoms of hemorrhagic phase |
|---|---|
| • **Integumentary:** Cyanosis, ischemic tissue necrosis, hemorrhagic necrosis<br>• **Respiratory:** Tachypnea, dyspnea, pulmonary emboli, and respiratory distress<br>• **Cardiovascular:** ECG changes, venous distention<br>• **GI:** Abdominal pain and paralytic ileus<br>• **Renal:** Kidney damage, oliguria and renal failure | • **Integumentary:** Pallor, petechiae, purpura, oozing of blood, venipuncture site bleeding, hematomas, and occult hemorrhage<br>• **Respiratory:** Tachypnea, hemoptysis, and orthopnea<br>• **Cardiovascular:** Tachycardia and hypotension<br>• **GI tract:** Bleeding of upper and lower GI tract, abdominal distention, and hematochezia<br>• **Renal:** Hematuria<br>• **Neurology:** Vision changes, dizziness, headache, mental status changes, and irritability<br>• **Musculoskeletal:** Pain in bones and joint |

**Table 14.9:** Laboratory findings in DIC.

| Test name | Changes in DIC | Normal range |
|---|---|---|
| Platelet count | Decreased | 150,000–450,000/mm³ |
| Prothrombin time (PT) | Elevated | 11–12.5 sec |
| Partial thromboplastin time (PTT) | Elevated | 23–35 sec |
| Thrombin time (TT) | Elevated | 8–11 sec |
| Fibrinogen | Decreased | 170–340 mg/dL |
| D-dimer | Elevated | 0–250 ng/mL |
| Fibrin degradation products (FDPs) | Elevated | 0–5 µg/mL |
| Euglobulin clot lysis | ≤1 hour | ≥2 hours |

**Table 14.10:** International society on thrombosis and hemostasis (ISTH) scoring system.

| Test name | Scores | Interpretation |
|---|---|---|
| Platelet count<br>• >100,000/mm³<br>• 50,000–100,000/mm³<br>• <50,000/mm³ | 0<br>1<br>2 | Score ≥5 = Overt DIC<br>Score <5 = Non-overt DIC |
| Fibrin markers (D-dimer and FDP)<br>• Normal<br>• Moderately increased<br>• Markedly increased | 0<br>2<br>3 | |
| Prothrombin time<br>• <3 sec<br>• 3–6 sec<br>• >6 sec | 0<br>1<br>2 | |
| Fibrinogen level<br>• >100 mg/dL<br>• <100 mg/dL | 0<br>1 | |

## Differential Diagnosis

- Massive blood loss
- Thrombotic microangiopathy
- Heparin-induced thrombocytopenia
- Vitamin K deficiency
- Liver insufficiency

## Management

### Medical Management

**Goal:**

- Treating the underlying cause of DIC
- Correct the secondary tissue ischemia through oxygenation, fluid replacement and vasopressor drugs

**Treatment includes:**

- Treatment of underlying cause—by fluid volume resuscitation, antibiotics and external cooling
- Thrombocytopenia (<50,000/mm³) and active bleeding will be managed by transfusion of platelet
- For prolonged prothrombin time (>1.5) and low fibrinogen (<100 mg/dL) transfusion of fresh frozen plasma (FFP) and vitamin K
- Cryoprecipitate is given to replace fibrinogen and factors V and VII
- Consider LMWH when thrombotic events dominate clinical picture (as heparin prevent formation of micro-clots and hence maintains the perfusion to various organs)
- Consider tranexamic acid for trauma-related DIC

## Nursing Management

The DIC is a medical emergency. Hence early identification of risk and prompt action is highly solicited both by the physician and nurses. Hence, the detailed nursing care plan for a client with DIC is discussed below. This includes nursing diagnosis, goal, expected nursing intervention with rationale of each and lastly expected outcome **(Table 14.11)**.

**Table 14.11:** Nursing care plan for a patient with DIC.

| Nursing diagnosis and goal | Nursing intervention | Rationale | Expected outcome |
|---|---|---|---|
| **Nursing diagnosis**<br>Potential for fluid volume deficit related to bleeding<br>**Goal**<br>To maintain the hemodynamic status | • To avoid strenuous activity which may increase intracranial pressure (ICP)<br>• Monitor vital parameters like hemodynamic status, urine output and abdominal girth, etc.<br>• Medications like aspirin, NSAIDs and beta-lactam antibiotics to be avoided<br>• Strict record of intake and output chart<br>• Use low pressure while suctioning<br>• Do oral hygiene carefully using salt and baking soda and avoid glycerine swabs | • To prevent intracranial bleeding<br>• To detect early sign of shock and hemorrhage<br>• Reduce the problems with platelet aggregation<br>• To know the exact hemodynamic status<br>• To prevent trauma and bleeding risk<br>• Glycerine based swans will dry the mucosa and will cause bleeding | • Stable state of consciousness<br>• CVP 5–12 cm $H_2O$, systolic BP ≥ 0 mm Hg<br>• Urine output ≥30 mL/hour<br>• Decreased bleeding<br>• Decreased oozing<br>• Clean and moist oral mucosa<br>• Absence of bleeding |
| **Nursing diagnosis**<br>Potential for impaired skin integrity secondary to hypoxia or hemorrhage<br>**Goal**<br>To maintain intact skin integrity | • Skin assessment with special attention to bony prominent areas and skin folds every 2 hourly<br>• Carefully change the position of the patient<br>• Use of pressure reducing mattress<br>• Maintain proper oral care | • Helps to early identify any broken skin early<br>• This prevents any further damage to skin<br>• To prevent the development of bed sore<br>• Prevents infection and injury to oral mucosa | • Integrity of skin remains intact with natural color<br>• Oral cavity is well protected |
| **Nursing diagnosis**<br>Potential for fluid volume excess secondary to increased cellular permeability<br>**Goal**<br>• To reduce edema<br>• To stabilize the breathing<br>• To tract intake and output | • Evaluate the degree of edema<br>• Auscultate breath sound for any abnormality<br>• Strict monitoring of intake and output chart<br>• Give diuretics if required | • Helps to take measure to reduce abnormal volume overload<br>• To evaluate any sign of abnormal breath sound and helps with the intervention<br>• Helps to maintain accurate body fluid balance<br>• Helps to reduce edema | • Reduction of edema<br>• Normally maintained breath sound<br>• Balanced body fluid intake and output |
| **Nursing diagnosis**<br>Potential for diminished tissue perfusion secondary to abnormal formation of clots<br>**Goal**<br>• To reduce hypoxia<br>• To ensure normal neurological state<br>• To normalize vitals | • Assessment of neurologic, pulmonary and circulatory status<br>• Evaluate for any sign of active internal or external bleeding<br>• Check for level of fibrinogen<br>• Evaluate the response of heparin therapy | • Early sign of thrombus formation can be ensured<br>• Helps to know when to start or stop the anticoagulant therapy<br>• To know how the body is responding<br>• To know the patient is responding to treatment positively or not | • Tissue perfusion well maintained<br>• No hypoxia with thrombus formation |

*Contd...*

*Contd...*

| Nursing diagnosis and goal | Nursing intervention | Rationale | Expected outcome |
|---|---|---|---|
| **Nursing diagnosis**<br>Potential for fear and anxiety secondary to disease progression and response to treatment<br>**Goal**<br>• To verbalize fear<br>• To create hope | • Teach patient how the coping strategy works<br>• Encourage patient to use coping mechanism<br>• Provide adequate and repeated explanation about the disease process, treatment options and what to expect as a patient<br>• Involve family in treatment process<br>• Assess the patient in need for more intense psychological counseling | • Helps to build confidence<br>• Helps reducing anxiety<br>• As familiar things creates less fear and anxiety<br>• Support system became stronger and the patient also will feel at ease<br>• Early identify before any unwanted event like progressing to depression, self-harm, discontinuation of treatment, etc. | • Patient develops strong coping strategy to handle the anxiety<br>• Family is more comfortable to support the patient |

## DRUG OVERDOSE AND POISONING

Emergencies like drug overdose and poisoning are crucial to consider as this calls for immediate identification and management to reduce the mortality and morbidity among the casualties. In developing natin like India due to various factors like poverty, easy access to poison, household disturbances, unemployment, depression, loneliness, domestic violence and history of addictions, the suicide rates are more. Apart from that those emergencies are the result of accidental intake secondary to lack of awareness and attention. Out if all sort of poisoning, pesticide poisoning is much prevalent in India due to more agricultural and houschold activities. Other means of poisoning are household agents, envenomation, and drugs. As estimated by World Health Organization (WHO) the incidence of pesticide induced poisoning are about 3 million/annum worldwide, leading to death of >220000 casualties. The current situation of COVID 19 also adds to this condition.

### Definition

A poison is considered as a substance which can cause harm or illness to a living being either upon contact or introduction to the body. On the other hand, poisoning is the harmful effect of a toxic substance known as poison, when introduced to the body in an amount capable of causing deleterious effect to various body systems.

"A drug overdose is defined as the ingestion or application of a drug in quantities much greater than the recommended dose. This may result with toxic state or death". The term drug overdose and poisoning of toxic substance including drugs often use interchangeably.

### Modes of Poisoning/Overdose

- Ingestion
- Inhalation
- Absorption
- Injection

### Substances Causing Poisoning/Overdose

- Household agents/chemicals like kerosene, bleaching.
- Industrial substances like methanol, ethylene glycol, cyanide and arsenic.
- Agricultural pesticides like organophosphorus (OP), organo-chlorines (DDT), rat poisons, etc.
- Drug overdose like paracetamol, aspirin, iron tablet, nifedipine, phenobarbitone, etc.
- Poisonous plants like toxic mushrooms, herbs, etc.
- Bites and stings by venomous animals like snake, scorpions, bees, spider, and other aquatic animals.

### Clinical Presentation

A clear tabular representation of clinical presentation for drug overdose and poisoning is shown in **Table 14.12**.

### Danger Signs of Poisoning/Overdose

- Apnea
- Abnormal breathing sounds

**Table 14.12:** Clinical picture of drug overdose and poisoning.

| Signs | Symptoms |
|---|---|
| • Pyrexia<br>• Dehydration<br>• Jaundice<br>• Change in pupil size may be squeezed or enlarged<br>• Unpleasant breathing smell<br>• Change in pulse rate<br>• Seizure<br>• Abdominal tenderness<br>• Discoloration of tongue | • Emesis<br>• Diarrhea<br>• Blisters and burns in mouth<br>• Upper abdominal pain<br>• Breathing difficulty<br>• Scanty urine<br>• Skin rashes<br>• Swelling of lips and other body parts<br>• Palpitation<br>• Bad mouth odor |

- Irregular pulse (tachy or bradycardia)
- No pupillary reaction
- Unconscious patient
- Episodes of seizure
- Temperature >38°C
- Anuria
- Severe abdominal tenderness

## Diagnosis

### Taking History

Collecting appropriate history while stabilizing patient is an important step to plan for specific treatment. This includes:
- Which drug/chemical was ingested?
- When it was taken?
- What amount of agent was taken?
- What was the route of exposure?
- Why it was taken?
- Was anything else taken along with the drug?

### Examinations and Monitoring

The overdose of drugs and poisoning has various sources to start with. For easy remembrance, a well schematic table with all details of examination and monitoring parameters were given. For this emergency condition, the emergency department staff should be ready with all the vital parameters measuring tools for pulse rate, respiratory rate, temperature, blood pressure along with a quick neurological examination, pupil examination, etc. **(Table 14.13)**.

### Laboratory Studies

- Serum electrolyte
- Differential count (DC) and total leukocyte count (TLC)
- Serum urea and creatinine
- Liver function test
- Blood glucose level
- ABG analysis
- Test of gastric aspirate to identify the toxic substance
- ECG
- Endoscopic examination
- X-ray and CT scan

## Management of Poisoning and Drug Overdose

### Management of Poisoning

*Initial Management*

Airway management
- Ensure and establish a patent airway.
- Check the airway for any foreign body or secretion obstructing it.
- Suction the airway to prevent aspiration.
- Check the need for intubation.
- Once ensure about the patency of airway the oxygenation should be maintained.
- Check the change in respiratory rate and abnormal breath sound (drugs like opiates, barbiturates and tricyclic antidepressant drugs decreases the respiratory rate).

Circulation
- Fluid volume is to be maintained by fluid infusion with large bored cannula
- Send investigations to evaluate need for transfusion
- Observe any sign of cyanosis
- Blood glucose level to be monitored
- Monitor vitals along with 12 lead ECG

Note
- Tricyclic antidepressants cases tachycardia, tachyarrhythmias, and low BP.
- Cocaine can also cause tachyarrhythmias and even MI.
- Bradycardia may be caused by organophosphate insecticides or β-blocker medication.

Neurological monitoring
- It is important to evaluate the neurological status for every drug overdoes and poisoning cases to detect early any sign of worsening.
- Some of the important GCS findings are "presence of reduced pupil diameter is a sign of narcotic overdose and dilated pupil is caused by cocaine, amphetamines, atropine, or tricyclic antidepressant".
- Episodes of seizure can be a sign of alcohol withdrawal.

*Specific Management*

Establishing core body temperature
- Both hypo and hyperthermia can be a result of drug overdose and poisoning.
- Hypothermia can result with certain drug overdose like barbiturates and phenothiazines. Management includes evaluation of rectal temperature followed by administration of warm IV fluids and covering with warm blanket to maintain the core body temperature.
- Similarly hyperthermia can be caused by drugs like amphetamines, cocaine, ecstasy, monoamine oxidase inhibitors (MAOIs), and theophylline. It can be managed by checking skin temperature followed by tepid sponging, maintaining adequate room temperature, giving loose cloths and adequate fluid to drink. And lastly antipyretic can be administered as per the need.

**Table 14.13:** Various assessment parameters of drug overdose and poisoning.

| Parameters | Findings | |
|---|---|---|
| Pulse rate | **Tachycardia** | **Bradycardia** |
| | • Anticholinergic<br>• Antihistamines<br>• Amphetamines<br>• Theophylline | • Propranolol<br>• Calcium channel blocker<br>• Clonidine<br>• Digoxin |
| Temperature | **Hyperthermia** | **Hypothermia** |
| | • Nicotine<br>• Antihistamines<br>• Aspirin<br>• Paracetamol<br>• Anticholinergics | • Carbon monoxide<br>• Opiates<br>• Oral hypoglycemics<br>• Alcohol<br>• Sedatives |
| Blood pressure | **Hypertension** | **Hypotension** |
| | • Cocaine<br>• Sympathomimetics<br>• Caffeine<br>• Amphetamines<br>• Nicotine<br>• Thyroid supplements | • Clonidine<br>• Antidepressants<br>• Sedatives<br>• Opiates<br>• Antihypertensive |
| Respiratory rate | **Tachypnea** | **Bradypnea** |
| | • Metabolic acidosis<br>• Pulmonary edema<br>• Pneumonitis | • Sedatives<br>• Alcohol<br>• Opiates<br>• Marijuana |
| Neurologic evaluation | **Altered mental status** | **Seizures** |
| | • Alcohol<br>• Intoxication<br>• Hypooxygenamia<br>• Tumor<br>• Trauma<br>• Shock | • Organophosphorus<br>• Ethanol<br>• Insulin<br>• Sympathomimetics<br>• Amphetamine<br>• Benzodiazepines withdrawal |
| Pupil examination | **Miosis** | **Mydriasis** |
| | • Sedatives<br>• Clonidine<br>• Opiates | • Antidepressant<br>• Atropine<br>• Cocaine |
| Odors | • Fruity<br>• Bitter almond<br>• Garlic<br>• Peanuts<br>• Carrots<br>• Rotten egg<br>• Gasoline | • Diabetic ketoacidosis, isopropanol<br>• Cyanide<br>• Arsenic, organophosphorus<br>• Rodenticide<br>• Water hemlock<br>• Sulphur dioxide<br>• Hydrocarbons |

## Decontamination of exposed body area

- In case of exposure to corrosive agents like pesticides, chemicals, etc, eyes should immediately be ringed with clean water for at least 10–15 min. The exposed skin should be washed with soap and water with special attention to the skin folds.
- In case the corrosive agent has been swallowed, the patient should be given enough fluid to flush out those chemicals and to reduce damage to the internal tissues and organs.

## Aspiration of gastric content

- Stomach wash or gastric lavage is a conventional method but yet used in current practice. In case of poison congestion with duration less than 1 hour, charcoal activated water suspension of given and either vomiting is induced or the content to be aspirated with the help of nasogastric tube. The dose is 25–50 g for an adult, and 1 g/kg body weight for a child. The calculation is one part poison to ten parts charcoal. Contraindication of charcoal aspiration is in case of poisoning with iron, lithium, alcohol, methanol, ethylene glycol, corrosive agents, acids, and alkalis, which requires oral antidotes or medication.

Psychological support and care

First of all, those patients with suicidal attempt need to be assessed by psychiatric team. Each patient should be approached in a sympathetic way and supportive manner. Every effort is made to help those patients and to identify the reason for such adverse event to prevent further bad consequences.

## Management of Drug Overdose

### Paracetamol

It is a commonly used and safe NSAID drug worldwide. The dose of >300 mg/kg is considered overdose as it may cause damage to both liver and kidney. In the 1st few hours, the patient will be asymptomatic and conscious with mild malaise, nausea and vomiting. After 2–3 days advanced signs appear like jaundice and elevated liver enzymes. Acetylcysteine is the drug of choice which is administered as an infusion over 60 min irrespective of the time of overdose and sign of hepatotoxicity.

### Salicylates

Salicylates like aspirin and other drugs overdose manifested with symptoms like vomiting, dehydration, tinnitus, deafness, sweating, warm extremities, and hyperventilation in mild case. Severe symptoms include coma, convulsions, pulmonary edema, and cardiovascular collapse. Management includes administration of oral activated charcoal within 1st hour of ingestion.

### Tricyclic Antidepressants

- Overdose symptoms include tachycardia, dilated pupils, cardiac arrhythmias and widened QRS complex, hypotension, hot dry skin, and dry mouth. Untreated and severe cases show convulsions, respiratory depression, and coma.
- Treatment includes cardiac monitoring up to 6 hours of ingestion and give oral activated charcoal within 1st hour of ingestion.

### Selective Serotonin Reuptake Inhibitors

Usually asymptomatic, even with large overdose ingestion. However, some patients may exhibit GI upset, drowsiness, tachycardia, muscle stiffness, and hypertension and in untreated and severe cases convulsions may occur. Activated charcoal is the antidote of choice.

### Benzodiazepines

Symptoms include drowsiness, ataxia, nystagmus, hypotension, respiratory depression, and coma, when benzodiazepines taken with alcohol or other CNS depressants. Flumazenil given as antidote.

### Iron Tablets

- Early symptoms include nausea, vomiting, abdominal pain, diarrhea and black stool. Severe symptoms include hematemesis and rectal bleeding progressing to coma and shock.
- Treatment involves evaluation of serum iron, gastric lavage, and deferoxamine treatment within few hours of ingestion.

### Cardiac Glycosides

- Includes drugs like digitoxin, digitalis, oleander. Overdose is considered when the plasma K+ concentration is >5.3 mmol/L.
- Symptoms include nausea, vomiting, cardiac arrhythmias, hypotension, and death. The treatment involves administration of activated charcoal.

# ACQUIRED IMMUNODEFICIENCY SYNDROME (AIDS)

Government of India (GOI) estimates that about 2.40 million Indians are living with HIV (1.93–3.04 million) with an adult prevalence of 0.31% (2009). Children (<15 years) account for 3.5% of all infections, while 83% are the in-age group 15–49 years. Of all HIV infections, 39% (930,000) are among women (2012). Recently on April 2022, World Bank collection of development indicators reported zero cases of AIDS in India. Hence, it is considered as a public health problem globally as it has no cure so far. But certain steps like prompt diagnosis, strong guideline of HIV prevention, awareness at grassroot level, easily accessible and affordable treatment enables people to live with HIV for long without any chronic deteriorated health problems. As a nursing personnel it is important to understand the problems of the people living with HIV. So that this will help them to care for those in a better way.

## What is HIV?
- **Human:** Can live/affect to only human
- **Immunodeficiency:** Damage to immune system
- **Virus:** Retrovirus (RNA).

## What is AIDS?
- **Acquired:** Gets infection from other source
- **Immune:** Weakens the immunity of the affected person
- **Deficiency:** Dysfunction of body immune system
- **Syndrome:** A group of clinical presentation.

## Definition
AIDS is a spectrum of conditions caused by infection with the human immunodeficiency virus (HIV) belong to the family of retrovirus. As the infection progresses it interferes with the bodies immune system and makes the body vulnerable for getting opportunistic infection **(Fig. 14.17)**.

## What is the difference between HIV and AIDS?
- HIV is a virus and AIDS is a disease.
- HIV develops into AIDS.
- AIDS is deficiency in the body's defense mechanism or immune system.
- AIDS is acquired, not hereditary.

## Clinical Presentation
The AIDS develops in four stages. The first stage is purely asymptomatic along with generalized lymphadenopathy, which makes the person unaware of the disease progression. The second stage is the initiation of further symptoms but in milder form like, loss of <10% of weight, recurrent respiratory infections, frequent oral ulcers, skin rashes, etc. The third stage is severe symptoms to second stage like weight loss of >10% of body weight, unexplained chronic diarrhea for >1 month, unexplained persistent fever. The last stage is the appearance of HIV wasting syndrome, pneumocystis pneumonia, recurrent severe bacterial pneumonia, esophageal candidiasis, etc., **(Table 14.14)**.

## Transmission
HIV is a pretty serious condition and more importantly can be prevented, only if you have knowledge on modes of transmission. The details of modes of transmission is given in the **Table 14.15**.

## Viral Replication Pathways
The replication of HIV-1 is a multi-stage process. It has a total of six steps **(Fig. 14.18)**.
1. HIV attaches to the CD4 cell and releases RNA and enzymes on entry.

**Table 14.14:** Clinical stages of HIV.

| Clinical staging | Clinical presentation |
|---|---|
| Stage 1 | • Asymptomatic<br>• Persistent generalized lymphadenopathy |
| Stage 2 | • Unexplained moderate weight loss (<10% of presumed or measured body weight)<br>• Recurrent respiratory tract infections (sinusitis, tonsillitis, otitis media, pharyngitis)<br>• Herpes zoster<br>• Recurrent oral ulceration<br>• Pruritic papular eruptions (PPE)<br>• Seborrheic dermatitis<br>• Fungal nail infections<br>• Angular cheilitis |
| Stage 3 | • Unexplained severe weight loss (>10% of presumed or measured body weight)<br>• Unexplained chronic diarrhea for longer than one month<br>• Unexplained persistent fever (above 37.5°C intermittent or constant for longer than one month) |
| Stage 4 | • HIV wasting syndrome.<br>• Pneumocystis pneumonia (PCP)<br>• Recurrent severe bacterial pneumonia<br>• Chronic herpes simplex infection (orolabial, genital or anorectal of more than one month's duration or visceral at any site)<br>• Esophageal candidiasis (or candidiasis of trachea, bronchi or lungs)<br>• Extrapulmonary tuberculosis<br>• Kaposi's sarcoma |

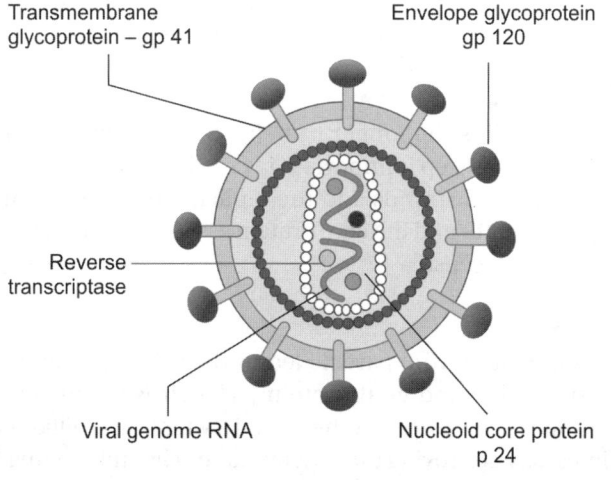

**Fig. 14.17:** HIV structure.

| Table 14.15: Modes of transmission of HIV. | |
|---|---|
| **HIV transmitted** | **HIV not transmitted** |
| Unprotected coitus | Touching, kissing/hugging |
| Sharing infected needle | Sharing food, toilet, clothing |
| Contact with infected blood and blood products | Mosquito bite |
| Vertically from mother to child perinatally and during breastfeeding | Bathing/swimming in the same pond/pool |
| Occupational exposure and reusing instruments | Contact with sweat, tears, urine or feces |

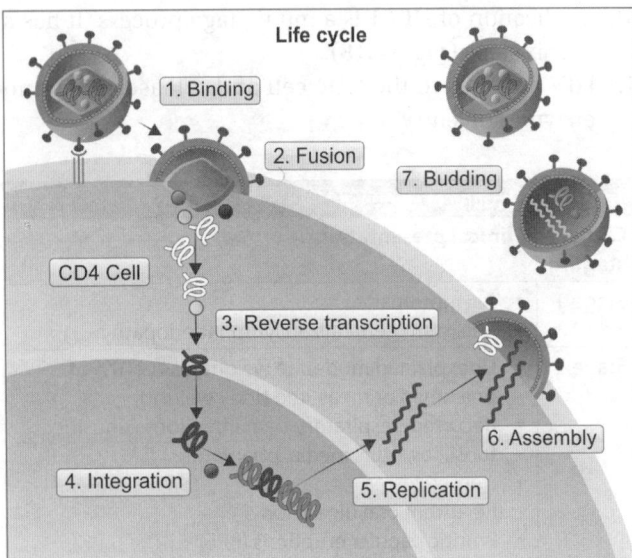

**Fig. 14.18:** HIV replication pathways.
*Source:* HIV Info. NIH. GOV, 2021.

2. The enzyme 'reverse transcriptase' makes a DNA copy of the viral RNA.
3. New viral DNA is then integrated using the enzyme 'integrase' into the CD4 cell nucleus.
4. New viral components are then produced, using the cell's machinery.
5. These are assembled together using the enzyme 'protease'.
6. The new viruses are released.

### Step 1

It is the infection of the suitable host cell such as a $CD_4$ positive T-Lymphocyte. Entry of HIV into the cell requires the presence of certain receptors and the cell surface. $CD_4$ receptors and the co-receptors such as $CCR_5$ or $CXCR_4$. These receptors interact with protein complexes which invaded in the viral envelop. These complexes are composed of 2 numbers of glycoproteins and extracellular GP-120 and a transmembrane GP-41.

When HIV approaches a target cell GP-120 binds to the CD-4 receptors. This process is called attachment. It promotes further binding to a co-receptor. Co-receptor binding results in a confirmational change in GP-120.

This allows GP-41 to unfold and insert its hydrophobic terminals into the cell membrane. GP-41 then folds back on itself. This brings the virus towards the cell and facilitates the fusion of their membrane.

The viral nucleocapsid enters the host cell and breaks open, releasing two viral RNA strand and three essential replication enzymes. Those enzymes are reverse transcriptase, integrase and protease.

### Step 2

Reverse transcriptase begins the reverse transcription of viral RNA. It has two catalytic domains such as Ribonuclease H active site and polymerase active site. Here single standard viral RNA is transcribed into an RNA DNA double helix.

### Step 3

Now integrase does its action. It cuts the ends of the DNA creating two sticky ends. Integrase then transfers the DNA into the cell's nucleus and facilitates its integration to the host cell genome. The host cell genome now contains genetic information of HIV. Activation of the cell induces transcription of pro-viral DN into messenger RNA.

### Step 4

The viral messenger RNA migrates into cytoplasm, where building blocks for a new virus are synthesized. Some of them has to be processed by the viral protease.

### Step 5

Protease clips the longer proteins into the smaller core proteins. This step is important in creating infectious virus. The viral RNS strands and the replication enzymes then come together and the core protein assemble around them forming the capsid.

### Step 6

This immature viral particle leaves the cell acquiring new host envelop and viral proteins. The virus matures and becomes ready to infect other cells. HIV replicates billions of times/day destroying the host immune cells and eventually causing disease progression.

## Diagnosis
- HIV antibody tests
  - HIV rapid test
  - ELISA
  - Western blot test (confirmatory test)
- HIV antigen tests
  - DNA PCR
  - P24 antigen

## Treatment

### Drugs
The treatment of choice is the antiretroviral drugs (ARVs). It is not a cure for AIDS and the patient has to take it for life long, but it dramatically improves the health and life expectancy of the patient living with HIV and AIDS (PLHIV/PLHA).

### How Antiretroviral Drugs Work?
The antiretroviral drugs act by interfering with key steps of the viral replication, hence stops the fatal process.

First of all, entry of the virus to the host cell can be blocked by fusion inhibitors drugs like nucleoside reverse transcriptase inhibitor (NRTI) and non-nucleoside reverse transcriptase inhibitor (NNRTI).

Similarly, the action of integrase can be blocked. And the multiplication of virus by protease can be blocked by protease inhibitor. Therefore, each blocked step in viral replication is a step towards better control of the disease.

### Drugs Included in ART
Antiretroviral drugs are effective treatments for HIV. It is advised to start ART immediately as soon as possible as it can reduce the risk of HIV-related complications, disease progression and prevent further transmission. The detailed classification of antiretroviral drugs, along with its action with examples were given in **Table 14.16**.

### Prevention of Opportunistic Infection
This can be achieved by maintaining hygiene and asepsis. Strict adherence and compliance with medication. Vaccination for preventable diseases should be considered. Isoniazid preventive therapy (IPT), is recommended for patients with HIV with no active TB infection. Prophylaxis against hepatitis (A and B) are advised for all people at risk or having HIV. Contraindicating breastfeeding for mothers infected with HIV. Some researchers also showed the benefit of Influenza vaccination and pneumococcal polysaccharide vaccine for the patients with HIV infection.

### Diet
The WHO recommended a well-balanced and nutrient rich diet for the people living with HIV. It suggests the inclusion of micronutrients and multivitamin supplements in diet.

**Table 14.16:** ART drugs with its action.

| Common class of art | Action of drugs | Included drugs |
|---|---|---|
| Nucleoside reverse transcriptase inhibitors (NRTIs) | NRTIs inhibit activity of reverse transcriptase, a viral DNA polymerase enzyme, that retroviruses need to reproduce | • Zidovudine (AZT, ZDV)<br>• Lamivudine (3TC)<br>• Stavudine (d4T)<br>• Didanosine (ddI)<br>• Abacavir (ABC)<br>• Tenofovir (TDF)<br>• Emtricitabine (FTC) |
| Non-nucleoside reverse transcriptase inhibitors (NNRTIs) | NNRTIs block reverse transcriptase by binding at a different site on the enzyme, compared to NRTIs | • Efavirenz (EFZ)<br>• Nevirapine (NVP) |
| Protease inhibitors (PIs) | Protease is a chemical, known as an enzyme, that HIV needs, in order to make new viruses and protease inhibitors prevents this action | • Nelfinavir (NFV)<br>• Lopinavir/Ritonavir (LPV/R)<br>• Saquinavir (SQV)<br>• Amprenavir (APV)<br>• Indinavir (IDV)<br>• Atazanavir (ATV)<br>• Ritonavir (RTV)—(recommended as booster only) |

**ARVs must be given in a 3-drug combination**
- This combination is referred to as the ARV regimen – also known as a triple drug combination
- Giving only 1 or 2 ARVs to treat HIV disease is incorrect and ineffective

But vitamin A, zinc and iron are to be avoided to prevent adverse outcomes in case of infected patient.

### Role of Alternative Medicines

Though no evidence has been established, in the US around 60% of patients with HIV adopts to complementary and alternative medicines like herbal medicines. Also, medical cannabis believes to be effective for improving appetite.

## Role of Nurse

Till date HIV carries a stigma and people fear and isolate the HIV infected persons in society. This is devastating for the patient and their family as well. Hence, the role of nurse is very important to create awareness among the societal people to support those who are in need. The role includes:
- Correct identification and referral of the cases to HIV testing centers.
- Keeping the test information absolutely confidential.
- Counseling for the people who are at risk, to make them encouraged to go for testing.
- Educating the patients with HIV infection regarding lifestyle changes, compliance and adherence with treatment and what to expect in reality.
- Also creating awareness regarding risk reduction strategy and palliative care for those who need it.
- Continuous follow up with creating help groups in society who will work for them.

# EYE INJURIES

## Epidemiology

Various types of eye or ocular injuries (**Fig. 14.19**) ranging from mild to severe one are commonly seen in clinical facilities in our daily practice as a healthcare professional.

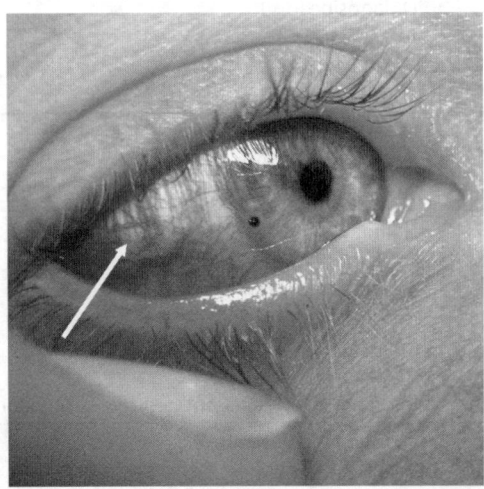

**Fig. 14.19:** Eye trauma.

Types of ocular injuries can be simple foreign body invasion to cornea to ruptured globe. India has reported an incidence of 2.4% of ocular trauma among urban population out of which about 11% became blind secondary to injury. Global data of United States that, about 2.0–2.4 million cases of eye trauma were reported to hospital each year and about 1 million of people have permanent visual impairment. Many reasons are there which may delay the early detection of eye trauma and initiation of treatment. Mostly eye trauma cases come to emergency department with other associated life-threatening conditions. Hence, this is mostly ignored leading to delayed identification of eye trauma. Other reasons which make it difficult to assess are swelling in periorbital areas, unconscious patients, etc. Hence, this part of the chapter is aiming to give adequate knowledge and exposure to the readers so that they can contribute towards early management of such emergencies.

## Classification

The eye injuries are very severe and delicate to handle, and the chances of complication development is much faster if not treated early. Hence, before knowing the possible management for the same, it is important to know the classification.

The eye injury is divided into two types, namely open globe and closed globe injury. In case of closed globe injury, the eye globe is intact. This further includes contusion and lamellar laceration.

On the other hand, open globe injury is the full thickness injury to the eye wall including both cornea and sclera. It is further divided into a ruptured globe (secondary to blunt trauma) and lacerated globe (is a full thickness injury to the globe caused by sharp object). The lacerated wound again can be either penetrating (the integrity of eye is disrupted by full thickness injury followed by prolapse of internal part of eye), perforating trauma (occurs when the external force enters and exits the eye. This trauma can be of two types like orbital fracture and muscle entrapment) and intraocular foreign body invasion (**Flowchart 14.25**).

## Management of Various Eye Injuries

### Gathering Relevant History

The information gathering following trauma should be very precise. It should include the type of injury, its severity, part of the eye affected and treatment given before bringing it to hospital.

### Tetanus Prophylaxis

It should be given in all cases of eye injury involving dirt exposure to eye and presence of laceration of eye.

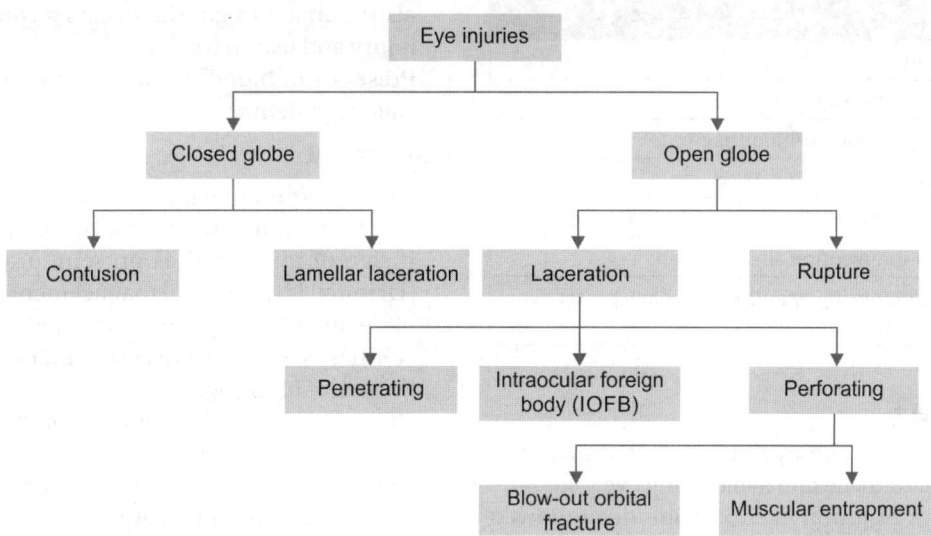

**Flowchart 14.25:** Types of eye injuries.

### Corneal Abrasions and its Management

- It is defined as the superficial lesion to the corneal epithelium of eye. The symptoms include pain, discomfort due to foreign body presence, decreased visual acuity/blurring sensation, epiphora (excess watering) and photophobia.
- **Diagnosis:**
  - Includes history and clinical assessment followed by specific treatment. History includes asking about any types of eye injury with associated pain and redness and all of the above symptoms suggest a corneal abrasion. It is also important to ask whether the patients wear contact lens which may deteriorate the abrasion and need to refer the patient to higher facility for treatment.
  - This follows the clinical examination. But before examination the eye should be instilled with 0.5% of tetracaine, topical anesthetic agent. The purpose is to make both patient and examiner comfortable and to alleviate pain. The clinical assessment should be done in a systematic way starting with the evaluation of visual acuity, sign of inflammation and trauma and any sign of foreign body presence. Then comes the examination of pupil change in size, reactivity.
  - The confirmatory test for corneal abrasion is stain the cornea with fluorescein and then to visualize with cobalt blue light. If that appears green, then abrasion is confirmed.
- **Management:**
  - It includes application topical antibiotic to prevent infection. The drug of choice is chloramphenicol 1% ointment or 0.5% drops (four times daily for 5 to 7 days). Other antibiotics like ciprofloxacin (0.3%) and ofloxacin (0.3%) may also be used.
  - Topical anti-inflammatory agents: being pain free is the right of every patient and the pain management also aids in the early recovery and also promotes the psychological wellbeing. Hence, the research suggests the use of NSAIDS topically like diclofenac (0.1%), ketorolac (0.5%) and indomethacin (0.1%).
  - Foreign body removal is highly advised as this may cause further damage to the cornea and increases the discomfort to the patient. Usual location of foreign body invasion is on the surface of cornea itself or under the upper eyelid. Hence, attempt should be made to remove this by eye irrigation.
  - Education to patient and routine follow up: The patient should be informed about the danger signs of treatment failure and when to seek medical attention. Also, the preventive measures of further damage.

### Penetrating/Open Injury of the Globe and its Management

It is evident that about 40% of the penetrating ocular trauma is complicated due to the presence of foreign agents and this may ends with vision loss. The management includes stabilizing the patient through resuscitation measures like ABCDE (airway-breathing-circulation-disability and exposure). Information should be gathered regarding usual medication, any allergy, etc.

**Note:** Remember to follow the pneumonic **"ATM IS TV"** during history collection **(Table 14.17)**.

**Table 14.17:** Pneumonic for data gathering in case of eye injury.

| A | **A**ge of patient |
|---|---|
| T | **T**ime and date of injury |
| M | **M**echanism (penetrating/blunt trauma) |
| I | **I**njuries sustained |
| S | **S**igns and symptoms (pain, redness, decreased vision) |
| T | **T**reatment or intervention already given |
| V | **V**isual status before injury and whether any protective eye wear was worn |

Actual management

- Apply eye shield to the eye before transporting to prevent further damage and avoid using eye pad.
- Administration of prophylactic antibiotics followed by analgesics to prevent infection and discomfort to patient resp.
- Give anti-emetics in case patient present with nausea or vomiting.
- Give tetanus toxoid injection.
- Keep the 'nil by mouth' status in case surgery may be planned.
- Careful documentation of all findings and actions taken.
- Avoid the evaluation of intraocular pressure measurements in patients with lacerations.
- Avoid any type of pressure to the eye and sclera.
- Do not attempt to pull out any foreign material that may be sticking out of the eye.
- Confirm the diagnosis with orbital X-ray and ultrasound, and CT scan. MRI is contraindicated in case of presence of metallic foreign body.

*Lid and Canalicular Lacerations with Management*

- Uncomplicated lacerations can simply be sutured. In case the lacerated area is infected due to the exposure to foreign particles, it should be cleaned immediately followed by administration of antibiotics. Delayed primary closure may be advisable.
- All medial canthus injuries cases should be evaluated for presence of tear to the lower canaliculus, and if found so, can immediately be referred to higher centres. So also, is the laceration of the eye lid margin need to be referred to a specialist immediately.

*Hemorrhage*

- A sub-conjunctival bleeding or hemorrhage is a usual complication seen post eye trauma. This is important to evaluate as this may be a sign of ruptured globe, when it is associated with a low intraocular pressure (IOP) and an abnormally deep anterior chamber. Dilated pupil can also be another sign. This occurs secondary to blunt eye injury and tear to iris.
- Presence of blood in the anterior chamber of eye is called hyphema.

Management

- Usually requires no advances management as it is self-limiting within 5-6 days with conservative treatment. If sign of raised IOP is present, oral acetazolamide (Diamox) is the drug of management. Surgical method of treatment is very rarely preferred.
- NSAIDs like aspirin are contraindicated as it increases the risk of bleeding.
- Do not forget to evaluate the sign of vitreous hemorrhage as this may be sign of serious intraocular trauma characterised by the loss of the red reflex.
- The indications for surgery are:
  - Corneal staining post to hyphema
  - Increased IOP for > 45 mm Hg for >4 days
  - Presence of sickle cell disease interfering with prognosis.

*Lens Damage*

The lens damage is defined as dislocation of lens secondary to any trauma. This happens when the supporting ligaments and accessory structures holding the lens is damaged. The symptoms include blurring of vision. Diagnosis can be confirmed by looking at the eye. In case difficult to diagnose, pupil can be dilated to see through this. This usually requires no management if the patient is stable. But if it is associated with other problems like retinal tear, severe dislocated and broken lens interfering with vision, treatment includes retinal repair and replacement of broken lens with artificial one resp.

*Burns to the Eye*

This is also an unfortunate but emergency condition demanding immediate attention. Burns may affect the eyelids, conjunctiva or cornea. This requires immediate and first aid management which include flushing of eye with cold water. Apply topical antibiotic ointment generously all over the conjunctiva, cornea and burned eyelids. Next to keep the cornea moist and free from exposure by applying eye shield. Avoid using eye pad as it may cause ulcerate the cornea. The patient may require skin grafting of the eyelids.

*Chemicals in the Eye*

- Immediately irrigate the affected eye with clean water for at least 15 minutes after instilling local anesthetic drops. Position the patient in flat supine position during the procedure. Next eye is examined for presence of

any corneal ulceration. If so present, administer topical antibiotics followed by eye pad application and daily follow-up.
- Casualty with alkali burns (e.g., ammonia) is more severe than acid burn. They require intensive topical steroids, tetracycline and vitamin C drops along with an ophthalmologic consultation.

*Eye Removal—Evisceration or Enucleation*

Enucleation is defined as the surgical removal of the entire eyeball leaving behind the lining of the eyelids and muscles of the eye. Whereas evisceration is only the removal contents of the eye, leaving the sclera and the eye muscles intact. The indication is when the eye is blind to light and severely damaged with no hopes of recovery. Out of the two methods evisceration is considered safe as it carries less risk, low chance of infection and cosmetically good. Commonly carried out under local anesthesia.

# NOSE INJURIES

## Epidemiology

Injury to the nose **(Fig. 14.20)** is quite common not only among adults but also among the pediatric group post to any accident. In every facial injury nose is the most vulnerable part to be traumatized. This is because it is a projected body part and hence more prone for trauma even with a mild facial injury. Nose injury can be of many types like nasal bone fracture, epistaxis, penetrating and blunt injuries, etc., out of all this nasal fracture is considered most common among of all facial fractures and are reported as 3rd most common fracture of the human skeleton. Research suggest about 40% of facial fracture involve breakage of nasal bone and 90% of all nasal fractures mostly involves septal injury. This requires immediate resuscitation measure as nasal fractures blocks airway. Hence, the patient must be attended with priority.

## Various Nasal Injuries and its Management

### *Nasal Fracture with its Management*

*Etiopathology of Nasal Fracture*

The following are the possible mechanism of nasal fracture:
- Nose is the most prominent and centrally placed structure in face making it vulnerable to trauma.
- Secondly nasal bones and underneath cartilages are brittle and hence with mild direct force high chance of breakage.
- According to research and low of forces, the breakage of nasal bone is considered as a protective mechanism to secure the neck, brain and eyes. As most intense impact of the direct force is neutralized by the nasal bone.
- Biomechanics or the direction of impact of nasal fracture in two ways such as lateral trauma (the nose is displaced towards the side of injury and away from the midline) and head-on trauma (the nasal bones are pushed up and spread wide in such a manner that the nasal bridge looks broad, and the height of the nose is collapsed called saddle-nose deformity). Deviated nasal septum is a common outcome in both cases.
- Every nasal bone consists of two parts namely the superior part which is thick and a inferior part which is thin. Both of these are separated by intercanthal line. The lower part is more prone for fracture as it is not supported by any structure. Whereas the upper part is supported by frontal bone and maxilla.

*Classification*

Stranc Robertson classification, 1978

This is based on the direction of force and the associated damage **(Fig. 14.21)**. Here damage to nasal bones and nasal septum is considered based on the clinical examination only and not the radiological findings.

**Harrison's classification:** This classification is according to the degree of damage and its management. It has a total of three divisions. The class I is the type of fracture occurs with very little force of 25–75 pounds/sq inch, the second class involves moderate type of fracture involving the nasal bone along with underlying frontonasal process of maxilla and nasal septum and the last type is the most severe one involving the orbit. The details is given in **Figure 14.22**.

Murray's classification

It is a pathological classification based on the damage suffered by the nasal septum. It has in total seven categories. The first type involves injury to the middle third of the

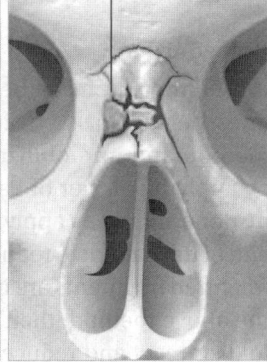

**Fig. 14.20:** Nasal trauma.

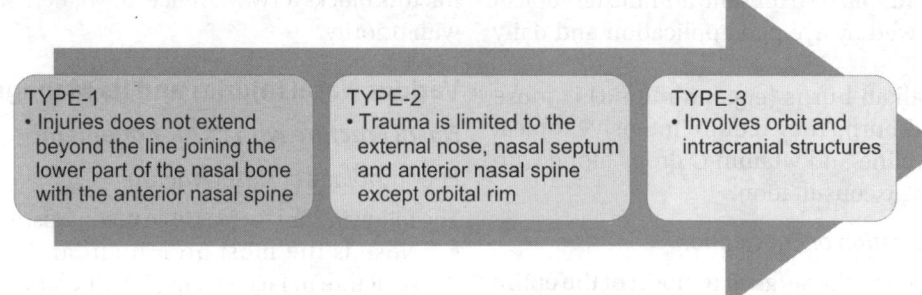

**Fig. 14.21:** Stranc Robertson classification.

**Class I**
- Fracture occurs with a little force of 25–75 pounds/sq inch
- Clinically seens as depressed fractures of nasal bones.
- Mild type with no deviation of nasal bone

**Class II**
- It is a moderate type of fracture involving the nasal bone + underlying frontonasal process of maxilla and nasal septum.
- Frontal traumatic force results in comminuted fracture of nasal bones and lateral impact causes deviation of septum.

**Class III**
- Most severe one results secondary to high velocity trauma.
- Also called ass naso-orbito-ethmoid fracture, as it involves orbit.

**Fig. 14.22:** Harrison's classification.

**Table 14.18:** Murray's classification.

| Types | Characteristics |
|---|---|
| 1 | Injuries involving middle third of face |
| 2 | History of bleeding from nose following injury |
| 3 | Edema over dorsum of nose |
| 4 | Tenderness and crepitus over nasal bone area |
| 5 | Eyelid edema |
| 6 | Subcutaneous emphysema involving eyelids |
| 7 | Periorbital ecchymosis |

face. Type 2 is about the history of bleeding nose post injury; the third type is development of edema over nasal dorsum. Similarly, the fourth type is little more severe that is feeling of tenderness and crepitus on nasal bone, with progressive development of eyelid edema in type five, leading to development of subcutaneous emphysema of eyelids in the next type and lastly the periorbital ecchymosis **(Table 14.18)**.

*Management*

Aim of treatment

The overall goal of treatment is to restore the function of nose to pre-traumatic stage as much as possible and to minimize the need for surgery. The management totally depends on the result of clinical assessment about its types, severity and intensity of damage.

The actual management includes closed reduction, open reduction and conservative management.

Conservative treatment

If the patient is receiving in emergency ward with active nasal bleeding, then bleeding to be arrested first by applying packing as it may interfere with the clinical assessment.

Apart from bleeding there is the possibility of swelling or edema to the dorsum of nose, interfering with assessment. Reduction of edema should be the second priority before proceeding for actual fracture treatment. This may take up to 3 weeks.

Closed reduction

**Indications:**
- Nasal bone fracture both unilateral/bilateral
- Nasal septum fracture with deviation of septum less than half width of nasal bridge

**Procedure:**
Closed reduction can be done using both local or general anesthesia. Class 1 fractures are treatment using this method and immobilization of the fracture part is done by applying plaster of Paris cast. Close reduction can also be done simply by applying digital pressure from the head end of the patient to reduce the fracture of nasal bone. If the fractured fragments are impacted and cannot be treated by the above method, then a Walsham's forceps can be used to disimpact and reduce the fracture. This procedure may cause epistaxis hence nasal packing needs to be given along with antibiotic ointment.

## Open reduction

**Indications:**
- Extensive fracture with bone and septum dislocated
- Deviated septum more than half width of nasal bridge
- Dislocation of caudal septum
- Open fracture with nasal septum

**Procedure:**

It is ideal for all types of class 3 nasal fracture. The problem with this type of reduction method is that the adjacent structures like components of the ethmoidal labyrinth do not support the nasal bone leading to failure. Hence, it is ideal to reconstruct and stabilize the anterior table of the frontal bone so that the nasal bone can be well supported. Traditional transnasal wires were replaced by plates and screws currently.

*Complications of Nasal Fracture*
- Cosmetic deformity
- Persistent deviation of nasal septum
- Leakage of CSF
- Edema of orbit
- Impaired nasal function

## Epistaxis with its Management

Epistaxis or nosebleed simply means bleeding from nose. Many times, it is not serious except for about 10% of cases. Children and elderly persons are mostly affected by this.

*Etiology*

Epistaxis is very common among all types of trauma to the face, so as its causes. The major etiologies are direct trauma, use of certain drugs, coagulation disorders and neoplastic conditions. The other details are listed below **(Fig. 14.23)**.

*Treatment*

Initial first aid management
- Make the patient sit in an upright position. Then tilt the patient forward and are due to blow out any blood clots. Tilting the patient helps to decrease the chance of nausea and airway obstruction. Then apply direct pressure for 5–20 min. This promotes blood clots.
- Vasoconstrictive medications such as oxymetazoline (Afrin) or phenylephrine can be given as initial management. These drugs are readily available over the counter.
- If the epistaxis continues for >20 min, seek immediate attention.

Nasal packing

This is the best one when the pressure and chemical cauterization fail. Traditional gauze packing has been

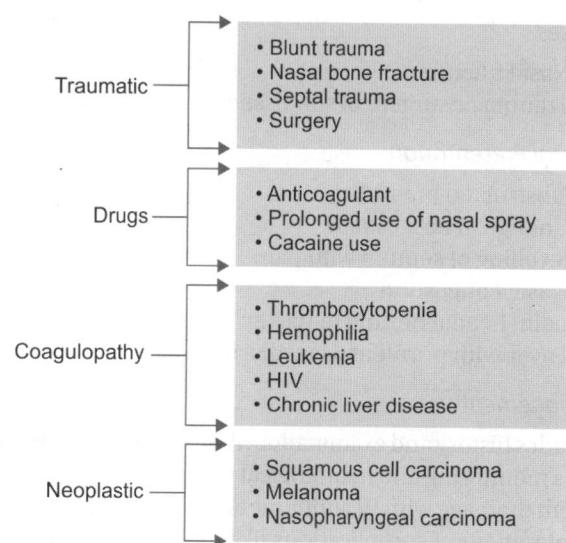

**Fig. 14.23:** Causes of epistaxis.

replaced with products like Merocel and the Rapid Rhino. Merocel is a synthetic foam polymer and is ideal for preventing spread of infection, whereas Rapid Rhino is a balloon catheter, made of carboxymethylcellulose, having a inflatable cuff to apply pressure to nasal cavity and stops bleeding. Nasal packing should be removed after 24–72 hours.

Tranexamic acid

It stops bleeding by clot formation. The routes are topical, oral or IV.

Cauterization

It is done by applying silver nitrate to nasal mucosa. It acts by creating local burns to arrest bleeding. Ideal for children with mild and visible bleeding sites. This may blacken the area due to the chemical reaction but will fade away spontaneously with time.

Surgery

The indication is active bleeding even with the above measures. This is done with endoscopic guidance to detect the site of bleeding and suturing. The possible vessels which may bleed are sphenopalatine, anterior and posterior ethmoidal arteries. This involves either intra-arterial embolization or ligation of the bleeding artery.

## Septal Hematoma and Abscess and its Management

*Definition*

"Nasal septal hematoma/abscess is a collection of blood/pus between the cartilaginous or bony septum and its adjoining mucoperichondrium or mucoperiosteum".

*Causes*
- Nasal fracture
- Trauma or surgery of soft tissue

*Clinical Presentation*
- Obstructed breathing
- Change in nasal shape
- Swelling of septum with pain
- Nasal congestion
- pain, headache, and malaise
- Fever with purulent nasal discharge

*Management*

Includes history and examination. Assessment involves vital signs monitoring and neurological evaluation. This requires urgent drainage with IV antibiotic administration to prevent development of complications like further tissue necrosis, airway obstruction, etc.

### Cerebrospinal Fluid Rhinorrhea

*Definition*

"The presence of thin, clear rhinorrhea after nasal trauma should be considered CSF leak until proven otherwise".

*Causes*
- Traumatic (post to nasal/skull fracture/trauma)
- Non-traumatic (carcinoma, infection, congenital problems)

*Diagnosis*
- Naked eye appearance of leakage of transparent fluid from nose
- **Beta-2**-transferrin assay test to confirms the diagnosis.

*Treatment*

Immediate hospitalization with quick decision of surgery is ideal to prevent the spread of infection to the meninges. Minimal invasive technique is mostly preferred over open one to reduce the chance of exposure and speedy the recovery. Conservative treatment include watchful waiting as minor leakage stops spontaneously.

## THROAT INJURIES

Throat injuries or neck trauma is an emergency condition as it increases the prevalence of morbidity and mortality. This accounts for 5–10% of death rates as it affects mostly the vital organs and impeding vital functions of body like obstructed airway, hypovolemic shock and acute neurologic injury. The patient may look stable in this type of injury but if not identified and evaluated early may increase the mortality. Hence, the knowledge regarding mechanism of injury, parts affected, relevant history, assessment, diagnosis and management should be known to the healthcare provider to tackle with this.

### Mechanism of Injury

#### Blunt Trauma
- Motor vehicle accidents
- Assault
- Hanging
- Clothes line injury
- Sports

#### Penetrating Trauma
- Stabbing
- Gun shot
- Animal bite
- Impalement

#### Strangulation
- Assault
- Criminal attempt
- Hanging/suicide

### Zones of Neck

From anatomical point the zones of neck are marked in three groups. That is zone I, II and III **(Fig. 14.24)**. The first zone extended from collarbones and sternum up to cricoid cartilage, the second zone is the space between cricoid cartilage to angle of the mandible and lastly the third zone is gap between the angle of the mandible to cranial base **(Table 14.19)**.

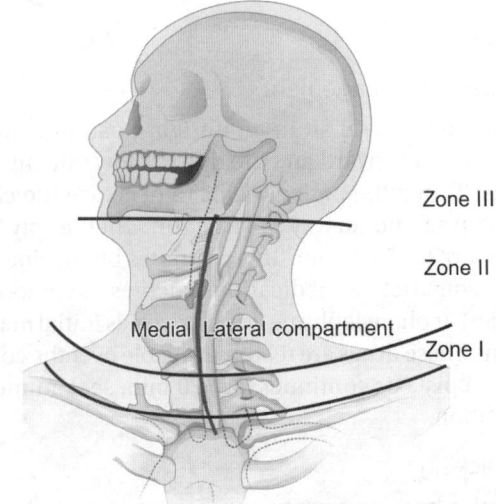

**Fig. 14.24:** Zones of neck.

**Table 14.19:** Anatomical zones of neck and the various structure involved in it.

| Zones | Anatomy | Structures involved |
|---|---|---|
| I | Extended from collarbones and sternum up to cricoid cartilage | Proximal cartilage, vertebral and subclavian arteries, innominate and jugular veins, spinal cord, recurrent laryngeal nerve and X cranial pair, trachea, esophagus and thoracic duct |
| II | Distance between cricoid cartilage to angle of the mandible | Carotid and vertebral arteries, jugular veins, spinal cord, recurrent laryngeal nerve and cranial X pair, hypopharynx and esophagus |
| III | Gap between the angle of the mandible to cranial base | Carotid and vertebral arteries, jugular veins, spinal cord, IX-XII cranial pairs and sympathetic trunk **(Fig. 14.24)** |

## Clinical Presentation

It is important to consider two types of signs before proceeding with management. These are hard and soft signs. The presence of hard sign indicates an absolute emergency needing immediate treatment. And that soft sign is not though that much panicking, gives some time in hand to manage.

### Hard Signs
- Active pulsatile bleeding
- Expanding hematoma
- Absence of carotid pulse
- Vascular murmur or thrill
- Cerebral ischemia

### Soft Signs
- History of bleeding at the scene
- Trauma in vascular territory
- Small non-pulsatile hematoma

## Diagnostic Tests
- History and examination of physical signs (includes questions like timing of injury, location of injury with its closeness to vital organs, mechanism and agent used for trauma and any existing medical conditions)
- Radiography of chest (for patient in zone 1 to look for hemothorax, pneumothorax, or pneumomediastinum)
- CT scan
- CT angiogram (done for injuries to the larynx, trachea, blood vessels and esophagus)
- Laryngoscopy
- Bronchoscopy
- Esophagoscopy (look for esophageal perforation)
- Color doppler flow study
- Arteriogram
- MRI

**Note:** Zone I: Angiogram, esophagogram, endoscopy and laryngoscopy, Zone II: Explored surgically, Zone III: Angiography.

## Management

The management of neck injury is decided according to the zone where the trauma has happened. But this comes after stabilizing the patient according to the protocol laid down by advanced trauma life support (ATLS). This is important to evaluate whether the patient is present with either hard sign or soft to determine the priority of care to be given and how much we can buy time.

The initial management involves "**ABC**".

### Airway Management
- Ensuring the airway patency
- Evaluate and provide needed oxygen
- Check on the condition of patient requiring immediate intubation like patient with apnea, unconscious and comatose, compromised respiration, massive airway bleeding and presence of hematoma in throat.

### Breathing Management

Breathing assessment done to evaluate for hemothorax or pneumothorax, particularly with penetrating zone 1 injuries.

### Bleeding Control
- Start rapid fluid of crystalloid solution with two large bore cannulas of 18 gauge
- Identify the source of active bleeding and do the needful to control it
- Remember certain points while controlling bleeding in neck trauma
  - Apply only local pressure
  - No torniquets
  - No pressure dressing.
  - No probing or blind clamping
- The above measures ensure adequate cerebral perfusion as about 10–30% of patients collateral circulation to cerebral tissue cannot be established due to various reasons.

### *Zone I: Neck Injury Management*

Injuries sustained in this zone has high mortality rate of about 12% as vital structures like mediastinum, large intrathoracic vessels and the tracheobronchial tree involved. And many times, these critical areas injuries can be un-noticed, hence proper diagnostic test should be chosen. For example, in stable patient Doppler ultrasound is recommended to rule out any vascular lesions, then to be confirmed by angiography if positive findings on Doppler came. Interventional radiology is proposed in case of vascular lesion, as this is difficult to reach area for surgery. The surgery options are middle sternotomy, anterior thoracotomy, clavicle resection or resection of the first rib.

In case of asymptomatic and stable patients with no evidence of injury, conservative management is indicated, like observation for 24–48 hours, suturing of wound followed by antibiotic and tetanus toxoid administration.

### *Zone II: Neck Injury Management*

This is the most commonly affected area. Surgery is proposed for all symptomatic cases. Doppler USG prior to surgery is a must.

In unstable patients exploration with positive diagnostic tests, surgical intervention is indicated. The affected area can be approached through cervicectomy parallel to the anterior edge of the sternocleidomastoid muscle.

### *Zone III: Neck Injury Management*

This is the sever one as this may cause central neurological sequelae such as coma, hemiparesis, aphasia and cranial nerve injuries.

If the patient is stable angiography is done to confirm the presence of vascular injury and once confirmed surgical intervention can be planned.

For unstable patients' surgical treatment are considered but with an aggressive approach for good exposure like horizontal incision to expose the cranial base, mandibular resection, mandibular dislocation and even craniotomy. In asymptomatic cases observation is advised for 24–48 hours, wound suture when necessary, and antibiotic coverage and tetanus vaccine similar to zone I treatment.

### *Complication*

- Airway obstruction
- Aspiration
- Vocal cord paralysis
- Perforated esophagus
- Severe vascular injury
- Necrotizing infection
- Stroke
- Air embolism
- Pneumothorax, hemothorax

### Nurses' Role in Managing Neck Trauma Patients

The neck trauma client care requires a team approach comprising of nurses, physical therapists, nutritionist, social workers, and occupational therapists. Apart from the medical management, there are various needs of the patient are there which can be fulfilled by nursing care. For say, neck trauma patients with neurological deficit may need to be in bed for longer, hence for daily basic care need can be approached by nursing personnel. Similarly, the nutritional need through tube feeding can be done by nurses for patients with esophageal injury. Also, the patients with tracheostomy need regular tracheostomy care to prevent infection. At the same time, the quality of life of patients are greatly affected post to injury. Hence, nurse can play an important role in psychological counseling and support. The communication is also an important aspect for the patient and their relatives to be at ease. Many patients sustaining neck trauma will have trouble verbalizing. In that case, the nurse should arrange something through which the patient can communicate his/her needs. The most importantly the nurse should inform about when they should return to hospital that is about the danger signs and the follow-up schedule.

 **Summary**

This chapter dealt with various emergency conditions with their medical and nursing management like how to assess and mechanism of injuries, various injuries like trauma to thorax, abdomen, pelvis, eye, nose and throat and complications of trauma, apart from those various types of shock with management, the relation between systemic inflammatory response syndrome and multiple organ dysfunction syndrome, DIC, drug overdose and lastly AIDS.

 **Points to Ponder**

### Thoracic Injury

- Minor chest wall injuries like rib fractures, can cause serious complications among elderly patients and patients with pre-existing pulmonary disease.
- Children are more susceptible to pulmonary contusion because of greater compliance of the chest wall.
- Unless there are abnormalities on the initial ECG, there is no need to go for diagnosis of myocardial contusion with more sophisticated tests.
- Many patients with myocardial rupture or traumatic aortic rupture survive to reach the hospital and can be salvaged with rapid diagnosis and intervention.
- Pericardial tamponade can be diagnosed accurately and early by standard cardiac ultrasound.

- Injury of the esophagus is relatively common with penetrating trauma of the chest or neck.

### Abdominal Trauma
- The accuracy of physical examination is limited in cases of blunt and penetrating trauma.
- The choice of diagnostic studies for abdominal trauma is based on clinical need first and foremost, as well as study availability and the accuracy of that study in a respective center.
- FAST and peritoneal aspiration are rapid methods of determining or excluding the presence of hemoperitoneum in the critically ill blunt or penetrating trauma patient.
- Clinical indications for laparotomy are more dependable in and more frequently applicable to cases of penetrating trauma than cases of blunt trauma.

### Pelvic Fracture
- Occurs with break to the bony structure to the pelvis.
- It can be both stable and unstable.
- This results from fall, collision of vehicle, crush injury, etc.
- Treatment includes resuscitation with immobilization, surgery and rehabilitation.

### DIC
- In disseminated intravascular coagulation (DIC), coagulation is usually activated when blood is exposed to tissue factor. In association with coagulation, the fibrinolytic pathway is also activated.
- DIC usually begins rapidly and causes bleeding and microvascular occlusion, leading to organ failure.
- DIC sometimes begins slowly and causes thromboembolic phenomena rather than bleeding.
- Severe, rapid-onset DIC causes severe thrombocytopenia, prolonged prothrombin time and partial thromboplastin time, a rapidly declining plasma fibrinogen level, and a high plasma D-dimer level.
- Immediate correction of the cause is the priority; severe bleeding may also require replacement therapy with platelets, cryoprecipitate (containing fibrinogen), and fresh frozen plasma (containing other coagulation factors).
- Heparin is useful in slow-onset DIC, but rarely in DIC of rapid onset (except in women with a retained dead fetus).

### AIDS
- HIV continues to be a major global public health issue, having claimed 36.3 million (27.2–47.8 million) lives so far.
- There is no cure for HIV infection. However, with increasing access to effective HIV prevention, diagnosis, treatment and care, including for opportunistic infections, HIV infection has become a manageable chronic health condition, enabling people living with HIV to lead long and healthy lives.
- There were an estimated 37.7 million (30.2–45.1 million) people living with HIV at the end of 2020, over two-thirds of whom (25.4 million) are in the WHO African Region.
- In 2020, 680 000 (480 000–1.0 million) people died from HIV-related causes and 1.5 million (1.0–2.0 million) people acquired HIV.

### Drug Overdose and Poisoning
- Worldwide, about 0.5 million deaths are attributable to drug use. More than 70% of these deaths are related to opioids, with more than 30% of those deaths caused by overdose.
- The medication naloxone can prevent death from an opioid overdose if administered in time.
- Poisoning is distinguished from hypersensitivity and idiosyncratic reactions, which are unpredictable and not dose-related, and from intolerance, which is a toxic reaction to a usually nontoxic dose of a substance.
- Recognizing a toxidrome (e.g., anticholinergic, muscarinic cholinergic, nicotinic cholinergic, opioid, sympathomimetic, withdrawal) can help narrow the differential diagnosis.
- Toxicity may be immediate, delayed (e.g., acetaminophen, iron, Amanita phalloides mushrooms causing delayed hepatotoxicity), or occur only after repeated exposure.
- Maximize recognition of poisoning and identification of the specific poison by considering poisoning in all patients with unexplained alterations in consciousness and by searching thoroughly for clues from the history.
- Consider other causes (e.g., central nervous system infection, head trauma, hypoglycemia, stroke, hepatic encephalopathy, Wernicke encephalopathy) if consciousness is altered, even if poisoning is suspected.
- Use toxicology testing (e.g., drug immunoassays) selectively because it can provide incomplete or incorrect information.
- Treat all poisoning supportively and use activated charcoal for serious oral poisoning and other methods selectively.

### Shock
- It is an emergency condition present with tachycardia, hypotension, cold and clammy skin, delayed capillary refill, etc.
- Types of shock includes hypovolemic, cardiogenic, neurogenic, anaphylactic, septic, endocrine, obstructive shock.
- Initial treatment includes ABC approach.

### Abbreviations
- RTA : Road Traffic Accident
- EMS : Emergency Medical Service
- ABCDE : Airway, Breathing, Circulation, Disability, Exposure
- ATLS : Advanced Trauma Life Support
- FAST : Focused Assessment using Sonography in Trauma

- GCS : Glasgow Coma Score
- SIRS : Systemic Inflammatory Response Syndrome
- PICS : Persistent Inflammation/Immunosuppression and Catabolism Syndrome
- USG : Ultrasonography
- CT Scan : Computed Tomography Scan
- ECG : Electrocardiography
- BPAP : Bilevel Positive Airway Pressure Device
- CPAP : Continuous Positive Airway Pressure
- ARDS : Acute Respiratory Distress Syndrome
- CPR : Cardiopulmonary Resuscitation
- VATS : Video-assisted Thoracoscopic Surgery
- ABG : Arterial Blood Gas
- HFNC : High Flow Nasal Cannula
- DPL : Diagnostic Peritoneal Lavage
- APC : Anterior-Posterior Compression
- AIS : Abbreviated Injury Scale
- DIC : Disseminated Intravascular Coagulation
- CAUTI : Catheter Associated Urinary Tract Infection
- NICE : National Institute for Health and Care Excellence
- CO : Cardiac Output
- qSOFA : Quick Sequential Organ Failure Assessment
- DAMP : Damage Associated Molecular Pattern
- PAMP : Pathogen Associated Molecular Pattern
- MODS : Multiple Organ Dysfunction Syndrome
- CVP : Central Venous Pressure
- COVID : Corona Virus Disease
- OP : Organophosphorus
- DDT : Dichlorodiphenyltrichloroethane
- TLC : Total Leukocyte Count
- MAOIS : Monoamine Oxidase Inhibitors
- AIDS : Acquired Immunodeficiency Syndrome
- HIV : Human Immunodeficiency Virus
- PCP : Pneumocystis Pneumonia
- PLHIV/PLHA : Patient Living with HIV and AIDS
- NRTI : Nucleoside Reverse Transcriptase Inhibitor
- NNRTI : Non-nucleoside Reverse Transcriptase Inhibitor
- IPT : Isoniazid Preventive Therapy
- IOFB : Intraocular Foreign Body
- IOP : Intraocular Pressure

### Short Answer Questions

1. What are the various techniques of assessment?
2. What is ABCDE approach?
3. Explain the mechanism of injury.
4. How to diagnose flail chest?
5. How to manage pulmonary contusion?
6. What is Beck's triad of cardiac tamponade?
7. How to manage blunt and penetrating abdominal trauma?
8. Explain the pelvic fracture classification by tiles.
9. What are the complications of trauma?
10. Explain SIRS criteria and its stages.
11. Explain the clinical features of multiple organ dysfunction syndrome.
12. Explain the DIC pathways.
13. Explain the nursing management of DIC.
14. Explain various antidots for drug overdose.
15. How the virus replicates in AIDS?
16. Explain the various classification of eye injuries.
17. Describe the various classification of nasal fracture diagnosis.
18. Explain the various zone of neck with involved structures.

### Long Answer Questions

1. What are the major types of thoracic injury? Explain the pathophysiology of blunt injury in detail.
2. Define chest injury. What is the clinical presentation of chest wall injury? Write differences between sternal and rib fracture.
3. Define pneumothorax. What are the various types of pneumothorax? Write about the management for the same.
4. How to manage hemothorax?
5. What is shock? Enumerate the various types of shock. Write in detail about the management of shock with suitable examples.
6. What do you mean by AIDS? Write various modes of transmission. Give a elaborated note on anti-retroviral drugs.
7. Classify eye injuries. Write in detail about the management of various eye injuries.
8. Enumerate various methods of trauma assessment. Write how the mechanism of injury work. Write briefly about the management of abdominal injury.

### Keypoints

- **Blunt injury:** Blunt trauma, also called nonpenetrating trauma or blunt force trauma, is an injury to the body caused by forceful impact, injury, or physical attack with a dull object or surface.
- **Penetrating injury:** Penetrating trauma is an injury caused by a foreign object piercing the skin, which damages the underlying tissues and results in an open wound.
- **Flail chest:** Defined as two or more contiguous rib fractures with two or more breaks per rib.
- **Pulmonary contusion:** A pulmonary contusion, also known as lung contusion, is a bruise of the lung, caused by chest trauma.
- **Pneumothorax:** This condition occurs when air leaks into the space between the lungs and chest wall.
- **Cardiac tamponade:** Compression of the heart caused by fluid collecting in the sac surrounding the heart.
- **FAST:** Focused assessment with sonography in trauma is a rapid bedside ultrasound examination performed as a screening test for blood around the heart or abdominal organs after trauma.

- **DPL:** Diagnostic peritoneal lavage or diagnostic peritoneal aspiration is a surgical diagnostic procedure to determine if there is free floating fluid in the abdominal cavity.
- **Open book pelvic injury:** Open book pelvic injuries result from an anteroposterior compression injury to the pelvis and result in a combination of ligamentous rupture and/or fractures to both the anterior and posterior arches.
- **Hypovolemic shock:** Hypovolemic shock is an emergency condition in which severe blood or other fluid loss makes the heart unable to pump enough blood to the body.
- **Cardiogenic shock:** Cardiogenic shock is a life-threatening condition in which your heart suddenly can't pump enough blood to meet your body's needs.
- **Anaphylactic shock:** Anaphylactic shock, is a serious allergic reaction that is rapid in onset and may cause death.
- **Neurogenic shock:** Neurogenic shock is a distributive type of shock resulting in hypotension (low blood pressure), often with bradycardia (slowed heart rate), caused by disruption of autonomic nervous system pathways.
- **Septic shock:** Septic shock is a potentially fatal medical condition that occurs when sepsis, which is organ injury or damage in response to infection, leads to dangerously low blood pressure and abnormalities in cellular metabolism.
- **SIRS:** Systemic inflammatory response syndrome (SIRS) is an exaggerated defence response of the body to a noxious stressor (infection, trauma, surgery, acute inflammation, ischemia or reperfusion, or malignancy, to name a few) to localize and then eliminate the endogenous or exogenous source of the insult.
- **qSOFA:** Quick sequential organ failure assessment is a score for detection of patients at risk of sepsis outside of intensive care units.
- **MODS:** Multiple organ dysfunction syndrome (MODS) is defined as the development of potentially reversible physiologic disarrangement involving two or more organ systems not involved in the disorders, resulted in ICU admission, and a potentially life-threatening physiologic insult.
- **DIC:** Disseminated intravascular coagulation (DIC) is a condition in which blood clots form throughout the body, blocking small blood vessels.
- **HIV:** Human immunodeficiency virus (HIV) is an infection that attacks the body's immune system, specifically the white blood cells called CD4 cells.
- **AIDS:** Acquired immunodeficiency syndrome (HIV/AIDS) is a spectrum of conditions caused by infection with the human immunodeficiency virus (HIV), a retrovirus.
- **Corneal abrasions:** It is defined as the superficial lesion to the corneal epithelium of eye.
- **Open reduction:** "Open reduction" means a surgeon makes an incision to re-align the bone.
- **Closed reduction:** Closed reduction is a procedure to set (reduce) a broken bone without cutting the skin open.
- **Epistaxis:** Epistaxis is bleeding from the nose.
- **Septal hematoma and abscess:** It is a collection of blood/pus between the cartilaginous or bony septum and its adjoining mucoperichondrium or mucoperiosteum.
- **Hard and soft sign:** The presence of hard sign indicates an absolute emergency needing immediate treatment. And that of soft sign is not though that much panicking, gives some time in hand to manage.

## Bibliography

1. Afacan G. Abdominal Trauma. In Trauma Surgery. 2018. Intech Open.
2. Alao T, Waseem M. Neck Trauma. 2017.
3. Anders CJ. Abdominal Injuries. Postgraduate Medical Journal. 1967;43(503):582.
4. Bajaj L, Hambidge S, Nyquist AC, Kerby G. Berman's Pediatric Decision-Making E-Book. Elsevier Health Sciences; 2011.
5. Balasubramanian T, Venkatesan U. Fracture Nasal Bones. Online Journal of Otolaryngology. 2013;3:1.
6. Baren JM. Pediatric Emergency Medicine. Elsevier Health Sciences; 2008.
7. Battle C, Hutchings H, Evans PA. Blunt Chest Wall Trauma: A Review Trauma. 2013;15(2):156-75.
8. Battle C, Lovett S, Hutchings H, Evans PA. Predicting Outcomes after Blunt Chest Wall Trauma: Development and External Validation of a New Prognostic Model. Critical Care. 2014;18(1):1-82.
9. Behera A, Singla N, Sharma N, Sharma N. Paradigm Shift in Pattern and Prevalence of Poisoning During COVID-19 Pandemic, Journal of Family Medicine and Primary Care: January 2022, Vol. 11, Issue 1 - p 208-214.
10. Bone RC, Grodzin CJ, Balk RA. Sepsis: A New Hpothesis for Pathogenesis of the Disease Process. Chest. 1997;112(1):235-43.
11. Butt MU, Zacharias N, Velmahos GC. Penetrating Abdominal Injuries: Management Controversies. Scandinavian Journal of Trauma, Resuscitation and Emergency Medicine. 2009;17(1):1–7.
12. Cerebrospinal Fluid Rhinorrhoea. [Wiki]. Available from: https://en.wikipedia.org/wiki/Cerebrospinal_fluid_rhinorrhoea. 2022.
13. Chakraborty RK, Burns B. Systemic Inflammatory Response Syndrome.
14. Choudhary D, Goykar H, Kalyane D, Desai N, Tekade RK. Dose, Dosage Regimen, and Dose Adjustment in Organ Failure. In Biopharmaceutics and Pharmacokinetics Considerations. Academic Press. 2021:29-82.
15. Coccolini F, Stahel PF, Montori G, Biffl W, Horer TM, Catena F et al. Pelvic Trauma: WSES Classification and Guidelines. World Journal of Emergency Surgery. 2017;12(1):1-8.
16. Dandona R, Kumar GA, Gururaj G, James S, Chakma JK, Thakur JS, et al. Mortality Due to Road Injuries in the States of India: the Global Burden of Disease Study 1990–2017. The Lancet Public Health. 2020;5(2):e86-98.

17. Dong SX, Shah N, Gupta A. Epidemiology of Nasal Bone Fractures. Facial Plastic Surgery and Aesthetic Medicine. 2022; 24(1):27-33.
18. Drug Overdose. [Wiki]. Available from: https://en.wikipedia.org/wiki/Drug_overdose. 2022.
19. Dumovich J, Singh P. Physiology, Trauma. InStatPearls [Internet] 2021; StatPearls Publishing.
20. Eye injury. [Wiki]. Available from: https://en.wikipedia.org/wiki/Eye Injury. 2022.
21. Grainger J, George A, Coulson C, De R. Nasal Injury Management: An Audit of Accident and Emergency Practice. European Archives of Oto-rhino-laryngology. 2009;266(12):1995-9.
22. Guthrie HC, Owens RW, Bircher MD. Fractures of the Pelvis. The Journal of Bone and Joint Surgery. British Volume. 2010; 92(11):1481-8.
23. Harna B, Arya S, Bahl A. Epidemiology of Trauma Patients Admitted to a Trauma Center in New Delhi, India. Indian Journal of Critical Care Medicine: Peer-reviewed, Official Publication of Indian Society of Critical Care Medicine. 2020;24(12):1193.
24. Harrison DH. Nasal Injuries: Their Pathogenesis and Treatment. British Journal of Plastic Surgery. 1979;32(1):57-64.
25. Hill B, Mitchell A. Hypovolaemic Shock. British Journal of Nursing. 2020;29(10):557-60.
26. Hoffmann JF. An Algorithm for the Initial Management of Nasal Trauma. Facial Plastic Surgery. 2015;31(03):183-93.
27. Iftikhar M, Latif A, Farid UZ, Usmani B, Canner JK, Shah SM. Changes in the Incidence of Eye Trauma Hospitalizations in the United States from 2001 through 2014. JAMA ophthalmology. 2019;137(1):48-56.
28. Kim L, Huddle MG, Smith RM, Byrne P. Nasal Fractures. In Facial Trauma Surgery. Elsevier. 2020:122-128.
29. Kostiuk M, Burns B. Trauma Assessment. InStatPearls [Internet] 2020; StatPearls Publishing.
30. Lecuona K. Assessing and Managing Eye Injuries. Community Eye Health Journal. 2005;18(55):101-4.
31. Lee PC, Lo C, Wu JM, Lin KL, Lin HF, Ko WJ. Laparoscopy Decreases the Laparotomy Rate in Hemodynamically Stable Patients with Blunt Abdominal Trauma. Surgical Innovation. 2014;21(2):155-65.
32. Lord JM, Midwinter MJ, Chen YF, Belli A, Brohi K, Kovacs EJ et al. The Systemic Immune Response to Trauma: An Overview of Pathophysiology and Treatment. The Lancet. 2014;384(9952):1455-65.
33. Marshall JC. The Multiple Organ Dysfunction Syndrome. In Surgical Treatment: Evidence-based and Problem-oriented. Zuckschwerdt. 2001.
34. Mitchell KJ, Schoster A, Auer JA, Stick J, Kümmerle JM, Prange T. Shock: Pathophysiology, Diagnosis, Treatment, and Physiologic Response to Trauma.
35. Mittal C, Singh S, Kumar MP, Varthya SB. Toxicoepidemiology of Poisoning Exhibited in Indian Population from 2010 to 2020: A Systematic Review and Meta-analysis. BMJ open. 2021; 11(5):e045182.
36. Munroe B, Curtis K. Assessment, Monitoring and Emergency Nursing Care in Blunt Chest Injury: A Case Study. Australasian Emergency Nursing Journal. 2011;14(4):257-63.
37. Mwangi N, Mutie DM. Emergency Management: Penetrating Eye Injuries and Intraocular Foreign Bodies. Community Eye Health. 2018;31(103):70-1.
38. Narayanan R, Kumar S, Gupta A, Bansal VK, Sagar S, Singhal M, et al. An Analysis of Presentation, Pattern and Outcome of Chest Trauma Patients at an Urban Level 1 Trauma Center. Indian Journal of Surgery. 2018;80(1):36-41.
39. Nasal Fracture. [Wiki]. Available from: https://en.wikipedia.org/wiki/Nasal_fracture. 2022.
40. Nasal Septal Hematoma. [Wiki]. Available from: https://en.wikipedia.org/wiki/Nasal_septal_hematoma. 2022.
41. Natarajan S. Ocular Trauma, an Evolving Sub Specialty. Indian Journal of Ophthalmology. 2013;61(10):539.
42. Nosebleed. [Wiki]. Available from: https://en.wikipedia.org/wiki/Nosebleed. 2022.
43. Petrone P, Velaz-Pardo L, Gendy A, Velcu L, Brathwaite CE, D'Andrea KJ. Diagnosis, Management and Treatment of Neck Trauma. Cirugía Española (English Edition). 2019;97(9):489-500.
44. Poisoning. [Wiki]. Available from: https://en.wikipedia.org/wiki/Poisoning. 2022.
45. Shahid SM, Harrison N. Corneal Abrasion: Assessment and Management. InnovAiT. 2013;6(9):551-4.
46. Shannon MW, Haddad LM. The Emergency Management of Poisoning. Clinical Management of Poisoning and Drug Overdose, 3rd edn. Philadelphia: WB Saunders. 1998:2-31.
47. Srivastava A, Peshin SS, Kaleekal T, Gupta SK. An Epidemiological Study of Poisoning Cases Reported to the National Poisons Information Centre, All India Institute of Medical Sciences, New Delhi. Human and Experimental Toxicology. 2005;24(6):279-85.
48. Stylianos S, Mazziotti MV. Abdominal Trauma. In Operative Pediatric Surgery. CRC Press. 2020:787-97.
49. Sukati VN. Ocular Injuries—A Review. African Vision and Eye Health. 2012;71(2):86-94.
50. Taha M, Elbaih A. Pathophysiology and Management of Different Types of Shock. Narayana Med J. 2017;6:14-39.
51. Tile M. Fractures of the Pelvis. In the Rationale of Operative Fracture Care. Springer, Berlin, Heidelberg. 2005:239-290.
52. Tolia J, Bhatt A. Prevalence of Chest Trauma at Tertiary Care Institute: A Cross Sectional Study. Academia Journal of Surgery. Vol 3 No 1. 2020.
53. Turner V, Buckler LT. Act Quickly with Chest Trauma. Nursing 2020 Critical Care. 2008;3(4):41-6.
54. Walker J. Pelvic Fractures: Classification and Nursing Management. Nursing Standard. 2011;26(10).
55. Yojana S, Mehta K, Girish M. Epidemiological Profile of Otorhinolaryngological Emergencies at a Medical College, in Rural Area of Gujarat. Indian Journal of Otolaryngology and Head and Neck Surgery. 2012;64(3):218-24.

# Chapter 15

# Psychiatric Emergencies and Crisis Intervention

*Suchismita Phantasingh*

## CHAPTER OUTLINE
- Psychiatric Emergencies
- Crisis Interventions

### Learning Objectives
At the end of the chapter, the students will be able to:
- Identify the prevalence and incidence of psychiatric emergency.
- Describe the principle of psychiatric emergency.
- List out and explain about the different types of psychiatric emergency.
- Prevent and manage psychiatric emergency.
- Define crisis.
- Enlist the characteristics of crisis.
- Explain the types and stages of crisis.
- Describe the different types of techniques used in crisis intervention.
- Explain crisis intervention.

## INTRODUCTION

Emergency seeks immediate and counteractive action as it is an acute, unpredicted, unforeseen alliance of upcoming events causing injury, loss of life, damage to the property and interference with the normal functioning.

A psychiatric emergency may result acute behavioral, thought or mood disorganization lead to harm, if remains untreated. The definition of psychiatric emergency varies from other medical emergencies which may harm to the society (Lunn and Day, 2017).

The psychiatric emergencies are most emergent types of psychiatric crisis causes sudden and severe disorganization in behavior or mood which, if it is not treated, causes severe harm to physical, emotional or social aspects. Example includes suicidal, homicidal attempts or emotional breakdown (Newhill, 1989).

## PREVALENCE AND INCIDENCE

In developed countries, a large proportion of people present with some sort of mental health issues seeking emergency services and treatment. As per report in emergency service unit psychiatric emergencies such as emergency related to trauma and neurological condition and among them 12% are emergency service attainders. Psychotic patients (12-29%), substance abuse related disorders (6-25%), bipolar mood disorders specially depressive disorders (2-23%), and disorders of personality (11-20%) are attending emergency services in developed countries (Nadkarni et al., 2015).

## PSYCHIATRIC EMERGENCIES

### Definition
A psychiatric emergency is a severe disturbance of mood, thought, or behavior that needs an immediate intervention (Nadkarni et al., 2015).

Psychiatric emergencies are conditions in which there is an acute changes in behaviors, emotion or thought seeking immediate attention and treatment. Psychiatric emergencies can be managed in psychiatric set up but it is commonly seen in hospital emergency unit. It is not necessary that all psychiatric emergency patients are suffering from only psychiatric disorders. They may be attending the emergency services unit due to medical conditions or conditions unrelated to medical field like disaster, rape and violence.

### Characteristics of Psychiatric Emergency
- It is acute and sudden in nature.
- It occurs when there is an imbalance between the subject and the environment.
- It is personal in nature but may affect others.

## Objectives of Psychiatric Emergency Intervention

See **Figure 15.1**.

## Basic Principles of Emergency Psychiatry

- A warm, direct and empathetic approach should be shown to the patient initially.
- Recognize the characteristics of the emergency condition and to initiate treatment a thorough and quick clinical evaluation must be done on the basis of severity.
- To understand the crisis and the patient's strength and abilities a thorough comprehensive history is essential
- Both from the patient and family member's psychiatric history must be gathered.
- A detailed clinical examination should be done which includes general, physical and neurological and mental status examination.
- In emergency file detailed history and clinical findings should be recorded and documented clearly.
- In order to save time in decision-making psychiatric examination should be modified and tailored.
- As per the understanding level of the patient's relative patient's condition and plan of management should be explained in simple language.
- General or categorical diagnosis should be made.
- Identify the supporting system of the patient which might assist in establishment of coping.

## Types of Psychiatric Emergencies

There are two types of psychiatric emergencies are there such as major and minor emergency. In major case, there is risk to the patient's life or other individual in his surrounding and minor emergency causes severe form of disintegration but without any threat to life.
- Suicide
- Stupor and catatonic syndrome
- Anger, aggression and violence
- Substance related emergencies
- Other psychiatric emergencies

## Suicide

In psychiatric emergencies, suicide is a most commonest type of emergency which causes death among psychiatric patients.

The word suicide breaks down into the Latin words "sui" and "caedere", which means "kill oneself".

### Definitions of Suicide

Self-inflicted death with evidence (either explicit or implicit) that the person intended to die (Kleber et al., 2006).

Suicide is death caused by injuring oneself with the intent to die (Centre for Disease Control, 2019),

Suicide is the act of deliberately killing oneself (World Health Organization, 2014).

### Prevalence and Incidence of Suicide

Approximately 804000 suicide mortality occurred worldwide in the year 2012 and annually in 100000 population the age-standardized suicide rate is 11.4 (15.0 for males and 8.0 for females). Among youth the rate of suicides are highest in some countries and suicide is the second leading cause of death worldwide in between 15–19 years of age (World Health Organization, 2014).

In India, the rate of suicide in 2002 was 11.2 per 100,000. Across the country suicide rate varies state-wise such as rate (30.8 per lakh ) was highest in Kerala in 2002 (Roy A, 2000).

Among youth aged 20–30 years in UK suicide is the common leading cause of death and when it is compared with women the rate is highest in men, and when it is taken into consideration, the suicidal death is around three times more among men. Men below 50 in UK suicide are the leading cause of death between 40 and 44 years of age with highest risk (24.1 deaths per lakh) (National statistics, 2017).

### Influencing/Risk Factor

Every 40 seconds someone loses their life due to suicide (Fitzpatrick, 2017).

Suicide has no single cause. Often an individual experiences despair and gloom when the stressor and

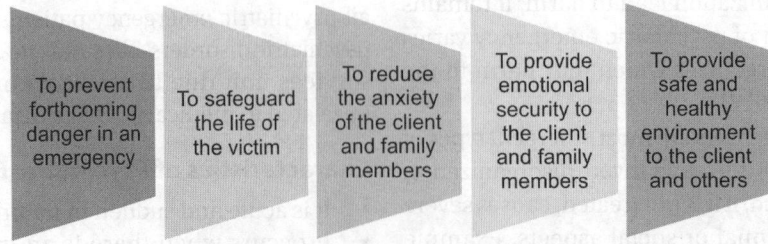

**Fig. 15.1:** Objectives of psychiatric emergency intervention.

health issues cluster and leads to suicide. Commonly suicide is associated with depression and oftentimes it is unrevealed or not treated. The suicide risk increases when certain mental health problems like depression, anxiety and substance related issues when unidentified. Yet it's important to note that most people who actively and effectively manage their mental health issues and move on to engage in life.

Over the last century, many theories of suicide have been developed which includes biological, sociological and psychological theories. These theories have conceptualized certain psychic escape phenomenon of suicide such as aversive self-cognizance, despair, emotional disintegration, perceived burdens, unsatisfactory relationship, and capability development for suicide defeat, entrapment and lack of social strength various diathesis-stress models and ideation to action frameworks (Franklin et al., 2017).

The major causes of suicide are family problems and illness which accounted for 27.6% and 15.8% during 2015 respectively from total suicides. Suicide related to marriage issues (4.8%), substance abuse and addiction (2.7%), love affairs and bankruptcy (3.3% each), employment issues and examination disappointment (2.0% each), property dispute (1.9%), poverty (1.3%) and career and professional issues (1.2%) are the major cause of suicides (National Crime Records Bureau, 2016).

A person when try to take his life or attempt suicide risk factors are the aggravating characteristics or conditions. Some of the risk factors are mentioned below:

- **Age:** Suicidal risk increases with age. At age 45 risk peaks among men and at age 55 among women. Among youth especially 15–24 ages the incidence of suicide are very high. Over the past decade, the suicidal cases has increased among 25–34 years of male. In USA among 15–24 years age group suicide is the principal reason of death by motor vehicle accident and homicide (Masango, Rataemane, and Motojesi, 2008).
- **Gender:** In comparison to females more males commit suicide whereas female attempts suicide more than males (Masango et al., 2008).
- **Divorced, widowed or separated** most often they attempt suicide.
- **Marital status:** Among married people the reported rates of suicide is 11/100000. Hence marriage acts as defensive factor against suicide. It is to be encouraged by having children and the marriage has to be stable (Masango et al., 2008).
- Recent valued losses or major stressful life situation.
- **Alcohol dependence:** For the increased risk of suicide alcoholism is an associated factor. In general population, the mortality rate of suicide for alcoholic increases six times approximately and it is second most frequent suicidal precursor (Kleber et al., 2006).
- History of previous suicide attempt and suicidal preoccupation
- Higher degree of aggressive behavior or impulsivity
- Health related issues like depression, schizophrenia and mood disorders from the research study it is clearly evident that the most significant risk factor of suicide is the presence of a major mood disorder (Kleber et al., 2006).

*Theories/Predisposing Factors of Suicide (Table 15.1)*

- **Biological theory:** Genetic, neurobiological risk factors and biochemical factors may be an important predisposition to suicide. Higher concordance rate between monozygotic twins than that between dizygotic twins.
- **Psychological theory:** Hopelessness, desperation and guilt, humiliation, stress, and frustration are associated with suicide behavior in adolescence and early childhood.

| Table 15.1: Theories and predisposing factors of suicide. | | |
|---|---|---|
| Biological theory | Psychological theory (Freud 1957) | Social theory (Durkheim 1951) |
| Genetic<br>Monozygotic twins | Anger turned inward | Egoistic suicide |
| Neurochemical factors<br>Serotonin deficiency | Hopelessness | Altruistic suicide |
| | Desperation and guilt | Anomic suicide |
| | Shame and humiliation | |
| | Aggression and violence | |
| | Developmental stressor | |

- **Sociological theory:** Durkheim (1951) studied the individual's interaction with the society in which he or she lived. The more cohesive the society and the more that individual felt an integrated part of the society, the less likely he or she was to commit suicide.

### Methods used for Suicide

The most easily accessible, adopted or effective means of suicide are jumping into the well, use of corrosive poison and the most aching means are strangulation, gun shooting and self-inflicted injuries, etc. Gun shoot is the most lethal means of suicide (National Crime Records Bureau, 2016).

The most common methods of suicides are ingestion of corrosive poison (34.8%), strangulation (32.2%), drowning (6.7%), suicide related to train or motor vehicle accident (3%) and most often men use more lethal means for committing suicide in comparison to women (NCRB, 2008).

The adopted methods of suicide has decreased during the year 2015 are drowning (in 2014 rate was 5.6% and reduced to 5.4% in 2015) and approaching moving train or motor vehicle (in 2014 rate was 2.6% and reduced to 2.5% in 2015) where asself burning (suicide rate was 6.9% in 2014 decreased to 7.2% in 2015), strangulation (in 2014 from 41.8% to 45.6% in 2015), 'By corrosive agent' (in 2014 from 26.0% to 27.9% in 2015) and 'by touching electric power wire' (in 2014 from 0.6% to 0.7% in 2015) have increased during 2015 over 2014 (National Crime Records Bureau, 2016).

### Myths and facts about suicide

Seven myths and facts about suicide, 2018 **(Table 15.2)**.

Misconception about suicide is very common and fatal because that stops us from identifying that someone is at risk. It can be preventable, and people can be helped also.

### Suicide vs Suicidal

See **Figure 15.2**.

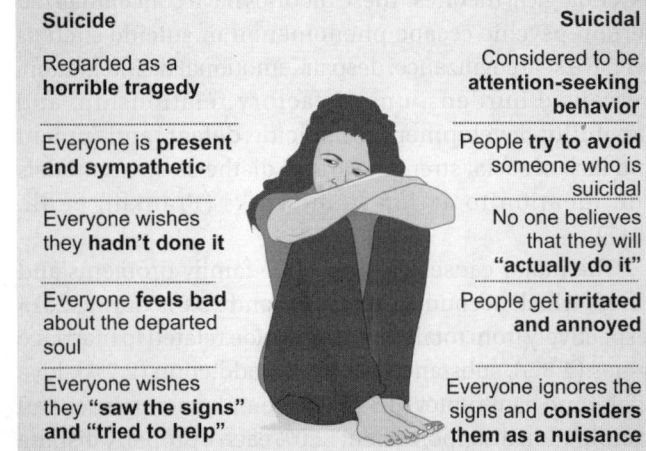

**Fig. 15.2:** Differences between suicide and suicidal.

| Table 15.2: Various myths and facts about suicide. | | |
|---|---|---|
| S. No. | Myths | Facts |
| 1. | Most of the individual will never commit suicide when they talk and threaten to kill themselves | Suicide committed people usually talk and gives clues about suicide. So, all the hints or threats should be taken seriously and carefully |
| 2. | The person who is going through depression is ideal not to discuss suicide | Discussing suicide facilitates the opportunity for free communication. At the initial phase, a simple inquiry can be done with the individual who is planning to bring an end to his life. However, whoever is discussing about suicide they should be under careful vigilance and prompt management |
| 3. | Mentally sick individuals are more likely to commit suicide | Everyone has suicide potential. The rate of suicide is more prevalent among clinically depressive client |
| 4. | A person will never a reattempt if he attempts suicide and survives | For further attempt suicide is regarded as an indicator. Further suicide attempt heightens the level of danger |
| 5. | During holidays like Christmas and thanksgiving suicide happens more frequently | The lowest suicidal rates are in December whereas during spring rate is very high |
| 6. | Nothing can stop a person when he is self-determined to commit suicide | Suicide is preventable. People can be helped. A suicidal crisis is acute and time limiting. |
| 7. | Very often Youngsters are having more potential or risk to commit suicide | Youths are more probable to commit suicide. Predominantly adults are at high risk between 45 and 54 as suicide death rate is 19.72 per lakhs, when compared with people over 85 it is about 19 per 100,000 and 13 per 100,000 in total population. Still, youngsters are in high-risk |

## Signs and Symptoms

The sign and symptoms of catatonic stupor are explained in **Figure 15.3** according to Gupta et al 2007.

## Management and Prevention of Suicide

Suicide is not a footstep towards death but a way to stay away from unbearable pain caused by mental illness, like bipolar disorder, which can be identified and managed (Bradley, 2016).

As part of routine assessment suicidal ideation need to be asked. For future suicidal attempts self-ruinous behaviors and past attempts are the most powerful forecaster. Asking about suicidal attempt is not influencing factor for committing suicide or instilling the idea of suicide.

Asking and explaining about the suicidal ideation as the part of an illness makes the patients to a state relieved (Lunn and Day, 2017).

These are certain measures can be taken towards the suicide prevention (Bradley 2016).

- Aware of the warning signs such as hopelessness, guilt, shame, anxiety, anger, difficulty in sleeping, depression or mania, eating difficult and that may lead to suicidal ideation.
- Identify your risk factors. Immediate after discharge or during the period of mania and depression patient may have suicidal ideation and may commit suicide.
- Never stop taking your medication without consulting a psychiatrist. If someone wants to bring any changes in medication seek advice from the psychiatrist to decrease the chance of recurrence, adverse effect of drugs and suicidal obsession.
- Remove potentially self-mutilating or self-injurious stimulants from environment. If someone is obsessed with suicidal thoughts, eliminate all the possible access to firearms, quantities of drugs, and other substance that could be used to for self-mutilation.
- Stay away from social separation. Discuss your suicidal thoughts with reliable friends or family member and list out their advice in seeking treatment.
- Collaborate with professional bodies. To prevent further suicidal ideation a psychiatrist can formulate a treatment plan.
- Ask for help. For easy communication during suicidal period add crisis hotline number to your phone and if you feel you may harm yourself move to your local emergency department.

*Guidelines for selecting a treatment setting for patients at risk for suicide or suicidal behaviors (Kleber et al. 2006)*

Psychiatric management consists of a wide range of therapeutic interventions that should be instituted for patients with suicidal thoughts, plans, or behaviors. Psychiatric management includes determining a setting for treatment and supervision, attending to patient safety, and working to establish a co-operative and collaborative physician-patient relationship **(Table 15.3)**.

## Catatonic Stupor

Catatonia is a motor dysregulation, and which is associated with numbers of illness. The term catatonia derived from the Greek word kata (down) and tonas (tension or tone) well described by Bellack (Wilcox and Duffy, 2015).

### Definition

Catatonia refers to a cluster of striking motor signs occurring with idiopathic psychosis (mood disorders, schizophrenia), intrinsic brain disease, metabolic disorders affecting brain function, and drug-induced syndromes. It may also be seen in many medical disorders including infections (such as encephalitis), autoimmune disorders, focal neurologic lesion (including strokes), metabolic disturbances, alcohol withdrawal (Sedain, 2014).

Catatonia exists in two subtypes, stuporous and excited catatonia (Gupta et al., 2007).

### Epidemiology

Prevalence of catatonia among psychiatric patients are from 7.6 to 38% and it is evident from various survey and studies (Gupta et al., 2007).

### Management of Catatonic Syndrome

Treatment

- Benzodiazepines
- ECT: If the patient is resistant to benzodiazepines and ECT then other medication can be given such as:
  - Mood stabilizing agents (e.g., carbamazepine)
  - Neuroleptics
  - NMDA antagonist (e.g., amantadine and memantine)
  - D2-agonist (e.g., bromocriptine)
  - Muscle relaxants (e.g., dantrolene), especially when NMS is suspected.

---

**Stuporous catatonia**
- Mutism
- Immobility
- Waxy flexibility
- Echophenomena
- Negativism

**Excited catatonia**
- Purposeless behavior
- Violent behavior
- Agitation or restlessness

**Fig. 15.3:** Signs and symptoms of catatonic based on their types.

**Table 15.3:** Guidelines for selecting a treatment setting for patients at risk for suicide.

| Admission generally indicated |
|---|
| After aborted suicide attempt or suicide attempt if:<br>• Client with psychotic thoughts<br>• Suicidal effort is very furious or aggressive, near fatal, or pre-intended<br>• Measures were chosen to abstain rescue or recovery<br>• Consistent plan of suicide and/or strong desire is present<br>• Client is stressed or weeps over his existence or survival<br>• A male patient has crossed 45 years and presenting with acute onset of mental sickness or obsessed with suicidal thoughts<br>• Client presenting low supporting system including lack of stable living relationship, aggressive behavior, poor decision-making capability, suicidal ideation with high brutality and suicidal intent |
| **Admission may be necessary** |
| Admission is usually suggested if suicidal ideation is present with:<br>• Psychotic thinking<br>• Mental illness (major type)<br>• Previous suicide attempts, especially if medically serious<br>• Suicide attempt specially due to certain medical illness (e.g., cancer, infection, acute neurological disorder)<br>• Lack of cognizance towards hospital or outpatient treatment<br>• Need for careful observation or clinical diagnostic evaluation which needs a structured set<br>• Lack of supporting systems<br>• Lack of an ongoing consultation with clinician or low accessibility to periodical outpatient follow-up<br>   Other than suicidal attempts or reported suicidal thoughts, during assessment if it is evident then it suggests an increased risk of suicide |
| **Discharge from emergency unit** |
| After suicide attempt or patient with suicidal ideation/plan follow-up recommendations may be given when:<br>• Precipitating events may cause suicide (e.g., failure in examination, unsatisfactory relationship), especially if the client's insights towards circumstances have distorted since moving to emergency unit<br>• Suicidal ideation/means and intent have low fatality<br>• Client with safe and supportive environment or family system<br>• Patient is able to cooperate with recommendations for follow-up |
| **Outpatient treatment may be more beneficial than hospitalization** |
| Outpatient psychiatric care is a continuous assessment, and it is required when a patient has chronic suicidal ideation/self-harming without any past serious attempts and when there is a stable and supportive living condition available |

Benzodiazepine is the drug of preference for catatonia. Patients who are resistant to benzodiazepines, electroconvulsive therapy (ECT) can be given as alternative.

### Anger, Aggression and Violent Behavior

Generally, for forensic mental health services, criminal justice system and for society anger, aggression and violence are major issues. The societal and financial costs of violence are huge. Apart from causing physical and psychological distress among patient and staff, violence can lead to poor morality, low job satisfaction, staff turnover and omission of therapeutic environment in which patient can be assisted to change and to enhance their well-being (Beck 1993).

### Definition of Anger, Aggression and Violence

- **Anger:** Anger can be defined as a strong, uncomfortable emotional response to an incitement that is unwanted and incoherent with a person's values, beliefs, or rights. It can also be categorized as rational (positive) or irrational (negative) (Hurskainen and Katainen, 2015).
- **Aggression:**
  – Aggression is any behavior directed toward another individual that is carried out with the proximate (immediate) intent to cause harm (Anderson and Bushman, 2002).
  – Aggression is a hostile behavior or threat of attack (Harwood, 2017).
- **Violence:**
  – All violence is aggression, but many instances of aggression are not violent. For example, one child pushing another off a tricycle is an act of aggression but is not an act of violence (Anderson and Bushman, 2002).

– Violence is the use of physical force, verbal abuse, threat or intimidation, which can result in harm, hurt or injury to another person (Harwood, 2017).

*Management of Aggressive and Violent Patient*

Health professionals often feel uncertain while handling a patient with violence and aggression. Sometimes the best action might ambiguous and the guidelines neither constantly applicable nor explicit by standing at the line between psychiatry, law and medicine. Sometimes violent, abusive or aggressive patient may behave criminally or anti-socially. In emergency medical setting it is seen that medical and mental health related issues or combination of this two is difficult to manage and contribution of each element is not clear. Problematic behavior occurs when there is communication distress or needs remain unmet. De-escalation and distressing situation can be prevented by developing the insight such as why it has created, identifying the causes and need and trying manage the situation (Harwood, 2017).

There are three significant steps for management of agression and violence.
1. Prevention
2. Escalating the situation
3. Managing crisis

### Prevention

Prevention sets priorities, validates good practice and challenges poor practices and which require skill and good leadership **(Fig. 15.4)**.

- Each individual should try to minimize the chances of upset, conflict or aggression.
- The professional should benonjudgmental, empathetic towards the patient.
- Fulfilling physical, psychological and emotional needs prevention focuses on good communication, and relationship-building.

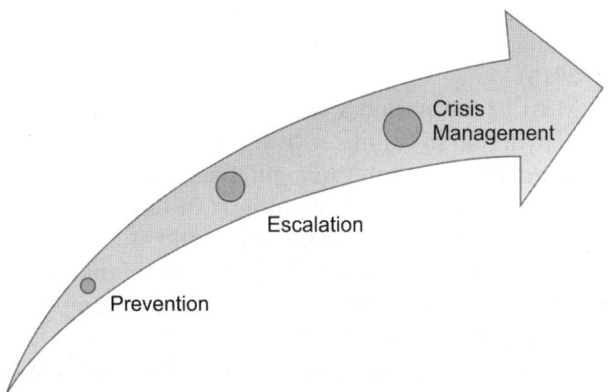

**Fig. 15.4:** Steps for aggression and violence management.

- Conduct mental status examination (MSE) for ensuring alertness, arousal, attention, anxiety, anger or any form of hallucination and delusion and which can make the patient more aggressive.
- When a patient is disoriented, and distraction must be done.
- Involve all family members in the therapeutic purpose or as useful allies.

### Escalating situations

- When a situation gets worse, there is need for 'de-escalation'. This is sometimes stated as 'nonpharmacologic' or 'behavioral' strategies.
- Target is to make the client stable and least distressed.
- Give some physical and emotional or private space and for a certain time leave the client alone (a 'leave and return' strategy).
- Remove the entire hazardous thing from patient's environment.
- Stay friendly and calm.
- Acknowledge the distress without making accusations.
- Ask and help the patient how to neutralize the condition and which is called 'positive engagement' in mental health practice.
- All staff should be skilled when a patient tries to help them rescue themselves is referred to as 'breakaway' techniques.
- If the situation is uncontrollable and the patient is with weapons, then call security staff.
- Medication helps in de-escalation.
- Drugs should be given as per the symptoms. In case of psychotic disorder, mania and delirium antipsychotic drug is preferred.
- Generally, in alcohol withdrawal, postictal seizure, Parkinsonism and lewy body dementia benzodiazepines are preferred.
- Aim to treat an identified problem rather simply aiming for sedation.

### Managing crisis

The patient who is very aggressive the aim is to take prompt action to manage the situation, safeguard those who are involved in the incident or who are present around and to minimize physical and emotional harm to the patient and others.

- Crowds should be cleared as gathering may aggravate the sense of danger.
- Call security staff for support.
- Bodily disconnection may be required immediately when a patient attacks other person in his environment.
- Physical or chemical restraints of the client may be needed to avoid any physical injury.

- Restraint the patient physically for a minimum period as per the requirement.
- Approach should be from back if the patient is restrained.
- Best restraint is done when a patient is on bed rest.
- Do not ground the patient; if it is not possible, restrain the patient in supine rather than prone and protect the head from injury.
- Monitor oxygen saturations and make sure that the airway is not obstructed.
- Combine physical restraint with first acting tranquilizer for sedating the patient. Within 30–60 minutes a patient needs to be controlled.
- Sedate the patient with Inj. Diazepam 10–20 mg I/V slowly but in case of psychotic disorder administer Inj. Serenace (Haloperidol) 20 mg I/M or Inj. Largactil (Chlorpromazine) 50–100 mg I/M.
- Peak or therapeutic effect of drugs may be achieved within 20–30 minutes. So, a gap may be given between the doses.
- Continuous monitoring of vital signs must be done.
- Benzodiazepines may cause respiratory depression and haloperidol may cause dystonia, so keep flumazenil and procyclidine available respectively.
- Lorazepam is a first line drug of choice in mental health and emergency department settings as haloperidol has the potential for causing extrapyramidal symptoms or side effects and arrhythmias.

### Substance Related Emergency (Substance Intoxication and Withdrawal)

Substance use disorders (SUD) are more common in emergency services (general emergency rooms—GER). In United States approximately 374,000 patients over 12 years aged were admitted due to SUD in emergency services in 2008. (Rev. Bras. Psiquiatr. vol. 32 supl. 2 São Paulo out. 2010).

Substance use disorder may present as a primary complaints or associate with a psychiatric disorder. The most commonly used substances are alcohol, cocaine and phencyclidine and lead to aggressive and violent behavior. During this period, patient should be placed in a secure room under close vigilance. Any kind of stimulation and attempt to talk with the patient is not advisable (Lunn and Day, 2017).

### Management

- Violent and aggressive patient may require sedation and physical restraints. The recommended dose of Lorazepam 2 to 4 mg stat or diazepam 10 to 20 mg stat is suggested to manage agitation (Lunn and Day, 2017).
- Generally, when a patient is having hyperthermia (>38.3°C or 101°F), severe symptoms, severe underlying somatic disorder and can't take enough fluids for hydration treatment in a hospital is safe and mandatory.
- Life-threatening condition may be occurred due to alcohol withdrawal and may associate with seizures.
- Delirium tremens is medical emergency which is an alcohol withdrawal syndrome, appears within 7 days of abstinence (usually 24 to 72 hours) and should be promptly treated in ICU.
- Withdrawal symptoms can be managed generally with increase benzodiazepines dose, intravenous thiamine and IV fluid for restoration of electrolyte balance.

### Other Psychiatric Emergency

Neuroleptic malignant syndrome (NMS) is potentially life-threatening neurologic rare emergency condition occurs due to the use of neuroleptic or antipsychotic drugs (Friedman and Fernandez, 2004).

*Definition*

Neuroleptic malignant syndrome is a rare but life-threatening, idiosyncratic reaction to neuroleptic/antipsychotic medication. It is characterized by fever, muscular rigidity, altered mental status, autonomic dysfunction and elevated creatine phosphokinase (Friedman and Fernandez, 2004).

*Management*

Neuroleptic malignant syndrome is a clinical emergency, if it is not treated timely can lead to death. NMS must be promptly identified and instant withdrawal of the neuroleptic agents is the initial step. Management of NMS includes specific psycho pharmacotherapy, supportive medical care and electroconvulsive therapy (ECT) (Friedman and Fernandez, 2004).

- Immediate withdrawal of antipsychotic agent must be combined with supportive medical therapy for better management of NMS (Djamashidian and O'Sullivan, 2015).
- Most of the patients with NMS in acute phase are dehydrated so volume revival should be aggressive.
- In extreme hyperthermia, physical cooling measures are highly essential, as long standing of elevated temperature may cause morbidity and mortality.
- In severe hyperthermia-hypothermic blankets, cold ice water, gastric lavage and under arm ice packets application and cold sponge bath are helpful to decrease the elevated body temperature. Antipyretics may be used to lower the temperature (Friedman and Fernandez, 2004).

- Clonidine is effective for lowering BP, if markedly elevated.
- First line treatment for acute NMS is Lorazepam, 1–2 mg IV starting dose, particularly who are having mild and primary catatonic symptoms (Djamashidian and O'Sullivan, 2015).

*Medicolegal Aspects of Psychiatric Emergency*

### Informed consent

The meaning of consent is voluntary agreement, compliance, or permission and the concept comes from issues of ethical aspects such as autonomy, individual integrity and self-determination (Swartz, 1987).

Generally, prior to any intervention it is essential to obtain consent. In cases of emergency, there is an important exception; sometimes a patient may be unable to give consent, in such cases, an alternate authoritative person, if available, should be approached. If that individual is unavailable, then here the responsibility of the doctor to do what is essential to save life of the patient even without consent.

Most of the courts has empowered the physician to treat in the absence of informed consent and even in the face of overt treatment denial in a genuine clinical emergency (Swartz, 1987).

### Refusal to treatment

The fundamental legal rights for psychiatric treatment are the right to refuse. During an emergency denial of all exceptions is possible. Exceptions are that right to refuse treatment will be denied. A doctor may provide involuntary treatment to control the emergency situation like medication through injection or by mouth—which, is stated as "an imminent danger to self or others." During emergency whatever the treatment is provided should be discontinued immediate after the threat has crossed, unless the patient agrees and gives informed consent.

### Suicidal act

Suicide and attempted suicide are the punishable offenses under the Indian Law. Section 309 of IPC (Indian Penal Court) states that "whoever attempts to commit suicide and does any act towards the commission of such offense, shall be punishable with simple imprisonment for a term which may extend to one year and shall also be liable to fine" (Ahuja Niraj, 2011).

## CRISIS INTERVENTION

"Crisis is part of life. Everybody has to face them, and it doesn't make any difference what the crisis is". (Jack Nicklaus).

At times stress in life can reach up to certain acute intense level and yielding more serious emotional distress, threats to one's security, make the individual to function less efficiently and extending an individual's ability to cope up to its limit. During these critical situations an individual may not detained himself for seeking help from mental health professionals or experts. To overcome from crisis immediate and active intervention must be given as a crisis intervention (Hannigan and Hertig, 2010).

A crisis situation require a expertise assessment and treatment by using different methods other than the non-crisis situation as it is more acute and overwhelming (Davanloo and Straker, 1980).

Due to the consequences of crisis an individual may adopt a maladaptive level of functioning or may achieve a pre-crisis functioning level by repressing crisis and other crisis inflicted psychological feelings.

So, the crisis intervention is highly essential to prevent the mental illness or mal adoptive behavior.

### Meaning of Crisis

The meaning of crisis in Greek word "krisis" is decision or turning point (Fano, 1988).

The Chinese language contains two character such as wei, means critical or dangerous situation, while another one is ji, means an opportunity for change and which connate the concept of crisis. Together this two word provides an opportunity for personality growth (Stevens and Ellerbrock, 1995).

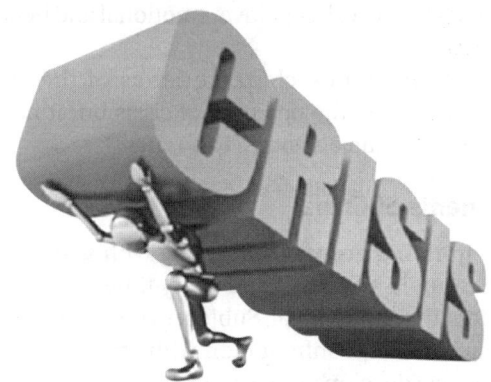

### Definitions

An emotional distress, arising from biological, psychological, situational, developmental, sociocultural, and/or spiritual entities. A temporary inability to cope by means of one's usual resources and coping mechanisms caused by emotional distress. Major disorganization occurs unless the stressors that precipitated the crisis are alleviated and/or the coping mechanisms are bolstered (Fujita, 2011).

"A perception or experiencing of an event or situation as an intolerable difficulty that exceeds the person's current resources and coping mechanisms" (Westerdal, Rights, and Copyright, 2002).

**Crisis** is a state of imbalance occurring from the interaction of an event with the individual's or family's coping mechanisms, which are not enough to meet the demands of the events, combined with the individual's or family's perception towards event (Kfir and Terner, 2014).

A **"crisis"** has been defined as an acute disruption of psychological homeostasis in which one's usual coping mechanisms fail and there exists evidence of distress and functional impairment (Roberts and Ottens, 2005).

**Crisis** experiencing an event or circumstance as an intolerable difficulty that go beyond the person's current resources and coping mechanisms (James and Gilliland, 2001).

A sudden event in one's life that disturbs homeostasis, during which usual coping mechanisms cannot resolve the problem (Lagerquist, 2001).

## Characteristics of Crisis (Kfir and Terner, 2014)

- Crisis is individualized.
- It is acute onset and will be resolved within certain period of time.
- Crisis continues for 4–6 weeks as it is self-limiting.
- Crisis experience is universal in nature.
- It occurs in its own predictable manner.
- At one point of time or other it happens in all individual.
- It causes biological, cognitive, emotional and behavioral disorganization.
- One's personality, characteristics of the stressor does not reflect the outcome of crisis but it has some influence on the outcome (Fano, 1988).

## Components of Crisis

- **Precipitating event:** Confronting with stressful situation is not itself a crisis and every time it is not clearly evident to an individual. Subject to personal and social circumstances, confrontation with stressor full blown crisis may develop or may not.
- **Perception of the event:** Subjective distress occurs when an individual starts to perceive the event. In the course of crisis subjective distress, the person may have more intense or overwhelming emotions or feelings and leave the client in a confusing state. When someone experiencing manageable stress that means subjective distress has not affected one's coping or general functioning and simultaneously it cannot be termed as crisis.
- **Usual coping methods:** An individual is not in a crisis until and unless he is emotionally, occupationally and interpersonally disorganized. Usual coping methods help to manage stress and prevent the crisis.

Nurses should recognize and identify these three components while handling the client with crisis to resolve or to help the client to find a best solution for the same.

## Types of Crisis

Two types of crisis were identified by Erikson in 1956 such as:

1. **Situational crisis:** Occurs when significant losses take place due to life hazards and leave an individual in a state of biological and behavioral upset (e.g., accident, job loss).
2. **Maturational or developmental crisis:** Everyone has to go through transitions in their life span. Adolescence, becoming a parent, getting married, and retirement, becoming an elder or dying are the major transitions. During this crucial period someone may not cope with changes and resulting crisis (Rosen, 1997).

Baldwin (1978) has developed six types of crisis situation causes emotional crisis:

1. **Dispositional crises** are acute response to external or stressful events can be resolved by appropriate interventions which include referral, education and information, change in administration, etc.
2. **Anticipated life transitional crisis**—individual has less or no control over normal life transitions, e.g., adolescence, marriage.
3. **Traumatic stress related crisis**, are unexpected, unanticipated, uncontrolled and overwhelming which are inflicted by external events or stressors, e.g., rape, robbery, terrorism.
4. **Maturational/developmental crises**, when the individual moves forward to successive stages in life often face distress. It is related as to how individual grows and moves toward maturity, e.g., adolescence, marriage, antenatal period, parenthood, retirement, etc. (Kfir and Terner, 2014).
5. **Crises reflecting psychopathology** in which crisis precipitated by pre-existing or current psychopathology, e.g., borderline personality disorder, schizophrenia and neurotic disorder.
6. **Psychiatric emergencies,** crisis occurs the individual is incapable to manage his personal responsibility and his general functioning is markedly impaired, e.g., suicide, addicts (Fano, 1988).

## Stages of Crisis

### *According to Rosen 1997*

*Stage I: Mounting Tension*

To restore equilibrium the person uses habitual or usual problem-solving measures.

*Stage II: Plateau of Disorganization*

- Anxious or agitated or chaotic feelings.
- Repeated failure attempt to accomplish problem-solving
- Repetitive behavior (e.g., "hitting head against a brick wall").
- Level of autonomy decreases and ventilation demand mounts.

*Stage III: Mobilization of All Internal and External Resources*

- Extreme agitation, need for suggestibility, increased demand for seeking good or poor advice becomes more prevalent at this stage.
- Novice problem-solving strategies and supporting measures can be identified and used to solve the problem.

*Stage IV: Adaptation or Maladaptation*

- **Crisis resolution:** New situational accommodation occurs by using novel adoptive skills or coping strategies. State of balance or equilibrium restored at equal or to a maximum level.
- **Maladaptation:** Treatment is required when there is surface "closure" or rectification of previous crises or continual medical symptoms. External and internal resources are exhausted to solve the problem leads to further disorganization.
- **Major disorganization:** If vulnerable, at this phase, crisis may move towards appearance of psychotic episodes or affective disorders (Rosen, 1997).

### *According to Caplan in 1964*

Stages of crisis reaction were first described by Caplan in 1964. Basing upon Caplan's work other theorist gave their contributions which were primarily consisted on a rephrasing of his stages. As per Caplan (1964) most crisis reactions occurs in four distinct phases:

1. **Stage I:** At the first phase, there is a threat to homeostasis as the person is confronted with the problem. Here the person uses the existing or habitual problem-solving measures to get rid from the increased tension and to restore the emotional integrity.
2. **Stage II:** Due to unsuccessful existing problem-solving strategies the tension increases which leads to persistent threat and problem. As the result of further increased tension the person senses emotional overwhelming and the general functioning becomes disorganized.
3. **Stage III:** Despite persistent failure of the individuals effort, a further increase in tension occurs which act as a call bell for the marshaling of emergency and adaptation of new problem-solving strategies. In third stage, the person redefines the issues and he may find a best possible solution or may give up himself to the problem.
4. **Stage IV:** The emotional stress or tension accelerates further threshold or pressure rises with time to breaking point if the problem continues. As an outcome major disorganization occurs in the areas individual's social, mental or general functioning and may be associated with psychotic symptoms (Fano, 1988).

## Signs and Symptoms of Crisis (Kfir and Terner, 2014) (Fig. 15.5)

### *Crisis Intervention*

Crisis intervention defines the techniques used to render instant or acute, help to those who confronts with the problem that produces emotional, mental, physical and/or behavioral distress (subjective distress) or problems. At the time of stress, it is an active and immediate step towards the life situation (e.g., divorce, rape or natural disaster) (Kfir and Terner, 2014).

### *Goals of Crisis Intervention (Kfir and Terner, 2014)*

- Decreases emotional stress
- Protect client from additional stress
- Assisting the client in organizing and mobilizing and adapting all internal or external resources
- Help the client to achieve a pre-crisis or higher level of functioning (Kfir and Terner, 2014)

### *Crisis Intervention Techniques*

See **Table 15.4**.

### *Principles of Crisis Intervention*

According to Puryear, crisis intervention is based on the following eight principles (Davanloo and Straker, 1980).

1. **Immediate intervention:** Crisis intervention should be immediate as an individual can't go through the crisis for long periods of time. The client needs or may request for treatment when the crisis is at peak and the individual is least defensive and more introspective.
2. **Action:** For resolving the crisis, the therapist actively engages himself into the problem and directs the activities to help the client.
3. **Limited goals:** Crisis intervention put emphasis on goals which are clearly defined and related to the event.

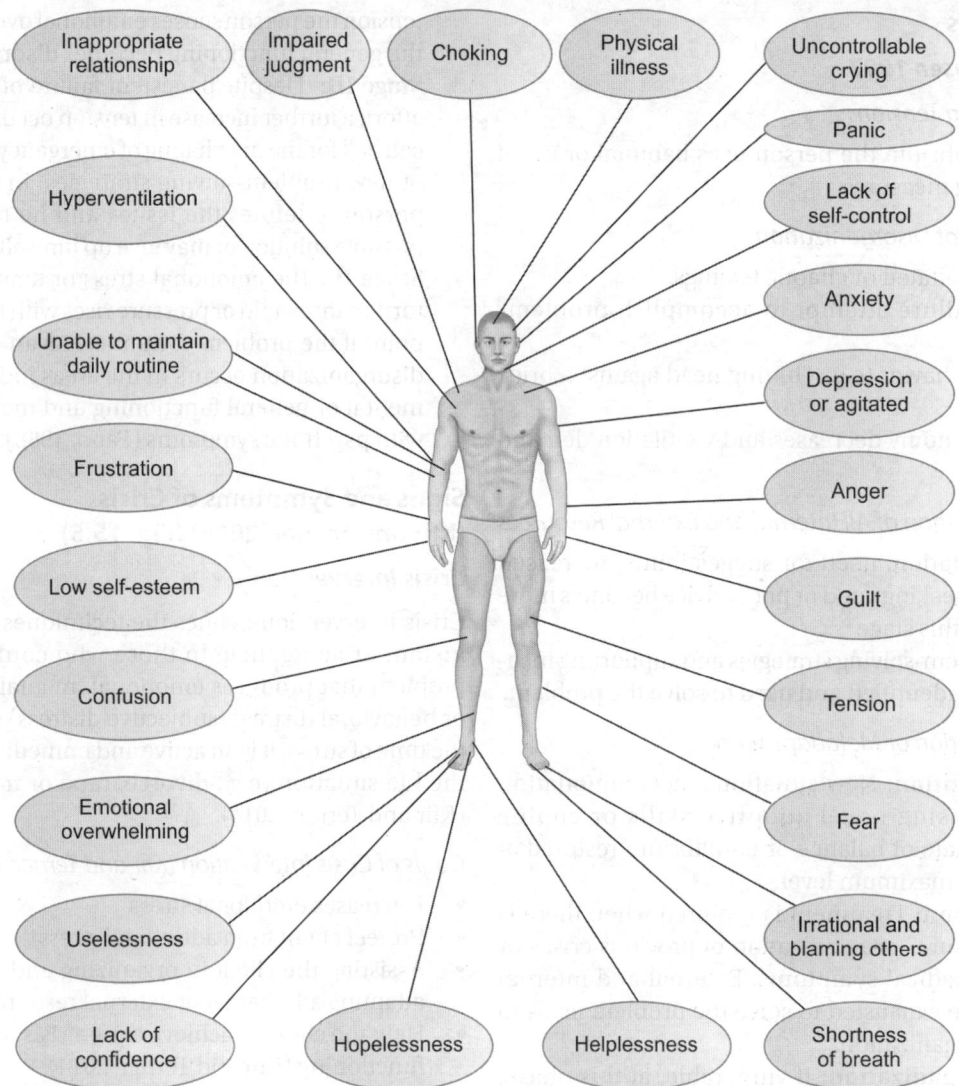

Fig. 15.5: Signs and symptoms of crisis.

4. **Hope and expectations:** Therapist should build up hopes and expectations that the crisis will be resolved because often people who are in crisis feel hopeless.
5. **Support:** Support is extremely required in crisis intervention because the lack of a supporting system is a contributing factor of crisis.
6. **Focused problem-solving:** Crisis interventions are problem oriented and emphasizes is on resolution of the problem(s) underlying the crisis.
7. **Self-image:** The client undergoing a crisis basically sees him/herself as inadequate and incapable. Therefore, to raise or protect the client's self-esteem the therapist should use the appropriate methods or approaches.
8. **Self-reliance:** From the onset of the crisis intervention, balance between support and fostering the client's self-reliance and independence must be maintained by the therapist (Davanloo and Straker, 1980).

Robertson's five stages of crisis intervention

Roberts (1991, 2000, 2005) has conceptualized the process of crisis intervention and identified seven critical stages for the crisis stabilization, resolution, and mastery through which every client has to pass (Roberts and Otten, 2005).
1. **Stage I—Biopsychosocial and lethality/imminent danger assessment:** Biopsychosocial assessment must be conducted by the crisis worker and this should assess

**Table 15.4:** Crisis intervention techniques.

| Intervention techniques | Explanation |
|---|---|
| Abreaction | It is the expression of emotional feelings that occurs when the client explains about emotionally charged areas, e.g., when a patient undergoes suicide the nurse encourages the client to explain how he perceives a particular incident or events by using different therapeutic techniques like paraphrasing, pin pointing |
| Clarification | It helps the client to clearly state the connection between the events and stressor. By this helps, the client to get an insight of his own emotional feelings and how these feelings turned into crisis |
| Suggestion | It helps the client to feel calm, less anxious and optimistic and which can be suggested by the nurses |
| Manipulation | Patient's emotions, wishes or values can be used to help the client in the therapeutic courses |
| Reinforcement of behavior | It can be insisted when the client shows adaptive or healthy behavior through positive response, e.g., patient can be reinforced through verbal praise or token economy |
| Support of defense | To maintain the emotional integrity, help the person to use healthy and acceptable behavior to cope up stressful events simultaneously discourage the maladaptive, unacceptable behavior, e.g., listening music, gardening, painting rather than taking substances or doing unsocial acts |
| Raising self-esteem | Self-esteem can be enhanced when the nurse help the client to get back his self-worth, e.g., self-esteem can be enhanced through active participation, effective communication, good listening skills, accepting his feelings with respect |
| Exploration of solutions | Help the client to find out the alternative solution for the acute problematic situation, e.g., the nurse and client actively and collaboratively find out best alternative solutions to resolve the crisis. For instance, when a patient is very aggressive and to make him calm down suggest the to drink glass of water, ventilate his emotion, sit quietly, etc. (Kfir and Terner, 2014) |

the person's supporting system and stressor, treatment requirement and medications, prevailing maladaptive use of any substances, internal and environmental coping strategies and resources (Roberts and Ottens, 2005).

2. **Stage II—Rapidly establish rapport:** Honesty, respect and acceptance of the client should be fostered by the counselor for facilitating the rapport (Roberts, 2005). During stage to gain trust and reliance the crisis worker must maintain intermittent eye contact, nonjudgmental acceptance, creativity, flexibility, positive healthy mindset, reinforcing small adaptive achievement, and resilience.
3. **Stage III—Identify the major crisis precipitants:** As the crisis intervention is problem focused and which are the precipitating factors of crisis. So the crisis worker must identify these contributing factors.
4. **Stage IV—Deal with emotions and feelings:** The therapist permits the individual to ventilate emotional feelings, and to elaborate her or his relation with the event. For understanding the relationship, the therapist must be familiar with certain skills like active listening, paraphrasing, reflecting, and probing (Egan, 2002).
5. **Stage V—Generate and explore alternatives:** In crisis intervention exploration of alternatives is difficult to accomplish. Alternative solutions are thought to be better when they are formulated collaboratively and selective alternatives are owned by the individual.
6. **Stage VI—Implement an action plan for restoring:** The client's equilibrium and emotional balance the concrete action plans taken at this stage are very essential. Therapist should implement the best chosen alternatives.
7. **Stage VII—Follow-up and booster sessions:** Follow-up schedule must set by the crisis worker after initial intervention to evaluate the post-crisis status of the client. Post-crisis evaluation includes physical health, appropriate cognition of the precipitating factor, assessment of general functioning, satisfaction and prognosis with ongoing treatment.

Role of nurse in crisis intervention

- **Phase I—Assessment:**
  - Assess the following:
    * Ability to perceive the problematic situation.
    * Identification of precipitating event and its relationship with the client.
    * Assess the client's supporting system, internal or external resources.
  - Identify the client's capabilities and in capabilities in dealing with the problem.

- Assess the client's immediate need.
- Assess the associated impact of crisis on the individual and family.
- Find out the behavioral problems which are associated with crisis, e.g., suicidal potentialities.
- Physical and mental status of the individual must assessed.
- History of previous exposure and habitual use of any coping strategies.
- Exploration of problematic situation.

- **Phase II:** After analyzing the gathered information through assessment nursing diagnosis is formulated to solve the immediate problems of the crisis situation.
- **Phase III:** In planning the short-term and long-term goals will be formulated with a specific and appropriate plan of activities, client's abilities or strengths, available resources for support, alternative solutions of the problem and methods for achieving the solutions has to be recognized during crisis intervention.
- **Phase IV:** Implementation of intervention described four levels of crisis intervention such as:
    1. *Environmental manipulation:* Directly modify client's physical or interpersonal environment to provides situational support, e.g., an individual may change his job from one place to another if his working environment is not comfortable.
    2. *General support:* While providing intervention to a crisis affected person render warmth, support, acceptance, empathy, caring, concern and reassurance.
    3. *Generic approach:* As soon as possible reach to the high-risk person. Debriefing a therapeutic intervention will be used to recall the traumatic events and to clarify painful experiences and to prevent maladaptive responses. Specific methods should be used who are in same problem.
    4. *Individual approach client's:* Specific psychodynamics has to be understood by the nurse which precipitates the crisis and specific intervention has to be adopted in response to the crisis.
- **Phase V—Evaluation of crisis resolution:** The nurse and client have to evaluate and reassess whether the intervention has resulted in a positive resolution of crisis; behavioral changes has been achieved or not; whether the client has returned to the normal level of functioning. If not achieved, modified strategies have to be initiated (Kfir and Terner, 2014).

Crisis intervention provides the opportunity and mechanisms for change to those who are experiencing psychological equilibrium, who are feeling overwhelmed by their current situation, who have exhausted their skills for coping and who are experiencing personal discomfort. To restore the equilibrium and to decrease the effect of crisis a mental health worker identifies, assesses, and intervenes with the individual in crisis. To reinforce the change the person need to connect him to the supporting resource. Crisis truly provides the opportunity for change.

 **Summary**

This chapter deals with different types of psychiatric emergencies and prompts management of those conditions. There are certain psychiatric emergencies are there like suicide, NMS which are life-threatening conditions and required constant supervision and immediate actions. Healthcare professionals should find skillful way to handle and manage the crisis and its related situation. A detailed and through assessment must be done to prevent further deterioration of the condition by safeguarding the life of the patient at the mean time and help the client to achieve a pre-crisis or higher level of functioning.

 **Points to Ponder**

- Psychiatric emergencies are conditions in which there is an acute changes in behaviors, emotion or thought seeking immediate attention and treatment.
- Suicide is the second leading cause of death worldwide in between 15–19 years of age.
- Discussing about suicide facilitate the opportunity for free communication.
- Benzodiazepine is the drug of preference for catatonia.
- Neuroleptic malignant syndrome (NMS) is potentially life-threatening neurologic rare emergency condition occurs due to the use of neuroleptic or antipsychotic drugs.
- Crisis is self-limiting and individualized in nature.
- Crisis is an opportunities for personality growth.
- Crisis intervention techniques used to provide instantaneous or acute, aid to those who confronts with the issues that creates emotional, physical and/or behavioral distress.

 **Abbreviations**

- NMS : Neuroleptic Malignant Syndrome
- IPC : Indian Penal Code
- ECT : Electroconvulsive Therapy
- ICU : Intensive Care Unit
- SUD : Substance Used Disorder
- GER : General Emergency Room
- MSE : Mental Status Examination
- NCRB : National Crime Records Bureau
- NMDA : N-Methyl-D-Aspartate

### Short Answer Questions

1. Explain in detail about principles of psychiatric emergency.
2. Define suicide and nurse's responsibility in suicide prevention.
3. Briefly explain about medicolegal aspects of psychiatric emergency.
4. Describe the stages of crisis.
5. Explain in detail about techniques used in crisis intervention.
6. Role of nurse in crisis intervention.

### Long Answer Questions

1. Define psychiatric emergencies. List out different types of psychiatric emergencies with their appropriate management.
2. Define crisis. List out the characteristics of crisis. Elaborate the role of nurse in crisis intervention.

### Bibliography

1. Ahuja N. A Short Textbook of Psychiatry. 2011;(7):224.
2. Anderson CA, Bushman BJ. Human Aggression. Annual Review of Psychology. 2002;53(1):27-51.
3. Beck JC. Review Essay: Aggression and Violence. Psychiatry. 1993;56(2):228-35.
4. Chaturvedi AN. Consent—Its Medico-Legal Aspects. Medicine Update. 2000:883-7.
5. Davanloo H, Strake M. Crisis Intervention: An Overview.1980: 221-236.
6. Dogra N, Cooper S. Defining Mental Health and Mental Illness. In Psychiatry by Ten Teachers, CRC Press: 2017: 15-25.
7. Fano U. Introduction to the Theory Symposium. In Fundamental Processes of Atomic Dynamics. Springer, Boston, MA; 1988:35-40.
8. Fitzpatrick JJ. World Mental Health Day. Archives of Psychiatric Nursing. 2017;1;31(6):531.
9. Franklin JC, Ribeiro JD, Fox KR, Bentley KH, Kleiman EM, Huang X, et al. Risk Factors for Suicidal Thoughts and Behaviors: A Meta-analysis of 50 Years of Research. Psychological Bulletin. 2017;143(2):187.
10. Fujita D. Crisis Intervention—Significance of Gradual Intervention. Seishin Shinkeigaku Zasshi= Psychiatria et Neurologia Japonica. 2011;113(6):601-4.
11. Gupta LN, Verma KK, Singhal AK, Dayal P, Jain V, Gupta P. Catatonic Syndrome–A Review, 10(1):19-25.
12. Hannigan MA, Hertig CA, Gilbride BP. Crisis Intervention. In The Professional Protection Officer, Butterworth-Heinemann; 2020: 219-228.
13. Harwood RH. How to Deal with Violent and Aggressive Patients in Acute Medical Settings. Journal of the Royal College of Physicians of Edinburgh. 2017;47(2):94-101
14. Hurskainen T, Katainen M. Anger, Aggression and Violence in Healthcare: Material for Nursing Education.
15. Kfir N, Terner. Crisis Intervention Verbatim. Taylor and Francis; 2014.
16. Kleber HD, Weiss RD, Anton RF, George TP, Greenfield SF, Kosten TR, el al. Treatment of Patients with Substance Use Disorders. American Journal of Psychiatry, 163 (8 SUPPL.). 2006:1-275.
17. Masango SM, Rataemane ST, Motojesi AA. Suicide and Suicide Risk Factors: A Literature Review. South African Family Practice. 2008;50(6):25-9.
18. Nadkarni A, Hanlon C, Bhatia U, Fuhr D, Ragoni C, de Azevedo Perocco SL, et al. The Management of Adult Psychiatric Emergencies in Low-income and Middle-income Countries: A Systematic Review. The Lancet Psychiatry. 2015;2(6):540-7.
19. Newhill CE. Psychiatric Emergencies: Overview of Clinical Principles and Clinical Practice. Clinical Social Work Journal. 1989;17(3):245-58.
20. Roberts AR, Ottens AJ. The Seven-Stage Crisis Intervention Model: A Road Map to Goal Attainment Problem Solving, and Crisis Resolution. Brief Treatment and Crisis Intervention. 2005;5(4):329-339.
21. Rosen A. Crisis Management in the Community. Med J Aust. 1997;167(11-12):633-8.
22. Sedain CP. Catatonia. Journal of Psychiatrists' Association of Nepal. 2014;3:34-7.
23. Seven Myths and Facts About Suicide, 2018.
24. Stevens BA, Ellerbrock LS. Crisis Intervention: An Opportunity to Change. ERIC Digest.
25. Swartz MS. What Constitutes a Psychiatric Emergency: Clinical and Legal Dimensions. Journal of the American Academy of Psychiatry and the Law Online. 1987;15(1):57-68.
26. Wilcox JA, Reid Duffy P. The Syndrome of Atatonia. Behavioral Sciences. 2015;5(4):576-88.
27. World Health Organization. Preventing Suicide Preventing Suicide. Preventing Suicide: A Global Imperative. 2014;92.

# Chapter 16

# Burns and Management

*Susan Konda*

## CHAPTER OUTLINE

- Classification and Pathophysiology of Burns
- Burn Assessment
- Fluid and Electrolyte Therapy
- Pain Management
- Wound Care
- Infection Control
- Prevention and Management of Burn Complication
- Grafts and Flaps
- Reconstructive Surgery
- Rehabilitation

### Learning Objectives

At the end of the chapter, the students will be able to:
- Recollect and learn about the classification and pathophysiology of burns.
- Assess and understand the burn assessment.
- Manage fluid and electrolyte therapy.
- Understand various types of pain management.
- Manage wound care.
- Have idea about the infection control.
- Gain knowledge about prevention and management of burn complication.
- Assess the grafts and flaps.
- Various types of reconstructive surgery.
- Gain an idea about rehabilitation in burns patients.

## CLASSIFICATION AND PATHOPHYSIOLOGY OF BURNS

Burn trauma continues to be immense challenge to care givers in the emergency department (ED). Every year in the United States, an estimated one million patients seek treatment for burn injury, and approximately one-third are treated in emergency department. In 2016, it was estimated that 486,000 patients received treatment for burn injuries. Approximately 40,000 patients were admitted to an acute care facility, with 60% admitted to 128 burn centers. Approximately 15,000 pediatric burn-injured patients were also admitted. Decreases in burn incidence and hospitalization are attributes to fire and burn prevention education, regulation of consumer products, and implementation of occupational safety standards. The decline in mortality is attributed to early care of the burn wound. Other factors contributing to the decline are management of patients with burns in specialty burn units, improved resuscitation, control of infection, and support of the hyper metabolic response. The survival rate at burn centers is reported as 96.8%. A significant portion of morbidity and mortality associated with burn injuries is caused by associated injuries. Pulmonary pathology from inhalation injury is the major cause of burn trauma death, with the majority of deaths at the extreme of age.

More than 90% of all burns are considered preventable. Education, particularly in the school-age population, combined with legislative efforts, is helping decrease the number of burn injuries. The American burn association has developed effective public education program. Legislation has been enacted requiring smoke alarms and sprinkler systems in public building, hotels, apartments, and new homes. For the caregiver, an accurate classification of injury, timely intervention, and rapid transport to an appropriate burn facility significantly reduces burn injury mortality and morbidity.

### Etiology

Not all burns are caused by fire. Tissue damage may be secondary to chemical, hot liquids, tar, electricity, lightning or frostbite. The location and duration of exposure to the source affects outcome, regardless of the specific source of burn injury. Specific mechanisms of burn injury are describes in the following sections.

### Thermal Burns

Thermal injuries represent the majority of all burns. They may result from flame, flash, steam, or scalding liquid.

### Scald Burns

Scalds from hot liquids are the most common cause of all burns. Exposure to water at 140°F (60°C) for 30 seconds can cause a deep partial-thickness or full-thickness burn. If water is 156°F (69°C), the same type of burn occurs in only 1 second. As a comparison, freshly brewed coffee is about 180°F (82°C). Tap water scalds occur within seconds and often happen during routine activities, involve large body surface area (BSA) burns, and are the most common source of scald-related deaths. Soups and sauces, which are a thicker consistency, remain in contact longer with the skin and cause deeper burns. Other liquids causing scalds are cooking oil and grease. When used for cooking, oil and grease may reach 400°F (204°C). Immersion burns are usually deep and severe because of prolong contact with a scalding liquid **(Fig.16.1)**.

Specific groups of patients at risk for scald burns include those with preinjury co-morbidities such as neurologic impairment, diabetes, and the extremes of ages. Adults older than 60 years disproportionately suffer burns from hot liquids. It is well documented that older patients are at high-risk for burn injury and experience worse prognoses than younger patients. This has been attributed to their compromised physical health status with chronic, debilitating conditions that increase the risk, exacerbate the extent of the injury, and impair recovery.

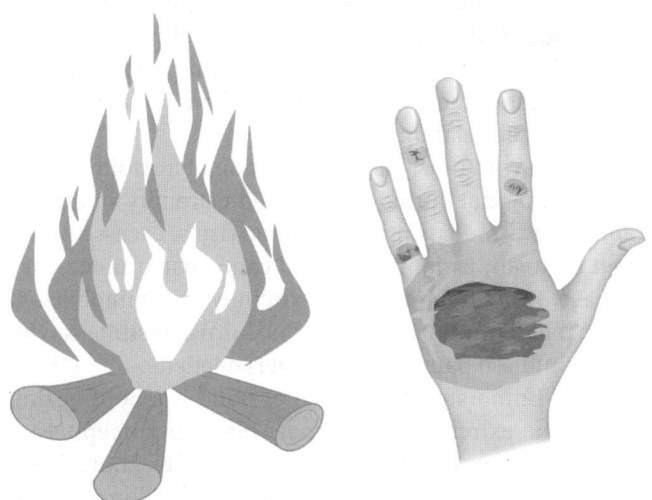

**Fig. 16.1:** Flame burns.

### Flame Burns

Burns from flames are the next common cause of burns. Fortunately, the number of house fires has decreased with increased use of smoke detectors. Most flame burns are caused by carless smoking, motor vehicle crashes, and clothing ignited from stoves or space heaters. Flame burns occurring outdoors are usually caused by misuse of cooking stoves fueled by white gasoline, lanterns in tents, smoking in a sleeping bag, and gasoline or kerosene used in a charcoal fire.

### Flash Burns

Explosions of natural gas, propane, gasoline, or other flammable liquids cause flash burns—the third most common type of thermal burn. The explosion causes intense heat for a very brief time. Flash burns are usually partial thickness, although depth is dependent on the amount and kind of exploding fuel. Flash burns can be large and are often associated with significant thermal damage to the upper airway.

### Contact Burns

Contact with a hot object such as metal, plastic, glass, or hot coals results in contact burns. The burns are usually not extensive but tend to be deep. People involved in industrial accidents often have contact burns associated with crush injuries from machine presses or hot, heavy objects. An increased incidence of contact burns has been seen in toddlers owing to the increased use of wood-burning stoves. The most common injury is to the palm when a child falls against the stove with hands outstretched.

### Electrical Burns

As electricity passes through the body and meets resistance from body tissues, it is converted to heat in direct proportion to amperage and the body's electrical. When electrical current pass through the skin cause entry and exit site. Muscles and nervous are easily damaged compare to bone and fat they are more resistant. The heart, lungs, and brain can sustain immediate damage. The nervous system is particularly sensitive to electrical burns. Damage to the brain, spinal cord, and myelin-producing cells causes devastating transverse myelitis. Autonomic dysfunction can cause pupils to appear fixed and dilated, but this finding should not cause resuscitation efforts to stop. The smaller the body part through which the electricity passes, the more intense the heat and the less it is dissipated. Consequently, extensive damage can occur in the fingers, hands, forearms, toes, feet, and lower legs. If the path is near or through the heart, damage to the heart's electrical conduction system can cause spontaneous ventricular fibrillation or other dysrhythmias. Alternating current is more likely to induce ventricular fibrillation than direct current.

Most lightning injuries do not traverse the body but flow around it, creating a shock wave capable of causing fractures and dislocations. Approximately 74% of patients who survive a lightning strike may have a permanent disability **(Fig. 16.2)**.

## Chemical Burns

Chemicals cause a denaturing of protein within the tissues or a desiccation of cells. Chemical concentration and duration of exposure determine extent of the burn. Alkali products usually cause more tissue damage than acids **(Fig. 16.3)**. A wet chemical should be removed as soon as possible by flushing with copious amount of water. Dry substances should be brushed off the skin before the area is flushed. Care must be taken not to expose the caregiver to the chemical during this procedure. All fluids used to decontaminate the patient should be contained; the fluid should not be allowed to drain into the general drainage system. Chemical burns can be deceiving as to depth; appearances can be similar in surface discoloration until tissue begins to slough days later. Consequently, all chemical burns should be considered deep partial thickness or full thickness until proven otherwise. After removal of chemical wounds are managed in the same manner as thermal burns.

## E-Cigarette Burns

Electronic cigarette use has increased, as have battery explosions causing burn injury. EC use has significantly increased among adolescents, with use reported up to 40% among middle and high school students. ECs have rechargeable lithium-ion batteries that provide nicotine into the inhalable vapor. Most EC explosions are caused by the battery. Lithium batteries can generate massive amount of thermal energy, causing spontaneous explosion. When the battery explodes, the contents, lithium-cobalt and lithium-manganese oxides, are released and may leak onto the skin and be absorbed by the body. The absorption of these elemental metals may lead to heavy metal poisoning. Toxicity from cobalt can affect the heart, skin, and nervous system and cause dysfunction of vision and hearing. Removal of the contents from the wound will decrease the incidence of toxicity. Burns from elemental metals can worsen when exposed to water. Before irrigation and debridement, a lithium test to identify alkali pH should be done and, if positive, the elemental metal should be removed with mineral oil or other nonaqueous solution.

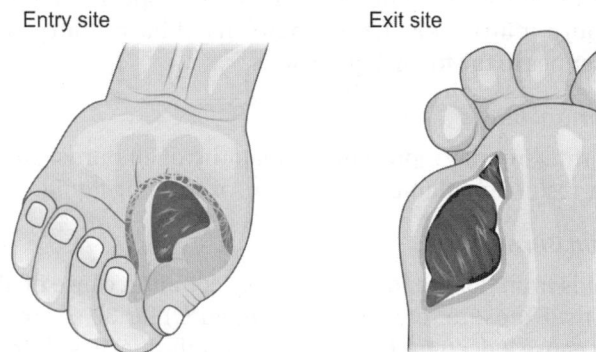

**Fig. 16.2:** Electrical burn.

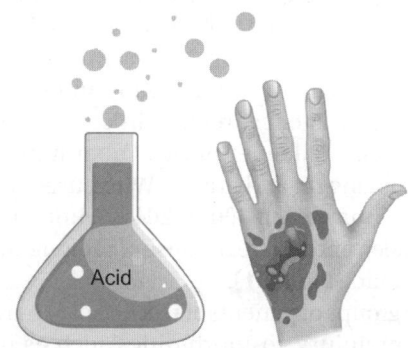

**Fig. 16.3:** Chemical burns.

## Frostbite

Frostbite is actual freezing of tissue from exposure to freezing or below-freezing temperature. In a cold environment, the body attempts to maintain heat by vasoconstriction of peripheral blood vessels to reduce heat exchange. The longer the period of exposure, the more peripheral blood flow is reduced. When extremities are left unprotected, intracellular and extracellular fluids can freeze, forming crystals that damage local tissues. Blood clots may form and impair circulation to the area.

Signs, symptoms, and classification of frostbite are the same as thermal burns. The effected extremity should be rapidly rewarmed using warm water. Use of excessive heat such as steam is dangerous and can cause unnecessary damage. Dress the rewarmed extremity and immobilize it with a padded splint. As with flame burns, frostbite can be very painful, so pain management is needed.

Cold immersion of the foot or hand is a nonfreezing injury. The extremity may appear black, but deep tissue destruction may not be present. Initially, there is an alternating arterial vasospasm and vasodilation with the tissue first cold and numb, progressing to hyperemia in 24 to

48 hours. As the injury progresses to hyperemia, the patient experiences an intense burning sensation and dysesthesia. Tissue damage occurs with resultant edema, blistering, redness, ecchymosis, and ulceration. Attention to hygiene will prevent local infection, cellulitis, or gangrene.

Patients who have exposure to chronic, repetitive, damp cold may develop chilblain, or pernio. This is a dermatologic condition, usually occurring on the face, dorsum of the hands and feet, or any area chronically exposed to a cold environment. Signs and symptoms include pruritic, reddened skin lesions. These lesions, with continued exposure, ulcerate or develop hemorrhagic lesions progressing to scarring, fibrosis, or atrophy with itching, tenderness, and pain. Symptoms are controlled by protection from further exposure and the use of antiadrenergics or calcium channel blockers **(Fig. 16.4)**.

## Pathophysiology

Burn injury occurs when skin is exposed to more energy than it can absorb. The cause of the burn may vary, but local and systemic responses are generally similar. To understand the pathophysiology of burn, one must first understand the functions of the skin, which consists of two layers—the epidermis and the dermis. The epidermis, the outer layer of the basement layer of cells, consists of cells that migrate upward to become surface keratin. The dermis, or inner layer, consists of collagen and elastic fibers and contains hair follicles, sweat and sebaceous glands, nerve endings, and blood vessels. The skin is the largest organ of the body and acts as an infection barrier, vapor barrier, and a heat regulator.

Three zones of tissue damage occur at the burn site. First is the central zone of coagulation, an area of irreversible damage. Concentrically surrounding this area is the zone of stasis, where capillary and small vessel stasis occurs. The ultimate fate of the burn wound depends on resolution or progression of the zone of stasis. Edema formation and prolonged compromised of blood flow to this area cause a deeper, more extensive wound; therefore depth and severity of burn wounds may not be known for 2 or more days after the initial injury. The third zone of damage is the zone of hyperemia, an area of superficial damage that heals quickly on its own.

The body responds to the burn injury with varying degrees of tissue damage, cellular impairment, and fluid shifts. A brief decrease in blood flow to the affected area is followed by a marked increase in blood flow to the affected area is followed by a marked increase in arteriolar vasodilation. Damaged tissues release mediators that initiate an inflammatory response. Histamine, serotonin, prostaglandin derivatives, and the complement cascade are all activated. Release of proinflammatory mediators combined with vasodilation causes increased capillary permeability, leading to intravascular fluid loss and wound edema. For burn injuries of less than 20% TBSA, these actions are usually limited to the burn site, with 90% of the edema present by 4 hours. The edema tends to reside within the dermis, and resorption is complete by 4 days, as the effected TBSA goes beyond 20%, local response becomes systemic. With large burns, the overwhelming inflammation, coagulation, and fibrinolysis can continue and constantly be reactivated. The cytokine activity creates a state of exaggerated or reactivated inflammation that includes organ involvement such as acute respiratory distress syndrome (ARDS), systemic inflammatory response syndrome (SIRS), and multiple organ dysfunction syndrome (MODS). Large burns cause a hypermetabolic state that has multiple harmful physiologic derangements associated with it. Derangements noted are muscle catabolism, hepatic dysfunction, and immunosuppression. Basal metabolic rate increases from insensible fluid loss, which, along with fluid shift, produce hypovolemia. Hypoproteinemia resulting from increased capillary permeability aggravates edema in nonburned tissue. Capillary permeability increase for 2 to 3 weeks, with the most significant changes occurring in the first 24 to 36 hours **(Flowchart 16.1)**.

Initially, blood viscosity increases when hematocrit rises secondary to vascular fluid shifts into the interstitium. Because of a marked increase in peripheral vascular resistance, decreased intravascular fluid volume, and increased blood viscosity, cardiac output falls. Capillary leakage and depressed cardiac output can depress central nervous system function, causing restlessness, followed by lethargy, and finally coma. Decreased cardiac output, decreased blood volume, and intense sympathetic response. Levels of thromboxane A2, a potent vasoconstrictor, are significantly increased in burned patients and contribute to mesenteric vasoconstriction and decreased splanchnic

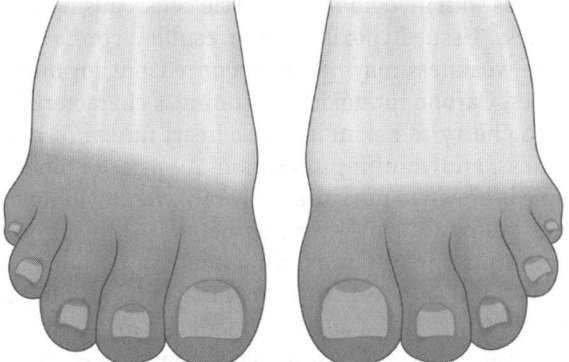

**Fig. 16.4:** Cold frost.

**Flowchart 16.1:** Pathophysiology of burn.

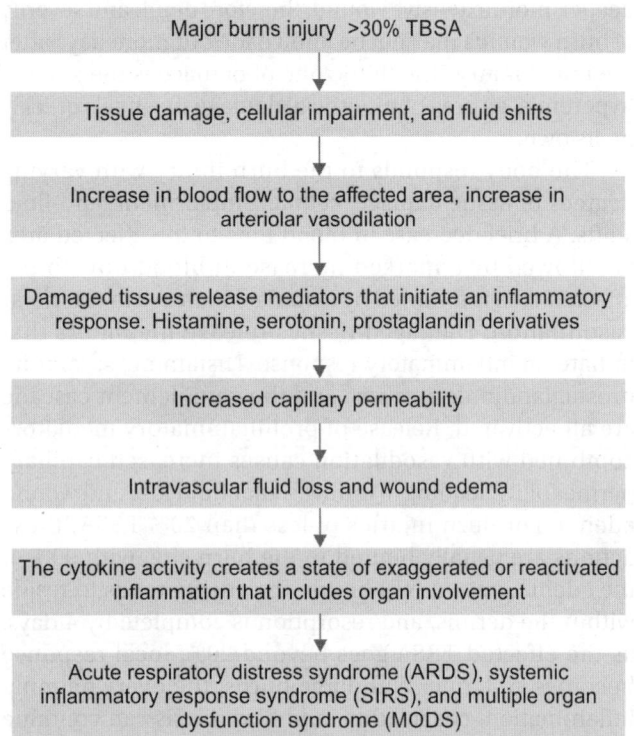

blood flow. Decreased flow can convert a zone of stasis to a zone of coagulation, which increased depth of the burn. Decreased circulating plasma with increased hematocrit can cause hemoglobinuria, which can lead to renal failure. Immediate hemolysis of red cells reduced by approximately 30% of normal. Platelet count and platelet survival time initially drop drastically and then continue to rebound increase for 5 days after injury. This period is followed by a rebound increase in platelets over the next 2 to 3 weeks.

Cardiovascular changes begin immediately after a burn. The extent varies with burn site and presence of additional injuries. Patient with an uncomplicated burn of less than 15% TBSA can usually be treated with oral fluid resuscitation. Patient with burns of the TBSA that surpass 20% have massive shifts of fluid and electrolytes from intravascular to extravascular spaces. This shift begins to resolve in 18 to 36 hours; however, normal extracellular volume is not completely restored until 7 to 10 days after the burn injury, if intravascular volume is not replenished, hypovolemic shock occurs. If untreated, the patient can die of cardiovascular collapse. Inadequate treatment may lead to renal failure from acute tubular necrosis.

The vasoconstriction of the mesentery mentioned previously predisposes the patient to gastric distention, aspiration, and ulceration (curling's ulcer). A patient with a burn of greater than 20% TBSA should have a gastric tube placed to decompress the stomach and avoid aspiration. Admission order will include medication to reduce gastric secretion and early enteral feeding (within 24 hours of injury) to meet basic energy needs.

The hypermetabolic response after burn trauma far exceeds the response seen in other forms of trauma. The patient's metabolic rate can increase as much as two to three times the normal rate. Release of catabolic hormones, including catecholamines, cortisol, and glucagon, initiates a persistent hypermetabolic response. This response causes accelerated breakdown of skeletal muscle, decreased protein synthesis, increased peripheral lipolysis, and increase utilization of glucose, which rapidly depletes glycogen stores. It manifests clinically as severe muscle wasting, decreased muscle strength, and increased liver fat with hepatomegaly and functional impairment. The hypermetabolic response is commensurate with the size of the burn. The adverse effects of the response are managed through nutritional and pharmacologic intervention to improve net nitrogen balance, preserve lean body mass, decrease cardiac work, and decrease hepatic fatty infiltration.

Inhalation injury or smoke inhalation is a syndrome comprising three distinct problems: carbon monoxide intoxication, upper airway obstruction, and chemical monoxide intoxication, upper airway and lung parenchyma. The majority of deaths from fire are caused by smoke inhalation rather than the burn injury or its sequelae. A burn injury with associated inhalation injury increases the mortality rate. Pulmonary complication, associated with inhalation injury directly contribute to death in up to 77% of patients with combined cutaneous and inhalation injury.

Carbon monoxide intoxication is the most common killer of victims of fire. Most people who die in a fire have been overcome by carbon monoxide before they sustain a burn injury. In the body, carbon monoxide has a 240 times greater affinity for hemoglobin than oxygen, which causes inadequate oxygen delivery to the tissues. Carbon monoxide combines with myoglobin in muscle cells, causing muscle weakness. Tissue hypoxia and the resultant confusion and muscle weakness may be the major reasons for most fire fatalities. Carbon monoxide poisoning is characterized by pink to cherry-red skin, increase heart rare and rhythm, dizziness, and vomiting sensation. An arterial blood gas sample is drawn to measure the carboxyhemoglobin level. Levels below 15% are rarely associated with symptoms of carbon monoxide poisoning and can be normal for a heavy smoker. Levels of 15 to 40% are associated with varying disturbances such as headache and confusion. Level greater than 40% are associated with coma. Reliance on pulse oximetry or an oxygen saturation of arterial blood

($SaO_2$) that is calculated from the partial pressure of oxygen ($PO_2$) rather than measured on a CO oximeter may result in failure to diagnose carbon monoxide poisoning. Most pulse oximeters cannot reliably differentiate between oxygenated hemoglobin and hemoglobin with carbon monoxide and will give a false high measurement. All patients with suspected carbon monoxide poisoning should receive 100% oxygen.

Cyanide poisoning may also occur during a fire and can rapidly result in death. Hydrogen cyanide is highly toxic and can be formed in high-temperature combustion from materials such as polyurethane, acrylonitrile, wool, cotton, and nylon. Cyanide binds to a variety of iron—containing enzyme, one of which plays a critical role in electron transport during oxidative phosphorylation. Even minute amount of bound cyanide can inhibit aerobic metabolism and rapidly result in death.

The patient with cyanide poisoning will rapidly develop coma, apnea, cardiac dysfunction, and severe lactic acidosis. Diagnosis can cyanide and still die owing to the combination. The two are synergistic because carbon monoxide primarily affects oxygen delivery and cyanide affects oxygen utilization.

Thermal injury associated with facial burns. Upper airway obstruction is the result of intrinsic or extrinsic edema that may lead to airway occlusion at or above the vocal cords. Edema progresses rapidly, totally occluding the airway in minutes to hours. This injury is primarily a thermal injury, resulting in tissue damage in the posterior pharynx. Upper airway edema will usually manifest within 24 hours of the injury. Management for airway edema is early intubation or tracheostomy if intubation is not possible. If the patient exhibits dyspnea, stridor, or cyanosis, suspect impending airway obstruction and be prepared to assist with intubation that may be difficult.

Thermal injury below the vocal, cords is rare because the posterior pharynx is such an efficient heat exchange system. Injuries that occur in an oxygen-enriched atmosphere or one in which the person was inhaling explosive gases (e.g., during inhalation anesthesia) also cause true thermal injury below the vocal cords. True thermal injury to the lungs is almost always fatal.

Chemical injury to the lower airway is a common problem with inhalation of smoke. Many lower-molecular-weight constituents of smoke are toxic to the mucosa and alveoli because of their pH or the ability to form free radicals. Chemical injury, from acids and aldehydes in the smoke, may damage the lung parenchyma. These chemical, attached to carbon particles in the smoke, are heavier than air, so they are readily inhaled and find their way down the bronchi into alveoli. Although the compounds produce acute neutrophilic airway inflammation, the symptoms (cough, bronchorrhea, dyspnea, and wheezing) may not appear for 12 to 26 hours. Many centers perform early bronchoscopy to determine whether there is injury to the lower airways. The bronchoscopy will reveal erythema, edema, carbonaceous debris, and ulceration of the airway. This condition may lead to rapid development of ARDS over 24 to 48 hours. Severe inhalation injury may increase the patient's fluid needs in the first 24 hours by as much as 50% of calculated values.

## BURN ASSESSMENT

Burn depth and extent are assessed to determine the severity of burn injury. In many case, final determination is not made for several days.

### Depth of Burn

Burns are described as partial thickness or full thickness. Identification of the depth of injury may be difficult initially because depth may actually increase over time as edema forms and circulation to the area of injury is compromised. This process usually peaks at 48 hours; therefore a more accurate determination of depth can be made between 48 and 72 hours. Depth determination is not a priority during initial resuscitation. Burns are classified into three main categories based on the severity of the injury and the depth of skin damage. These categories are first-degree burns, second-degree burns, and third-degree burns (**Fig. 16.5**).

### *First-degree Burns*

First-degree burns are considered the least severe type of burn. They only affect the outer layer of the skin (the

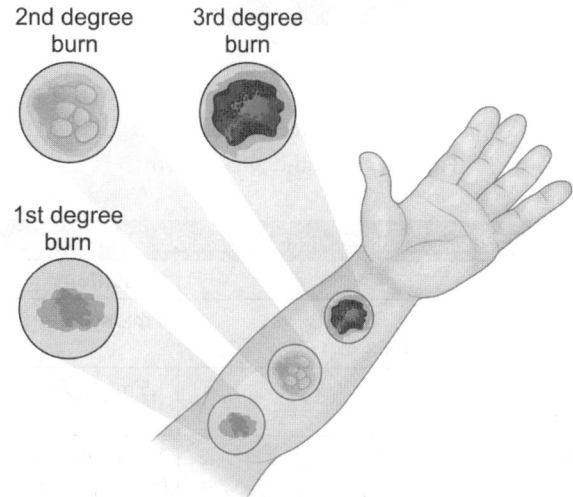

**Fig. 16.5:** Stages of burns.

epidermis) and cause redness, swelling, and pain. The affected area may also be slightly dry or itchy. These burns can usually be treated at home with first aid measures like cooling the burn with cool water, applying aloe vera gel, and taking pain relievers. These burns typically heal within a week without scarring.

### *Second-degree Burns*

Second-degree burns are more severe and involve damage to the outer layer of skin (the epidermis) and the underlying layer of skin (the dermis). Symptoms include pain, redness, swelling, and the formation of blisters. These burns may require medical attention to prevent infection and promote healing. Treatment typically involves cleaning the wound, applying dressings and creams to prevent infection, and possibly administering pain medication. Healing time for second-degree burns can range from a few weeks to several months, depending on the severity of the burn and the patient's overall health **(Fig. 16.6)**.

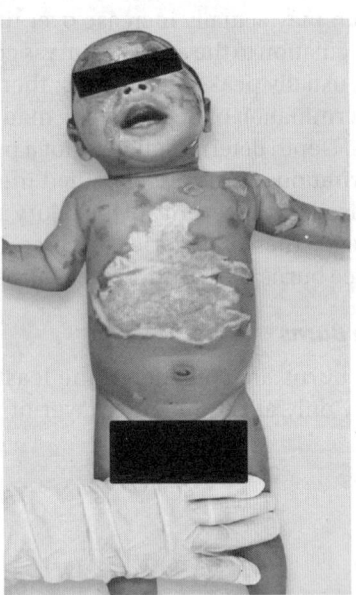

**Fig. 16.6:** Second-degree of burns.

### *Third-degree Burns*

Third-degree burns are the most severe type of burn and involve damage to all layers of the skin, including the underlying tissues and possibly the bones and organs. Symptoms include charred or blackened skin, numbness or tingling, and severe pain or discomfort. Third-degree burns require immediate medical attention and typically require hospitalization and specialized burn care. Treatment may involve debridement (removal of dead tissue), skin grafting, and long-term wound care. The recovery time for third-degree burns can be lengthy and may require physical therapy or rehabilitation to regain full function. In severe cases, permanent disfigurement or disability may occur.

### *Extent of Burn*

Extent of injury for thermal and chemical injuries is assessed by using formulas such as the rule of nines, Brooke formula, or Lund and Browder table **(Table 16.1)**. The caregiver should remember to modify the rule of nines for children; the head and neck of an infant represent 18% of BSA, whereas the legs represent 14% for each lower extremity. To correct for age, 1% is subtracted from the head for each year of age through 10 years, and 0.5% is added to each lower extremity. To calculate burn surface area palm method is also been used. The palm is visualized over the burned areas. To obtain a more accurate estimate of the extent of burns, both burned and unburned areas are calculated. The two estimates should then be compared. If the total is more or less than 100%, the areas should be reestimated. Assessing extent of injury in electrical burns is more difficult because surface damage is minimal compared with underlying damage. When discussing an electrical injury, describing the injury anatomically is more important than calculating percentage of BSA burned **(Fig. 16.7)**.

## Severity of Burn

The severity of burn injury is based on assessment of extent and depth of injury, patient age, and presence of concomitant injuries, smoke inhalation, and pre-existing

| Table 16.1: Fluid calculation for burn patient. | | |
|---|---|---|
| **Formula** | **Crystalloid** | **Colloid** |
| Parkland (Baxter and Shires) 1968 | 4 mL/Kg/% | |
| Brooke (Reiss et al) | 1.5 mL/Kg/% | 0.5 mL/Kg/% |
| Evan's | 1 mL/Kg/% NS | 1 mL/Kg/% |
| Galveston | 5000 mL/ TSA burned + 1500/TSA | |

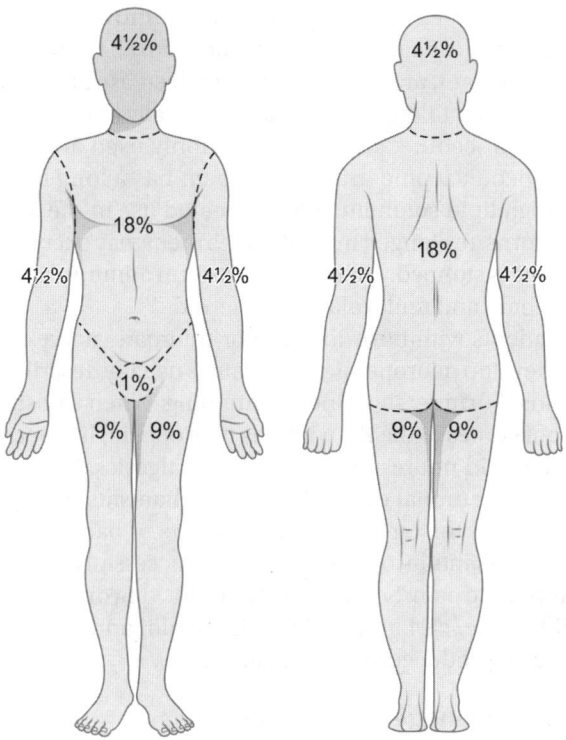

**Fig. 16.7:** Rule of nine.

disease. Care of patients with burns of different severity is determined by availability of specialized care facilities. Initial stabilization of the patient with a burn should be available in any community hospital with 24-hour emergency capabilities. Patient with minor burns may be treated as outpatient or admitted to the community hospital. Patients with moderate burns may be treated in a community hospital with appropriate staff and facilities to deliver burn care or transferred to a specialized burn care facility. Patient with major burns require care in a specialized burn care facility. Transfer agreements with special-care units should be develop in advance to facilitate timely and uneventful transfer. Any patient with concomitant trauma is at increased risk for morbidity or mortality and should be treated in a trauma center until he or she is stable and then transferred to a burn center as appropriate.

# FLUID AND ELECTROLYTE THERAPY

## Fluid Balance

Water is the most abundant fluid medium in the body, composing 65% of total body weight for the average adult, 75% in a full-term infant, and as little as 45% in an older adults. In a healthy physiologic state, this fluid medium has a constant balance of electrolytes controlled by a unique system of checks and balance. Fluid and electrolyte abnormalities may be caused by burns, gastrointestinal (GI), urologic, cardiac, respiratory, and endocrine disease, as well as many forms of traumatic injury.

- Fluid loss greater in children
- Normal blood volume
  - Neonate 90 mL/Kg
  - Children 80 mL/Kg
  - Adult 70 mL/Kg
- Resuscitation formula may result in sub-optimal resuscitation because of difference in BSA in comparison to adult.

### IV Fluid: Parkland Formula

- Only RL
- Total amount of fluid in 24 hours: 4 mL*Kg*% TBSA
- Time starts from time of burn: Half in 1st 8 hours another half next 16 hours
- Additional maintenance fluid for children <15 Kg.

### Principles of Fluid Correction

- Maximum fluid given in first 8 hours of burn because of capillary leakage which gets restored within 8 to 12 hours
- **First day:** Only crystalloid (RL) is given
- **Second day:** Colloid is given to reduce edema

Total amount of fluid to be given in 1st 24 hour:
- **Adult:** 2 mL*Kg*%TBSA RL
- **Pediatric (below 15 Kg):** 2 mL* kg*% TBSA

Formulas are guidelines only resuscitation should be individualized and described in **Table 16.1**.

### Assessment of Resuscitation

- Capillary refill
- Heart rate
- Mental status
- ABG
- BP
- Urine output (1–2 mL/kg/hour)

### Nursing Management

Nurses play a crucial role in the management of fluid and electrolyte therapy in burns. The nursing management of fluid and electrolyte therapy in burns involves several key steps:

- **Assessment:** The nurse must assess the patient's fluid and electrolyte status to determine the appropriate treatment. This includes monitoring vital signs, urine output, and laboratory values such as serum electrolytes, blood gases, and hematocrit.

- **Monitoring:** The nurse must monitor the patient's fluid intake and output, including intravenous fluids, oral fluids, and urine output. This helps to ensure that the patient is receiving adequate hydration and electrolyte replacement.
- **Documentation:** Accurate and timely documentation of fluid and electrolyte intake, output, and laboratory values is essential for effective communication between healthcare providers and for tracking the patient's progress.
- **Administration of IV fluids:** Nurse must administer IV fluids as ordered, ensuring that the infusion rate is appropriate and that the IV site is properly maintained. Nurse must also monitor the patient for signs of fluid overload or electrolyte imbalances.
- **Patient education:** The nurse must educate the patient and family members about the importance of fluid and electrolyte management, including the signs and symptoms of dehydration and electrolyte imbalances, and the need for regular monitoring.
- **Collaboration:** The nurse must collaborate with other members of the healthcare team, including physicians, pharmacists, and dietitians, to develop and implement a comprehensive plan of care that addresses the patient's fluid and electrolyte needs.

Overall, the nursing management of fluid and electrolyte therapy in burns requires careful assessment, monitoring, documentation, administration of IV fluids, patient education, and collaboration with the healthcare team.

## PAIN MANAGEMENT

Burn wound are exquisitely painful and deserve special consideration. The pain of primary tissue damage and nerve damage may be worsened by primary and secondary hyperalgesia. Intravenous opioid administration should be the prime treatment for burn pain. During initial resuscitation, analgesics or anesthetic should be titrated to effect. After 24 hours, decreased plasma protein levels increase bioavailability of free drugs, especially those that are protein bound. Giving pain medication as needed may increase the patient's awareness of pain and other symptoms. Administering opioids on a schedule, based on drug half-life or by continuous infusion, can facilitate the patient's ability to cope with the pain. The opioid of choice has been IV morphine at 25 to 50 mcg/kg per hour, titrating to avoid respiratory depression. Fentanyl may also be used for some patients. For the burn-injured patient, pain can be made worse by fear of pain or disfigurement, anxiety related to loss of control, and distress over losing family members or material possessions at the time of injury. Anxiety decreased pain tolerance. Reducing anxiety minimizes interplay between acute pain and sympathetic arousal. For the burn-injured patient, anxiolytics may help decrease anxiety and improve pain tolerance. They are especially helpful during painful procedure. The most commonly used anxiolytics are benzodiazepine drugs. Diazepam has a long half-life and high lipid solubility. After repeated use in the patient with burns, prolonged mental impairment may occur when the drug is stopped. Therefore short-term administration of lorazepam and midazolam is preferred.

Patients with burn-induced or traumatic nerve injury may develop neuropathic pain. Pain is usually described as tingling, burning, shooting, or numbing. When a postburn patient comes to the ED with this type of pain, it is because the pain did not respond to opiate analgesics. Drugs that decrease neuronal excitability by mechanisms other than opiate receptors are useful for this type of pain. Tricyclic antidepressants in low doses are often successful in relieving neuropathic pain. Sodium channel-blocking drugs such as IV lidocaine, carbamazepine, phenytoin, and mexiletine have also produced successful analgesia.

### Nursing Management in Pain

Pain management is an essential aspect of nursing care for patients with burn injuries, as these patients can experience severe pain that can impact their physical and emotional well-being. The nursing management of pain in burn patients includes several key steps:

- **Assessment:** The nurse must assess the patient's pain intensity, location, and quality, as well as any factors that may exacerbate or alleviate the pain. This helps to develop an individualized pain management plan.
- **Nonpharmacological interventions:** The nurse can use nonpharmacological interventions such as distraction, relaxation techniques, and positioning to help alleviate pain.
- **Pharmacological interventions:** The nurse can administer pain medications as ordered by the physician, including opioids, nonsteroidal anti-inflammatory drugs (NSAIDs), and acetaminophen. The nurse must closely monitor the patient for adverse effects of these medications, such as respiratory depression or gastrointestinal bleeding.
- **Wound care:** Proper wound care can help reduce pain and discomfort in burn patients. The nurse can help to manage wound pain by using topical analgesics, such as lidocaine, and by providing wound care education to the patient and family members.
- **Patient education:** The nurse can educate the patient and family members about the importance of pain management, the side effects of pain medications,

and nonpharmacological interventions that can help alleviate pain.
- **Collaboration:** The nurse must collaborate with other members of the healthcare team, including physicians, pharmacists, and physical therapists, to develop and implement a comprehensive plan of care that addresses the patient's pain management needs.

Overall, the nursing management of pain in burn patients requires careful assessment, nonpharmacological interventions, pharmacological interventions, wound care, patient education, and collaboration with the healthcare team. The nurse must prioritize pain management to help the patient recover from burn injuries and improve their overall quality of life.

## WOUND CARE

Wound care should be delayed until the patient's condition is stabilized; however, initial management must include removal of jewelry and constrictive clothing. Wound must be kept covered with clean sheets until more definitive care can be provided. All patients with full-thickness burns are assessed for circulatory problem. Capillary refill and the presence of paresthesia are evaluated with distal pulses checked by Doppler ultrasonography. Because burn tissue does not stretch, swelling beneath burned tissue compromised circulation because of lack of elasticity. If the patient has signs of compromised, escharotomy are indicated. Significant bleeding that occurs with escharotomy can be controlled with an electrocautery unit or small hemostats. After the procedure is completed, a topical antibacterial agent is applied to the open wound, a light pressure dressing is applied, and the extremity is slightly elevated.

- **Thermal burns:** Thermal burns may be secondary to flame, flash, scalds or hot objects. Thermal burns are cleaned with mild soap and water. The use of skin disinfectant, such as povidone-iodine (Betadine), has been shown to inhibit the healing process and is discouraged. Ruptured blisters should be removed, but intact blisters may be left alone and should never be aspirated with a needle because of this chance of infection. The wound is covered immediately with a topical antibacterial agent such as silver sulfadiazine (Silvadene) or bacitracin. Burns of the face should be left open and covered be a topical antibiotic ointment such as bacitracin, which is reapplied every 6 hours after gently washing the skin.
- **Chemical burns:** Chemical burns should be immediately irrigated with tap water or normal saline for at least 5 to 10 minutes to remove the chemical. Clothing and jewelry are removed, and unburned areas adjacent to the burned areas are rinsed. These areas can be injured but may not hurt, blister, or turn red immediately. If the chemical dry, it can be brushed from the patient before irrigating. After the wound is thoroughly irrigated, it is treated like a thermal burn. Chemical burns of the eye are an ophthalmologic emergency. The eye must be irrigated thoroughly with water.
- **Electrical injuries:** Electrical injuries are different from thermal and chemical burns. These wounds may be present beneath normal-looking skin or minor to severe exit wounds. Wounds should be cleaned gently with a 0.25% povidone-iodine solution using sterile water or 0.9% sodium chloride; they rarely need immediately debridement. Topical agents such as mafenide acetate (sulfamylon) solution that deeply penetrate tissue are used to cover the wound. Light dressing may be applied to cover these often grotesque wounds; however, dressing must not interfere with assessment for circulation compromise and possible compartment syndrome. High-voltage injuries are associated with severe muscle contractions, so radiographs of the cervical spine may be indicated.

Electrical injuries of the extremities cause significant damage that leads to tissue swelling. Consequently, these patients are at risk for compartment syndrome. Symptoms associated with this condition include pain, pallor, paresthesia, pulselessness, paralysis, and pressure in the affected areas. Fasciotomies are used to relieve compartment syndrome.

- **Tar or asphalt burns:** Tar or asphalt burns may be deep or superficial depending on the temperature of the tar, which may range from 150°F to more than 600°F, as well as the length of time the skin was in contact with it. Immediate treatment of a tar burn is to cool the tar, but do not try to peel it off the patient's skin. Using mineral oil, petroleum jelly, or a solvent such as Medi-sol-loosens the tar. In areas where the burn is not circumferential, oil or ointment is applied and the burn is covered with a light dressing. Dressing is removed in 4 to 12 hours, oil or ointment is applied and the burn is covered with a light dressing. Dressings are removed in 4 to 12 hours, oil or ointment is reapplied, and a new dressing is applied. For areas with circumferential tar, oil or ointment can be applied with light dressing and changed every 20 to 30 minutes until tar is removed. After the tar is removed, the burn is treated as a thermal injury.

### Equipment

- Wash with savlon and saline
- Debride blisters

- Antiseptic dressing with silver sulphadiazine 1%
- Thick layer of oint
- Gauge pad/roller
- Compressive bandage

### *Dressing for Special Sites*
- **Face:** Neosporin eye oint only
- **Ear:** Occlusive fluffy dressing
- **Hand:** Splintage in position of function
- **Wrist:** Extension
- **MP joint:** Flexion
- **IP joint:** Extension
- **Thumb:** Abduction

## Diagnostic Procedure

Diagnostic procedure that may assist during the resuscitation of the burn patient are the following:

### *Laboratory*
- Complete blood count with differential
- Serum electrolytes
- Carboxyhemoglobin
- Type and crossmatch/screen blood
- Urinalysis, pregnancy test in females of childbearing age
- Arterial blood gas

### *Radiography*
- Chest
- Other X-ray examinations as indicated for associated trauma

### *Other Special Studies as Indicated for Associated Trauma*
- Focused assessment sonography for trauma (FAST)
- Computed tomography (CT) scan as indicated by assessment findings
- Possible peritoneal lavage
- 12-lead electrocardiogram (ECG) if electrical or lightning injury

## Nursing Management in Burn Wound

Wound care is a critical aspect of burn management, as the severity of burn injuries can cause significant damage to the skin and underlying tissues. The goals of wound care in burns are to promote healing, prevent infection, and minimize scarring. The nursing management of wound care in burns includes the following steps:

- **Assessment:** The nurse must assess the extent, depth, and location of the burn injury, as well as any associated injuries or medical conditions that may affect wound healing.
- **Cleansing:** The nurse must cleanse the burn wound using sterile saline or other appropriate wound cleansing solutions to remove debris, bacteria, and other contaminants. The nurse must use gentle pressure and avoid scrubbing the wound, which can cause further damage.
- **Debridement:** In some cases, the nurse may need to debride the wound, which involves removing dead tissue and debris to promote healing. This can be done through surgical debridement or through the use of enzymatic or mechanical debridement agents.
- **Dressing:** The nurse must apply appropriate wound dressings to promote healing and prevent infection. The type of dressing used will depend on the extent and depth of the burn injury, as well as any associated medical conditions.
- **Pain management:** Proper pain management is essential for wound care in burns. The nurse can use topical or systemic analgesics, such as opioids or non-steroidal anti-inflammatory drugs (NSAIDs), to help alleviate pain.
- **Patient education:** The nurse can educate the patient and family members about the importance of proper wound care, including dressing changes and infection prevention. The nurse can also provide education about the signs and symptoms of wound infection and when to seek medical attention.
- **Collaboration:** The nurse must collaborate with other members of the healthcare team, including physicians, wound care specialists, and physical therapists, to develop and implement a comprehensive plan of care that addresses the patient's wound care needs.

Overall, the nursing management of wound care in burns requires careful assessment, cleansing, debridement, dressing, pain management, patient education, and collaboration with the healthcare team. The nurse must prioritize wound care to promote healing, prevent infection, and improve the patient's overall outcome.

## INFECTION CONTROL

Infection commonly occurs because it affects our immune system. Due to burns, it loss the protection on skin, risk for exposure of outside germs from the environment, and the cell that protect from entry of microorganism are damage. As a nurse some measure to be taken to prevent infection this is the huge risk in acute phase.

- **Protective isolation:** Hand hygiene, whenever giving care to severe burns must wear hair cover, gloves, gown, mask, and shoe covering in order to prevent infection.
  - When doing room care should use sterile gloves
  - Sterile lines, covers and gloves for wound care.

- Patients should last tetanus shot for more than 5 to 10 years, because there is risk of developing illness and infection.
- **Temperature regulation loss:**
  - Patients with severe burns will lose the ability to temperature regulation, especially if hypodermis is affected.
  - The room temperature should be 85–100°F, monitor patient if shivering keeps in warm temperature.
- **Pain management:** IV route is the best for medication and have proper absorption.
- **Wound care:** There are two types of wound care open and closed wound care. Pre medicate before performing wound care. Cleaning of burn are by hydrotherapy or shower is painful procedure. Debridement must remove necrotic tissue.

## Nursing Management in Infection Control

Infection control is a critical aspect of nursing care for patients with burn injuries, as these patients are at increased risk of developing infections due to compromised skin barriers and weakened immune systems. The nursing management of infection control in burns patients includes the following steps:

- **Hand hygiene:** The nurse must perform frequent hand hygiene using soap and water or alcohol-based hand sanitizer to prevent the spread of microorganisms.
- **Personal protective equipment (PPE):** The nurse must wear appropriate PPE, such as gloves, gowns, and masks, when caring for burns patients to prevent the spread of infections.
- **Environmental cleanliness:** The nurse must ensure that the patient's environment, including their room and equipment, is kept clean and disinfected to prevent the spread of infections.
- **Isolation precautions:** The nurse may need to implement isolation precautions, such as contact or airborne precautions, if the patient has a known or suspected infection.
- **Wound care:** Proper wound care is essential for infection control in burns patients. The nurse must ensure that the burn wounds are cleaned, dressed, and monitored for signs of infection.
- **Antibiotic therapy:** The nurse must administer antibiotics as ordered by the physician to treat or prevent infections in burns patients. The nurse must monitor the patient for adverse effects of antibiotics and ensure that they complete the full course of treatment.
- **Patient education:** The nurse can educate the patient and family members about the importance of infection control, including hand hygiene, wound care, and antibiotic therapy.
- **Collaboration:** The nurse must collaborate with other members of the healthcare team, including physicians, infection control specialists, and pharmacists, to develop and implement a comprehensive plan of care that addresses the patient's infection control needs.

Overall, the nursing management of infection control in burns patients requires careful attention to hand hygiene, PPE, environmental cleanliness, isolation precautions, wound care, antibiotic therapy, patient education, and collaboration with the healthcare team. The nurse must prioritize infection control to prevent the spread of infections and improve the patient's overall outcome.

## PREVENTION AND MANAGEMENT OF BURN COMPLICATION

The majority of complications are due to delays in the identification of problem in early stages. Prevention of scars and post burn changes over the vital organs and special sense organs and deformities involvement in muscle, ligaments and bones. Prevention of complication is an major integral section of burns management. Usually all burn patient should be under the constant physiotherapy support, and able to use appropriate pressure or compression garment soon after the surgery and splints in order to avoid scars and able to maintaining the positioning and function of the vital organs like extension, rotation of the neck movements simultaneously alignment with the thorax, abduction and adduction of all the joints in propitiate with the ligament of the mid-point of the body.

When the joints are healed at all areas, they must be lubricated, and appropriate splints should used in order to avoid the contractures formation. Constant massage at the burn scar site with nonirritant lubricant like coconut oil reduces in preventing hypertrophy. Finally, should provide psychological support to burn patients.

Burns can result in a range of complications, including infection, scarring, and reduced mobility. Prevention and management of these complications are crucial to ensure optimal healing and recovery.

### Tips on Preventing and Managing Burn Complications

- **Infection prevention:** Burns can create an environment for bacteria to grow, leading to infection. To prevent infection, keep the burn clean and covered with a sterile dressing. Use a topical antibiotic cream or ointment as prescribed by your healthcare provider. Watch for signs of infection, such as increasing pain, redness, swelling, or drainage, and report them to your healthcare provider immediately.

- **Scar management:** Burns can lead to scarring, which can be unsightly and limit movement. To manage scarring, keep the burn area moisturized with a non-fragranced lotion or cream. Massage the area to prevent stiffness and contractures. Use silicone sheets or gels, or other scar management products as prescribed by your healthcare provider.
- **Pain management:** Burns can be painful. To manage pain, use over-the-counter pain relievers or prescription pain medication as prescribed by your healthcare provider. Relaxation techniques, such as deep breathing or guided imagery, can also help reduce pain.
- **Physical therapy:** Burns can limit movement, especially in joints. Physical therapy can help improve mobility and prevent contractures. Your healthcare provider can recommend a physical therapist who can work with you to develop an exercise program.
- **Nutrition:** Burns can increase your body's need for nutrients. Eat a well-balanced diet that includes plenty of protein, which is essential for healing.
- **Emotional support:** Burns can be emotionally challenging. Seek emotional support from family, friends, or a mental health professional. They can provide emotional support and help you develop coping strategies.

By following these tips, you can prevent and manage burn complications and promote healing and recovery. Remember to always follow your healthcare provider's recommendations and seek medical attention if you have concerns about your burn or its healing.

## GRAFTS AND FLAPS

Skin is the best dressing material. In 3rd degree and 4th degree burns skin grafting is required. There are different types of skin grafting example autografts, isograft, allografts, xenograft. Types of autograft are sheet and meshed. Sheet graft id used in cosmetic areas like face, neck, hands. Meshed graft often used to cover larger wound. In split thickness skin graft, epidermis and dermis is involved but in full thickness skin graft all three layers are involved epidermis, dermis and subcutaneous **(Fig. 16.8)**. In composite graft two tissue elements are included they are skin and cartilage. The indications for grafting are flame burns, frictional burns and chronic leg ulcers. The nursing management in preoperative preparation is consent from both donor and recipient, hemogram, plain radiograph, wound care and antibiotics. Intraoperative management—anesthesia care, positioning, commonly supine, and depends on the site, cleaning and draping the donor site first and harvesting, graft preparation and dressing. After care in split thickness skin graft donor site should be inspect for 2 weeks and recipient site 5th day

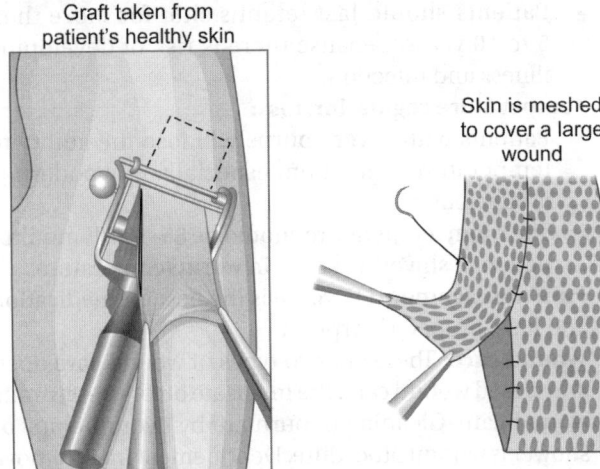

**Fig. 16.8:** Grafts and flaps.

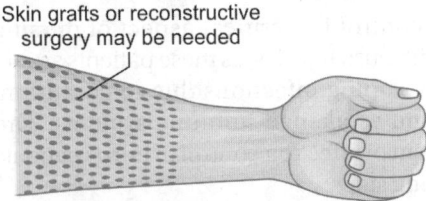

**Fig. 16.9:** Reconstructive surgery.

and in full thickness skin graft donor site and recipient site for 1 week and depends on the site, observe for skin changes. Advantages of full thickness grafting are most resembles normal skin, minimal secondary contraction, resistant to trauma, good sensation. Disadvantages are poorest survival, donor site must be closed surgically, donor sites are limited. Complications such as donor site morbidity, graft loss, hyperpigmentation, poor cosmesis.

In grafts and flaps absolute indication must be met, meticulous procedure is required postoperative care is important. Sin substitutes are also used in grafting they are synthetic bio-substitutes, e.g., presterilized sheets like Tegaderm or opsite they are best for partial thickness burns as they control evaporative water loss and also helps in formation of dermal bed. The skin substitutes use for full thickness burns are integra, therafoam, biobrain, omniderm, trancyte, etc. However, they are cost effective and rarely used **(Fig. 16.9)**.

Grafts and flaps are commonly used in the treatment of burn injuries to promote wound healing and improve functional outcomes. The nurse plays an important role in the nursing management of patients who have undergone grafts and flaps, and their responsibilities include:

- **Preoperative care:** The nurse must ensure that the patient is adequately prepared for the graft or flap procedure. This may involve educating the patient about the procedure, ensuring that they are fasting appropriately, and administering any preoperative medications as ordered.

- **Intraoperative care:** The nurse may be responsible for assisting the surgical team during the graft or flap procedure, ensuring that the patient is positioned appropriately and monitoring their vital signs.
- **Postoperative care:** The nurse must monitor the patient closely in the immediate postoperative period to assess for complications such as bleeding, infection, or graft or flap failure. The nurse must also manage the patient's pain and ensure that they are comfortable.
- **Wound care:** The nurse must ensure that the graft or flap site is appropriately dressed and monitored for signs of infection. The nurse may also be responsible for assisting with wound care procedures such as dressing changes or debridement.
- **Mobilization and functional rehabilitation:** The nurse must work closely with the physiotherapist and occupational therapist to ensure that the patient is mobilized appropriately, and that functional rehabilitation is initiated as soon as possible following the graft or flap procedure.
- **Patient education:** The nurse must provide the patient and family members with education about the graft or flap procedure, wound care, and any necessary lifestyle modifications following the procedure.
- **Collaboration:** The nurse must collaborate closely with the surgical team, physiotherapist, occupational therapist, and other members of the healthcare team to ensure that the patient receives comprehensive care that addresses all aspects of their recovery.

Overall, the nurse plays a critical role in the nursing management of patients who have undergone grafts and flaps, and their responsibilities include preoperative care, intraoperative care, postoperative care, wound care, mobilization and functional rehabilitation, patient education, and collaboration with the healthcare team.

## RECONSTRUCTIVE SURGERY

Reconstructive surgery is performed to correct the function to some extent and also improve body appearance. Few common reconstructive surgeries are facial in burns cases, hand repair, breast reduction or breast reconstruction after mastectomy **(Fig. 16.10)**.

## REHABILITATION

The rehabilitation phase starts after the acute phase and often runs for years after surgery. In this phase, the patient

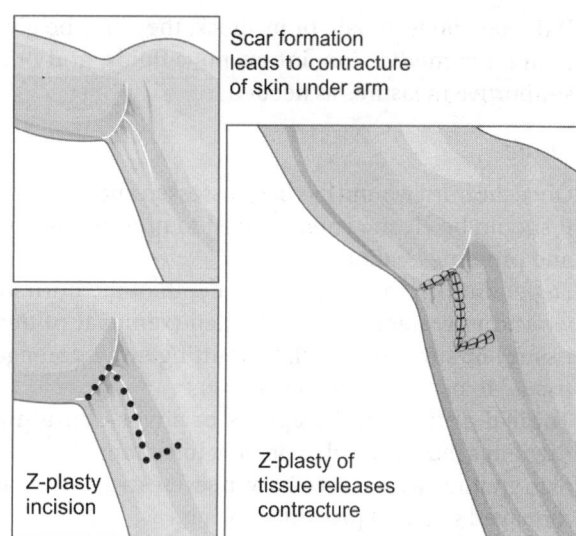

**Fig.16.10:** Z-plasty and Y-plasty to release.

mostly focuses on self-image and lifestyle. Nurses have to focus on wound healing, psychosocial support and restoration of maximum functional activities of organs. During this rehabilitation phase, the body undergoes maximum changes as it heals and the patient may face new complications such as contractures, wound breakdown, gait deviations, hypertrophic scarring and joint instability. Patients are instructed about wound care and close monitored about the pain management, nutritional support and prevention of complication. Inform about the specific exercise and use of specific pressure garments. Family is taught about to recognize about any specific abnormal signs.

## Medical Management

It involves several stages, including initial assessment and treatment, wound care pain management, infection prevention, and rehabilitation.

### Initial Assessment and Treatment

The first step in treating a burn is to assess the severity and extent of the injury. This involves evaluating the depth, size, and location of the burn, as well as any other injuries or underlying medical conditions that may affect treatment.

- The person's airway, breathing, and circulation should also be evaluated and managed as necessary.
- The burn wound should be cooled with cool (not cold) running water for at least 20 minutes to minimize tissue damage and relieve pain.
- Clothing and jewelry should be removed from the affected area, unless they are stuck to the skin.

- If the person is in pain or in shock, they may be given pain relief medication, intravenous fluids, and other supportive measures as needed.

*Woodcare*

- Once the burn wound has been assessed and stabilized, it should be cleaned and dressed to prevent infection and promote healing.
- Depending on the severity and depth of the burn, the wound may need to be debrided (removal of dead tissue) or surgically excised (cutting away damaged tissue) to promote healing.
- Topical antimicrobial agents or silver-containing dressings may be used to prevent infection.
- Skin grafting may be necessary in severe cases to replace damaged skin and promote healing.

*Pain Management*

- Burn injuries can be very painful, so pain relief medication should be given as needed. Nonsteroidal anti-inflammatory drugs (NSAIDs) and opioids may be used, depending on the severity of the pain.
- Pain management strategies may also include distraction techniques, such as music or guided imagery.

*Infection Prevention*

- Burn wounds are highly susceptible to infection, so measures should be taken to prevent infection, such as administering antibiotics, cleaning and dressing the wound, and maintaining good hygiene practices.
- The person should also be monitored closely for signs of infection, such as fever, redness, swelling, or drainage from the wound.

*Rehabilitation*

- After the initial treatment phase, the person may require ongoing rehabilitation to promote healing and restore function.
- This may include physical therapy, occupational therapy, or psychological counseling to address any emotional or psychological effects of the burn injury.
- Supportive measures such as pressure garments or silicone sheets may also be used to minimize scarring and promote healing.

## Nursing Management

It involves several key areas, including assessment, wound care, pain management, infection control, nutrition, and psychosocial support. Here are some important considerations for each area:

*Assessment*

- Assess the extent and severity of the burn injury using a standardized burn assessment tool.
- Evaluate the patient's airway, breathing, and circulation (ABCs) to determine if there are any immediate life-threatening injuries.
- Assess the patient's pain level and comfort.
- Determine if there are any associated injuries or conditions that may impact burn care.

*Wound Care*

- Cleanse and debride the burn wound to remove any necrotic tissue and reduce the risk of infection.
- Apply dressings to protect the wound and promote healing.
- Monitor for signs of infection, such as increased redness, swelling, or drainage from the wound.
- Consider the use of topical antimicrobial agents or systemic antibiotics as needed.

*Pain Management*

- Administer pain medication as ordered and monitor the patient's response.
- Use nonpharmacological interventions, such as distraction techniques, relaxation exercises, or guided imagery, to help manage pain.
- Re-evaluate pain management regularly and adjust the treatment plan as needed.

*Infection Control*

- Use standard precautions, including hand hygiene, personal protective equipment (PPE), and isolation precautions, to prevent the spread of infection.
- Monitor for signs of infection and promptly initiate treatment as needed.
- Educate patients and their families on proper hand hygiene and infection control measures.

*Nutrition*

- Assess the patient's nutritional status and provide appropriate nutritional support, such as enteral or parenteral feeding.
- Monitor fluid and electrolyte balance to prevent complications such as dehydration or electrolyte imbalances.
- Consider the use of supplements such as vitamin C and zinc to promote wound healing.

*Psychosocial Support*

- Assess the patient's emotional and psychological needs and provide appropriate support and counseling.

- Involve the patient and their family in the care plan and provide education on burn care and self-care.
- Consider the need for referral to a mental health professional if the patient is experiencing significant emotional distress or symptoms of depression or anxiety.

## Nursing Diagnosis

Nursing management and nursing diagnosis for burns involve a comprehensive approach to the patient's care, which includes the assessment, treatment, and prevention of complications. Here are some nursing management and nursing diagnosis for burns:

- Acute pain related to tissue damage, and nursing management includes:
  - Assess the patient's pain level and characteristics.
  - Administer analgesics and other pain management strategies as prescribed.
  - Monitor the patient's response to pain management and adjust the treatment plan as needed.
  - Provide emotional support to the patient to alleviate anxiety and fear associated with pain.
- Impaired skin integrity related to tissue damage, and nursing management includes:
  - Assess the extent and severity of the burn injury.
  - Provide wound care and dressings as prescribed to promote healing and prevent infection.
  - Monitor the wound for signs of infection or other complications.
  - Encourage proper nutrition and hydration to support tissue repair and growth.
- Risk for infection related to tissue damage and loss of skin barrier, and nursing management includes:
  - Monitor the wound for signs of infection, such as redness, swelling, warmth, or discharge.
  - Follow strict infection control protocols, including hand hygiene and wearing gloves during wound care procedures.
  - Administer prophylactic antibiotics as prescribed to prevent infection.
  - Educate patients on wound care and hygiene practices to reduce the risk of infection.
- Risk for hypothermia related to fluid and heat loss, and nursing management includes:
  - Monitor the patient's body temperature and prevent further heat loss.
  - Provide warm blankets and heating devices to maintain the patient's body temperature.
  - Administer IV fluids and electrolytes to restore fluid and electrolyte balance.
  - Encourage the patient to stay warm and dry to prevent hypothermia.
- **Imbalanced nutrition:** Less than body requirements related to increased metabolic demands and nursing management includes:
  - Assess the patient's nutritional status and dietary habits to develop a nutrition plan.
  - Collaborate with the dietician to develop a dietary plan that meets the patient's nutritional needs.
  - Provide enteral or parenteral nutrition support, if necessary, to prevent malnutrition and promote wound healing.
  - Monitor the patient's laboratory values, such as albumin and pre-albumin, to evaluate the effectiveness of the nutrition plan.
- Disturbed body image related to physical disfigurement and nursing management includes:
  - Provide emotional support and counseling to the patient to cope with physical changes and disfigurement.
  - Encourage the patient to participate in self-care activities, such as bathing and dressing, to promote self-esteem and independence.
  - Provide education on scar management and wound care to promote healing and reduce scarring.
  - Refer the patient to support groups or resources for burn survivors to provide peer support and resources.

Overall, nursing management and nursing diagnosis for burns aim to promote wound healing, prevent complications, and improve the patient's quality of life.

## Prognosis of Burns

The prognosis of a burn injury depends on several factors, including the severity and extent of the burn, the age and overall health of the person, the location of the burn, and the promptness and effectiveness of medical treatment.

Superficial burns that affect only the outer layer of the skin (epidermis) usually heal within a few days to a week without scarring. However, deeper burns that affect the underlying layers of the skin (dermis) or other tissues may require more extensive medical treatment and take longer to heal. Severe burns can also lead to complications such as infections, scarring, and disfigurement.

In general, the larger and more severe the burn, the higher the risk of complications and the longer the recovery time. However, with prompt and appropriate medical care, many people are able to recover fully from their burn injuries and return to their normal activities. Rehabilitation and support from healthcare professionals and loved ones may also be necessary to help with physical and emotional healing.

##  Summary

Burn wounds heal best in moist—not wet—environments that promote re-epithelialization and prevent cellular dehydration. This environment is best created by applying a topical agent or occlusive dressing to reduce fluid loss. Topical agents provide pain control, promote healing, and prevent wound infection and desiccation. Patients with burns to the face also should be referred, because these burns can result in significant psychological trauma and identity issues.

##  Points to Ponder

- Most burns only affect the skin (epidermal tissue and dermis). Tissue destruction results from coagulation, protein denaturation, or ionization of cellular contents.
- The skin and the mucosa of the upper airways are the site of tissue destruction.
- Exposure to water at 140°F (60°C) for 30 seconds can cause a deep partial-thickness or full-thickness burn.
- Flash burns can be large and are often associated with significant thermal damage to the upper airway.
- Chemical injury to the lower airway is a common problem with inhalation of smoke.
- Three zones of tissue damage occur at the burn site. First is the central zone of coagulation, an area of irreversible damage.
- Large burns cause a hypermetabolic state that has multiple harmful physiologic derangements associated with it.
- Burn depth and extent are assessed to determine the severity of burn injury.
- Extent of injury for thermal and chemical injuries is assessed by using formulas such as the rule of nines.
- Intravenous opioid administration should be the prime treatment for burn pain.
- Full-thickness burns are assessed for circulatory problem.
- The wound is covered immediately with a topical antibacterial agent such as silver sulfadiazine (Silvadene) or bacitracin.
- Chemical burns should be immediately irrigated with tap water or normal saline for at least 5 to 10 minutes to remove the chemical.
- Skin substitutes are also used in grafting they are synthetic bio-substitutes, e.g., presterilized sheets like Tegaderm or opsite they are best for partial thickness burns.
- Management for airway edema is early intubation or tracheostomy.

##  Abbreviations

- EC : Electronic Cigarette
- TBSA : Total Body Surface Area (Burn)
- FAST : Focused Assessment with Sonography in Trauma
- ABG : Arterial Blood Gas
- ECG : Electrocardiogram
- BSA : Body Surface Area
- ARDS : Acute Respiratory Distress Syndrome
- SIRS : Systemic Inflammatory Response Syndrome
- MODS : Multiple Organ Dysfunction Syndrome
- $SaO_2$ : Saturation of Arterial Blood

##  Short Answer Questions

1. Burn assessment.
2. Fluid and electrolyte therapy.
3. Pain management.
4. Wound care.
5. Infection control.
6. Grafts and flaps.

##  Long Answer Questions

1. What do you mean by burn injury? Classify the burns and its etiological factors. Describe the clinical manifestations of burns. What will be the management of patients having partial thickness injury?
2. Describe in detail about the prevention and management of burn and its complication.
3. Explain different types of reconstructive surgery. Explain in detail about plastic surgery and its indication. Add a note on rehabilitation care for severe burns.
4. What are the emergency management of burn injury? How will you assess the burn injury?

##  Bibliography

1. American Burn Association. Burn Incidence and Treatment in the United States. https//:ameriburn.org. Published 2016. Accessed 2018.
2. American Burn Association. Burn Injury Fact sheet, https//:ameriburn.org. Accessed, 2018.
3. Burn Foundation. Pediatric Burn Fact sheet. https//www.burnfoundation.org. Accessed 2018.
4. Capek KD, Sousse LE, Hundeshagen G, et al. Contemporary Burn Survival. J Am Coll Surg. 2018;226(4):453-63.
5. Hefferman JM, Comeau OY. The ABCDEs of Emergency Burn Care. Am Nurse Today. 2015;10(10). https://american-nursetoday.com. Accessed 2018.
6. ISBI Practice Guidelines Committee. ISBI Practice Guidelines for Burn Care. Burns, 2016:42(5):953-21.
7. Maraqa T, Mohamed AT, Salib M, Morris S, Mercer L, Sachwani-Daswani GR. Too Hot for Your Pocket! Burns from Care Res. 2018;39(6):1043-47
8. Pinto DS, Clardy PF. Environmental and Weapon-related Electrical Injuries. Up To Date website.http://www.uptodate.com/contents/environmental-and-weapon-related-electricalinjuries?search=Environmental%20and%20 20weaponrelated%20el ectricall%20injuries.

9. Rice PL Jr, Orgill DP. Emergency Care of Moderate and Severe Thermal Burns in Adult.
10. Schraga ED. Emergent Management of Thermal Burns. Medscape Website. https://emedicine.medscape.com/article/ 769193-overview. Accessed 2018.
11. Stoppler MC. Frostbite. https://wwwemedicinehealth.com Accessed 2019.
12. Texas EMS Trauma Andamp; Acute Care Foundation (TETAF) Trauma Division. Burn Clinical Practice Guideline. TETAF wensite. http://tetaf.org/wp-content/uploads/2016/01/burns.
13. Valles LJ, Plourde BD, Wentz JE, Nelson-cheesemom BB, Abraham JP. A review of scald burn injuries. Int Med Rev 2017;3(3):1-17.
14. Vorstenbosh J. Thermal Burns. Medscape Website. http://www.ebmedicine.medscape.com /article//1278244-print. Updated December 29, 2017. Accessed June 28, 2018.

# Chapter 17

# Legal and Ethical Issues in Critical Care

 Suchismita Phantasingh

## CHAPTER OUTLINE

- Principles of Critical Care
- Ethical Issues in Critical Care Unit
- Principles of Bioethics
- Legal Issues in Critical Care

### Learning Objectives

At the end of the chapter, the students will be able to:
- Describe the principles of critical care.
- List and explain about legal and ethical issues of critical care nursing.
- Describe the nurse's responsibility in legal and ethical issues in critical care nursing.

## INTRODUCTION

An central part of hospital care is the intensive care unit (ICU), the critical care unit where the most higher technological treatment are given to the patient (Curtis and Vincent, 2010). The ICU is a multifaceted setting which encompasses a distinctive cluster of physical health care supplier who are assigned to provide the care for the seriously sick clients. Everyday decision-making related to critical care is based on the ICU care giver's values, attitude, behavior and actions. Literature and facts have recommended that in ICU care dilemmas are very usual and deleterious. Both the nurses and physicians may have ethical issues. Even though the nursing personnel and doctors are the member of the similar squad and run after the similar objective of care, but they may have distinct perspective of ethical dilemmas such as end-of-life (EOL) care and life-sustaining treatment (LST) decision. Critical care nurse acts avital role in harmonizing and integrating the ICU care supplier's want that devote the maximum amount of time with patients and families (Park and Moon et al., 2015).

As nurses are likely to work in an ethical way and ethical competencies are required and which are governed by regulatory bodies and the pertinent ethical codes through the demonstration. Development of 'moral competence' is important for the nurses in their workplace, so that they are able to discuss and implement issues concerning ethics and rights of human. Ethical issues present in a given clinical situation can be identified by moral competence and ethical action and is helpful to take ethical measures if and when essential, and an individual obligation to accomplish moral outcomes. Being a part of the critical care team, this assorted knowledge of ethics is supreme to nurses of critical care, whose patient is a particularly vulnerable one. So, in order to offer precision in relation to attainment of their ethical responsibilities' nurses working in critical care unit are stimulated to discuss ethics and its educational opportunities.

## PRINCIPLES OF CRITICAL CARE

Critical care unit is designed specifically and set with skillful human resources to offer efficient and protected care for life-threatening or potentially life-threatening dependable patients. The critical care nursing principles are the following:

### Anticipation

Anticipation is the first and foremost principle in critical care. One has to identify and anticipate the high-risk patients and their needs and consequences and get ready to face any emergency. Smooth running of the unit depends upon the proper organization of the unit with all necessary equipment and supplies.

### Early Detection and Prompt Action

Improvement of the patient depends on the early identification of variation, quick and proper steps to be taken to prevent or fight against complications. The most important assessment is monitoring of cardiorespiratory function.

### Collaborative Practice

Critical care which has developed as technological sub-specialized body of understanding, has emerged into a extensive practice demanding a very specialize body of knowledge for the doctors and nurses in decision-making of critical care unit through joint venture and assures high quality and humanitarian care to the patient. Then other discipline collaborative care practice is highly required for critical care.

### Communication

Smooth running of critical care units requires multi-disciplinary, interdepartmental and interpersonal communication. The mutual approach model, unlike the conventional practice model enhances better results as far as patient, nurse, doctor and hospital are focused. This representation focuses on the client, promotes individualized decision-making, and uses included hospital records and combined review of care.

## ETHICAL ISSUES IN CRITICAL CARE UNIT

Conflicts relevant to ethics between collaborators occur more commonly in the intensive care unit and also the ICU is the most usual place for death. Hence, ICU caregivers ought to be capable enough in every decision-making in ethical perspective. Behavioral issues such as vocal cruelty or lack of communication between doctors and nursing personnel and concern related to end-of-life care includes disrespect for the client's autonomy are key source of conflicts in critical care unit (Jae Young Moon, 2015).

Ethics have always been an important part of nursing on a everyday basis. Burnout or resignation becomes more prevalent among critical care nurses due to frequent exposure to moral and ethical conflicts. Nursing has developed its own ethical codes which elucidate the right and wrong philosophy along with offering quality standards for professional behavior, so as to safeguard the well-being of the people (Mahajan, 2006).

Moral issues, principles, responsibilities and obligations of nurses are clarified through ethical analysis and offer a sufficient ethical validation for any choice made or measures taken.

### Meaning of Ethics

Bioethics is the trust between a doctor and his/her patient by applying moral principles which are accepted as appropriate behavior.

Universal ethical principles may varies from culture to culture, individual to individual and they follow a common fashion across most cultures, namely beneficence, justice, nonmaleficence and the dignity of persons (Hardcastle, 2010).

The philosopher and ethicist Immanuel Kant during the 18th century believed that one's duty may reflect someone's behavior. He believed that, the meaning of well-being is the freedom to get the autonomy (self-determination), not used as a way to an end, being treated with dignity, and having the competence to think logically.

The code of ethics for the nurse practitioner has been developed and published by some countries like the USA and the UK based on the draft of the International Council of Nurses' Code for Nurses, 1993. The code for the use of critical care nurses has further specified by the Critical Care Nurses Association (CCNA) in US (Balachandran, 2001). ANA code of ethics has supported by other regulatory association such as "American Nurses Association (ANA) of critical care nurses" (AACN) **(Table 17.1)**.

### American Nurses Association Code of Ethics for Nurses 2015

*See* **Table 17.1**.

## PRINCIPLES OF BIOETHICS

Within biomedical sciences ethical conflicts and decision-making made within the biomedical sciences, including patient care, healthcare delivery, health care of public, and biomedical research is called as bioethics and these principles are more frequently used to ethical issues or dilemmas in critical care (Neurosurgical et al., nd). Principles of bioethics are depicted in **Figure 17.1**.

- **Nonmaleficence:** Nonmaleficence is an obligation not to harm another deliberately. Both the ethical and legal practices of health care nonmaleficence have been sustained. Utilitarian principles are used for the benefit of procedure is balanced against the harm. The action is considered as an ethical if the benefit is higher (Introduction, nd). Nurses can prevent harming the patient through nonmaleficence principle.
  As Jarneton notes, "taken literally this principle would be impracticable, since only the easiest forms of treatment do no harm."

**Table 17.1:** ANA code of ethics for nurses.

| | |
|---|---|
| Provision 1 | The nurse practices with compassion and respect for the inherent dignity, worth, and unique attributes of every person |
| Provision 2 | The nurse's primary commitment is to the patient, whether an individual, family, group, community, or population |
| Provision 3 | The nurse promotes, advocates for, and protects the rights, health, and safety of the patient |
| Provision 4 | The nurse has authority, accountability and responsibility for nursing practice; makes decisions; and takes action consistent with the obligation to provide optimal patient care |
| Provision 5 | The nurse owes the same duties to self as to others, including the responsibility to promote health and safety, preserve wholeness of character and integrity, maintain competence, and continue personal and professional growth |
| Provision 6 | The nurse, through individual and collective effort, establishes, maintains, and improves the ethical environment of the work setting and conditions of employment that are conducive to safe, quality health care |
| Provision 7 | The nurse, in all roles and settings, advances the profession through research and scholarly inquiry, professional standards development, and the generation of both nursing and health policy |
| Provision 8 | The nurse collaborates with other health professionals and the public to protect human rights, promote health diplomacy, and reduce health disparities |
| Provision 9 | The profession of nursing, collectively through its professional organizations, must articulate nursing values, maintain the integrity of the profession, and integrate principles of social justice into nursing and health policy |

*Source:* American Nurses Association 2015. Code of ethics with interpretative statements. Silver Spring, MD.

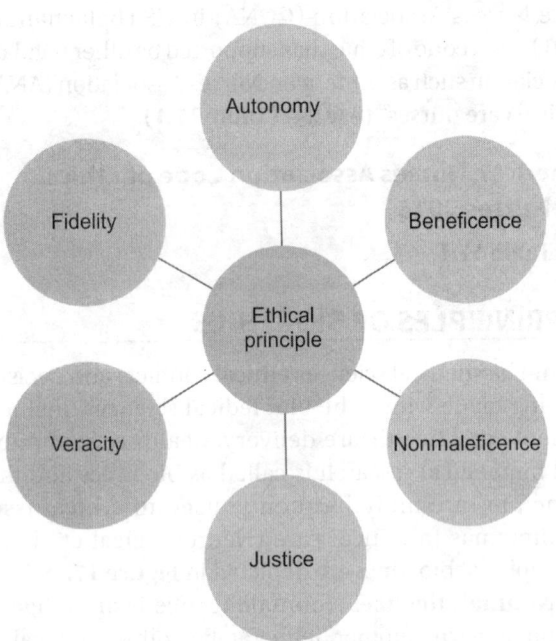

**Fig. 17.1:** Principles of bioethics.

As an alternative, not to harm anyone believe whether the medical procedures cause no pain and discomfort, on balance, exceed by benefits patients receive. The pledge of nineteenth-century Florence Nightingale is to "abstain from whatever is deleterious and mischievous and devote myself to the welfare of those committed to my care" (Jecker, 2017).

- **Beneficence:** An obligation to enhance other's well-being, to capitalize the benefits and reduce harm to the patient is called beneficence. The principle of beneficence emphasizes the end result of nursing measures and emphasizes that the utmost fundamental objective of nursing is to lend a hand to the patient. In critical care unit health care worker can enhance the overall benefit readily or decrease treatment load and prioritize more intently on promoting distinct functional effects on different parts of the body" (Jecker, 2017).
- **Respect for autonomy:** An obligation to respect, and not to get involved with, the choices and actions of self-governing individuals (i.e., those capable of self-determination). Autonomy signifies the right of the patient to be fully informed about the disease and the consequences of treatment, and equally focuses on the patient's right to accept or deny the planned treatment. In critical care practice the principle of autonomy may be used with proper modification. Critically ill patients are mostly incapable of making decisions, hence in discussion about the treatment goal most commonly the family members involve. Most of the critically ill patients are unable to make decisions; the family mostly get involved in decisions about the care goals and many a times express the patient's values and preferences. Often the decision of the family member varies according to the countries and cultures. The decision of the family member varies as per the country and culture. On the other hand, irrespective of location in ICU accurate

exchange of information between the physician and family is crucial for end-of-life quality care (Curtis and Vincent, 2010).

- **Justice:** Justice is an obligation to have fair distribution of loads, social services and welfare such as healthcare service or nursing service.

  It may be stated as impartial, reasonable and right action in support of what is owing to a significant person. The distributive justice is defined as the reasonable, fair and proper supply of health services, decided by acceptable policies or protocols (Ethics, nd).

- **Veracity:** Veracity is a conformity to the accurate facts or an obligation to tell the truth.
- **Fidelity:** To keep promises and fulfill commitments is known as fidelity. The nurse keeps the promises and commitment of the nursing profession and that promise making is the principle of fidelity. The basic principle of nurse patient relationship is fidelity and faithfulness towards patients care (Carolyn M Hudak).

## Ethical Dilemmas

An ethical dilemma is a situation where between two equally unfavorable alternatives an individual to makes a choice. Mostly an individual while taking decision or choice go through the conscious conflict (Townsend).

Every day in many areas of nursing or clinical practice nurse are confronted with ethical dilemmas. Ethical dilemmas are the challenging issues for the nurses when they provide clinical care to clients, when collaboratively they work with clinicians (healthcare providers) or when they perform their duty with other nursing personnel. In Intensive care unit along with other health care providers nurses also face ethical dilemmas. Nurses in every day practice come across issues or challenges which require ethical resolution. Dilemmas of the nurses may arise due to advancement of technology and increase demand of consumers for high quality nursing service. Nurses in an ICU exposed to ethical dilemmas which emerge from treatment withdrawal and withhold, utilization higher technology, distribution of insufficient supplies, and breach of privacy or from withholding of information and truth telling (Suttharangsee and Yai, 2004).

## Ethical Decision-making

In critical care practice the most fundamental character and vital part of being a nurse is critical care decision-making. Only the nurse may involve in these decision-making, while other decision-making would comprise healthcare personnel and other health team member. Decisions which are taken by the critical care nurses fluctuate between usual and critical moral decisions (Braganza et al., 2017).

It is very difficult to get the resolution for ethical dilemmas. Decision-making in ethical dilemmas are very difficult because of undeniable reasons exist between two or more alternative actions. Right actions can be taken through systematic application of available codes of ethics and ethical principles which may the healthcare team and ethical committee to recognize ethical obligations and meet these obligations. Satisfactory resolution of ethical issues is also very critical through multidisciplinary collaboration and dialogue.

Ethical decision-making models is a process of systematic and thoughtful way of investigating a dilemma, clinch before taking action subject think about every significant portions of a circumstance critically and carefully (Neurosurgical et al., nd).

### Ethical Decision-making Model (Flowchart 17.1)

- Collect the pertinent information and recognize the choice maker(s) and the associates.
- Find out the moral dilemma(s), in decision-making engage others and seek appropriate discussion of physical resources or professionals.

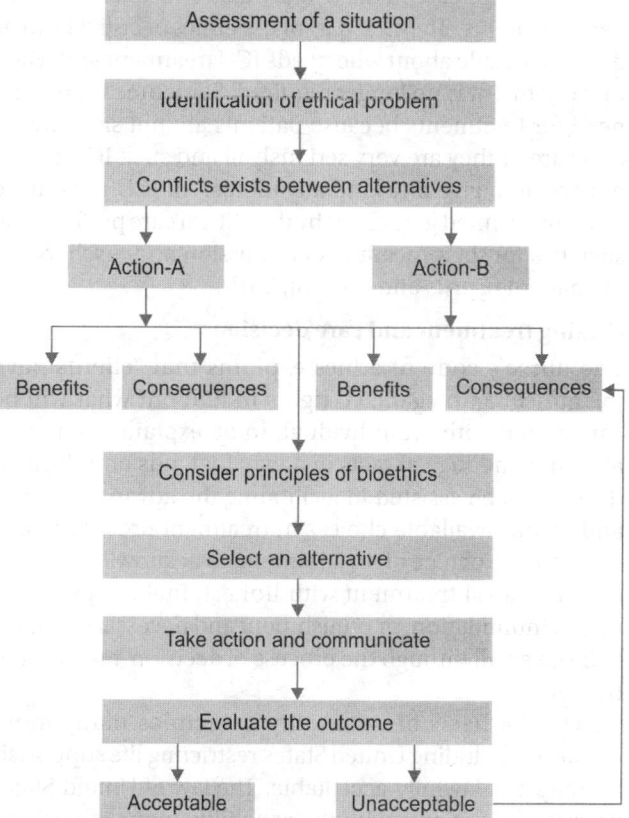

**Flowchart 17.1:** Ethical decision-making model.

- Critical analysis of the issues by using resources and principles of ethics.
- In the light of ethical principles make out substitute actions, select the most appropriate measure and validate the alternative.
- Appraise and replicate the action or decision (Neurosurgical et al., nd).

## Ethical Dilemmas in Critical Care Unit

### Admissions and triage decisions or allocation of beds

At any given time, the number of patients that can be cared for on the critical care unit is sorted or restricted both by the number of beds and the availability of competent staff to provide care. Often critical care use triage for making decision about admitting or discharging patients and to enhance the effectual and proficient resource utilization (Neurosurgical et al., nd).

Considerably different countries have different availability of ICU resources and accordingly triage, admission and end-life-care decision also varies. For example, ICU care is not readily available in developing countries and in rural part of developed countries. The part of hospital beds that are beds of ICU varies between centers, even where ICU care is available. The decisions about need for care in the ICU are also affected by the ICU bed availability. The vital part of the ethics of critical care is decisions made about who needs ICU treatment and when that treatment is no longer required. Sometime there is no need for treatments because patients are not sickly for ICU care or they are very seriously ill and such ICU care is not going to give any kind advantage. All ICU must have clear and printed guidelines by the critical care professional societies for the procedure of admission and discharge of the patient (Curtis and Vincent, 2010).

### Making treatment and care decisions

The nurse's code of ethics explains that "clients have the ethical and legal civil rights to find out what will be carried out with an individual, to be explained enough, absolute and logical facts in a way that aids an informed decision to be assisted in facilitating the advantage, loads and readily available choices in treatment process, which includes the choice of no treatment, to acknowledge, deny or withdrawal treatment with honest, include pressure, threat, intimidation, or punishment and necessary support to be given all through the process of decision-making and treatment.

On the basis of autonomy principles many more countries including United States restricting life supportsis morally and lawfully acceptable. The law of United States permits the patients with the capability to make decision have the right to say no to some and every treatment, as well as those that preserve the life. However in ICU this protocol is challenging as around 95% of patients may unable to take life decisions because of either their ill health or sedateness. On behalf of patient decisions are taken by surrogates or legally acceptable representative (LAR), when they cannot make decisions for themselves. Hence all the information should be communicated in ways that are delicate to the client's culture, religion, and needs of communicative language and enough time must be given to the patients and families to make end-of-life decisions (Alparslan, 2007).

### Withholding or withdrawing life support

Always ICU will be a stimulating zone for withdrawal of treatment and care of end-of-life calling for a personalized treatment approach to each and every patient. In ICU numbers of ethical principles are used for treatment withdrawal. Often in ICU either due to the use of tranquilizers/sedatives or due to the consequence of the primary disease condition patients are too desensitized and incapable to involve in important discussions made about withdrawal of treatment (Braganza et al., 2017).

In some cases, especially at the end-of-life, a patient or substitute decision maker may make a decision to withhold or take out a treatment. Withholding specifies not at all annoying/introducing an action, whereas withdrawal of treatment means to stop a treatment once progressed. The difference between not progressing a treatment and withdrawal the treatment has no ethical meaning; what focuses most is whether the treatment decision is supported with the client's wishes and choices. Ideally treatment preference discussions take place when the patient is aware and has a realistically clear consciousness. The critical care nurse helps to make sure that the patient receives enough treatment information, has the capability to be aware of available options, and can make a purposeful healthcare related decision. A legally authorized representative is called to give consent when patient is not capable enough to make decision. The client or substitute person must be aware of what the treatment entails and most likely how it will put an impact on disease condition and quality of life, prior to make a deliberate and informed decision to allow or to deny any treatment (Neurosurgical et al., nd).

### Brain death and organ donation

Every year, dramatically people have safeguarded their lives through organ donation. Organs can only be safely transplanted very soon after someone has died, and the donated organs need to be in a suitable condition to. Those people have died in ICU, or accident and emergency department can only be the donor.

After a diagnosis of death organ donation can only takes place.

Following a decision to diagnose death using neurological criteria or to consider withdrawal of life sustaining treatment (and before undertaking the tests/withdrawal of life sustaining treatment), the intensive care team caring for the patient will make a referral to the organ donation service. A medical team will conduct an initial assessment.

**Counseling for organ donation**

The most distressing and emotional intensive conversation occurs during the family counseling and conversations on organ donation. As the loss of a loved one is devastating supporting family in this toughest time is highly essential. Family must be handled with sensitivity and empathy while offering for organ donation.

- If the patient found to be a fit organ donor following further assessment offering specialist nurse for organ donation (SN-OD) will work meticulously with the doctors and nurses to support the family, through the confirmation of death using neurological criteria (if occurring)
- The SNOD will try and ensure that the option of donation is only raised when the grieving family are ready and able to consider it.
- The family will be given an opportunity to consider any other family members that may want to be present for the breaking bad news conversation.
- During the discussion, the SNOD will provide information about any decision their family member may have made on the organ donor register (ODR), whether it was to donate some/all organs, or not to donate any organs.
- If the family supports an existing organ donation decision or gives consent for donation to proceed, the SNOD will provide them with information regarding what happens next and the process.
- Formal/legal paperwork needs to be completed with the family and the consent/authorization form will be signed at this point.
- A copy of the consent form can be given to the family if they wish.

### End-of-Life Issue, DNR Order

Most of the patients come to the ICU with the terminal illness approaching to death, even the acutely ill patient also moves towards terminally ill condition. There are many reasons or conditions where the patient progressing to terminal illness may be the condition of patient itself or patient not able to afford the needed money to pay for the entire care and some cases are there where the doctor may order for do-not-resuscitate (DNR) when there is a diagnosis made for permanent brain damage that is irreversible. Therefore, it may not be dignified simply perfusing the organs, ventilating the lungs or keeping the body in a vegetative state. So, the patient may give consent to end-of-life or to have a peaceful death. Here, the role of a nurse is to identify the DNR order, root cause, and follow the order.

### Limits to Treatment and Futility of Care

Futility care includes the hospital services which is having curative effects and that is ineffective or inadequate. The term "futile care" in 1980 was first defined and it is used in the texts of medical ethics in 1990 (Gabbay, Calvo-Broce, Meyer, Trikalinos, Cohen, and Kent, 2010).

The meaning of futility care varies in the light of patient's health status and the individualized nurse's value (Palda, Bowman, McLean, and Chapman, 2005).

In some cases healthcare workers would like to treat patients against their wishes, whereas in some other cases a client and their family member, or proxy wishes for the treatment where as the physicians, nurses, or other members of the health team feels it ineffectual or even futile. Particularly for dying patient critical care is considered as "excessive" and is a major cause of concern among care providers, especially critical care nurses. When a patient's wish for treatment is denied because of futility, then there will be immense consultation occurs among ethicists, healthcare members, and patients' proxy or family members. Futility is a complex idea that can be understood or perceived in at least one of two different ways: (1) when an action would be unsuccessful at producing its desired effect and (2) when an intervention might be physiologically effective but is unlikely to give a significant benefit. Some facilities allow a physician to write a DNR order or withhold certain treatments without the consent of the patient, under carefully delineated conditions and after discussion with other health care team members (Neurosurgical et al., nd).

### Euthanasia

It is stated as a direct cut to end life with a primary intention. Euthanasia it is considered as illegal in many states, some countries have legalized euthanasia, best attempt to save the patient's life is made and method of euthanasia is intended to dignify the patient's death when all the extra measures taken to continue the life of the patient is unsuccessful and especially in ICU euthanasia is very rare. For instance, a patient has irreversible brain damage, choice for euthanasia is made, but not compulsory chance, before euthanasia decision patient's consent, and advanced directives are received.

## Advance Directives

End-of-life decision-making most frequently occurs at ICUs. In ICU decision-making should be carried out by desires of the patient, and advance directives (AD) are the single means, where end-of-life decision can be made by the patient (Scherer, Jezewski, Graves, Wu, and Bu, 2006). A set of documents where patient expresses how their death will be or at the end-of-life how to be treated, with the motive to dignify their wishes is known as advance directives or living wills (AD/LW) (advance directives in intensive care: Health professional competences, 2016).

It is a kind of living wills, healthcare surrogates, DNR orders, and powers of attorney with durability. Medical members take a vital part in the patient's cognition and completion of advance directives.

Preferably, before an acute illness advance directive should be completed, in a less chaotic and stressful environment. Advance directive in ICU helps family member of the patient to conceptualize and deal with end-of-life choice making (Scherer et al., 2006).

### Types of Advance Directives

Basically, there are two types of advance directives—instructive and proxy.

Living wills are coming under instructive ADs and proxy in health care includes a durable power of attorney. AD must be signed by two witnesses as well as the individual to whom it is applied. Instead of two witnesses in some states living wills may be signed by a Notary public (Robreta Kaplow, 2007).

### Accountability

Refers to being answerable to what is being done. It is valued related to the social responsibilities of nursing and to the moral and legal requirements of nursing practice. The value of accountability is seen, as superior moral standard in nursing that provides foundation for the relationship required in critical care nursing and the basis for high quality care (Jaya Kuruvilla, 2007).

### Advocacy

According to the Oxford dictionary advocacy, is 'one who pleads or speaks for another'. Browne claims that 'advocacy is a means of transferring power back to the patient'.

For nurse's advocacy comprises suggesting, linking, communicating the information, giving guidance, and helping the patients to make decisions. It also includes standing in support of the patient if he/she denies health care or takes away the consent (Balachandran, 2001).

## LEGAL ISSUES IN CRITICAL CARE UNIT

Major areas of law:

### Informed Consent

The three important elements of informed consent are: the consenting person must be capable, informed and be proficient in making decisions. During an emergency condition authentic informed consent must be obtained for the treatment purpose and it should be taken before the treatment is started.

An informed consent is issued to a person with multiple injuries or in a state of coma as soon as medical personnel offer emergency treatment. Because patients as a result of their injury are notable to react to health care members and in such cases the informed consent is dealt in a general way. For providing necessary medical treatment the law finds that absolutely the consent must be obtained from the injured party (Sundaram, 2007).

### Implied Consent

It allows medical treatment to be provided during an emergency with no fear of liability and without the consent of the patient. During emergency there is need for treatment to the affected individual for saving life or limb and for this condition implied consent can be applied with limited treatment. The principle of implied consent does not administer, once the crisis treatment is no longer required (Sundaram, 2007).

### Confidentiality (Breach of Privacy)

Nurses in their professional role are exposed to various moral and legal responsibilities and also liable to protect the privacy and confidentiality of the patients. About confidentiality regulation nurses of critical care must be responsive, as well as conditions where the secured health information are permitted to use and revelation.

Clinicians, nursing personnel and other healthcare team members in ICU share and make constant communication about the patient's condition, improvement of health condition and all through how to care for the patient especially when a patient is critically ill. Communication can be made with various groups such as the family members, peers, the legal bodies, the community and the media. Effectively and reliably the information can be shared with the multidisciplinary healthcare team members, as well as the nurses and those who are accountable for patient care.

Often, the seriously sick clients are unable to verbalize, so the patient's family member turn into the representative in these cases. The family members in the absence of doctor for information are mostly dependent on nurses of

ICU regarding the condition and prognosis of the patients. Information sharing commonly impacts upon the privacy and confidentiality of the patient's health status. Nurses have a moral obligation to maintain confidentiality or not to disclose the patient's health information to anyone and anywhere.

Confidentiality is the private information about a patient whether from the internal or external practice sources should not to be disclosed if not the patient wishes to give permission, legal validation is required for revelation or where actual threat of severe damage, or harm prevails (Matlakala, 2016).

- Confidentiality safeguarding should expand not only to medical reports or documents, but also to other personal particular health information, which includes record of scientific research, verbal testimony, pictures or figures and psychotherapy interpretation. These constraints should be established in the clinical situation and in all other areas (Of and Position, 2015).
- The patient should receive written, clear information of how their health records are used if his personal identifiable health information is revealed to third parties (Of and Position, 2015).
- Appropriate administrative, physical and technological protections must be developed by the organization and are necessary to guard the confidentiality, veracity and availability of individually identifiable health information (Of and Position, 2015).
- Strong and enforceable remedies must be taken for violations of confidentiality protection and health care professionals who report violations should be protected from retaliation/revenge (Of and Position, 2015).

## Standing Order

Standing orders are the policies made by the hospital management in relation to administration of medication/treatment procedures without the already written medical orders at the time of emergency and otherwise. Every critical care unit should have it and made available for nurses thereby the nurses are protected, and patients are ensured safe care (Jaya kuruvilla, 2007).

## Medicolegal Case

Police must be notified through the proper channel when a patient is admitted after accidents, suicide attempts, burns, assaults and are considered as medicolegal case. In such case after police clearance only dead body can be handed over. For discharge of a medicolegal case this principle is also applied.

## Nursing Negligence in Critical Care

A nurse may assert with negligence that any kind of care action or malfunction causes harm to the patient.

Malpractice lawsuits may happen due to an unintentional failure to adhere to a standard of clinical practices.

The "**Joint Commission on Accreditation of Healthcare Organizations (JCAHO)** defines negligence as a "failure to use such care as a reasonably prudent and careful person would use under similar circumstances."

"**JCAHO** describes malpractice as" "improper or unethical conduct or unreasonable lack of skill by a holder of a professional or official position; often applied to physicians, dentists, lawyers, and public officers to denote negligent or unskillful performance of duties when professional skills are obligatory."

Various components are responsible to the augment the malpractice numbers and negligence counter to nurses such as:
- Failure to follow standards of care
- Failure to communicate
- Improper documentation
- Failure to act as advocate
- Allocation
- Early discharge
- Shortage and downsizing of nurses
- Advanced technology
- Increased responsibility, work load and autonomy of nurses (Croke, 2003)

## Issues Involve Life Support Measures in Critical Care Units

End-of-life issues are potential landmines for intensive care physicians. Legal guidelines regarding end-of-life decision-making are less clear when patients without capacity lack an appropriate surrogate. Some states allow physicians to make decisions for such patients based on wishes expressed to the physicians when the patients have capacity. However, no state explicitly allows physicians to make decisions based on their view of the best interests of the patient.

Self-determination of patients relating to medical decisions is not well articulated in Indian Constitution. Indeed, the position of the law with respect to death in dignity is unclear, as Indian courts have only addressed appeals for Euthanasia. In India legal opinion is yet to fully explore the issue of terminal care (Mani RK, 2012).

### Role of Nurse in Legal and Ethical Issues in Critical Care Nursing

*Provide Secure, Empathetic, Skilled and Ethical Care*
- Nurses provide compassionate care through understanding and empathizing health care needs of the

patients and also through their verbal communication and concerned body language.
- Nurses develop reliable relationships with patients as the basis of significant therapeutic communication, recognizing that developing these relationships demands a conscious endeavor. Such relationships are vital to perceive people's needs and concerns.
- Nurses shore up each other in providing individual-centered care.

*Promoting the Health and Well-being of the Client*
- Nurses provide directed initial and primary care after identifying and applying the standards and principles of primary health care towards the health and well-being of individuals receiving treatment.
- To maximize health benefits and meeting the needs of persons receiving care nurses collaborate with other healthcare providers.

*Promoting and Dignifying Informed Decision-making Nurses*
- Nurses identify value and support an individual's right to be informed about the condition and make genuine decisions.
- Nurses respect the wishes of the patient receiving care to refuse or to obtain information about their health condition.
- Nurses must make sure that with the person's informed consent nursing care is provided. Nurses should know and stand for enable individual's right to say no or the distinction between take out consent at any point of time for care or treatment.

*Honoring Dignity*
- Nurses should support maintaining the dignity and integrity of the persons getting treatment.
- A nurse honors and maintains the confidentiality of persons receiving care by providing care in a tactful way and by minimizing invasion.
- Nurses encourage an ethical society in which ethical values and issues can be explicitly discussed and supported.

*Supporting Individual's Privacy and Confidentiality*
- Nurses support the importance of patient's privacy and confidentiality as well as protection of family, individual, and community details put together in the perspective of professionalism.
- She/he should recognize guidelines that safeguard and protect the privacy of persons receiving care, including technological safeguard of information.

*Promoting Justice*
- For protecting individual's right nurses support principles of justice, impartiality and by promoting the public good.
- On the ground of a person's race, customs, traditions, political and religious values, communal or marital status, gender, gender identity, sexual orientation, age, health status, place of birth, standard of living, psychological or physical capability, financial background, or any other characteristics nurses do not differentiate.

*Promoting Accountability*
- Nurses are to be answerable for their care actions and for their professional performance they are legally responsible.
- Nurses are truthful and work with honesty in all of their professional connections. Nurses symbolize themselves undoubtedly with respect to name, designation and function (Peter and Storch, 2008).

# CONCLUSION

ICU is the site where clients are cared for through scientifically higher life supporting treatments and care of critically ill patients is a central goal of medical service. Nurses are expected to render services which are ethically and lawfully unharmed. All health care experts should have sufficient understanding in the legal and ethical contexts to provide comprehensive care to the patients. Thus, they can protect themselves and the clients from the legal and ethical issues or challenges (Nurses, 2016).

### Summary

This chapter deals with legal and ethical issues of critical care units. Nurses are expected to have the knowledge about legal and ethical aspects of critical care unit, so that they can safeguard patient's life from any kind of negligence and malpractice along with they can protect themselves. Hence legal and ethical aspects have a significant role in critical care unit.

### Points to Ponder

- Nonmaleficence is an obligation not to harm another deliberately.
- Police must be notified through the proper channel when a patient is admitted after accidents, suicide attempts, burns, assaults and are considered as medicolegal case.
- Confidentiality safe guarding should expand not only to medical health documents, but also to other personal identifiable health information, including scientific

research records, pictures or figures and psychotherapy interpretations.
- Negligence due to any care action or malfunction causes harm to the patients.

### Abbreviations

- ICU : Intensive Care Unit
- LST : Life-sustaining Treatment
- EOL : End-of-Life
- CCNA : Critical Care Nurses Association
- AACN : American Nurses Association of Critical Care Nurses
- ANA : American Nurses Association
- LAR : Legally Acceptable Representative
- DNR : Do-Not-Resusciate
- AD : Advance Directives
- LW : Living Wills
- JCAHO : The Joint Commission on Accreditation of Health Care Organizations
- SNOD : Specialist Nurse for Organ Donation

### Short Answer Questions

1. What are the different types of advance directives?
2. What are the principles of critical care?
3. Explain ethical dilemmas in critical care unit.

### Long Answer Question

1. Define ethics. Explain the role of nurse in legal and ethical issues in critical care nursing.

### Bibliography

1. ANA. Source: American Nurses Association. 2015.
2. Advance Directives in Intensive Care: Health Professional Competences. Medicina Intensiva (English Edition). 2016;40(3):154-62.
3. Balachandran S. Patient Autonomy, Advocacy and the Critical Care Nurse. Issues in Medical Ethics. 2001;9(3):82-3.
4. Butts JB, Rich KL. Nursing Ethics Across the Curriculum and in to Practice.
5. Curtis JR, Vincent JL. Ethics and End-of-life Care for Adults in the Intensive Care Unit. The lancet. 2010;376(9749):1347-53.
6. Hardcastle TC. The Ethical and Medico-legal Issues of Trauma Care. South African Journal of Bioethics and Law. 2010;3(1):25-7.
7. Hudak CM, Gallo BM. Critical Care Nursing: A Holistic Approach. Lippincott Williams and Wilkins; 1986.
8. Introduction I (nd). Nonmaleficence and Beneficence. 47–64.
9. Issues, L. Patients' Confidentiality. 2012;32(5):61-4.
10. Jae Young Moon. Ethics in the Intensive Care Unit. Uberc Respir Dis (Seoul). 2015;78(3):175-79.
11. Jaya Kuruvilla. A Textbook of Essentials of Critical Care Nursing. 2007;(1):8-11.
12. Jecker NS. Principles and Methods of Ethical Decision-Making in Critical Care Nursing. Critical Care Nursing Clinics of North America. 1997;9:29-34.
13. Kumaş G, Öztunç G, Nazan Alparslan Z. Intensive Care Unit Nurses' Opinions About Euthanasia. Nursing Ethics. 2007;14(5):637-50.
14. Mahajan RP. Principles of Critical Care. Principles of Critical Care. FE Udwadia (Ed). Published by Oxford University Press, New Delhi, India. Pp. 747; indexed; illustrated.
15. Mani RK, Amin P, Chawla R, Divatia JV, Kapadia F, Khilnani P, Myatra SN, Prayag S, Rajagopalan R, Todi SK, Uttam R. Guidelines for End-of-life and Palliative Care in Indian Intensive Care Units' ISCCM Consensus Ethical Position Statement. Indian J Crit Care Med. 2012;16(3):166-81.
16. Matlakala MC. Sharing the Critically Ill Patient's Information with the Family: Reflections and Lessons Learned. Journal of Nursing Education and Practice. 2015;5(10):115.
17. Mayall RM. Substance Abuse in Anaesthetists. Bja Education. 2016;16(7):236-41.
18. Morton PG, Fontaine DK, Hudak CM, Gallo BM. Critical Care Nursing: A Holistic Approach. Philadelphia: Lippincott Williams and Wilkins; 2005.
19. Park DW, Moon JY, Ku EY, Kim SJ, Koo YM, Kim OJ, el al. Ethical Issues Recognized by Critical Care Nurses in the Intensive Care Units of a Tertiary Hospital During Two Separate Periods. Journal of Korean Medical Science. 2015;30(4):495-501.
20. Peter E, Storch JL. The CNA Code of Ethics for Registered Nurses. Nursing Leadership (Toronto, Ont.). 2008;21(2):28-33.
21. Robreta K, Sonya RH. A Textbook of Critical Care Nursing. 2007;(1):720-1.
22. Scherer Y, Jezewski MA, Graves B, Wu YW, Bu X. Advance Directives and End-of-life Decision-Making: Survey of Critical Care Nurses' Knowledge, Attitude, and Experience. Critical Care Nurse. 2006;26(4):30–40.
23. Setiawan S, Chaowalit A, Suttharangsee W. Ethical Dilemmas Experienced by Nurses in Providing Care for Critically Ill Patients in Intensive Care Units, Medan, Indonesia. Songklanagarind Medical Journal. 2004;22(4):221-9.
24. Sundaram AM. Medicolegal Aspects of Critical Care Medicine. Indian Journal of Anesthesia. 2007;51(4):344-6.
25. The Journey Through Intensive Care and the Gift of Organ Donation, nd.
26. Verghese D, Latha T, Jomon C. Knowledge on Legal and Ethical Aspects in Patient Care Among Critical Care Nurses. Int j health sci res. 2016;6(3):197-201.

# Chapter 18

# Quality Assurance in Critical Care

*Bishnupriya Mohapatra*

## CHAPTER OUTLINE

- Quality Assurance
- Standards of Critical Care Unit
- Protocols and Policies of Critical Care Unit
- Nursing Audit
- Staffing of Critical Care Unit
- Design of Critical Care Unit

### Learning Objectives

At the end of the chapter, the students will be able to:
- Describe the steps and cycle of quality assurance.
- Enumerate different levels of critical care unit (CCU).
- Implement various protocol and policies in their respective critical care settings.
- Perform the nursing audit as per the various steps mentioned.
- Enumerate various factors affecting nursing audit.
- Explain regarding staffing pattern of CCU.
- Provide various suggestions regarding the design of CCU.

## INTRODUCTION

Critical care the term encompasses intensive care, intensive therapy and high dependency units. Critical care is essential for the clients who need specialized monitoring and attention for their life-threatening illness or injury.

A critical care nurse is responsible for ensuring those acutely and critically ill patients and their families for receiving optimal care through quality assurance, continuous nursing audits and various standards of CCU, which are very important components for the critical care nurses.

## QUALITY ASSURANCE

**Meaning of quality assurance (QA):** It refers to a program for monitoring and evaluating the aspects of a project, services and facilities in a systematic manner to ensure that standards of quality are being met (Black N,1990).

### Principles of Quality Assurance

- Focus on client needs.
- Focus on systems and process.
- Focus on data bases for decision-making.
- Focus on team approach to problem solving and quality improvement.

### Steps of Quality Assurance

Quality assurance consists of different steps to assist the organization in fulfilling the demands and expectations of clients. It also refers to the processes and procedures implemented to ensure that its services meet a certain level of quality. All the steps are explained in detail under the following **(Flowchart 18.1)**:

#### Step 1: Plan

The criteria and procedures that will ensure and also verify the data that will fulfill the precise objectives are defined in the plan.

#### Step 2: Set Standards

Documents that give rules, specifications, guidelines, or characteristics that can be applied consistently to ensure that materials, products, processes, and services are appropriate for their intended use are referred to as quality standards.

#### Step 3: Communicate Standards

Effective communication is a big issue in terms of both safety and quality, yet it is necessary for providing safe patient care. Failures in communication can result in

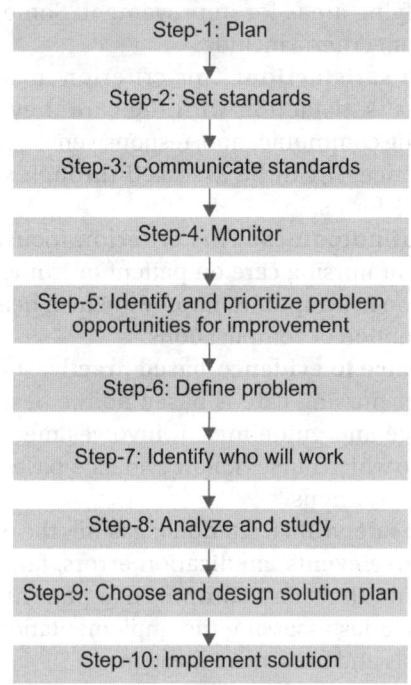

**Flowchart 18.1:** Steps of quality assurance.

- Do any of the issues pose a risk that the business won't be in conformity with regulations?
- Which issues are most detrimental to the operation's long-term financial stability?
- Which issues have an immediate effect on the operation's stability?
- Since there is only one issue at hand—a lack of a regular ration—prioritization is not required.

### Step 6: Define Problem

Uneven calibration of the evaluation process may lead to issues with quality assurance initiatives. Standards must be applied uniformly throughout. All assessors must be knowledgeable and unbiased. One of the main reasons for problems with quality assurance programs is allegations of favouritism.

### Step 7: Identify Who Will Work

In the absence of an effective implementation plan, quality control is challenging to establish. The management is in charge of developing these measures and educating healthcare professionals about them. Making major investments in the staff's training in a range of skills, such as coaching, delegation, and communication, is necessary as a result. The healthcare industry requires managerial education. It is crucial to give managers and staff the right training on how to use cutting-edge medical technologies as technology advances.

errors, inaccurate diagnoses, inappropriate treatments, and inferior care outcomes, as can inadequate or poorly documented clinical information. It goes without saying that informal interaction will occur while a patient is being cared for.

### Step 4: Monitor

An organization can maintain constant and unbiased listening to and analysis of customer interactions by implementing programs like quality monitoring. The development of a quality assurance plan, which should clearly identify the quality of the data required and describe in detail the planned actions to give confidence that the program will meet its stated objectives, is one of the most crucial aspects of quality assurance in a monitoring program.

### Step 5: Identify and Prioritize Problem Opportunities for Improvement

If there are multiple issues, you must rank them in order of importance so that you can concentrate on the most pressing issues first. To organize the issues so that the ones with a greater importance are at the front of the list, ask the following questions:
- Which issue could have detrimental effects on the health of cows or employees?

### Step 8: Analyze and Study

A high standard of service is ensured and upheld by QA in a number of healthcare systems. When a healthcare provider's service matches the patients' expectations, it is deemed to be of a high standard. The rise of quality assurance (QA) in healthcare delivery, on the other hand, is related to the need to contain rising healthcare costs in the face of limited resources and to guarantee high-quality patient care in a shifting healthcare environment where the power dynamic between patients and doctors is shifting in favour of patients.

### Step 9: Choose and Design Solution Plan

The blueprint for your analytics project is called a solution design document, also known as a solution design reference or business requirements document.

### Step 10: Implement Solution

One of the most important benefits of a thorough healthcare quality assurance program is the opportunity to quickly identify problems that may endanger patient care or safety and implement immediate adjustments. That can necessitate further staff training in some cases. In some circumstances, it could be required to upgrade obsolete medical equipment or modify rules that make it challenging for your staff to provide high-quality care. Cycle of quality assurance is depicted in **Flowchart 18.2**.

Cycle of quality assurance focuses about the quality care for which is possible by maintaining the standard care, document the problem with solutions and proper assessment. Also, committees give various recommendations for any change with suspected problem area which will enhance the quality of care.

**Quality of care:** The possibility that intended health outcomes will occur as a result of individual and population health interventions is referred to as quality of care. It is crucial for establishing universal health coverage and is based on professional knowledge supported by evidence. All actions that define, create, evaluate, monitor, and enhance the standard of care are considered to be part of quality assurance (QA). An increasingly significant component of the administrative management of the intensive care unit (CCU) is quality assurance. This helps in efficient resource use in addition to improving clinical procedures and patient outcomes.

### Standards of Care

There is evidence that an CCU's organization and structure can affect the outcome. It is crucial for members of the healthcare team to work together. The quality of patient care in the ICU is significantly improved by a multidisciplinary approach and the addition of a full-time intensivist, as well as by the presence of clinical chemists and critical care nurses with adequate staffing ratios. Clinical procedures are increasingly being used, and solid evidence supporting their application has improved care for critically ill patients.

### Measurement Criteria

Measurement criteria in quality of care in nursing are used to assess and evaluate the effectiveness, safety, and patient-centeredness of nursing care. These criteria help in measuring the quality of care provided by nurses and identifying areas for improvement. Some common measurement criteria include:

- **Patient satisfaction:** This criterion measures the patients' satisfaction with the care they received, including communication, responsiveness, and overall experience. It can be assessed through surveys or feedback forms.
- **Clinical outcomes:** This criterion focuses on the impact of nursing care on patient outcomes, such as reduction in symptoms, improvement in health status, or prevention of complications.
- **Adherence to evidence-based practices:** It assesses whether nursing care is based on the best available evidence and guidelines. It involves measuring the extent to which nurses follow evidence-based protocols and interventions.
- **Patient safety:** This criterion measures the occurrence of adverse events, medication errors, falls, or other incidents that may compromise patient safety. It also includes assessing the implementation of safety protocols and preventive measures.
- **Care coordination:** This criterion evaluates the effectiveness of nursing care in coordinating with other healthcare providers and ensuring seamless transitions of care.
- **Timeliness:** It assesses the timeliness of nursing care delivery, including prompt response to patient needs, medication administration, and timely communication with other healthcare team members.
- **Continuity of care:** This criterion measures the continuity and consistency of nursing care provided to patients across different settings or healthcare encounters.

### Assessment

A continuous process, quality assurance is centered on recognizing issues with a specific health service and setting standards and criteria in regard to such issues. Data gathering and analysis are used in quality assessment

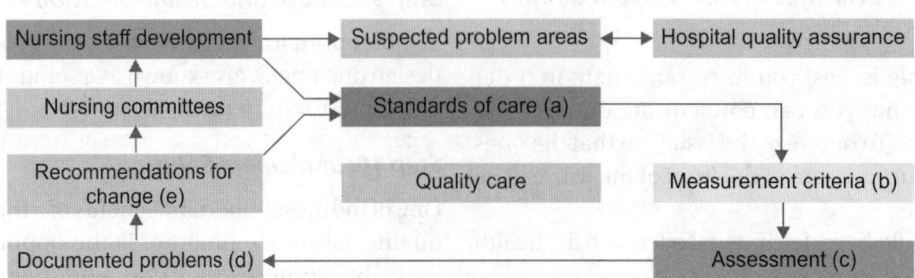

**Flowchart 18.2:** Cycle of quality assurance.

to demonstrate how closely something complies with established standards and criteria.

## Documented Problems

The documentation of issues in the CCU is crucial for quality assurance since nurse performance is frequently judged on the basis of the appropriateness of the care they provided and the standard of their service. A nurse's knowledge and clinical judgment are demonstrated through proper documentation, which also helps with funding and resource management. Regarding patient data that may be used as evidence, nursing documentation is crucial for legal purposes. Safe, high-quality, and evidence-based nursing practice requires documentation that is clear, accurate, timely, and accessible. Medication errors are just one of many unfavorable outcomes that might result from incomplete, inaccurate, delayed, illegible, or altered documentation. Nursing documentation is crucial for education, research, and quality control, among other things.

## Recommendations for Change

One recommendation is for hospitals to increase the number of CCU beds as much as possible by increasing CCU capacity and moving CCUs to new locations. For these expanding areas, hospitals should have the requisite beds and monitors. To exert control over resources, establish management systems with control groups at facility, local, regional, and/or national levels. Create a framework for the CCU and important interfacing departments to cooperate, communicate, and plan. A strategy for gaining access to, coordinating, and expanding labor resources is needed, along with a comprehensive list of all clinical and non-clinical workers. Delegate tasks that are outside the normal range of what your employees do. Ensure that there is an appropriate supply of drugs, supplies, and vital medical equipment. Utilize infection control procedures and policies that support occupational health to safeguard patients and staff. Keep the staff's faith.

## Nursing Committees

Nursing committees in quality care are groups of healthcare professionals, specially nurses who work together to ensure the delivery of high-quality patient care. These committees focus on improving patient outcomes, enhancing safety measures and implementing evidence-based practices within healthcare settings. So some common types of nursing committees in quality care include:

- **Quality improvement committee:** This committee focuses on identifying areas for improvement in patient care, developing action plans and monitoring the effectiveness of implemented changes.
- **Patient safety committee:** This committee aims to prevent and reduce medical errors, adverse events and other safety risks. They develop strategies, policies and protocols to enhance patient safety.
- **Evidence-based practice committee:** This committee promotes the integration of research evidence into clinical practice. They review current literature, develop guidelines, and educate nursing staff on evidence-based practices.
- **Infection control committee:** This committee is responsible for preventing and controlling healthcare-associated infections. They develop policies, monitor infection rates and implement preventive measures.
- **Education and training committee:** This committee focuses on providing ongoing education and training to nursing staff to enhance their knowledge and skills. They develop educational programs, organize workshops and ensure staff competency.
- **Ethics and training committee:** This committee address ethical dilemmas and issues related to patient care. They provide guidance and support to healthcare professionals in making ethical decisions.

## Nursing Staff Development

Nursing staff development in quality care refers to the ongoing training and education of nursing personnel to ensure they have the necessary knowledge, skills, and competencies to provide high-quality care to patients. It involves continuous professional development, updating clinical knowledge, improving communication and teamwork, and staying updated with the latest evidence-based practices. Some agencies and associations are there for the development of nursing staff like:

- **American Nurses Association (ANA):** This page provides information on various continuing education opportunities for nurses, including webinars, conferences, and online courses.
- **National League for Nursing (NLN):** NLN offers resources, workshops, and conferences for nursing educators and professionals to enhance their teaching and leadership skills.
- **Agency for Healthcare Research and Quality (AHRQ):** AHRQ's team program focuses on improving teamwork and communication among healthcare professionals, including nurses, to enhance patient safety and quality of care.
- **Joint Commission:** The Joint Commission provides resources and guidance on nursing education and staff development to promote safe and effective care delivery.

## Suspected Problem Areas

### Problem

Infections like ventilator-associated pneumonia, catheter-associated bloodstream infections, and urinary tract infections, venous thromboembolism, delirium, myopathies and neuropathies linked to critical illness, and stress ulcers are significant complications of care in the CCU. Acute respiratory distress syndrome (ARDS) and other critical illnesses survivors' long-term effects are receiving more and more attention. Muscle weakness, cognitive and neuropsychiatric issues, and mortality rates are high among patients in the CCU who are severely sick, and these conditions can lower quality of life. Many of these patients will not recover to resume their prior level of functional status.

### Identify the Goal

In order to apply evidence-based prevention interventions where possible, assess patients for complications after an CCU stay, and educate dialogues with patients and families regarding treatment objectives, hospital staff members should be informed of the key difficulties associated with CCU care.

### Describe a Step-by-Step Approach to this Problem

The major complications of critical illness and ICU care include the following:
- Even if the patient recovers from the original critical episode, this should be taken into account in goals-of-care discussions with families since they might not always understand the long-term effects of a protracted stay in the CCU. Comparing CCU survivors to population controls of same age and sex, death rates are two to five times higher.
- In severely ill patients who are mechanically ventilated, take into account early physical and occupational treatment. An increase in return to independent functional status, a reduction in delirium duration, and an increase in ventilator-free days were all observed in a randomised controlled trial in which mechanically ventilated patients received early physical and occupational therapy [including activities of daily living (ADL) and walking if tolerated] during interruptions of sedation while on mechanical ventilation.
- CCU patients frequently develop bloodstream infections linked to central venous catheters and urinary tract infections linked to urine catheters. When possible, think about inserting central venous catheters in the subclavian vein because it has a decreased risk of infection. Other precautions include washing the skin with chlorhexidine after placing a central venous catheter and removing the catheter as soon as it is no longer necessary.

### Quality Assurance in Hospital

The main goals of healthcare quality assurance are consumer happiness, ongoing organizational improvement, and faster and better service delivery. When people hear the term "quality assurance," they frequently envision stern inspectors scrutinizing components on a manufacturing line. This image is not entirely inaccurate. QA is related to the production process of a product. However, it unmistakably does not represent the position of a QA officer at a hospital or healthcare organization accurately. You must concentrate on particular procedures created to result in positive patient outcomes when it comes to healthcare quality assurance. QA teams can review a variety of procedures related to the patient experience, such as:
- Giving medical care evaluations
- Determining the appropriateness of external referrals
- Scheduling appointments
- Medical devices and technology
- Facilities and provisions of third-party payers

## STANDARDS OF CCU

Critical care unit is a specially designed and equipped facility staffed by skilled personnel to provide effective and safe care for dependent patients with a life-threatening problem.

### Models of CCU

The open model allows a variety of medical staff members to handle patients in the CCU, whereas the closed model restricts all patients' care to CCU-certified physicians. The hybrid model, it is the combination of both open and closed models by arranging the staffing pattern of the CCU with an attending physician and team to work efficiently (Critical Care Medicine, 1988).

### Classification of CCU

- **Level I:** It comes under the high dependency, where close monitoring, resuscitation, and short-term ventilation <24 hours has to be performed.
- **Level II:** It can be located in general hospital, undertake more prolonged ventilation. Must have resident doctors, nurses, access to pathology, radiology, etc.
- **Level III:** It refers to a major tertiary hospital, which is a referral hospital. It should provide all aspects of critical care is required.

## Levels of CCU

### Level I—Recommended for Hospitals including Nursing Homes up to 50 Beds

- Number of beds—6 to 8.
- Should be able to perform cardiopulmonary resuscitation including intubation, short-term cardiorespiratory support including, noninvasive ventilation, and defibrillation.
- Provision for short-term mechanical ventilation (desirable).
- Have syringe pumps/infusion pumps.
- Have multipara monitors with $SPO_2$, HR and ECG, NIBP, temperature facility.
- Access to ABG facility.
- Access to ultrasound, X-ray and basic clinical lab (CBC, blood sugar, electrolytes, LFT and RFT).
- Desirable to have access to CT scan and microbiology.
- Access to ambulance (ACLS desirable) and trained manpower for safe transport of the patients to higher level centers.
- Doctors should be encouraged to participate short-term training courses/workshops like ACLS/mechanical ventilation, etc.
- Access to 24 × 7 blood bank/pharmacy/nutrition.
- Provision for telemedicine consultations.
- At least one book and one journal of critical care medicine should be available as ready reckoner.
- General infection control and, patients and staff safety measures should be observed.

### Level II—Recommended for Larger General Hospitals up to 100 to 150 Beds

It includes all recommendations of Level I in addition to the following requirements:
- Number of beds—8 to 12.
- HOD/director/in-charge of the CCU should be an intensivist and be qualified/trained/certified in critical care.
- Facility for multisystem organ support.
- Central nursing station (CNS)/central monitoring facility.
- Provision of both invasive and noninvasive ventilation (preferably up to half to two-thirds of bed strength).
- Access to renal replacement therapy (RRT).
- Transcutaneous pacing facility.
- Microbiology support with facility for fungal identification (desirable).
- Nurses and duty doctors are trained/certified in critical care.
- Should have ABG, bedside X-ray and ultrasound 24 × 7.
- Access to CT and MRI.
- Protocols and policies for CCUs must be there and are observed.
- Research should be encouraged.
- Should have access to super-specialties of medicine and surgery.

Level III (for tertiary care hospitals >150 beds including medical colleges and corporate hospitals). It includes all recommendations of Level II in addition, must have following facilities/provisions.

### Level III

- Critical care unit should preferably be a closed CCU.
- Protocols and policies are defined.
- Must have provision of advanced cardiorespiratory monitoring—both invasive and noninvasive.
- Intra-and inter-hospital transport facilities available.
- Multisystem care and referral available round the clock.
- Should become lead centre for teaching and training in critical care.
- Ultrasound and echocardiography in the CCU 24 × 7.
- In-house blood bank, pharmacy and canteen services 24 × 7.
- In-house CT scan and MRI facilities strongly recommended.
- Bedside flexible bronchoscopy facility is desirable.
- Bedside renal replacement therapy (RRT).
- Continuous renal replacement therapy (CRRT) and plasma exchange facility are recommended.
- Optimum patient/nurse ratio (1:1 on patients on organ support, e.g., mechanical ventilation, RRT, multiple inotropes; and 1:2 at least when patient is on noninvasive ventilation and/or requires less intense monitoring).
- Should follow guidelines of a professional body of critical care (ISCCM) or equivalent in terms of ICU structure.
- Should act as a center for research, training and teaching, including tele-consultations and telemedicine center.
- Should be equipped for both long-term acute care and palliative care.
- Team should be well versed with transplant critical care.

### Structure

- Safe, easy, fast transport of a critically sick patient should be priority in planning for location of CCU.
- Ground floor should be avoided for CCU location.
- First floor is the ideal location in close proximity of emergency and operation theater.

- Higher floors are suitable if elevators are available close to CCU.
- Corridors, lifts and ramps should be spacious enough to provide easy movement of bed/trolley (crisscross passage of two beds/trolleys simultaneously).
- Close/easy proximity is also desirable to diagnostic facilities, blood bank, pharmacy, etc.

## DESIGN OF CCU

### Dormitory-like CCU

Space per bed has been recommended from 150 to 200 sq ft in the patient care area. Some recommendations have placed it even higher up to 250 sq ft per bed. In addition, there should be 100 to 150% extra space to accommodate nursing station, storage, patient/doctors/staff movement area, equipment area, doctor's and nurse's rooms, teaching area, relative's area and toilets to include all the four zones of ICU.

A buffer/bare area is desirable between relative's area and doctor's area.

1. However, in Indian circumstances and, after reviewing and receiving feedback from various CCUs in our country, it may be satisfactory to suggest an area of at least 150 square feet per bed be provided in patient care area (zone 1) for comfortable working with a critically sick patient where all the paraphernalia including monitoring systems, ventilators and other machines like bedside X-ray, ultrasounds, etc. Single accommodation cubicles/rooms.
   - Patient care area should be 200 to 250 sq ft. It may be prudent to make one or two bigger rooms or areas, depending upon needs like for bariatric patients and bedside procedures.
   - It is recommended to have 10% (one to two) isolation rooms where immunocompromised/infected patients may be treated. These rooms should have 20% extra space. Need for lamellar flow in isolation room in CCU has not found favor.
2. **Partition between two rooms/cubicles/beds:**
   - It is recommended that there should be a partition between rooms for patient's privacy.
   - Standard curtains soften the look and are placed commonly between two patients in most Indian CCUs, however, curtains may become unclean or get displaced and breach the privacy.
   - Two rooms may be separated by unbreakable fixed or removable partition which may be of aluminum, wood or fiber. However permanent partitions may take away the flexibility of increasing floor space temporarily when required.
3. **Isolation rooms (positive and negative pressure):**
   - To provide protective environment for patients at highest risk of infection, e.g., neutropenic and post-transplant. These rooms should have greater supply of air than exhaust air.
   - Pressure differential of 2.5–8 Pka, preferably 8 Pka. Positive airflow relative to the corridor (i.e., air flows from the room to the outside adjacent space).
4. **Number of CCU beds:**
   - Brainstorming sessions should be held to decide how many CCU beds are needed for the CCU.
   - The number of CCU beds requirement depends on the hospital's total bed strength, available need assessment data and future requirement.
   - Various issues like available space, trained manpower and budget are also important factor for consideration in deciding number of CCU beds.
   - In a tertiary care hospital, number of CCU beds requirement may vary from 5 to 25% of the total hospital beds according to the focus of the hospital. However, it is recommended that the number of CCU beds in any hospitals should not be less than 5% of total hospital beds.
   - CCUs having <6 beds are not cost-effective and may not provide enough clinical experience and exposure to staff of the CCU. At the same time CCU with bed strength of >12 is difficult to manage. Recommendations suggest that efficiency may be compromised once total number of beds crosses 12 in CCU.
   - It is recommended that total bed strength of CCU should be between 8 and 12. To have more CCU beds, it is recommended that number of ICUs be increased rather than increasing numbers of beds in one CCU.

### Zones of ICU

ICU area can be categorized into four different zones:
1. **Zone 1:** Patient care zone
2. **Zone 2:** Observation area
3. **Zone 3:** Support area
4. **Zone 4:** Family support zone

### Zone 1: Patient Care Zone

It includes the area around patient's bed.

#### Pendant vs Head-end Panel

- One of the most important decisions is how to plan bedside design.
- Two approaches are usually practiced [head-end wall panel or free-standing/hanging systems

(power columns) usually from the ceiling]. Each can be fixed or moveable and flexible. It can be on one or either side of the patient.

- Flexibility is usually desirable. Panels on head wall systems do not allow for free movements on the head end of the patients because of hanging wires and tubes.
- Though the hanging pendants look much more scientific, but our survey indicates most of our CCUs in India have head-end panels. However, new CCU planners may give a critical look at pendants rather than head-end panels.
- Adaptable power columns can move from side to side or rotate. Mounts on power columns are also usually adjustable.
- Flexible systems are expensive and counterproductive if the staff never move or adjust them.
- Ceiling-mounted, moveable, rotatory systems may reduce clutter on the floor and make a lot of work space available. However, this may not be possible if the weight of the power column cannot be structurally supported.
- A usual problem observed in CCU is getting access to the head of the bed in times of emergency and therefore keep bed 2 feet away from head-end wall. This can be achieved effectively by placing a 2 ft wide, 6 inches high wooden plank between the wall and head end.
- Lines may be routed through a fixed band.

### Height of Monitoring System

Monitoring system should be placed at the eye level. Doctors and nurses may have chronic head tilting leading to cervical neck discomfort and disorders otherwise.

### Zone 2: Observation Area

It includes central nursing station, nursing and doctor's station/computer area/immediate investigation area like ABG analysis/drug trolleys, chairs and other support system needed at the nursing station.

### Central Nursing Station

- This is the nerve center of CCU, despite lots of development, the old standard of a central station still holds good and is endorsed by most guidelines and regulations regardless of today's practice needs.
- It is the station where all the resident doctors, nurses and other support staff come together to share information and keep records. All computers and digital information system, stationery material, registers, etc., are kept here. It provides moments of discussion, relaxation and center of administration.
- All/near-all monitors and patients must be observable from there, either directly or through the central monitoring system. Most CCUs use the central station, serving six to twelve beds arranged in an L or U fashion. Patients in rooms may be difficult to observe and therefore should be placed on remote television monitoring. These monitors may satisfy regulatory requirements but do not really provide adequate patient safety if the clarity of the picture is poor.
- Some CCUs have unit pods of about four or five beds, each served by a separate workstation, nurses assigned to patients in the pod form a team, a monitor technician is also required. Ensure adequate space planning, also, new equipment purchased over the next decade will probably increase the amount of desk and shelf space required.
- At times of high use, the number of people in the central station can increase several folds. Having enough space and chairs to meet needs during such times should be provided for. The space should accommodate computer terminals and printers. A large number of communication cables may be required per bedside to connect computers and faxes to other departments, as well as to other institutions and offices, adequate space for charting on the platform is absolutely important.
- Patients must be easily visible from the charting area whether the nurse is sitting or standing, taller chairs are often necessary. In case of space constraint, collapsible desktops or shelves that can flip up off the wall can be planned. Space allotted for storage of the previous charts of patients currently in the unit should also be provided It is also important that a storage space is provided for equipment, linen, instruments, drugs, medicines, disposables, stationery and other articles to be stored at the nursing station must be provided. All these cupboards should be labelled. The latest generation of monitoring systems allows access to patient data from any bedside; this means that the doctor who is busy caring for one patient can monitor others without leaving that bedside. Consoles can be programmed to automatically display critical events from one bedside at several sites without personnel calling for it.

### Zone 3: Support Area

It includes offices, doctor's duty room, nurses' room, stores, toilets, discussion and teaching rooms including library. Three important store levels are recommended in a busy ICU.
1. By the bedside/a portable trolley
2. At the nursing station
3. Nursing stores

*Remote Central Store*

- Those items used repeatedly and in emergencies should be readily available and easy to access. Storage of large inventory can be costly and also waste of personnel time. Making items more easily available may increase their use. Some overcautious or clever staff may decide to hoard or hide them. Cost-effective and efficient designs are needed.
- Staff nurses can always give useful ideas about improvement of systems, which they develop while working with patients. Their opinion can be invaluable.
- Bedside supply carts that are stocked for different subsets of patients can make storage in the room more efficient, e.g., surgical, medical, trauma, and cardiac patients where needs are different.
- Staff nurses may be specifically trained for such care and work determining what supplies are placed near but not at the bedside is based on the size of the unit, the grouping of patients and the patterns of practice, although many units organize supplies by the department that restocks them (central services, nutrition, pharmacy, respiratory therapy, etc.).
- It is worth considering grouping supply by activity, like chest tray, central line tray, skin care tray, catheterization tray, intracranial pressure tray, etc.

### Zone 4: Family Support and Remote Area

It includes waiting area, relaxation area, prayer area, food, beverages, water, rest rooms, pharmacy and social workers area/counseling area/CCU central stores.

*Floor*

- The ideal floor should be easy to clean, non-slippery, able to withstand abuse and absorb sound while enhancing the overall look and feel of the environment, carts and beds equipped with large wheels should roll easily over it.
- In Indian context vitrified non-slippery tiles seem to be the best option which can be fitted into reasonable budgets, easy to clean and move on and may be stain-proof vinyl sheeting is another viable option, it can be nonporous, strong and easy to clean.
- The life of vinyl flooring is not long and a small damage in one corner may trigger damage of entire flooring and make it accident-prone. It may require frequent replacement making it to be inconvenient choice.

*Walls*

- Durability, ability to clean and maintain, flame retardance, mildew resistance, sound absorption and visual appeal are the major requirements.
- It has been very useful to have a height up to 4 to 5 feet finished with similar tiles as of floor for similar reasons. For rest of the wall soothing paint with glass panels on the head end at the top may be good choice.
- Wooden panelling has also found favor with some architects, but costs may go high.
- Door stoppers and handrails should be placed well to reduce abuse and noise to minimum, it helps patient movement and ambulation.

*Ceiling*

- Ceiling surface is most commonly seen by patient. Bright spotlights or fluorescent lights can cause eye strain, ceiling should be soiling and break-proof due to leaks and condensation.
- Tiles may not be the most appealing or soothing surface, but for all practical purposes, it is easier to remove individual or few tiles for repairs over ceiling in times of need.
- Ceiling design may be enhanced by varying the ceiling height, softening the contours, griddled lighting surfaces, painting it with a medley of soft colors (yellow, sky-blue, light grey) rather than a plain background color, or decorating it with patterns or murals, to make it more patient- and staff-friendly.
- It is recommended that no lines or wires be kept or run over ceiling or underground because damages do occur once in a while and, therefore, it should be easy to do repairs if the lines and pipes are easily explorable without hindering patient care.

*Furniture and Furnishings*

- The counters and furniture should be tough to withstand a lot of heavy use, easy to clean and maintain, connections should be made of metal-to-metal fasteners.
- Cabinet-quality wood construction should also be tough and strong, surfaces for counters should be solid, nonporous and stain-resistant, fabrics should be durable, color fast and flame- and static-resistant, if possible.
- Bedside clocks, calendars and bulletin boards help the conscious patient to get well-oriented and in better moods.
- Providing the patient with a place to keep a few small personal items of their own make the environment more familiar and personalized.
- **Chair number and types:** Individual units should decide about the number, usually enough number to accommodate the care-giving staff/doctors and nurses and additional chairs may be stored and used whenever needed. Individual units should decide whether they

want to allow the relative to sit by the side (short or long time) of the patient in the CCU. However, a chair/sofa-type chair on wheels with safety belt or vault is recommended for mobilizing the patient and making him sit during recovery.

*Electrical Services*
- The main electrical circuit breaker panel should branch out to individual feeder line for each CCU.
- The emergency power source like electricity generator power should quickly take over in case of city power failure.
- Each patient cubicle should have at least seven duplex grounded receptacles 5/15 amp. The location of these receptacles can be either on wall, bed head panel, ceiling-suspended pendant units or vertical column based on choice from hospital team.
- It is strongly suggested to have at least 50% of electrical receptacles connected to uninterrupted power supply (UPS) with proper label. Each receptacle or cluster within an CCU should be serviced by its own circuit breaker in the electrical panel preferably located in utility room of CCU.
- The lighting distribution illumination control should be planned based on routine physical examination (around 350 lux), during procedure of patient (around 1000 lux), during nighttime (around 5 lux). The lighting distribution board should be separate from power distribution board. The emergency lighting should be connected to few light fixtures to avoid a complete black out scenario. The energy conservation aspect like LED lights and more natural daylight should also be considered.

*Environmental Requirements*
- Heating, ventilation and air-conditioning (HVAC) system of CCU.
- The CCU should be fully air-conditioned which allows control of temperature, humidity and air change. If this may not be possible, then one should have windows which can be opened ('tilt and turn' windows are a useful design). Suitable and safe air quality must be maintained at all times.
- Air movement should always be from clean to dirty areas. It is recommended to have a minimum of six air changes per room per hour, out of which two air changes per hour composed of outside air. Where air-conditioning is not universal, cubicles should have fifteen air changes per hour and other patient areas at least three per hour. The dirty utility, sluice and laboratory need five changes per hour, but two per hour are sufficient for other staff areas.
- In negative pressure isolation rooms (isolation of patients infected/suspected to be infected with organisms spread via airborne droplet nuclei <5 μm in diameter), the windows do not open. They have greater exhaust than supply air volume. Pressure differential of 2.5 Pa. Clean to dirty airflow, i.e., direction of the airflow is from the outside adjacent space (i.e., corridor, anteroom) into the room. Air from room preferably exhausted to the outside but may be re-circulated provided it is through HEPA filter.
**NB:** Re-circulating air taken from areas intended to isolate a patient with TB is a risk not worth taking and is not recommended.
- Central air-conditioning systems and re-circulated air must pass through appropriate filters. It is recommended that all air should be filtered to 99% efficiency down to 5 microns. Smoking should not be allowed in the CCU complex.
- Heating should be provided with an emphasis on the comfort of the patients and the CCU personnel. For critical care units having enclosed patient modules, the temperature should be adjustable within each module to allow a choice of temperatures from 16 to 25°C.

*Lighting*
- Access to outside natural light is recommended by regulatory authorities in USA. This may improve the staff morale and patient outcome.
- Data suggests that synthetic artificial daylight use in work environment may deliver better results for nighttime workers. It may be helpful in maintaining the circadian rhythm.
- Natural lighting in the unit can decrease power consumption and the electrical bill which is so relevant to Indian circumstances. Access to natural light also means one may have access to viewing external environment which may be developed into green and soothing.
- **Light for procedures:** High illumination and spot lighting is needed for procedures, like inserting central lines, etc. They can descend from the ceiling, extend from the wall/panel, or be carried into the room. Spot lighting should be shadow free with 150 footcandles (fc) strength.
- Light required for general patient care should be bright enough to ensure adequate vision without eye strain.
- Overhead lighting should be at least 20 footcandles.
- Higher frequency fluorescent lights and coated phosphorus lamps may be good for assessing skin color and tone
- Patients may need rest and quiet surroundings during the day, blackout curtains or blinds or individual eye

may be used. This may be helpful when the staff requires a high level of lighting at the bedside while the patient is resting.
- Lights that come on automatically when cupboard doors or drawers are opened are useful.
- Floors lighting may be important for safety at the bedside and in the hallways at night and should be about 10 fc. Glare created by reflected light should be diffused.
- Light switches should be strategically located to allow some patient control and adequate staff convenience.
- A second remote control can be turned on/off by the nurses/doctors to observe patients intermittently at night without entering the room and disturbing the patient.

### Noise Level in CCU

The International Noise Council recommends that the noise level in an ICU be under 45 dBA in the daytime, 40 dBA in the evening and 20 dBA at night. For example, 16 A watch ticks at about 20 dBA, normal conversation is at about 55 dBA, vacuum cleaner produces about 70 dBA.

## Critical Care Unit Equipment

Client monitoring, respiratory and cardiac support, pain management, emergency resuscitation devices, and other life support equipment are all part of critical care unit (CCU) equipment, which is used to care for seriously injured patients, life-threatening illness, or have undergone a major surgical procedure and require 24-hour care and monitoring **(Fig. 18.1)**.

### CCU Equipment

- Patient monitoring
- Emergency resuscitation devices
- Diagnostic devices

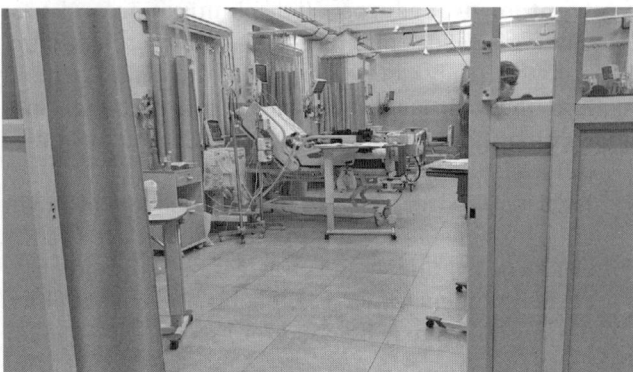

**Fig. 18.1:** Emergency resuscitation equipment with CCU setup.

### Patient Monitoring Equipment

- Physiological monitoring system
- Pulse oximeter
- ICP monitor
- Apnea monitor

### Emergency Resuscitative Equipment

- Ventilator
- Infusion pump
- Crash cart
- Intrathoracic balloon pump

### Diagnostic Devices

For early diagnostic evaluation the devices are used like-mobile X-ray, portable devices and blood analyzer, etc.

## PROTOCOLS AND POLICIES OF CCU

Protocol defines a set of operational procedures to ensure that there is a well-defined manner of doing a given task. Policy is typically a set of rules designed to achieve certain goals as part of an organization's growth (Lane H et al., 2020).

### Purpose

To delineate the policies for guiding regarding the care of patient in CCU and HDU.

### Policy

- The treating doctor/in charge of the CCU will decide on admission and discharge. Each patient must be cared for by a nurse, with a patient-to-nurse ratio of 2:1 at all times. Infection control procedures must be followed in intensive care areas. The quality assurance programme must be followed by intensive care units (Citrome L et al.).
- Visitors are not permitted in high dependency areas, except in exceptional circumstances where close relatives may be admitted during visiting hours.
- In scarcity of beds, people who are normal condition will be relocated to the wards, and emergency patients will be given priority.
- At-least one empty bed must available at all times for emergency clients requiring CCU admission.
- In CCUs, a quality assurance system has been implemented and is being followed.
- Bionil disinfectant will be used to clean the floors, workstations, and other areas.

### Procedure

Admission and discharge in CCU will be decided by the treating doctor/CCU charge nurse. A nurse must be present

with each patient at all times, with a patient-to-nurse ratio of 2:1. In CCU, infection control protocols must be followed:
- If there are not enough beds, normal individuals will be sent to the wards, and emergency patients will be prioritized.
- Admission criteria in CCU based on the patient who needs critical care services. At the consultant's request, patients who meet all the criteria, will be admitted to the CCUs. While we make every effort to meet admission requirements, we do make exceptions for consultants who believe a patient would benefit from extensive monitoring in the CCU.

### Infection Control

Nosocomial infection prevention document, which includes instructions and best practices for patient care, is a valuable resource. The committee should evaluate, approve and update (Rosenthal VD et al., 2004).

### Education of Health Care Staff

The need of an infection control program should be stressed to health officials. They should have knowledge on infection control and also have efficient skill to perform the activities. Health team should:
- Evaluate staff programs and give necessary training through programs, in-service education, and training during the job period.
- Arrange staff training programs for critical care.
- Re-train or orient staff on a regular basis, and assess the effect of training.

### Infection Control Practices

Infection control protective measures are divided into standard measures which should be followed by all the patients in all times regardless of any disease and patient condition can prevent and control infection transmission in healthcare facilities (Caddell A, 2020).

### Quality Precautions

Educate all the patients in a hospital about the "standard" precautions necessitates the use of work practices that are critical which can enhancing the level of protection to patients, healthcare personnel, and relatives. These are some of them (WHO).

Use of personal protective clothing when handling blood, bodily substances, excretions, and secretions; appropriate handling of patient care equipment and dirty linen.
- Avoiding needlestick and sharp injury
- Environmental clean-up and spill clean-up
- Waste management that is appropriate.
- Proper hand hygiene can reduce the number of microorganisms on the hands acquired through daily tasks.
- To avoid cross-contamination between distinct body sites between tasks and treatments on the same patient.
- Immediately after taking off the gloves.
- Using a simple soap with an antimicrobial agent, such as an alcoholic handrub or a waterless handwash.

### Use of PPE

- Personal protection equipment (PPE) acts as physical barrier between microbes and the wearer. It can protect by means of preventing microbes from infecting objects.
- It is informed to other patients and staff are being informed (about PPE).

The following individuals should wear personal protection equipment:
- Healthcare professionals whose who are giving treatment to patients and work in environments when they come into touch with soiled linens, bodily fluids.
- Lab personnel who handle patient specimens; and family members and may come into touch with blood, body fluids, secretions, or excretions. Personal protective equipment (PPE) guidelines personal protective equipment minimises the danger of infection but does not totally remove it. It is critical that it is used properly, accurately, and at all times when patients' blood and bodily fluids are involved **(Fig. 18.2)**.

### PPE Guidelines

#### Gloves

When handling of contaminated objects and body fluids use sterile or clean gloves. When working with various patients, change gloves. To avoid cross-contamination across various body sites. Before attending another patient,

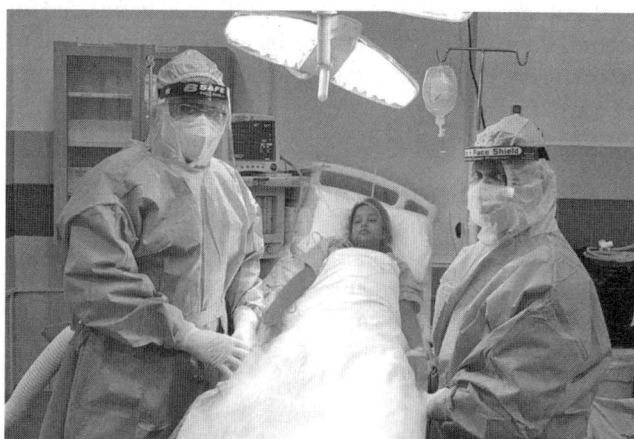

**Fig. 18.2:** Handling of patient by using PPE.

remove gloves immediately after use. After removing the gloves, immediately wash your hands. Use a simple soap, an antimicrobial, waterless antiseptic. Disposable gloves should be disposed away according to hospital practice.

## Masks

When performing procedures that may result in splashes of body fluids, use mask to protect the mouth and nose. Instead of using cotton or gauze masks, use surgical masks. Surgical masks are made of several materials that resist fluids to varied degrees. Disposable masks should never be used again. They should be disposed of in accordance with the hospital's procedures. When dealing with a patient's blood, body fluids, excretions, or secretions, it's critical to utilise personal protective equipment properly, accurately, and at all times.

## Protective eyewear/goggles/visors/face shield

When performing procedures there may be chances of splitting of bodily fluids so use face shield or googles to protect the eyes. If disposable, dispose of it properly. If they're reusable, follow the manufacturer's recommendations for decontamination.

## Gowns or aprons

Wear gown during procedures to protect yourself from soiling. Gowns that are impermeable are preferred. As quickly as possible, remove a filthy or wet gown. To protect against blood, body fluids, secretions, and excretions, a plastic apron can be put over the gown. If gowns and aprons are reusable, wash them according to the hospital's instructions. Disposable gowns should not be reused and disposed according to the hospital's policies.

## Cap and shoe covers

Caps and boots/shoes to be used when there is risk of contamination. And these types of PPE need to be used for second time, use it by washing it by following the standard instructions. Disposable caps and shoe covers should not be reused.

## Patient care items

Handling of the patient care equipment that has been soiled with contaminated body fluids with caution to avoid skin and mucous membrane exposure, as well as clothing and the environment. Before using reused equipment on another patient, make sure it is thoroughly cleaned and reprocessed.

## Linen

Handling, transporting, and processing of contaminated linen with caution to avoid fluid leakage.

## Prevention of needle stick/sharps injuries

When utilizing needles or other sharp items, exercise caution. Dispose of discarded disposable syringes in a PPC with a cover that latches and is close to where the item is used. Reusable devices use with extreme caution. Never twist or recap needles. Sharp instruments must be disinfected and/or disposed of according to national regulations or guidelines.

## Management of biomedical waste

It is very important to maintain control over the bio-medical waste to prevent a higher range of infections.

### *Additional (Transmission-based) Precautions*

Additional safeguards: Airborne, droplet, contact infection precautions.

### For Airborne Related Precautions

The measures are intended to limit disease transmission via the airborne route. Droplet nuclei (evaporated droplets) microns cause airborne transmission. These droplet nuclei can be present in air for some minutes to hours. Droplet can be ranging from 1 to 5 micron. Droplets are produced by an infected person coughing, sneezing, talking, or when health care providers perform operations like tracheal suctioning precautions should be taken.

**Implement of standard precautions**

- Place the patient in a "negative pressure room," which is a single room with a monitored negative airflow pressure.
- Keep doors shut.
- Anyone entering the room they should wear a specific mask (e.g., N 95) with high filtration.
- Only relocate and transport the patient out of the room when absolutely necessary. If transportation is required, mask the patient with a surgical mask to prevent droplet nuclei from dispersing. For ensuring that negative airflow pressure is maintained, it is critical to secure the assistance of engineering services.

### For droplet related precaution

When droplets (> 5 microns) come into touch with immune suppressed person, droplet transmission occurs. 7 Droplets are produced by infected people when they cough, sneeze, talk, or when healthcare providers perform treatments like tracheal suctioning. Precautions should be taken as follows:

**Implementation of standard precautions**

- Isolate the client.
- Distance should be maintained that is 1–2 meters of a patient, there you can wear a surgical mask.
- While transporting, cover the patient with a surgical mask.

- No special air handling or ventilation is necessary to avoid infection transmission via droplets.

### For contact related precautions

Organisms which are resistant to antibiotics, GI infection, and dermatological infections are all diseases spread by this route. Precautions should be taken as follows:

### Implementation of standard precautions

- Isolate the client. When deciding where to send patients, keep in mind the disease's epidemiology and the patient population.
- Where there is risk of exposure wear a clean or non-sterile gown.
- Keep patient mobility and transport to a minimum; patients should only be transported for medical reasons. If transportation is necessary, take care to reduce the chances of infection.
- Patients must be placed appropriately or selectively to limit the infection in hospital during transportation. The ideal distance between two beds is 1–2 meters.

## NURSING AUDIT

The word "audit" comes from the Latin word "auditus" a hearing. It used to mean hearing facts and arguments about a topic in order to ascertain the truth.

Nursing auditing is the practice of gathering information about patient care through nursing reports and other written evidence and evaluating it using quality assurance procedures.

A nursing audit is a thorough examination and evaluation of selected clinical data by qualified professionals in order to assess nursing care quality.

### Meaning

**Quality** is a judgment of what constitutes good or bad. **Audit** is a systemic methodical and critical analysis that is used to verify something.

### Nursing Audit

It is a method of assessing the quality of nursing care that employs and the use of a record to aid in the evaluation of patient care.

**Medical auditing** is a systematic, critical analysis of the quality critical care, encompassing diagnostic and treatment methods, resource utilization, and patient outcomes and quality of life (Saranto K et al, 2012).

### Definition

"The term "nursing audit" refers to the evaluation of clinical nursing quality (Elison).

A nursing audit is a test to see if excellent nursing practices are being followed. The audit is a tool that allows nurses to create standards from their perspective and describe actual nursing practice (Goster Walfer).

### Purposes of Nursing Audit

- The patient's nursing treatment is being evaluated.
- Achieves a level of nursing care that is both deserved and possible.
- Encourages better records.
- It focuses on the care given rather than the giver.
- Contributes to evidence-based practice research.

### Essential Characteristics of Nursing Audit

- Written nursing care standards to review.
- Proof that real practice was compared to these criteria.
- Review and analyzed the findings.
- Evidence of therapeutic action.
- Proof that corrective action was effective.
- Accurate audit program documentation.

### Types of Nursing Audit

- **Internal auditing:** It is a control technique performed by an external auditor who is an employee of the organization. He makes an independent appraisal the policies, plans and points the deficits in the policies or plans and give suggestions for deficits.
- **External auditing:** It is an independent appraisal of the organizations financial account and statements. The external auditor is a qualified person who has to certify the annual profit and loss account and prepare a balance sheet after careful examination of the relevant books of accounts and documents.

### Audit Committee

An audit committee of at least five members should be created before an audit is conducted.

### Methods for Nursing Audit

Two methods are used for:

*Retrospective View*

It is an in-depth evaluation of the quality care after discharge of the patient, using the patient's records as the source of data. Retrospective auditing is a method of assessing the quality of nursing care by looking at the nursing care as it appears in discharged patients' medical records. Specific behaviors are detailed in this form of audit, then convert into questions, the examiner searches the record for responses,

e.g., the examiner goes over the patient's documents and asks:
- Was the problem-solving approach applied to nursing care planning?
- Is patient information obtained in a systematic way?
- Did you include a description of the patient's pre-hospital routines?

*Concurrent Review*

This is based on the assessments which is made for the patients who are still receiving the treatment. It entails monitoring the patient at the bedside against predetermined criteria, interviewing the caregivers, and analyzing the patient's medical record and treatment plan.

## Steps of Audit Cycle

*Selecting a Topic*
- At the outset, significant consideration and planning are required.
- Attempting to audit an uncommon condition with an insignificant outcome seems pointless.

*Planning Audit*
- Include everyone who is affected.
- Schedule time and resources.
- Obtain evidence and data.
- The methodology to be used.
- Pilot project.
- Make a report for action.
- Re-audit every action should be recorded.

*Developing Criteria*
- Establish a patient population.
- Establish a time schedule for evaluating care outcomes.
- State patient outcome criteria and identify regularly recurrent nursing difficulties presented by the described patient group. Indicate the information's source.

*Keypoints to be Remembered*
- Quality control must be prioritized. Those are in charge not only utilize a tool, but also conduct a periodic program.
- Quality assurance activities should be developed and evaluated by a coordinator. It is necessary to assign roles and tasks.
- Nurses must be informed on the program's methodology and outcomes.
- Data must be trustworthy, e.g., data collecting must be properly oriented.

*Measuring Level of Performance*
- The information gathered should be precise, complete, and adequate.
- To be included in the user group immunization status of pregnant mothers, for example. Keep it basic and brief by not trying to acquire too many objects.
- Information saved on computers, medical records, surveys, questionnaires, and interviews, focused groups, prospective data is recording to obtain the necessary information and compare the performance.

*Making Improvements Identifying Barriers to Change*
- Misunderstanding
- Low morale
- Poor communication
- Uncertainty about the outcome.

*Systematic Approach*
- Identifying local change hurdles
- Altering the culture
- Encouragement of teamwork
- Employing a variety of specialized techniques such as delegation and accountability

*Sustaining Improvement Monitoring*
- Organized strategy to altering the practice, should include goals to track and assess progress.
- Keep the transformation going on and reinforce it.

*Reinforcing Improvement*
- Management-provided reinforcement or motivation.
- Auditing is integrated.
- Effective management by strong leadership.

*Re-audit*
- Examine the evidence.
- Evaluate efficiency.
- Establish a schedule for re-auditing.
- Continuous monitoring of the process.
- Unfavorable outcomes.

## Merits of Nursing Audit
- It is used as a measurement tool in all aspects of nursing.
- Evaluates the efforts of everyone involved in the documentation of care.
- In regions where accurate records of care are preserved. Also included is a biographical index of each patient's nursing quality.
- It will provide useful and relevant information to the employees, including improvements in nursing quality as well as strengths and shortcomings in nursing service.

- Improved nursing note quality will lead to better collaboration and communication among nurses and other members of the healthcare team.
- It will aid in the self-evaluation of each professional nurse.

## Demerits of the Nursing Audit
- It evaluates nursing process.
- Many of the components overlap, making it difficult to analyze. Takes a long time.
- Trained auditors are required.
- It compacts with lot of data and is viewed as a source of punishment by the professional community.

## Quality Care Through Nursing Audit

### Dyssy's (Dynamic Standard-Setting System) Quality Assurance Cycle

Phases
- **Describing phase:**
  - Select topic
  - Identify care group
  - Write standard statement
- **Audit phase:**
  - Agree on standard and implement studies
  - Define criteria
  - Design audit tool
  - Collect audit data
  Evaluate results (either compliance or non-compliance)
- **Taking action phase:**
  - Identify problems (action plan for quality improvement)
  - Plan, implement and action
  - Re-evaluate result

### Writing Standard Statement
Adopt RUMBA technique

**R**—**R**elevant
**U**—**U**nderstandable
**M**—**M**easurable
**B**—**B**ehaviorally stated
**A**—**A**chievable

- Nursing standard like admission, OT, ITU postoperative care in ITU and late postoperative care.
- Touch the aspects of structure, process and outcome.

*Structure: Which? Setting in Which Patient Care Provided*

**Example:** Staff, knowledge, protocol, equipment, records and environment, etc.

*Process: How?*

Process of care and the way the care was carried out and it is task oriented.

**Example:** Direct nurse client interaction, supervision of client, observation of symptoms and reacting and reporting and recording.

*Outcome: What Results? It is the End Results of Care*

- **Example:** Measure the quality of hospital care includes mortality, morbidity and length of hospital stay
- **Writing standard statement:**
  - *Topic:* Basic nursing
  - *Sub topic:* IM Injection
  - *Care group:* Staff nurses
  - *Standard statement:* All patients receive IM injection following proper technique to prevent injection abscess **(Table 18.1)**.

*Implement the Standard by*

- Audit topic
- Audit objective
- Auditors
- Date of audit
- Area: CCU
- Audit tool: Questionnaire regarding proper IM injection practice **(Table 18.2)**.

**Table 18.1:** Questionnaire on structure, process and outcome regarding IM injection with following proper technique to prevent injection abscess.

| Structure | Process | Outcome |
|---|---|---|
| Knowledge on complication of IM injection | Hand washing with appropriate technique | No pain |
| Adequate sterile syringes | Maintaining sterilization | No manifestation of infection |
| Adequate 24 gauze needles | Using 24 gauze needle or not | No abscess |
| Written drug protocol available in unit | Maintaining protocol for IM inj. | No drug error |
| Availability of registered nurses with experience | IM procedure is explained by RN to patient prior to procedure or not | No ethical problem was findout |

**Table 18.2:** Audit questionnaire on IM injection practice.

| Code no. | Audit questions | 1 | 2 | 3 | 4 | 5 | 6 | 7 | 8 | 9 | 10 |
|---|---|---|---|---|---|---|---|---|---|---|---|
| $S_1$ | Does the staff has knowledge on complications of IM inj? | Y | N | Y | Y | N | N | Y | N | Y | Y |
| $P_1$ | Did she wash her hand with appropriate steps of handwashing? | Y | Y | Y | N | N | N | N | N | N | Y |
| $S_2$ | Are adequate sterile syringes are available? | | | | | | | | | | |
| $O_4$ | Whether any drug error occurred during administration? | | | | | | | | | | |
| $S_5$ | Whether experience registered nurses are available in that ward? | | | | | | | | | | |
| $P_5$ | Does staff explained the IM procedure to patient before administration? | | | | | | | | | | |

### Role of Nurse in Quality Assurance and Audit Cycle

Nursing audit team include:

- **Nursing administrator:** Audits the charges on medical bills; conducts managed care defence audits; conducts under/over charge audits; reviews charge-related patient complaints; reviews denied charges; recommends appeals and where appropriate, facilitates the resolution of root causes; communicates audit findings. Under direction, performs specialized administrative tasks pertaining to hospital billing and reimbursement activities.
- **Nursing service:** Nursing audit is the assessment of the quality of nursing care and uses a record as an aid in evaluating the quality of patient care. Nursing Audit is an important component of medical audit. Nursing documentation is an important part of multi-professional patient care. The standard of information that all healthcare workers have access to determines the ability to provide high-quality treatment and communicate effectively regarding patient care. Nursing education. The purpose of a nursing audit is to identify, analyze, or verify the performance of specific specified components of nursing care using established criteria.
- **Nursing specialist:** Clinical nurse specialists are qualified to request tests, offer some diagnoses, carry out simple procedures, and, in some states, write prescriptions for drugs. Beyond this, they could offer knowledge and assistance to a group of nurses, give direct patient care, work as knowledgeable consultants for nursing staffs, and actively participate in enhancing health care delivery systems. Clinical nurse specialists frequently hold management positions and may also create policies and procedures independently or as part of a team.
- **Clinical nurses:** The purpose of a nursing audit is to identify, analyze, or verify the performance of specific specified components of nursing care using established criteria. It entails a thorough assessment and evaluation of selected clinical data by qualified professional staff.

The practice of gathering data from nursing reports and other sources of written evidence concerning patient care and evaluating the quality of care using quality assurance programs is known as nursing audit.

### Role of Nurse Administrator in Implementing Quality Assurance

- **Initiator:** Creates an awareness or sensitizes the nurses about the importance of quality assurance.
- **Facilitator:** She facilitates to develop, implement, monitor and evaluate standards for nursing practice at all times.
- **Coordinator:** She coordinates the different units of quality assurance program and coordinates the activities with the hospitals quality assurance program.
- **Educator:** She gives orientation to nursing personnel regarding the need for standards and auditing of nursing service.
- **Leader:** She communicates the quality message to all the staff members.
- **Evaluator:** She evaluates the implementation of standards for nursing practice.
- **Supervisor:** She supervises the activities of different committees. She supervises the nurses at first and second level leadership positions.

### Utilization of Results of Nursing Audit

- **For nursing care services:**
  - Changing nurse care plans for a specific patient demographic, including discharge planning.
  - Putting in place a program to improve nursing care documentation through better charting policies, procedures, and forms.
  - Concentrating supervisory attention on identified weakness, such as a single nursing staff.
- **For nursing administrators:**
  - Conduct evaluations of specific programs, such as employee orientation or the implementation of a patient teaching program.

- Assist with accreditation and funding requests for specific programs.
- Assist in identifying areas of strength and weakness in nursing programs as a whole, in individual aspects of the program, and in diverse contexts where a program is offered.
- Assess the impact of various staffing arrangements.
- It can be used to determine cost-effectiveness. Studies comparing the quality of care obtained by patients in various scenarios with varying staffing expenses, for example.
- **For supervisor and head nurse:**
  - Identify areas where patient care could be improved.
  - Provide a foundation for developing an in-service education program.
  - Determine the training and supervision requirements for workers who provide direct patient care.
- **For staff nurse:**
  - Conduct a self-evaluation of care in their particular nursing unit or location.
  - Determine which sorts of care will require greater knowledge and skill on the part of the personnel to enhance.
  - Identify specific types of care for which enhanced attention and consciousness could improve practice.

*Factors Affecting Quality Assurance in Nursing Care*

- **Lack of resources:** Insufficient resources, infrastructures, laws or torts in the hospital settings are equipment, funds to meet the minimum needs of the patients, are major factors which may affect the quality of care.
- **Lack of qualified nursing personnel:** Lack of qualified skilled nurses, lack of motivation, indisciplined organizational climate may affect the quality care.
- **Unreasonable patients and relatives:** Illness anxiety, absence of immediate response to treatment, sometimes lead to uncooperative attitudes from patient and significant others which ultimately affect quality care.
- **Improper maintenance:** The building especially leakage of roofs, cleaning of bathroom, toilets, and wards have to be maintained properly otherwise patient may develop hospital acquired infections.
- **Absence of well-informed populace:** To improve quality nursing care, it is surveys necessary that the people become knowledgeable and assert their right to quality care. This can be achieved through continuous health education program.
- **Absence of accreditation laws:** Accreditation laws keep check over quality care by:
  - Inspecting hospitals and ensuring that basic requirements are met.
  - Enquiring into major incidence of negligence.
  - Taking action against health professionals involved in malpractices.
- **Legal readers:** Laws or torts in the hospital settings are very less applicable to the nursing profession for their quality of care and do not exist practically. Thus the professional behavior may affect the quality of care.
- **Lake of incident review procedures:** The critical incidents may be:
  - Delayed attendance by physicians, surgeon, nurse.
  - Barriers assisting out of faculty procedures.
  - Death in a corridor with no physician/nurse accompanying the patient.
- **Lack of good hospital information system:**
  - Workload, statistic, admission, bed occupancy, procedure, length of stay.
  - Activity, audit, scheduling of procedures, cost list/procedures in critical areas.
  - These information should be accurately informed.
- **Absence of conducting patient satisfaction:** Surveys come out through questionnaires or interviews by social worker, hospital management trainers and consultant groups, e.g., delay in attendance by doctors/nurses, incidents or incorrect treatment.
- **Lack of nursing care records:**
  - Details of the patient condition should be documented.
  - For information regarding response to treatment nurses should use problem-oriented record system.
- **Miscellaneous factors:**
  - Lack of good supervision.
  - Substandard education and training.
  - Lack of policy and administrative manuals.

## STAFFING OF CCU

### Staffing

It is the ongoing process of locating, choosing, reviewing, and creating a working relationship with current or prospective employees. The size of the hospital necessitates a larger crew (Follath F et al., 2011).

The staffing levels of critical care environments is one of the most important factors in the delivery of higher levels of care. The ratios of both medical and nursing staff to patients are standardized by the faculty of intensive care medicine and the intensive care society guidelines.

### Medical Staff

- Senior medical staff should be appointed to the CCU are carrier intensivists, and he or she will be the director.

- Other experts with clinical commitments elsewhere, such as anesthesia, medicine, and chest, are less chosen.
- Trainees in critical care, trainees from other disciplines make up the junior staff.

## Nursing Staff

The level of patient care required in terms of organ system support dictates the nursing staff to patient ratio. There should also be a supernumerary nurse in charge to co-ordinate care and participate in the daily ward rounds. Additionally, larger intensive care units should have extra supernumerary 'floating' nurses to assist with patient care, allowing for surge capacity and cover for staff meal breaks. The numbers required depend upon the size of the unit but is recommended to be:

- **11–20 beds** = 1 additional supernumerary registered nurse.
- **21–30 beds** = 2 additional supernumerary registered nurses.
- **31–40 beds** = 3 additional supernumerary registered nurses.

At least 50% of the nurses (but ideally most if not all) should have a post registration award in critical care nursing. Similar to the medical staff there should be a senior nurse who has overall managerial responsibility for each CCU, i.e., a matron.

- The primary tertiary education institution critical-care nurses will be required in the CCU.
- Having an in-house critical care nursing training program could be ideal.
- For such units, a 1:1 nurse-to-patient ratio is appropriate.
- They may need two nurses per patient in more difficult scenarios.
- The trained nurses should be calculated based on the kind of CCU, workload.

## Requirements for Director of Unit

- CCU clinical, administrative, and educational direction requires training, enthusiasm, and time availability.
- Requirement of critical care medicine board certification.
- Access to the unit 24 hours a day, 7 days a week (either the director or a suitably trained surrogate) for clinical and administrative problems. Participation in local and national critical care organizations. Participation in critical care medicine-related continuing education programs.
- Permission to undertake invasive operations in the hospital. Active participation in the overall organization of care for critically ill patients in the community. And reviewing the proper utilization of CCU resources.

## Nurse as a Manager

- A nurse practitioner have the degree—critical care certification or comparable graduate study.
- Able to verify that critical care nursing practise which meets the standards. A complished with health information systems, quality improved management initiatives.
- Establish a co-operative attitude when it comes to the training of health workers regarding the treatment of medical-surgical unit patients.
- Continuing nursing education classes. Current developments in the field of critical care knowledge regular attendance should be checked out.
- Participate in strategic planning.

## CCU Nursing Requirements

- A skilled critical care nurse able to give all patient care under supervision.
- Before taking full responsibility for patient care, all nurses working in CCU should complete critical care course.
- Before taking on patient care responsibilities, you must complete a unit orientation.
- Written hospital policies should dictate nurse-patient ratio based on patient acuity.
- Continuing education is required for all critical care nurses.
- Educate the nurses in advanced techniques for early diagnosis and immediate treatment which enhancing the prognosis of the disease condition.
- They should be aware about the risks associated with advanced techniques and therapies.

### Requirements for Respiratory Care

- This services should be offered 24 hours per day, seven days in a week, and the unit should always have an adequate number of respiratory therapists with specific expertise. Staffing levels are based on acuity. Before giving treatment to CCU patients, therapists must complete a unit orientation.
- The therapist must be familiar with mechanical ventilators and their varied modes of operation.
- Experience of transporting a critically ill patients is necessary.
- Respiratory therapist participate in quality improvement and ongoing education relating to their activities.

- Ideally, in-house coverage should be given 24 hours a day who are solely focused on the treatment of CCU patients and have no competing obligations.
- The ratio should be based on delicacy, complexity, and welfare of clients in hospitals.
- Within 30 minutes, the following specialists should be available and competent to offer patient care.

### Physician of Different Specialists

There are different specialists are required to provide the treatment and quality care such cardio, nephro, neuro, etc. Some other health personnels are playing an important role in CCU **(Table 18.3)**.

### Other Personnel

Other personnel may make a substantial contribution to the CCU's efficient operation.

Clerical staff, skilled nurses, physician in speciality wise, dietician, biomedical waste management superior are among these professionals.

### Laboratory Services

A clinical laboratory should be open 24-hours a day, 7 days a week to perform hematologic, chemical and toxicological studies. Laboratory tests must be provided quickly, in certain cases instantly. Next to the CCU or quick transport systems are "STAT" or "bedside" laboratories.
- CCU patients should have access to diagnostic and therapeutic radiologic procedures around the clock.
- In critically ill patients, portable chest radiographs influence decision-making.

## Design of CCU

A strategy for designing, fashioning, executing, or constructing a structure for a certain purpose (Hasin Y et al., 2005).

### Definition

A specific goal or objective pursued by an individual or a group.
- It necessitates meticulous planning. The hospital's need and location must be kept in mind. Medical CCU, surgical ICU, CCU, burns ICU, trauma ICU, and other units may be planned by an institute and managed separately by single discipline specialists' beds in hospitals typically range from 1 to 10 per 100 in total hospital beds. Interdisciplinary programs necessitate about more beds than single-specialty programs. CCU with less beds are inefficient, whereas those with more than twenty beds are unmanageable. OT, imaging logy, wards, and the casualty should all be within close proximity of the CCU. There should be enough elevators available to transport these severely ill individuals to various locations (Gao F et al.) **(Fig. 18.3)**.

### Bed Space

Each open bed should be 150–200 square feet, with 8 feet between them. In a single room, 225–250 square feet per

| S. No. | Therapist | Functions |
|---|---|---|
| 1. | Physiotherapist | Treats chest issues, aids mobilization, protects immobile patients from contractures |
| 2. | Pharmacists | In patients with hepatic or renal impairment, advice on drug adverse effects, as well as drug dosing |
| 3. | Dieticians | • Provide nutritional guidance and feed recommendations<br>• Assess the calorific and nutrient requirements of both short-and long-term critical care patients and advise on specialist feed regimes for specific conditions (e.g., complex GI or renal disease)<br>• Organize total parenteral nutrition as required alongside the pharmacy team |
| 4. | Microbiologists | Treatment and infection control advice |
| 5. | Technicians | Operating monitors, emergency and other items |
| 6. | Healthcare assistants | Support the nursing staff and therapy teams in patient care |
| 7. | Speech and language therapists | Assess patients' ability to swallow and re-start oral feeding as well as assisting with the communication difficulties of patients who remain intubated or with tracheostomies. |
| 8. | Legal services | Important for the families of patients who have long-term conditions or short-term incapacity to deal with their own legal or financial affairs. Legal services provide help and support to enable mortgages and bills to be paid and allow access to funds that are solely in the name of an incapacitated patient |
| 9. | Occupational therapists | Work closely with the physiotherapy team to provide patient support and aids to enhance rehabilitation |

Table 18.3: Different therapists and their functions.

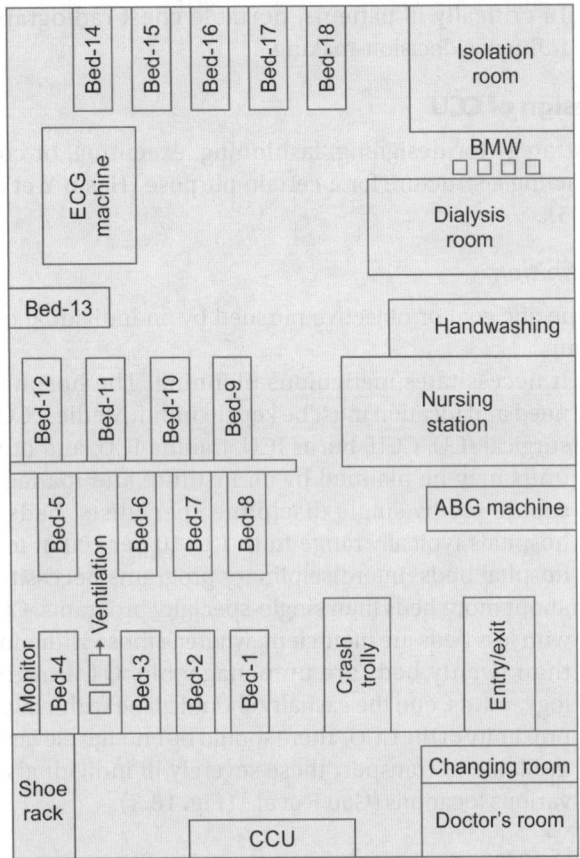

**Fig. 18.3:** Design pattern of CCU.

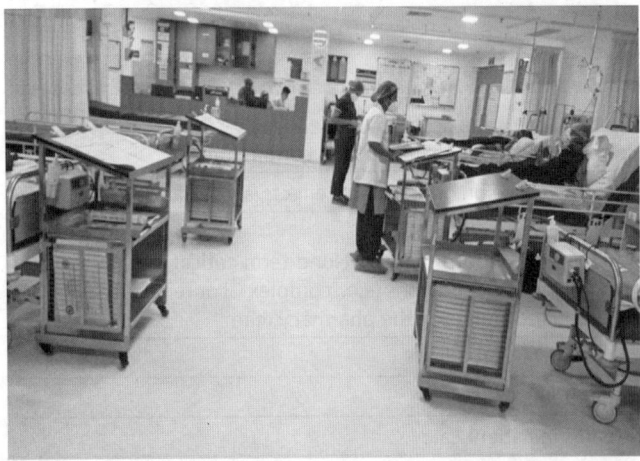

**Fig. 18.4:** Physical setup of CCU.

bed. Beds should have side rails and wheels for adjustment, but no head board **(Fig. 18.4)**.

## Physical Setup of 5 Beded in CCU

See **Figure 18.4**.

### CCU Therapeutic Elements

- Natural vistas through windows and art can relieve stress, speed recuperation, lower blood pressure, and lessen the need for pain medication.
- Participation by the entire family, including overnight accommodations and nice waiting areas.
- Adjustable curtains, shades, easy bed controls, and TV, VCR, CD players provide a level of privacy and personal control.
- Computerized pagers and silent alarms help to reduce noise.
- The ability for one medical staff to accompany a patient during his or her entire stay.

### CCU Team

Interdisciplinary team composed of:
- CCU chief medical
- CCU nurse
- Architecture and technicians
- Staff should approach CCU design and environmental designer

### Floor Planning and Design

Floor planning and design of a critical care unit play a crucial role in providing optimal care for critically ill patients. Here are some considerations for the floor and design of a CCU:

- **Patient rooms:** CCUs typically have individual patient rooms to ensure privacy, infection control, and space for medical equipment. These rooms should be spacious enough to accommodate necessary medical equipment, monitoring devices, and provide easy access for healthcare providers. Adequate space for family members or visitors should also be considered.
- **Centralized nursing station:** A centralized nursing station allows nurses to have a clear view of all patient rooms, facilitating constant monitoring and quick response to emergencies. The station should be designed to provide a comfortable and efficient workspace for nurses, with easy access to necessary supplies and equipment.
- **Patient visibility:** The layout should allow healthcare providers to maintain visual contact with patients from the nursing station. This can be achieved through the use of glass walls or windows in patient rooms or through strategically placed observation windows.
- **Support spaces:** CCUs require various support spaces, such as medication rooms, storage areas for medical supplies, clean and dirty utility rooms, and staff break rooms. These spaces should be designed to optimize workflow, ensure easy access to supplies, and maintain infection control standards.

- **Equipment and technology integration:** The floor design should consider the integration of medical equipment and technology. This includes provisions for electrical outlets, data ports, and appropriate infrastructure for medical gas supply and ventilation systems.
- **Infection control:** CCUs should have proper infection control measures in place, including hand hygiene stations, isolated rooms for patients with contagious conditions, and appropriate ventilation systems to minimize the risk of airborne infections.
- **Accessibility and safety:** The floor design should ensure easy access for patients, staff, and emergency equipment. It should also incorporate safety features such as non-slip flooring, proper lighting, and clear signage.

From a practical standpoint, eight to twelve beds per unit is ideal. Positive and negative pressure isolation rooms in the CCU should be considered. It will depend mainly upon-patient population and department of public health requirements in the state. Each CCU should be a geographically distinct area within the hospital, when possible, with controlled access. And areas like:

- **Patient areas:** Positioning of the patient should be maintained in such a way that healthcare providers can see them directly or indirectly. This allows for both normal and emergency monitoring of the patient's condition. The central area of nursing station should have a clear line of sight. Visible of the patients from their nurse substations in a CCUS with a modular architecture. This design is made easier by sliding glass doors and dividers, which allow for easier recognition to the area in an emergency.
- **Recommended ranging of noise:** The sensory overload in CCU is exacerbated by the signals from patient call systems, monitors, and telephones. Noise levels in hospital should not exceed 45 decibels (A) during day time, 40 decibels (A) in the evening time and 20 decibels (A) at night, according to the International Noise Council. In most hospitals, noise levels vary from 50 to 70 decibels (A) in hospital setting (Baker CF, 1993).
- **Prime station:**
  - A main station should large enough to accommodate all required employees in a pleasant environment.
  - In a modular CCU, each nurse substation is situated in a place which should be able to perform, if it is not all of the functions of a central station.
  - There should be ample overhead and task lighting, as well as a wall-mounted clock.
  - When using automated systems, having enough room for computer terminals and printers is critical.
  - Patient records should be available at all times.
  - Provide enough surface space and chairs for both physicians and nurses to chart medical records.
  - Medical records and forms are must be stored in shelving, filing cabinets, and other locations that are easily accessible by all workers who need them.
- **For X-ray viewing area:** Each CCU or CCU cluster should have its own room or space where patient radiographs can be examined and kept. An illuminated viewing box/carousel with sufficient size should be present to enable the viewing of serial radiographs simultaneously.
- **Working areas and storage:** A separate medication are having atleast 50 sq ft with a refrigerator for medications, a double locking safe for regulated substances, and a basin with hot and cold running water should be there. Countertops for medication preparation should be provided, and cabinets for medication and supply storage should be available.
- **Receptionist area:**
  - Each CCU include a receptionist area to monitor visitor access.
  - Receptionist able to communicate within CCU(s) by phone or other means.
  - A separate visitors' entry from the one used by healthcare personnel is desirable.
- **Special rooms for procedures:**
  - Procedure rooms are positioned within CCU.
  - A single special procedures room can accommodate many CCUS in close proximity.
  - Ease of access of patients for being evacuated from outside the CCU which must be considered.
  - Monitor capabilities, items, services, and safety considerations which has to compare with those provided in the CCU, and the room size should be sufficient for accommodate necessary equipment and the employees.
  - Work surfaces and storage rooms must be large enough to accommodate all necessary materials and allow staff to conduct all requested processes without leaving the room.
- **Utility room/dirty rooms:**
  - These rooms are separate rooms with no connections, be suitably temperature managed, and the dirty utility room's air supply must be exhausted.
  - To make cleaning easier, floors are covered with materials with no seams.
  - All clean and sterile materials should be stored in the utility room, which can used to store clean linen. Storage shelving and cabinet must situated at high enough off the floor to provide easy access to the floor underneath for cleaning.

– Hot and cold mixing faucets in the clinical sink and hopper must be provided in the dirty utility room, as well as separate covered containers for waste products.
– There should be approved disposal mechanisms for things compromised by bodily fluids and chemicals.
- **Equipment storage:**
  – There should be enough space to allow for quick access, convenient location of necessary equipment.
  – There should be sufficient grounded electrical outlets in the storage area to allow for the recharging the battery of operated devices.
- **Nourishment area:**
  – For feeding preparation space should be identified. A refrigerator, prep surfaces, an ice maker, a hot and cold running water sink.
  – Laboratory specimens should not be stored in the refrigerator.
- **Lounge for staffs:** Each CCU must have a staff loupe on or near it to give a private, pleasant, and soothing atmosphere. Locker rooms, showers, and toilets should all be available.
- **Conference room:**
  – It is easily accessible to CCU physicians and personnel.
  – This room must be connected by phone or other means to each relevant CCU and alarms for cardiac arrest must be audible across the room.
  – Ongoing education and training for staffs, multidisciplinary patient care conferences are all possible uses for the conference room.
  – The preservation of medical and nursing resources and reference materials, as well as computerised interactive and self-paced learning technology, is perfect in a conference room **(Fig. 18.5)**.
- **Visitors' waiting room:**
  – Each CCU should have a visitors' waiting area, and visitor access and monitored from the receptionist area. Each critical care bed should have one and a half to two seats.
  – Visitors must have access the telephones. There should be available of television and music.
  – Public restrooms must within or immediately next to the lounge area.
  – The carpet, indirect soft lighting, and windows all looks like attractive.
  – It's also a good idea to have a range of seating options, such as upright, lounge, and reclining chairs.
  – Educational resources should be available.
  – It is strongly suggested about separate family consultation room be set up.

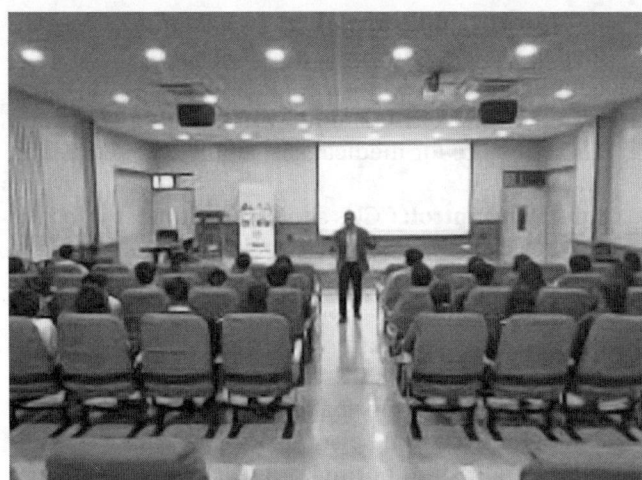

**Fig. 18.5:** Conference room of CCU.

- **Supply and service corridors:**
  – For supplying and servicing each CCU, a corridor has simple entrance and departure. soiled objects and rubbish should also be removed along this corridor.
  – The corridor should be at least 8 feet wide to avoid any disturbance of patient care activities, to reduce unwanted noise. For easy and unhindered movement of items and supplies, each CCU's doorways, apertures, and tunnels must be at least 36 inches wide.
- **Patient modules:**
  – Each isolation room should have at least 250 sq ft of floor area and with atleast 20 sq ft for gowning/gloving and storage.
  – Each bed in CCU should have at least 225 sq ft of free floor space.
  – Width of 15 ft, excluding auxiliary space, should be provided in a CCU with individual patient modules (assuming one patient per room) (anteroom, toilet, storage).
  – Every bedside in the CCU must have emergency alarm button. From the alarm should sounds coming automatically. The source of these alerts must be identified.
  – Computer terminals and space for patient documentation and surfaces.
  – Each patient's personal items and supplies, bedding, and toiletries must be stored. If syringes and drugs are kept at the bedside, draw lockers and cabinets must be employed.
  – Do not keep personal valuables in the CCU. Rather, hospital security should keep these until the discharge of patient.

- Every effort should promote a stress-free atmosphere for patients and staff. As a result, natural lighting and views should be considered when designing.
- Windows are a crucial part of sensory orientation, windows in all rooms which reinforces about day and night orientation.
- Drapes are made of fireproof cloth which used for window coverings and sound absorbers.
- **Sensory orientation improvement:**
  - A clock, calendar and pillow speaker connected to radio/television are some other techniques to assist individuals with sensory orientation.
  - If at all possible, each room should have a telephone.
  - Methods for establishing patient privacy should be included in comfort considerations. The patient's interaction with his or her environment should be controlled via shades, blinds, curtains, and doors.
  - Portable or folding chairs must be available at the bedside to enable for family visits. A room's color palette, which promotes rest and calming impact, is an extra comfort concern.
- **Utilities:** Each CCU must have electrical power, water, oxygen, compressed air, vacuum, lighting, and environmental control systems that meet or exceed accreditation agency norms and requirements (Bartley J, 2001).
- **Electric supply:**
  - Within few feet of each clients bed, grounded 110 v electrical outlets with 30 amp circuit breakers should be installed. A total of sixteen outlets per bed is ideal.
  - To enable connection, way out at the top of the bed should be situated roughly 36 inch above the floor.
  - Pull the power cord instead of the plug to prevent disconnection.
  - To avoid tripping over electrical cords, way out sides and foot of the bed should near to the floor.
- **Water supply:**
  - If hemodialysis is to be done, the supply of water must come from are liable source.
  - Pipes entering each CCU must have zone stop valves installed to allow service to be switched off in the event of a line break.
  - To minimise the splitting sink should be deep and broad for hand wash and at the entrances of the patient modules or in between every 2 patients.
- **Lightning in CCU:**
  - Lighting controls should be placed on variable control dimmers located slightly outside the room, and total brightness of 30 foot-candles is recommended.
  - For continuous use, light should not exceed 6.5 fc in night time, or 19 fc for short periods.

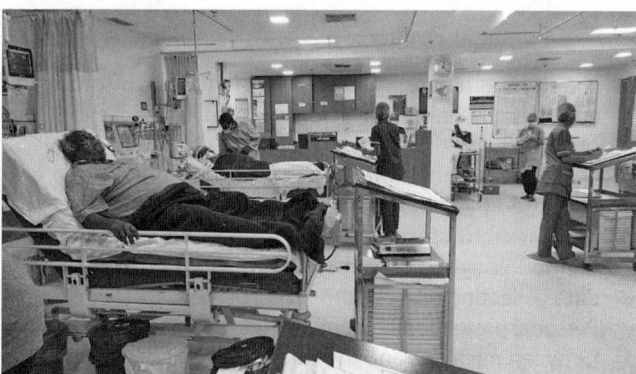

**Fig. 18.6:** Lighting of CCU.

  - Emergency and procedure lighting should be situated in the ceiling above the patient and at least 150 fc of illumination like shadow free should be provided **(Fig. 18.6)**.
- **Systems for environmental control:**
  - Each room must have a minimum of six total air changes per hour, two of which must be outside air.
  - Outside air should be used to meet the toilet exhaust of 75 cubic ft per min in rooms with toilets.
  - Recirculated air and central air conditioning systems must use adequate filters.
  - Patient comfort should be prioritized while providing air cooling and heating.
  - In critical care units with enclosed patient modules, the temperature of each module should be changeable.
  - In enclosed CCU patient modules, temperature can be changed.
- **Computerized documentation:** These technologies will enable for "paperless" management of data, data entry, and nurse/physician documentation. Which helps them to remain in bedside during the critical or monitoring of the patient for documentation. And they can access the data for further diagnosis or assessment.

## Other Facilities

Facilities like voice intercommunication, physician on call rooms, administrative offices and satellite labs.

## Summary

Quality, policy and infection control is important in health organization for providing quality and evidenced-based practice and cost-effective care to the clients. So quality care increases the probability of positive outcomes and reduce the chances of undesired outcomes also given the current state of knowledge and expand the body of knowledge.

**Points to Ponder**

- Quality assurance in health care is the monitoring the activities of client care to determine the degree of excellence of implemented activities.
- Quality assurance activities should be developed and evaluated by a coordinator. It is necessary to assign roles and tasks. Nurses must be informed on the program's methodology and outcomes. Data must be trustworthy, e.g., data collecting must be properly oriented.
- Personal protection equipment (PPE) acts as physical barrier between microbes and the wearer. It can protect by means of preventing microbes from infecting objects.
- When handling of contaminated objects and body fluids use sterile or clean gloves. When working with various patients, change gloves.
- When performing procedures that may result in splashes of body fluids, use mask to protect the mouth and nose.
- The distance between the beds should be enough between each bed in open plan wards to prevent the danger of cross infection. The ideal distance between beds is 1–2 meters.
- CCU beds in hospitals typically range from 1 to 10 per 100 in total hospital beds.
- A single special procedures room can accommodate many CCUS in close proximity.
- Ease of access of patients for being evacuated from outside the CCU which must be considered.
- Monitor capabilities, items, services, and safety considerations which has to compare with those provided in the CCU, and the room size should be sufficient for accommodate necessary equipment and the employees.
- Each CCU should have a visitors' waiting area, and visitor access and monitored from the receptionist area. Each critical care bed should have one and a half to two seats.
- Each isolation room should have at least 250 sq ft of floor area and with at least 20 sq ft for gowning/gloving and storage.
- Each bed in CCU should have at least 225 sq ft of free floor space.
- Width of 15 ft, excluding auxiliary space, should be provided in a CCU with individual patient modules (assuming one patient per room) (anteroom, toilet, storage).
- Every bedside in the CCU must have emergency alarm button. From the alarm should sounds coming automatically. The source of these alerts must be identified.
- Visitors must have access the telephones. There should be available of television and music.
- Lighting controls should be placed on variable control dimmers located slightly outside the room, and total brightness of 30 foot-candles is recommended.
- For continuous use, light should not exceed 6.5 fc in night time, or 19 fc for short periods.
- Emergency and procedure lighting should be situated in the ceiling above the patient and at least 150 fc of illumination like shadow free should be provided.

 **Abbreviations**

- CCU : Critical Care Unit
- ICU : Intensive Care Unit
- ICP : Intracranial Pressure
- IM : Intramuscular
- QA : Quality Assurance
- HDU : High Dependency Unit
- PPE : Positive Protective Equipment
- Dyssy's : Dynamic Standard-setting System

 **Short Answer Questions**

1. Methods of nursing audit.
2. Factors affecting quality assurance in nursing care.
3. Role of nurse administrator in implementing quality assurance.
4. Infection control practices.
5. Utilization of results of nursing audit.
6. Design of CCU.

 **Long Answer Questions**

1. Define quality assurance in health care. Explain briefly about the standards organization of CCU.
2. What do you mean policy and protocol? Describe in detail regarding policies and protocols followed in CCU.
3. Define audit. List out the different types of nursing audit. Also enumerate the audit cycle.
4. What is staffing? Explain briefly about the staffing pattern in CCU.
5. Define design of CCU. Explain in detail regarding designing of CCU.

 **Bibliography**

1. Baker CF, Garvin BJ, Kennedy CW, Polivka BJ. The Effect of Environmental Sound and Communication on CCU Patients' Heart Rate and Blood Pressure. Research in Nursing and Health. 1993;16(6):415-21.
2. Bartley J, Bjerke NB. Infection Control Considerations in Critical Care Unit Design and Construction: A Systematic Risk Assessment. Critical Care Nursing Quarterly. 2001;24(3):43-58.
3. Black N. Quality Assurance of Medical Care. Journal of Public Health Medicine. 1990;12(2):97-104.
4. Caddell A, Belliveau D, Pottinger L, Moeller A. Multi-disciplinary Simulation to Enhance Safe Care of Critically Ill Covid-19 Patients in the Coronary Care Unit. Canadian Journal of Cardiology. 2020;36(10):S41.
5. Citrome L. Practice Protocols, Parameters, Pathways, and Guidelines: A Review. Administration and Policy in Mental Health and Mental Health Services Research. 1998;25(3):257-69.

6. Follath F, Yilmaz MB, Delgado JF, Parissis JT, Porcher R, Gayat E et al. Clinical Presentation, Management and Outcomes in the Acute Heart Failure Global Survey of Standard Treatment (ALARM-HF). Intensive Care Medicine. 2011;37(4):619-26.
7. Gao F, Liang H, Zhang K, Li Y. Safety Enhancement Design Method and Control Strategy for CCU of High-speed Train. Advances in Mechanical Engineering. 2022;14(4): 16878132221089806.
8. Gast PL, Baker CF. The CCU Patient: Anxiety and Annoyance to Noise. Critical Care Nursing Quarterly. 1989;12(3):39-54.
9. Hasin Y, Danchin N, Filippatos GS, Heras M, Janssens U, Leor J et al. Recommendations for the Structure, Organization, and Operation of Intensive Cardiac Care Units. European Heart Journal. 2005;26(16):1676-82.
10. https://www.freepik.com/free-photos-vectors/ppe
11. https://www.slideshare.net/ravindrajha10/planing-and-organization-of-intensive-cares
12. Lane H, Maidstone K. Operational Policy and Procedure for the Critical Care Units. Policy. 2020.
13. Mykkänen M, Saranto K, Miettinen M. Nursing Audit as a Method for Developing Nursing Care and Ensuring Patient Safety. InNI 2012: 11th International Congress on Nursing Informatics. Montreal, Canada. 2012. American Medical Informatics Association.
14. Rosenthal VD, Guzmán S, Crnich C. Device-associated Nosocomial Infection Rates in Intensive Care Units of Argentina. Infection Control and Hospital Epidemiology. 2004;25(3):251-5.
15. Thomas L, Culley EJ, Gladowski P, Goff V, Fong J, Marche SM. Longitudinal Analysis of the Costs Associated with Inpatient Initiation and Subsequent Outpatient Continuation of Proton Pump Inhibitor Therapy for Stress Ulcer Prophylaxis in a Large Managed Care Organization. Journal of Managed Care Pharmacy. 2010;16(2):122-9.
16. World Health Organization. Rational Use of Personal Protective Equipment for Coronavirus Disease (COVID-19): Interim Guidance. World Health Organization, 2020.

# Review Questions

 **Multiple Choice Questions**

1. Common causes of antepartum hemorrhage:
   a. Placenta previa
   b. Uterine rupture
   c. Placental abruption
   d. Vasa previa
   e. All of the above

2. What is placenta previa?
   a. Early separation of placenta
   b. Partial or total covering of the cervix by the placenta
   c. High blood pressure during pregnancy
   d. High blood sugar during pregnancy

3. Which of the following is a symptom of placenta previa?
   a. Quickening
   b. Nausea and vomiting
   c. Bright red, painless vaginal bleeding
   d. Dizziness

4. Placenta previa is associated with all except the following:
   a. Bulky placenta
   b. Previous scar due to CS
   c. Primipara mother
   d. Previous history of placenta previa

5. Which of the following are true regarding placenta previa?
   a. The majority of 'low-lying' placentas diagnosed at 20 weeks will remain so at term
   b. Placenta previa is typically more painful than an abruption
   c. Placenta previa complicates about 0.6% of pregnancies at term
   d. Complications of placenta previa include need for cesarean section, hemorrhage, placenta accreta, placenta percreta and hysterectomy.

6. True statement regarding abruption:
   a. Occurs between 20 weeks of gestation to prior to birth
   b. Bleeding into the decidua basalis leads to separation of the placenta
   c. Retroplacental blood penetration leads to Couvelaire uterus
   d. All of the above

7. Which of the following should be done after placental abruption is first suspected?
   a. Check maternal clotting studies
   b. Check maternal serum calcium
   c. Obtain blood cultures and begin antibiotics
   d. Give Rh immune globulin

8. Signs of placenta abruption include increased uterine resting tonus and sudden vaginal bleeding.
   a. True
   b. False

9. Most placental abruptions occur after labor has started.
   a. True
   b. False

10. Increase the risk for placenta abruption *except*:
    a. Hypertensive disorders of pregnancy
    b. Maternal cocaine use
    c. A woman's first pregnancy
    d. Maternal abdominal trauma

11. Pre-eclampsia can cause disseminated intravascular coagulopathy (DIC).
    a. True
    b. False

12. Use of low dose aspirin does not lessen pre-eclampsia.
    a. True
    b. False

13. What is eclampsia?
    a. A possible complication of pre-eclampsia
    b. A condition that places the mother and baby's health at great risk and can cause death in either or both
    c. A condition of pregnancy causing high blood pressure and seizures
    d. All answers are correct

14. Arrest can occur during which phase of labor?
    a. Latent phase
    b. Active phase
    c. Either latent or active phase

15. Ineffective uterine contractions, cephalo disproportion and occipito-posterior position are main causes of:
    a. Obstructed labor      b. Normal labor
    c. Prolonged labor       d. None of the above

16. Which of the following amounts of blood loss following birth can cause postpartum hemorrhage?
    a. More than 100 mL
    b. More than 300 mL
    c. More than 600 mL
    d. More than 500 mL

17. All of the following are the signs of obstructed labor, *except*:
    a. Non-engagement of presenting part even if good contraction
    b. Rapid dilatation of cervix
    c. Dehydration
    d. Formation of retraction ring

18. Eclampsia is least likely to occur at:
    a. Antepartum
    b. After 48 hours postpartum
    c. Immediately postpartum
    d. Intrapartum

19. Any infection during pregnancy, childbirth, postpartum or post-abortion can develop into maternal sepsis.
    a. True
    b. False

20. Maternal sepsis is one of the important causes of maternal mortality at the worldwide.
    a. True
    b. False

21. What is an early sign of tension pneumothorax?
    a. Tracheal deviation
    b. Respiratory distress
    c. Increased cardiac output
    d. Epistaxis

22. Flail chest is defined as:
    a. Multiple rib fractures with subsequent subcutaneous emphysema
    b. Chyle in the pleural space
    c. Excess fluid in pericardium
    d. Two or more ribs fractured at two points

23. A nasogastric tube was inserted in a trauma patient. A follow-up chest radiograph shows abdominal contents in the chest cavity. The nurse should be suspicious of:
    a. Diaphragmatic rupture
    b. Chylothorax
    c. Pleural effusion
    d. Tension pneumothorax

24. What is the most appropriate immediate nursing intervention for a patient who has pulled out their chest tube?
    a. Restrain patient and place bed in Trendelenburg position
    b. Cover site with a dressing and contact the physician
    c. Apply oxygen per face mask and order chest X-ray
    d. Monitor for air leaks and report subcutaneous emphysema

25. What is a significant nursing intervention to reduce morbidity in the patient with rib fractures?
    a. Aggressive pulmonary toilet
    b. Monitoring supplemental oxygen
    c. Application of sequential stockings
    d. Administering cough suppressant medication

26. The abdominal organ most susceptible to injury in blunt trauma is the:
    a. Spleen
    b. Small bowel
    c. Esophagus
    d. Pancreas

27. Pain that is referred to left shoulder due to peritoneal irritation is:
    a. Chvostek's sign
    b. Ballance's sign
    c. Cullen's sign
    d. Kehr's sign

28. A driver in a motor vehicle accident arrives in the emergency department complaining of diffuse abdominal pain, nausea and vomiting. His vital signs are stable, and serial hemoglobin and hematocrit measurements are unremarkable. His serum amylase is elevated. You suspect he has sustained a:
    a. Gastric injury
    b. Splenic injury
    c. Pancreatic injury
    d. Small bowel injury

29. A priority nursing diagnosis for the patient who develops an intestinal fistula is:
    a. Impaired skin integrity
    b. Pain
    c. Infection
    d. Fluid imbalance

30. The innominate, or hip bones, are composed of the:
    a. Symphysis pubis, ileum and acetabulum
    b. Ilium, ischium and pubis
    c. Sacrum, coccyx and pubic symphysis
    d. Tibia, fibula and patella

31. An unstable pelvic fracture is one in which:
    a. One pelvic bone is broken and the bone is not displaced
    b. The broken bone is reduced externally by having the patient rest
    c. Two or more bones in the pelvic ring are broken and the bones are displaced
    d. The broken bone is exposed

32. An open reduction is a procedure in which:
    a. External traction is applied
    b. No incision is made
    c. A surgical incision is made and the bones are realigned internally
    d. The broken bones are reduced while the patient is still out in the open

33. All of the following areas are commonly involved sites in pelvic fracture, *except*:
    a. Pubic rami
    b. Alae of ileum
    c. Acetabulum
    d. Ischial tuberosities

34. A previously fit 35-year-old man presents to emergency ward with septic shock secondary to arm cellulitis. He is cold peripherally and slightly confused. His HR is 125/min NSR, BP 60/30 mm Hg, RR 25/min. The most appropriate first step in his management should be to:
    a. Give 100% oxygen, establish IV access and administer 500 mL of Gelofusine
    b. Insert central line to guide fluid therapy
    c. Start a peripheral vasopressor to increase afterload and improve BP
    d. Use a noninvasive cardiac output monitor

35. The main neurotransmitter for the sympathetic nervous system is:
    a. Dopamine
    b. Noradrenaline
    c. Adrenaline
    d. Acetylcholine

36. All following drugs can be used in pure cardiogenic shock, *except*:
    a. GTN infusion
    b. Adrenaline
    c. Dopamine
    d. Noradrenaline
    e. Dobutamine

37. Noradrenaline has no effect on β1 adrenergic receptors.
    a. True
    b. False

38. Which of the following clinical signs is not typical for a classic presentation of shock?
    a. Cool extremities
    b. Weak pulses
    c. Systemic hypertension
    d. Tachypnea

39. In shock, which of the following statements is true relative to oxygen consumption?
    a. Oxygen demand exceeds oxygen delivery
    b. Oxygen delivery and oxygen demand are determined by stroke volume
    c. Because $DO_2$ is greater than $VO_2$ in shock situations, anaerobic metabolism results in formation of lactate
    d. As long as $VO_2$ is greater than $DO_2$, anaerobic metabolism will be minimal and blood lactate levels will remain normal

40. Which of the following clinical findings is often a result of activation of the sympathetic nervous system?
    a. Decreased inotropy
    b. Increased heart rate
    c. Decreased arterial tone
    d. Increased liver enzymes

41. What causes decreased BP in neurogenic shock?
    a. Movement of fluid into the cells
    b. Movement of fluid into the vasculature
    c. Disrupted SNS communication
    d. Polyuria

42. What class of drug is typically used to treat neurogenic shock?
    a. Beta-blocker
    b. Calcium-channel blocker
    c. Loop diuretic
    d. Vasopressor

43. What type of sensitivity reaction is anaphylactic shock?
    a. Type I, immediate hypersensitivity disorder
    b. Type II, antibody-mediated disorder
    c. Type III, immune complex-mediated disorder
    d. Type IV, cell mediated hypersensitivity disorder

44. What is the preferred treatment for an anaphylactic shock?
    a. Epinephrine
    b. Placing the patient in a sitting position and administer oxygen
    c. Preventing the reaction from occurring through patient teaching
    d. Placing a bag of ice on the area, administer antihistamines and corticosteroids

45. What is the primary cause of septic shock?
    a. Bleeding
    b. Medication allergy
    c. Infection
    d. Poison

46. A 30-year-old man is admitted to the emergency ward with sudden onset of severe shortness of breath, no chest pain, diffuse wheezing, cyanosis, and a BP of 70/30, pulse = 100. This event occurred soon after a meal. What is the likely diagnosis?
    a. Acute pulmonary embolism
    b. Tension pneumothorax
    c. Anaphylaxis
    d. Myocardial infarction

47. In a shock patient with low body temperature, cold and clammy extremities, low urine output, and elevated lactic acid level in the blood, the most likely cause of shock is:
    a. Asthma
    b. Pulmonary embolism
    c. Sepsis
    d. CHF

48. A 82–year-old diabetic is involved in an automobile accident, with severe thoracic and abdominal traumatic injuries. He is rushed to the hospital and placed in the intensive care unit. After a few hours, there is the rapid onset of myocardial dysfunction, hypotension, disseminated intravascular coagulation, and coma. This sequence of events most closely mimics what type of shock?
    a. Septic (distributive)   b. Cardiogenic
    c. Anaphylactic            d. Neurogenic

49. The CO is normal or elevated in which of shock types:
    a. Hypovolemic shock
    b. Cardiogenic shock
    c. Distributive shock
    d. Obstructive shock

50. Sequential organ failure assessment (SOFA) is defined as:
    a. An aide in the diagnosis and treatment of sepsis in the infectious patient
    b. A test that advises the providers on the best medication to treat the infection
    c. A tool to assist physicians track progress and predict risk in patients with sepsis
    d. A program that gives the nursing staff the best care plan for the patient with sepsis

51. Part of diagnosing multiorgan dysfunction syndrome (MODS) involves seeing an increase in what type of cell in the blood?
    a. White blood cell
    b. Red blood cell
    c. Plasma cells
    d. Hemoglobin

52. What can be done nutritionally to help manage complications associated with multiorgan dysfunction syndrome (MODS)?
    a. Limiting all fluids a person consumes
    b. Feeding a person a high carbohydrate diet
    c. Providing a person enteral feeds
    d. Giving person a high dose of vitamin C supplementation

53. Which of the following may be an underlying condition that leads to DIC?
    a. Trauma
    b. Cancer
    c. Liver disease
    d. Complication of pregnancy
    e. All of these conditions could lead to DIC

54. Which of the following set of finding is seen in DIC?
    a. Increased fibrinogen, increased antithrombin III, increased thrombin–antithrombin III complexes
    b. Increased FDP, decreased PT, increased antithrombin III
    c. Increased FDP, prolonged PT, increased thrombin-antithrombin complexes
    d. Increased FDP, prolonged PT, reduced platelets

55. Nurse Ejay is assigned to telephone triage. A client called who was stung by a honeybee and is asking for help. The client reports pain and localized swelling but has no respiratory distress or other symptoms of anaphylactic shock. What is the appropriate initial action that the nurse should direct the client to perform?
    a. Removing the stinger by scraping it
    b. Applying a cold compress
    c. Taking an oral antihistamine
    d. Calling 911

56. Which of the following is not a side effect of digoxin toxicity?
    a. Bradycardia
    b. Yellow vision changes
    c. Scooping of the T segment on ECG
    d. Hypokalemia
    e. Gynecomastia

57. Which of the following is true with regard to acetaminophen toxicity?
    a. The Rumack-Matthew Nomogram may be used for both acute and chronic ingestions
    b. The APAP level should ideally be checked within 1–4 hours of ingestion
    c. The Rumack-Matthew Nomogram applies for ingestions up to 48 hours post-ingestion
    d. N-Acetylcysteine (NAC) should be started within 8 hours of ingestion if an APAP level cannot be obtained
    e. Activated charcoal should be used for all sustained-release ingestions

58. All of the following are treatment options for toxic alcohol poisoning, *except*:
    a. Fomepizole
    b. Hydroxocobalamin
    c. Thiamine
    d. Folic acid
    e. Pyridoxine

59. Which of the following is a symptom of AIDS?
    a. Fever
    b. Lymph node swelling
    c. Tiredness
    d. All of the above

60. The first ever instance of AIDS was reported in:
    a. USA
    b. France
    c. Russia
    d. None of the above

61. HIV parasitizes:
    a. Y-helper cells
    b. T-helper cells
    c. K-helper cells
    d. None of the above

62. HIV is a:
    a. Lentivirus
    b. Capripoxvirus
    c. Gallivirus
    d. Papillomavirus

63. A person has AIDS when which of these occurs?
    a. Exposure to HIV
    b. HIV antibodies are found in the blood
    c. The CD4+ count is lower than 200 or opportunistic infections develop in an HIV-infected person
    d. A person has HIV for 5 years

64. HIV attacks a certain kind of cell in the immune system. Which is it?
    a. Red blood cells
    b. White blood cells called T-cells
    c. Platelets
    d. Epithelial cells

65. What is the CD4 T-cell count at which AIDS is considered to have developed?
    a. Below 1,000 per cubic milliliter
    b. Below 500 per cubic milliliter
    c. Below 200 per cubic milliliter
    d. Below 50 per cubic milliliter

66. Irrespective of the etiology of a corneal ulcer, the drug always indicated is:
    a. Corticosteroids
    b. Cycloplegics
    c. Antibiotics
    d. Antifungals

67. What are the three common types of ocular trauma?
    a. Forced, direct and progressive
    b. Indirect, stabbing and splashing
    c. Blunt, chemical and sharp
    d. Hemorrhage, bruising and twitching

68. Name three symptoms of blunt trauma to the eye.
    a. Constricted pupil, swelling and hemorrhage
    b. Redness, dilated pupil and increased intraocular pressure
    c. Subcutaneous emphysema, cloudy cornea and vision loss
    d. Distorted pupil, blepharospasm and glaucoma

69. What is hyphema?
    a. Swelling of the eye causing it to remain shut
    b. Bulging of the eyes causing dryness
    c. Loss of intraocular pressure causing tearing
    d. Pooling of blood between the cornea and iris causing vision loss

70. A 25-year-old male presents with a stab wound to the left side of the neck. All of the following indicate a need for aggressive airway management, *except*:
    a. Massive subcutaneous emphysema of the neck
    b. Trachea midline
    c. Expanding neck hematoma
    d. Zone II wound

71. A 30-year-old male presents with a stab wound to the left side of the neck. He is alert but has active bleeding. He is in a resuscitation cubicle. You would address this bleeding by:
    a. Placing 2 large bore IV cannula and giving O-negative blood
    b. Apply pressure to the site
    c. Clamp the bleeding vessels to obtain stasis
    d. Locally explore the wound and locate the bleeding point

72. What is the most common medical intervention required for patients with thoracic trauma?
    a. Decompression and chest tube
    b. Thoracotomy
    c. Pericardiocentesis
    d. Insertion of nasogastric tube

73. A common complication of nasal fractures that must be urgently treated is:
    a. Loss of sense of smell
    b. Septal hematoma
    c. Periorbital edema
    d. Subcutaneous edema

74. Which model of CCU allows a variety of medical staff members to handle patients in CCU?
    a. Open
    b. Hybrid
    c. Closed
    d. Both (a) and (b)

75. What is the average free floor space in each bed in CCU?
    a. 230 sqft
    b. 240 sqft
    c. 275 sqft
    d. 300 sqft

76. Which level of CCU is a major tertiary hospital?
    a. Level I
    b. Level III
    c. Level II
    d. Level IV

77. Which acts as a physical barrier between microbes and wearer?
    a. Gloves/gown
    b. Mask
    c. PPE
    d. PPC

78. What is the ideal distance between bed in CCU?
    a. 1–2 meters
    b. 3–4 meters
    c. 2–3 meters
    d. 5–6 meters

79. Which method in nursing audit is used for assessing the quality of nursing care by looking at the nursing care as it appears in discharged patient's medical record?
    a. Retrospective view
    b. Prospective view
    c. Concurrent view
    d. Internal view

80. In which types of auditing external auditor has to certify the annual profit and loss account and prepare a balance sheet after careful examination of the relevant books of accounts and documents.
    a. Internal auditing
    b. External auditing
    c. Re-auditing
    d. Concurrent view

81. Pain is unpleasant sensory and ………………… associated with actual or potential tissue damage or described in terms of such damage.
    a. Emotional experience
    b. Physical
    c. Emotional
    d. Spiritual

82. ………………… pain arises from skin and muscle.
    a. Somatic
    b. Visceral
    c. Neuropathic
    d. All of the above

83. The pain which is longer than expected is called as …………
    a. Acute pain
    b. Chronic pain
    c. Ischemic pain
    d. All of the above

84. The theory which is explained about the emotion is called as …………………
    a. Specific theory
    b. Gate control theory
    c. Biophysical model
    d. Pattern theory

85. Narcotics relieve pain and produce a sense of ………… effect.
    a. Euphoria
    b. Metaphoria
    c. Utopia
    d. All of the above

86. Cutaneous simulation creates the release of …………
    a. Morphine
    b. Narcotic
    c. Endorphine
    d. All of the above

87. ………… are used to relax specific muscle relaxation.
    a. Muscle
    b. TENS
    c. Biofeed back
    d. Music

88. ………… is a energy focus which heals through touch.
    a. Heat
    b. Cold
    c. TENS
    d. Reiki

89. The layer protects the heart:
    a. Epicardium
    b. Myocardial tissue
    c. Endocardium
    d. Pericardium

90. Which side of the body apex of heart is pointed?
    a. To left
    b. To right
    c. Posteriorly
    d. Different for males and females

91. Which layer consist of cardiac muscle tissue?
    a. Epicardium      b. Myocardium
    c. Endocardium     d. Pericardium

92. Though which structure does blood pass from right atrium to the right ventricle?
    a. Bicuspid valve
    b. Tricuspid valve
    c. Ascending aorta
    d. Intraventricular septum

93. From left ventricle, where does blood pass?
    a. Right atrium
    b. Right ventricle
    c. Aortic semilunar valve
    d. Pulmonary trunk

94. Which of the below prevent blood from following back from the lungs?
    a. Pulmonary valve    b. Pulmonary vein
    c. Bicuspid valve     d. Tricuspid valve

95. This heart structure carries deoxygenated blood:
    a. Left atrium
    b. Left ventricle
    c. Right atrium and ventricle
    d. Right ventricle

96. Which term used to describe hard for the heart to deliver blood to the body and lead to heart failure?
    a. Cardiomyopathy    b. Myocarditis
    c. Pericarditis      d. Cardiomegaly

97. Which of the following is most common symptom of MI?
    a. Chest pain     b. Edema
    c. Dyspnea        d. High heart rate

98. The amount of blood pumped by each ventricle per beat is called:
    a. Heart beat     b. BP
    c. Pulse          d. Stroke volume

99. A side effect of too rapid administration of magnesium sulfate is ...........
    a. Hypotension
    b. Cardiac arrest
    c. Respiratory depression
    d. All of these

100. The most effective management for eclamptic seizures is ...........
    a. Administration of calcium gluconate
    b. Administration of normal saline
    c. Administration of magnesium sulfate
    d. Administration of midazolam

101. You are managing a 20-year-old female patient, 36/40 gestation with severe PV bleeding, hemodynamically unstable but with no abdominal pain. She is most likely suffering from ...........
    a. Placental abruption
    b. Vasa previa
    c. Placenta accreta
    d. Placenta previa

102. Eclampsia is defined as ...........
    a. Severe hypertension during pregnancy
    b. Seizure activity superimposed on pre-eclampsia
    c. Hypertensive crisis resulting in cerebral hemorrhage in pregnancy
    d. None of these selections

103. ........................... is a sign of an inevitable miscarriage.
    a. Lower back pain and abdominal cramping
    b. Vaginal bleeding prior to 20 weeks
    c. Rupture of the fetal membranes
    d. Prolonged abdominal pain

### Answer Key

| 1. | (a) | 2. | (b) | 3. | (c) | 4. | (c) | 5. | (d) |
|---|---|---|---|---|---|---|---|---|---|
| 6. | (d) | 7. | (a) | 8. | (a) | 9. | (b) | 10. | (c) |
| 11. | (a) | 12. | (b) | 13. | (d) | 14. | (b) | 15. | (a) |
| 16. | (d) | 17. | (b) | 18. | (a) | 19. | (a) | 20. | (a) |
| 21. | (b) | 22. | (d) | 23. | (a) | 24. | (b) | 25. | (b) |
| 26. | (a) | 27. | (d) | 28. | (c) | 29. | (a) | 30. | (b) |
| 31. | (c) | 32. | (c) | 33. | (d) | 34. | (b) | 35. | (d) |
| 36. | (a) | 37. | (b) | 38. | (c) | 39. | (a) | 40. | (b) |
| 41. | (c) | 42. | (d) | 43. | (a) | 44. | (a) | 45. | (c) |
| 46. | (c) | 47. | (c) | 48. | (a) | 49. | (c) | 50. | (a) |
| 51. | (a) | 52. | (c) | 53. | (e) | 54. | (d) | 55. | (a) |
| 56. | (d) | 57. | (d) | 58. | (b) | 59. | (d) | 60. | (a) |
| 61. | (b) | 62. | (a) | 63. | (c) | 64. | (b) | 65. | (c) |
| 66. | (b) | 67. | (d) | 68. | (c) | 69. | (d) | 70. | (b) |
| 71. | (b) | 72. | (b) | 73. | (b) | 74. | (a) | 75. | (a) |
| 76. | (b) | 77. | (c) | 78. | (c) | 79. | (a) | 80. | (b) |
| 81. | (c) | 82. | (a) | 83. | (b) | 84. | (c) | 85. | (b) |
| 86. | (d) | 87. | (c) | 88. | (d) | 89. | (d) | 90. | (a) |
| 91. | (b) | 92. | (b) | 93. | (c) | 94. | (a) | 95. | (c) |
| 96. | (a) | 97. | (a) | 98. | (d) | 99. | (d) | 100. | (c) |
| 101. | (d) | 102. | (b) | 103. | (b) | | | | |

# Review Questions

## Fill in the Blanks

1. ........................... ethical principle ensures that patients make their own choices about their care.
2. DNR stands for ...........................
3. End of life decision-making is called as ...........................
4. The pain is also referred as ........................... mechanism.
5. The pain which arises from abdomen is called as ...........................
6. An example of phantom pain are ...........................
7. The theory which results in perception of pain and summation of impulses is called as ...........................
8. ........................... is the fifth vital sign.
9. An example for a antagonist are ...........................
10. The therapy which consist of battery powered device is called as ........................... which provide electric impulses.
11. The outer layer of heart is called as ...........................
12. ........................... regulates blood flow between right atrium
13. Duration of cardiac cycle is ...........................
14. The upper chamber of heart is known as ...........................
15. The cavities of cardiac chamber are line by ...........................
16. Pulmonary orifice lead from ...........................
17. The amount of blood pumped out by each ventricle into the circulation per minute is ...........................
18. The entire heart enclosed by ...........................
19. Heart has ........................... chamber.
20. Arotic orifice leads from ...........................
21. The maximum volume of the air exhaled from the point of maximum inspiration is called as ...........................
22. Vital capacity performed with a maximally forced expiratory effort is termed as ...........................
23. Volume of air exhaled in the specified time during the performance of forced vital capacity is called as ...........................
24. Total lung capacity of an adult is ...........................
25. Amount of gas left in the lungs after a maximal exhalation is called as ...........................
26. Increased anteroposterior diameter as a result of increased air trapping is called as ...........................
27. An opening into the thorax through pleura is the procedure called as ...........................
28. Procedure of removal of the entire lung is called as ...........
29. Resection of a small well circumscribed lesion of lung is known as ...........................
30. The total number of alveoli present in the human lungs is estimated to be around ...........................

### Answer Key

| 1. | Autonomy |
|---|---|
| 2. | Do not resuscitate |
| 3. | Advance directives |
| 4. | Defense |
| 5. | Somatic pain |
| 6. | Spinal cord injury |
| 7. | Gate control theory of pain |
| 8. | Pain |
| 9. | Naloxone |
| 10. | TENS |
| 11. | Epicardium |
| 12. | Tricuspid valve |
| 13. | 0.8 sec |
| 14. | Atrium |
| 15. | Endocardium |
| 16. | Left ventricle to right ventricle |
| 17. | 5 to 6 per min |
| 18. | Pericardium |
| 19. | 4 |
| 20. | Left ventricle to aorta |
| 21. | Vital capacity (VC) |
| 22. | Forced vital capacity |
| 23. | Timed forced expiratory volume (FEV1) |
| 24. | 6 liter |
| 25. | Residual volume (RV) |
| 26. | Emphysema |
| 27. | A thoracotomy |
| 28. | A pneumonectomy |
| 29. | Segmental lung resection |
| 30. | 600–800 million |

# Index

Page numbers followed by *f* refer to figure, *fc* refer to flowchart, and *t* refer to table.

## A

ABCDE assessment 214*t*
Abdomen 102, 125, 515
    quadrant, four 102*f*
Abdominal cavity 100
Abdominal examination 399, 419
Abdominal injury 114, 526
    clinical presentation of 527*t*
    types of 526
Abdominal pain 74, 101, 125, 132, 404, 409, 415
    severe 426
Abdominal radiograph 481
Abdominal surgery 131
Abdominal trauma 124, 131, 132, 500, 563
    causes of 114
    clinical presentation of 116*t*
Abruptio placentae 396, 402, 403*f*
    complications of 404
    management of 405*fc*, 407
Abscess 559, 565
    prevent injection 625*t*
Absolute refractory period 172
Absorption atelectasis 333
Accessory muscle during breathing, use of 308
Aceclofenac 58
Acetaminophen 83, 85, 119
Acetazolamide 64
Acetylcholine receptor 204
    antibodies 204
Acetylcholinesterase
    enzyme 204
    inhibitors 205
Acetylcysteine 58
Acetylsalicylic acid 45
Achilles tendon 179
Acid 54
Acid-base
    balance 141
    imbalance 272
        different conditions of 312*t*
Acidosis 213, 287
    cause of 74
Acidotic state 183
Acquired drug resistance 328
Acquired immunity 89
Acquired immunodeficiency syndrome 550, 551, 563, 565
Activin A level 468
Activity restriction 401
Acupuncture 84
Acute care physiologic monitoring system 10
Acute coronary syndrome 247, 255
Acute kidney injury 144, 164
Acute myocardial infarction 259
Acute pancreatitis 123, 124, 126
    interpretation of 126*t*

Acute renal failure 143, 144
    pathophysiology of 144*fc*
    stages 143
Acute respiratory distress syndrome 27, 333, 338, 339*t*, 492
    pathophysiology of 340*fc*
Acute tubular necrosis 150
    causes of 150
    pathophysiology of 151*fc*
Acyanotic heart disease 474
Addition's crisis pathway 390*fc*
Adenosine 56
Adequate oxygenation, provide 471
Adjuvant analgesics 83
Administer morphine
    contraindications of 42
    sulfate 476
Adopt RUMBA technique 625
Adrenal crisis 388
    case of 390
    management of 390, 391
Adrenal fatigue syndrome
    signs of 389*f*
    symptoms of 389*f*
Adrenal gland 370
Adrenal insufficiency
    diagnosis of 390, 391*fc*
    management of 390, 391*fc*
Adrenal medulla, stimulation of 223
Adrenaline 55
Adrenergic inhibitors 254
Adsorbent 495
Advance directives, types of 606
Advanced maternal age 398
Advanced trauma life support teamwork 514*f*
Adynamic obstruction 128
Afferent sensing 222
Aggression 572
    and violence management, steps for 573*f*
Aggressive and violent patient, management of 573
Agitation 213
Agonists 41
    full 83
    mixed 83
    partial 41
Agranulocytosis 62
Airborne related precautions 622
Airway 214, 513, 528
    complete obstruction of 498
    difficulty, causes of 350
    location of 314*f*
    management 194, 317, 342, 343, 349, 353, 387, 503, 548, 561
        basic techniques of 349*fc*
    obstruction 441
    partial obstruction of 498
    support 200

Alanine aminotransferase 209
Albumin 69
Albuminuria 150
Albuterol 57
Alcohol 54, 73, 124, 198, 207, 272
    avoidance 414
    consumption 211
    dependence 569
    metabolic complication of 74
    pancreatitis 126
    use 257
    withdrawal 74, 199
Alcoholic cirrhosis 74
Alcoholic ketoacidosis 74
Aldehydes 54
Aldosterone 2
Alkanones 47
Alkaptonuria 462, 462*fc*
Allergy 44
Alprazolam 59
Alveolar
    dead space 302
    ventilation 302*f*
Alzheimer's dementia 377
Amantadine 571
Amikacin 49
Amiloride 64
Amino acid 139
    maintain 122
    metabolism defect 457
Aminoglycosides 48, 49, 488
    administration of 50
Aminosalicylic acid compounds 124
Amiodarone 56, 273, 275
Amitriptyline 60
Ammonia 207, 227
Amnesia, post-traumatic 214
Amniotic fluid embolism 432
Amniotomy 419
Amphetamine drug abusers 259
Amphotericin 92, 488
Ampicillin 488
    resistant strains 51
Amrinone 55
Amyloidosis 263
Analgesia 187
Analgesics 41, 133
Anaphylactic shock 433, 537, 565
    pathophysiology of 538*fc*
Anaphylaxis 432, 442
Anatomical dead space 301
Anemia 280
    severe 213, 266
Anesthesia
    considerations 411
    induction 383
Anesthetic agents 119

Aneurysm 276, 276f
  clipping of 191
Aneurysmal rupture 188
Aneurysmal subarachnoid hemorrhage,
    nursing management of 190
Angina 257, 263, 271, 272
  decubitus 257
  pathophysiology of 257, 257fc
  recurrent 289
  types of 257
Angiodysplasia 110
Angiography 111, 533
Angiotensin 281
  converting-enzyme inhibitor 147, 254, 260
Anidulafungin 92
Aniline dye 54
Animal-assisted therapy 35
Ankle jerk 179
Ankylosing spondylitis 47
Annular pancreas 124
Annuloplasty 294
Anomie 43
Anorectal malformation 482f, 506
Anorexia 101, 102, 144
Anosmia 211
Anoxic encephalopathy 210
Antacid 45
Antagonists 41
Antenatal care and monitoring 410
Antenatal corticosteroids 473
Antenatal management 410
Antenatal period 399
Antepartum factors 430
Antepartum hemorrhage 397
  causes of 397, 397fc
  classification of 397t
  management of 400fc
Anterior cord syndrome 218
Anthranilic acid derivatives 47
Anthropometric measurements 248
Anti-arrhythmic medications 475
Antibacterial classification 48
Antibiotic 48, 122, 127, 133, 334, 473, 478
  resistance 91
  resistant infections 91
  therapy 117, 423, 427, 431, 593
  use of 53
Antibody 205
Anticipated life transitional crisis 576
Anticoagulants 234
Anticoagulation 477
  management 162
  therapy 269, 336
Anticonvulsant 60
Antidiarrheals 63
Antidiuretic hormone 65, 139, 143, 168, 281, 392
  dysfunction 392
  function and action of 392f
Antidote 496, 496t
Antidysrhythmic agents 260, 269
Antiembolic stockings 234
Antiemetics 133
Antiepileptic drugs, first line 456

Antihistamines 57, 253
Antihypertensive agent 147
Antihypertensive therapy 411
Antiliteral temporal lobe focus 196
Antimicrobial therapy 343, 345
Antimicrobial treatment 471
Anti-mycobacterial agents 52
Antiretroviral drugs work 553
Antiretroviral therapy
  common class of 553
  drugs 553, 553t
Antiseptic 53
  kills 53
Antispasmodics 63
Antithrombotic therapy 290
Antithyroid
  antibody, levels of 208
  medications 66
  stimulating hormone receptor antibody 384
Antituberculosis medications, first line 329t
Anxiety 35, 145
  assessment 26
Aorta
  ascending 251
  overriding 474
Aortic aneurysm, abdominal 276
Aortic dissection 247, 253
Aortic regurgitation 247, 249
Aortic root aneurysm 276
Aortic stenosis 247, 252, 263
Aortic valve 268
  regurgitation 268
    pathophysiology of 269, 269fc
  stenosis 268
    pathophysiology of 268, 268fc
Apgar score 443t
Aphasia 173
  expressive 193
  global 193
  receptive 193
Apnea
  monitor 11
  test 229
Appendix, ruptured 132
Arachnoid mater 169f
Aromatherapy 34
Arrhythmia 207, 262
Arterial blood gas 126, 311
  analysis 209
Arterial dissection 188
Arterial laceration 109
Arterial pulse 249
Arteriovenous fistulas 148f
  and grafts, internal 147
Arteriovenous
  graft 148
  hemodialysis, continuous 161, 162
  malformation 188
Arylacetic acid derivatives diclofenac 46
Ascites, abdominal 264
Aseptic techniques 95
Aspartate aminotransferase 209
Asphyxia neonatorum 442

Aspiration
  devices 289
  pneumonia 315
Aspirin 40, 45-47, 234, 258, 260
  decrease effects of 45
  prophylaxis 414
  toxicity 45
Assisted vaginal delivery techniques 420
Asterixis 208
Asystole 275f
Ataxia 193, 208
Atelectasis 332
  acute 320, 333
  chronic 333
  non-obstructive 333
  nursing management of 334
  rounded 333
Atenolol 55, 258
Atherosclerosis 255f
  development 255
  stages of 256f
Atonic seizure 197, 456
Atorvastatin 260
Atria, evolution of 240
Atrial contraction, premature 272, 273f
Atrial depolarization 245
Atrial diastole 245
Atrial fibrillation 61, 273, 273f, 292
Atrial flutter 61, 273, 273f, 292
Atrial natriuretic hormone 142
Atrial septal defects 476
Atrial systole 245
Atrial tachycardia 292
Atrioventricular block
  first degree 270
  types of second degree 271fc
Atrioventricular canal, evolution of 240
Atropine 56, 272
Attapulgite 63
Audit Committee 623
Audit cycle 626
  steps of 624
Audit questions 626
Auricle, right 243
Auscultation 102, 252, 310
Auscultatory gap 250
Autoimmune 203
  disease 101, 150
    history of 389
  pancreatitis 124
  response 201
Automated external defibrillator 292
Autonomic cardiovascular dysfunction, severe 203
Autonomic disturbances 203
Autonomic dysfunction 202
Autonomic dysreflexia 222
Autonomic nervous system 167, 170
  division of 171
Autoregulation 183
Axon 167
  injured 217
Axonal injury, diffuse 212
Azactam 48
Azathioprine 124, 205

# B

B lymphocytes 90
Babinski's reflex 179
Bachmann's bundle 245
Bacillus anthracis 48
Bacitracin 48
Bacteremia 94
Bacteria 278, 429
Bacterial cell wall biosynthesis, inhibitor of 48
Bacterial endocarditis 280
Bacterial entry 429
Bacterial infection 276
Bacterial metabolism, inhibitors of 48, 51
Bacterial protein synthesis, inhibitors of 48, 49
Bag-valve-mask 498
Balloon
   atrial septostomy 477
   gastrostomy 106
   tamponade 113
Band ligation 113
Barbiturate 59
   coma 188
Barium sulfate 131
Baroreceptors stimulate 141
Barrel chest 309
Basal metabolic rate 223
Basic life support algorithm 285fc
Basilar skull fracture 231
Battle's sign 213
B-cell 90, 202, 205
   immunity 90
Becker asthma severity assessment score 502
Bed
   rest 133, 401
   space 629
Bedside 373
Behavioral coping, active 36
Belly laugh 34
Benzodiazepine 59, 72, 119, 200, 207, 550
Benzoic acid 54
Benzthiazide 64
Best motor response 175
Beta 2 agonists 503
Beta adrenergic blockers 260, 269
Beta antagonists 253
Beta blocker 56, 62, 258, 273, 475
   therapy, long-term 277
Bicarbonate 227
   ions 304
Bicuspid aortic valve 276
Bigeminal pulse 249
Bile 131
Bilevel positive airway pressure 350
Biliary spasm 44
Biliary tract
   anatomy of 100f
   disease 123
Bilirubin 209
   clearance 450
   levels, irregular 27
   metabolism 450, 451fc
Binge drinking 74
Bioethics, principles of 601, 602f

Biologic porcine heterograft 294
Biological theory 569
Biomedical waste, management of 622
Biopsy forceps 498
Biot's respiration 308
Biphasic defibrillator 292f
Birth
   defects 40
   spacing 402
Black urine disease 462
Bladder 193
   cancer 164
   drainage 153
   incontinence 218
   injury
      causes of 153
      mechanism of 153
   loss of 415
   management 221
   palpation 103
   trauma 153
Bleeding
   abnormal 426
   assessment and management 401
   control 533, 561
   excessive 422
   prolonged 422
   signs of 434
Blood 69, 117, 373
   borne 90
   brain barrier 169
   cells, levels of 51
   chemistry 209
   clots 424
      large 422
   component 69
      transfusion 117
   count, evaluation of 209
   cross-matching 422
   culture 431, 470
   flow 40, 179, 265f
   glucose, determining levels of 378
   hypercoagulability of 265
   investigations 209
   products 231
   studies 214, 215
   sugar management 194
   supply, disruption of 404
   test 144, 196, 335, 459
   type 422
   urea nitrogen 5, 147
Blood loss
   amount of 397
   measurement of 422
Blood pressure 234, 250, 253, 549
   augments 56
   control 190, 417
   high 56
   management 190, 194, 408, 410, 411, 413
   monitoring 412
   severe elevation of 255
   systolic 250
Blood transfusion 345, 405, 427, 534
   preparation 400

Blood volume 143
   decreased 433
   increase in 184
Bloodstream 39
   infections 94
Blunt abdominal trauma, management of 528, 529fc
Blunt injury 115, 156, 526, 527, 564
   mechanism of 341, 517, 517fc
   pathophysiology of 517, 517fc
Blunt trauma 341, 517, 560
Blurred vision 208, 254
Body
   circadian system, controlling 25
   image, enhancing 106
   mass index 248
   osmotic balance 392
   systems, drugs in 56
   temperature 222, 224
Bone 343
   and joints infection 48
   marrow depression 51
Boric acid 54
Bowel 193
   control, loss of 415
   habits 102
   injury
      large 117
      small 117
   management 221
   movement, impaired 534
   obstruction, large 130
   sounds, periodic assessment of 221
Bowman's capsule 139
Brachioradialis 178
Bradycardia 7, 221, 264, 271, 549
Bradykinesia 122
Bradypnea 308, 549
Brain 167, 169f, 188f
   cells 213
   connection 171
   damage, irreversible 291
   hemorrhage, types of 212, 212f
   little 169
   parts of 168f
   structures of 232
   swelling 233
   tissue, anoxia of 207
   to pituitary action, relationship of 371f
   volume, increase in 184
Brain dead patient 28
   caring for 229
Brain death 156, 228, 604
   clinical signs of 228
   determination of 228
   diagnosed 229
   mimic 228
Brain herniation 231
   types 231f
Brain injury 44, 211, 223
   traumatic 211, 233
Brainstem 167, 168
   function 228
Breast milk 40

Breath
  examination of 225
  shortness of 272
  sound, abnormal 249, 310
Breathing 194, 200, 214, 500, 514, 528
  control 302
  difficulty 475
  exercise, role of 526
  ineffective 211, 222
  management 561
  mechanism 301
  pattern 308, 345
  slow 225
Breathlessness 306
  causes of 307$t$
  progression of 307
Broca's aphasia 193
Bromhexine 58
Bromocriptine 571
Bronchi, location of 339$f$
Bronchial hygiene 354
  therapy, indication of 354
  types of 354
Bronchodilator 57, 334
Bronchopneumonia, acute 490
Bronchoscopic lung volume reduction 362$f$
Bronchoscopy 312, 344
  complication of 313
Bronchospasm
  acute 57
  early 502
Brown-Séquard syndrome 218
Bruises, multiple 225
Bulbar muscle weakness 206
Bulbus cordis 240
Bullectomy 325, 361
Bundle of His 245
Buprenorphine 41, 42
Burn 442, 582
  asphalt 591
  assessment 587
  chemical 584, 584$f$, 591
  classification of 582
  complication
    management of 593
    prevention of 593
  contact 583
  depth of 587
  E-cigarette 584
  electrical 583, 584$f$
  extensive 3
  extent of 588
  first-degree 587
  flame 583, 583$f$
  flash 583
  management 582
  pathophysiology of 582, 586$fc$
  patient, fluid calculation for 588$t$
  prognosis of 597
  scald 583
  second-degree of 588, 588$f$
  severity of 588
  stages of 587$f$
  tar 591

thermal 583, 591
third-degree 588
wound 592
Burnout
  causes of 35
  syndrome 35
Burr hole 232

## C

Caffeine 272
Calcitonin 142
Calcium 70, 142, 147
  channel blockers 62, 258, 273, 277
  ions triggers 217
  supplements 5, 414
Campylobacter 53, 124
  jejuni 201
Canalicular laceration 556
Cancer 101, 208
Candida infections 57
Capillary refill 250
Carbamates 73
Carbamazepine 60, 571
Carbamino compound 304
Carbohydrate metabolism defect 457
Carbon dioxide 1, 142, 227
  partial pressure 229
  transportation 304
Carbon monoxide 73
Carbon tetrachloride 118
Carbonic anhydrase 64
  inhibitor 64
Carboxymethyl cellulose 206
Carcinogenesis 40
Cardiac arrest 7, 55, 156
Cardiac arrhythmia 44, 272
Cardiac assessment 251
Cardiac auscultation 251$f$
Cardiac catheterization 263, 269, 476, 478
Cardiac chambers 243, 243$f$
Cardiac chest pain and discomfort, causes of 247
Cardiac complications 191
Cardiac conditions 272
Cardiac conduction system 245
Cardiac contraction 284
Cardiac cycle 245
  starts 245
Cardiac decompensation 254
Cardiac disease 143
Cardiac emergencies 440, 441
Cardiac enlargement 383
Cardiac events 432
Cardiac glycosides 61, 73, 550
Cardiac myocardium 284
Cardiac output 245
Cardiac problems 249
Cardiac surgeries 293
  complications after 294
  nursing management of 295
Cardiac tamponade 522, 524$f$, 564
  pathophysiology of 525$fc$
Cardiac tissues, nerve supply to 244
Cardiac transplantation 294

Cardiac vein
  anterior 243
  middle 244
Cardio toxic agents 262
Cardiogenic area 239
Cardiogenic pulmonary edema 331$f$
Cardiogenic shock 262, 433, 536, 565
  pathophysiology of 537$fc$
  risk factors of 536$fc$
Cardiomyopathy 262, 262$f$, 270
  causes of 74, 262
  classification of 262, 262$fc$
Cardiopulmonary resuscitation 284
Cardiovascular agent 147
Cardiovascular assessment 246
Cardiovascular changes 155
Cardiovascular diseases 255
Cardiovascular disorders 158, 246
Cardiovascular effects 231
Cardiovascular emergencies 239
Cardiovascular history collection 246
Cardiovascular management 239
Cardiovascular status 345
Cardiovascular system 218, 239, 415
  anatomy of 239
  assessment of 246
  disorders 292
    management modalities for 284
  drugs in 61
  physiology of 244
Cardioversion 273, 290
Care
  continuing 128
  continuity of 612
  coordination 612
  futility of 605
  goals of 31
  intermediate 8
  long-term 8
  lower costs of 13
  postoperative 402
  preconception 402
  standards of 612
  supportive 425, 428, 431, 435, 503
  surgical 429
Caregiver's role strain 28
Carnitine deficiency 458
Carotid endarterectomy 194
Cartilage 343
Carvedilol 258
Caspofungin 92
Catatonic based, signs of 571$f$
Catatonic stupor 571
Catatonic syndrome, management of 571
Catecholamine 55, 201
Catharsis 495
Catheter
  embolism 109
  insertion 94, 161
  obstruction 159
  sepsis 109
Catheter-associated urinary tract infection,
  prevention of 94
Cauda equina syndrome 218

Causative microorganism 278
Causative organism 132, 279
Caustic chemicals 73
Cauterization 559
Celecoxib 47
Cell
    body 167, 171
    membrane 40
    types of 167
Cellular oxygen deprivation 433
Central catheters, peripherally inserted 108
Central control 223
Central cord syndrome 218
Central cyanosis 248
Central nervous system 373, 415
    stimulants 59
Central nursing station 617
Central parenteral nutrition 107
Central pontine myelinolysis 393
Central sensitization 79
Central venous access devices, types of 108
Centralized nursing station 630
Cephalosporin 48, 49
    administering 49
    side effects of 49
Cerebellar examination 178
Cerebellar tonsillar herniation 230
Cerebellum 167, 169
Cerebral
    angiography 181, 189
    autoregulation 187
    blood
        flow 179, 187, 213
        vessel, clot in 192f
    causes 195
    cortex 167
    edema 184, 187, 231
    function 228
    ischemia 213
    medulla 167
    metabolism 183, 213
    perfusion pressure 179, 228
    salt wasting syndrome 228
    vasospasm, delayed 190
Cerebrospinal fluid 169, 179
    analysis 202
    disturbance 233
    drainage 188
    leakage 213
    rhinorrhea 560
    volume, increase in 184
Cerebrovascular accident 156
Cerebrovascular disease 188
Cerebrum 167
Certified brain stem death 229
Cervical
    cord injury 218
    injury 218
    spine trauma 500
    vertebra 169
Cesarean
    delivery 400, 411
    section 420
Cetirizine 57

Chemo regulation 183
Chemoreceptors 303
Chemotherapy 208
Cherry red discoloration 225
Chest 515
    compression 448
        maintain 448f
    configuration 309
    percussion 355
    physiotherapy 206, 334, 343, 355
    radiography 311
    tube insertion 345
    vibration 355
    X-ray 312, 342, 475, 476
Chest injury 517
    emergency management of 345
    penetrating 516f
    risk score 518t
    score 518
Chest pain 125, 247, 268, 305
    managing 536
Chest trauma 341
    pathophysiology of 341fc
    severe 344
    types of 341, 341fc
Chest wall
    dysfunction of 338
    injury 517
    pain 305
Cheyne-Stokes respiration 308
Chief cells 100
Chitosan 160
Chlamydia 51, 132
Chloramphenicol 48, 51
Chlordiazepoxide 59, 63
Chlorhexidine 54
Chloride 70, 139, 142, 227
Chlorothiazide 64
Chloroxylenol 54
Chlorpheniramine 57
Cholera 53
    shigellosis 53
Chromosomal abnormalities 475
Chronic kidney disease 146, 164
    classifying stages 146
    stages of 146f
Chronic obstructive pulmonary disease 322
    pathophysiology of 323fc
    stages of 324f, 324t
    symptoms of 323f
Cibenzoline 55
Ciprofloxacin 48, 52, 53, 65
Circadian rhythm 168
Circulation 284, 500, 528
    airway, breathing, defibrillate 284
Cisapride 62
Cisplatin 488
Classic maple syrup urine disease 461
Clear airway 446
    infection 325
Cleft
    lip 505
    palate 505
Clindamycin 48

Clinical nurses 626
Clonazepam 59, 60
Clonic seizure 197, 456
Clonic stage 416
Clonidine 55, 253
Clopilet 258, 260
Clostridium 132
Clotting, abnormal 202
Coagulation abnormalities 430
Coagulation disorders 421
Coagulation management 406
Coagulation profile 422
Coagulation support 423
Coagulation system 415
Cocaine 73, 259
    abuse 188
Codeine 83
    phosphate 235
Cold caloric test 228
Cold frost 585f
Colitis 110
Collaborative practice 601
Collagen
    tissue disorders 270
    vascular diseases 253
Colloid 69, 588
    common 69, 69t
Coma 226, 254
    stage of 416
Common congenital disorders 505
Common respiratory emergency disorders 313
Communication 9, 12, 86, 601
    barriers 82
    difficulties 207
    problems 193
Community-acquired pneumonia 314
Compensatory mechanisms, activation of 433
Complementary therapy 325
Complete blood count 202, 470
Complete cord lesion 218
Compression atelectasis 333
Compression fractures, causes 217
Computerized documentation 633
Conception, retained products of 421
Conference room 632
Configurational isomerization 452
Confusion 125, 226, 254
Congenital disorders 474
Congestive heart failure 56, 320
Conjunctiva-suggest alcoholism 225
Consciousness 224
    altered 415
    disturbances in 122
    level of 175, 185, 215, 225, 234
    normal 225
    state of 225-227
Conservative therapy 127
Constipation 74
Consultation and multidisciplinary care 423, 425
Contraception counseling 412
Contraceptive jellies, use of 140
Contralateral stimulation 84
Contusion 212

Conus medullaris syndrome 218
Cool and clammy extremities 257
Copartial agonists 83
Cord lesion, incomplete 218
Cord prolapsed 397
Corneal abrasions 555, 565
Corneal reflex 176
Coronary angiography 258, 260, 261
Coronary artery 243, 255f, 260
    bypass graft 293
    right 243
Coronary artery disease 247, 255
    classification of 255, 256fc
    management of risk factors of 258
    pathophysiology of 255, 256fc
Coronary atherectomy 289
    directional 289
Coronary circulation 239, 243, 244f
Coronary revascularization 258
Coronary sinus 243, 244
Coronary stents 289
Correct systemic hypotension 231
Corticosteroid 57, 124, 221, 410, 493, 503
    related complications 158
    side-effects of 205
Cough 304
    assess 304
    causes of 304
    etiquette 93
Counter regulatory mechanism 280
Coup-contrecoup injury 212f
Cranial nerve 170, 171, 171t
    examination 176
Cranial neuropathy 213
Cranioplasty 188
Craniosacral division 171
Craniotomy 188, 188f, 216, 232
Crash cart 11
C-reactive protein 126, 209
Creatinine 209
    clearance 147
Cresol 54
Crigler Najjar syndrome 450
Crisis 576
    characteristics of 576
    cholinergic 206
    components of 576
    developmental 576
    dispositional 576
    managing 573
    maturational 576
    meaning of 575
    myasthenic 205
    reflecting psychopathology 576
    resolution 577
        revaluation of 580
    signs of 577, 578f
    situational 576
    symptoms of 577, 578f
    types of 576
Crisis intervention 9, 567, 575, 577, 578
    principles of 577
    role of nurse in 579
    techniques 577, 579t

Critical care
    environment 10, 28
        components of 24
        impact of 24
    family 24
    nurse 10, 28
    nursing negligence in 607
    principles of 600
    psychosis 27
    purpose of 8
    quality assurance in 610
Critical care nursing 1, 9, 14, 607
    concept of 8
    future of 14
    practice 14, 23
        evidence-based 13
    principles of 9
    scope of 9
Critical care unit 25, 34, 78, 89, 91, 93, 95, 604, 607
    classification of 614
    design pattern of 630f
    disinfection in 95
    documentation in 11
    equipment 620
    ethical issues in 601
    legal issues in 606
    levels of 615
    models of 614
    nursing requirements 628
    pain assessment in 81
    psychosis 27
    setup 10
    staffing of 627
    standards of 614
    sterilization in 95
    team 630
    therapeutic elements 630
Critical illness 24
Critically ill patient 10, 89
Critically sick patients 8
Crushing effect 115
Crushing injury 3
Crystalloid 68, 68t, 231, 588
    solution, common 68
Cullen's sign 134
Cushing's syndrome 248
Cushing's triad 185
Cutaneous stimulation 83
Cyanide poisoning 225
Cyanosis 475
    peripheral 248
Cyanotic heart
    disease 474
    lesions 441
Cyclizine 57, 235
Cyclooxygenase-1 45
Cyclophosphamide 205
Cycloserine 48
Cytomegalovirus 201
Cytotoxic edema 184

## D

Dairy products 207
Dantrolene 571

D-dimer level 335
Deafness 72
Deceased donor 156
Decerebrate posturing 185
Decidua formation, reduced 398
Decompressive craniectomy 188, 194, 216, 233
Decorticate posturing 185
Deep breathing 34
    exercise 354
Deep tendon reflexes 178
Deep vein thrombosis 216, 265, 265f
    prophylaxis 203
    risk factors of 265
    types of 265fc
Defibrillation 291, 291f
Defibrillators, types of 292
Deficient fluid, risk for 155
Deficit fluid volume 211
Dehydration 64, 72, 266, 481, 484
    based on osmolarity, types of 484
    based on severity, types of 484
    management of 485
    mild 484
    moderate 484
    severe 484, 485
    severity of 484
    signs of 155
Delirium 125
    tremens 74
Delivery 417
    mode of 411
Demeclocycline 50
Dementia, occurrence of 27
Demyelination 202f
Dendrites 167
Dendritic cells 90
Dental procedures 278
Deoxyribonucleic acid
    analysis 460
    binding agents 52
Depression 62
Dermatitis 52
Desmopressin 65
Destot sign 501
Dextran 69
Dextropropoxyphene 41
Diabetes 90, 258, 289
    insipidus 154, 215
    mellitus 257
        drug therapy for 66
        type 2 377
Diabetic acidosis, symptoms of 380
Diabetic ketoacidosis 2, 74, 379
    classification of 381t
    coma 225
    resolution of 382
Diagnostic devices 620
Diagnostic equipment 11
Diagnostic peritoneal lavage 565
Dialysate 148
Dialysate prescription 161
Dialysis 147, 462, 496
    complications of 208
    disequilibrium syndrome 208

fluid, composition of 148
  prescription 160
  principles of 147
Dialyzer 148, 148f, 161f
Diamorphine 41
Diaphragm muscle 116
Diaphragmatic breathing, goal of 354
Diaphragmatic tear 116
Diarrhea 50, 62, 74, 164
  aggravating foods 207
Diastolic failure, pathophysiological changes in 280fc
Diazepam 59
Diclofenac 46
  sodium 58
  stops production 46
Dicyclomine hydrochloride 63
Didanosine 124
Diencephalon 167, 168
Diet 553
  restriction 147
  therapy 460
Dietary history 101, 174
Dietary management 2, 4-6
Dietary restriction 462
Dieulafoy's lesions 110
Diffusion 147
Digestive system
  accessory organs of 98
  anatomy of 99f
  basic functions of 99
  physiology of 100
Digestive tract
  histology of 99
  organs of 98
Digoxin 55, 61, 273
  discontinue 271
Dihydrocodeine 41
Dilated cardiomyopathy 262, 263
Diltiazem 258
Diminish gastric acid 63
Dinitrophenylhydrazine test 460
Diphenhydramine 57
Diphenoxylate hCl 63
Diplopia 193, 204
Dirty rooms 631
Disability 214, 514, 528
Discharge planning 400, 402
Disequilibrium syndrome 208
Disopyramide 55
Disseminated intravascular coagulation 543, 545t, 546t, 565
  clinical presentation of 545t
  pathophysiology of 544fc
  risk factors of 545f
Distress 29
Diuresis 144
Diuretic 64, 151, 344, 475, 476
  classification of 64
  therapy 6
Diverticulitis 132
Diverticulosis 110
Diving seal reflex 444
Dizziness 45, 47, 48, 211, 263, 268, 271-273

Dobutamine 55
Documentation, proper 12
Donor
  preparation 156
  selection 294
  sources 156
Dopamine 55
Doppler ultrasound 478
Doxepin 60
Doxycycline 50
Drowning 442
Drowsiness 47, 48, 62, 185, 226
Drug
  absorption 40
  abusers 269
  action of 553
  administration 40
  antiarrhythmic 56
  antibiotic 279, 325
  anticholinergic 63, 228, 503
  antifungal 92t
  antihypertensive 277
  anti-inflammatory 41, 57
  antiplatelet 133, 194, 258
  biochemical effects of 39
  biotransformation 40
  cardiac 61
  cardiotonic 61
  distribution 40
  doses 64
  excretion 40
  illicit 73
  induced 203
  interactions 329
  life-saving 56
  management, acute 261
  misuse 73
  overdose, management of 548, 550
  physiological effects of 39
  resistance
    primary 327
    secondary 328
  review of 39
  therapy 258, 266, 279t
  toxicity 199
  transport across membranes 40
Drug overdose and poisoning 71, 547, 563
  clinical picture of 547t
  parameters of 549t
Drug-drug interactions 253
Drug-food interactions 253
Dual-lumen catheters 159
Dubin Johnson syndrome 450
Duloxetine 221
Duodenal cause 109
Duodenal ulcer 63, 110, 131
Duodenum 127
Dura mater 169f, 188f
Dysarthria 193, 204
Dysmenorrhea 47
Dysphagia 193, 203, 206
Dysphasia 495
Dysphoria 44

Dyspnea 257, 263, 264, 268, 272, 273
  degree of 307, 307t
Dysrhythmias 280
Dyssy's quality assurance cycle 625
Dystonia, sign of acute 62

# E

Ear 515
Earle sign 501
Echinocandins 91
Echocardiogram 475, 476
Echocardiography 193
Eclampsia 253, 396, 407, 414, 432, 445
  clinical features of 415
  management of 416fc
  maternal complications of 416
Ecstasy 73
Ectopic pregnancy 396
Eczema 54
Edema 10, 250, 415
  dependent 264
Edrophonium chloride test 204
Education 86
  and support 160, 161
  and training 93
  committee 613
Efferent sensing 223
Efficient coding 12
Efficient program maintenance 13
Eisenmenger's syndrome 248
Electrical alternans 525
Electrical injuries 591
Electrical services 619
Electrocardiogram 193, 475, 476
Electrocardiography 258
Electrodes 284
Electroencephalogram 196
Electroencephalography 180
Electrolyte 70, 209, 471
  balance 141, 150, 418
  disturbances 486
Electrolyte imbalance 4, 163, 195, 270, 287, 481
  cause of 74
  management of 162
  risk for 155, 163
Electromyography 182, 202
Elevated cardiac biomarkers 289
Elevated intracellular calcium 192
Emboli protection device 289
Embryo, mesodermal layer of 239
Embryogenic form 242
Emergency
  care 115, 194, 393
  delivery 405
  department 138
  laparotomy 428, 528
  management 112, 214, 220
  psychiatry, basic principles of 568
  resuscitation equipment 11, 620, 620f
  stabilization measures 495
  treatment 523
  unit, discharge from 572
Emergent surgical intervention, prepare for 476

Emotional support 86, 401, 594
    and comfort 418
    and communication 406, 420, 425
    and education 432
Enalapriland captopril 258
Encephalopathy 207, 208, 209$t$
    chronic 207
    diagnosis of 208
    type of 208
End diastolic volume 245
End systolic volume 245
Endocardial tubes 240
Endocardium 243
Endocrine
    assessment, symptoms-centered 369
    associated encephalopathy 210
    disease 143
    disorders 208, 350
    disturbance 208
        clinical features of 372$t$
    dysfunction 150
    emergencies 440, 441
    glands 368
Endocrine system 368, 369$f$
    anatomy of 368
    assessment of 369
    drugs in 66
    emergencies 368
    examination of 369
    management of 368
    physiology of 368
End-of-life issue 605
Endomyocardial fibrosis 263
Endoscopic procedure 105$t$
Endoscopic retrograde
        cholangiopancreatography 124
Endoscopic sclerotherapy 113$f$
Endoscopy 111, 113
Endothelial damage 265
Endothelial dysfunction 408, 409, 415
Endothelin production 281
Endotoxin effects 430
Endotracheal intubation 227
Endotracheal tube 175
Endovascular coiling 191
End-tidal carbon dioxide monitoring 311
Energy failure
    primary 444
    secondary 444
Enoxacin 52
Enoximone 55
Enteral feeding, complications of 106, 107$t$
Enteral nutrition 105
Enteritis 128
Enterobacter 470
Enterococcus 429
Enterotomy 130
Environmental cleaning 93
Environmental cleanliness 593
Environmental control, systems for 633
Environmental emergencies 440, 442
Environmental factors 474
Environmental requirements 619
Environmental stressors, decrease 32

Epicardium 242
Epidural hematoma 212
Epilepsy 44
Epinephrine 55, 56
Epispadias 506
Epistaxis 559, 565
    causes of 559$f$
    management 559
Epstein-Barr virus 201
Equipment 591
    and supplies 10
    and technology integration 631
    storage 632
Erythromycin 48
Erythropoietin 468
Escalating situations 573
Escherichia coli 429
Esophageal atresia 480, 506
    types of 480$f$
Esophageal cancer 110
Esophageal cause 109
Esophageal injury 116
Esophageal ulcer 110
Esophageal varices 110
Esophagitis 110
Esophagus 99
Estrogens 124
Ethambutol 319, 328, 329
Ethic
    and training committee 613
    meaning of 601
Ethical decision-making 603
    model 603, 603$fc$
Ethical dilemmas 603, 604
Ethnicity 257
Etidronate disodium 6
Euglycemic diabetic acidosis 382
Eustress 29
Euthanasia 605
Evidence-based practice committee 613
Evolutionary theory 80
Exacerbation, risk of 53
Exchange technique 161
Exchange transfusion 453
Excitotoxicity 213, 217
Exercise 277
    history 101, 174
    stress test 258
Exhalation 301
Exogeneous contamination 132
Exotoxin effects 430
Expiration 301
Exposed body area, decontamination of 549
Extra diastolic sounds 252
Extra systolic sounds 252
Extracardiac fontan 477
Extracellular fluid volume
    deficit 2
    excess 2
    shift, pathophysiology of 3$fc$
Extracranial causes 224, 225
Extracranial injuries 211
Extremities trauma 501
Exudative effusions 320

Eye 248, 515
    burns to 556
    chemicals in 556
    decontamination 495
    movement 176
    opening 175
    trauma 554$f$
Eye injury 554
    case of 556$t$
    management of 554
    types of 555$fc$
Eye removal 557
    enucleation 557
    evisceration 557

**F**

Fabry's disease 458
Facial nerve 168, 176
Facial palsy 203
Facilitate social support 32
Factor Xa inhibitor 266
Factors influencing cardiac output 245
Failure to thrive 475
Family 28
    history 101, 174, 247
    issues 28
    perception 24
    teaching 29
Farber's disease 458
Fascicle
    anterosuperior 245
    posteroinferior 245
Fatigue 62, 206, 211, 257, 263, 264, 433, 475
Fatty streak 256
Feeding
    long-term 106
    short-term 105
Female newborn 482
Fenamates 47
Ferric chloride test 460
Fetal abnormalities 418
Fetal complications 399, 404, 405, 410
Fetal consequences 426
Fetal distress 404, 419, 427
Fetal factors 403, 418
Fetal lung maturation 410
Fetal macrosomia 418
Fetal monitoring 434
Fetal surveillance 410
Fetal well-being 406
Fetor hepaticus 118
Fetus 419
Fever 74, 187, 191, 213
    extrapelvic causes of 430
Fiber electromyography, single 204
Fibreoptic bronchoscopy 334
Fibrinoid necrosis, development of 208
Fibrinolytic therapy 261
Fibrosis incorrect lead position 287
Fibrous pericardium 242
Fibrous plaque 256
Fingers and toes, clubbing of 475
Finger-to-finger test 178
Finger-to-nose test 178

First kidney transplantation 156
First-aid
    management, initial 559
    treatment 523
Fissure 110, 168
Flail chest 342, 343f, 520, 564
    pathophysiology of 343fc, 520fc
Flank and back 515
Flecainide 55
Fluconazole 92
Fluid
    and nutrition management 413
    correction, principles of 589
    disturbances 150, 483
    infusion 533
    maintain 471
    resuscitation 488, 535
    therapy 537
Fluid and electrolyte
    management 431
    therapy 589
Fluid balance 143, 162, 418, 493, 589
    altered 2
Fluid electrolyte
    balance, altered 2
    disturbance 483
Fluid intake 151
    monitor 151
    restriction 147
Fluid volume
    deficit, risk for 152
    disorders of 154, 155
    management 342
    treatment for 154
Flunitrazepam 73
Flushing 45
Focal neurologic deficits 185, 213
Focal seizure 455, 456
Foley catheters 11
Folic acid 51, 174
Folinic acid 51
Fontan shunt 477
Food poisoning 74
Forced diuresis 495
Forceps delivery 420
Foreign body
    aspiration 497
    management of 498
Formaldehyde 54
Formoterol 57
Fosphenytoin 200
Fracture, category of 532
Frequent hemodynamic monitoring 536
Frostbite 584
Fulminant hepatic failure 117
    pathophysiology of 118fc
Functional nephrons, loss of 150
Functional obstruction 128
Fungal infection, treatment of 91
Funnel chest 309
Furosemide 64

## G

G cells 100
Gabapentin 221
Gag reflex 177
Gait, shuffling 122
Galactokinase deficiency 463
Galactose epimerase deficiency 463
Galactosemia 462
    biochemical pathway of 463fc
    classic 463
Gallbladder 100
Gallstone pancreatitis 127
Gamma-glutamyl transpeptidase 209
Gas exchange
    impaired 155
    risk for impaired 330
Gastric cancer 110
Gastric cause 109
Gastric content, aspiration of 549
Gastric injury 117
Gastric irritation, less 47
Gastric juice 131
Gastric lavage 72
Gastric motility 100
Gastric origin 125
Gastric secretory cells 100
Gastric ulcer 110, 221
    prophylaxis 216
Gastric varices 110
Gastrin 100
Gastritis 110
Gastroenteritis 53
Gastroesophageal reflux disease 63
Gastrointestinal bleeding 109, 110
    presentation of 109
    severity of 112, 112t
Gastrointestinal complaints 101
Gastrointestinal decompression 133
Gastrointestinal decontamination 495
Gastrointestinal disease 143
Gastrointestinal disorder 101
Gastrointestinal emergencies 440, 441
Gastrointestinal perforation 132
Gastrointestinal stimulation, lack of 109
Gastrointestinal system 102, 172, 218
    anatomy of 98
    assessment of 101
    diagnostic evaluation of 104
    drugs in 62
Gastrointestinal tract 50
    bleeding 109f
Gastrojejunostomy 106
Gastroschisis 507
Gastrostomy
    device, low profile 106
    radiologically inserted 106
    surgically placed 106
Gate control theory 79
Gaucher's disease 458
Gender 569
Gene 461
Generalized convulsive status
        epilepticus 199
Genetic abnormality 450
Genetic disorder 156
Genetic factors 408, 415, 474, 480
Genital tract infection 132
Genitalia 515
    external 140
    male external 140
Genitourinary system 219
    parts of 138
Gentamicin 49
Gentian violet 54
Gestational hypertension 407, 408, 445
Ghon complex 326
Gilbert syndrome 450
Gingival hyperplasia 60
Glasgow coma scale 175, 175t, 211, 214
Glenn shunt 477
Glomerular filtrate 142
Glomerular filtration rate 139
Glomerular injury and loss 150
Glomerulonephritis 207
Glossopharyngeal nerve 177
Gloves 621
Glucocorticoid therapy 387
Glucose 139
Glucose 6 phosphate dehydrogenase
        deficiency 464
Glutamate 192
Glycemic control 378
Glycopyrrolate 63
Gonococcus 132
Gonorrhea 48
Graft
    and flaps 594, 594f
    rejection 294
Gram-negative bacteria 53
Gramoneg 52
Gram-positive bacteria 53
Grand mal
    epilepsy 60
    seziure 197
Graphesthesia 178
Grave's disease 66
Gray baby syndrome 51
Great arteries, transposition of 477
Great cardiac vein 244
Grey turner's sign 134
Group A streptococcus 429
Guillain-Barré syndrome 201
    diagnostic criteria for 202
Gunshot wounds 344, 521
Gut integrity 109
Gyri 168

## H

Hallucinogens 73
Hand hygiene 93, 94, 593
    and aseptic technique 471
Harrison's classification 557, 558f
Hashimoto's thyroiditis 387
Head 248, 515
    trauma 500
Head injury 199, 211, 214
    adult 211
    causes for 211
    nursing management of 216
    surgical management of 216
Headache 45, 74, 185, 208, 211, 254, 409, 415

Healing
    art for 34
    environment 31, 32
Health
    care staff, education of 621
    history, collection of 101
    status, present 371
    teaching 198
Health education 319, 353
    and discharge planning 418
Healthcare
    associated infections, risk of 92
    professionals 27, 28
    providers 9
    research and quality, agency for 613
    setting 35
    specialist 91
Healthy diet 277
Healthy lifestyle choices 402, 413
Hearing
    existence of 27
    loss 25
Heart 239
    anatomy of 240, 243*f*
    attack 45
    burn 101
    conduction system of 240, 244
    embryology development of 241*f*
    layers of 242, 242*f*
    lymphatic circulation of 244
    normal 524*f*
    pacemaker of 243
    part of 242*t*
    rates 56
    transplantation 294
    tube 240
    venous circulation of 244
Heart block 270
    complete 271
    types 270*f*
Heart disease 282
    classification of congenital 474
    congenital 474
Heart failure 61, 154, 263, 270, 271, 279, 283
    causes of 280, 280*fc*
    clinical manifestations of 281
    compensatory mechanisms in 280, 281*fc*
    pathological mechanism in 280
    signs of 289
    symptoms of 289
    types of 280, 282*fc*
Heart sound
    first 252
    second 252
Heartbeats, irregular 56
Heel-to-knee test 178
HELLP syndrome 253
Hematemesis 109
Hematochezia 109, 134
Hematocrit level 422
Hematogenous spread 132
Hematuria 140
    microscopic 140
Hemiclamshell thoracotomy, bilateral 359*f*

Hemiparesis 193
Hemiplegia 193
Hemobilia 110
Hemodialysis 147, 159*f*, 160
    complication of 148
    technique 160
Hemodilution 190
Hemodynamic instability 427
Hemodynamic stability 215
    maintenance of 471
Hemodynamic support 428
Hemoglobin level 422
Hemolytic causes 449
Hemoperfusion 496
Hemophilus influenza 201
Hemoptysis 305
    causes of 306*t*
Hemorrhage 10, 154, 426, 432, 556
    accidental 402
    extradural 466
    primary postpartum 421, 423
    secondary postpartum 421, 423
    splinter 249
    subconjunctival 249
    subdural 467
Hemorrhagic phase, symptoms of 545
Hemorrhagic stroke 191, 192, 194
    causes of 192*t*
Hemorrhoid 110
    treatment of 56
Hemostasis 428
Hemosuccus pancreaticus 110
Hemothorax 344, 346, 522, 524*f*
    management of 524*fc*
    pathophysiology of 346*fc*
    physiologic resolution of 346
    unresolved 346
Henle's loop 139
Hepatic coma 225
Hepatic congestion 248
Hepatic damage 50
Hepatic encephalopathy 120, 207, 209, 210
    grading of 121
    pathophysiology of 121*fc*
Hepatic myelopathy 122
Hepatic system 415
Hepatitis
    B 95
        virus 117
    E 201
Hepatotoxicity 47
    drug-related 117
Hereditary pancreatitis 124
Herniation syndrome 229, 230
    management of 231
    types of 229, 230*t*
Heroin 73
Hexachlorophene 54
Hexobarbitone 59
Histamine 127
    H2 antagonists 63
Hoarseness 57, 308
Holistic caring 23
Holter monitoring 263

Homan's sign 251*f*
    positive 266
Home care 8
Homograft 294
Homonymous hemianopsia 193
Honoring dignity 608
Hormonal control 2
Hormonal factors 480
Hormonal imbalances, symptoms of 118
Hormonal thermogenesis 223
Hormones 370
    major 370*t*
Hospital, quality assurance in 614
Hospital-acquired pneumonia 314
Human blood, components of 69*t*
Human chronic gonadotrophins 373
Human immunodeficiency virus 551, 565
    clinical stages of 551*t*
    modes of transmission of 552*t*
    replication pathways 552*f*
    structure 551*f*
    transmitted 552
Human-animal bond 35
Hunt and Hess grading 189*t*
Hydralazine 411, 412
Hydration 194, 462
Hydrocephalous 190, 213, 229
Hydrochloride 63
    thiazide 64
Hydrochlorothiazide 64
Hydrogen 139
    ions 142
    peroxide 54
Hydroxychloroquine 488
Hydroxyzine 57
Hyper bilirubin anemia 26
Hyper encephalopathy 208
Hyperbilirubinemia 126
    predicting severe 452
Hypercalcemia 6, 70, 124, 142, 162
Hypercapnia 213
Hypercapnic failure 337
Hyperchloremia 71
Hypercholesterolemia 64, 276
Hyperemia 225
Hyperextension injuries 217
Hyperflexion 217
Hyperglycemia 191, 213, 215, 376-379
    differential diagnoses of 379
    pathogenesis of 378*fc*
    treatment of 379, 380*t*, 381*f*
Hyperglycemic encephalopathy 209, 210
Hyperhomocysteinemia 266, 276
Hyperkalemia 5, 70, 162, 489
Hyperlipidemia 248
Hypermagnesemia 6, 71, 162
Hypernatremia 4, 162, 213, 487
    acute 487
    chronic 488
    correction of 488
Hyperosmolar therapy 187
Hyperperistalsis movement 102
Hyperphenylalaninemia, mild 459
Hyperphosphatemia 7, 71

Hyperpyrexia 224
Hypersensitivity reactions 48
Hypertension 27, 90, 101, 187, 190, 208, 225, 257, 258, 263, 276, 294, 403, 409, 415, 549
    pregnancy-induced 407
Hypertensive crisis 253, 253f, 254, 255
    pathophysiology of 254fc
Hypertensive emergencies 254
Hypertensive encephalopathy 208-210, 254
Hypertensive urgencies 255
Hyperthermia 200, 215, 223, 225, 549
    malignant 223
Hyperthyroidism 224, 385f
Hypertriglyceridemia 124
Hypertrophic cardiomyopathy 247, 263
Hypertrophic pyloric stenosis, congenital 480
Hyperventilation 187, 308
Hypervolemia 190, 280
Hypoalbuminemia 126
    severe 320
Hypocalcemia 5, 70, 142, 162, 202
Hypocapnia 213
Hypochloremia 70
Hypoglossal nerve 177
Hypoglycemia 200, 208, 213, 373
Hypoglycemic coma 227
Hypoglycemic encephalopathy 208-210
Hypokalemia 4, 56, 64, 70, 162, 488
Hypomagnesemia 6, 71, 162
Hyponatremia 4, 64, 162, 191, 200, 213, 215, 486
Hyponatremic dehydration 143
Hypo-osmolar edema 185
Hypophosphatemia 7, 71
Hypospadias 505
Hypotension 7, 56, 64, 125, 202, 213, 221, 225, 272, 433, 549
    risk of 235
Hypothalamus 168, 370
    anterolateral 143
Hypothermia 223, 225, 549
Hypothyroidism 280
Hypotonic dehydration 143
Hypoventilation 308
Hypovolemia 2
    signs of 422
Hypovolemic shock 433, 535, 565
    pathophysiology of 535fc
Hypoxemia 183, 213
Hypoxemic failure 337
Hypoxia 206, 272, 287, 409
    duration of 207
Hypoxic encephalopathy 207, 209, 210
Hypoxic ischemic encephalopathy 228, 442
Hysteroscopy 424

## I

Ibuprofen 47, 58, 83, 85
Idiopathic hyperhidrosis 54
Illness
    past history of 101, 174
    present history of 101, 173

Imipenem 48
Imminent respiratory distress 203
Immobilization 84, 220
Immune
    maladaptation 408
    system 89fc
        abnormalities in 414
Immunity, types of 89
Immunization 174
    history of 101
Immunocompromised host 315
Immunosuppressive agents 205
Immunosuppressive therapy 158
Impaired skin
    integrity 293
    risk for 157
Implantation abnormality 398
Implied consent 606
Inadequate insulin therapy 208
Inadequate nutrition 534
Inadequate tissue perfusion 141, 433
Incontinence 93
Indomethacin 58
Ineffective airway 195
    clearance 329
Infantile spasm 456
Infarction 260
Infection 124, 233, 280, 350, 421, 430
    cause of 74
    chronic 156
    free of 159
    prevention of 9, 108, 353
    risk factors for 90, 90f
    risk for 145, 149, 154, 157, 160, 328, 345
    spreading 430
Infection control 89, 431, 592, 593, 596, 621, 631
    committee 613
    practices 621
    protocols 93
Infection prevention 95, 160, 161, 593, 596
    and control 96
Infective emergencies 440, 442
Infective endocarditis 277, 277f
    pathophysiology of 278, 278fc
Inflammation 45, 409
    routes of 132
Inflammatory bowel disease 110
Inflammatory conditions 217
Inflammatory demyelinating polyneuropathy, acute 201
Inflammatory diseases 276
Inflammatory heart disease 248
Inflammatory phase, late 502
Inflammatory response 430
Influenza 95
    virus 201
Informed consent 575, 606
Infusion pump 11
Inguinal lymph nodes palpation 103
Inhalation 301, 325
Inhibits bacterial protein synthesis 51
Injection sclerotherapy 113

Injury
    classification of 516fc
    location of 211
    penetrating 521, 526, 527, 564
    primary 212, 217
    secondary 213, 217
    severity of 211
    traumatic 93
Innate immunity 90
Inotropics 55
Inspiration 301
Insulin
    cloudy 67
    detemir 67
    glargine 67
    intermediate acting 67
    long acting 67
    pharmacologic 67
    regular 67
    therapy 382
    uses of 66
Intensive care 8, 431
Intensive care unit 10, 23, 203, 384
    conference room of 632f
    lighting of 633f
    physical setup of 630f
    psychosis
        management of 28
        prevention of 28
    zones of 616
Interatrial septum
    development 241f
    evolution of 240
Intercostal drainage 342, 355
Interleukin 542
Interstitial edema 184
Interstitial lung disease 318
Interventricular septum 240
Intestinal injury 116
Intestinal ischemia 110
Intestinal obstruction 3, 128
    classification of 129t
    pathophysiology of 129fc
Intestine, large 100
Intra-aortic balloon pump 11, 290, 290f
    complications of 291
Intracellular calcium, prevents 223
Intracellular fluid 143
    volume excess 3
Intracerebral hemorrhage 212, 229
    surgery for 195
Intracerebral parenchymal hemorrhage 467
Intracranial causes 224, 225
Intracranial hematomas 232
Intracranial hemorrhage 466
    classification of 466f
Intracranial hypertension 214, 232, 233
    management of 232
Intracranial pressure 179, 229
    assessment of 185, 232
    causes of increased 184t
    etiology of increased 184
    increased 179, 191, 213
    management 215

monitoring 10, 185, 214
regulation of 179
signs 189
symptoms of 189
Intracranial region 212
Intramuscular injection 42
Intranatal management 410
Intranatal period 399
Intraoperative nursing care 364
Intraoperative support 402
Intrapartum factors 430
Intraperitoneal dialysis 131
Intravascular cooling
    device 224
    strategies 221
Intravenous access 200
Intravenous calcium, administration of 145
Intravenous devices 278
Intravenous fluid 67, 431
    resuscitation 405, 434
Intravenous immunoglobulin 202, 205
Intravenous injection 42
Intravenous therapy 68
Intraventricular hemorrhage 467
    classification of 468
Intubation 133, 447
Intussusception 134, 441
Invasive brain monitoring 179
Invasive devices, management of 96
Invasive mechanical ventilation 351
Ionized calcium, less 5
Iron tablets 72, 550
Irrigation 94
Irritability 475
Isavuconazole 92
Ischemia 150, 212
Ischemic cardiomyopathy 247
Ischemic encephalopathy 207
Ischemic stroke 191, 192, 192$f$, 194, 228
    causes of 192$t$
Isoenzyme 126
Isolation precautions 93, 593
Isoniazid 329
Isoprenaline 55
Isovolumic contraction 245
Isovolumic ventricular relaxation 245
Itraconazole 55

## J

Janeway's lesion 249, 278
Jaundice 248
    pathological 449, 450$t$
    physiological 450$t$
Jejunostomy 106
Joint commission 613
Jugular vein, right 249
Jugular venous pulse 249
    monitoring 251$f$
Juxtaglomerular apparatus 139

## K

Kanamycin 49
Kehr's sign 103, 134

Ketoacid dehydrogenase complex, branched chain 461$t$
Ketogenic diet 198
Kidney 2, 56, 138
    artificial 146
    biopsy 144
    dialysis 151
    disease, end-stage 320
    disorder 156
    palpation 103
    stones 164
    transplant
        causes of 156
        recipient 157
    transplantation 156
    with renal arteries, structure of 139$f$, 140$f$
Klebsiella 132, 429
    pneumoniae 470
Knee jerk 179
Korotkoff sound 250
    phases of 250
Korsakoff's psychosis 74
Krabbe's disease 458
Krickenbeck classification 482
Kyphoscoliosis 309

## L

Lab results, monitoring of 471
Labetalol 411, 412
Labor
    and delivery, obstetrical emergencies during 397
    augmentation of 419, 426
    during 410
    induction and augmentation 411
    obstructed 418, 426
    prolonged 419, 426, 445
Lacosamide 196
Lactic acid 169
Lahshal classification 505, 505$f$
Laparoscopy 528
Laryngopharynx 298
Larynx 298
Late ventricular diastole 245
Leaflet valve 294
Left atrium 243
    evolution of 240
Left bundle branches 245
Left coronary artery 243, 244
Left trunk 244
Left ventricle 243
Left ventricular changes 262$f$
Leg pain
    bilateral 218
    unilateral 218
Legal and ethical issues, role of nurse in 607
Legionellae 314
Lens damage 556
Leopold's maneuvers 399
Leprosy, treatment of 52
Lesions, complicated 256
Leukocytes 169
Leukocytosis, peripheral 201
Levetiracetam 196, 200

Levofloxacin 65
Levosimendan 55
Levothyroxine 66
Lidocaine 56
Life support 11
    withdrawing 604
Lifestyle modification 277
Ligament of Treitz 134
Lightheadedness 268
Limb
    movements 234
    weakness 213
Limbic system 224
Linen 622
Liothyronine 66
Liotrix 66
Lipid metabolism defect 458
Liposomal amphotericin 92
Live donor 156, 158
Liver 56, 100, 116
    anatomy of 99$f$
    cirrhosis 320
    disease 46, 132, 141
    failure 101
    function, assessment of 412
    injury 117
    metabolism in 46
    palms 118
    palpation 103
    transplantation 113, 119
Lobe
    frontal 168
    occipital 168
    parietal 168
    temporal 168
Lobectomy 334, 360
    types of 360$f$
Locked-in syndrome 227
Log-rolling movement 220
Loop 64
    diuretics 64
Loperamide 63
Lorazepam 59
Low molecular weight heparin 266
Lower abdominal discomfort 422
Lower extremity cyanosis 266
Lower gastrointestinal bleeding 109, 110
    cause of 110
    management of 114
Lower limb
    paresthesia 218
    weakness 206
Lower respiratory tract 297
Lumbar puncture 180, 196, 470
Lumbar surgeries 93
Lung 2, 299
    cancer 56, 306
    capacities of 301$t$
    disorders 56
    injury 339$t$
        direct 339
        indirect 339
    location of 314$f$, 322$f$, 339
    mechanism of breathing of 302$f$
    normal 322$f$

Index  657

parenchyma, dysfunction of 338
parts of 300f
structure of 299
transplantation 325
types of abnormal sounds of 310t
volume reduction surgery 325, 362
wedge resection of 361f
Lysergic acid diethylamide 73
Lysol 54

## M

Macrophages 90
Magnesium 70, 71, 142, 191, 503
    sulfate 411
        therapy 410
Maladaptation 577
Malignancy 276
Mallory-Weiss tear 110
Malnutrition 215, 266
Malpresentation 418
Mannitol 64, 69, 231
    administration of 231
Mantoux test 326
Maple syrup urine disease 457, 460
    biochemical pathway of 461fc
    intermediate 461
    intermittent 461
    types of 461
Marfan's syndrome 249, 276, 278
Marital status 569
Mask 622
    ventilation 231
Mass lesions, resection of 188
Massage 35, 84
Mast cell stabilizers 57
Maternal and fetal monitoring, continuous 411
Maternal complications 399, 404, 410
Maternal consequences 426
Maternal discomfort 419
Maternal exhaustion 419
Maternal factors 408, 418
Maternal health 475
Maternal hypoxia 443
Maternal immune 414
Maternal risk factors 403
Maternal stabilization 406
McBurney's sign 103, 103f, 134
Mechanical assistive devices 537
Mechanical obstruction 128
    causes of 129t
Mechanical ventilation 334, 340, 350, 473
    common modes of 352t
    purposes of 350
Mechanical ventilators
    cycles of 351
    modes of 352
    settings on 351, 351t
Meconium-stained amniotic fluid 445
Median sternotomy incision 358
Medical staff 627
Medication 86, 400
    administration 413, 417, 425, 431, 503
    management 96, 162

Medicines, role of alternative 554
Medicolegal case 607
Meeting nutritional needs 106
Meigs's syndrome 320
Melena 109
Memantine 571
Membranes, premature rupture of 397
Memory
    deficits 211
    loss 173
Meningeal irritation, signs of 189
Meningeal layers 169f
Meninges 169
Meningitis, treatment of 52
Mental clouding 211
Mental status 174
    altered 208, 415, 433, 549
    examination 174
Meperidine 41, 43
Mercaptopurine 124
Meridian therapy 34
Mesenteric artery syndrome, severe superior 110
Metabolic abnormalities 199
Metabolic alkalosis 5, 64
Metabolic conditions 118
Metabolic diseases 263
Metabolic disorders 457
    nursing management of 465
Metabolic encephalopathies 207
Metabolic imbalance 122, 195
Methadone 41
Methamphetamine 73
Methenamine 65
Methicillin-resistant Staphylococcus aureus 94
    infections, types of 94
Methotrexate 205
Methyldopa 124, 411, 412
Methylenedioxy 73
Methylxanthines 503
Metoclopramide 62
Metoprolol 258
Micafungin 91, 92
Micro transducer devices 185
Microbial factors 91
Midazolam 59
Midbrain 168
Middle lobe, atelectasis of 332f
Miller Fisher syndrome 201
Milrinone 55
Mineral metabolism defect 458
Minimally conscious state 227
Minimally invasive direct coronary artery bypass 293
Minocycline 50
Miosis 549
Mitochondrial diseases 458
Mitral area 251
Mitral commissurotomy 294
Mitral insufficiency 251
Mitral regurgitation, pathophysiology of 268

Mitral valve 267
    prolapse 268
    regurgitation 268
        pathophysiology of 268fc
    stenosis 267
        pathophysiology of 267, 267fc
Monoamine oxidase inhibitors 253
Monro-Kellie hypothesis 179
Mood and perception, affecting 26
Morphine 41-43, 85, 235
    doses of 42t
    poisoning, acute 44
    sulphate 260
        opioid 235
    therapeutic effects of 42
Motor and sensory neuron, functions of 170f
Motor axonal neuropathy, acute 201
Motor deficits 193
Motor function 176, 220
Motor sensory axonal neuropathy, acute 201
Motor strength assessment 177
Mounting tension 577
Mouth 515
Movement, neck range of 215
Mucolytic agents 334
Mucolytics 58, 325
Mucous
    cells 100
    solution 101
Muddy brown cast 151
Multi-dimensional assessment 82
Multidrug resistance 328
Multifocal myoclonus 208
Multiparity 398
Multiple organ dysfunction syndrome 541, 541fc, 565
    clinical manifestation of 543f
    pathophysiology of 542fc
Multiple pregnancies 403
Murmur 252
    classification of 252
    grading of 252, 252t
Murphy's sign 103, 134
Murray's classification 557, 558t
Muscle 343
    mass 177
    rigidity 415
    specific receptor tyrosine kinase 204
    strength 177, 206
    tone 177
    twitching 208
    weakness 6, 201
Muscular contractions 200
Muscular organ 240
Musculoskeletal exam 515
Musculoskeletal injuries 201
Musculoskeletal pain, acute 46, 47
Musculoskeletal system 249
Mushrooms, types of 73
Music therapy 34, 353
Mutagenesis 40
Myambutol 329
Myasthenia gravis 203, 204
Mycobacterium tuberculosis 124

Mycophenolate mofetil 205
Mycoplasma 51
   pneumonia 124, 201
Mydriasis 549
Myelin sheath 202f
Myelogram 181
Myocardial cells, working 242
Myocardial infarction 259
   classification of acute 259fc
   complications of 262
   pathophysiology of 259, 259fc
Myocardial perfusion imaging 258, 260
Myocardial rupture 262
Myocarditis 263, 270
Myocardium 242
Myoclonic seizure 197, 456
Myoclonic status epilepticus 199
Myoepicardial mantle 240
Myoglobinuria 208
Myxedema 320, 385
Myxedema coma 386
   management of 387
   signs of 386
   symptoms of 386

## N

N-acetylcysteine 119
Nails, clubbing of 250f
Nalidixic acid 48, 52, 65
Naloxone 41, 43, 44
   uses of 44
Naltrexone 41, 44
Naproxen 58
Narcotic analgesics 43, 58
Nasal cavity 298
Nasal field 193
Nasal fracture
   complications of 559
   etiopathology of 557
Nasal injuries, various 557
Nasal packing 559
Nasal steroids 325
Nasal trauma 557f
Nasogastric lavage 112
Nasogastric suctions 127
Nasogastric tube 215
   feeding 105
   insert 228
Naso-jejunal feeding 105
Nasopharynx 298
Natriuretic peptides 280
Natural killer cells 90
Nausea 41, 50, 74, 101, 102, 125, 144, 185, 208, 211, 254, 257, 409
   mild effects of 47
Nebulization therapy 354
Neck 515
   injury management 562
   zones of 560, 560f
Necrotizing enterocolitis 441
Negative-pressure ventilators 351
Neisseria gonorrhea 48
Neomycin 49
Neonatal emergencies 439, 440

Neonatal jaundice, clinical assessment of 451
Neonatal management 439
Neoplasia 110
Neoplastic tumor 263
Nephritic syndrome 266, 320
Nephron, structure of 139f
Nephrotoxins 207
Nerve conduction studies 182, 202
Nervous system
   anatomy of 167
   assessment of 173
   drugs in 58
   emergencies and management 166
   enteric 167, 172
   physiology of 172
Nervous tissue 167
Neural pathways 224
Neuroemergency 232
Neurogenic shock 221, 538, 565
   pathophysiology of 539fc
Neurohormonal performance 281
Neuroleptic malignant syndrome 224
Neurologic assessment 190, 215, 229
Neurologic deficit 416, 500
   permanent 233
   temporary 233
Neurologic examination 174, 225, 515
Neurologic function 224
Neurologic morbidity 207
Neurological changes 122, 155
Neurological disorders 222
Neurological emergencies 440
Neurological monitoring 72, 548
Neurological symptoms 173t, 415
Neuromatrix 80
   hypothesis 80
   theory 80
Neuromuscular blocking agents 50
Neuron 172f, 173
   depolarization of 213
   parts of 167f
Neuronal dysfunction 224
Neuropsychological test 122
Neurosurgical approaches, management modalities of 232
Neurotoxin 207
   induced demyelination 208
Neutral thermal environment, maintain 471
Neutrophils 90
Newborn, male 482
Niacin 174
Nicardipine 412
Niemann Pick disease 458
Nifedipine 258, 411, 412
Nil per oral status 221
Nimesulide 47, 58
Nimodipine 190
Nitrazepam 59
Nitric oxide 280
Nitrofurantoin 52, 65
   norflox 48, 52
Nitrogenous load, decrease of 122
Nitroglycerin 258, 261f

N-methyl-d-aspartate 213
   receptor 200
Nocturnal angina 257
Nodal cells 243
Nodes of Ranvier 201
Noise 25
   volume of 25
Noncardiac chest pain and discomfort, causes of 247
Non-cardiogenic pulmonary edema 331f
Nonconvulsive status epilepticus 199
Noncoronary artery disease 247
Non-intensive care unit 380
Noninvasive brain monitoring 179
Noninvasive mechanical ventilation 350
Noninvasive ventilation, complication of 350
Non-narcotic analgesics 44, 45, 58
Nonopioid 83
   analgesic 44, 46, 83
Nonoptical forceps 498
Nonpharmacological interventions 86
Nonpharmacological pain management 83
Nonresistant bacteria 91
Nonspecific clinical manifestations 470
Non-ST-elevation myocardial infarction 261
Nonsteroidal anti-inflammatory drugs 44, 383
   mode of actions of 45
Non-surgical interventions 419
Non-traumatic causes 346
Non-traumatic conditions 186
Nontunneled central catheters 108
Nonvariceal bleeding 109
   management of 112
Nonverbal pain scale 81
Noradrenaline 55
Norepinephrine 55
Normoactive bowel sound 102
Nose 298, 515
   function of 298
   injuries 557
Nosocomial infection 91, 93, 278
Nourishment area 632
Noxious stimuli 187
Nuclear medicine scans 111
Numerical rating scales 81
Nurse
   administrator, role of 626
   ethics for 602t
   responsibility 62, 288, 292
   role of 31, 74, 554, 562, 626
Nursing
   administrator 626
   assessment 72
   committees 613
   practice, highly qualified 9
   process assessment 47
   responsibility 186
   service 626
   specialist 626
Nursing audit 623, 624
   demerits of 625
   essential characteristics of 623
   methods for 623
   purposes of 623

types of 623
utilization of results of 626
Nursing care 24, 313
  records, lack of 627
Nursing interventions 72
  types of 34
Nursing staff 628
  development 613
Nutrition 122, 203, 325, 493, 594, 596
  altered 160
  and hydration management 96
  for all, effectively use 33
  imbalanced 330
  management 162
  risk for imbalanced 149
  therapy 340
Nutritional deficiency 280
Nutritional management 127, 258
Nutritional status, assessment of 206
Nutritional support 160, 161, 206, 478
Nutritional therapy 117, 147
NYHA classification 282

# O

Obesity 257, 258
Obscure origin 110
Obstetric shock 397
  diagnosis of 434
  types of 433
Obstetrical emergency 396
  types of 396
Obstructive atelectasis 332
Obstructive uropathy 320
Obturator's sign 103, 134
Occult gastrointestinal bleeding 109
Occupational history 101, 174
Octreotide 113, 124
Ocular muscle weakness 206
Oculocephalic reflex 228
Oculovestibular reflex 228
Odors 25, 549
Off pump coronary artery bypass 293
Ofloxacin 52
  enoxacin 48
Olfactory nerve 176
Oliguria 125, 143
Omeprazole 64
Ondansetron 235
Open bulla resection 362*f*
Opening snaps 252
Ophthalmoplegia 208
Opiates 228
Opioid 41, 41*t*, 73, 207
  agonist-morphine 42
  analgesics 41, 58
    administering 43
  antagonists naloxone 44
  receptors 42
  strong 83
  therapy 43
  types of 42
  weak 83
Opportunistic infection, prevention of 553
Optic nerve 176

Optical forceps 498
Optimal nutrition, maintaining 108
Oral antiplatelets 290
Oral cavity 99
  complete 102
Oral contraceptives 266
Oral hygiene care 89
Oral ingestion 127
Oral mucous membrane, impaired 163
Oral nutrition 194
Oral steroid drugs 325
Orem's theory 23
Organ affected 116
Organ donation 604
  counseling for 605
Organ dysfunction 430, 433
Organ failure 224
Organophosphates 73
Oro-gastric feeding 105
Oropharyngeal irritation 57
Oropharynx 298
ORS requirement 485*t*
Osler's node 249, 278
Osmosis 147, 185
Osmotic
  dieresis 154
  diuretic 119, 235
  fluids 215
Osteoarthritis 46, 47
Outpatient
  care 8
  treatment 572
Oxazepam 59
Oxicams 47
Oxidative stress 150, 409
Oxidizing agents 54
Oxycodone 85
Oxygen
  administration 340
  partial pressure of 229
  saturation
    maintenance of 470
    measurement 478
  supplementary 127, 446
  therapy 263, 325, 334, 473, 477
Oxyhemoglobin dissociation curve 303, 303*f*
Oxymetazoline hydrochloride nasal spray 58
Oxytocin 168

# P

P wave 245
Pacemaker 272, 278, 284
  codes 287
  malfunction of 287
  spikes 284
  temporary 284, 287
Paget's disease 280
Pain 101, 203, 213, 590
  acute 79, 230, 258
  and symptom management 96
  assessment of 353
  back 218, 404, 422
  cancer 79
  causes of 307*t*

center 80
characteristic of 102
chronic 79
dental 47
epigastric 47
functional 41
inflammatory 79
killer 46
management 78, 127, 343, 345, 428, 432, 526, 534, 590, 593, 596
  ABCDE for 81
mediastinal 306
moderate 45
neuropathic 79, 221
nociceptive 78
nursing management for 86
phantom 79
pleural 305
psychogenic 41, 79
receptors 78
recurrent 44
referred 41, 79
sensation 177
somatic 79
theories of 79
types of 78, 305
visceral 79
Pallor 248, 257
Palmar erythema 118
Palpable olive-like mass 481
Palpation 103, 251, 533
Palpitation 263, 268
Pancreas 100, 116, 370
  developmental abnormality of 124
  divisum 124
Pancreatic enzyme, premature activation of 124
Pancreatic injury 117
Pancreatic secretions 131
Pancreaticoduodenectomy 127
Pancreatitis 132
  risk factors of acute 125*t*
Pancytopenia 51
Pantoprazole 64
Papilledema 185, 254
Paracentesis 133
Paracetamol 46, 58, 72, 117, 235, 550
  dose of 46
  overdose, management of 72
Paradoxical movement 343
Paraplegia 217, 218
  chest with 218
Parasympathetic nervous system 170, 171
Parathyroid
  glands 370
  hormone 142, 208
Parental support 471
Parenteral feeding, complications of 108
Parenteral nutrition 105, 107
  complications of 108*t*
  peripheral 107
Paresthesia 193
Parietal cells 100
Parkinson's disease 233

Parkland formula 589
Paroxysmal atrial tachycardia 61
Paroxysmal nocturnal dyspnea 263
Paroxysmal supra ventricular tachycardia 273
Patchy atelectasis 333
Patient
    and family education 96, 402
    areas 631
    context 82
    discharge planning 406
    education 48, 86, 406, 593
    family 29
    modules 632
    monitoring equipment 10, 620
    perception 23
    placement 93
    rooms 630
    safety 612
        committee 613
    satisfaction 612
    screening 93
    selection 288
    teaching 63
    under mechanical ventilators, nursing care of 352
    visibility 630
Patient care
    appraisal of 31
    evaluation of 30
    items 622
Pectus carinatum 309
Pectus excavatum 309
Pediatric emergencies 439, 440, 483
Pediatric management 439
Pelvic abnormalities 418
Pelvic examination 430
    abnormal 419
Pelvic fracture 93, 529, 563
    classification 530, 530$t$, 531$f$, 532$f$, 532$t$
    nursing management of 534
    previous 418
Pelvic inflammatory disease 418
Pelvic injury, open book 565
Pelvic surgeries, previous 418
Pelvic trauma 501
Pelvis
    anatomy of 530$f$
    X-ray of 533
Pendant vs. head-end panel 616
Penetrating abdominal trauma, management of 529, 529$fc$
Penicillin 48
    administration of 48
    beta-lactam and thiazolidine 48
    derivatives 48
    G 119
    types of 48
Pentamidine 124
Pentazocine 41, 42, 44
Pentobarbitone 59
Pentose phosphate pathway 465$fc$
Peptic ulcer 101
    perforated 3
Percutaneous coronary intervention 261$f$, 288
    anticoagulation treatment for 290

Percutaneous endoscopic gastrostomy 106
Percutaneous transluminal balloon valvuloplasty 269
Perforated colon 132
Perfusion pressure 179
Pericardial cavity 242
Pericardial friction rub 253
Pericardial heterograft 294
Pericarditis 262
Pericardium 242
Perinatal asphyxia 442, 445
    management of 445
Perineal anesthesia 218
Peripheral nervous system 167, 170
Peripheral vascular
    disease 276
    system 250
Peritoneal chemotherapy 131
Peritoneal dialysis 132, 159, 161, 320
Peritoneal lavage 133
Peritonitis 128, 159
    infected 131
    noninfected 131
    pathophysiology of 132$fc$
    perforated 131
    primary 131
    secondary 131
    signs of 427
Permanent pacemaker 271, 284, 287
Persistent hunger 481
Personal protection equipment guidelines 621
Personal protective equipment 93, 94, 593, 621$f$
    use of 621
Personality, changes in 122
Petechiae 41, 278
Pethidine 42
    hydrochloride 43
Petit mal epilepsy 60
Petrosal sinus sampling, inferior 373
Pharmacologic management 133, 200
Pharmacologic therapy 147, 328, 340
Pharmacological interventions 427
Pharmacological management 4, 334
Pharmacological pain management 84$f$
Pharmacological therapy 119, 460
Pharmacotherapy, role of 536
Pharynx 99, 298
Phenelzine 60
Phenobarbitone 59, 60
Phenol 54
    derivatives 54
Phenylalanine
    ammonia lyase 460
    biochemical pathway of 462$f$
    metabolism pathway 458$fc$
Phenylephrine hydrochloride 58
Phenylketonuria 458
    classic 459
    types of 458
Phenytoin 60, 200
Pheochromocytoma 253
Phlebitis 45
Phosphate 70, 71, 142

Phosphodiesterase inhibitors 55, 61
Phosphorus 142
    binders 147
Photo-oxidation 453
Photophobia 211
Phototherapy
    mechanism of 453$fc$
    role of nurse in 453
    unit, types of 453
Physical activity, encouraging 108
Physical examination 475
Physical infrastructure 33
Physical mobility
    impaired 222
    risk for impaired 157
Physical therapy 594
Physiology gas exchange 302
Physiotherapy 203
Pia mater 169$f$
Pigeon chest 309
Pineal gland 370
Piroxicam 47
Pitting edema 250$f$
Pituitary gland 370, 371$f$
Placebo
    advantages of 85
    controlled experiments 85
    effect 84
    quick information about 85
Placenta accreta 397
Placenta previa 396, 397, 399
    complications of 399
    management of 401$fc$
    pathophysiology of 398$fc$
    types of 399$f$
Placental detachment 404
Placental dysfunction 408, 414
Placental factors 409, 444
Placental implantation, abnormal 398
Placental ischemia 409
Placental separation 406
Placental site, subinvolution of 421
Placental tissue, retained 421, 424
Placental vessel disruption 398
Planning audit 624
Plasma 69
    amylase 126
    exchange 202
    filtration of 139
    half-life 41
    lipase 126
    phenylalanine level 459
    protein, normal 143
Plasmapheresis 205
Plateau of disorganization 577
Platelets 69
Pleural effusion 319, 319$f$, 321, 321$fc$
    causes of exudative 320
Pleural fluid, thoracentesis aspiration of 321$f$
Pneumococcus 132
Pneumonectomy 360
Pneumonia 94, 313, 314$f$, 315, 490
    grading of 490
    label diagram of 314$f$

pathophysiology of 315*fc*
severe 490, 491
symptoms of 315*f*
Pneumothorax 109, 344, 347, 522, 564
classification of 347, 347*fc*
closed 523, 523*f*
management modalities of 349
open 523, 523*f*
primary 347, 348
secondary 348
traumatic 347
types of 347, 348*fc*, 523*t*
with management, types of 522
Poisoning 270, 272, 494
agent 494
common 494
danger signs of 547
management of 548
modes of 547
Pons and medulla oblongata 168
Poor cardiac function 43
Poor placental perfusion 414
Poor weight gain 481
Position sense 177
Positive airway pressure, continuous 350
Positive end-expiratory pressure 187, 229
Positive pressure ventilation 351, 447
Positron emission tomography 181
Postcraniectomy 236
Postcraniotomy 236
Posterior cord syndrome 218
Postictal state 415
Post-intensive care syndrome 28
Postnatal period 399
Postpartum
management 412
obstetrical emergencies during 397
Postpartum care 417
and monitoring 420
Postpartum hemorrhage 397, 420
diagnosis of 422
management of 424*fc*
Post-resuscitation management 448
Postural drainage 355
different positions of 356*f*
Potassium 64, 70, 139, 142, 227
permanganate 54
sparing 64
therapy 382
Potent catecholamine 56
Potential progression 408
Potential reversible syndromes 228
Pott's spine 217
Practicing silver catheter 94
Pre-anesthetic agent 43
Prebiotics 122
Preburnout indicators 36
Pre-eclampsia 396, 403, 407, 408, 412*t*, 432
complications of 410
diagnostic criteria of 409
etiology for 408
preceding symptoms of 415
risk factors for 408
severe symptoms 412*t*

Pregabalin 196, 221
Preganglionic neurons 171
Pregnancy 263, 266
Pre-hospital assessment 513
Prenatal care 402
Prenatal hypertension 195
Prenatal screening 475
Pressure
increased 398
sore 221
ulcer, risk of 534
Pressure-cycled ventilators 351
Pressure-volume changes 183
Preterm baby 485
Previous cesarean sections, management of 402
Priftin 329
Primitive ventricle 240
Prinzmetal's angina 257
Probiotics 122
Procainamide 56
Procalcitonin 126
Progressive patient care 7
advantages of 8
Progressive weakness 204
Projectile vomiting 481
Promethazine 57
Prophylactic antibiotic therapy 269
Prophylactic therapy 279
Prophylaxis 95
Propionic acid derivatives 47
Propofol 200
Propranolol 113
Proprioception 177
Prostaglandin 45
E1 475, 476
administration 477
infusion 478
Prostate, enlargement of 140
Prosthetic valvular surgery 294
Protective eyewear 622
face shield 622
goggles 622
visors 622
Protective isolation 592
Protein 169
restriction 151
Proteinuria 150, 409, 415
absence of 408
Proton pump inhibitor 63, 127
Pseudo aneurysm 276
Pseudocyst, percutaneous drainage of 127
Pseudoephedrine 383
hydrochloride 58
Pseudomonas aeruginosa 314
Pseudo-obstruction 128
Psoas's sign 103, 134
Psychiatric emergency 567, 574, 576
characteristics of 567
intervention 568, 568*f*
medicolegal aspects of 575
types of 568
Psychogenic polydipsia 393
Psychological education 412

Psychological states 257
Psychological status 371
Psychological support 412, 550
Psychological theory 569
Psychomotor epilepsy, control 60
Psychosocial care 72, 550
issues 30
Psychosocial disorders 156
Psychosocial support 429, 596
Ptosis 204
right sided partial 204*f*
Puerperal pyrexia 431
Puerperal sepsis 397, 429
risk factors of 430
Puerperium 410
Pulmonary angiography 312
Pulmonary area 251
Pulmonary artery 251
Pulmonary complications 191, 416
Pulmonary contusion 343, 344*f*, 520, 521*f*, 564
pathophysiology of 344*fc*, 521*fc*
severe 344
Pulmonary edema 231, 331, 331*f*
pathophysiology of 332*fc*
Pulmonary embolism 280, 334, 335*f*
acute 247
risk factors of 335*t*
Pulmonary embolus 221
Pulmonary function test 311
Pulmonary hypertension 56, 247
Pulmonary injuries 522
Pulmonary resections 359, 360*f*
Pulmonary stenosis 269, 474
Pulmonary thromboendarterectomy 336*f*
Pulmonary tuberculosis 326, 326*f*
pathophysiology of 327*fc*
Pulmonary valve 269
disease 269
pathophysiology of 269, 269*fc*
repair 475
replacement 475
Pulmonary volume, normal 301*t*
Pulmonic ejection sounds, causes of 252
Pulse 234
generator 284
oximeter 10, 310
rate 549
Pulseless electrical activity 275
Pulsus
bisferiens 249
paradoxus 249
Pupil examination 549
Pupillary changes 185
Pupillary reaction 176
Pupillary reflex 228
Purkinje cells 243
Purkinje fibers 245
Pursed-lip breathing, goal of 354
Pyelonephritis 207
Pyloromyotomy 481
Pyrazinamide 329
Pyrimethamine 51
Pyrimidine metabolism defect 458

## Q

qSOFA 565
  score 539*fc*
Quadriplegia 201, 217
Qualitative tests 464
Quality assurance 610, 626
  cycle of 612*fc*
  principles of 610
  steps of 610, 611*fc*
Quality improvement committee 613
Quality precautions 621
Quantiferon-TB gold test 326
Quantitative test 464

## R

Rabeprazole 64
Raccoons eyes 213
Radiation exposure 263
Radioactive iodine therapy 383
Radiofrequency ablation 292
Radiological procedure 113
Radionuclide 264, 373
Ranson score 126
Rapid acting insulin 67
Rapid alternating movements 178
Rapid breathing 225
Rashes 47
Rashkind procedure 477
Re-audit 624
Rebleeding 190
Recipient selection 156
Reconstructive surgery 594*f*, 595
Recovery room care system 1
Rectum 515
Red blood cell 69, 169, 465*fc*
Red orange feces 52
Reduced blood 444
  flow 476
Re-exposure, prevention of 496
Reflex 178
  abnormal 179
  activity 170
  return 219
  superficial 178
Refractory epilepsy 199
Refractory status epilepticus 199
Refsum's disease 458
Regular prenatal care 413
Rehabilitation 534, 595, 596
Reinforcing improvement 624
Reliable tools 81
Remote central store 618
Remove mucus 325
Renal artery 138
Renal biopsy 147, 151
Renal concentration test 147
Renal disease 141, 289
  end-stage 138, 156, 157
  history of 49
Renal encephalopathy 207-210
Renal failure 143, 164, 416
  chronic 146, 149, 150, 207
  pathophysiology of chronic 146*fc*
Renal function
  assessment of 412
  impaired 145
  preserve 150
Renal hypoperfusion 150
Renal impairment 27
Renal inflammation 150
Renal injury 201
  cause for 156
Renal insufficiency 254
Renal pelvis 140
Renal perfusion, restoration of 150
Renal replacement therapy 27, 158, 159*f*
Renal system 415
  anatomy of 138
  assessment of 140
  disorders 164
    management modalities for 158
  emergencies 138
  management 138
  physiology of 139
Renal transplantation 156
Renal vein 138
Renin 2
  angiotensin aldosterone system 281
Reperfusion therapy 261
Repetitive nerve stimulation 204
Residual scar 336*f*
Residual symptoms, management
  of 412
Respiration 234, 300
  center of 302
  external 303
  internal 303
  pattern of 308*t*
  rate, abnormal 222
  support 133
Respirator 11
Respiratory alkalosis 141
Respiratory care 127
  requirements for 628
Respiratory center 303*f*
Respiratory depression 44
Respiratory disease 143
Respiratory distress 434
  syndrome 472
    assessment of severity of 472
Respiratory drive, decreased 337
Respiratory emergency 440
  diseases 297
Respiratory failure 201, 217, 218, 337
  acute 337
  classification of acute 337*fc*
Respiratory function 203
  regular monitoring of 203
Respiratory groups 303*f*
Respiratory hygiene 93
Respiratory management 187
Respiratory muscle weakness 204, 206
Respiratory rate 549
Respiratory status 345
  assessment of 305*t*
  steps to maintain 526
Respiratory symptoms 52
Respiratory system 3, 218, 297
  anatomy of 297
  drugs in 56
  parts of 298, 299*f*
  physiology of 300
Respiratory tract infection 128
Respiratory muscle weakness, 386
Resting membrane potential 172
Restlessness 264
Restrain mast cell activity 57
Restraints, use of 27
Restrictive cardiomyopathy 247, 263, 264
Resuscitation
  anticipating need of 445
  assessment of 589
  equipment for 446
  initial steps of 446
  primary treatment with 533
Reticular activating system 224
Reticulocytopenia 51
Retinopathy 254
Retroperitoneal injury 116
Rheumatic fever 269
Rheumatic heart disease 248
Rheumatoid arthritis 46, 47
Rib fracture 342, 344*f*, 518, 518*f*, 520
  multiple 343
Ribonucleic acid synthesis inhibitor rifampicin
  52
Rickettsia 51
Rifampicin 48
Rifampin 52, 329
Rifaximin 122
Right atrium 243, 244
  evolution of 240
  obstructed flow from 476
Right bundle branches 245
Right marginal vein 243
Right middle lobe syndrome 333
Right vats thymectomy incisions 363*f*
Right ventricle 243, 476
Right ventricular
  dysplasia 248
  hypertrophy 474
Rinne's test 176
Road traffic accident 513*f*
Robertson's five stages of crisis intervention
  578
Robotic surgery 363*f*
Robotic thoracic surgery 363
Rofecoxib 47
Rohypnol 73
Romberg test 178
Rotational coronary atherectomy 289
Roth's spot 278
Rotor syndrome 450
Roux sign 501
Rovsing's sign 103, 134
Rule of Nine 589*f*
Rupture, causes of 426
Ruptured uterus 397, 425
  medical management of 427
  nursing management of 428
  surgical management of 428

# Index

## S

SA node 244
Salbutamol 57
Salicylates 58, 72, 228, 383, 550
Salicylic acid 54
Salmonella 53, 124
Sapropterin dihydrochloride 460
Sarcoidosis 263
Scalp 169*f*
    injury 211
    laceration 211
Sedation 187
    level, assessment of 353
Sedative 59
Sedentary life style 257
Segmental colectomy 114
Segmental pulmonary emboli 336*f*
Segmental resection 334
Segmentectomy 361
Seizure 62, 185, 191, 233, 254, 415, 440, 549
    absence 197, 456
    activity 187
        phases of 455
    atypical absence 197
    complex partial 196
    control 416
    disorder 195
    during 198
    generalized 196, 455, 456
    initiation, mechanism of 195
    mixed 60
    monitoring of 471
    neonatal 455
    partial 196
    post-traumatic 216
    precautions 417
    prevention of 187
    prophylaxis 411
    simple partial 196
    treatment of 471
    types of 196*t*, 197*t*, 456
    unclassified 455
    unknown onset 455
Selective serotonin reuptake inhibitors 550
Self-care 8
Self-esteem, promote positive 198
Semi-fowler's position 155
Sensation deficits 173
Sensory
    deficit 193
    disturbances 202
    examination 177
    function 176, 220
    neurons 170
    orientation improvement 633
Sepsis 208, 266, 432, 442
    diagnosis of 27
    early onset 469
    mimics 53
    neonatal 469
    screen 470
Septal hematoma 559, 565
Septic encephalopathy 208-210

Septic shock 433, 539, 565
    pathophysiology of 540*fc*
Septicemia 48, 131, 202, 383
Septum primum
    appearance of 240
    fusion of 240
Serotonin syndrome 224
Serous pericardium 242
Serum
    cardiac markers 260
    chemistries 151
    concentration 487
    cortisol level 373
    creatinine 5
    levels of glucose 227
    lipid
        elevated 258
        values, increased 257
    osmolarity 69
    potassium 5
Service corridors 632
Sexual history 174
Shaken baby syndrome 440
Sharp injury 115
Shigella 53
    infection 53
Shock 141, 154, 207, 217, 534, 541, 541*fc*, 563
    classification of 535
    clinical features of 433
    electric 272
    hemorrhagic 231, 433
    obstetrical 432
    signs of 404, 422
Shoulder dystocia 397
Simple blisters 3
Sinoatrial node 243
Sinus
    bradycardia 272, 272*f*
    tachycardia 272, 272*f*
Skin 2, 248
    care, providing 106
    change 118, 385*f*
    decontamination 495
    examination of 225
    infections 94
    integrity, risk for impaired 154
Skull 169*f*
    bone 232
    fracture 211
        depressed 214
        piece removed 188*f*
    X-ray 214
Sleep deficiency 30
Sleeve lobectomy 360, 360*f*
Small intestine 100, 127
Smoking 27, 198, 257, 398
    cessation 277, 414
Sociological theory 570
Socrates 102
Sodium 46, 70, 139, 141, 227
    bicarbonate 145
    channels 172
    chloride 215
    deficit 487

    imbalance 215
    intoxication 487
    levels 141
    nitroprusside 254, 412
        infusion 277
Soft sign 565
Somatic nervous system 167
Somatosensory evoked potential 210
Somatostatin 113
Sotalol 56
Space occupying lesions 184
Species, evolution of 80
Specific antidote administration 495
Sphincterotomy 127
Spinal accessory nerve 177
Spinal cord 169, 217, 221
    and brain 78
    disorders 253
    end of 218
    regions 169*f*
    syndromes 219*f*
Spinal cord injury 217, 219, 222
    causes of 217
    diagnosis of acute 219
    mechanisms of 217
    nontraumatic 217
    traumatic 217
Spinal injury 217
Spinal nerve 170
    pairs of 170
Spinal shock 221
Spinal surgeries 93
Spinal X-ray 220
Spirometry 323, 334
Spironolactone 64
Spleen 116
    injury 117
    palpation 103
Spontaneous causes 346
Sprain 3
Sputum
    analysis 306*t*
    production 305
Stab wounds 344, 521
Stable angina 247, 257
Standard defibrillator 292
Staphylococci 48
Staphylococcus
    albus 470
    aureus 429, 470
Statin treatment 194
Status asthmaticus 317, 502
    nursing management of 317
Status epilepticus 198, 199
    management of 199
ST-elevation myocardial infarction 261
Stereognosis 178
Sterile
    drainage, closed 94
    techniques 95
Sternal fracture 342, 519, 520, 520*t*
Steroids 188, 207
Stimulants 198
Stimulus 284

Stomach 100
    injury 116
    ulcer 132
Stool softener or enemas 43
Stranc Robertson classification 557, 558f
Streptomycin 49
Stress 29, 35, 258
    disorder, post-traumatic 35
    echocardiography 258, 260
    reduction 9
    related crisis, traumatic 576
Strict bed rest 400
Strict immobilization 220
Stridor 308
Stroke 45, 101, 191
    nursing management of 195
    surgical management of 194
    volume 245, 249
Structural isomerization 453
Stupor 226, 254
Subarachnoid hemorrhage 188, 189t, 212, 229, 467
    grading of 189
Subarachnoid space 169
Subcutaneous emphysema 344f
Subcutaneous infusion repeatedly, continuous 42
Subcutaneous injection 42
Subdural hematoma 212
Subfalcine herniation 230
Subsegmental pulmonary emboli 336f
Substance
    abuse 403
    causing poisoning 547
    intoxication 574
    related emergency 574
    withdrawal 574
Subtotal colectomy 114
Suicidal Act 575
Suicidal behaviors, risk for 571
Suicide 568, 570, 570f, 570t
    behaviors, risk for 571
    incidence of 568
    management of 571
    methods used for 570
    predisposing factors of 569, 569t
    prevalence of 568
    prevention of 571
    risk for 572t
Sulcus 168
    terminalis 243
Sulfadiazine 65
Sulfamethoxazole 65
Sulfonamides 51, 124
    metabolic effect of 51
    primarily 51
Sulindac 124
Sulphonamide 65
Sunitinib 55
Super infection
    signs of 49
    symptoms of 49
Superior nursing skills 13
Supplemental oxygen administration 503

Support spaces 630
Supportive management 119
Supportive therapy 385f, 473, 496
Supportive treatment 117, 122
Surface cooling device 224
Surfactant therapy 473, 493
Surgery 221, 559
    timing of 479
    types of 294
Surgical approach 479
Surgical correction 478
Surgical management 113
Surgical portosystemic shunts 113
Surgical procedure 124, 157, 482
Surgical site infection 94
    prevention of 94
Surgical therapy 127
Swallowing 194
Sweating 41, 72, 257
Sympathetic nervous system 170, 171, 281
Synapse 167
Syncope 263, 271-273
Syndrome of inappropriate antidiuretic hormone 228
Syphilis 48, 276
Systematic approach 624
Systemic complications 415
Systemic inflammatory response syndrome 540, 541, 541fc, 565
    criteria 539fc
    etiology of 540fc
    stages of 541fc
Systemic lupus erythematosus 248
Systolic diastolic timing 252
Systolic failure, pathophysiological changes in 280fc

# T

T lymphocyte 90
T4 test 373
Tachycardia 5, 45, 125, 140, 433, 549
Tachypnea 140, 308, 549
Tacrolimus 205
Tactile stimulation 446
Tapentadol 83
Target organ damage 253
Target population 352
Taste sensation 176, 177
Tay-Sachs disease 458
T-cell 90, 205
    immunity 90
Tears, artificial 206
Telangiectasis 225
Temperature 248, 549
    regulation loss 593
    sensation 177
    testing 223
Temporal field 193
Temporary vascular access 148
Tenderness 132
Tendon xanthoma 248
Tension
    pneumocephalus 232
    pneumothorax 348, 349, 523, 523f

Terbutaline 57
Terlipressin 113
Term baby 485
Testes 370
Tet spell 441, 475
    management of 476
Tetanus 95
    prophylaxis 554
Tetracycline 48, 50, 124
Tetralogy of Fallot 474
Thalamus 168
Thallium scan 264
Theophylline 488
Therapeutic actions 46
Therapeutic communication 352
Therapeutic environment
    background of 31
    maintaining 31
    purposes of 31
Therapeutic hypothermia 221
Therapeutic sounds 34
Therapeutic tones 34
Therapeutic touch 35
    purpose of 35
Thermoregulation 470
    mechanism of 222
Thermoregulatory center 223
Thermoregulatory sweat test 223
Thiamine 227
    therapy 462
Thiazide 6, 64
Thiopentone 59
Thoracentesis 321, 321f
Thoracic aortic aneurysm 276
Thoracic incisions 357
Thoracic injury 515, 562
    causes of 515
    mechanism of 517f
    nursing management of 525
Thoracic palpation 309
Thoracic percussion 310
Thoracic region, examination of 309
Thoracic surgery 357
    complications of 364
    patient undergoing 364
    video-assisted 362
Thoracic trauma 500
Thoracoabdominal incision 358, 358f
Thoracolumbar division 171
Thoracosternotomy 358
Thoracotomy
    anterior 357
    posterolateral 357
Threshold stimulus 173
Threshold value 173
Throat injuries 560
Thrombectomy 289
Thrombin inhibitors, direct 266
Thromboembolism 432
Thrombolysis 194, 336
Thrombophlebitis 251
Thromboprophylaxis 221
Thrombotic phase, symptoms of 545
Thrombotic thrombocytopenic purpura 208

Thymectomy 205
Thymoma 204
Thymus 370
   hyperplasia 204
Thyroid
   desiccated 66
   gland 370
   hormone 66, 224, 383
      monitoring of 387
      replacement 387
   increases, overactive 224
   medications 66
   storm 383, 384, 384fc, 385f
Thyroid-stimulating hormone 373
Thyrotoxicosis 66, 280, 384, 441
Thyroxine 384
Tile, classification by 530
Tilting disc valve 294
Time-cycled ventilators 351
Tinnitus 72, 211
Tips procedure 134
Tissue
   damage, actual 80
   oxygenation, maintaining adequate 536
Tobacco 257, 272, 276
   use 258
Tobramycin 49
Tonic clonic seizure 197, 456
Torsades de pointes 274
Torsemide 64, 124
Total body water 143
Total parenteral nutrition 127
Touch sensation 177
Toxicity 40
Toxin 124, 195, 496
   enhancing excretion of 495
   related hepatotoxicity 118
   removal of 495
Trachea 299
   location of 339f
Tracheoesophageal fistula 480, 506
   types of 480f
Tracheostomy tube 175
Tramadol 83
Tranexamic acid 559
Trans myocardial laser revascularization 293
Transcalvarial herniation 230
Transcranial Doppler sonography 182
Transcutaneous electrical nerve stimulation 79, 84
Transfuse blood 112
Transfusion 435
Transient blindness 254
Transmural bacterial translocation 132
Transudative pleural effusion 319
   causes of 320
Transverse thoracosternotomy 358
Transverse uterine rupture 426f
Trauma 276, 350, 403, 421, 432, 499, 592
   assessment 512
      of severity of 499
   complications of 534
   patient, role of 534
   penetrating 344, 560

Traumatic brain injury, mild 211
Traumatic causes 346
Traumatic conditions 186
Travelers' diarrhea 53
Tremor 122, 208
Triazolam 59
Tributaries 243
Triceps 178
Tricuspid area 251
Tricuspid atresia 476
Tricuspid valve 243
   disease, pathophysiology of 269, 269fc
   stenosis 269
Tricyclic antidepressants 72, 199, 253, 550
   overdose of 72
Trigeminal nerve 176
Triiodothyronine 384
Trimethoprim 51
Triple-H therapy 190
Trophoblastic invasion, abnormal 398, 408
Troubleshooting problems 287
True aneurysm 276
Truncus arteriosus 240
Trunk 213
   right 244
Tube care, providing 106
Tuberculin test 326
Tuberculosis
   symptoms of 328f
   treatment of 52
Tubular necrosis, acute 151
Tubulointerstitial fibrosis 150
Tumor 10, 124, 306
   necrotic factor 542
Tunnel fontan, lateral 477
Tunneled central catheters 108
Two-point discrimination 178
Tylenol 83
Tyramine 253

## U

Ultrafiltration 147
Ultrasonography 527
Umbilical cord, prolapsed 445
Unconscious patient, caring for 227
Unconsciousness 224
   extracranial causes of 225t
   intracranial causes of 225t
Unstable angina 257, 261
Unusual urea levels 27
Upper gastrointestinal bleeding 109
   management of 112
Upper gastrointestinal series 481
Upper limb weakness 206
Upper respiratory tract 297
Urea 227
Uremia 225
Uremic encephalopathy 207, 208
Uremic neurotoxins 208
Ureters 138
Urethra 138
Urinalysis 151

Urinary
   antiseptics 65
   bladder 138
   catheter 11, 133
   elimination, impaired 154
Urinary system 515
   drugs on 64
   structure of 139f
Urinary tract infection 65, 164
   catheter related 93
Urine
   alkalizer 45
   culture 470
   infection 534
   osmolality 147
   output 145
      decreased 433
   test 144, 460
Urologic disease 143
Uterine
   abnormalities 398, 418
   anomalies 426
   artery embolization 424
   atony 421
   contractions 404
      ineffective 419
   factors 403, 418
   firmness, abnormal 422
   inertia 418
   injury 426
   massage 423
   overdistension 426
   repair 428
   rupture 426
   stimulants 423
   surgeries, previous 398, 425
   tenderness 404, 427
   trauma 426
   wall integrity 426
Utility room 631

## V

Vaccination 93
Vacuum extraction 420
Vagal nerve stimulation 197
Vagal stimulation 273
Vaginal bleeding 404
Vaginal delivery 411
Vaginal examination 399, 419
Vagus nerve 177
Valid tools 81
Valproic acid 124, 200
Valve therapy 362f
Valvular diseases 263, 267, 267f
Valvular heart disease
   classification of 267fc
   diagnosis of 269
Valvular surgery 293
Valvuloplasty 294
Vancomycin 48
Variant angina 257
Variceal bleeding 109
   management of 113
Varicose vein 251

Vascular abnormalities 124
Vascular access site, assessment of 162
Vascular causes 118
Vascular malformation 110
Vascular spiders 118
Vasculitis 188
Vasculopathy 294
Vasodilators 254
Vasogenic edema 184
Vasopressin 56
Vasopressors, taking 27
Veau classification 505
Vegetative state 226
Vena cava
    inferior 243
        filter 266f, 336, 336f
    superior 243
Venae cordis minimae 243
Venous stasis 265
Venous thromboembolisms, prevention of 534
Venous thrombosis 188, 265
    large 3
    types of 265
Venovenous hemofiltration, continuous 158
Ventilation 300, 471, 493
    controlled 231
    creating ineffective 343
Ventilation-perfusion
    relationship 300
    scan 313
Ventilator 11
    appropriately, weaning from 353
    classification of 351
    modes and setting 353
    settings, types of 351
    weaning from 352
Ventilator-associated pneumonia 93
    prevention of 89, 93
Ventilatory management 350
Ventilatory support 215
Ventricular aneurysms 262
Ventricular contraction, premature 273, 274f
Ventricular diastole 245
Ventricular ejection phase 245
Ventricular fibrillation 56, 275, 275f
Ventricular septal defect 474, 476
    closing 475

Ventricular systole 245
Ventricular tachycardia 56, 274, 274f, 289, 292
Ventricular thrombus 263
Verapamil 55, 258, 488
Verbal response 175
Vestibulocochlear nerve 168, 176
Vibration sensation 177
Violence 572
Violent behavior 572
Viral hepatitis 117
Viral replication pathways 551
Virus 278
Visible peristalsis 481
Vision, disturbed 416
Visitors' waiting room 632
Visual acuity 176
Visual analog scale 81
Visual deficit 193
Visual disturbances 409, 415
Visual field 176
Visual injury 27
Visual tasks, enabling performance of 25
Vital organs
    anatomy of 2
    physiology of 2
Vital sign 215, 220
    continuous monitoring of 162
    monitoring 387, 427, 434
        continuous 277
Vitamin 142, 325
    B12 174
    D 140
        metabolism 26
        supplements 6
    K antagonists 266
Volume-cycled ventilators 351
Volvulus 134
Vomiting 50, 72, 101, 102, 125, 144, 164, 185, 208, 254, 257, 409
Voriconazole 92

## W

Walking test 178
Warm extremities 72
Watch test 176
Water

depletion 154
excess 154
intoxication 486
pills 64
Water deficiency 487
    signs of 154
    symptoms of 154
Water-soluble molecules 40
Watson's theory 23
Weak pulse indicates 249
Weakness 264, 273, 433
Weber test 177
Wedge resection 361
Weight loss 101, 481
Wenckebach heart block 271
Wernicke's aphasia 193
Wernicke's encephalopathy 74, 208, 210
Wheezing 308
Whipple procedure 127
White blood cell 69
    type of 90
Whole bowel lavage 72
Wintomylon 52
Withdrawal syndrome 253
Wolf-Parkinson-White syndrome 292
Woodcare 596
Worsening mitral regurgitation 289
Wound
    care 92, 431, 591, 593, 596
    drainage 431
    infection, postoperative 92
    management 429

## X

Xanthelasma 257
Xanthoma 248

## Y

Y-plasty 595f

## Z

Zellweger's syndrome 458
Zika virus 201
Zollinger Ellison syndrome 63
Zonisamide 196
Z-plasty 595f